Harris Methodist
Health Sciences Library
1301 Pennsylvania Ave.
Fort Worth, TX 76104

AF681741

Marc E. Lippman, M.D.
Head, Medical Breast Cancer Section
Medical Branch
National Cancer Institute
Bethesda, Maryland

Clinical Professor of Medicine and
Pharmacology
Uniformed Services University of the
Health Sciences
Bethesda, Maryland

Allen S. Lichter, M.D.
Professor and Chairman
Department of Radiation Oncology
University of Michigan Medical Center
Ann Arbor, Michigan

David N. Danforth, Jr., M.S., M.D.
Senior Investigator
Surgery Branch
National Cancer Institute
Bethesda, Maryland

Diagnosis and Management of BREAST CANCER

1988
W.B. SAUNDERS COMPANY
Harcourt Brace Jovanovich, Inc.
Philadelphia London Toronto
Montreal Sydney Tokyo

W. B. SAUNDERS COMPANY
Harcourt Brace Jovanovich, Inc.

West Washington Square
Philadelphia, PA 19105

Library of Congress Cataloging-in-Publication Data

Diagnosis and management of breast cancer.

1. Breast—Cancer. I. Lippman, Marc E., 1945–
II. Lichter, Allen S. III. Danforth, David N.
[DNLM: 1. Breast Neoplasms—diagnosis. 2. Breast Neoplasms—therapy. WP 870 D5355]

RC280.B8D436 1988 616.99'449 87–9680

ISBN 0–7216–1958–4

Editor: Dean Manke
Designer: Terri Siegel
Production Manager: Bob Butler
Manuscript Editor: Gina Scala
Illustration Coordinator: Lisa Lambert
Indexer: George Vilk

Diagnosis and Management of Breast Cancer ISBN 0–7216–1958–4

© 1988 by W. B. Saunders Company. Copyright under the Uniform Copyright Convention. Simultaneously published in Canada. All rights reserved. This book is protected by copyright. No part of it may be reproduced, stored in a retrieval system, or transmitted in any form or by any means, electronic, mechanical, photocopying, recording, or otherwise, without written permission from the publisher. Made in the United States of America. Library of Congress catalog card number 87-9680.

Last digit is the print number: 9 8 7 6 5 4 3 2 1

CONTRIBUTORS

R. MARSHALL AUSTIN, M.D, PH.D.

Department of Gynecologic and Breast Pathology, Armed Forces Institute of Pathology, Washington, D.C.

Gross and Microscopic Pathology of the Female Breast

CAROLINE STOKES BAGLEY, R.N., M.S.N.

Research Nurse Specialist, National Cancer Institute, Bethesda, Maryland.

Nursing Care of the Patient with Breast Cancer

DAVID N. DANFORTH, JR., M.S., M.D.

Senior Investigator, Surgery Branch, National Cancer Institute, Bethesda, Maryland.

The Diagnosis of Breast Cancer; Surgical Treatment of Breast Cancer

TERESA M. D'ANGELO, R.N., B.S.N.

Nurse Clinician, Cancer Nursing Service, National Institutes of Health, Bethesda, Maryland.

Nursing Care of the Patient with Breast Cancer

NANCY E. DAVIDSON, M.D.

Assistant Professor of Oncology, Johns Hopkins University School of Medicine; Staff Physician, Johns Hopkins Hospital, Baltimore, Maryland.

Adjuvant Therapy for Breast Cancer; Treatment of Metastatic Breast Cancer

BRENDA K. EDWARDS, PH.D.

Statistical Considerations in the Design and Interpretation of Clinical Trials

PEGGIE A. FINDLAY, M.D.

The Jewish Hospital, Cincinnati, Ohio. Fort Hamilton-Hughes Memorial Hospital, Hamilton, Ohio.

Radiation Therapy as Definitive Treatment of Breast Cancer; Radiation Therapy as an Adjuvant to Surgery in the Treatment of Operable Breast Cancer

GLORIA FRANKL, M.D.

Clinical Professor of Radiology, University of Southern California School of Medicine; Associate Clinical Professor of Radiology, University of California, Los Angeles, School of Medicine; Staff Radiologist, Kaiser Permanente Medical Center, Los Angeles, California.

Screening and Detection of Breast Cancer

LYNN H. GERBER, M.D.

Adjunct Associate Professor, George Washington University, Washington, D.C.; Chief, Department of Rehabilitation Medicine, Clinical Center, National Institutes of Health, Bethesda, Maryland.

Rehabilitation of the Patient with Breast Cancer

CATHERINE RICE GORRELL, R.N., M.S.N.

Cancer Nursing Consultant, Cancer Nursing Service, National Institutes of Health, Bethesda, Maryland.

Nursing Care of the Patient with Breast Cancer

SANDRA M. LEVY, PH.D.

Associate Professor of Psychiatry and Medicine, University of Pittsburgh School of Medicine; Program Director, Behavioral Medicine in Oncology, Presbyterian University Hospital, Pittsburgh, Pennsylvania.

Psychologic Response to Breast Cancer: Direct and Indirect Contributors to Treatment Outcome

ALLEN S. LICHTER, M.D.

Professor and Chairman, Department of Radiation Oncology, University of Michigan Medical School, Ann Arbor, Michigan.

The Diagnosis of Breast Cancer; Technical Aspects of the Treatment of Breast Cancer with Radiation Therapy; Radiation Therapy as an Adjuvant to Surgery in the Treatment of Operable Breast Cancer; Special Situations in the Treatment of Breast Cancer

MARC E. LIPPMAN, M.D.

Head, Medical Breast Cancer Section, Medicine Branch, National Cancer Institute; Clinical Professor of Medicine and Pharmacology, Uniformed Services University of the Health Sciences, Bethesda, Maryland.

Epidemiology of Breast Cancer; The Diagnosis of Breast Cancer; Surgical Treatment of Breast Cancer; Locally Advanced Breast Cancer; Intraepithelial Carcinoma of the Breast: LCIS and DCIS; Steroid Hormone Receptors and Mechanisms of Growth Regulation of Human Breast Cancer; Adjuvant Therapy for Breast Cancer; Treatment of Metastatic Breast Cancer; Special Situations in the Treatment of Breast Cancer

HAROLD D. MCDONALD, M.D., F.A.C.S.

Assistant Professor of Surgery, Uniformed Services University of the Health Sciences; Senior Investigator, Surgery Branch, National Cancer Institute, Bethesda, Maryland.

Reconstruction of the Breast

SHAHLA MOSHIRI, M.D.

Cytopathology Fellow, Department of Pathology, National Institutes of Health, Bethesda, Maryland.

Gross and Microscopic Pathology of the Female Breast

HENRY J. NORRIS, M.D.

Clinical Professor of Pathology, Uniformed Services University of the Health Sciences, Bethesda, Maryland; Chairman, Department of Gynecologic and Breast Pathology, Armed Forces Institute of Pathology, Washington, D.C.

Gross and Microscopic Pathology of the Female Breast

CHERYL M. REICHERT, M.D., PH.D.

Pathologist, Columbus Hospital, Great Falls, Montana; Consultant, Surgery Branch, National Cancer Institute, Bethesda, Maryland.

Gross and Microscopic Pathology of the Female Breast

WENDY S. SCHAIN, ED.D.

Adjunct Clinical Professor, Georgetown University School of Medicine, Washington, D.C.; Medical Care Consultant, National Institutes of Health, Bethesda, Maryland.

Psychologic Response to Breast Cancer: Direct and Indirect Contributors to Treatment Outcome

JEFFREY SCHLOM, PH.D.

Adjunct Professor, Graduate Faculty in Genetics, George Washington University, Washington, D.C.

Future Prospects in Breast Cancer Research and Management

RICHARD A. SORACE, M.D., PH.D.

Staff Radiation Oncologist, University Community Hospital, Tampa, Florida.

Locally Advanced Breast Cancer

SANDRA M. SWAIN, M.D.

Medical Breast Cancer Section, Medicine Branch, National Cancer Institute, Bethesda, Maryland.

Intraepithelial Carcinoma of the Breast: LCIS and DCIS

MARGARET N. WESLEY, PH.D.

Statistical Considerations in the Design and Interpretation of Clinical Trials

CAROL WOOD, B.S., R.P.T.

Retired—Physical Therapy Coordinator, Rehabilitation Department, National Cancer Institute, Bethesda, Maryland.

Rehabilitation of the Patient with Breast Cancer

PREFACE

During the past decade, the approach to the patient with breast cancer has undergone dramatic changes. These changes have arisen through major advances in tumor biology, prospectively designed trials exploring many aspects of clinical care, improved diagnostic and therapeutic techniques, and increased use of multimodality approaches. Given this rapidly changing and complicated field, there is a need, in our opinion, for a concise and completely up-to-date text providing the clinician with a therapeutically oriented manual of breast cancer care.

For the past decade, our group of physicians and other health care providers practicing and conducting research together at the National Cancer Institute has felt the need to document these developments in breast cancer care and provide the rational basis for our treatment strategies for the patient with breast cancer. For these reasons, we have decided to prepare what is essentially a manual for breast cancer treatment that provides a detailed rationale for the treatment choices we have made. Because of the complexity of modern breast cancer treatment, which involves so many disciplines, it has been our opinion that no single source has adequately provided completely up-to-date information with respect to local treatment modalities, systemic therapy, and rehabilitation. For this reason, we have tried to provide detailed information on aspects of care that range widely, including modern radiotherapeutic treatment planning strategies and physical and psychologic rehabilitation. We have also included detailed information concerning unusual and particularly difficult clinical situations, paying particular attention to stage III breast cancer, including inflammatory breast cancer and intraductal disease.

Though, admittedly, many treatment situations are controversial, such as intraductal disease and indications for adjuvant therapy in some patient subgroups, we have presented firm recommendations for management after attempting to fairly present the current literature.

There are many individuals who have contributed to our training and knowledge and to the preparation of this book, and it would be difficult adequately to thank them all. We would particularly like to thank Ms. Phyllis Rand for her tireless efforts to help assemble, type, and edit most of the chapters in this book. We wish to acknowledge the many colleagues and clinical fellows whose dedication and care of our patients over the years have permitted the assembly of the clinical information that has gone into this book.

Finally, we would like to dedicate this book to the many women who, in a sense, made this book possible by their courage and dedication, manifested by their willingness to participate in our clinical research program.

MARC E. LIPPMAN
ALLEN S. LICHTER
DAVID N. DANFORTH, JR.

CONTENTS

Epidemiology of Breast Cancer

MARC E. LIPPMAN, M.D.

In 1986, breast cancer continued to be the leading cause of death from cancer in women. For 1987, approximately 120,000 newly diagnosed cases of breast cancer are expected in the United States, and approximately 40,000 of these will eventually prove fatal. Since the median age for developing breast cancer is 57 years, it is certain that even more women would eventually die of metastatic disease if they survived long enough. Enormous attention has been focused upon the critical role of endocrine factors in the etiology of this disease. Given the current limitations of successful control of both localized and systemic breast cancer, rational endocrine approaches to disease prevention are of obvious interest. In this chapter we will summarize some of the epidemiologic data that pertain to breast cancer risk, paying particular attention to endocrine factors. As will become clear, the time may well be ripe to entertain the initiation of endocrine or dietary trials.

The epidemiology of breast cancer has been studied extensively and while many controversies remain to be resolved, a variety of important risk factors are widely agreed upon.[1–3] Among the most important predictors of risk are sex, age, height, weight, age at menarche and menopause, age at first parturition, country of origin, dietary factors, and a family history of breast cancer. In addition, certain exogenous factors such as hormone exposure are clearly of great importance. Many of these risk factors are interdependent and it appears likely that the majority are mediated through endocrine pathways. A summary of many of these risk factors is presented in Table 1–1.

An understanding of the mechanism by which these various risk factors increase breast cancer incidence is of extraordinary importance, as prophylactic endocrine measures of real significance might result. Unfortunately, though the impact of these risk factors is great, no risk factor, taken either by itself or in combination with others, is sufficiently discriminatory at the present time to identify women in whom special therapeutic intervention is warranted. This is particularly significant given the fact that therapeutic intervention is presently limited to prophylactic mastectomy in one of its various forms. The only exception may be certain very-high-risk kindreds or women with first-degree relatives (mothers or sisters) with bilateral

1

TABLE 1–1. Risk Factors for Breast Cancer in Females

Factor	*High Risk*	*Low Risk*	*Magnitude of Risk Differential**
Age	old age	young age	>>>
Location of country of residence	North America, northern Europe	Asia, Africa	>>>
Socioeconomic class	upper	lower	>>
Marital status	never married	ever married	>
Place of residence	urban	rural	>
Place of residence	northern U.S.	southern U.S.	>
Race	white	black	>
Age at first birth	older than 30	younger than 20	>>
Oophorectomy	no	yes	>>
Body build	obese	thin	>>
Menarche	early	late	>
Menopause	late	early	>
Family history of premenopausal bilateral breast cancer	yes	no	>>>
History of cancer in one breast	yes	no	>>>
History of fibrocystic disease	yes	no	>>
Any first-degree relative with breast cancer	yes	no	>>
History of primary cancer in ovary or endometrium	yes	no	>>
Radiation to chest	large doses	minimal exposure	>>

*>>> Denotes relative risk of greater than 4.0. >> Denotes relative risk of 2.0–4.0. > Denotes relative risk of 1.1–1.9. (Modified from Kelsey JL: A review of the epidemiology of human breast cancer. Epidemiologic Reviews, Vol. 1, 1979.)

premenopausal breast cancer, for whom the risk of breast cancer in the related individual may be as high as 65 percent. Furthermore, the absence of any known risk factors is not sufficient to rule out the possibility of breast cancer in a woman with a suspicious lump. Therefore, at this time, the diagnostic approach to patients should be almost entirely without regard to a history of risk factors. All too often biopsies are not performed for otherwise suspicious lumps because the patient is thought to be too young or to lack a family history. Eighty-five percent of all breast cancer occurs in women without meaningful family histories of breast cancer.

Information will be provided concerning four general groupings of risk factors, in which endocrine influences almost certainly play a substantial role. These are reproductive history, international variation, familial clustering, and endocrine environment.

REPRODUCTIVE AND MENSTRUAL HISTORY

Reproductive and menstrual history has been examined in numerous studies. Age at menarche is an important determinant of breast cancer risk. Women who begin menstruating at an earlier age have a higher risk of breast cancer. Thus, if onset of menses at age 13 or older is assigned a relative risk of 1, then menstruation beginning before age 12 has nearly a twofold increase in relative risk.[4] In addition, the interval from menarche to the establishment of regular cycles is important. Women who take longer to establish regular menses have a decreased risk of breast cancer compared with women who develop regular cycles sooner.[5] This is an extremely interesting point in that it argues against the "estrogen window" hypothesis, to be discussed shortly, and is supportive of the notion that unlike the case of the endometrium, progestins may not exert an antimitotic effect on the breast.

Similarly, age of menopause is also an important factor in breast cancer risk. It has been estimated by Trichopolous and colleagues[6] that women whose natural menopause occurs before age 45 have only one half of the breast cancer risk of those whose menopause occurs after age 55. Surgical menopause is protective against breast cancer in proportion to the reduction in years of menstrual life. It is appropriate to consider risk ratios in the context of total disease incidence. While a risk ratio of 7 may be highly significant for a specific carcinogen in leukemogenesis (as for combined chemo- and radiation therapy for Hodgkin's disease), the total number of cases may remain very low if the control incidence is very low. In breast cancer, reduction of risk ratios by 0.5 would eliminate 55,000 cases.

Parity is also of critical importance in estimating breast cancer risk. If one arbitrarily assigns a relative risk of 1 to nulliparous women, then a nearly threefold variation in the risk of breast cancer can be seen (varying from 0.5 for women who have their first child before age 20 to 1.4 for women who give birth to their first child after age 37).[7] Alternative hypotheses have suggested that the protective effect of early pregnancy is due either to a permanent pregnancy-induced alteration in the mammary gland or to a chronic post-partum alteration in circulating hormone levels. Study of this issue is critical because identification of the source of this substantial protection against breast cancer risk provided by early first birth might allow prophylactic endocrine manipulations in young women. Generally, it has not appeared likely that this protective effect is due to lactation per se,[8, 9] although one study in women who nursed their children on only one breast showed a highly significant reduction in breast cancer on that side.[10] Significantly, this protective effect of early age at first birth is maintained throughout life, even among women aged 70 and older. This is a particularly alarming observation, given the fact that there is such a widespread trend toward delay in having children for many American families, coupled with a rise in infertility.

Pike and colleagues[4] have made the disturbing observation that a first-trimester abortion, whether spontaneous or induced, that occurs prior to a full-term pregnancy is associated with a substantial increase in breast cancer risk, whereas abortions after the first full-term pregnancy do not alter the risk of breast cancer. The combined effect of parity, menarche, and menopause on breast cancer risk had not been fully appreciated until Pike and colleagues proposed a means to explain international variation in incidence on this basis. In their proposal, early menarche and the length of menstrual life prior to first pregnancy are particularly important risk factors.[11] In this model, three intervals of time are defined: menarche to first full-term pregnancy; first full-term pregnancy to menopause; and menopause to current age.

In the model defined by Pike and colleagues, the incidence of a given cancer at a particular time (I(t)) is a function of time.

Thus, $I(t) = at^k$ will fit the data for colorectal cancer; the exponent "k" is between 4 and 5. For breast cancer

$$I(t) = a(d(t))^k$$

where d(t) is the relevant tissue age. For breast cancer, they used as estimators of d(t) the following numbers:

$$\begin{aligned} d(t) = {} & (\text{time from menarche to FFTP} + 4) \\ & + 0.7\ (\text{time from (FFTP} + 4) \text{ to (menopause} - 3)) \\ & + 0.115\ (\text{time from (menopause} - 3) \text{ to } (t - 1)) \end{aligned}$$

Fascinatingly, when data for menarche, age at first full-term pregnancy, and menopause are supplied for various countries, this equation can account for approximately 85 percent of the international variation in breast cancer. Since dietary practices are also likely to influence height and weight and thereby the onset and regularity of menses, this is an attractive means of incorporating multiple risk factors into a single hypothesis.

DeWaard and colleagues have demonstrated the important relation of height and weight on breast cancer risk.[12] Of great interest is their observation that while an increased body weight (greater than 70 kg versus less than 60 kg) can approximately double the breast cancer risk, this increase is limited exclusively to postmenopausal women and increases with age.[3, 13] These data are consistent with the general view that the etiology of pre- and postmenopausal breast cancers may be somewhat different, with the latter having the greater dependence upon external endocrine factors. Such a view is supported by the observation that the international variation in premenopausal breast cancer is very much less than that for older women (see below).

INTERNATIONAL VARIATION

International variation is an enormously important epidemiologic finding from numerous studies on breast cancer risk around the world.[3, 13] For example, the incidence of breast cancer is about six times higher in the United States than in Japan or Taiwan for women aged 50. For postmenopausal women, the difference increases to nearly 20-fold. While this might initially be interpreted as evidence for a genetic basis for breast cancer risk, this hypothesis is untenable. In observations on the descendants of Chinese and Japanese people living in Western nations, these second-generation Japanese and Chinese have a breast cancer risk equivalent to that of the white individuals living in surrounding communities.[14] In Japan, the incidence of breast cancer is increasing rapidly. This would fit the hypothesis of Pike and colleagues,[11] in which altered dietary habits that have clearly led to increased height and weight and early onset of menstruation could result in increased breast cancer risk. These kinds of data lead one to the inescapable conclusion that environmental factors, most probably diet in the broadest sense, are responsible for nearly 90 percent of all the breast cancer cases seen in the United States.

Studies of international variation also emphasize the potential difference between pre- and postmenopausal breast cancer. In those countries in which a high incidence of breast cancer has been observed, there is a continued increase with age such that by age 50 the breast cancer risk in the United States is approximately 80 per 100,000 women but by age 70 has risen to 350 per 100,000.

In low-risk countries the rate of development of breast cancer decreases after menopause. This is further evidence in support of deWaard's observations that pre- and postmenopausal breast cancer may have different etiologies and that the chronic effects of some endocrine factor mediated through diet, height and weight, and menstrual history may alter the incidence of postmenopausal breast cancer.[12]

FAMILY HISTORY

Family history is a major contributor to breast cancer risk.[15] Many patients and physicians overinterpret these data and mistakenly presume that any relative with a history of breast cancer or even unrelated malignancy substantially influences the patient's likelihood of eventually developing breast cancer. Breast cancer risk is primarily determined by a history of breast cancer in first-degree relatives. While the increase in risk is approximately two- to threefold for women with a single postmenopausal first-degree relative with breast cancer, it may rise to ninefold (approximately 65 percent) in cases in which the first-degree relative is premenopausal and has bilateral breast cancer. It is not clear how much of this increase in familial risk may be attributed to shared environmental factors or genetic predisposition. Unfortunately, efforts to study these patients from an endocrine point of view, with respect to differences in the levels of, for example, prolactin, gonadotrophins, and estrogens, have been almost completely negative. This may reflect either the long-term effects of relatively minor differences in concentrations of previously measured hormones or the failure to as yet appreciate the significance of some alternative growth factor or metabolite. Finally, recent data have been most consistent with an autosomal dominant mode of inheritance.[16]

What is clearly inarguable is the central role of hormonal factors in the genesis of breast cancer. One can identify at least three sites of action of hormones that are likely to be important in the eventual development of gross malignancy. First, there is direct evidence that steroidal and nonsteroidal estrogens may function as true carcinogens. That is, they are capable of forming covalent adducts to DNA and by this primary modification of the DNA structure, as well as the resultant repair process set in motion, induce mutations that may lead eventually to a heritable expression of a malignant phenotype. Second, hormones clearly can function as promoters of some previously occurring carcinogenic event. There are many examples both in animal models and from epidemiologic studies that suggest that if hormonal stimulation is withdrawn following exposure to a carcinogen, a tumor will not appear. Third, it is likely that hormones play a permissive role in allowing carcinogenic events to occur. In this scenario, unless the target tissue is under hormonal stimulation, the carcinogen is ineffective. This may conceivably result from alterations in chromatin structure following hormonal stimulation, which render growth-regulating genes that are under hormonal control accessible to carcinogenic action. A straightforward illustration of these processes is provided by carcinogen-induced breast cancers in rats. In this situation, the carcinogen dimethylbenzanthracene is ineffective if given to sexually immature animals. It is similarly ineffective if castration is performed following administration to sexually mature animals. Tumors are seen only when sexually mature animals are treated with a carcinogen followed by continuous physiologic exposure to sex steroids. Thus separate carcinogenic, promoter, and permissive actions of sex steroids in the evolution of cancer can be identified.

THE ENDOCRINE ENVIRONMENT

If endocrine factors are important in the etiology of breast cancer, one would expect either that important endogenous differences in hormone levels would exist or that exogenous hormone administration would be an important risk factor for patients developing breast cancer compared with normal controls.

Since a relationship between breast cancer and estrogen seems likely, the measurement of urinary estrogens was undertaken by several groups; there were, however, no consistent or reproducible differences between women with breast cancer and those in the normal population. These studies may be criticized in that estrogens should have been measured at the time of carcinogenesis rather than at some stage of clinical disease. Further, the large fluctuations of estrogens during the menstrual cycle and the alterations in route of metabolism with disease or with drugs make interpretation difficult. A review of this subject generally concludes that hormonal patterns of presumptively high-risk groups of women do not differ from those of the normal population.[17]

As a result of some previous work suggesting that estriol was an estrogen antagonist, considerable attention has been given to data showing a decreased risk of breast cancer in women with a high urinary excretion of estriol.[18] In support of this hypothesis was the finding that Japanese women (a low-risk group) had higher urinary estriol excretion than did Australian women.[19] However, the hypothesis is not very likely to have merit for the following reasons. First, estriol is an estrogen whose receptor-binding characteristics make it act as an antagonist only when it is given intermittently with simultaneous administration of more potent estrogens.[20] When given continuously, it is a potent estrogen and will act as a promoter of mammary gland carcinogenesis in experimental systems. Second, continuous exposure to estriol can be shown to directly stimulate hormone-responsive human breast cancer cells in long-term tissue culture.[21] Third, urinary estriol levels have no relationship to plasma estriol concentrations or production rates.[22] Further, the ratio of estriol to estrone plus estradiol is not related to differences between estrogen blood levels and production rates in normal women or in women with breast cancer. Henderson and colleagues have found that teenage daughters of patients with breast cancer had estradiol and estrone concentrations that were significantly elevated compared with age-matched controls.[23] Differences were quantitatively small but the impact of such differences summed over decades is difficult to assess.

Other work has supported the idea that abnormalities in estrogen contribute to the development of breast cancer. Korenman has suggested that unopposed estrogen action is a major risk factor.[24] His "estrogen window" hypothesis is based on five premises:

1. Human breast cancer is induced by carcinogens in a susceptible (that is, a hormone-primed) mammary gland.
2. Unopposed estrogenic stimulation favors tumor induction.
3. There is a long latency between tumor induction and clinical disease.
4. The duration of the estrogen window is proportional to breast cancer risk.
5. Inducibility declines with establishment of normal ovulatory menses and becomes very low during pregnancy.

Brown has reviewed daily endocrine profiles in young women entering puberty, during normal menstrual life, and at menopause.[25] These studies document multiple anovulatory cycles at either extreme of menstrual life and provide some biologic basis for the hypothesis of Korenman just mentioned. This hypothesis does not fit well with the epidemiologic data of Pike and colleagues, previously described, who found irregular (and presumably anovulatory) menses to be associated with a decreased breast cancer risk.[4]

Finally, Siiteri and colleagues have reexamined the question of serum estrogen concentrations in breast cancer.[26, 27] They found that while total serum estrogen concentrations may be normal in women with breast cancer, abnormally high concentrations of free estrogen occur because of decreased plasma binding. The latter results from a decrease in sex hormone–binding globulin (SHBG) or possibly, in some cases, because of an abnormal SHBG. More recently it has been suggested that these differences are due to sample storage. Further developments in this area should be closely followed. In addition, the failure to detect major effects of postmenopausal estrogen therapy goes against the Korenman hypothesis. It is, however, concordant with other observations such as breast cancer risk and obesity, breast cancer risk and endometrial cancer risk, and a host of biologic data.

The exact role of prolactin in the etiology of human breast cancer remains enigmatic. Some investigators have found abnormalities in prolactin in patients with breast cancer[4, 28] as well as their daughters.[29] Others have failed to detect significant abnormalities.[30] One excellent review of the subject[31] concluded that prolactin abnormalities probably were associated with breast cancer risk, but whether causally or not remains to be determined.

As will be discussed later, there is, however, virtually no evidence that a significant subset of established breast cancers is dependent on prolactin as a trophic hormone.

Abnormalities of thyroid function, usually goiter or hypothyroidism, have been reported to be increased in patients with breast cancer. However, at least two critical reviews of this area[3, 32] have failed to support these contentions. At present, little evidence links any thyroid abnormality to an altered breast cancer risk.

Androgens have also been felt to play an etiologic role in breast cancer. Bulbrook has shown that a higher excretion of androgen metabolites was correlated with a greater likelihood of response to adrenalectomy or hypophysectomy.[33] The use of this discriminant function has markedly decreased because of the much higher predictability of estrogen receptors. Of greater interest was the finding in a prospective trial that urinary etiocholanolone (an androgen metabolite) excretion was lower in women who subsequently developed breast cancer.[34] In a more recent study, the same group showed that women at high risk for breast cancer had the lowest plasma levels of androgens.[35] Attention has been focused on other androgens; urinary testosterone excretion[36] and plasma testosterone levels[37] were higher in women with early breast cancer. Other conflicting data do not inspire confidence that important endocrine abnormalities separating normal women from those at high risk for breast cancer have been delineated, since in other hands such discriminants appear to have little validity.[38] Most of the data regarding the hormonal milieu relate to hormones present in plasma or in urine. However, Adams and Wong[39, 40] reported that human breast cancer tissue could metabolize dehydroepiandrosterone to androstenedione and possibly to estriol. Cholesterol was converted to C-19 steroids. Breast cancer tissue can also aromatize steroids. Estrone and estradiol can be isolated after incubation of breast cancer samples with C-19 steroids. Thus, the breast cancer cell has the potential to create its own microenvironment and thereby may defeat efforts to lower estradiol levels in the surrounding medium. Some breast cancers have the capacity to sulfurylate various steroids, and the absence of sulfokinase was correlated with a lack of response to adrenalectomy. Recent studies of the ability of a metabolite of dehydroepiandrosterone, androstenediol, to compete with estradiol for receptors[40] suggest a mechanism for relating androgen metabolism to the clinical response to hormonal therapy.

Although most benign breast diseases are not considered to be premalignant, there is strong evidence to suggest that women with benign breast disease have a substantially increased risk (up to four times in one well-studied series) of developing breast cancer.[41, 42] While other explanations are possible, it is likely that benign and malignant breast disease share common etiologic factor(s) related to the endocrine milieu. Thus, an examination of the effects of exogenous sex hormones on benign breast disease is of interest. There is now strong evidence from both retrospective analyses [42–47] and prospective studies[48, 49] that oral contraceptive use diminishes the incidence of clinically significant benign breast disease. Generally, those studies show a greater protective effect against cystic disease as compared with fibroadenoma. In addition, protection is greater in "long-term users" as compared with "ever users," an important point in favor of a causal relationship. There was some evidence showing the incidence rates for benign breast disease to be inversely related to the amount of progestogen in the contraceptive preparation. Confirmation of this observation is provided by surveys of women using noncontraceptive estrogen preparations in which no protection against benign breast disease was demonstrated.[43, 48] However, certain forms of benign breast disease such as intraductal papilloma and fibrosing adenosis, as well as severe atypia of the ductular lining cells, have been associated with a particularly high likelihood of subsequent malignancy.[49, 50] Effects of oral contraceptives on women with these specific histologic features have not been assessed; therefore, it should not be concluded that the effectiveness of oral contraceptives in reducing benign breast disease is equivalent to a protection against breast cancer. The possibility exists that in particular subsets of women with benign breast disease, estrogen use increases the risk.

A recent development in the management of benign breast disease is the observation that danazol (17α-Pregna-2,4-dien-20-yno.[2,3-d] isoxazol-17-ol) can induce worthwhile objective and symptomatic improvement in greater than 90 percent of patients.[51, 52] This drug is also active in the management of advanced breast cancer.[53] It might therefore be hoped that chronic danazol administration might be protective against breast cancer, but no information on this point is available yet.

EXOGENOUS HORMONE ADMINISTRATION

Studies of exogenous hormone administration have also been confusing. Multiple retrospective case control studies have failed to reveal a significant overall increase in risk of developing breast cancer among oral contraceptive users.[44, 48, 54, 55] However, several observations prevent a totally sanguine view of this conclusion. In general, the time required for tumor promotion in humans is long, and there may not be sufficient experience as yet for firm conclusions. Two studies of younger women showed a relative risk ratio of 1.7 for users of oral contraceptives for more than eight and five years, respectively,[56, 57] although this increase was not statistically significant. Two other studies have failed to show an increase in risk with the passage of time.[44, 48] However, in one of these studies[48] oral contraceptives increased the risk of breast cancer in three subsets of patients: nulliparous women, women using the pill prior to the birth of their first child, and women with a history of benign breast disease.

Three major exceptions may exist. Women with previous benign breast disease may have striking increases in breast cancer risk following oral contraceptive use.[4, 58] Henderson and colleagues[14] and others[59, 60] have shown that oral contraceptive use at either the beginning or the end of menstrual life may dramatically increase breast cancer risk. Thus, the relative risk for women using oral contraceptives between ages 46 and 50 was 2.4 and 4 in the three studies cited. For women using oral contraceptives for more than eight years prior to the first full-term pregnancy, the relative risk was 3.5. These data are badly in need of confirmation. They would appear to be in direct conflict with the estrogen window hypothesis and would imply an important promotional role for progestins. This would fit the data of Fergusson and Anderson, who found that cell division in the human breast is higher during the luteal phase.[61] This area of research should be watched closely. These biologic data are also in need of confirmation, although it has long been appreciated that progestins augment the effectiveness of estrogens as tumor promoters after DMBA carcinogenesis.

There have been many retrospective analyses of women using estrogens after menopause, and few show a significant association between use and breast cancer risk.[48, 55–57] In one large retrospective study,[62] a relative risk ratio of 1.3 (of borderline statistical significance) was found for estrogen users. More alarmingly, risk was related to duration of administration, with a doubling of this risk ratio after 12 years of use. No follow-up of oral contraceptive users of this duration is available. A recent National Institutes of Health (NIH) study revealed a significant dose-dependent increase in breast cancer among users of menopausal estrogens.[63] The risk was greatest in women who took the highest-strength preparation, although it was not related to duration of use. Several recent well-done studies have suggested small but significant (1.3 to 2) relative risk increases in long-term and high-dose users.[59, 62, 64, 65] Many have advocated discontinuation of therapy, cyclical therapy with or without intermittent progestins, or low-dose therapy. None of these recommendations has been proved to either increase or decrease risk, nor is it possible to assess alternative effects of such therapeutic interventions on such conditions as osteoporosis and cardiovascular disease. The critical topic on which information is badly needed is the role of progestins combined with estrogens.

Several drugs have been shown to be efficacious in objectively and symptomatically lessening the severity of benign breast disease. These are danazol, bromocriptine, and antiestrogens (generally tamoxifen). The first and last are clearly effective for some patients with metastatic breast cancer, whereas bromocriptine is clearly ineffective. The role of chronic administration of these drugs in breast cancer risk reduction is not known, but given the general lack of toxicity, randomized clinical trials should probably be undertaken.

REFERENCES

1. MacMahon B, Cole P, Brown J: Etiology of human breast cancer: A review. J Natl Cancer Inst 50:21, 1973.
2. Miller AB: An overview of hormone-associated cancer. Cancer Res 38:3985, 1973.
3. Kelsey JL: A review of the epidemiology of human breast cancer. Epidemiol Rev 1:74, 1979.
4. Pike MC, Henderson BE, Casagrande JT, et al.: Oral contraceptive use and early abortion risk factors for breast cancer in young women. Br J Cancer 43:72, 1981.
5. Henderson BE, Pike MC, Casagrande JT: Breast cancer and the oestrogen window hypothesis. Lancet 2:363, 1981.
6. Trichopolous D, MacMahon B, Cole P: The menopause and breast cancer risk. J Natl Cancer Inst 48:605, 1972.
7. MacMahon B, Cole P, Lin TM, et al.: Age at first birth and breast cancer risk. Bull WHO 43:209, 1970.
8. MacMahon B, Feinleib M: Breast cancer in relation to nursing and menopausal history. J Natl Cancer Inst 24:733, 1960.
9. Abramson JH: Breastfeeding and breast cancer. A study of cases and matched controls in Jerusalem. Isr J Med Sci 12:457, 1966.
10. Ing R, Hoe JHC, Petrakis NL: Unilateral breastfeeding and breast cancer. Lancet 2:124, 1977.
11. Pike MC, Henderson BE, Casagrande JT: The epidemiology of breast cancer as it relates to menarche, pregnancy and menopause. *In*: Pike MC, Siiteri PK, Welsch CW (eds.): Hormones and Breast Cancer. Cold Spring Harbor, NY: Cold Spring Harbor Publishing, 1981, pp. 3–20.
12. deWaard F, Cornelis JP, Aoki K, et al.: Breast cancer incidence according to weight and height in two cities of the Netherlands and in Aichi Prefecture, Japan. Cancer 40:1269, 1977.
13. Doll R, Payne P: Cancer Incidence in Five Continents. Berlin: Springer-Verlag, 1966.
14. Henderson BE, Pike MC, Ross RM: Epidemiology and risk factors. *In*: Bonadonna G (ed.): Breast Cancer: Diagnosis and Management, Vol. 1. New York: John Wiley & Sons, 1984, pp. 15–33.
15. Anderson DE: Breast cancer in families. Cancer 40:1855, 1977.
16. King MC, Go RCP, Elston RC, et al.: Allele increasing susceptibility to human breast cancer may be linked to the glutamate-pyruvate transaminase locus. Science 208:405, 1980.
17. Zumoff B: Abnormal plasma hormone levels in women with breast cancer. *In*: Pike MC, Siiteri PK, Welsch CW (eds.): Hormones and Breast Cancer. Cold Spring Harbor, NY: Cold Spring Harbor Publishing, 1981, pp. 143–168.
18. Lemon HM, Wotiz HH, Parsons L, et al.: Reduced estriol excretion in patients with breast cancer prior to endocrine therapy. JAMA 196:1128, 1966.
19. MacMahon B, Cole P, Brown J, et al.: Oestrogen profiles of Asian and North American women. Lancet 2:900, 1971.
20. Anderson JN: Estrogen-induced uterine responses and growth: Relationship to receptor estrogen binding by uterine nuclei. Endocrinology 96:160, 1975.
21. Lippman ME, Monaco ME, Bolan G: Effects of estrone, estradiol and estriol on hormone-responsive human breast cancer in long-term tissue culture. Cancer Res 37:1901, 1977.
22. Longcope C, Pratt JH: Relationship between urine and plasma estrogen ratios. Cancer Res 38:4025, 1978.
23. Henderson BE, Gerkins V, Rosario I, et al.: Elevated serum levels of estrogen and prolactin in daughters of patients with breast cancer. N Engl J Med 293:790, 1975.
24. Korenman SG: Reproductive endocrinology and breast cancer in women. *In*: Pike MC, Siiteri PK, Welsch CW (eds.): Hormones and Breast Cancer. Cold Spring Harbor, NY: Cold Spring Harbor Publishing, 1981, pp. 71–82.
25. Brown JB: Hormone profiles in young women at risk of breast cancer: A study of ovarian function during thelarche, menarche and menopause and after childbirth. *In*: Pike MC, Siiteri PK, Welsch CW (eds.): Hormones and Cancer. Cold Spring Harbor, NY: Cold Spring Harbor Publishing, 1981, pp. 33–54.
26. Siiteri PK, Hammond GL, Nisker JA: Increased availability of serum estrogens in breast cancer: A new hypothesis. *In*: Pike MC, Siiteri PK, Welsch CW (eds.): Hormones and Breast Cancer. Cold Spring Harbor, NY: Cold Spring Harbor Publishing, 1981, pp. 87–101.
27. Moore JM, Clark CMG, Bulbrook RD, et al.: Serum concentrations of total and non–protein-bound estradiol in patients with breast cancer and in normal controls. Int J Cancer 29:17, 1981.

28. Hill P, Wynder EL, Kuman J, et al.: Prolactin levels in populations at risk for breast cancer. Cancer Res 36:4102, 1976.
29. Levin PA, Malarkey WB: Daughters of women with breast cancer have elevated mean 24-hour prolactin (PRL) levels and a partial resistance of PRL to dopamine suppression. J Clin Endocrinol Metab 53:179, 1981.
30. Fishman J, Fukushima D, O'Connor J, et al.: Plasma hormone profiles of young women at risk for familial breast cancer. Cancer Res 38:4006, 1978.
31. Henderson BC, Pike MC: Prolactin—an important hormone in breast neoplasia? *In*: Pike MC, Siiteri PK, Welsch CW (eds.): Hormones and Breast Cancer. Cold Spring Harbor, NY: Cold Spring Harbor Publishing, 1981, pp. 115–127.
32. Bulbrook RD, Thomas BS, Fantl VE, et al.: A prospective study of the relation between thyroid function and subsequent breast cancer. *In*: Pike MC, Siiteri PK, Welsch CW (eds.): Hormones and Breast Cancer. Cold Spring Harbor, NY: Cold Spring Harbor Publishing, 1981, pp. 131–140.
33. Bulbrook RD: Prediction of response of breast cancer to treatment. *In*: Holland JF, Frei E (eds.): Cancer Medicine. Philadelphia: Lea & Febiger, 1973, pp. 907–911.
34. Bulbrook RD, Hayward JL: Abnormal urinary steroid excretion and subsequent breast cancer. Lancet 2:519, 1967.
35. Wang DY, Bulbrook RD, Hayward JL: Plasma androstenedione levels in women with breast cancer. Eur J Cancer 13:187, 1977.
36. Grattarola R, Secreto G, Recchione C: Androgens in breast cancer III. Breast cancer recurrence years after mastectomy and increased androgenic activity. Am J Obstet Gynecol 121:169, 1975.
37. McFayden IJ, Prescott RJ, Groom RV, et al.: Circulating hormone concentrations in women with breast cancer. Lancet 1:1100, 1976.
38. Masnyk IJ, Silverman DT, Hankey BF: Prediction of response to adrenalectomy in the treatment of advanced breast cancer. J Natl Cancer Inst 60:271, 1978.
39. Adams JB, Wong MSF: Paraendocrine behaviour of human breast carcinoma: In vitro transformation of steroids to physiologically active hormones. J Endocrinol 41:41, 1968.
40. Adams JB, Archibald L, Clarke C: Adrenal dehydroepiandrosterone and human mammary cancer. Cancer Res 38:4036, 1978.
41. Kelsey J: A review of the epidemiology of human breast cancer. Epidemiol Rev 1:74, 1974.
42. Kelsey JL, Holford TR, White C, et al.: Oral contraceptives and breast disease. Am J Epidemiol 107:236, 1978.
43. Nomura A, Comstock GW: Benign breast tumor and estrogenic hormones: A population-based retrospective study. Am J Epidemiol 103:439, 1976.
44. Paffenbarger RS, Fasal E, Simmons ME, et al.: Cancer risk as related to the use of oral contraceptives during fertile years. Cancer 39:1887, 1977.
45. Vessey MP, Doll R, Sutton PM: Oral contraceptives and breast neoplasia: A retrospective study. Br Med J 3:719, 1972.
46. Ravnihar B, Seigel DG, Lindner J: An epidemiologic study of breast cancer and benign breast neoplasias in relation to oral contraceptive and estrogen use. Eur J Cancer 15:395, 1979.
47. Ory H, Cole P, MacMahon B, et al.: Oral contraceptives and reduced risk of benign breast diseases. N Engl J Med 294:419, 1976.
48. Boston Collaborative Drug Surveillance Programme. Lancet 1:1399, 1973.
49. Black MM, Barclay TH, Cutler SJ, et al.: Association of atypical characteristics of benign breast lesions with subsequent risk of breast cancer. Cancer 29:338, 1972.
50. Kodlin D, Winger EE, Morganstern NL, et al.: Chronic mastopathy and breast cancer. A follow-up study. Cancer 39:2603, 1977.
51. Mansel RE, Wisbey JR, Hughes LE: The use of danazol in the treatment of painful benign breast disease: Preliminary results. Postgrad Med J 55:61, 1979.
52. Madanos AE, Farber M: Danazol. Ann Intern Med 96:625, 1982.
53. Coombes RC, Dearnaley D, Humphreys J, et al.: Danazol treatment of advanced breast cancer. Cancer Treat Rep 64:1073, 1980.
54. Kelsey JL, Holford TR, White C, et al.: Oral contraceptives and breast disease. Am J Epidemiol 107:236, 1978.
55. Sartwell PE, Arthes FG, Tonascia JA: Exogenous hormones, reproductive history and breast cancer. J Natl Cancer Inst 59:1589, 1977.
56. Casagrande J, Gerkins V, Henderson BE, et al.: Brief communication: Exogenous estrogens and breast cancer in women with natural menopause. J Natl Cancer Inst 56:839, 1976.
57. Craig TJ, Comstock GW, Geiser PB: Epidemiologic comparison of breast cancer patients with early and late onset of malignancy and general population controls. J Natl Cancer Inst 53:1577, 1974.
58. Brinton L, Williams R, Hoover R, et al.: Breast cancer risk factors among screening program participants. J Natl Cancer Inst 62:37, 1979.
59. Jick H, Walker AM, Watkins RN, et al.: Oral contraceptives and breast cancer. Am J Epidemiol 112:577, 1980.
60. Lippman ME, Huff K, Bolan G, et al.: Interactions of R5020 with progesterone and glucocorticoid receptors in human breast cancer and peripheral blood lymphocytes *in vitro*. *In*: McGuire WL, et al. (eds.): Progesterone Receptors in Normal and Neoplastic Tissues. New York: Raven Press, 1977, pp. 193–210.
61. Fergusson DJP, Anderson TJ: Morphological evaluation of cell turnover in relation to menstrual cycle in the "resting" human breast. Br J Cancer 44:177, 1981.
62. Hoover R, Gray LA, Cole P, et al.: Menopausal estrogens and breast cancer. N Engl J Med 295:401, 1976.
63. Brinton LA, Hoover RN, Szkio M, et al.: Menopausal estrogen use and risk of breast cancer. Cancer 47:2517, 1981.
64. Hoover R, Glass A, Findle WD, et al.: Conjugated estrogens and breast cancer risk in women. J Natl Cancer Inst 67:815, 1981.
65. Ross RK, Hill AP, Gerkins VR, et al.: A case-control study of menopausal estrogen therapy and breast cancer. JAMA 243:1635, 1980.

Screening and Detection of Breast Cancer

GLORIA FRANKL, M.D.

Breast cancer screening, the detection of breast cancer before it is palpable in asymptomatic women, is a technique that saves lives. Early detection permits a better outcome and even allows breast-preserving treatment.

New data and recent reports from the Netherlands suggest a 50 to 70 percent reduction in the number of deaths due to breast cancer among women screened by mammography. These data dramatically support the famous Health Insurance Plan (HIP) trial conducted in New York, which showed a one-third reduction in mortality from breast cancer among women offered screening by mammography and physical examination. Since the HIP study, mammography has advanced in two important ways: Modern equipment can detect smaller cancers than those detected in the past and the amount of radiation employed has decreased considerably.

The numerous ways of detecting breast cancer are discussed, and each is evaluated as a screening or detection method.

METHODS OF DETECTION

Physical Examination

Breast self-examination is an inexpensive, noninvasive method of cancer detection that can be taught successfully to patients. Some reports suggest that this tool can be effective in reducing breast cancer mortality.[43] The author's data from the Los Angeles Kaiser Permanente Medical Center are less optimistic. Although 60 percent of the breast cancers were self-discovered, perhaps it is more important to note that among patients with palpable lesions who died because of their disease, 79 percent of the deaths occurred in those who had self-detected lesions. By the time the patient noted the tumor, it often was too late; there already were axillary node metastases.

Although there obviously are degrees of competency, proficiency, and thoroughness, approximately 75 percent of all breast cancers are found by the examining clinician. While detection itself is vital, assessment of the stage at which the cancer is found is of equal importance. Almost 50 percent of women

2

with palpable infiltrating ductal carcinomas already have axillary node metastases at the time the cancer is discovered.

Mammography

Mammography is an x-ray study of the breast. There currently are two main systems of mammographic examination, film-screen and xeroradiography. Controversy suggests that there is no clear or definite advantage of film-screen mammography over xeroradiography. All agree that the mammography must be of optimum diagnostic quality and must be interpreted by a qualified reader who is trained in mammography.

The author prefers xeromammography because the images permit clear visualization of all breast structures, including skin, ducts, calcifications, masses, tumor spiculations, and vessels, and the chest wall. Excellent resolution and the unique edge-enhancement effect of xeroradiography contribute to an accuracy rate reported to be as high as 92.1 percent.[8] A good diagnostic xeroradiographic examination is comfortable and convenient for the patient and for the technologist. Although the delivered radiation dose is not as low as in some film-screen systems, modern xeroradiography is a safe, low-dose technique. (Risk-benefit ratios and theoretical risks will be considered in the next section.)

As shown in a series analyzing 4625 breast cancer biopsies performed at the Los Angeles Kaiser Permanente Medical Center, where a panel of 14 radiologists interprets xeroradiographic studies, physical examination and xeroradiography are complementary procedures (Table 2–1). Findings derived from this table show the following: (1) 88 percent of the cancers were correctly identified by the radiologist; (2) 96 percent of the cancers were imaged by the xeroradiography system; (3) the radiologists' false-positive rate was 48 percent, versus the clinicians' false-positive rate of 75 percent; (4) 27 percent of the 1435 cancers were occult, found only with xeromammography; (5) a palpable mass not imaged with mammography must never be ignored.

TABLE 2–1. Pathology Correlations: 4625 Biopsies

Pathology	*+XRO, +PE*	*+XRO, −PE*	*−XRO, +PE*
Cancer	873	387	112 misinterpreted 63 not imaged
Benign	741	794	1655

+XRO = Suspicious or + xeromammogram
+PE = Suspicious or + physical examination

Mammography can be performed either with a modified general-purpose overhead x-ray tube or with an x-ray system that is specifically designed for breast imaging, a "dedicated" mammography unit. Although satisfactory mammograms can be produced with general-purpose equipment, only dedicated systems combine the features that can provide optimum imaging geometry, compression devices, positioning features, and exposure factors that result in images of the highest quality. Numerous manufacturers currently make dedicated mammography units.

Risks and Benefits of Mammography

Feig has shown that the known benefits from early detection of breast cancer outweigh by far any theoretical risk from exposure to currently used low-dose radiation methods of screening.[13] To place in perspective the proposed risk of incurring an excess number of breast cancers as a consequence of screening, theoretically, examination of 1 million women at age 40 could result in ten excess (beyond the natural or background) cancers over the lifetimes of these patients. However, this risk must be considered along with the natural incidence of 800 breast cancers in this group of women, noting that with screening mammography most of the cancers could be detected at a curable stage.[3, 6]

Whatever the theoretical risk may be, for women over 35 years of age at the time of exposure, there is a real and definite reduction in the possible hazards of radiation. A study of patients in Canadian sanitaria found no increased risk for women x-rayed and fluoroscoped multiple times if the exposures occurred when the patients were more than 40 years of age.[19] In addition, a review of Japanese women found no excess breast cancer risk among women aged 30 or over at the time of exposure when the dose received was less than 99 rads.[42] The benefit-risk ratio for women more than 35 years of age definitely is favorable; one study fixed the ratio at 6:1 with currently used techniques.[26]

Chiacchierini and Lundin used life-table models to evaluate the risk-benefit ratio as a function of an annual radiation dose.[10] Using 1 rad as the dose delivered per examination, analyses showed two clear benefits of mammography: (1) A large number of person years was to be gained and (2) the number of breast cancer deaths averted greatly exceeded the radiation risk. In a similar fashion, Fox and colleagues described a model for estimating the benefit-risk ratio for mammography in screening populations of asymptomatic, randomly selected women.[15] Their numbers were based on five annual screenings and also showed that significant benefit was manifested in terms of breast cancer deaths averted.

Data from the 27 National Breast Cancer Detection Demonstration Projects indicate that mammography can detect early, small cancers prior to their being evident on physical examination.[5] With appropriate therapy, a ten-year survival rate of 95 percent or greater can be expected in Stage 0 cancers, 72 percent in Stage I, and only 40 percent in Stage II.[25] This information clearly demonstrates the importance of early diagnosis.

Current guidelines established by the U.S. Department of Health and Human Services state that a routine two-view mammographic examination of the breast should deliver a total of 1 rad or less to the midbreast.[45]

Mammography in Diagnosis

There are two uses for mammography: (1) for the evaluation and assessment of a clinically noted abnormality and (2) for the detection of occult (nonpalpable) cancers in asymptomatic screenees.

In a woman with a palpable tumor, mammography could replace a biopsy procedure if the x-ray study demonstrates a rather definite benign process at the site of the proposed biopsy. Lesions typically having a benign appearance include lipofibroadenomas or calcifying degenerating fibroadenomas, both of which have characteristic appearances radiographically. The lipofibroadenoma mass usually is oval and sharply outlined and has an internal cauliflower-like appearance, with areas of sharp density and areas of lucency. The calcifying degenerating fibroadenoma is an oval or gently lobulated circumscribed mass that contains large irregular calcifications. Sometimes, if the fibroadenoma is embedded in a fatty area, there will be a lucent halo around it.

Mammography should always precede breast biopsy for several reasons:

1. To evaluate the contralateral breast.
2. To look for occult lesions elsewhere in the ipsilateral breast.
3. To check for possible dermal lymphatic invasion by the cancer, which often can be detected radiographically before clinical findings are evident.
4. To defer or cancel biopsy if the palpable lesion is quite definitely benign in its mammographic appearance. If breast biopsy is canceled or deferred on the basis of radiographic findings, follow-up mammography or ultrasonography may be appropriate.

(Figures 2–1 through 2–6 demonstrate these features and principles.

Mammography in Screening and Detection

There is now a great deal of evidence showing that the examination of asymptomatic women with screening mammography will help to reduce mortality from breast cancer. Earlier detection will add years to the patient's life, and detection of cancers found early in their development (minimal cancers) can permit breast-conserving treatment.[33, 34, 46]

Detection at the earliest possible stage demands excellent technique and interpretation by a skilled, trained mammographer. In addition to the usual radiographic signs of breast cancer—a spiculating mass and clustered microcalcifications—the more subtle signs are important, especially in the diagnosis of breast cancer at an early stage. These less obvious signs of carcinoma include a single isolated duct or ductal asymmetry, focal architectural distortion, and asymmetry in breast density where none previously existed.[40] Figures 2–1 through 2–4 are xeroradiographic examples of occult, nonpalpable cancers.

Detection of cancer when it is small and confined to the breast dramatically improves survival. As reported by McLelland, the vast majority of early minimal cancers are found by screening mammography.[30] In the author's data, the term minimal cancer is based on histologic criteria. Minimal cancers are infiltrating ductal carcinomas 0.5 cm or less in diameter, intraductal carcinomas, and lobular carcinomas in situ. One hundred eight occult (nonpalpable) minimal cancers were found with xeromammography in a 13-year

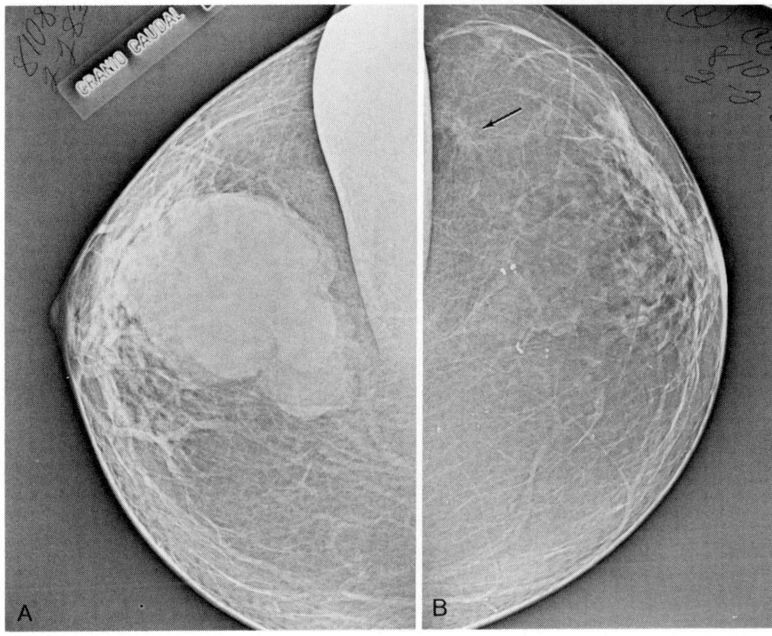

FIGURE 2–1. Bilateral cancers. *A*, Palpable cancer (craniocaudal view, left breast). *B*, Occult cancer in opposite breast (arrow).

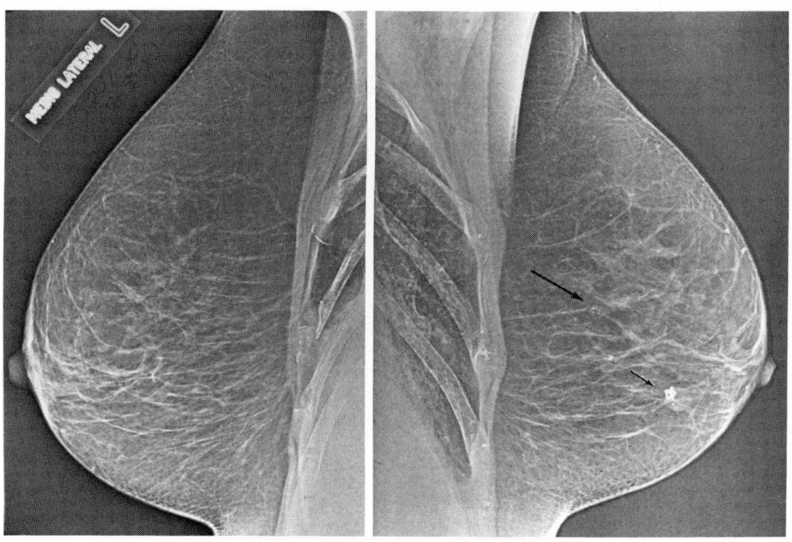

FIGURE 2–2. Xeromammography, performed prior to a planned biopsy of a palpable mass that proved to be benign (small arrow), revealed the presence of an otherwise undetected occult cancerous lesion (large arrow).

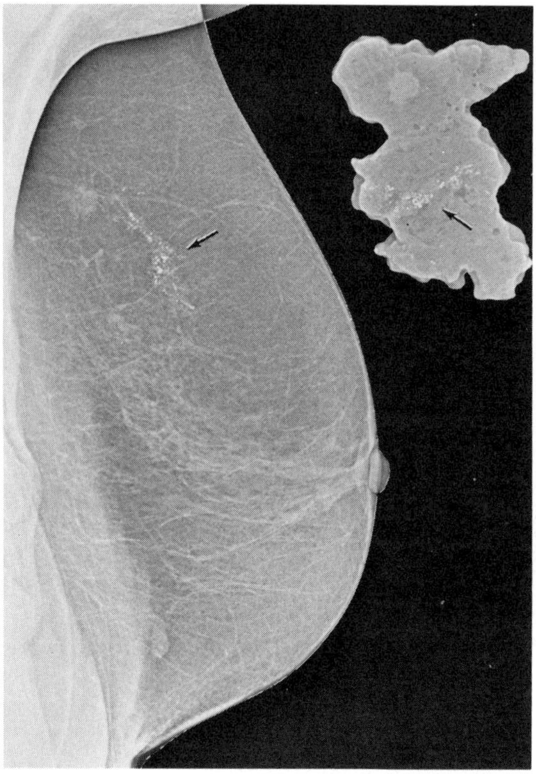

FIGURE 2–3. Two radiographic manifestations of cancer: occult spiculating cancerous mass with adjacent intraductal comedocarcinoma. Spiculating, invasive mass is obvious on mammography, but not palpable. Nests of microcalcifications (arrows) are typical of comedocarcinoma.

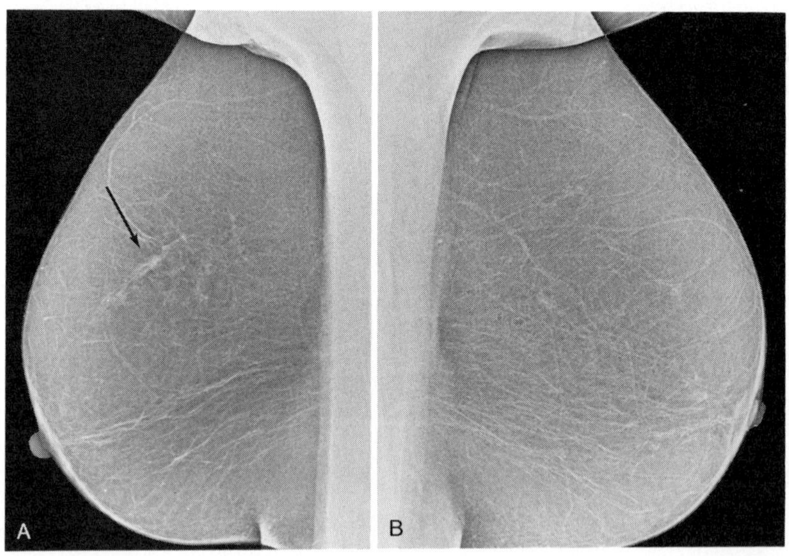

FIGURE 2–4. Asymmetry and distortion (arrow) as signs of breast cancer. Note the asymmetric increased density and parenchymal distortion (*A*), when compared with the same area in the opposite breast (*B*). Biopsy revealed adenocarcinoma.

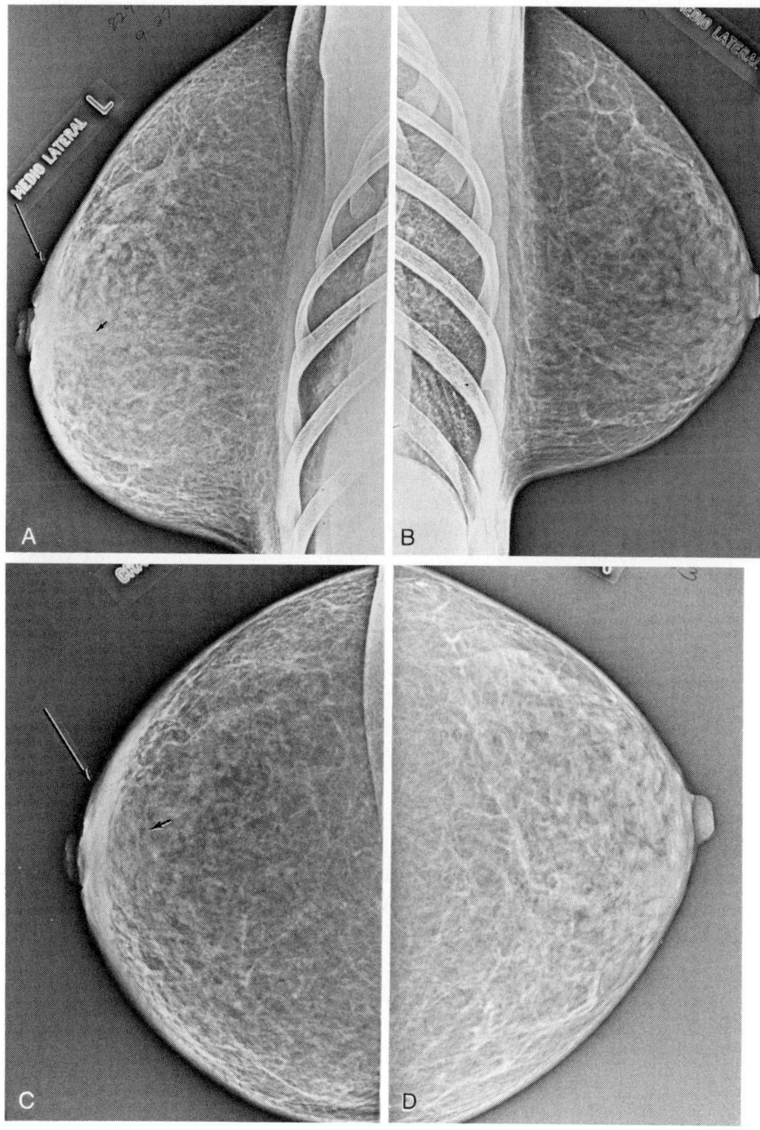

FIGURE 2–5. Occult invasion of the dermal lymphatics (mediolateral, *A* and *B*, and craniocaudal, *C* and *D*, views of left and right breasts). A mass, strongly suspicious for cancer, was clearly evident on palpation, but no skin changes were seen. Xeroradiography shows dermal lymphatic invasion (large arrows) as well as the palpable cancer mass density (small arrows).

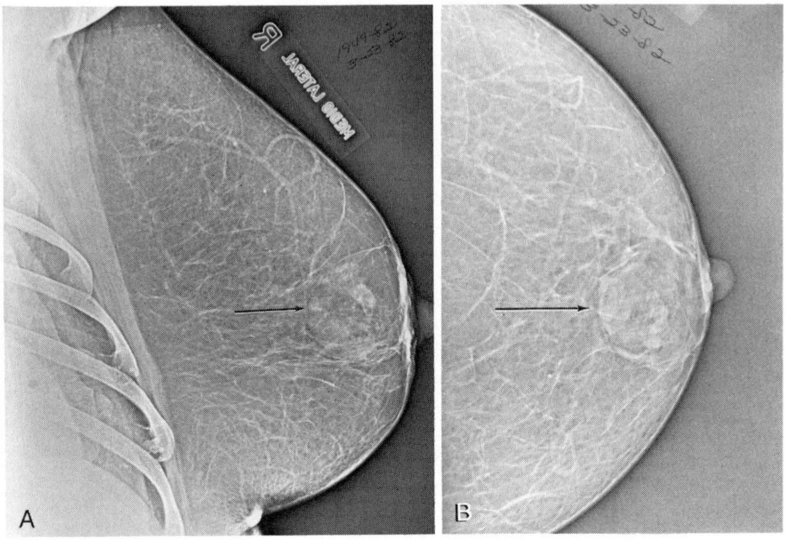

FIGURE 2–6. Lipofibroadenoma—an example of a typically benign process (mediolateral, *A*, and craniocaudal, *B*, views). Sharply circumscribed encapsulated mass (arrows) has a mixture of fat and connective tissue and epithelial components, resulting in the characteristic cauliflower-like appearance that is pathognomonic of lipofibroadenoma.

period (Table 2–2). Follow-up of this group revealed that only one treated patient with minimal cancer died of metastatic breast disease in this span of time.

As indicated in Tables 2–2 and 2–3, the mortality rates and positive axillary node rates are significantly higher in women with palpable breast cancers. Table 2–2 summarizes and compares the outcome data of three breast cancer patient populations: those with occult minimal cancers, those with other occult cancers, and those with palpable cancers.

Axillary node status also is improved if the breast cancers are occult rather than palpable. Among 1435 patients followed by the author at the Los Angeles Kaiser Permanente Medical Center, there is a greater than twofold difference in positive axillary node rates when the palpable and occult cancer patient populations are compared (Fig. 2–7).

In 1971, Shapiro and colleagues[36] reported results from the Health Insurance Plan (HIP) trial of screening for breast cancer, a study in which women randomly selected for screening by physical examination and mammography in four successive years were compared with a control group. There was a one-third reduction in breast cancer mortality attributable to screening, and the benefit was shown to continue on long-term follow-up.[37] Since this HIP study, widely different viewpoints on the value of screening have been published.[2, 3] In addition, several trials have been set up[32, 35, 41, 44] to test the HIP findings regarding the benefit of screening and to answer additional questions, such as whether it is efficacious to screen women under the age of 50 and whether it is necessary to use both clinical examination and mammography. Results from these studies and from the National Cancer Institute–American Cancer Society Breast Cancer Detection Demonstration Projects (BCDDP)[3] show that modern mammography is a more sensitive screening test than is clinical evaluation, may be more cost-effective,[17] and involves an almost negligible radiation hazard.[18]

These kinds of data have led to the increasing interest in and acceptance of screening mammography. Two studies reported from the Netherlands in June 1984 offer factual confirmation of the benefits of screening.[11, 47] These studies were not originally intended to test the effect of screening on mortality and therefore lack control groups. They differ from the volunteer screening programs such as the BCDDP in that they included defined

TABLE 2–2. Outcomes (%) in Three Groups of Breast Cancer Patients

Cancer Group	*5-Year Follow-Up*	*Positive Nodes*	*Alive, No Evidence of Disease*	*Died, With Breast Cancer*
Occult minimal (n = 108)	38	1	95	2
Other occult, not minimal (n = 279)	42	23	69	17
Palpable (n = 1048)	37	43	56	25

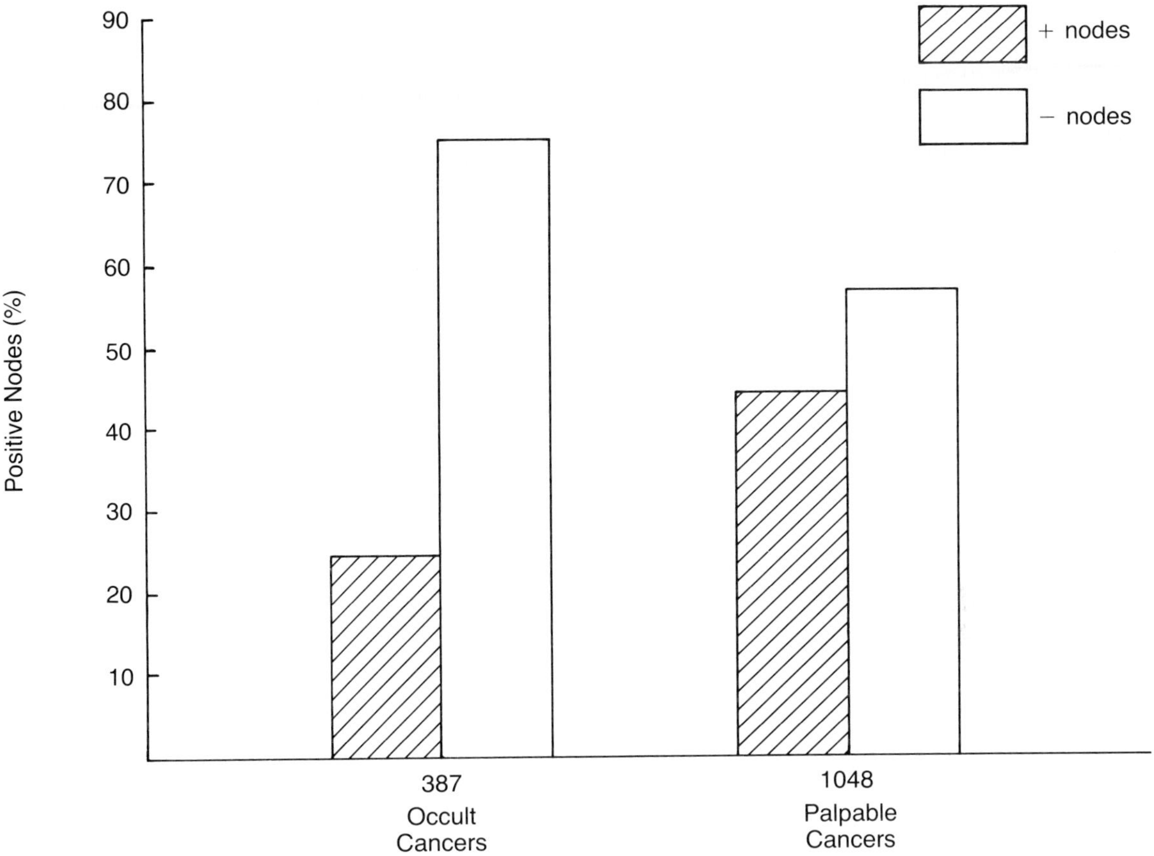

FIGURE 2–7. Axillary node status: palpable versus occult cancers.

populations, and all of those who were screened were invited to participate. In each study, the cancer incidence and mortality were recorded. The well-known case-control epidemiologic method was used to evaluate the effect of interventional screening by comparing women with breast cancer with controls who did not suffer from breast cancer. Mortality reductions of 50 to 70 percent were shown in screened women in Nijmegen and Utrecht. These studies showed that the protective factor between the two groups was the history of having been screened. Also, the Nijmegen study, which screened using only mammography without clinical examination, provided evidence that screening by mammography alone may be effective in reducing the risk of dying of breast cancer.

Guidelines for the Use of Mammography

The American College of Radiology has developed and published guidelines for screening with mammography that also have been fully endorsed by the American Cancer Society:[1, 29]

1. Symptomatic women: Mammography is an essential part of the diagnostic workup
2. Asymptomatic women:
   a. Women should be taught breast self-examination and should have an annual breast examination after age 35.
   b. Baseline mammography should be performed between the ages of 35 and 40, then annually or biennially between ages 40 and 49, and annually after age 50.

Wolfe's work shows that certain patterns of breast anatomy, as delineated on the mammogram, are predictors of an excessive susceptibility to breast cancer.[48] His studies also support the value of baseline mammography in women near 35 years of age.[49] Wolfe's recommendations for routine serial mammography differ slightly from the guidelines suggested by the American College of Radiology and the American Cancer Society. His guidelines for interval screening studies

TABLE 2–3. Parenchymal Pattern and Breast Cancer Risk (%)

Parenchymal Pattern Assignment	Population Studied	Cancers on First Mammography	Subsequent Cancers
Low Risk N1, P1	66	32	20
High Risk P2, Dy	34	68	80

are: fatty breasts (N1), every three to five years; slight ductal prominence (P1), every two to three years; and severe ductal prominence (P2) or dysplasia (DY), every year. The author's data corroborate the validity of Wolfe's description of parenchymal patterns as predictors for susceptibility to breast cancer (Table 2–3).

Since Wolfe's work was first published, there have been many articles confirming and many denying the validity of parenchymal patterns as a predictor of breast cancer risk. Contradictory results from 17 English language medical literature reports were reviewed by Boyd and colleagues.[7] These authors found a strong association between the standards adopted by a particular study and the results obtained. It appears that the methodological differences among the studies contribute greatly to the controversy. However, the studies that conformed to the usual scientific methods used in the epidemiologic investigation of risk have confirmed, in general, that an association does exist between mammographic patterns and the risk of breast cancer.

Computed Tomographic Mammography

In the 1970's, Chang and colleagues investigated the use of computed tomographic (CT) mammography.[9] The examination was long and rigorous and delivered a moderately high dose of radiation. According to Kopans and Meyer,[22] the best and most appropriate use of CT breast imaging stems from the cross-sectional nature of the scans, the ability to image the extreme medial and lateral portions of the breast tissue as well as the tissue immediately adjacent to the chest wall, and the ability to localize those rare lesions that are visible only in the mediolateral mammographic projection.

Nuclear Magnetic Resonance Imaging

The newest cross-sectional digital imaging system is nuclear magnetic resonance imaging (NMR). There are only limited data on the efficacy of NMR in the breast.[23] An obvious advantage of NMR is the omission of any radiation dose. Additional potential advantages of NMR include the ability to differentiate between benign and malignant lesions, thereby reducing the biopsy rate. Also, NMR may permit preoperative staging of breast cancer.[23] Some disadvantages are its high cost and its inability to detect microcalcifications, which are so important in the x-ray detection of early breast cancer.

NMR provides a potential for chemical analysis of breast tissue; however, thus far, it only represents a new way of demonstrating the morphology of breast lesions. Although NMR has promise, until its true efficacy is demonstrated, it still must be considered experimental in the field of breast analysis.

Fossel, Carr, and McDonagh[50] reviewed another possible use for NMR, studying the water-suppressed proton nuclear magnetic resonance spectroscopy of plasma. They showed that the narrowing of lipoprotein-lipid resonances in those patients with cancer (consistent with the response of a host to tumor growth) differs from the resonances in those patients without malignant tumors. The presented preliminary results demonstrate that water-suppressed proton NMR spectroscopy is a potentially valuable approach to the detection of cancer and the monitoring of therapy.

Digital Mammographic Imaging

Digital mammographic imaging, a technology under development and testing, will result in high resolution with a very low dose of radiation. The system will use a solid-state detector with a thick scintillator, achieving high detector efficiency, without sacrificing resolution quality, and eliminating radiation scatter. By obtaining a digital image, computer manipulation can be applied. Thus, in addition to inherently lower radiation doses because of high detector efficiency, there will be a computer compensation capability, which will eliminate underexposed and overexposed images that necessitate repeated patient exposures.

Ultrasound

Ultrasound is not suitable for breast cancer screening and should not be used as a detection modality. Ultrasound cannot accurately differentiate benign from malignant solid lesions. Its primary role is the differentiation of cystic from solid lesions and as an adjunctive guide for needle aspiration and localization procedures.[21, 38] It sometimes may be a useful adjunct for further evaluation of lesions that already have been detected by either mammography or physical examination.

Because of its composition, breast tissue is not well suited to evaluation by ultrasound imaging. Virtually all cancer masses in the breast are hypoechoic; they often are irregular in shape and are not homogeneous in density. The scattered fat and glandular and fibrous tissues in the breast produce irregularities that mimic cancer. For example, fat in the breast tends to be hypoechoic relative to the surrounding denser tissues. The classic posterior acoustic shadowing described in the literature concerning breast ultrasound often is absent in malignant lesions,[20] and benign lesions also can demonstrate similar posterior acoustic shadowing.[31]

An additional limitation of breast ultrasound is its inability to consistently image microcalcifications, which are so important in the diagnosis of breast cancer. It is no surprise that Sickles and colleagues reported that small cancers (less than 1 to 2 cm) rarely were detected by ultrasound.[38]

Thermography

Thermography is a direct method of measuring temperature. Numerous kinds of thermographic technique have been proposed for evaluation of the breast:

1. Telethermography measures infrared rays emitted from the skin and converts these measurements into a skin temperature map.
2. Liquid crystal thermography uses esters of cholesterol that are encapsulated in Mylar sheaths and reflect polarized light and change color in response to temperature changes when placed in direct contact with the skin.
3. Computer-assisted thermography uses temperature measurements from multiple standardized locations on each breast; these measurements then are analyzed by a computer to provide an index of the likelihood of malignancy.
4. Graphic stress thermography uses computer-assisted interpretation of temperature readings taken before and after patients have undergone the stress of immersing their hands in ice water for 15 seconds. The rationale for the stress test is that normal vasoconstriction does not occur in areas of malignancy.
5. Microwave thermography measures normal microwave radiation emitted from the breast and has the theoretical advantage of providing deep, as well as superficial, thermal information.

Most of the early thermographic work was performed using telethermography; in most of the more recent work, liquid crystal thermography has been used. The other techniques described have been less well studied, but with all techniques, the results generally have been poor.

Studies of symptomatic patients indicate that thermography operates at a high level of predictability only for large (5-cm or greater) cancers.[12, 14, 24, 27] Thermography cannot be used to detect clinically occult cancer; it is not an acceptable tool for screening asymptomatic women; and it is not an effective "pre-screener" to determine which women need further study by mammography. In the Breast Cancer Detection Demonstration Project, the breast cancer detection rate for thermography was only 42 percent, which is especially unacceptable when compared with the rates of 57 percent for physical examination and 91 percent for mammography.[3, 19]

Some studies have indicated a possible prognostic role for thermography because breast cancers with grossly abnormal thermograms may be associated with substantially higher than expected mortality rates.[16, 28] However, the results are considered unproven and, therefore, experimental because of incomplete documentation and flaws in the design of the studies (e.g., no correction for tumor size or histologic grading).

The fact that thermography does not employ ionizing radiation does not by itself justify its use. Adding thermography to physical examination and mammography provides little meaningful information, may engender a false sense of security, and increases the cost of medical care. According to a policy statement issued in 1984, the American College of Radiology has concluded that breast thermography has no established clinical indications and that its use should be limited to properly controlled prospective studies designed to test its clinical efficacy.

Diaphanography

Diaphanography involves transillumination of the breast by either infrared or visible light. The major finding associated with carcinoma is a dark area, an area of light attenuation that is asymmetric when compared with the contralateral breast. Other less definite findings relate to the effect of the cancer on surrounding tissue: hypervascularity, abrupt changes in vessel diameter, and an asymmetric increase in the number of vessels when compared with the opposite breast.

Although studies by Bartrum and Crow[4] and by Sickles[39] show that diaphanography can demonstrate large tumors, only 19 to 44 percent of small lesions (1 cm or less in diameter) could be found with this modality. Based on these studies, it is apparent that diaphanography should not be used as a screening procedure, nor can it be relied upon without associated mammography.

DISCUSSION

Breast self-examination and physical examination by the clinician are proven methods of breast cancer detection; however, using only these methods, the cancers often are not discerned before there has been spread out of the breast, worsening prognosis and impairing treatment. Mammography provides an important supplement to physical examination, and its value in early breast cancer detection is now universally accepted. With the low levels of radiation currently required for quality studies, the benefit-risk ratio for mammography is substantially favorable for women over 35 years of age. Only mammography has proved capable of detecting early, small cancers prior to their detection by physical examination.

Although it may have some other uses in breast analysis, ultrasound is not a suitable screening device and should not be used for detection of breast cancer. In addition, the other modalities described in this chapter must be considered unproven or experimental.

Early cancers have an improved prognosis, with decreased rates of axillary node metastasis and decreased mortality rates. Not only is the prognosis influenced by the detection of occult, nonpalpable cancers, but treatment also may be altered if the cancer is detected in the earliest stage of development. There is now good evidence that in selected cases it may be appropriate to treat minimal cancers with breast-conserving therapy.[15, 16]

CONCLUSION

X-ray mammography is the only imaging device with a proven capability of detecting early-stage breast cancer. In the past, there was little success in reducing the mortality rate of patients with breast cancer, and the early detection of breast cancer continues to be a major goal in the health care of women. With screening mammography, occult breast cancer often can be found in asymptomatic women, when it still is confined to the breast. The established benefit of this early detection is an improved outcome.

REFERENCES

1. American College of Radiology Guidelines for Mammography. ACR Bull 38:6, 1982.
2. Bailar JC: Mammography: A contrary view. Ann Intern Med 84:77, 1976.
3. Baker LH: Breast Cancer Detection Demonstration Project: Five-year summary report. CA 32:194, 1982.
4. Bartrum RJ, Crow HC: Transillumination lightscanning to diagnose breast cancer: A feasibility study. AJR 142:409, 1984.
5. Beahrs OH, Shapiro S, Smart C: Report of the Working Group to Review the NCI/ACS Breast Cancer Detection Demonstration Projects. Sept. 6, 1977.
6. Beahrs OH, Shapiro S, Smart C: Report of the Working Group to Review the National Cancer Institute–American Cancer Society Breast Cancer Detection Demonstration Projects. J Natl Cancer Inst 62:640, 1979.
7. Boyd NJ, O'Sullivan B, Fishell E, et al.: Mammographic patterns and breast cancer risks: Methodologic standards and contradictory results. J Natl Cancer Inst 72:1253, 1984.
8. Castiglione V, et al.: Diagnostic accuracy of xeromammography. Tumor (Milan) 67:447, 1981.

9. Chang CHJ, Nesbit DE, Fisher DR, et al.: Computed tomographic mammography using a conventional body scanner. AJR 138:553, 1982.
10. Chiacchierini R, Lundin F: Benefit-risk in mammography. Presented at the Eighth National Conference on Radiation Control. Springfield, Illinois, May 2–7, 1976.
11. Collette HJA, Rombach JJ, Day NE, et al.: Evaluation of screening for breast cancer in a non-randomized study (The DOM Project) by means of a case-control study. Lancet 1:1224, 1984.
12. Dodd GD: Heat-sensing devices and breast cancer detection. *In*: Feig SA, McLelland R (eds.): Breast Carcinoma: Current Diagnosis and Treatment. New York: Masson, 1983, pp. 207–225.
13. Feig SA: Low-dose mammography and the question of radiation risk. Syllabus for the Categorical Course on Mammography, pp. 101–116. Presented at the Annual Meeting of The American College of Radiology, Los Angeles, 1948.
14. Feig SA, Shaber GS, Schwartz GF, et al.: Thermography, mammography, and clinical examination in breast cancer screening. Radiology 122:123, 1977.
15. Fox S, Moskowitz M, Saenger E, et al.: Benefit/risk analysis of aggressive mammographic screening. Radiology 128:359, 1978.
16. Gautherie M, Gros CM: Breast thermography and cancer risk prediction. Cancer 45:51, 1980.
17. Gravelle HSE, Simpson PR, Chamberlain J: Breast cancer screening and health service costs. J Health Econ 1:185, 1982.
18. Howe GR, Sherman GJ, Semenciw RM, et al.: Estimated benefits and risks of screening for breast cancer. Can Med Assoc J 124:399, 1981.
19. Howe GR: Epidemiology of radiogenic breast cancer. *In*: Boice JD, Jr., Fraumeni JF, Jr. (eds.): Radiation Carcinogenesis: Epidemiology and Biological Significance. New York: Raven Press, 1984, pp. 119–120.
20. Kopans DB, Meyer JE, Steinbock RT: Breast cancer: The appearance as delineated by whole breast water bath ultrasound. J Clin Ultrasound 10:313, 1982.
21. Kopans DB, Meyer JE, Lindfors KL, et al.: Breast sonography to guide cyst aspiration and wire localization of occult solid lesions. AJR 143:489, 1984.
22. Kopans DB, Meyer JE: Computed tomography guided localization of clinically occult breast carcinoma. Radiology 145:211, 1982.
23. Kopans DB: Digital mammography and magnetic resonance imaging. Syllabus for the Categorical Course on Mammography, pp. 149–161. Presented at the Annual Meeting of The American College of Radiology, Los Angeles, 1984.
24. Lapayowker MS, Revesz G: Thermography and ultrasound in detection and diagnosis of breast cancer. Cancer 46:933, 1980.
25. Leis HP, Jr.: Selective and reconstructive surgical procedures for carcinoma of the breast. Surg Gynecol Obstet 148:1, 1979.
26. Lester RG: A radiologist's view of the benefit/risk ratio of mammography. *In*: Logan WW (ed.): Breast Carcinoma: The Radiologist's Expanded Role. New York: John Wiley & Sons, 1977, pp. 29–33.
27. Libshitz HI: Thermography of the breast: Current status and future expectations. JAMA 238:1953, 1977.
28. Lloyd-Williams K: Thermography in the prognosis of breast cancer. Bibl Radiol 5:62, 1969.
29. Mammography guidelines 1983: Background statement and update. CA 33:255, 1983.
30. McLelland R: Screening for breast cancer. Syllabus for the Categorical Course on Mammography, pp. 117–124. Presented at the Annual Meeting of The American College of Radiology, Los Angeles, 1984.
31. Meyer JE, Kopans DB, Oot R: Mammographic visualization of breast cancer in patients under 35 years of age. Radiology 147:93, 1983.
32. Miller AB, Howe GR, Wall C: The national study of breast cancer screening. Protocol for a Canadian randomized controlled trial of screening for breast cancer in women. Clin Invest Med 4:227, 1981.
33. Montague ED, Paulus DD, Schell SR: Selection and follow-up of patients for conservation surgery and irradiation. Front Radiat Ther Oncol 17:124, 1983.
34. Moskowitz M: Mammography to screen asymptomatic women for breast cancer. AJR 143:457, 1984.
35. Roberts MM, Alexander FE, Anderson TJ, et al.: The Edinburgh randomized trial of screening for breast cancer. Br J Cancer (In press, 1985).
36. Shapiro S, Strax P, Venet L: Periodic breast cancer screening in reducing mortality from breast cancer. JAMA 215:1777, 1971.
37. Shapiro S, Venet W, Strax P, et al.: Ten- to fourteen-year effects of breast cancer screening on mortality. J Natl Cancer Inst 69:349, 1982.
38. Sickles EA, Filly EA, Callen PW: Breast cancer detection with sonography and mammography. AJR 140:843, 1983.
39. Sickles EA: Breast cancer detection with transillumination and mammography. AJR 142:841, 1984.
40. Sickles E: Mammographic features of "early" breast cancer. AJR 143:461, 1984.
41. Tabar L, Gad A: Screening for breast cancer—the Swedish trial. Radiology 138:219, 1981.
42. Tokunaga M, Land CE, Yamoto T, et al.: Breast cancer among atomic bomb survivors. *In*: Boice JD, Jr., Fraumeni JF, Jr. (eds.): Radiation Carcinogenesis: Epidemiology and Biological Significance. New York: Raven Press, 1984, pp. 45–56.
43. Turner J, Roy D, Irwin G, et al.: Does a booklet on breast self-examination improve subsequent detection rates? Lancet 1:337, 1984.
44. UK Trial of Early Detection of Breast Cancer Group: Trial of early detection of breast cancer: Description of method. Br J Cancer 44:618, 1981.
45. U.S. Dept. HEW Publication No. (NIH) 77-1400. Washington, D.C., March 1977.
46. Unzeitig G, Frankl G, Ackerman M, et al.: Analysis of the prognosis of minimal and occult breast cancer. Arch Surg 118:1403, 1983.
47. Verbeck LM, Holland R, Sturmans F, et al.: Reduction of breast cancer mortality through mass screening with modern mammography. Lancet 1:1222, 1984.
48. Wolfe JN: Risk for breast cancer development determined by mammographic parenchymal patterns. Cancer 37:5, 1976.
49. Wolfe JN: Xeroradiography of the Breast, 2nd ed. Springfield, Illinois: Charles C Thomas, 1983, p. 112.
50. Fossel ET, Carr JM, McDonagh J: Detection of malignant tumors. N Engl J Med 315:1369, 1986.

Gross and Microscopic Pathology of the Female Breast: Prognostic Variables and Current Approaches to Primary Breast Cancer Diagnosis

CHERYL M. REICHERT, M.D., Ph.D.
SHAHLA MOSHIRI, M.D.
R. MARSHALL AUSTIN, M.D., Ph.D.
HENRY J. NORRIS, M.D.

Fundamental to an understanding of the difference between benign and malignant breast lesions is a knowledge of the phylogeny, anatomy, embryology, physiology, and histology of the normal female breast. It is therefore appropriate that this chapter on pathology of the breast begin with an introduction to normal findings.

3

NORMAL FINDINGS

The breast is a complex network of milk-producing glands and ducts, embedded in a supporting matrix of fibroadipose tissue, lymphatics, blood vessels, and nerves. Approximately ten to 15 percent of the breast mass consists of the epithelial component; the remainder is stroma. Mammary glands are unique to the division of vertebrate animals that suckle their young, Mammalia (mammals). In the seven-week-old human embryo, the ectoderm-derived breast tissue appears as a band-like thickening of epidermis that extends from the axilla to the zroin (milk line). In humans, most of this tissue regresses shortly after its formation, but in the thoracic areas bilaterally, small portions persist, form downgrowths, and perforate the underlying mesenchyme. Subsequently, epithelial sprouts bud and eventually canalize to form the major lactiferous ducts of each breast.[1] In one to five percent of women, the regression of nonthoracic breast tissue is incomplete, resulting in an accessory nipple(s) with or without residual functioning breast tissue that is susceptible to the same disease processes as is the normal breast. The finding of polymastia in humans was cited by Darwin as an example of an atavism, in support of his theory of evolution.[2]

Using the nipple as a reference point, each breast is divided into upper-inner, lower-inner, upper-outer, and lower-outer quadrants. In the normal adult female, the breast tissue extends from the midline to the edge of the latissimus dorsi laterally and from the clavicle superiorly to the sixth cartilage inferiorly. The fascia of the pectoralis major, external oblique, serratus anterior, and portions of the rectus abdominis form the deep border of the gland. Projections of fibrous tissue (Cooper's ligaments) extend from the deep muscular fascia to the fibrous tissue of the dermis. These bands of fibrous tissue, which serve to support the breast, are important pathologically because of the communication that they establish between the breast and the skin. This communication leads to skin retraction overlying some infiltrating carcinomas of the breast.

The two breasts are frequently of unequal size. Much of the mammary tissue is in the upper-outer quadrant, accounting for the observation that more benign and malignant processes affect this sector than any other. A "tail" of breast tissue commonly extends into the axilla. The areolae (darkly pigmented rings of epithelium surrounding the nipples) and the nipples contain smooth muscle, the contraction of which facilitates the expulsion of milk. Large, specialized sebaceous glands (Montgomery's glands) are found at the perimeter of the areolae.

Histologically, each breast is divided into 15 to 20 *lobes* or *segments*. Because these segments are distinct, diseases that affect the ramifying processes of one ductal segment do not necessarily affect other lobes. Approximately 5 to 9 *collecting ducts* extend from the surface of the nipple into corresponding lactiferous sinuses; the remainder of the epithelial pits are thought to terminate in blind pouches.[3] A *lactiferous sinus* collects secretions from an underlying *segmental duct*, which in turn receives its contents from several *subsegmental ducts* (Fig. 3–1). Smaller interlobular *ductules* link the subsegmental ducts and intralobular ductules. The basic structural unit of the breast is the *lobule*, which contains the epithelial units responsible for milk production. Each lobule contains 10 to 100 or more *acini* (alveoli, or saclike glands), arranged around a central *intralobu-*

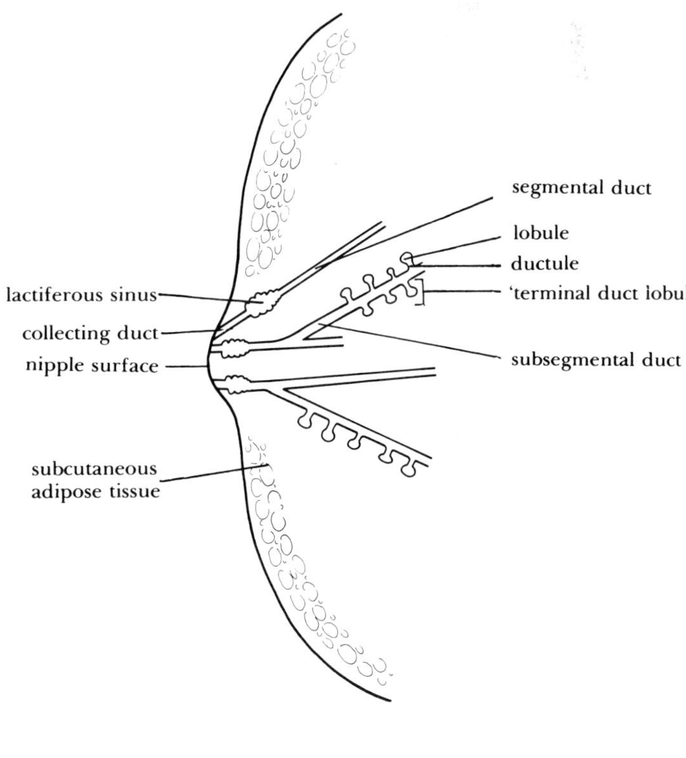

FIGURE 3–1. Normal breast structures. (With permission from Azzopardi JG, Ahmed A, Millis RR: Problems in Breast Pathology. Philadelphia: W. B. Saunders Co., 1979.)

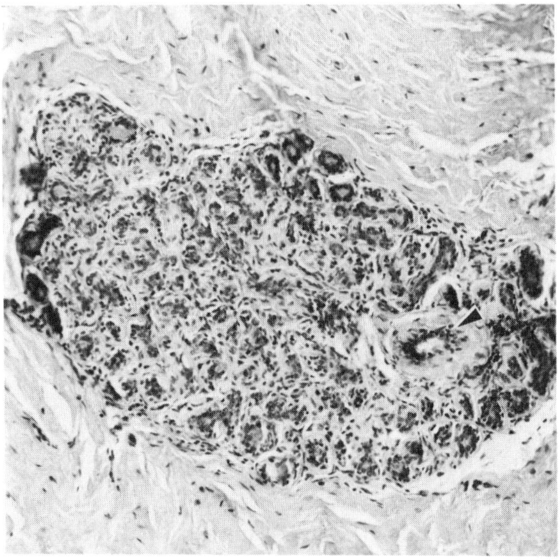

FIGURE 3–2. A normal nonlactating mammary lobule and intralobular ductule (arrowhead) from a premenopausal woman (H & E × 130).

lar ductule (Fig. 3–2). Taken together, the lobule and the intralobular ductule form the *terminal duct–lobular unit*. Because of the controversy as to whether the nonlactating breast contains true acini or only terminal ductules (secretory tubules), the glandular portion of nonlactating breast tissue has been termed the lobular epithelial unit by Azzopardi and colleagues.[3] Male breasts typically consist of only ducts, without lobules or alveoli. A knowledge of the normal breast architecture is helpful to an understanding of disease, since certain pathologic processes affect the lobule and others affect the ducts (Fig. 3–3).

In the premenopausal woman, collagen within the lobule is loose and finely reticular, as opposed to the more dense, hyalinized collagen of the interlobular stroma (Fig. 3–4). Elastic tissue is normally found around the ducts and is absent from the lobules.[4] The amount of elastic tissue roughly correlates with parity.[5]

The glandular elements of the breast contain two cell layers: an inner epithelial layer capable of milk secretion and an outer myoepithelial layer that provides a mechanism for oxytocin-stimulated milk ejection from the acinus (Fig. 3–5). A complete basement membrane envelops each acinus. By light microscopy, the myoepithelial cells are distinguished by their clear cytoplasm and the orientation of their nuclei next to the basement membrane. By electron microscopy, these cells contain myofibrillar elements, substantiating their similarity to smooth muscle cells, and desmosomes of epithelial origin.[6,7] An appreciation of this basic repetitive two-cell architectural pattern is crucial to making

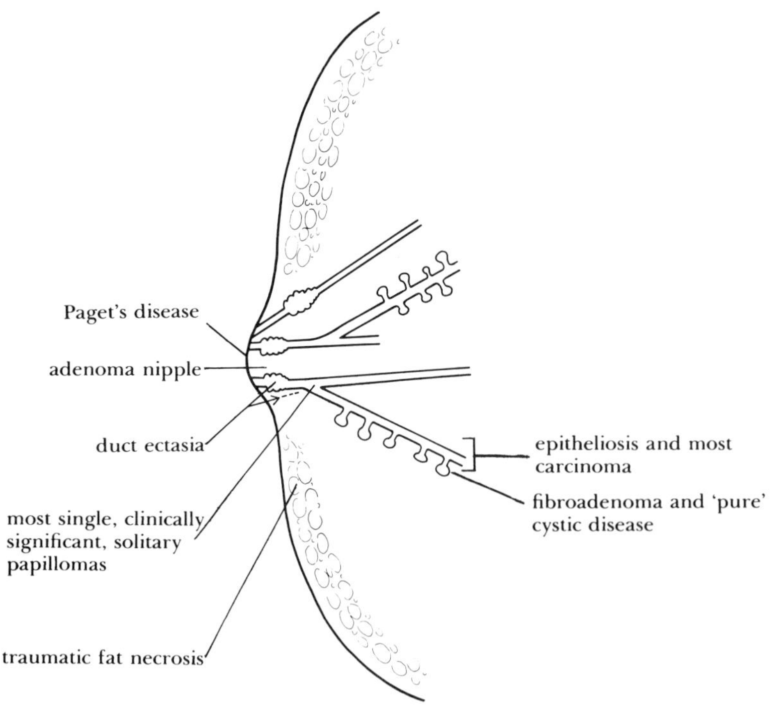

FIGURE 3–3. Localization of various disease processes within the breast. (With permission from Azzopardi JG, Ahmed A, Millis RR: Problems in Breast Pathology. Philadelphia: W. B. Saunders Co., 1979.)

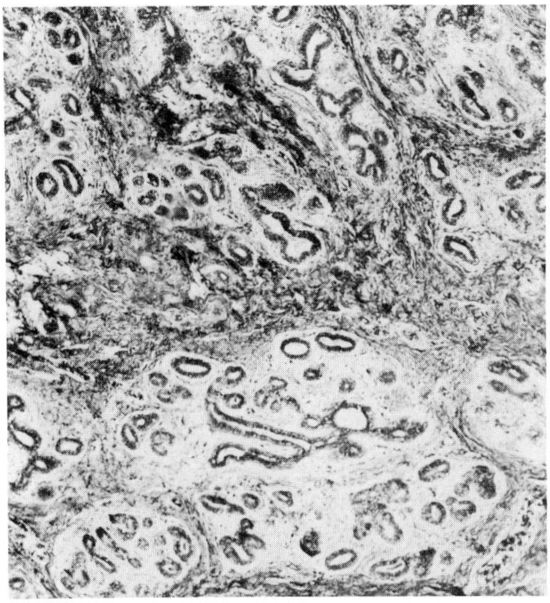

FIGURE 3–4. Premenopausal nonlactating breast lobules. Note the pale, delicate reticular collagen of the lobule in comparison with the coarse collagenous bands of the interlobular stroma (H & E × 54).

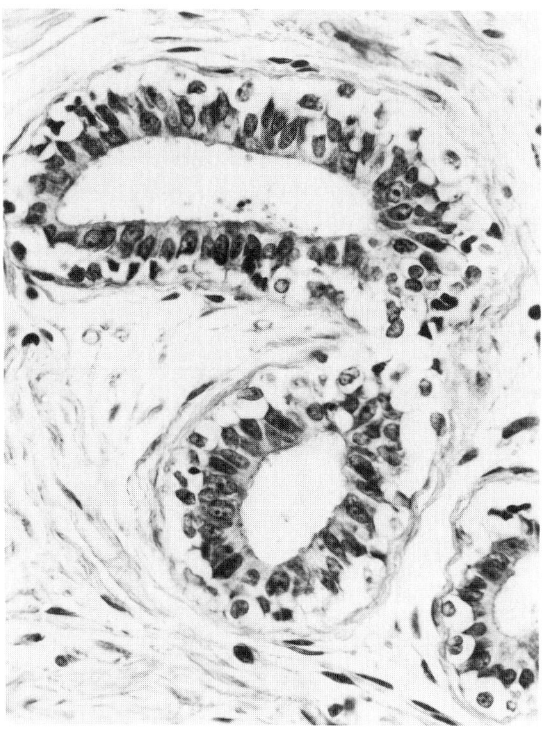

FIGURE 3–5. Two cell–layer glandular architecture of the breast. Note the inner epithelial layer, oriented around the lumen, and the outer myoepithelial layer consisting of cells with clear cytoplasm. A basement membrane envelops each acinus (H & E × 540).

the histologic distinction between benign epithelial proliferations and carcinomas.

In the process of evaluating a patient with a breast abnormality, it is important for the physician to avoid mistaking normal physiologic phenomena for breast disease. The consistency of the breast changes with the menstrual cycle. Increased nodularity and engorgement may be noted several days prior to the onset of menses. These changes are often most pronounced in nulliparous, premenopausal women. Although the underlying histologic correlate has not been conclusively established, these alterations are thought to be due to accumulation of fluid rather than cyclical epithelial proliferation and regression.[2]

Dramatic histologic changes accompany pregnancy and lactation. There is an increase in the size of the mammary lobule and in the numbers of gland fields (Fig. 3–6). There is frequently variation in degree of development among the lobules or even within an individual lobule. The epithelial cells lining the glandular lumina show vacuolization and evidence of secretion. Lipid droplets pass to the apex of the cell, where they are pinched off with a small portion of the plasmalemmal membrane.[8] Following the cessation of lactation, retained secretion is gradually removed by phagocytosis.

With menopause comes normal involution

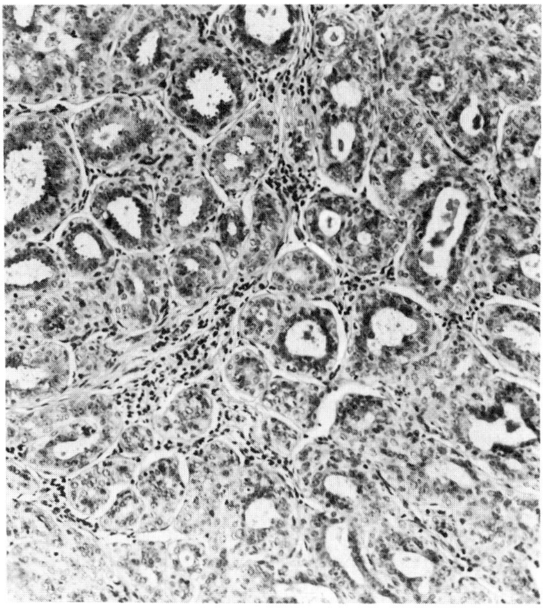

FIGURE 3–6. Numerous secretory glands of the lactating breast (H & E × 130).

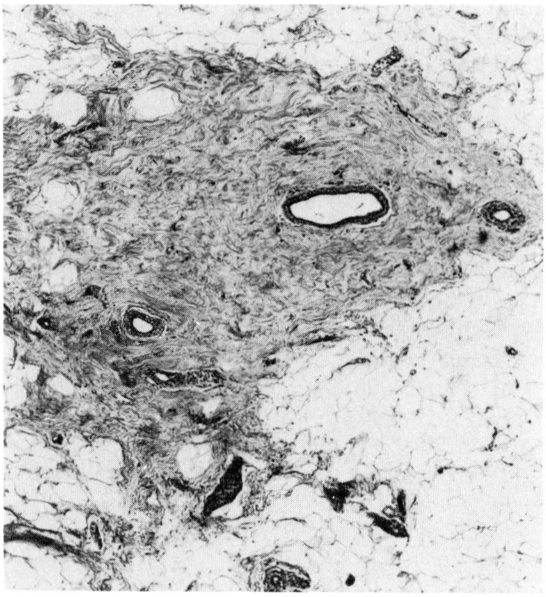

FIGURE 3–7. Postmenopausal breast tissue exhibits a combination of fat, densely hyalinized stroma, atrophic lobules, and residual ducts (H & E × 54).

of both epithelial and stromal elements (Fig. 3–7). The basement membrane of the acini becomes thickened, the two-layer epithelium atrophies, and the loose connective tissue of the lobule gradually converts to dense hyaline collagen that merges with the interlobular stroma. Eventually, adipose tissue replaces most of the collagenous stroma. This physiologic involutionary process, which is typically nonuniform, may result in palpable differences in consistency in the breasts of postmenopausal women.

BENIGN BREAST DISEASE

A variety of benign epithelial proliferations, cysts, and stromal alterations are encompassed within the spectrum of "fibrocystic disease." Because this process occurs clinically in 50 percent and histologically in 90 percent of women, there is some question as to whether such a widespread phenomenon should be considered a "disease."[9, 10] Some clinicians still include all benign breast epithelial proliferation under the rubric of "fibrocystic disease"; however, because of substantial differences in the relative risk of subsequent malignancy, Dupont and Page and others recommend that the histologic lesions of benign breast disease be separated into three categories: lesions with no appreciable proliferative activity (nonproliferative), proliferative disease without atypia, and atypical hyperplasia.[11] Each component element should be specified in the microscopic section of the pathology report. In this manner, the clinician is better able to interpret the significance of the histologic findings to the patient.

NONPROLIFERATIVE LESIONS

Nonproliferative lesions, including cysts, minimal hyperplasia, epithelium-related calcification, and apocrine metaplasia, convey no increased risk of malignancy.[11] These lesions are typically bilateral and characteristically occur in nulliparous women during the premenopausal years. In contrast with duct ectasia (see later), there is no nipple discharge. During the normal menstrual cycle, cysts may enlarge prior to the onset of menses and become painful and tender. Involvement of breast tissue may be extensive (Fig. 3–8). Contrary to popular belief, cysts arise within the lobules rather than the ducts. Ductular tissue contains elastic fibers at the periphery; elastic stains of dilated cysts fail to reveal elastic fibers.[3] Apocrine metaplasia is a frequent and easily recognizable component of nonproliferative breast disease (Fig. 3–9). The identification of apocrine metaplasia within an unusual proliferative lesion of the breast warrants caution in the interpretation of its malignant potential. Fibrosis, a common ingredient of benign breast disease, is included among nonproliferative lesions.

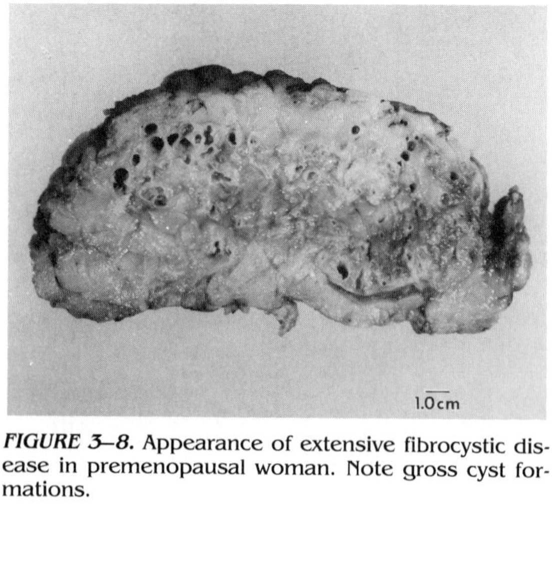

FIGURE 3–8. Appearance of extensive fibrocystic disease in premenopausal woman. Note gross cyst formations.

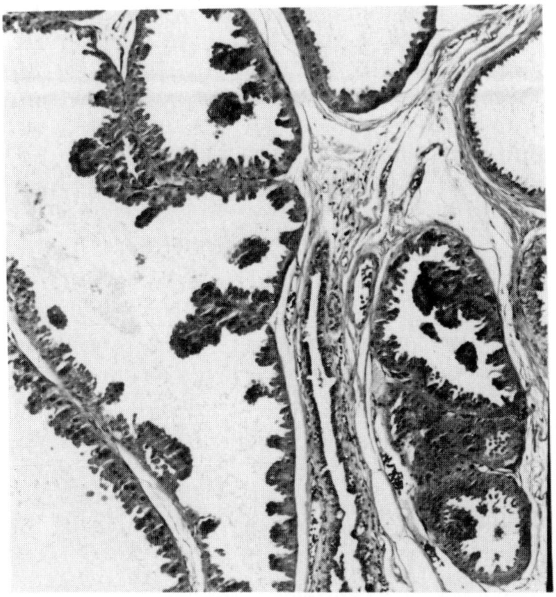

FIGURE 3–9. Apocrine metaplasia is a frequent component of nonproliferative benign lesions of the breast. The cells typically possess generous eosinophilic cytoplasm, small central nuclei, and cytoplasmic "snouts" that project into the lumen. These findings convey no risk of malignancy (H & E × 80).

Proliferative Lesions

Proliferative lesions include a variety of benign epithelial alterations, moderate or florid, that lack cytologic or architectural atypia. Women with such lesions are at slightly increased risk for subsequent malignancy, approximately twice that of the general population.[11] Unfortunately, there is no uniform terminology for classifying all the histologic variants. Whereas British pathologists frequently describe benign epithelial proliferations of the lobules and small ducts in terms of "epitheliosis," American pathologists are more likely to employ terms such as lobular hyperplasia, and intraductal papillomatosis (Fig. 3–10) to describe benign proliferation within the lobule and ducts, respectively.

Several benign epithelial lesions deserve special mention, by virtue of their potential misinterpretation as malignant processes. Blunt duct adenosis (proliferation of two-layered acini within the mammary lobule) and sclerosing adenosis (presence of individual benign acinar units within the stroma) are pseudoinfiltrative processes. Acinar tissue may also track along tissue planes of decreased resistance and produce benign epithelial inclusions in perineural and perivascular sites. Benign sclerosing papillary lesions and radial scars may be particularly difficult to distinguish from infiltrating carcinoma.[12] The pathologist must be aware of these deceptive lesions that mimic malignancy, especially in frozen sections or in material that is less than optimally processed.

Atypical Hyperplasias

On occasion, the epithelial proliferations will possess a mixture of benign and malignant features. These lesions are classified as *atypical hyperplasias* and may be either ductal or lobular in origin.[13] Atypical hyperplasia frequently falls into one of the following categories: (1) an intraductal lesion that exhibits significant cytologic atypia but lacks one of the recognizable architectural patterns of intraductal malignancy, (2) an *isolated*, noninvasive ductal lesion that is recognizable as intraductal carcinoma but is quantitatively insufficient to establish a diagnosis of malignancy, and (3) lobular proliferation of neo-

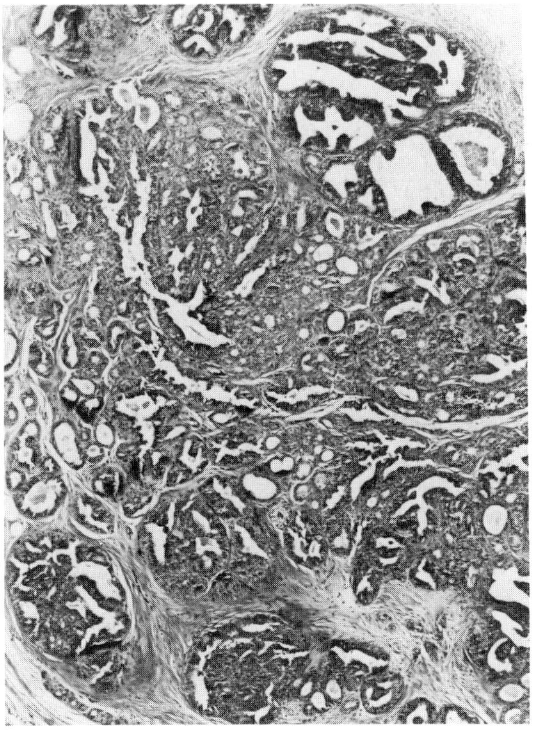

FIGURE 3–10. Adenosis and intraductal papillomatosis are common components of benign breast lesions. Note the expansion of the lobules, the increased cellularity, and the complex glandular pattern in comparison with normal breast tissue (see Fig. 3–4) (H & E × 54).

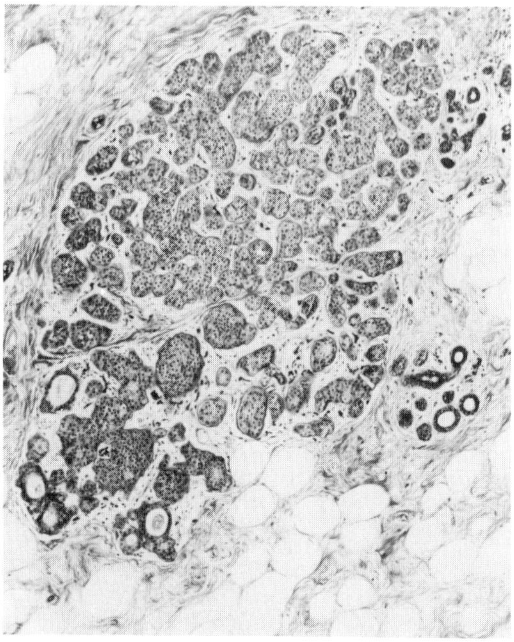

FIGURE 3–11. Atypical lobular hyperplasia, as evidenced by proliferation of epithelial cells to varying degrees in many but not all acini within the mammary lobule. Before this histologic diagnosis can be rendered, a thorough search of the specimen must be made to rule out fully developed *in situ* or invasive malignancy at adjacent sites (H & E × 64).

plastic cells that affects some but not all acini within a mammary lobule (Fig. 3–11) or that affects all acini of a lobule but is limited to a solitary focus. With atypical hyperplasias, the pathologist should thoroughly evaluate all of the available material. It is necessary for the clinician to closely monitor this group of patients because the risk of subsequent infiltrating malignancy is increased fivefold in the presence of atypical intraductal or lobular hyperplasia. By combining histologic diagnosis with clinical factors such as age and family history, it is possible to calculate an even more precise relative risk factor (for example, women with atypical hyperplasia and a positive family history have an 11-fold increased risk over women with normal breasts and a negative family history).[11]

Mammary Duct Ectasia

Mammary duct ectasia is a benign inflammatory process involving the subareolar and segmental ducts rather than the lobules. The disease is thought to arise as a complication of periductular inflammation (periductal mastitis) (Fig. 3–12) in parous women.[2] Nipple discharge is common. The process may eventuate in nipple inversion, periductal fibrosis, and calcifications. Although excision of the major duct system is sometimes required to eliminate bothersome nonbloody discharge, this lesion is not commonly biopsied.

Adenomas

Fibroadenomas are discrete, usually solitary, palpable lesions that typically occur in patients between the ages of 20 and 35. Usually less than 3 cm in diameter, these lesions are sharply demarcated from the adjacent normal breast tissue by gross and microscopic examination. Probably of lobular origin, fibroadenomas are composed of characteristic glandular formations in a homogeneous, collagenized stroma (Fig. 3–13). Although the epithelial component may show florid hyperplasia, there is usually no significant atypia or necrosis. Older lesions may ossify or calcify. Fibroadenomas may increase in size during pregnancy; these lesions typically regress as the patient ages. Occasionally, the presence of a persistent fibroadenoma goes unnoticed until the adjacent breast tissue undergoes the normal involutional changes of aging; thus, a patient may first present

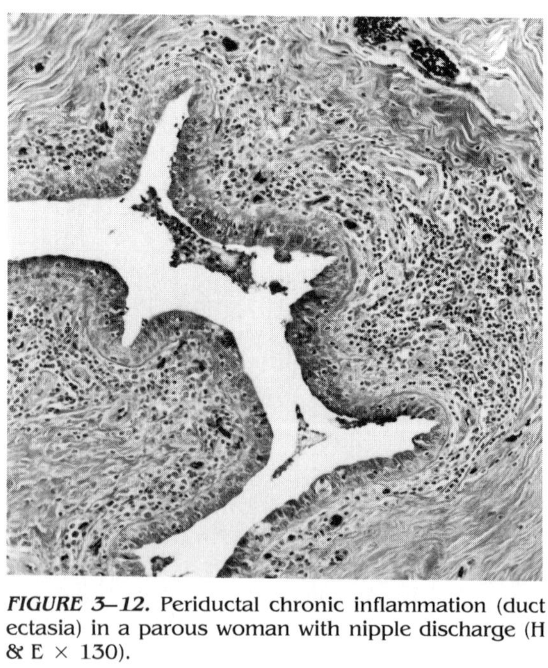

FIGURE 3–12. Periductal chronic inflammation (duct ectasia) in a parous woman with nipple discharge (H & E × 130).

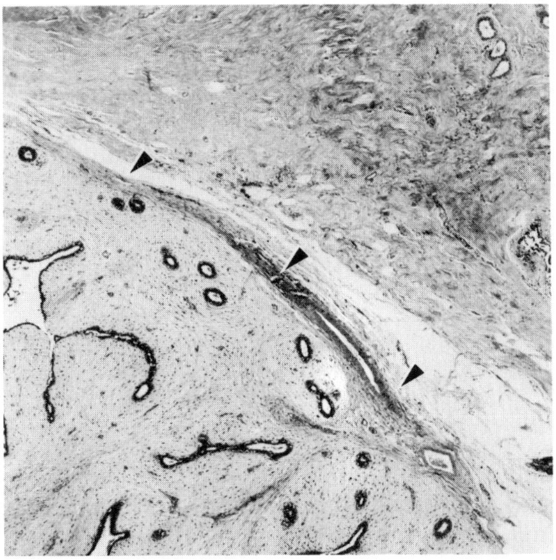

FIGURE 3–13. Fibroadenoma (arrowheads at edge), characterized by glandular formations in a homogeneous collagenized stroma. The adjacent breast tissue is normal (H & E × 38).

with a fibroadenoma during the menopausal years.

Tubular adenomas and *cellular adenofibromas* are uncommon benign neoplasms seen in young women.[14, 15] For these and other benign breast processes, the patient's age is an important factor for the pathologist to consider in the histologic interpretation of a lesion.

Lactating adenomas occur during pregnancy or the puerperium. These generally well-circumscribed, actively secreting lesions represent a localized focus of hyperplasia in the lactating breast.

Nipple duct adenoma appears clinically as a subareolar mass, frequently accompanied by nipple discharge. Histologically, there is a marked epithelial proliferation, easily mistaken for an infiltrating carcinoma on frozen section, especially if the pathologist is not informed that the mass was located directly beneath the nipple or areola.

Papilloma

A discrete intraductal papilloma may be as large as several centimeters in diameter. This lesion consists of an arborizing fibrovascular stalk, with a terminal benign epithelial proliferation that projects into the lumen of a dilated duct or cyst (Fig. 3–14). An important clue to the benign nature of the lesion is the detection of two cell types—epithelial and myoepithelial. Because of the papilloma's cellularity and architectural complexity, the diagnosis may be particularly difficult from frozen section, especially if the pathologist does not have the entire lesion. On permanent sections, the significance of a papilloma lies in its distinction from papillary carcinoma (see following section on intraductal carcinoma.)

Traumatic Fat Necrosis

This lesion may produce a palpable abnormality. Although diagnosis of this lesion from frozen section can be challenging, especially if the pathologist is not given a history of trauma, its appearance on permanent section is seldom confused with that of a malignant process (Fig. 3–15). The histologic differential diagnosis includes (1) duct ectasia, when there has been extrusion of contents into the adjacent stroma, and (2) fat necrosis secondary to the surgical trauma of a previous biopsy.

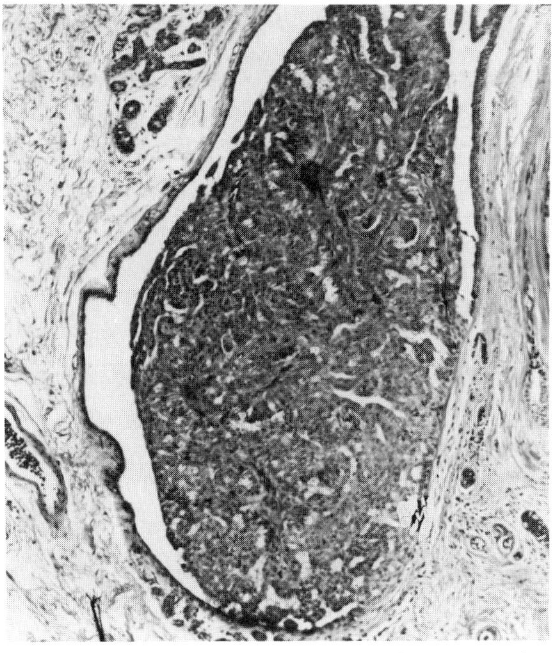

FIGURE 3–14. A small intraductal papilloma, consisting of a benign epithelial proliferation that forms a complex papillary network within a dilated duct or cyst (H & E × 80).

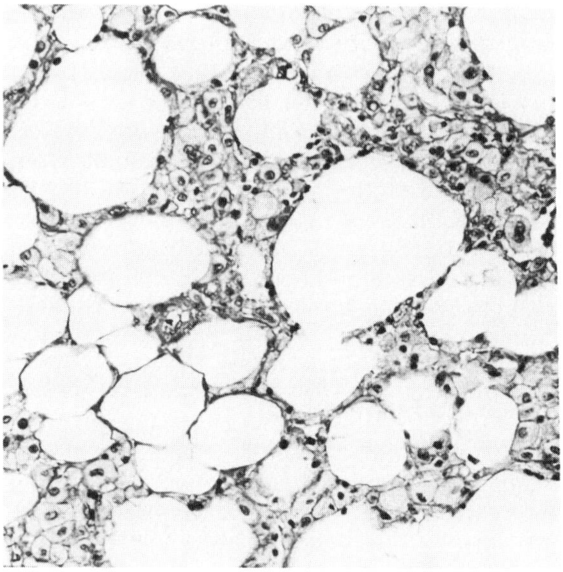

FIGURE 3–15. Fat necrosis within the breast. Numerous foamy macrophages are scattered among necrotic adipocytes (H & E × 220).

PRIMARY BREAST CANCER

Noninvasive (In Situ) Primary Breast Cancer

In situ carcinoma is divided into intraductal and lobular carcinoma subtypes. The conceptual evolution of these two lesions, recently reviewed by Rosen,[16] has evolved over more than a century. This is discussed in detail in Chapter 10.

TABLE 3–1. Histologic Classification of Primary Malignant Epithelial Breast Tumors

Noninvasive (intraepithelial)
- Intraductal carcinoma
- Lobular carcinoma *in situ*

Invasive
- Common
  - Infiltrating ductal carcinoma
  - Infiltrating lobular carcinoma
- Rarer
  - Medullary carcinoma
  - Tubular (well-differentiated) carcinoma
  - Mucinous (colloid) carcinoma
  - Papillary carcinoma with invasion
  - Secretory (juvenile) carcinoma
  - Adenoid cystic carcinomas
  - Carcinoma with metaplasia (squamous cartilaginous, osseous, spindle, mixed)
  - Others

Paget's disease of the nipple

Adapted from International Histological Classification of Tumors, No. 2. *In:* Histological Typing of Breast Tumors. Geneva: World Health Organization, 1981.

Intraductal Carcinoma

Intraductal carcinoma arises within mammary ducts and is confined within the limits of the basement membrane that separates the epithelium from the stroma. It is important to emphasize that a pathologic diagnosis of "intraductal" carcinoma refers to a *noninvasive* lesion. This term is not to be confused with "infiltrating ductal" carcinomas, which are *infiltrating* malignancies with metastatic potential. Intraductal carcinoma ranges from an early microscopic focus, detected incidentally or via mammography, to an extensive, clinically palpable dominant mass that ramifies throughout the ducts of one or more segments of the breast. Over half of the lesions are centrally located, and approximately a fourth of patients with intraductal carcinoma have nipple discharge.[17] Histologically, preinvasive carcinoma is frequently multicentric.[18]

There are five histologically recognizable *architectural* patterns of intraductal carcinoma:

1. Cribriform—sheets of neoplastic cells, perforated by round, sievelike or "cartwheel" spaces that fill ductular lumina (Fig. 3–16).

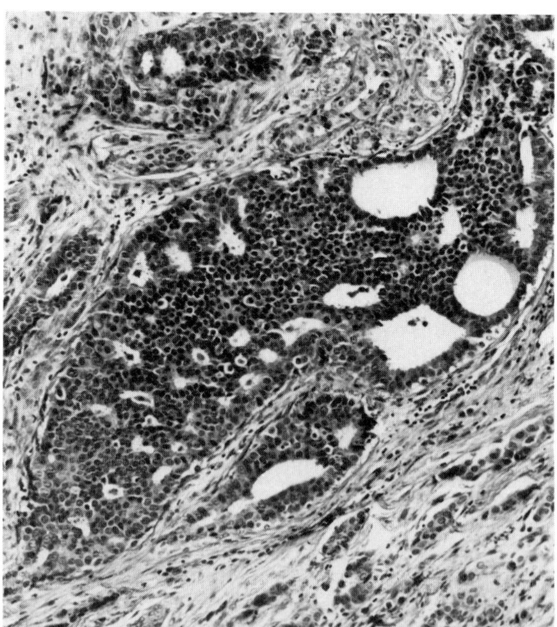

FIGURE 3–16. A cribriform (sievelike pattern) of intraductal carcinoma. (This tumor also showed foci of invasion.) (H & E × 130.)

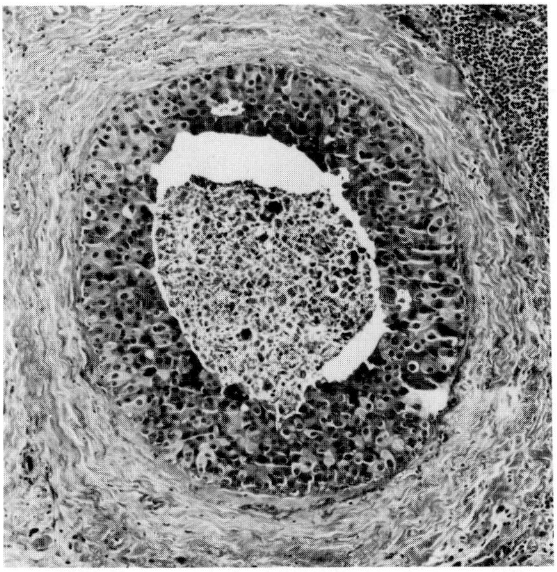

FIGURE 3–17. Intraductal comedocarcinoma. Note the neoplastic rim of viable tumor and the central comedo-like necrosis (H & E × 105).

2. Comedocarcinoma—sheets of atypical cells within ducts, exhibiting central, comedolike necrosis (Fig. 3–17).

3. Micropapillary—epithelial papillary projections "clinging" from duct walls into empty lumina, frequently forming Roman archlike configurations (Fig. 3–18).

4. Solid—solid sheets of tumor cells filling the ducts.

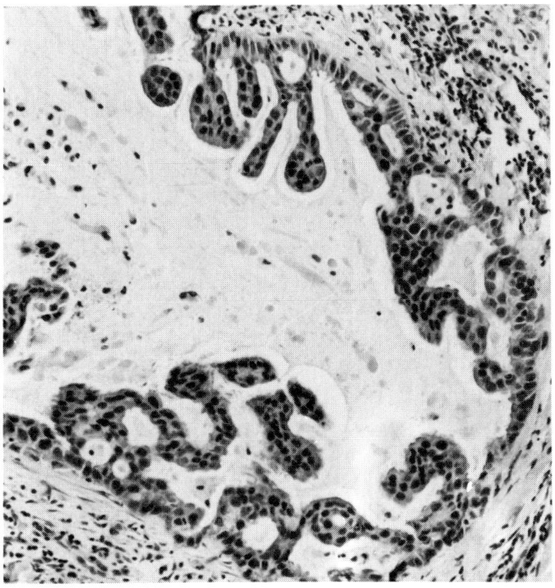

FIGURE 3–18. Micropapillary (clinging) pattern of intraductal carcinoma (H & E × 170).

5. Noninfiltrating papillary carcinoma—fingerlike projections of fibrovascular cores covered by relatively uniform malignant epithelial cells that proliferate and expand a ductular lumen (Fig. 3–19). This rare form of noninvasive breast cancer usually appears as a discrete, circumscribed, solitary mass, confined to a cystically dilated duct. Careful histologic examination of the adjacent breast tissue is warranted to rule out extension of the tumor into small ducts and the presence of invasion, which alters prognosis and therapy.[19]

Mixtures of these patterns often occur. The tumors may extend from the ducts into the mammary lobules (cancerization of the lobules) (Fig. 3–20). This growth pattern must be distinguished from lobular carcinoma *in situ*, which may extend from the lobules into the ducts (see later). On occasion, intraductal carcinoma colonizes the cysts of previously existing benign breast disease (intracystic carcinoma).

Intraductal carcinoma usually possesses *cytologic* features that also can be used to distinguish it from benign proliferations. The malignant cell population of intraductal carcinoma is composed of a single cell type, in contrast with the two-cell, epithelial-myo-

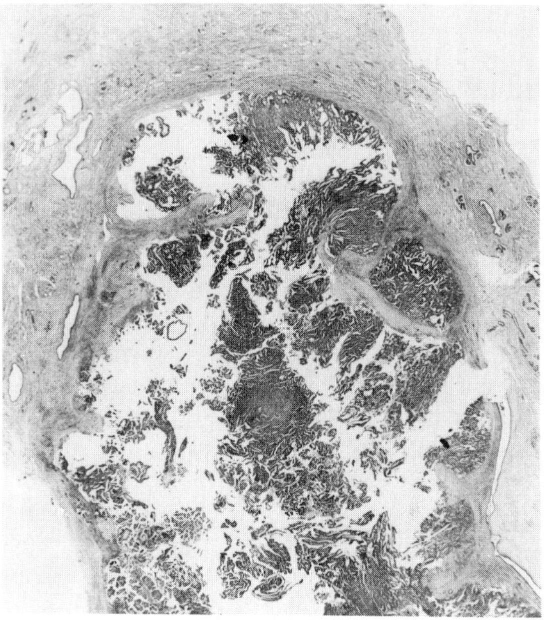

FIGURE 3–19. Papillary carcinomas, evidenced by projection of neoplastic epithelial cells on a fibrovascular stalk extending into an expanded ductular lumen. This tumor is distinguished from a benign papilloma on the basis of its cytologic features (H & E × 130).

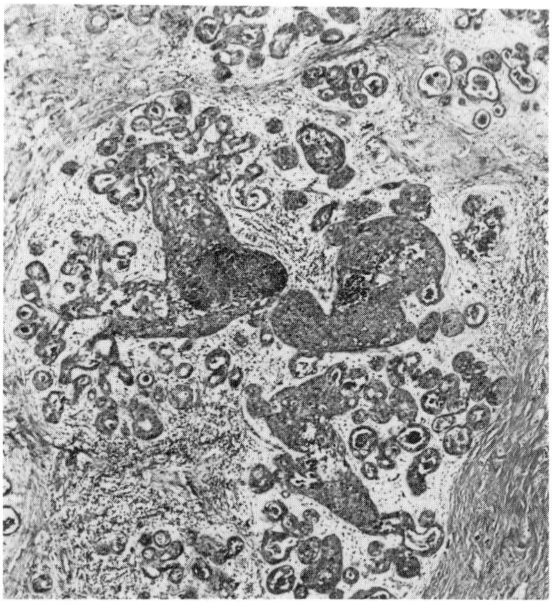

FIGURE 3–20. Cancerization of the mammary lobule. An intraductal (comedo-type) carcinoma is seen extending into the acini of several lobules (H & E × 40).

epithelial composition of benign lesions. Necrosis, not commonly a feature of benign lesions, is frequently present in intraductal carcinomas. Another helpful feature in distinguishing intraductal carcinoma from benign hyperplasia is the presence of cellular pleomorphism, in the form of nuclear enlargement, irregularities in the nuclear membrane and chromatin pattern, altered nuclear:cytoplasmic ratio, and increased mitotic activity. However, about 10 percent of intraductal carcinomas lack atypia or necrosis and can be identified only by the monomorphic cell population forming cribriform, papillary, or micropapillary patterns.[20] Since architectural and cytologic clues are often subtle, intraductal carcinomas are not reliably distinguished from benign and atypical hyperplasia on frozen section. In such cases, histologic diagnosis is best deferred from frozen to permanent sections.

Intraductal carcinoma is thought to be a precursor of invasive disease. Ductal carcinoma, unlike lobular carcinoma, seems to have a very transitory preinfiltrating phase,[21] and most often intraductal carcinoma is seen in association with infiltrating malignancy. Thus, pure intraductal carcinomas have a relatively low incidence (4 to 5 percent).[16, 21] Women with pure intraductal carcinoma appear to have a virtually normal life expectancy after therapy.[21] Before rendering a diagnosis of intraductal carcinoma, pathologists are obligated to sample extensively the tissue to search for microscopic foci of infiltration that may alter prognosis and the therapeutic approach. Failure to identify stromal invasion does not rule it out. A small percentage of patients with intraductal carcinomas (usually less than 3 percent) are found to have axillary nodal metastases.[17] The occasional disparity between the identification of a "noninvasive" intraductal carcinoma and the detection of metastasis to regional lymph nodes is reconciled by the inherent limitations of histologic sampling, the static rather than dynamic nature of the process that is captured on histologic sections, and the disruption of the lamina basalis and penetration of the basement membrane by individual malignant cells that can be demonstrated by electron microscopy.[7]

Mastectomy will cure virtually all patients with intraductal carcinoma.[16] Page and colleagues reported on a group of women with "pure" intraductal carcinoma who were treated by biopsy only. For 25 patients whose follow-up included at least three postbiopsy years, invasive carcinoma was observed in seven (28 percent)[22] (see discussion of clinical management of noninvasive breast cancer in Chapter 10).

Lobular Carcinoma In Situ (LCIS, Lobular Neoplasia)

In 1941, Foote and Stewart introduced the term lobular carcinoma *in situ*. This lesion is a noninvasive epithelial neoplasm that originates within the mammary lobule rather than the duct. Because it usually does not produce clinical signs or symptoms, it is typically discovered as an incidental finding in a biopsy that was performed for some other benign or malignant process. In some instances, biopsy is prompted by mammographic detection of stippled calcifications.

Lobular carcinoma *in situ* is not evident grossly. Microscopically, LCIS is composed of a relatively uniform population of noncohesive, small epithelial cells that fill and distend the acini within mammary lobules (Fig. 3–21). There are few mitoses. Necrosis is rare. The cells usually possess a central nucleus and sufficient cytoplasm to prevent overlap of nuclei; signet-ring forms may also be present. Microcalcifications may be iden-

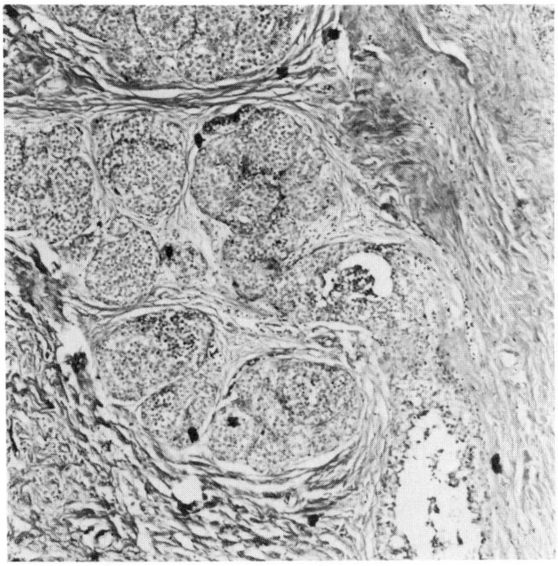

FIGURE 3–21. Lobular carcinoma in situ (LCIS). Uniform populations of small epithelial cells fill and distend all the acini within multiple mammary lobules (H & E × 64).

tified histologically; however, these calcified spherules are more often associated with residual uninvolved lobules than with the tumor itself. There may be accompanying pagetoid spread from the lobules into adjacent ducts (neoplastic cells "sandwiched" between the myoepithelium–basement membrane and attenuated residual epithelium of the duct) (Fig. 3–22). Clinical Paget's disease of the nipple is not a feature of LCIS. When pagetoid spread is detected in the ducts in the absence of lobular involvement, these intramural lesions serve as a signal to the pathologist to process additional material, in search of the typical lobular lesions of LCIS.[23] Although distinction is not always easy, it is usually possible for the pathologist to differentiate pagetoid spread of LCIS from intraductal carcinoma with secondary involvement of acini. The distinction is of some importance clinically, because of the greater incidence of bilateral and multicentric breast malignancies in association with lobular carcinoma *in situ* (up to 58 percent) in comparison with intraductal carcinoma (up to 30 percent).

Because the number of untreated women with biopsy-proven LCIS is relatively small and follow-up is limited, the risk of developing invasive cancer has not been conclusively established for these patients. Therefore, treatment of LCIS is controversial, ranging from "watchful waiting" to bilateral prophylactic mastectomy (see discussion of clinical management of noninvasive breast cancer in Chapter 10).

Paget's Disease of the Nipple

Paget's disease of the breast typically begins as slowly progressive reddening and thickening of the nipple.[24] With erosion of the surface epithelium there may be oozing of serum. Nipple discharge of ductular contents is not a feature of this process. Paget's disease of the nipple is associated with an underlying malignancy of the breast, most often a nonpalpable intraductal carcinoma. However, if a definite mass is present beneath the diseased nipple, the underlying tumor is likely to be invasive. Clinical management and prognosis are largely dependent upon the intraductal versus infiltrating nature of the underlying carcinoma rather than upon the presence of Paget's disease.

Histopathologically, Paget's disease is an intraepithelial adenocarcinoma, to be distinguished from Bowen's disease (squamous cell carcinoma *in situ*) or *in situ* melanoma. Tumor cells are seen individually and in small clusters within the epithelial layer of the nipple (Fig. 3–23). The neoplastic cells usually contain PAS-positive, diastase-resistant glycoproteins, a useful diagnostic fea-

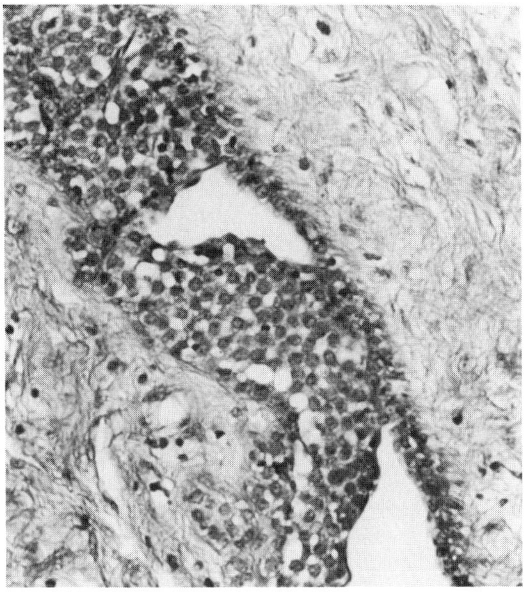

FIGURE 3–22. Pagetoid spread of LCIS within a mammary duct (H & E × 256).

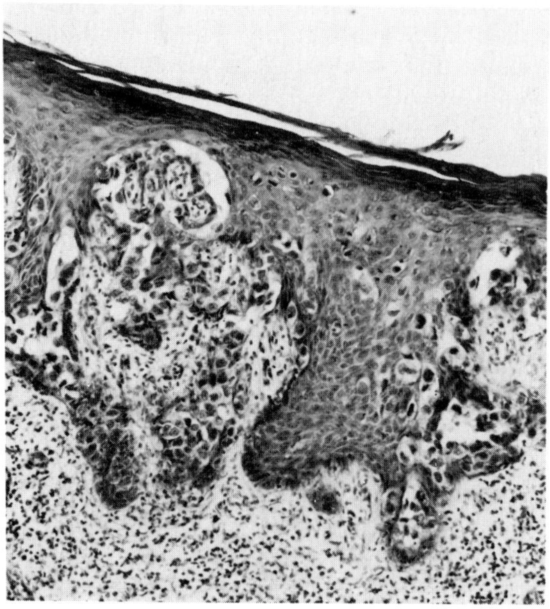

FIGURE 3–23. Paget's disease of the nipple. Tumor cells are seen individually and in clusters within the epidermis of the nipple. The subepithelial connective tissue is chronically inflamed (H & E × 130).

ture. S-100 immunohistochemical staining (positive for melanoma and negative for Paget's disease) and electron microscopy may also be helpful in the histologic differential diagnosis. The peculiar intraepithelial location of neoplastic cells is thought to be secondary to direct extension of tumor cells along the mammary ducts. With adequate sampling, it is usually possible to demonstrate the underlying intraductal malignancy, with or without an invasive component. Paget's disease is not limited to a specific histologic type of breast cancer; however, it is always associated with tumors of epithelial origin.

Invasive Primary Breast Cancers

INFILTRATING DUCTAL CARCINOMA

The most common form of breast cancer, constituting 70 to 80 percent of invasive primary breast neoplasms, infiltrating ductal carcinoma usually appears as a solitary, palpable breast mass. Upon gross pathologic examination, it appears firm, gritty, irregular, and gray-white with yellowish flecks and streaks (Fig. 3–24). Jackson and Orr[25] and Azzopardi and Laurini[4] have shown that the streaks are periductal and perivenous elastic tissue and not, as commonly believed, necrosis or chalky calcium deposits. Tumors that range from several millimeters to several centimeters in diameter typically radiate from the central mass into the adjacent breast tissue. Infiltrating ductal carcinoma often incites a desmoplastic reaction that is responsible for the scirrhous (Greek *skirrhos*, hard) nature of the mass, which cuts with the consistency of an unripe pear. Biochemical analysis of the desmoplastic matrix reveals increased collagen deposition, with a relative increase in collagen Type V.[26] The desmoplasia is thought to reflect a host response to invasive carcinoma. Desmoplasia rather than malignant epithelial proliferation gives breast carcinoma its distinctive palpatory characteristics.

Microscopically, the tumor is variably composed of cords, nests, primitive tubules, glandular formations, and sheets of malignant epithelial cells that infiltrate a collagenized stroma (Fig. 3–25). Often, an accompanying intraductal component is detected, especially if histologic sampling is generous.

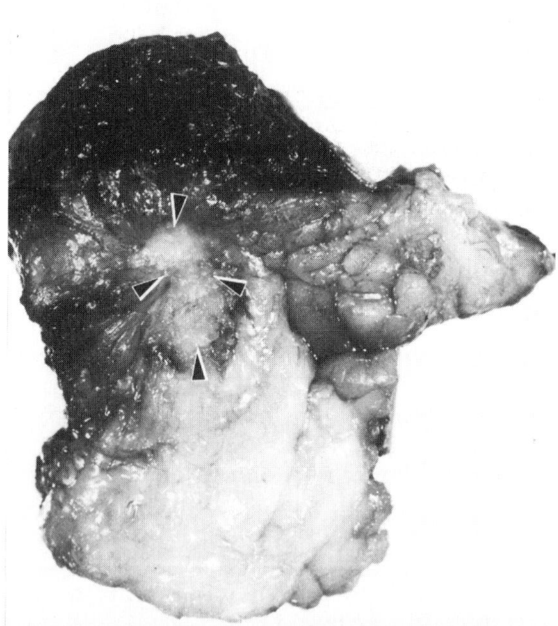

FIGURE 3–24. Gross photograph of a small infiltrating ductal cancer. Note the central depression and the irregular stellate borders (arrowheads).

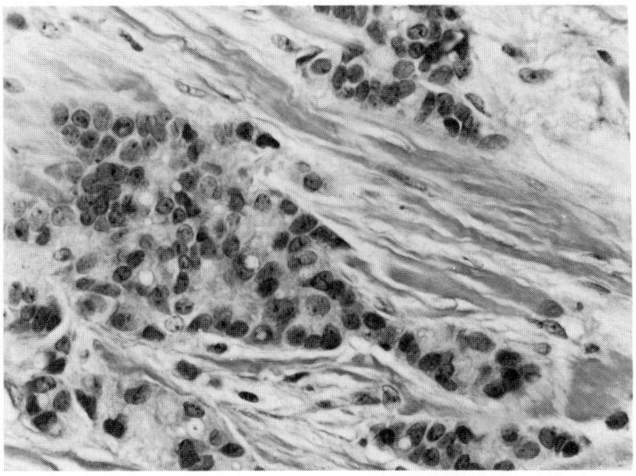

FIGURE 3–25. Typical infiltrating ductal carcinoma. Cords and nests of cells form abortive tubular structures within a densely collagenized (desmoplastic) matrix (H & E × 330).

The cells are relatively large and the nuclear characteristics are variable. Nucleoli are usually prominent. Mitotic figures are typically detected with ease, and necrosis is common, particularly within residual intraductal disease. There is often an accompanying lymphocytic infiltrate, most prominent at the tumor periphery. Immunohistologic studies of the lymphocytes have revealed a disproportionally increased population of T lymphocytes bearing the cytotoxic-suppressor phenotype.[27] Infiltrating ductal carcinoma may be mixed with other histologic findings. Considerable effort has been made to subdivide infiltrating ductal carcinomas into prognostically significant categories (see following section on pathologic variables and prognosis in breast cancer).

Infiltrating Lobular Carcinoma

Infiltrating lobular carcinoma accounts for approximately 5 percent of invasive breast cancers.[28] In its clinical and mammographic presentations, this form of breast cancer is indistinguishable from infiltrating ductal carcinoma. The importance of the infiltrating lobular histologic type resides in its increased frequency of multicentricity, bilaterality, and tendency for bone and meningeal spread. In addition, the recognition of this form of invasive breast cancer as a distinct clinicopathologic entity serves to alert the pathologist to its characteristic and sometimes subtle histologic pattern of invasion.

On gross examination infiltrating lobular carcinoma is an irregular, firm, gray-white mass, indistinguishable from infiltrating ductal carcinoma. Several histologic criteria are helpful in establishing the diagnosis. Infiltrating lobular carcinoma is thought to be the invasive component of lobular carcinoma *in situ*, inasmuch as the tumor cells share similar cytologic features and the two lesions are frequently seen in association.[29] Thus, the finding of residual LCIS, while not essential to establishing the diagnosis of infiltrating lobular carcinoma, is a useful clue.[30] To some extent, the frequency of detection of LCIS within infiltrating lobular carcinoma is dependent upon the thoroughness of the histologic sampling. In one study, Newman found an *in situ* lobular component in 72 of 73 examples of infiltrating lobular carcinoma.[31] Another helpful histologic feature is the diffuse tumor cell infiltration of the stroma by monotonous small tumor cells that characteristically penetrate the fibrous background in a single file ("Indian file"). As the tumor cells infiltrate the stroma around residual normal ducts, they are arrayed in concentric formations in so-called targetoid patterns (Fig. 3–26). Because the tumor cells are typically small, they may be confused with fibroblast or lymphocyte nuclei, especially in frozen sections. Mucin stains may be helpful in this regard, since a high proportion of lobular carcinomas are positive for intracytoplasmic mucin. By electron microscopy, intracytoplasmic lumina may be a prominent feature. Given the presumed origin of this

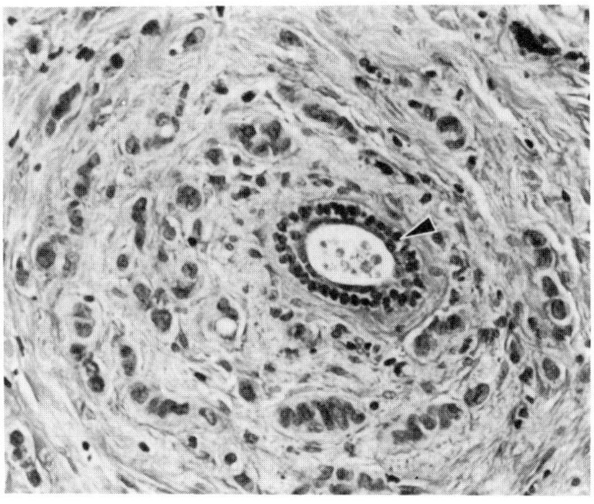

FIGURE 3–26. Infiltrating lobular carcinoma. The tumor cells are arrayed in a concentric fashion (targetoid) around a residual normal duct (arrowhead). Note the tendency of the tumor cells to align one after the next in characteristic "Indian file" pattern (H & E × 256).

tumor within the mammary lobule, it is not surprising that milk-related proteins such as casein and lactalbumin may be detected within some of these tumors.[32]

There appear to be several histologic variants of infiltrating lobular carcinoma. Most pathologists consider the signet-ring carcinoma, with its abundant intracytoplasmic mucin, to be of lobular origin. Some invasive lobular tumors may exhibit limited trabecular differentiation, which makes it difficult to distinguish them from infiltrating ductal carcinomas. This may be further complicated by the recognition of bona fide mixed lobular-ductal carcinomas, as well as transitional forms. In rare instances, the distinction between lobular and ductal types cannot be made with certainty. The propensity of infiltrating lobular carcinomas to form sheets of poorly cohesive cells in axillary nodal metastases is well documented, where on occasion these tumors masquerade as lymphoma or amelanotic melanoma. The relationship of the solid variant of infiltrating lobular carcinoma to the recently described argyrophilic, carcinoid-like primary breast tumor is still under investigation.[33, 34]

Medullary Carcinoma

Representing approximately 3 percent of malignant mammary tumors, this tumor appears as a soft, well-circumscribed, gray-white mass on gross inspection. Histologically, the tumor is composed of sheets of malignant cells that exhibit no significant tendency for tubular or glandular formation. There is prominent lymphocytic infiltration. The tumor borders are "pushing" rather than infiltrating into the adjacent breast stroma (Fig. 3–27). Cytologically, the tumor cells are large and pleomorphic, with prominent nucleoli. Mitotic figures are frequent. Despite its poor architectural differentiation and aggressive cytologic appearance, pure medullary carcinoma has a higher survival rate than infiltrating ductal carcinoma, according to most studies.[35–38]

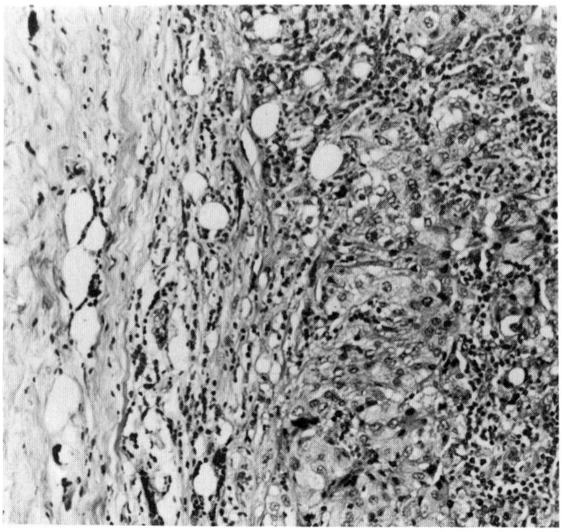

FIGURE 3–27. Medullary carcinoma. Sheets of malignant cells, accompanied by prominent lymphocytic infiltration, possess "pushing" rather than irregularly infiltrating borders (H & E × 150).

Mucinous (Colloid) Carcinoma

These unusual tumors (about 2 percent of all breast cancers) are distinguished grossly and histologically by copious extracellular mucin production.[39, 40] Small clusters and strands of cells float in a gelatinous lake of mucin (Fig. 3–28). The prognosis for patients with these tumors is better than that for patients with invasive ductal carcinoma, provided that the mucinous carcinomas are not mixed with a more aggressive component.[41]

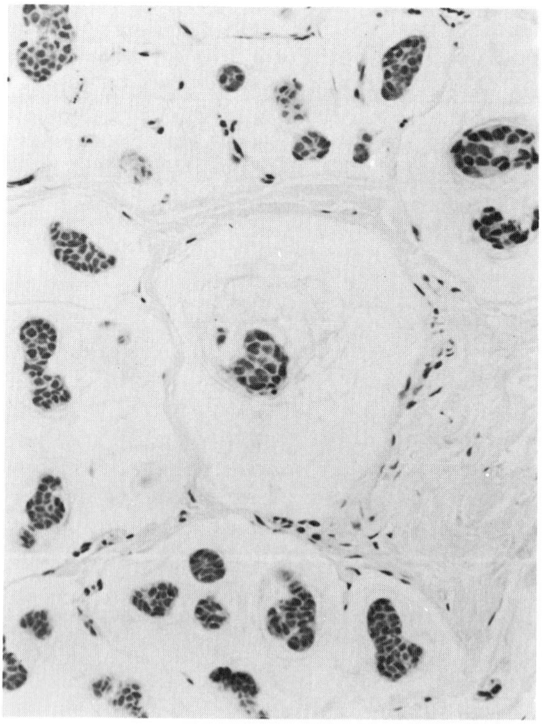

FIGURE 3–28. Mucinous (colloid) carcinoma. Clusters of epithelial cells float in gelatinous lakes of mucin (H & E × 240).

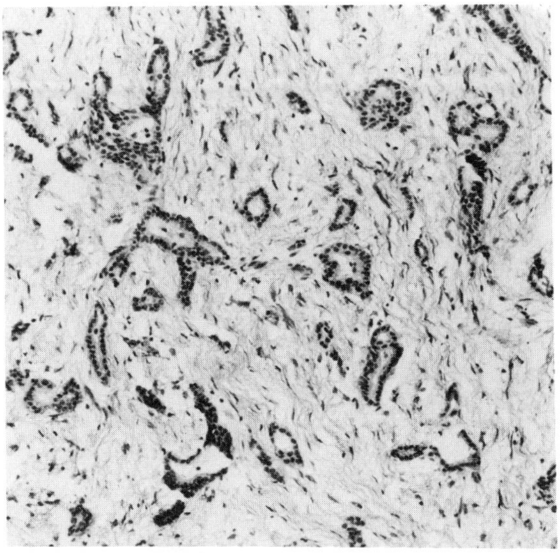

FIGURE 3–29. Tubular carcinoma. Irregular angulated glandular structures formed by a single layer of epithelial cells infiltrate the stroma (H & E × 130).

Tubular Carcinoma

This neoplasm consists of proliferations of small, irregular tubules that infiltrate a desmoplastic stroma (Fig. 3–29).[42, 43] The malignant glands are distinguished by (1) the haphazard manner in which they infiltrate the interlobular stroma, (2) their open lumina, (3) their angulated, "teardrop" edges, (4) the presence of a single layer of malignant cells that lack a normal biphasic epithelial-myoepithelial relationship, and (5) the absence of a basement membrane (best appreciated by electron microscopy). Necrosis is absent, and mitotic figures are difficult to find. Histologically, this process may be "deceptively innocent" and must be distinguished from sclerosing adenosis.[42] Tubular carcinoma is synonymous with "well-differentiated carcinoma," which refers to a specific histologic type rather than a histologic grade (see discussion of factors related to prognosis, in the following section). Because the differentiating features may be subtle, the diagnosis of tubular carcinoma should be established on permanent sections rather than on frozen sections.

Tubular carcinoma is a rare histologic finding, constituting approximately 1 percent of all breast cancers. There is an increased incidence of multicentricity and bilaterality for this histologic subtype.[44] When this tumor appears in its pure form, the prognosis is very favorable with a more than 90 percent cure rate.[45] Axillary nodal metastases occur but apparently do not have an adverse impact on prognosis to the same extent as other forms of breast cancer.[42] To the extent that there is an accompanying infiltrating ductal component, survival is diminished.[44, 45] Coexisting lobular neoplasia occurs in 10 percent of cases of tubular carcinoma.[45, 46]

Secretory Carcinoma

Carcinoma of the breast in prepubertal females is extremely rare.[47] Secretory carcinoma, also known as juvenile carcinoma, is characterized by its abundant intracellular and extracellular matrix. A few cases have been reported in adults.[48–50] Axillary metastases may occur, but distant metastases are rare, and the prognosis is excellent.[51]

Adenoid Cystic Carcinoma

This very rare, slowly growing variant of ductal carcinoma accounts for less than 1 percent of all breast cancers.[52, 53] First described by Foote and Stewart in 1941, the tumor is histologically identical to certain tumors of the salivary glands and bronchi.[54] Microscopically, the tumor is characterized by cystic spaces lined by tumor cells arrayed in a honeycomb arrangement. This pattern of infiltrating malignancy is to be distinguished from intraductal tumors with a cribriform pattern. The prognosis is good in comparison with other breast cancers and with similarly appearing tumors in other anatomic locations.[55]

Inflammatory Carcinoma

Inflammatory carcinoma has an incidence of about 1 to 2 percent in patients with breast cancer.[56] Inflammatory carcinoma of the breast is not a specific histologic subtype; rather, it is a clinicopathologic entity.[57] By definition, at least a quarter of the involved breast shows signs resembling a localized acute inflammatory process: redness, swelling, and warmth. An underlying palpable mass may or may not be present. Although clinically the process may simulate mastitis, the histologic correlate is not inflammation but rather is widespread dermal lymphatic invasion by breast carcinoma, accompanied by edema of the dermis and vascular dilatation.[58] Typically, these highly aggressive infiltrating malignancies are poorly differentiated and have a high nuclear grade. Axillary metastases are almost always present; in some cases, there is massive involvement of nodes.

Mastectomy is inadequate for gaining local control over this aggressive form of breast cancer. However, combination chemotherapy with or without local radiation therapy has met with some success in treating inflammatory carcinoma of the breast. Rebiopsy after systemic chemotherapy has demonstrated histologic regression of biopsy-proven inflammatory carcinoma. Inflammatory breast cancer is considered in greater detail in Chapter 9, Locally Advanced Breast Cancer.

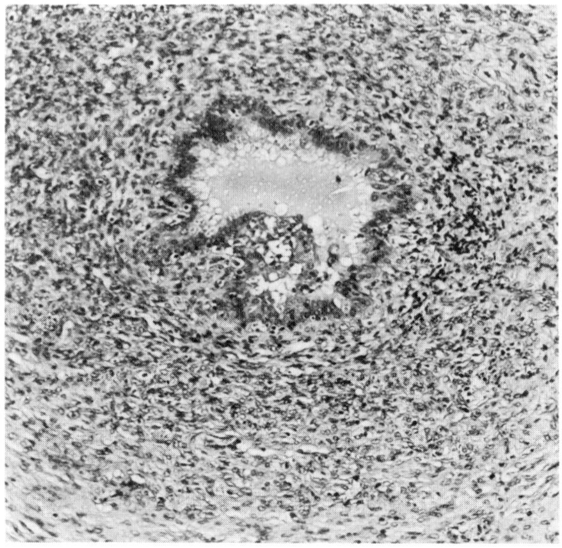

FIGURE 3–30. Cystosarcoma phyllodes. Although this tumor shares some histologic similarities with fibroadenoma (see Fig. 3–13), the stroma is much more cellular and atypical (H & E × 130).

Other Breast Cancers

Cystosarcoma Phyllodes

This tumor is a large, solitary, palpable breast mass, frequently with a history of recent rapid growth. The overlying skin may be stretched and taut. The tumor takes its name from the gross appearance of the specimen (Greek *phyllon,* leaf), in which leaflike lobulations of tumor project into long, epithelium-lined clefts and cystic cavities. This tumor has both mesenchymal and epithelial components. Its distinction from fibroadenoma is based primarily on the greater cellularity of the stromal component seen in cystosarcoma. In addition, in contrast to fibroadenoma, cystosarcoma is usually larger, is less likely to be multiple, and appears in an older age group (mean age 45, roughly two decades older than that for fibroadenoma).[59] The distinction is important, inasmuch as the cystosarcoma will recur locally if not completely excised, and the higher grades have metastatic potential.

Because of the difficult and sometimes arbitrary histologic division among benign, borderline, and malignant variants of this tumor, Norris and Taylor[59] and, more recently, Azzopardi and colleagues[3] recommend using a histologic prognostication of behavior based upon the characteristics of the stromal component, that is, cellularity, mitotic activity, atypia, infiltrating margins, size, and disproportional overgrowth of the stromal elements relative to the benign epithelial component (Fig. 3–30). In this manner, the pathologist avoids unduly alarming the patient and clinician with a diagnosis of cystosarcoma in those cases with histologically bland features, while acknowledging the sometimes unpredictable nature of this tumor.

When cystosarcoma phyllodes tumors do metastasize, they usually do so within the first two years after presentation. The malignant variants disseminate hematogenously, as do other sarcomas, to the lungs and bones. Only the malignant mesenchymal element (usually fibrosarcoma or liposarcoma) is seen in the metastases. Because these tumors infrequently metastasize to the regional lymph nodes, axillary dissection is not usually performed, unless there is clinical suspicion of nodal involvement. Ordinarily, the tumor is excised locally, with generous margins, to minimize the risk of local recurrence.

Sarcomas

These unusual malignant breast mesenchymal tumors lack an epithelial component. They characteristically appear as a solitary large mass. On gross examination, they typically are firm, gray-white lesions with a "fish-flesh" appearance. Hemorrhage and necrosis are correlated with aggressive be-

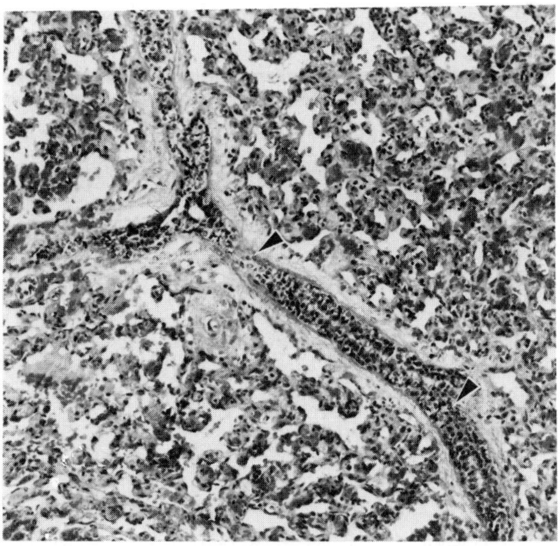

FIGURE 3–31. Angiosarcoma of the breast. Note the stroma is replaced by irregular vascular channels. A normal residual ductular structure remains (arrows) (H & E × 130).

havior. Because sarcomas disseminate hematogenously rather than by lymphatics, they are treated by wide excision–mastectomy without axillary nodal dissection. There are a variety of histologic subtypes, corresponding to the normal mesenchymal elements of the breast. Several deserve special mention.

Angiosarcoma may arise *de novo* or perhaps from a benign perilobular angioma, a lesion occurring in 3 percent of breasts as an incidental finding. Angiosarcomas can be graded; patients with poorly differentiated lesions have a poor prognosis.[60] Histologically, the tumor consists of spindle-shaped cells that to varying degrees exhibit a tendency for blood vessel formation. Some angiosarcomas are remarkably well differentiated, and care must be taken to avoid a benign interpretation of a deceptively bland lesion. Others show, in addition to vascular differentiation, solid sheets of tumor cells, often with hemorrhage and necrosis (Fig. 3–31).

Other patterns of sarcoma include fibrosarcoma and liposarcoma.[61] Rarely, rhabdomyosarcomatous differentiation may occur.[61–63] In the presence of apparent osteosarcoma or chondrosarcoma, the distinction from a metaplastic carcinoma may be difficult.[3] True carcinosarcomas of the breast (with malignant epithelial and malignant mesenchymal components) have also been reported.[64]

Tumors Metastatic to the Breast

Metastatic tumors masquerading as primary breast tumors are unusual.[65] The most common is carcinoma that has metastasized from a contralateral breast cancer, presumably as a result of transthoracic lymphatic spread. A relatively high proportion of metastatic neoplasms are leukemias and lymphomas (see later). Other histologic types include metastatic oat cell carcinoma of the bronchus, melanoma, gastric cancers, and renal cell carcinoma.[65–67]

Lymphomas and Leukemias

It is most unusual for a lymphoma to present as a mass in the breast (approximate incidence is 1 in 1000 breast cancers).[20, 68] It is much more common for breast involvement to be a manifestation of generalized lymphoreticular-hematopoietic disease. Grossly, the tumor appears as a soft, graytan mass within the breast parenchyma. The lesions may be multicentric, bilateral, or both. As with lymphoma and leukemia presenting elsewhere, there are a variety of histologic subtypes (Fig. 3–32) that must be distinguished from benign inflammatory processes. Immunocytochemical markers may be helpful in determining the clonality

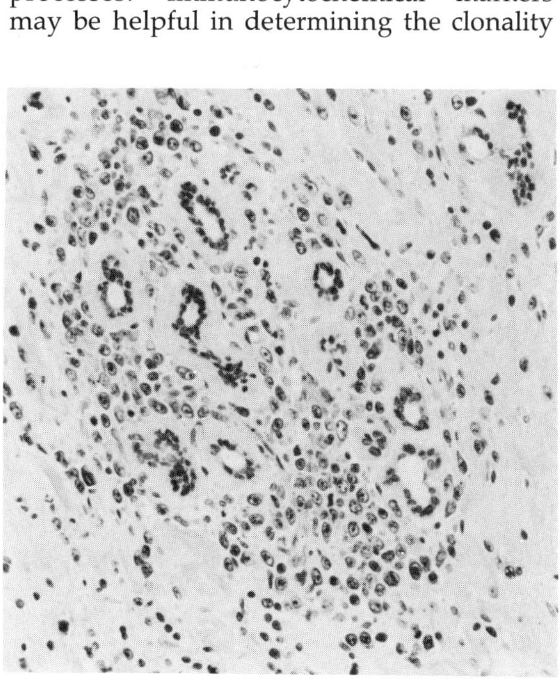

FIGURE 3–32. Diffuse large-cell lymphoma involving the breast. Note the infiltration of mammary tissue by single noncohesive cells. Several residual sclerotic acini are present (H & E × 220).

of a lymphoid infiltrate, and a von Leder chloroacetate esterase stain may be useful in evaluating a possible leukemic infiltrate (chloroma). Prognosis is related to the tumor's histologic type.

PATHOLOGIC VARIABLES AND PROGNOSIS IN BREAST CANCER

There is a large body of literature that establishes the correlation of certain pathologic findings with clinical outcome. These factors include (1) invasiveness, (2) tumor size, (3) axillary nodal status, (4) nipple and skin involvement, (5) histologic type, and (6) kinetic analysis of cell division.

Invasiveness

Noninvasive (*in situ*) carcinomas almost never metastasize.[17, 21] Noninfiltrating lesions are cured by mastectomy; local excision alone is followed by recurrence in 25 to 75 percent of cases.[22, 69] However, distinguishing between recurrence and multifocality and multicentricity is not easy, which makes interpretation of such statistics very difficult.

Tumor Size

Once the cancer ruptures through the basement membrane and infiltrates the stroma, *size* becomes an important indicator of prognosis, since size directly correlates with the likelihood of metastasis. Invasive carcinomas that are less than 1 cm in diameter (minimal carcinoma) metastasize in only about 15 percent (5 to 25 percent) of cases, and five- and ten-year survival rates are in the range of 90 percent.[70–72] Invasive neoplasms between 1 and 2 cm in diameter have an approximately 30 percent likelihood of metastasis; lesions 2 to 2.5 cm in diameter have a metastatic rate of 40 percent and a five-year survival rate of 65 percent.[73] Tumor size and axillary lymph node involvement, although highly correlated, are independent prognostic variables for survival.

Axillary Nodal Status

The presence of *axillary nodal metastases* reduces the overall survival rate. Increasing numbers of positive axillary nodes are associated with a progressively greater incidence of treatment failure. In most studies, axillary nodal status is indicated by placing the patient into one of three groups: negative nodes, one to three positive nodes, four or more positive nodes. Although the prognosis worsens with each successive positive node, patients with four or more nodes appear to have a much worse prognosis than those with negative nodes or those with one to three positive nodes.[74, 75] The size of the nodal metastasis may be of significance. Among those patients with only one positive lymph node, patients with a micrometastasis (less than 2 mm in diameter) appear to have a better prognosis than patients with a macrometastasis (greater than 2 mm in diameter).[76] A solitary nodal metastasis greater than 2 cm in diameter is the equivalent of three or more positive nodes not grossly enlarged by tumor.[77] The location of the involved nodes (Level I, adjacent to the breast; Level II, beneath the pectoralis minor muscle; Level III, superior to the pectoralis minor muscle) does not appear to be as predictive as the number of involved nodes.[78] However, because Level I nodes are usually involved first in breast cancers arising in the upper outer quadrant, positive Level III nodes are a poor prognostic indicator for these patients. Clinical assessment of nodes is unreliable, with 24 percent false-positive findings and 39 percent false-negative findings in one study.[79]

Histologic Type

Invasive breast cancers can also be divided into favorable and unfavorable types, depending upon histologic classification.[80, 81] Favorable histologic types include tubular carcinoma, mucinous (colloid) carcinoma, adenoid cystic carcinoma, secretory (juvenile) carcinoma, and perhaps medullary carcinoma (see earlier). Unfortunately, these histologic classifications constitute only a small fraction of all carcinomas of the breast. Unfavorable types include inflammatory carcinoma and undifferentiated carcinoma. The vast majority of invasive breast cancers are

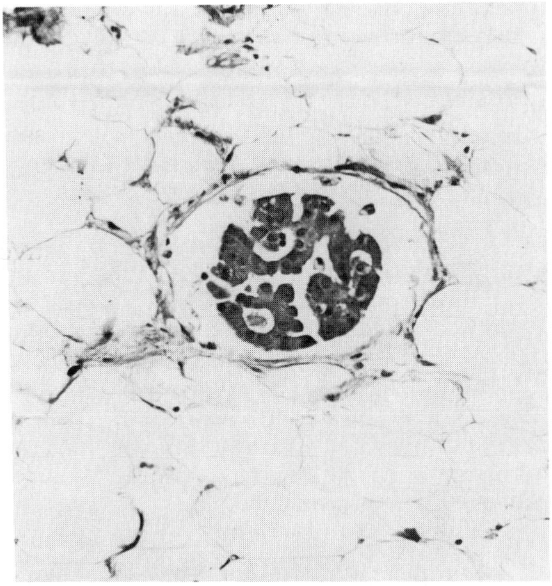

FIGURE 3–33. Intramammary lymphatic invasion. Note the tumor embolus in a dilated, partially obstructed lymphatic channel (H & E × 220).

of the intermediate-prognosis infiltrating ductal type. A variety of histologic parameters have been examined in an attempt to predict outcome among patients in this large group. Prognostic factors such as intramammary lymphatic invasion[82] (Fig. 3–33) may help to identify node-negative (Stage I) patients with infiltrating cancer, who are at increased risk for recurrence and, therefore, might reasonably be considered for adjuvant chemotherapy programs. In addition, certain pathologic findings, such as extensive intraductal involvement, may be useful in identifying a subgroup of patients treated by lumpectomy and local radiation therapy who are at increased risk for local recurrence.[83] Other prognostic variables that have been examined singly and in various combinations include nuclear grade (see later), differentiation (see later), blood vessel invasion,[79, 84, 85] tumor necrosis,[79] host immune response,[86] circumscription of tumor margins,[79] location of the tumor within the breast,[73] hormone-receptor status,[87] expression of various biologic markers,[88] and intensity of T-lymphocyte infiltration.[89]

Histologic grading schema[90, 91] encompass an assessment of nuclear features (nuclear size, nuclear:cytoplasmic ratio, pleomorphism, hyperchromatism, regularity of nuclear membranes, prominence of nucleoli, and mitotic activity) and the degree of differentiation (tubule, duct, and gland formations). In evaluating these studies, it is important to note that the nuclear grading suggested by Black and Speer[92] employed a scale (0 to 3, worst to best) that is the exact opposite of the one currently in use, which is based upon the studies of Bloom and Richardson:[93] irregularity of size, shape, or staining of nuclei (1, 2, or 3 points, well-differentiated, intermediate, or poor); hyperchromatic nuclei and mitoses (1, 2, or 3 points, few, moderate, or many); and tubule formation (1, 2, or 3 points, many, moderate, or none), with Grade I equal to 3 to 5 points, Grade II equal to 6 to 7, and Grade III equal to 8 to 9.

Most authorities agree that there is a meaningful correlation between histologic grading and clinical outcome that is useful in the analysis of follow-up data from groups of patients. Unfortunately, most of these schema are of less value in judging prognosis for the individual patient at the time of diagnosis, because of inter- and intraobserver variability and the limited discriminatory power of these variables in predicting recurrence.[86, 91, 94]

These shortcomings have been addressed in the work of Stenkvist and colleagues,[86, 95] who utilize computerized nuclear morphometric analysis; Sharkey and co-workers,[96] who employed quantitative morphometric analysis of differentiation; and Auer and colleagues,[97] who performed automated microspectrophotometric determinations of DNA content to obtain more objective and reproducible methodologies for grading breast cancers. In addition, improved statistical methodologies (computerized linear discriminant analysis and recursive partitioning) have been useful in the identification of those prognostic factors of greatest predictive value.[86, 98] In this manner, Stenkvist and colleagues evaluated the prognostic value of 435 cytochemical, cytometric, morphologic, epidemiologic, and clinical variables in a prospective study of 179 breast cancer patients followed for five years after mastectomy.[86] During the first two and a half years, recurrence rates correlated with mitotic frequency, size of the primary tumor and axillary metastases, degree of differentiation in fine-needle aspiration biopsies,[99] and numbers of lymphocytes around the tumor. The combination of variables that had the most discriminatory power in predicting recurrence during the second two-and-a-half-year period included variance of DNA content, numbers of lymphocytes around the tumor, multicentricity, and occurrence of breast cancer among relatives. Although other factors also positively correlated with recurrence, they did not increase the predictive value of the aforementioned variables. Using this quantitative approach, the recurrence rate during the first follow-up period was predicted with an impressive 90 percent accuracy.[86]

Kinetic Analysis of Cell Division

Kinetic analysis of tritiated thymidine uptake by replicating breast cancer cells has also been used as an independent objective indicator of prognosis.[100] In this technique, tissue sections are pulse-labeled for one to two hours with tritiated thymidine, which is incorporated into the DNA of cells in the S phase. The specimen is then exposed to photographic emulsion, and after a suitable interval (usually about one week) the autoradiographs are developed and stained with hematoxylin and eosin. Cells in the S phase are marked by silver grains over their nuclei. Since the duration of the S phase greatly exceeds the duration of the M phase (mitosis), this technique is considered more reliable than counting mitoses.[100]

By this method, the mean labeling index for breast cancer is calculated to be about 5 percent, meaning that after a brief exposure to radioactive thymidine, 5 percent of the tumor cells are labeled. However, the range is broad. Well-differentiated tumors, tumors with high estrogen content,[101] and tumors with low nuclear grade tend to have a low labeling index, whereas tumors with high nuclear grade and little tendency toward tubule or gland formation tend to have a high labeling index.[100] Of interest, the *in vitro* labeling index may be modified by hormonal factors.[102] The thymidine index shows a tendency to increase between primary treatment and relapse.[103]

S phase can also be quantitated by flow cytometry, using a DNA-specific dye.[100] This technique has the advantage of immediate availability of results; however, the specific cell type is not identified, as with autoradiography. If the tumor cells are aneuploid, they can easily be distinguished from nonmalignant cell types. Both the thymidine-labeling index and the flow cytometric analysis of DNA content show promise in identifying women at increased risk for recurrence.

TECHNIQUES OF PATHOLOGIC EVALUATION

Core Needle Biopsy

With this technique a small, cylindrical core of intact breast tissue is removed using a needle equipped with a special cutting edge. Most often, a disposable Tru-Cut needle is used. The needle has a wider bore diameter than the "skinny" needle used for fine-needle aspiration biopsy (see later). The procedure requires local anesthesia and can be readily performed in an outpatient setting. In some hospitals, this technique has gained wide acceptance for use in patients with palpable breast masses. In this patient population, the technique provides a cost-effective means for establishing diagnosis prior to definitive surgery. It is usually not performed for clinically benign lesions or for small, nonpalpable abnormalities detected radiographically. While it has the advantage over fine-needle aspiration biopsy of preserving the architectural integrity of the specimen, cytologic features are not as well seen in paraffin-embedded tissue as in the aspirates, there are frequently crush artifacts, and the core biopsy may not provide as representative a sampling. Distinction can be made between *in situ* and infiltrating carcinomas, and often the histologic type of the tumor can be determined. When compared with the results of open biopsy, this technique provides the correct interpretation in 67 to 98.5 percent of cases.[104]

Needle Aspiration of Cysts

The majority of breast cysts collapse after needle aspiration. The diagnostic value of aspiration in distinguishing a solid mass from a cystic lesion is considerable. Typically, with the aspiration of a cyst a small amount of clear fluid is obtained in a syringe; the fluid is essentially acellular or contains only a sparse number of duct cells, histiocytes, and apocrine cells. In such circumstances, cytologic examination of the aspirated fluid is usually unrewarding. In 1982, Dohrmann and colleagues reviewed a series of 169 patients who developed 220 cysts, all treated by needle aspiration. In this study, cytologic examination of the cyst was performed in all women presenting for the first time; in no case were the cytologic findings suggestive of a malignancy.[105] However, whenever the aspirated fluid is turbid or blood stained, or there is skin fixation or nipple retraction, or residual tumor is palpated after aspiration, cytologic evaluation of the fluid is indicated.

Fine-needle Aspiration

Various reports have demonstrated the value of fine-needle aspiration (FNA) in the diagnosis of primary breast masses.[104, 106–109] This technique has been evolving as a diagnostic method for several decades.[110] Although usually performed for palpable lesions, in some institutions FNA of nonpalpable lesions visualized by mammography is carried out under stereotaxic control.[111, 112] In addition, FNA can be used to evaluate enlarged lymph nodes and local recurrence following mastectomy.

FNA differs from needle aspiration of fluid-filled cysts and tissue core needle biopsy in that the aspirated mass is solid and the specimen consists of cell clusters and isolated cells that are examined cytologically. Thus, the technique represents a hybrid between exfoliative cytologic examination and routine histologic testing. The aspiration is performed using a specially adapted syringe that can be held in one hand while the other hand immobilizes the lesion.[106] A fine (20 to 25 gauge) needle is employed. The mass is aspirated under suction generated by a 10 to 20 ml syringe. During the procedure the needle is maneuvered up and down (*not* laterally) to maximize sampling from different aspects of the lesion. The vacuum is gently released before the needle is withdrawn. A new needle may then be reinserted at different angles to ensure representative sampling. Microscopic fragments of tissue and individual cells are sucked into the hub of the needle. Following aspiration, the needle is removed from the syringe, and air is sucked into the syringe. The needle is then reattached to the syringe, after which the specimen is directly expelled onto a glass slide by rapidly depressing the plunger. The cells are gently smeared with a coverglass or another glass slide. The material is usually air-dried and stained with a May-Grünwald–Giemsa stain. Additional material may be stained with Diffquik, a modified Wright stain. Some pathologists simultaneously fix one or more slides in alcohol and stain using the method of Papanicolaou. Washings of the needle can also be submitted for evaluation by cytocentrifuge, sedimentation, or cell block.[113] FNA has the advantages of safety, good patient acceptance, low cost, rapid diagnosis, and expediency. With respect to possible tumor dissemination, no deleterious effect of FNA on long-term survival has been noted.[106, 114]

The overall cellularity of the specimen, the architectural arrangement of the cells within groups, the nuclear features of the individual cells, and the monomorphism of the neoplastic cells are all utilized to interpret the material (Fig. 3–34). Because of the relative loss of cellular cohesiveness seen with a malignancy, the presence of detached cells with abnormal nuclear features and with intact cytoplasm is of diagnostic value. The degree of differentiation may be expressed by the tendency of cancer cells to dissociate, and nuclear abnormalities of size, shape, and

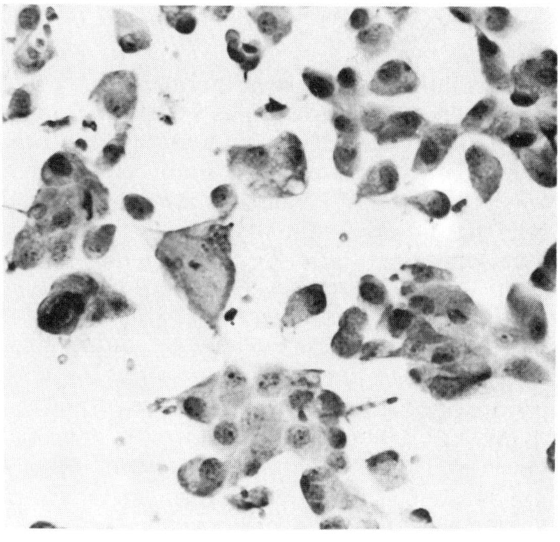

FIGURE 3–34. Fine-needle aspiration cytology of biopsy-proven infiltrating ductal carcinoma. Note the cellularity of the specimen, the loss of cohesiveness, and the presence of individual cells with intact cytoplasm, increased nuclear size, irregular chromatin pattern, and prominent nucleoli. One cell possesses an intracytoplasmic "acinus" (H & E × 320). (Courtesy of Sibley Memorial Hospital, Washington, D.C.)

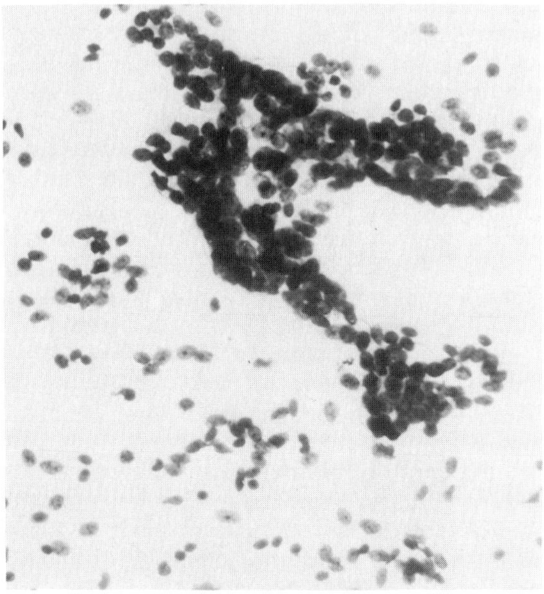

FIGURE 3–35. Fine-needle aspiration cytology of biopsy-proven fibroadenoma. Note the ramifying ductular pattern of the cellular aggregate, the uniformity of nuclear size, and the presence of numerous individual "naked" nuclei (H & E × 320). (Courtesy of Sibley Memorial Hospital, Washington, D.C.)

density can be quantitated.[86] However, the cytologic features of malignant cells in some forms of breast cancer can be deceptively bland.

The histogenesis of several benign lesions can be established by this technique. Benign lesions are usually less cellular, with the exception of fibroadenomas and papillomas. Fibroadenomas characteristically are composed of a dual population of clusters of small bland epithelial cells and individual cells with naked bipolar nuclei, possibly of myoepithelial origin (Fig. 3–35). The clusters of cells often exhibit a branching ductular pattern; each cell within the aggregate maintains a uniform distance from neighboring cells, creating a "honeycomb" effect. Benign proliferations often contain apocrine cells and foam cells, as well as ordinary epithelial cells. However, the finding of a negative FNA in the presence of a palpable mass or mammographically suspicious lesion requires further diagnostic interventions, since it is possible that the aspirated material is not representative.

There are limitations to the procedure. Noninfiltrating carcinomas cannot be distinguished from invasive carcinomas. Complex intraductal processes, lobular carcinomas, well-differentiated (tubular) carcinomas, and unusual and mixed histologic findings are not as easily interpreted by this technique; indeed, sometimes a routine excisional biopsy that preserves all the diagnostic clues may prove exceedingly difficult to interpret. In addition, rare false-positive diagnosis of malignancy is a major concern. The authors believe that open biopsy with confirmatory frozen section immediately prior to mastectomy is indicated. This also ensures that appropriate tissue is promptly sent for hormone-receptor analysis.

The effective application of this technique requires good communication among clinician, surgeon, and pathologist. The diagnosis of malignancy by FNA leads to better planning of the surgical strategy, thereby reducing operating time and cost. Major deterrents to its widespread application in the United States have been the lack of physicians trained in the aspiration procedure and in the interpretation of the specimens. Recent interest in this technique has been stimulated both by the development of increasingly sophisticated imaging technologies, used to localize lesions in various organ sites, and by an increased awareness of cost-effectiveness in the planning of diagnostic strategies. Future applications of FNA are likely to extend diagnostic capabilities by computerized morphometric analysis of nuclei and cell clusters, hormone-receptor analysis performed directly on aspirates, and immunoperoxidase analysis of the smears for tumor-related antigens.

Open Excisional Biopsy

Currently, the conventional approach to the management of a clinically suspicious, palpable breast mass is excisional biopsy of the lesion under local anesthesia. This procedure is typically carried out in the operating room as part of a two-stage approach to the diagnosis and treatment of breast cancer. Once the mass is resected, it is placed in an appropriately labeled container and sent for frozen section analysis. In handling these specimens, it is important for the pathologist to measure the overall dimensions of both the specimen and the tumor mass. If conservative therapy is planned, attempts should be made to assess the gross surgical margins as well. A frozen section is then obtained to provide a preliminary diagnosis and to ensure that representative tumor is promptly sent for hormone-receptor analysis. When a diagnosis cannot be established by frozen section, the pathologist submits the entire specimen for fixation and permanent histologic sections.

A nonpalpable lesion is first localized mammographically and marked for excision by the injection of dye or via needle localization.[115, 116] Once resected, the specimen is immediately radiographed and then evaluated in conjunction with the specimen xeromammogram, to ensure that the mammographically suspicious region has been removed and appropriately sectioned for histologic evaluation. (Radiographic examination can also be performed directly on the paraffin blocks.)

When mastectomy is chosen, it is carried out at a subsequent date, thereby allowing time for the patient to evaluate various treatment options and time for the pathologist to confirm the diagnosis on permanent histologic sections. The delay between excisional biopsy and mastectomy does not appear to unfavorably influence prognosis. Potential disadvantages of this two-stage approach include (1) hematoma formation, which theoretically may contaminate the adjacent normal breast with miscroscopic deposits of residual tumor; (2) infection of the biopsy site; and (3) possibly, poor orientation of the biopsy incision, should the patient desire plastic surgical reconstruction after mastectomy. Rarely, if clinically warranted, is a biopsy carried out under general anesthesia; if a frozen section is positive for malignancy, mastectomy is performed without delay.

When excisional biopsy with local radiation therapy is the treatment of choice, the excisional biopsy serves to remove all visible and palpable evidence of disease prior to radiation therapy. It is clear that excisional biopsy is inadequate to control local disease, unless coupled with radiation therapy. In a prospective trial of excisional biopsy with local radiation versus mastectomy, the authors have histologically evaluated breast tissues from excisional biopsies in those patients who subsequently underwent mastectomy. When three or more histologic sections were obtained from the excisional biopsy site, microscopic residual disease was detected in more than a third of cases.

When a biopsy fails to reveal evidence of malignancy, it is important that the pathologist and the clinician discuss the case to determine if the histologic findings explain the palpable or mammographic abnormalities that originally brought the patient to their attention. If not, it may be necessary for the pathologist to process additional tissue or obtain levels on the paraffin blocks; on occasion, it may be necessary for the surgeon to repeat the biopsy to be certain that the suspicious lesion has been excised and appropriately evaluated.

Mastectomy and Axillary Nodal Dissection

Modified radical mastectomy is still the conventional surgical approach for Stages I and II breast cancer. If a maximum of information is to be derived from the specimen, the following data should be made available to the pathologist prior to specimen processing: the side of the mastectomy, the quadrant of the malignancy, previous diagnostic procedures, and whether or not hormone-receptor analysis has already been performed. If information is desired about the axillary nodes by level, these should be separately tagged or otherwise identified by the *surgeon* (Level I, lateral to the pectoralis minor muscle [low]; Level II, beneath the pectoralis minor muscle [middle]; Level III, superior to the pectoralis minor muscle [high, apex]). In the National Institutes of Health primary breast cancer protocol, a complete axillary dissection is performed for all patients, regardless of whether the patient is treated by mastectomy or excisional biopsy with local radiation therapy. However, some institutions limit axillary sampling to low lymph nodes for those patients treated by excisional biopsy and local radiation therapy, even though this approach is likely to underestimate node positivity.[117]

In evaluating the mastectomy specimen, Breast Cancer Task Force recommendations are used.[118] The pathologist routinely obtains at least three sections at the tumor or biopsy site, a random sampling of each of the uninvolved breast quadrants, a section of the nipple, and a section of skin overlying the tumor. The axillary fat is carefully searched for palpable or visible lymph nodes. If the fat itself is grossly involved by tumor, a representative section is taken as well.

Lymph nodes smaller than 3 mm in thickness are submitted intact; a representative longitudinal section is embedded for each larger node. In this manner, each lymph node is represented only once in the microscopic sections (lymph node counts are performed directly on the slides). During microscopic examination, special attention is directed toward the subcapsular sinuses of the nodes, where tumor emboli are first deposited by the efferent lymphatics. A typical complete axillary dissection contains an average of 22 lymph nodes (range 9 to 44). Additional nodes may be visualized after "clearing" the adipose tissue with Carnoy's solution; however, the additional data gained by this procedure have not been demonstrated to provide clinically useful information beyond that obtained by routine examination.[119] Because of the therapeutic implications and prognostic significance of metastasis to axillary lymph nodes (see previously), it is essential that the pathologist conduct a thorough dissection of all palpable lymph nodes within the specimen, as well as a careful microscopic examination of each node.

ACKNOWLEDGMENTS

The authors wish to thank Drs. Ernest V. deMoss, Thomas A. Fleury, Cecil H. Fox, Marc E. Lippman, Carlos Restrepo, and Björn Stenkvist for their various contributions to the content of this manuscript. In addition, the authors are most appreciative of the efforts of photographers Mr. Larry K. Ostby, Mr. Gary Best, and Mr. James R. Banks and histotechnologists Ms. Ruby M. Howard, Mrs. Margaret W. Duvall, and Ms. Sarah E. DeLay and of the expert secretarial assistance provided by Ms. Kathleen Moore.

REFERENCES

1. Langman J: Medical Embryology. Baltimore: Williams & Wilkins Co., 1969, p. 367.
2. Haagensen CD: Diseases of the Breast. Philadelphia: W.B. Saunders Co., 1971, pp. 1–67, 190–201.
3. Azzopardi JG, Ahmed A, Millis RR: Problems in Breast Pathology. Philadelphia: W.B. Saunders Co., 1979, pp. 8–91, 346–378.
4. Azzopardi JG, Laurini RN: Elastosis in breast cancer. Cancer 33:174, 1974.
5. Davies JD: Hyperelastosis, obliteration and fibrous plaques in major ducts of the human breast. J Pathol 110:13, 1973.
6. Ozzello L: Ultrastructure of the human mammary gland. *In*: Sommers SC (ed.): Pathology Annual, Vol. 6. London: Butterworth, 1971, pp. 1–59.
7. Ozzello L: Benign and malignant proliferations of the mammary epithelium: Ultrastructural observations. *In*: McDivitt RW, Oberman HA, Ozzello L, et al. (eds.): The Breast. Baltimore: Williams & Wilkins Co., 1984, pp. 105–138.
8. Copenhaver WM, Bunge RP, Bunge MB: Bailey's Textbook of Histology. Baltimore: Williams & Wilkins Co., 1971, pp. 617–618.
9. Love SM, Gelman RS, Silen W: Fibrocystic "disease" of the breast: A non-disease. N Engl J Med 307:1010, 1982.
10. Hutter RVP: Goodbye to "fibrocystic disease." N Engl J Med 312:179, 1985.
11. Dupont WD, Page DL: Risk factors for breast cancer in women with proliferative breast disease. N Engl J Med 312:146, 1985.
12. Oberman HA: Benign breast lesions confused with carcinoma. *In*: McDivitt RW, Oberman HA, Ozzello L, et al. (eds.): The Breast. Baltimore: Williams & Wilkins Co., 1984, pp. 1–33.
13. Page DL, Dupont WD, Rogers, LW, et al.: Atypical hyperplastic lesions of the female breast. Cancer 55:2698, 1985.
14. Hertel BF, Zaloudek C, Kempson RL: Breast adenomas. Cancer 37:2891, 1976.
15. Pike AM, Oberman HA: Juvenile (cellular) adenofibromas. Am J Surg Pathol 9:730, 1985.
16. Rosen PP: Lobular carcinoma *in situ* and intraductal carcinoma of the breast. *In*: McDivitt RW, Oberman HA, Ozzello L, et al. (eds.): The Breast. Baltimore: Williams & Wilkins Co., 1984, pp. 59–105.
17. Ashikari R, Hadju SI, Robbins GY: Intraductal carcinoma of the breast (1960–69). Cancer 28:1182, 1971.
18. Alpers CE, Wellings SR: The prevalence of carcinoma *in situ* in normal and cancer-associated breasts. Hum Pathol 16:796, 1985.
19. Carter D, Orr SL, Merino MJ: Intracystic papillary carcinoma of the breast. Cancer 52:14, 1983.
20. McDivitt RW, Stewart FW, Berg JW: Tumors of the breast. *In*: Atlas of Tumor Pathology, second series, fascicle 2. Washington, D.C.: Armed Forces Institute of Pathology, 1968, pp. 9–149.
21. Silverberg SG, Chitale AR: Assessment of significance of proportions of intraductal and infiltrating tumor growth in ductal carcinoma of the breast. Cancer 32:830, 1973.
22. Page DL, Dupont WD, Rodgers LW, et al.: Intraductal carcinoma of the breast: Follow-up after biopsy only. Cancer 49:751, 1982.
23. Fechner RE: Epithelial alterations in the extralobular ducts of breasts with lobular carcinoma. Arch Pathol 93:164, 1972.
24. Paget J: On disease of the mammary areola preceding cancer of the mammary gland. St Barth Hosp Rep 10:87, 1874.
25. Jackson JG, Orr JW: The ducts of carcinomatous breasts, with particular reference to connective tissue changes. J Pathol Bacteriol 74:265, 1957.
26. Barsky SH, Rao CN, Grotendorst GR, et al.: Increased content of Type V collagen in desmoplasia of human breast carcinoma. Am J Pathol 108:276, 1982.
27. Giorno R: Mononuclear cells in malignant and

benign human breast tissue. Arch Pathol Lab Med 107:415, 1983.
28. Fisher ER, Fisher B: Lobular carcinoma of the breast: An overview. Ann Surg 185:377, 1977.
29. Haagensen CD, Lane N, Lattes R, et al.: Lobular neoplasia (so-called lobular carcinoma *in situ*) of the breast. Cancer 42:737, 1978.
30. Fechner RE: Infiltrating lobular carcinoma without lobular carcinoma *in situ*. Cancer 29:1539, 1972.
31. Newman W: Lobular carcinoma of the female breast: Report of 73 cases. Ann Surg 164:305, 1966.
32. Eusebi V, Pich A, Macchiorlatti E, et al.: Morphofunctional differentiation in lobular carcinoma of the breast. Histopathology 1:301, 1977.
33. Cubilla AL, Woodruff JM: Primary carcinoid tumor of the breast—a report on eight patients. Am J Surg Pathol 1:283, 1977.
34. Clayton F, Sibley RK, Ordonez NJ, et al.: Argyrophilic breast carcinomas: Evidence of lactational differentiation. Am J Surg Pathol 6:323, 1982.
35. Moore OS, Foote FW, Jr.: The relatively favorable prognosis of medullary carcinoma of the breast. Cancer 2:635, 1949.
36. Richardson WW: Medullary carcinoma of the breast: A distinctive tumor type with a relatively good prognosis following radical mastectomy. Br J Cancer 10:415, 1956.
37. Blood HJG, Richardson WW, Field JR: Host resistance and survival in carcinoma of the breast: A study of 104 cases of medullary carcinoma in a series of 411 cases followed for 20 years. Br Med J 3:181, 1970.
38. Ridolfi RL, Rosen PP, Port A, et al.: Medullary carcinoma of the breast: A clinicopathologic study with 10-year follow-up. Cancer 40:1365, 1977.
39. Saphir O: Mucinous carcinoma of the breast. Surg Gynecol Obstet 72:908, 1941.
40. Silverberg SG, Kay S, Chitale AR, et al.: Colloid carcinoma of the breast. Am J Clin Pathol 55:355, 1971.
41. Norris HF, Taylor HB: Prognosis of mucinous (gelatinous) carcinoma of the breast. Cancer 18:879, 1965.
42. Taylor HB, Norris HJ: Well-differentiated carcinoma of the breast. Cancer 25:687, 1970.
43. Carstens PHB, Huvos AG, Foote FW, Jr., et al.: Tubular carcinoma of the breast: A clinicopathologic study of 35 cases. Am J Clin Pathol 58:231, 1972.
44. Cooper HS, Patchefsky AS, Krall RA: Tubular carcinoma of the breast. Cancer 42:2334, 1978.
45. Deos PH, Norris HJ: Well-differentiated (tubular) carcinoma of the breast. Am J Clin Pathol 78:1, 1982.
46. McDivitt RW, Boyce W, Gersell D: Tubular carcinoma of the breast. Am J Surg Pathol 6:401, 1982.
47. Byrne MP, Fahey MM, Gooselaw JG: Breast cancer with axillary metastasis in an eight-and-one-half-year-old girl. Cancer 31:726, 1973.
48. Oberman HJ: Secretory carcinoma of the breast in adults. Am J Surg Pathol 4:465, 1980.
49. Akhtar M, Robinson C, Ali MA, et al.: Secretory carcinoma of the breast in adults. Light and electron microscopic study of three cases with review of the literature. Cancer 51:2245, 1983.
50. Tavassoli FA, Norris HJ: Secretory carcinoma of the breast. Cancer 45:2404, 1980.
51. Sullivan JJ, Magee HR, Donald KJ: Secretory (juvenile) carcinoma of the breast. Pathology (Sydney) 9:341, 1977.
52. Friedman BA, Oberman HA: Adenoid cystic carcinoma of the breast. Am J Clin Pathol 54:1, 1970.
53. Cavanzo FJ, Taylor HB: Adenoid cystic carcinoma of the breast: An analysis of 21 cases. Cancer 24:740, 1969.
54. Foote FW, Jr., Stewart FW: Lobular carcinoma *in situ*: A rare form of mammary carcinoma. Am J Pathol 17:491, 1941.
55. Galloway JR, Woolner LB, Clagett OT: Adenoid cystic carcinoma of the breast. Surg Gynecol Obstet 122:1289, 1966.
56. Robbins GF, Shah J, Rosen P, et al.: Inflammatory carcinoma of the breast. Surg Clin North Am 54:801, 1974.
57. Droulias CA, Sewell CW, Mcsweeney MB, et al.: Inflammatory carcinoma of the breast: A correlation of clinical, radiologic, and pathologic findings. Ann Surg 184:217, 1976.
58. Ellis DL, Teitelbaum SL: Inflammatory carcinoma of the breast: A pathologic definition. Cancer 33:1045, 1974.
59. Norris HJ, Taylor HB: Relationship of histologic features to behavior of cystosarcoma phyllodes: Analysis of 94 cases. Cancer 20:2090, 1967.
60. Merino MJ: Angiosarcoma of the breast. Am J Surg Pathol 7:53, 1983.
61. Norris HJ, Taylor HB: Sarcomas and related mesenchymal tumors of the breast. Cancer 22:22, 1968.
62. Bird CC: A breast sarcoma containing rhabdosarcomatous and other metaplastic elements. J Pathol 101:286, 1970.
63. Barnes L, Pietruszka M: Sarcomas of the breast: A clinicopathologic analysis of ten cases. Cancer 40:1577, 1977.
64. Harris M, Persaud V: Carcinosarcoma of the breast. J Pathol 112:99, 1974.
65. Sandison AT: Metastatic tumours in the breast. Br J Surg 47:54, 1959.
66. McIntosh IH, Hooper AA, Millis RR, et al.: Metastatic carcinoma within the breast. Clin Oncol 2:393, 1976.
67. Hajdu SI, Urban JA: Cancers metastatic to the breast. Cancer 29:1691, 1972.
68. DeCosse JJ, et al.: Primary lymphosarcoma of the breast: A review of 14 cases. Cancer 15:1264, 1962.
69. Betsill WL, Jr., et al.: Intraductal carcinoma: Long-term follow-up after treatment by biopsy alone. JAMA 239:1863, 1978.
70. Bedwani R, Vana J, Rosner D, et al.: Management and survival of female patients with "minimal" breast cancer: As observed in the long-term and short-term surveys of the American College of Surgeons. Cancer 47:2769, 1981.
71. Say CC, Donegan WL: Invasive carcinoma of the breast: Prognostic significance of tumor size and involved axillary nodes. Cancer 34:468, 1974.
72. Fisher ER, Fisher B, Sass R, et al.: Pathologic findings from the National Surgical Adjuvant Breast Project XI. Cancer 54:3002, 1984.
73. Nemoto T, Vana J, Bedwani RN, et al.: Management and survival of female breast cancer: Results of a national survey by the American College of Surgeons. Cancer 45:2917, 1980.
74. Fisher B, Baver M, Wickerham DL, et al.: Relation

of number of positive axillary nodes to the prognosis of patients with primary breast cancer, a National Surgical Adjuvant Breast Project Update. Cancer 52:1551, 1983.
75. Rosen PP, Saigo PE, Braun DW, et al.: Prognosis in stage II ($T_1N_1M_0$) breast cancer. Ann Surg 194:576, 1981.
76. Rosen PP, Saigo PE, Braun DW, et al.: Axillary micro- and macrometastases in breast cancer. Ann Surg 194:585, 1981.
77. Huvos AG, Hutter RV, Berg JW: Significance of axillary macrometastases and micrometastases in mammary carcinoma. Ann Surg 173:44, 1971.
78. Smith JA, Gamez-Araujo JJ, Gallager HS, et al.: Carcinoma of the breast; analysis of total lymph node involvement versus level of metastasis. Cancer 39:527, 1977.
79. Fisher ER: The pathologist's role in the diagnosis and treatment of invasive breast cancer. Surg Clin North Am 58:705, 1978.
80. Gallager HS: Pathologic types of breast cancer: Their prognoses. Cancer 53:623, 1984.
81. Fisher ER, Gregorio RM, Fisher B, et al.: The pathology of invasive breast cancer. A syllabus derived from findings of the National Surgical Adjuvant Breast Project (Protocol No. 4). Cancer 36:1, 1975.
82. Nime FA, Rosen PP, Thaler HT, et al.: Prognostic significance of tumor emboli in intramammary lymphatics in patients with mammary carcinoma. Am J Surg Pathol 1:25, 1977.
83. Schmitt SJ, et al.: Pathologic predictors of early local recurrence in stage I and II breast cancer treatment by primary radiation therapy. Cancer 53:1049, 1984.
84. Nealon TF, Nkongho A, Grossi C, et al.: Pathologic identification of poor prognosis stage I ($T_1N_0M_0$) cancer of the breast. Ann Surg 190:129, 1979.
85. Kister SJ, Sommers SC, Haagensen CD, et al.: Reevaluation of blood-vessel invasion as a prognostic factor in carcinoma of the breast. Cancer 19:1213, 1966.
86. Stenkvist B, Bengtsson E, Dahlqvist B, et al.: Predicting breast cancer recurrence. Cancer 50:2884, 1982.
87. McCarty KS, Jr., Barton TK, Fetter BF, et al.: Correlation of estrogen and progesterone receptors with histologic differentiation in mammary carcinoma. Cancer 46:2851, 1980.
88. Walker RA: Biologic markers in human breast cancer. J Pathol 137:109, 1982.
89. Shimokawara I, Imamura M, Yamanaka N, et al.: Identification of lymphocyte subpopulations in human breast cancer tissue and its significance: An immunoperoxidase study with anti-human T and B sera. Cancer 49:1456, 1982.
90. Scarff RW, Torloni H: Histological typing of breast tumors. International Histological Classification of Tumors, no. 2. Geneva: World Health Organization, 1968.
91. Stenkvist B, Westman-Naeser S, Vegelius J, et al.: Analysis of reproducibility of subjective grading systems for breast carcinoma. J Clin Pathol 32:979, 1979.
92. Black MM, Speer FD: Nuclear structure in cancer tissues. Surg Gynecol Obstet 105:97, 1957.
93. Bloom HJG, Richardson WW: Histological grading and prognosis in breast cancer. A study of 1409 cases, of which 359 have been followed for 15 years. Br J Cancer 11:359, 1957.
94. Stenkvist B, Bengtsson E, Eriksson O, et al.: Histopathological systems of breast cancer classification: Reproducibility and clinical significance. J Clin Pathol 36:392, 1983.
95. Stenkvist B, Westman-Naeser S, Holmquist J, et al.: Computerized nuclear morphometry as an objective method for characterizing human cancer cell populations. Cancer Res 38:4688, 1978.
96. Sharkey FE, Pavlak RJ, Greiner AS: Morphometric analysis of differentiation in human breast carcinoma. Tumor grading. Arch Pathol Lab Med 107:406, 1983.
97. Auer GU, Caspersson TO, Wallgren AS: DNA content and survival in mammary carcinomas. Anal Quant Cytol 2:161, 1980.
98. Armitage P, Gehan A: Statistical methods for the identification and use of prognostic factors. Int J Cancer 13:16, 1974.
99. Stenkvist B, Bengtsson E, Eriksson O, et al.: A morphometric expression of differentiation in fine-needle biopsies of breast cancer. Cytometry 1:292, 1981.
100. Meyer JS: Cell kinetic analysis of human breast carcinomas. *In*: McDivitt RW, Oberman HA, Ozzello L, et al. (eds.): The Breast. Baltimore: Williams & Wilkins Co., 1984, pp. 45–58.
101. Meyer JS, Bauer WC, Rao BR: Subpopulations of breast carcinoma defined by S-phase fraction, morphology, and estrogen receptor content. Lab Invest 39:225, 1978.
102. Lippman ME, Osborne CK, Knazek R, et al.: *In vitro* model systems for the study of hormone-dependent human breast cancer. N Engl J Med 296:154, 1977.
103. Meyer JS, Lee JY: Relationship of S-phase fraction of breast carcinoma in relapse to duration of remission, estrogen receptor content, therapeutic responsiveness, and duration of survival. Cancer Res 40:1890, 1980.
104. Millis RR: Needle biopsy of the breast. *In*: McDivitt RW, Oberman HA, Ozzello L, et al. (eds.): The Breast. Baltimore: Williams & Wilkins Co., 1984, pp. 186–203.
105. Dohrmann PJ, Hughes ES, McDermott FT, et al.: Aspiration of breast cysts. Aust NZ J Surg 52:605, 1982.
106. Linsk JA, Franzen S: Breast aspiration. *In*: Linsk JA, Franzen S (eds.): Clinical Aspiration Cytology. Philadelphia: J.B. Lippincott Co., 1983, pp. 105–137.
107. Franzen S, Zajicek J: Aspiration biopsy in the diagnosis of palpable lesions of the breast: Critical review of 3479 consecutive biopsies. Acta Radiol 7:241, 1968.
108. Kline TS, et al.: Fine-needle aspiration of the breast: Diagnosis and pitfalls; a review of 3545 cases. Cancer 44:1458, 1979.
109. Frable WJ: Thin Needle Aspiration Biopsy. Philadelphia: W.B. Saunders Co., 1983.
110. Martin HE, Ellis EB: Biopsy by needle puncture and aspiration. Ann Surg 42:169, 1930.
111. Hennig K, Johanssen H, Rimsten A, et al.: X-ray

and fine-needle biopsy in the diagnosis of nonpalpable breast lesions. Acta Cytol 19:7, 1975.
112. Bolmgren J, Jacobson B, Nordenström B: Stereotaxic instrument for needle biopsy of the mamma. AJR 129:121, 1977.
113. Karnauchow PN, Bonin RE: Cell block technique for fine-needle aspiration biopsy. J Clin Pathol 35:688, 1982.
114. Robbins GF, Brothers JH, Eberhart WF, et al.: Is aspiration biopsy of breast cancer dangerous to the patient? Cancer 7:774, 1954.
115. Meyer JE: Occult breast abnormalities: Percutaneous preoperative needle localization. Radiology 150:335, 1984.
116. Homer MJ: Localization of nonpalpable breast lesions: Technical aspects and analysis of 80 cases. AJR 140:807, 1983.
117. deMoss EV, et al.: Complete axillary lymph node dissection before radiotherapy for primary breast cancer. *In*: Harris JR, Hellman S, Silen W (eds.): Conservative Management of Breast Cancer. Philadelphia: J.B. Lippinoctt Co., 1983, pp. 163–182.
118. Breast Cancer Task Force: Standardized management of breast specimens recommended by Pathology Working Group. Am J Clin Pathol 60:789, 1973.
119. Morrow M, Evans J, Rosen PP, et al.: Does clearing of axillary lymph nodes contribute to accurate staging of breast carcinoma? Cancer 53:1329, 1984.

The Diagnosis of Breast Cancer

DAVID N. DANFORTH, JR., M.D.
ALLEN S. LICHTER, M.D.
MARC E. LIPPMAN, M.D.

4

The diagnosis of breast cancer involves differentiating benign from malignant changes in the breast and determining the nature and extent of those changes that are malignant. The diagnostic approach to breast cancer patients includes the systematic evaluation of breast changes, beginning with the history and physical examination and concluding with assigning an appropriate stage to the cancer and making treatment recommendations. The history defines the chronology and character of the breast complaint and identifies any risk factors, including genetic and hormonal factors and exposure to carcinogenic agents, that may increase the likelihood that the changes in the affected or contralateral breast are malignant. The physical examination defines the location and extent of the breast changes and whether they are associated with any abnormalities in regional tissues, especially lymph node–bearing areas, or distant sites, including lung, bone, and liver.

The history and physical examination, by defining the breast changes, will indicate the additional studies to be performed to further characterize the abnormalities. These studies may be noninvasive or invasive and may be directed at the breast or at distant organs and tissues. Noninvasive studies evaluating the breast include mammography, galactography, ultrasonography, thermography, and computerized tomography. These studies differ in their sensitivity for detecting certain lesions but, in general, may identify malignant changes in the suspicious area, ductal pathologic conditions, cystic versus solid lesions, and suspicious changes in the remaining tissue of the affected or contralateral breast.

Invasive procedures are almost always necessary to establish the diagnosis of the breast abnormality and are performed after noninvasive procedures are completed. Available invasive procedures include fine-needle aspiration and cytologic analysis, percutaneous needle biopsies, and open incisional or excisional biopsies. Selection of a particular procedure will depend upon the nature of the lesion (occult versus a large palpable mass) and the information desired (cytologic, histologic, or steroid receptor content). If a malignancy is confirmed, the possibility of spread to distant organs and tissues can be evaluated by a second group of noninvasive studies, including hepatic and bone serum enzymes, plasma CEA or other biomarkers, chest and skeletal x-rays, radionuclide scans, and computerized tomography. As with breast imaging studies, these procedures vary in their sensitivity for detecting malignant disease. Procedure selection will be determined by the findings on history and physical examination and by the local or regional extent of the breast cancer.

Information acquired at each step of the evaluation of a breast cancer patient should be summarized according to one of the commonly used staging classifications. Staging accurately defines the extent of the malignancy and indicates the treatment options that are appropriate and offer the best chance for cure. We recommend the American Joint Commission on Cancer TNM Classification as being the most accurate and informative and the most widely used. Each of the methods employed to evaluate the patient suspected of having breast cancer will be discussed in detail later. It should be emphasized that all these methods necessarily complement each other and are designed to define the local, regional, and metastatic extent of the malignancy. A systematic and thorough evaluation of the breast cancer patient will allow the malignancy to be most effectively treated.

For many women, local treatment for breast cancer will be curative. The probability of developing recurrent disease is directly related to the stage of the malignancy at presentation. All women with breast cancer, however, should be followed for a considerable period of time after treatment. While the history and physical examination are an essential part of any follow-up examination, many of the noninvasive studies previously noted are also used routinely in the follow-up of patients with breast cancer. Use of noninvasive studies is indicated by the findings on history and physical examination and is directly related to the stage of breast cancer at the time of presentation. The role of these studies, along with their indications, sensitivity, and likelihood of providing useful information, will also be discussed in this chapter. Appropriate follow-up of patients with breast cancer should allow timely detection of lesions in the vast majority of those women who fail initial treatment.

STAGING CLASSIFICATIONS FOR BREAST CANCER

The stage of a breast malignancy describes the extent to which the malignancy involves the breast tissue locally and the extent to which it has spread to regional lymph nodes and to distant organs and tissues. The importance of any staging classification lies in its ability to define the treatment options that are appropriate and effective for a given patient. Surgery or radiation therapy may be curative for tumors localized to the breast without advanced changes, whereas systemic therapy is required for disseminated disease. Terms such as "early stage," "operable" or "inoperable," and "locally advanced" breast cancer should be avoided, unless it is clear to what stage they are referring. What is operable and what is potentially curable by surgery alone are not necessarily one and the same. Defining the stage will make this distinction. Accurate staging will, in addition, allow for the uniform reporting of treatment results.

A breast cancer patient may be staged on the basis of clinical or pathologic information, or both. The clinical stage represents the summary of an evaluation based on the physical examination (including primary tumor size and mobility, associated skin changes, enlargement and mobility of regional lymph nodes, and any signs or symptoms of distant metastases), x-rays, and radionuclide scans. The pathologic stage refers to that stage established by pathologic review of the primary breast tumor, specimens of regional lymph nodes, and (when applicable) tissue from distant sites thought to contain metastatic disease. The stage of breast cancer, however, is to be distinguished from the grade, which refers only to the degree of histologic differentiation of a given sample of tumor, whether it be the primary tumor or a metastasis. In most staging classifications, the grade of the tumor does not affect the stage, although it does have an important bearing on prognosis.

While both the clinical and the pathologic stages provide essential information for the management of the patient, they may not always be in complete agreement. Inflammatory changes of the breast skin do not always represent inflammatory carcinoma. Clinical estimation of axillary lymph node status (whether negative or positive) is inaccurate in approximately one third of cases.[1] Bone and liver scans cannot always distinguish benign, unrelated conditions from metastatic disease. Nevertheless, accurate clinical staging, especially of the breast, can best be accomplished before any invasive procedures are performed. To attempt to determine accurate tumor measurements or to evaluate adjacent skin changes after a recent breast biopsy may be difficult at best.

Several staging classifications have been proposed for breast cancer; however, three classifications have been most widely used. These are the American Joint Commission on Cancer (AJCC) TNM Classification,[2] the Columbia Clinical Classification (CCC),[3] and the Manchester Classification.[4] Each of these classifications stages the breast cancer patient according to the characteristics of the primary tumor and the presence or absence of lymph node involvement and distant metastases. All histologic types are included. While all three classifications allow for staging based on clinical information (clinical stage), only the TNM Classification includes pathologic information as well. The classifications also differ with regard to the criteria each uses to describe a given stage. In the TNM Classification, the size of the primary tumor is an important characteristic used to determine stage; tumor size is not used in the CCC or the Manchester system. The TNM Classification places all patients with locally advanced breast cancer in Stage III, with a subclassification (Stage III_a or III_b) according to the degree of local or regional involvement. The CCC and Manchester systems place locally advanced tumors in one of two stages (Stage C or D and Stage III or IV, respectively), according to the degree of local involvement by the primary tumor. Stage IV of the TNM Classification includes only patients with distant metastases, whereas Stage D and Stage IV in the other two classifications include patients with localized as well as disseminated disease.

The TNM Classification is the one most widely used today and the one we recommend. It defines more accurately the local extent of the malignancy and includes clinical as well as pathologic information. Historically, each of these three classifications has been used to report a considerable body of information on breast cancer. Because long-term follow-up is essential for the evaluation of any treatment regimen, each of these classifications will continue to be used to report results of trials conducted in the past. An understanding of these classifications is essential so that information from these trials can be properly interpreted. The classification selected should be used consistently both throughout the management of the patient and in reports of any treatment results. Every patient should be accurately staged, and the stage of the tumor should be determined only upon completion of the evaluation. For the TNM Classification, whether the stage is clinical or pathologic should be clearly specified. This approach emphasizes the importance of evaluating all aspects of the patient's malignancy, indicates clearly to others involved in her care the extent of her disease, and facilitates decisions regarding appropriate and effective treatment.

AJCC TNM Classification

The AJCC TNM classification was initially proposed in 1979. In 1983, this classification underwent a minor revision, with locally advanced cancer (Stage III_b) being placed in Stage III instead of Stage IV (as it was in the 1979 classification). The 1983 classification was otherwise unchanged. In 1986, the TNM classification underwent major changes, described later. In the interest of completeness, both the 1983 and the 1986 AJCC TNM classifications are presented and discussed in the following section.

The 1983 AJCC TNM Classification[2] stages patients according to the characteristics of the primary tumor (T), nodal involvement (N), and distant metastases (M) (Table 4–1). The stage of any given patient is described as the clinical-diagnostic stage (cTNM), the surgical-evaluative stage (sTNM), or the post–surgical resection pathologic stage (pTNM), depending upon the source of the information used. Regardless of whether a clinical, surgical, or pathologic stage is being used, the basic criteria for determining the categories T, N, and M are the same.

The TNM Classification has four stages, I, II, III and IV. Stages I and II tumors are considered operable breast cancer; Stage III, locally advanced breast cancer; and Stage IV, distant metastatic disease. Stages I, II, and III tumors are also distinguished according to size ($\leq$ 2 cm, greater than 2 cm but less

TABLE 4–1. 1983 TNM Classification

Primary Tumor (T)

Definitions for the primary tumor (T) for the clinical-diagnostic classification are the same as those for the post–surgical resection pathologic classification.

- T_X Minimum requirements to assess primary tumor cannot be met.
- T_0 No evidence of primary tumor
- TIS *In situ* cancer (*in situ* lobular and pure intraductal cancer, and Paget's disease of the nipple without palpable tumor)
- T_1 Tumor 2 cm or less in greatest dimension
  - T_{1a} No fixation to underlying pectoral fascia or muscle
  - T_{1b} Fixation to underlying pectoral fascia or muscle
    - i tumor less than or equal to 0.5 cm
    - ii tumor greater than 0.5 but less than or equal to 1.0 cm
    - iii tumor greater than 1.0 but less than or equal to 2.0 cm
- T_2 Tumor greater than 2 cm but not more than 5 cm in its greatest dimension
  - T_{2a} No fixation to underlying pectoral fascia or muscle
  - T_{2b} Fixation to underlying pectoral fascia or muscle
- T_3 Tumor greater than 5 cm in its greatest dimension
  - T_{3a} No fixation to underlying pectoral fascia or muscle
  - T_{3b} Fixation to underlying pectoral fascia or muscle
- T_4 Tumor of any size with direct extension into chest wall or skin (chest wall includes ribs, intercostal muscles, and serratus anterior muscle, but not pectoral muscle)
  - T_{4a} Fixation to chest wall
  - T_{4b} Edema (including peau d'orange), ulceration of the skin of the breast, or satellite skin nodules confined to the same breast
  - T_{4c} Both of the above

Nodal Involvement (N)

The definition of N categories varies somewhat as to time period of staging, as follows.

DEFINITIONS FOR CLINICAL-DIAGNOSTIC STAGE

- N_X Regional lymph nodes cannot be assessed (not removed for study or previously removed).
- N_0 No evidence of homolateral axillary lymph node involvement
- N_1 Metastases to homolateral axillary nodes not fixed to one another or to other structures
- N_{1a} Micrometastases less than or equal to 0.2 cm in lymph node(s)
- N_{1b} Gross metastases in lymph nodes
  - I Metastases greater than 0.2 cm but less than 2.0 cm in one to three lymph nodes
  - II Metastases greater than 0.2 cm but less than 2.0 cm in four or more lymph nodes
  - III Extension of metastases beyond the lymph node capsule (less than 2.0 cm in largest dimension)
  - IV Metastases in lymph node 2.0 cm or more in largest dimension.
- N_2 Metastases to homolateral axillary lymph nodes that are fixed to one another or to other structures
- N_3 Metastases to homolateral supraclavicular or infraclavicular lymph node(s), or edema of the arm. Edema of the arm may be caused by lymphatic obstruction, and lymph nodes may not then be palpable.

DEFINITIONS FOR SURGICAL-EVALUATIVE AND POST–SURGICAL RESECTION PATHOLOGIC CLASSIFICATION STAGE

- N_X Regional lymph nodes cannot be assessed (not removed for study or previously removed).
- N_0 No evidence of homolateral axillary lymph nodes metastasis
- N_1 Metastasis to movable homolateral axillary nodes (not fixed to one another or to other structures)
  - N_{1a} Micrometastasis less than or equal to 0.2 cm in lymph nodes(s)
  - N_{1b} Gross metastasis in lymph node(s)
    - I Metastasis greater than 0.2 cm but less than 2.0 cm in one to three lymph nodes
    - II Metastasis greater than 0.2 cm but less than 2.0 cm in four or more lymph nodes
    - III Extension of metastasis beyond the lymph node capsule (less than 2.0 cm in greatest dimension)
    - IV Metastasis to lymph node 2.0 cm or more in greatest dimension
- N_2 Metastases to homolateral axillary lymph nodes that are fixed to one another or to other structures
- N_3 Metastasis to homolateral supraclavicular or infraclavicular lymph node(s). Homolateral internal mammary nodes considered to contain growth are also included in N_3. Edema of the arm may be caused by lymphatic obstruction, and lymph nodes may not then be palpable.

Distant Metastasis (M)

All time periods

- M_x Minimum requirement for assessing the presence of distant metastasis cannot be met.
- M_0 No (known) distant metastasis
- M_1 Distant metastasis present
  Specify*____________________

*Specify sites according to the following notations:

Pulmonary—PUL	Bone marrow—MAR
Osseous—OSS	Pleura—PLE
Hepatic—HEP	Skin—SKI
Brain—BRA	Eye—EYE
Lymph nodes—LYM	Other—OTH

Table continued on following page

TABLE 4–1. 1983 TNM Classification Continued

Stage Groupings
Always indicate time of classification.
CLINICAL-DIAGNOSTIC (cTNM), SURGICAL-EVALUATIVE (sTNM), AND POST–SURGICAL RESECTION PATHOLOGIC (pTNM) STAGING

Stage	
Stage TIS	*In situ*
Stage X	Cannot stage
Stage I	T_{1ai}, N_0, M_0
	T_{1aii}, N_0, M_0
	T_{1aiii}, N_0, M_0
Stage I	T_{1bi}, N_0, M_0
	T_{1bii}, N_0, M_0
	T_{1biii}, N_0, M_0
Stage II	T_0, N_{1a}, N_{1b}, M_0
	T_{1a} or T_{1b}, N_{1a} or N_{1b}, M_0
	T_{2a} or T_{2b}, N_0, M_0
	T_{2a} or T_{2b}, N_{1a} or N_{1b}, M_0
Stage III_A	T_0, N_2, M_0
	T_{1a} or T_{1b}, N_2, M_0
	T_{2a} or T_{2b}, N_2, M_0
	T_{3a} or T_{3b}, N_0, M_0
	T_{3a} or T_{3b}, N_1, M_0
	T_{3a} or T_{3b}, N_2, M_0
Stage III_B	Any T, N_3, M_0
	Any T_4, any N, M_0
Stage IV	Any T, any N, M_1

than 5 cm, and greater than 5 cm, respectively). Stages I and II tumors both are subclassified according to whether there is fixation of the primary tumor to pectoral fascia or muscle, or both. Fixation to the chest wall, however, is Stage III disease. Fixation of axillary lymph nodes (to each other or to adjacent structures), but not their size, will change the stage, according to the TNM Classification. Only distant metastases are included in Stage IV.

In 1986, the AJCC executive committee approved another modification that simplifies the TNM classification. The modified classification, which replaces the classification adopted in 1983, is given in Table 4–2. The basic changes are as follows. (1) The breast cancer is classified according to a clinical stage or a pathologic stage. The clinical-diagnostic, surgical-evaluative, and post–surgical resection pathologic stages are no longer used. (2) Fixation of the primary tumor to pectoral fascia or muscle, or both, is no longer used. The subcategories "a" and "b," as they were used to classify the primary tumor, are therefore deleted. (3) Tumors ≤2.0 cm in diameter (T_1) are subclassified according to size (T_{1a}, 0.5 cm or smaller; T_{1b}, larger than 0.5 cm but not larger than 1.0 cm; T_{1c}, larger than 1.0 cm but not larger than 2.0 cm). (4) Guidelines have been introduced for the classification of patients with multiple, simultaneous primary tumors. (5) Tumors larger than 5.0 cm, but without locally advanced signs (e.g., edema and ulceration), are now included under Stage II (Stage II_b). (6) Inflammatory carcinoma has been designated as a separate category (T_{4d}). (7) Axillary lymph node metastases are now subclassified according to their anatomic location within the axilla (Level I, II, or III). (8) Axillary lymph node metastases are also classified according to the number of involved nodes (one to four vs. five or more). The subclassification of axillary nodes according to fixation to one another or to other structures has been deleted. (9) Metastases to supraclavicular, cervical, or contralateral internal mammary lymph nodes are now classified as distant metastases (M_1) rather than as N_3, as in the former classification. It should be emphasized that T_3, N_0 lesions are still locally advanced tumors, despite the fact that they have been placed in Stage II. Therefore, modifications of the staging system do not necessarily reflect changes in treatment recommendations.

Columbia Clinical Classification

The CCC,[3] as stated, is a clinical classification (Table 4–3). Patients are staged on the

TABLE 4–2. 1986 TNM Classification

Measuring the Size of the Primary Cancer

The tumor size is a measure of the invasive component. If there is a large *in situ* component (e.g., 4.0 cm) and a small invasive component (e.g., 0.5 cm), the tumor is coded T_{1a}.

Multiple, Simultaneous Cancers

The following guidelines should be used when staging multiple, simultaneous primary (grossly measurable, infiltrating) cancers within the same breast. These criteria do not apply to multiple microscopic lesions (since they may represent intramammary spread).

Use the largest primary cancer to stage the case.

Enter on the record that the case is one of simultaneous, multiple primary cancers in one breast. These cases should be analyzed separately.

Include in breast checklist (pathology) simultaneous, multiple, primary infiltrating cancers.

Simultaneous *bilateral* breast cancers: Each should be staged independently.

Inflammatory Carcinoma

Inflammatory carcinoma of the breast is characterized by diffuse, brawny induration of the skin, with an erysipeloid edge, usually with no underlying palpable mass. This clinical presentation is due to tumor embolization of dermal lymphatics. The tumor of inflammatory carcinoma is coded T_{4d}.

Primary Tumor (T)

The size of the intact tumor should be measured before any tissue is removed for special studies, such as estrogen-binding studies.

T_x The primary tumor cannot be assessed
T_o No evidence of primary tumor
TIS Carcinoma *in situ*: intraductal carcinoma, lobular carcinoma *in situ*, or Paget's disease of the nipple with no tumor. Paget's disease associated with a tumor is classified according to the size of the tumor.
T_1 Tumor is 2.0 cm or smaller in greatest dimension.
- T_{1a} 0.5 cm or smaller
- T_{1b} Larger than 0.5 cm but not larger than 1.0 cm
- T_{1c} Larger than 1.0 cm but not larger than 2.0 cm

T_2 Tumor is larger than 2.0 cm but not larger than 5.0 cm in greatest dimension.
T_3 Tumor is larger than 5.0 cm in greatest dimension.
T_4 Tumor of any size with direct extension to chest wall or skin. (Chest wall includes ribs, intercostal muscles, and serratus anterior muscle, but not pectoral muscle).
T_{4a} Extension to chest wall
T_{4b} Edema (including peau d'orange), ulceration of the skin of the breast, or satellite skin nodules confined to the same breast.
T_{4c} Both a and b, above.
T_{4d}* Inflammatory carcinoma (as defined in introductory comments).

Note: Dimpling of the skin, nipple retraction, or other skin changes, except those in T_4, may occur in T_1, T_2, and T_3 without affecting the classification.

Regional Lymph Node Stations (N)

Axillary (ipsilateral) and interpectoral (Rotter's nodes): lymph nodes along the axillary vein and its tributaries, which may be divided into the following levels:

Level I (low axilla): lymph nodes located lateral to the lateral border of the pectoralis major muscle.

Level II (mid axilla): lymph nodes located between the medial and lateral borders of the pectoralis minor muscle and the interpectoral (Rotter's) lymph nodes.

Level III (apical axilla): lymph nodes medial to the medial margin of the pectoralis minor, including those designated as the subclavicular, infraclavicular, or apical lymph nodes.

Intramammary lymph nodes are coded as axillary lymph nodes

Internal mammary (ipsilateral): lymph nodes located in the intercostal spaces along the edge of the sternum in the endothoracic fascia.

All other lymph node metastases are coded as distant metastases (M_1), including supraclavicular, cervical, or contralateral internal mammary lymph nodes.

N—REGIONAL LYMPH NODES

N_x The regional lymph nodes cannot be assessed (e.g., clinical staging: previously removed; pathologic staging: previously removed, or not removed for pathologic study).
N_0 No regional lymph node metastases
N_1 Metastases in four or fewer ipsilateral axillary lymph nodes, none larger than 3.0 cm in greatest dimension.
- N_{1a} Only micrometastases (none larger than 0.2 cm)
- N_{1b} Metastases in 1–3 axillary lymph nodes, any one larger than 0.2 cm, but none larger than 3.0 cm

N_2 Metastases in four or more ipsilateral axillary lymph nodes, and/or in any axillary lymph node larger than 3.0 cm, or in any ipsilateral internal mammary lymph node(s)
N_{2a} Metastasis in five or more axillary lymph nodes, or any ipsilateral axillary metastasis larger than 3.0 cm
N_{2b} Metastasis in any ipsilateral internal mammary lymph node(s)

*If the skin biopsy is negative and there is no localized, measurable primary cancer, the T category is pT_x when pathologically staging a clinical inflammatory carcinoma, cT_{4d}.

Table continued on following page

TABLE 4–2. 1986 TNM Classification Continued

Distant Metastasis (M)

M_x	Distant metastasis cannot be assessed
M_0	No distant metastasis
M_1	Distant metastasis

Clinical Staging

Clinical staging includes the following: physical examination, including careful inspection and palpation of the skin, the mammary glands, and the lymph nodes (axillary, supraclavicular and cervical). Pathologic examination of the breast or other tissues to establish the diagnosis of breast cancer. The extent of tissues examined pathologically for clinical staging is less than that required for pathologic staging (see Pathologic Staging below). Appropriate operative findings are elements of clinical staging, including size and chest wall invasion of the primary cancer and the presence or absence of regional or distant metastasis.

Pathologic Staging

Pathologic staging includes the following:

- All data used for clinical staging
- Surgical resection and pathologic examination of the primary cancer, including not less than excision of the primary carcinoma with no tumor in any margin of resection by *gross* pathologic examination. A case can be included in the pathologic stage if there is only microscopic, but not gross, involvement in a margin. If there is tumor in the margin of resection by gross examination, it is coded T_x.
- Resection of at least 5 ipsilateral axillary lymph nodes.

Stage Groupings

Stage 0		TIS	N_0	M_0
Stage I		T_1	N_0	M_0
Stage II				
	II_a	T_0	N_1	M_0
		T_1	N_1†	M_0
		T_2	N_0	M_0
	II_b	T_2	N_1	M_0
		T_3	N_0	M_0
Stage III				
	III_a	T_3	N_1	M_0
		T_1,T_2,T_3	N_2	M_0
	III_b	T_4	Any N	M_0
Stage IV		Any T	Any N	M_1

†The prognosis of patients with N_{1a} is similar to that of patients with N_0.

basis of clinical evaluation, including x-rays and other imaging studies, but excluding pathologic information from biopsies, lymph node dissections, or other procedures. When pathologic information becomes available, it does not change the original stage.

The CCC includes four stages, A, B, C, and D. Stages A and B were considered by Haagensen (the originator of the CCC) and by others to be operable breast cancer. Stages C and D were seen as inoperable by virtue of locally advanced characterisics or distant metastatic disease, or both. Haagensen's clarification of the grave signs of breast cancer represented a major contribution to the understanding and treatment of this malignancy. High local recurrence and poor survival rates are associated with treatment by radical surgery alone of patients with any grave sign in Stage C or with more advanced local characteristics in Stage D (see Chapter 5, Table 5–8).

The CCC does not distinguish tumors according to size. Tumors of any size may therefore be staged A or B (depending upon clinical axillary nodal status) if they are not associated with any grave sign. The size of axillary lymph nodes is, however, important. Patients with clinically palpable axillary nodes have Stage A or B tumors, depending upon whether the nodes are less than or greater than 2.5 cm, respectively. There is no subclassification for involvement of pectoral fascia or muscle, only for the chest wall (ribs, intercostal muscles, or serratus anterior muscle). The advantage of the CCC lies in the simplicity with which a patient can be staged. The failure to include all information about the patient, however, has significantly limited its use.

Manchester Classification

The Manchester system[4] was introduced in 1940 by the Holt Radium Institute in Man-

TABLE 4–3. Columbia Clinical Classification

Stage A	No skin edema, ulceration, or solid fixation of tumor to chest wall. Axillary nodes not clinically involved
Stage B	No skin edema, ulceration, or solid fixation of tumor to chest wall. Clinically involved nodes, but less than 2.5 cm in transverse diameter and not fixed to overlying skin or deeper structures of axilla
Stage C	Any one of five grave signs of advanced breast cancer: Edema of skin of limited extent (involving less than one third of the skin over the breast) Skin ulceration Solid fixation of tumor to chest wall Massive involvement of axillary lymph nodes (measuring 2.5 cm or more in transverse diameter) Fixation of the axillary nodes to overlying skin or deeper structures of the axilla
Stage D	All other patients with advanced breast cancer, including: A combination of any two or more of the five grave signs listed under Stage C Extensive edema of the skin (involving more than one third of the skin over the breast) Satellite skin nodules The inflammatory type of carcinoma Clinically involved supraclavicular lymph nodes Internal mammary metastases, as evidenced by a parasternal tumor Edema of the arm Distant metastases

chester, England (Table 4–4). This classification is similar to the CCC in that breast cancer patients are staged solely on the basis of clinical evaluation. Pathologic information is not included, nor does this information change the stage of the patient. Patients are placed in one of four stages (Stage I, II, III, or IV), based on the extent of local involvement by the primary tumor, the presence and mobility of the axillary lymph nodes, and the presence of distant metastases.

It can be seen that tumor size is not included in the classification. The absence or presence of palpable, nonfixed axillary nodes is the principle criterion for distinguishing Stage I cancer from Stage II. Stage IV represents patients with distant metastases. The criteria for assigning a stage to the patient with locally advanced breast cancer are not well defined. Skin involvement may be present, but if it is limited, the patient may still be considered to have Stage I disease. No classification is specified for patients with skin edema, arm edema, a parasternal mass, or inflammatory carcinoma. In contrast with the TNM Classification, fixation to pectoral fascia or muscle represents Stage III disease. Because of the limitations of this classification, the Manchester system is infrequently used today.

HISTORY AND PHYSICAL EXAMINATION

The evaluation of any patient suspected of having breast cancer must begin with a complete history and physical examination. The history should determine the chronology and characteristics of the patient's breast symptoms and the presence or absence of any factors known to increase the risk of breast cancer. The presence of risk factors not only

TABLE 4–4. Manchester Classification

Stage I	The growth is confined to the breast. Involvement of the skin directly over and in continuity with the tumor does not affect staging, provided the area involved is small in relation to the size of the breast.
Stage II	The growth is confined to the breast, but there are palpable, mobile lymph nodes in the axilla.
Stage III	The growth extends beyond the corpus mammae. Signs: The skin is invaded or fixed over an area that is large in relation to the size of the breast or is ulcerated. The tumor is fixed to the underlying muscle or fascia. Axillary glands may or may not be palpable, but if glands are present, they must be mobile.
Stage IV	The growth has extended beyond the breast area, as shown by: Fixation or matting of the axillary nodes Complete fixation of tumor to chest wall Secondary lymph nodes in supraclavicular region Secondary deposits in skin wide of tumor Secondary deposits in the opposite breast Distant metastases

may increase the probability that a specific breast symptom represents a malignancy but also emphasizes the importance of examining the remaining breast tissue and the contralateral breast. The review of risk factors should be systematic and should include familial, endocrine, and reproductive factors, pathologic changes noted on previous biopsies, prior radiation exposure, and associated malignancies (e.g., uterine or ovarian). Each of these factors is discussed in detail in Chapter 1. Certain risk factors, however, may influence the selection of treatment of malignancies. Previous radiation treatment or a prior history of lobular carcinoma *in situ* would indicate surgery as the primary treatment modality for Stage I or II breast cancer. Should the patient's symptoms prove to represent benign disease, the presence of certain risk factors will influence the nature and frequency of follow-up examinations.

All breast symptoms should be defined in terms of chronology, location, and periodicity. The increased awareness of breast cancer among women and the emphasis on self-examination should allow a reliable history of a breast mass or breast changes to be obtained in most cases. The signs and symptoms of breast cancer and their frequency are listed in Table 4–5. The history should begin with the date of onset of the symptom; whether it is persistent, intermittent or progressive; and whether there have been prior episodes of similar symptoms. The appearance of a painless palpable mass is the most common presenting symptom in women with breast cancer. The persistence of any breast mass should increase concern. Many studies have been conducted to determine the doubling time of breast cancer. These studies have found, however, a wide range in the time interval—from a few days to more thân a year—that may be required for a tumor to double in size.[8] Therefore, because this interval may be long, the absence of a noticeable change in the size of a mass does not argue against its malignancy. Similarly, because the practice of self-examination is not universal, the recent detection of a large breast mass does not imply that it is benign. Approximately 50 to 60 per cent of women who present with breast cancer have tumors larger than 2 cm in diameter.[9]

Any tenderness or skin change associated with the mass should be noted. These may represent an infectious etiology, especially in the post-partum period; however, inflammatory carcinoma needs to be considered. Pain is not a common symptom of breast cancer. In Haagensen's and Donegan's series of patients with breast cancer, only 3.1 percent of patients had pain as their primary symptoms.[6, 10] This is not to suggest, however, that the presence of breast pain should be disregarded. The evaluation of patients with breast pain as their only symptom may result in the detection of occult cancers. Preece and colleagues found that, among 17 patients with occult malignancy, pain was the single most common symptom leading to investigation and diagnosis.[11] Therefore, while the vast majority of women who have pain as their only symptom will have benign disease, this symptom should always be evaluated and defined. Pain is more often present with a locally advanced tumor and is usually focal, constant, and nonradiating and is not related to the menstrual period. Pain from fibrocystic disease, on the other hand, is usually bilateral and diffuse, radiates to the axilla, and is more prominent at the time of the menstrual period.

Any nipple discharge should be characterized according to its frequency, whether it is unilateral or bilateral, and whether it is bloody. This will be discussed in detail later;

TABLE 4–5. Frequency of Signs and Symptoms of Breast Cancer

Sign or Symptom	*Frequency (%)*
Palpable mass	73.5
Pain in breast	6.1
Nipple discharge	4.4
Nipple retraction	2.9
Skin dimpling	2.8
Nipple erosion	1.9
Axillary tumor	1.6
Skin edema	1.3
Skin erythema	1.2
Breast enlarged	1.1
Tenderness on pressure over breast	0.7
Nipple itching	0.6
Breast abscess	0.6
Generalized hardness of breast	0.4
Skin ulceration	0.3
Breast shrunken	0.2
Skin ecchymoses	0.2
Swelling of arm	0.2
Total	100.0

Adapted from Donegan WL: Diagnosis. *In:* Donegan WL, Spratt JS (eds.): Cancer of the Breast, 2nd ed. Philadelphia: W.B. Saunders Co., 1979, p. 50; and Haagensen CD: Diseases of the Breast, 2nd ed. Philadelphia: W.B. Saunders Co., 1971, p. 467.

however, any association with other breast abnormalities should be noted, as this may help in finding the cause of the discharge. Finally, information from previous evaluations should be carefully reviewed, including mamograms, previous attempts at aspiration, cytologies from aspirations or secretions, biopsy material, and the response to any treatment regimens. In this manner, the diagnosis of breast changes can be facilitated and unnecessary repetition of procedures avoided.

The physical examination will define the location and extent of the breast changes and whether they are associated with any abnormalities in regional tissues or distant sites. The entire breast and adjacent lymph node–bearing areas should be examined for all breast complaints. The adage "Proceed from the known to the unknown" is just as appropriate for breast as for other physical examinations. Accordingly, the area of concern should be examined after adjacent breast tissue and the contralateral breast have been examined. Breast tissue extends from the second or third rib superiorly to the sixth or seventh costal margin inferiorly and from the lateral border of the sternum to beyond the anterior axillary fold. Both breasts should be systematically inspected and palpated in the supine and sitting positions (Figs. 4–1 and 4–2). Certain maneuvers, discussed later, may be used to accentuate changes noted in these two positions. Any asymmetry, skin edema, erythema, and retraction or previous biopsy scars should be noted as well as any nipple retraction or excoriation. Skin retraction represents focal shortening of Cooper's ligaments by a parenchymal process. Skin retraction may become evident when the patient is placed in the sitting position with her arms raised (Fig. 4–3). Any indentation in the skin should be noted. Skin retraction signs may also be accentuated by retraction of the pectoral muscles (Fig. 4–4). The patient, in the sitting position, places her hands on her hips and presses inward. This maneuver will also accentuate breast changes associated with fixation of a mass to pectoral fascia or muscle.

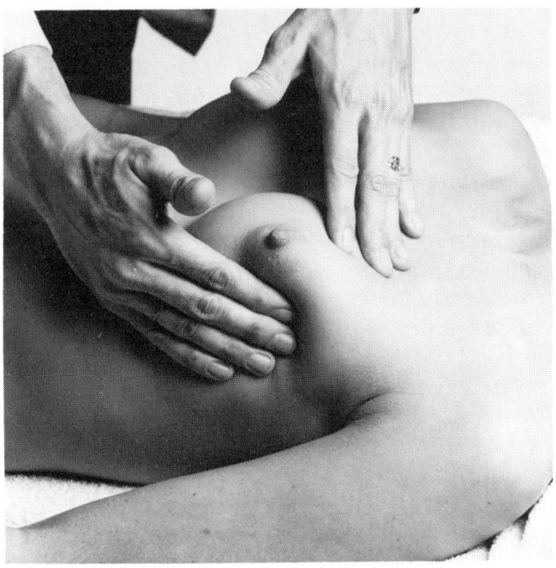

FIGURE 4–1. Examination of the patient in the supine position. The skin and nipple should be inspected first to detect any abnormalities. All quadrants of the breast should be systematically palpated. Palpation of a mass against the chest wall in the supine position will help to define its size and consistency.

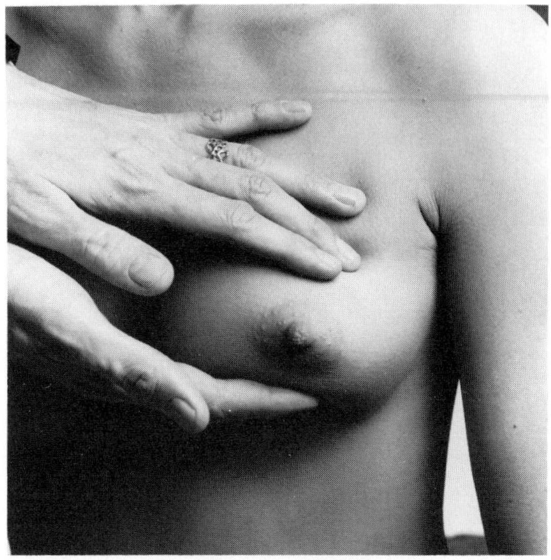

FIGURE 4–2. Examination of the patient in the sitting position. Inspection may reveal asymmetry, skin or nipple retraction, venous dilatation, inflammatory changes of the skin, or prominence of a mass in the upper quadrants. This position may also facilitate palpation of superficial masses.

Nipple retraction may represent focal involvement of the mammary ducts by a malignancy (the history will exclude congenital nipple retraction or retraction secondary to previous biopsies). Nipple retraction may be accentuated by examining the patient in the sitting position and having her bend forward (Fig. 4–5).[12] Dependency of the breasts will increase the prominence of the nipple retraction. Subtle changes in the nipple, in addition to retraction, may be a manifestation of ma-

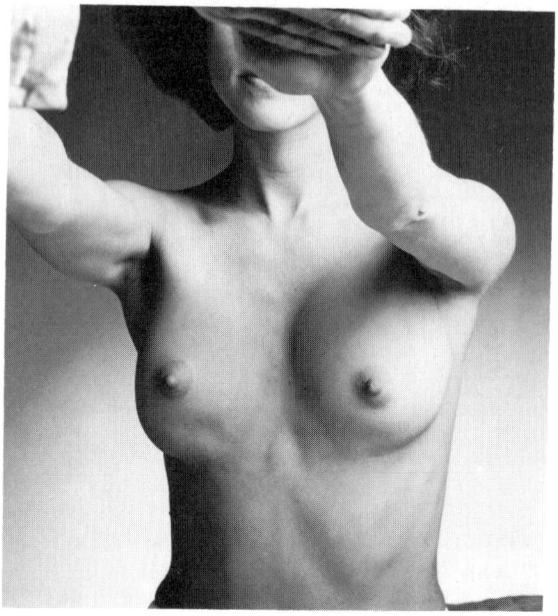

FIGURE 4–3. Examination of the patient with arms raised. This maneuver will accentuate skin retraction caused by a mass.

lignancy (Paget's disease). These changes may include eczema, scaling, crust formation, erosion, ulceration, and a bloody nipple discharge. A palpable tumor in the breast may be present in 25 to 44 percent of such cases.[13–15] These changes are thought to rep-

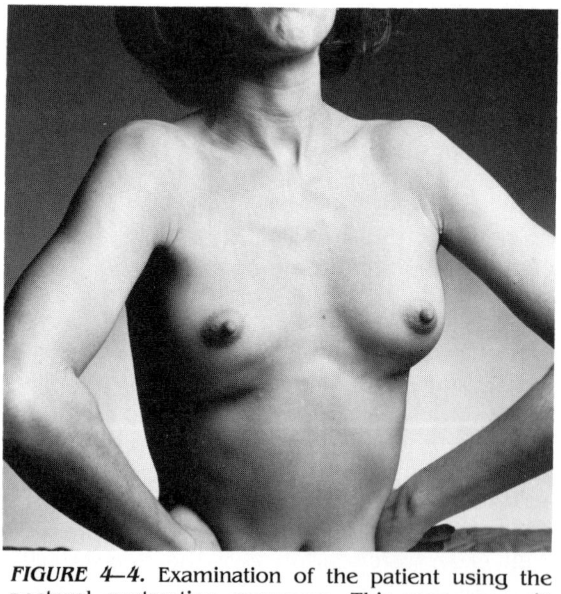

FIGURE 4–4. Examination of the patient using the pectoral contraction maneuver. This maneuver will accentuate skin dimpling, especially by those masses that involve the pectoralis fascia or muscle.

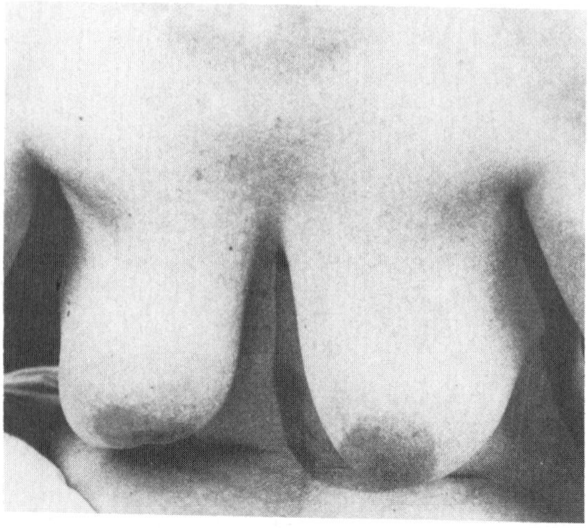

FIGURE 4–5. Examination of the patient in the forward-bending position. This position accentuates nipple retraction caused by a carcinoma in the right breast. (From Haagensen CD: Diseases of the Breast, 3rd ed. Philadelphia: W. B. Saunders Co., 1986.)

resent secondary extension of cancer cells from the underlying ductal cancer to the epidermis by way of the lactiferous ducts.[16] Unfortunately, in many women with these nipple changes, the possibility of breast carcinoma is not considered, and the changes are treated wih topical applicants. The time course of benign dermatitis of the nipple and areola, however, is frequently much more rapid than that for Paget's disease.[13] Within a few weeks, benign dermatitis may extend to involve a large portion of the areola. Paget's carcinoma evolves slowly, and many months may be required for Paget's erosion to extend over as wide an area. Haagensen considered all erosions and dermatitis-like lesions that involved only the nipple to be carcinomatous.[13] Lesions that involve the areola and the nipple epithelium and, sometimes, the skin of the breast are usually carcinomatous but occasionally are due to dermatitis. Erosions of the areola or the skin of the adjacent breast that leave the nipple uninvolved are not Paget's disease. Carcinoma should therefore be considered in the differential diagnosis of any eczematoid lesion of the nipple. Suspicious lesions that occur in the absence of palpable abnormalities of the breast should be biopsied with a deep wedge of the nipple and the underlying major ducts. Because the majority of women with Paget's disease who do not have palpable abnormalities of the breast will have noninfiltrating intraductal carcinoma, permanent rather than frozen section diagnosis of the biopsy specimen should be performed. Paget's disease of the breast is discussed further in Chapter 14.

The characteristics of any palpable breast mass should be determined and accurately recorded. As noted in the discussion of the staging classification, the size and mobility of the mass and whether it is associated with skin ulceration, inflammation, or satellite nodules are major determinants for tumor (T) classification. Masses in the lateral aspects of the breast may be more easily delineated by placing the patient in the opposite-side-down position. This will allow palpation of the lesion against the chest wall and will minimize the amount of intervening breast tissue. The size, contour, consistency, and mobility of the mass as well as any associated skin changes should be noted. The initial examination preceding any invasive studies is clearly the best time to evaluate any breast changes. Such timing of evaluation will ensure accurate clinical staging. Several points regarding the characteristics of a mass should be emphasized.

1. Fixation of the mass to pectoralis fascia or muscle (which does not alter the stage according to the TNM Classification) should be distinguished from fixation to the chest wall (ribs, intercostal muscles, or serratus anterior muscle). Thus, a 2 cm tumor with fixation to only pectoral fascia is still a Stage II tumor, whereas a tumor with fixation to the chest wall is Stage III_b. This distinction must be made on clinical grounds and can be noted by assessing the relative mobility of the lesion. Masses that are fixed to the chest wall are completely immobile, in which case, as has often been stated, "the patient will move with the mass." Masses involving only the pectoral fascia have some relative mobility, but their movement is restricted with maneuvers that contract the pectoralis major muscle (see earlier). Examination of the patient in the forward-bending position will also identify fixation of the mass by revealing asymmetry in the dependency of the breasts.

2. The tumor should be accurately measured in both dimensions with a ruler. The distinction between a 4 cm and a 6 cm mass is an important one and can have a major influence on treatment options. Measurements should be done at the time of presentation. It may be impossible to accurately determine the dimensions of the mass if one waits until after a percutaneous or incisional biopsy is performed.

3. The skin changes associated with inflammatory carcinoma may be subtle and are not always immediately adjacent to the mass. Any skin changes can be easily biopsied with a 3 to 4 mm skin punch, which will provide adequate tissue for the determination of the presence of tumor in the subdermal lymphatics.

Breast cancer frequently metastasizes to regional lymph nodes, including axillary, internal mammary, and supraclavicular areas. Approximately 20 percent of patients with T_1 lesions and 40 to 50 percent of patients with T_2 lesions will have metastases to axillary lymph nodes at presentation (see Chapter 5, Table 5–29).[17, 18] Examination of these areas is important for staging purposes and for detecting evidence of locally advanced disease. The axilla is best examined with the patient in the sitting position and the arm relaxed (Fig. 4–6).[19] The patient's arm is flexed at the elbow and supported by the physician, allowing optimum relaxation of the axillary tissue and placing the lower axillary contents in a dependent position. The presence of any palpable lymph nodes, their size, and whether they are thought to be matted or fixed should be noted. While the presence of axillary metastases represents, at a minimum, Stage II disease, lymph nodes that are fixed or matted or larger than 3.0 cm constitute locally advanced (Stage III_a) disease. Contralateral axillary metastases represent Stage IV disease. The distribution of axillary metastases and the role of axillary lymph node analysis in the treatment of early stage breast cancer are discussed in Chapter 5, in the section on axillary lymph node dissection.

Metastases to the internal mammary lymph nodes, generally less common than axillary metastases, have an incidence range from 2 to 5 percent for outer quadrant lesions with negative axillary nodes to 43 to 59 percent for inner quadrant lesions with axillary metastases (see Chapter 5, Table 5–11). The internal mammary nodes are protected by the pectoralis major muscle, fascia, and intercostal tissues, and thus are not accessible to physical examination. Rarely, they may enlarge to the point that a parasternal mass is evident; in this case, they are most often present in the second or third intercostal space. This finding is significant because it

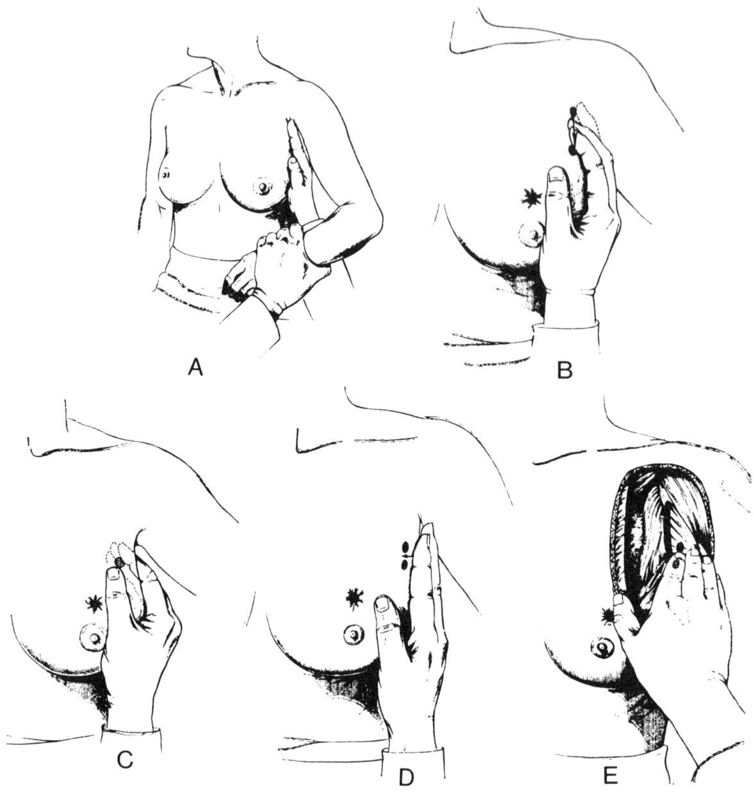

FIGURE 4–6. Examination of the axilla. *A,* The patient is examined in the sitting position, with the arm slightly abducted and supported by the examiner. This will place the axillary contents in a dependent position. *B,* Examination begins in the superior portion of the axilla and proceeds inferiorly, allowing retraction of superiorly placed lymph nodes. Axillary lymph nodes can be further defined by palpation against the posterior aspect of the pectoralis major muscle (*C*), the lateral chest wall (*D*), or the subscapularis muscle (*E*). (From Jessiman AG: The breast. *In*: Warren R (ed.): Surgery. Philadelphia: W. B. Saunders Co., 1963.)

represents inoperable (Stage III_a) breast cancer. Metastases to supraclavicular lymph nodes also occur with breast cancer, and their incidence is related to the stage of the disease and the presence or absence of axillary and internal mammary lymph node metastases (see the discussion on superradical mastectomy, in Chapter 5). The finding, at presentation, of clinically palpable supraclavicular lymph node metastases is uncommon; however, their presence represents advanced disease (Stage IV). The supraclavicular regions are best examined with the patient in the sitting position. Each supraclavicular region is examined with the physician first in front of, then in back of, the patient.

The history and physical examination should also include an evaluation for distant metastatic disease. Approximately 10 percent of patients with breast cancer will have distant metastases at presentation.[9] The most common sites for metastases from breast cancer are, in order of decreasing frequency, lung, bone, liver, and the adrenal gland.[20] Signs or symptoms of distant metastases noted on history and physical examination will serve as indicators for specific imaging studies (including x-rays and radionuclide scans) and will identify areas for which local treatment may be helpul. Accordingly, any evidence of bone pain or tenderness (especially in the pelvis, spine, ribs, or long bones), abdominal pain, hepatic enlargement, jaundice, or pruritus should be documented as an indication for further staging procedures. The history, with its notation of any medical problems of the patient, will also facilitate interpretation of any abnormalities noted on these studies.

In summary, the diagnosis of breast cancer requires sensitivity to a variety of changes in the breast tissue. The minority of breast cancer presents as a locally advanced lesion. Subtle signs or symptoms may be the only manifestation of malignancy. Haagensen has succinctly summarized the most common reasons for missed diagnoses of breast cancer[21]; the authors have added two other common errors. These are listed in Table 4–6. All of these errors involve failure to consider carcinoma in the differential diagnosis of a breast problem, failure to apply the basic principles of the history and physical examination, or failure to use simple methods of

TABLE 4–6. Diagnostic Errors in the Evaluation of Breast Complaints

Failure to examine a breast containing an obvious tumor while treating the patient for an unrelated disease
Failure of the physician, in palpating the breast, to feel the tumor that the patient had discovered and for which she sought medical attention
Mistaking a carcinomatous tumor of the breast for a breast infection
Wrongly diagnosing a carcinomatous tumor of the breast as a benign lesion, and failing to recommend biopsy or excision
Disregarding a history of sharp pain in the breast
Disregarding a definite retraction sign
Failure to determine the cause of a nipple discharge
Relying upon negative aspiration biopsy
Relying upon mammography rather than palpation
Disregarding an eczematoid nipple eruption
Failing to perform a biopsy on a palpable mass because a mammogram is considered to be normal

Modified from Haagensen CD, Bodian C, Haagensen DE: Breast Carcinoma: Risk and Detection. Philadelphia: W.B. Saunders Co., 1981.

diagnosis. The importance of appreciating these common errors cannot be overemphasized. Avoiding a needless delay in diagnosis is one of the best means for improving survival in breast cancer.

EVALUATION OF THE PALPABLE BREAST MASS

The appearance of a mass in the breast signifies pathologic changes in the breast tissue that should be carefully evaluated. The etiology of these changes will vary with the age of the patient. In this chapter, the discussion of breast masses will be concerned with those that occur in women over the age of 20. Breast carcinoma in adolescents is extremely rare. Several excellent reviews discuss the evaluation and management of breast lesions in children and adolescents.[22–25] The reader should consult these reviews for further information about breast disorders in this age group.

A variety of histologic changes may be responsible for a breast mass. Fibrocystic disease, carcinoma, and fibroadenoma are responsible for the vast majority of palpable lesions. The frequency with which any given histologic entity is responsible for a breast mass will vary with age, with some overlap between the different age groups (Fig. 4–7).[26] Fibroadenoma is the most common cause of breast masses in the younger age group (15 to 35 years). Fibrocystic disease predominates in the 35 to 50 year group. Carcinoma is the most common cause in women aged 50 years and older. The majority of palpable breast masses are found to be benign on histologic examination. Fibrocystic disease is the most common cause of breast masses overall, accounting for, on the average, 45 percent (range 29 to 63 percent) of all breast masses.[27–31] While masses representing fibroadenoma or carcinoma are almost exclusively solid tumors (see discussion of cystic carcinoma, later), masses associated with fibrocystic disease are predominantly cystic, either microcystic or macrocystic. Fibrocystic disease, unfortunately, has been used to designate a variety of histologic patterns, including macrocysts, microcysts, adenosis, apocrine change, fibrosis, fibroadenomas, and ductal hyperplasia.[32] Fibrosis or adenosis

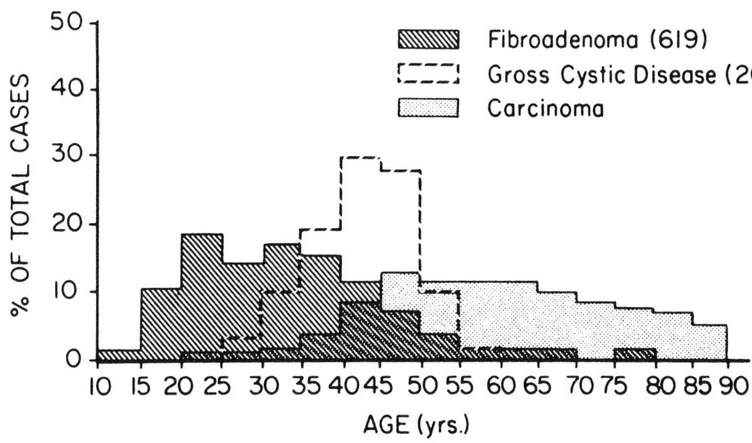

FIGURE 4–7. The three most common breast tumors and their distribution according to age. Each tumor may occur over a wide age range. There is overlap in incidence between the three tumor types; however, fibroadenoma predominates in the 20- to 35-age group, fibrocystic disease in the 35–50 age group, and carcinoma predominates in women over 50 years of age. (From Donegan WL: Diagnosis. *In*: Donegan WL, Spratt JS (eds.): Cancer of the Breast, 2nd ed. Philadelphia: W. B. Saunders Co., 1979.)

TABLE 4–7. Histologic Types of Breast Cancer

Histologic Type	Frequency (%)
Infiltrating ductal carcinoma	74.0
Lobular invasive carcinoma	6.0
Intraductal carcinoma	3.5
Lobular carcinoma *in situ*	3.0
Medullary carcinoma	2.7
Cystosarcoma	2.5
Paget's disease	2.3
Mucinous carcinoma	2.0
Papillary carcinoma	1.5
Inflammatory carcinoma	1.5
Sarcomas	1.0
Miscellaneous	2.0
Total	100.0

Source: Hermann RE, Esselstyn CB, Crile G, Jr., et al.: Results of conservative operations for breast cancer. Arch Surg 120:746, 1985; and Haagensen CD: Diseases of the Breast, 2nd ed. Philadelphia: W.B. Saunders Co., 1971.

may be a prominent component of fibrocystic masses, and for this reason, they may present as solid tumors. Other benign histologic entities that form palpable masses include duct ectasia, fat necrosis, infections, multiple papilloma, nonepithelial neoplasms (e.g., lipoma and leiomyoma), gynecomastia, and galactocele.

The frequency with which a biopsied mass represents a carcinoma will vary with the age of the patient and the biopsy criteria used by the surgeon. The incidence of carcinoma among three series ranged from 21 to 42 percent.[33–35] The majority of malignant lesions are of the invasive ductal type (Table 4–7; see also Chapter 3). Invasive lobular and medullary carcinomas are next in frequency, followed by a variety of other histologic entities. Noninvasive lesions are uncommon; however, their incidence is increasing as a result of the emphasis on screening mammography and more effective biopsy methods for occult lesions.[37] While most noninvasive lesions are occult, they may, on occasion, present as a palpable mass. Conversely, the absence of a palpable mass does not exclude the possibility of invasive carcinoma (see the section on evaluation of occult abnormalities detected by mammography). Finally, breast malignancies are almost always of breast origin. Chest wall sarcomas extending into breast tissue are uncommon, and metastasis to the breast from other (nonbreast) malignancies is rare.

Noninvasive Studies

While the history and physical examination will provide information about the nature of the breast mass, noninvasive studies are useful for further defining the mass and the remaining breast tissue. These studies include mammography, ultrasonography, thermography, and computerized tomography. The decision to obtain these studies and the determination of the most useful study depend on the character of the mass, the age of the patient, and the presence or absence of associated risk factors. Optimum information from these studies is obtained when they are performed prior to invasive procedures. Reactive changes from a biopsy may distort the breast architecture and make the delineation and interpretation of subtle changes much more difficult. Sickles and associates[38] reviewed mammograms of 58 patients with solid masses who recently had a needle aspiration of their mass. In 17 cases, the mass was considered suspicious on mammography but found to be benign histologically. All of these false-positive interpretations occurred when aspiration preceded mammography by less than two weeks; no such diagnostic error occurred when mammography was delayed for two weeks or more after aspiration.

Breast Mammography

Mammography (either conventional plain films or xeroradiography) has been the most widely used noninvasive procedure and the one in which the greatest experience has been gained. The use of mammography for screening and detection is discussed in Chapter 2. Later in the present chapter, the management of occult mammographic lesions is discussed. The present section reviews the use of mammograms for evaluation of abnormalities found on physical examination.

Table 4–8[39] summarizes breast lesion abnormalities suggestive of malignancy that are detected by mammography, as well as the reliability of these findings. The major characteristics are illustrated in Figure 4–8. The overall false-negative rate for mammography of palpable masses ranges from 3.3 to 31.5 percent (average 15.7 percent), and the false-positive rate ranges from 0.6 to 15.7 percent (average 9.3 percent).[40–47] The incidence of a

TABLE 4–8. Predictive Value of Certain Mammographic Signs for Identifying Breast Cancer in the Presence of a Positive Clinical Examination

Mammographic Sign	*Number of Cancers Found by This Sign Alone*	*Rate of False-Positive Findings (%)*	*Predictive Value of This Sign Alone**
Punctate calcification	8	38	5.16
Mass, probably malignant	13	30	10.65
Mass, definitely malignant	7	1	100.0
Mass, benign	6	79	1.86
Mass, questionable	4	25	3.88
Vein dilatation	1	2	9.00
Skin thickening	0	0	0.0
Nipple retraction	2	5	9.09
Duct dilatation	1	22	1.00

*Predictive value represents percentage of cases in which any single sign is accurate in diagnosing breast cancer.
Source: Moskowitz M: Minimal breast cancer redux. Radiol Clin North Am 21:93, 1983.

false-negative or false-positive diagnosis varies according to the criteria used, the quality and technique of the films, the age of the patient, and the familiarity of the radiologist with mammographic studies. The increased density of breast tissue in younger women may compromise interpretation of the films, especially the identification of a small mass within glandular tissue.[47] The reliability of mammography for detecting carcinoma in women under 45 years of age is approximately 60 percent, compared with an accuracy rate of 90 percent in women over 60.[47] While calcifications may be an important sign of malignancy, they are more frequently associated with benign disease. Benign lesions that have been shown to contain calcifications include sclerosing adenosis, fibrocystic disease, papillomatosis, ductal and lobular hyperplasia, galactoceles, and fibroadenomas.[47, 48] In general, the area of the individual clusters and the number of calcifications tend to be greater and the clusters tend to be less dense in carcinomas than in benign lesions. Colbassani and colleagues[48] noted that in the clusters containing more than 30 calcifications, the incidence of malignancy was 80 percent, whereas in a cluster of less than nine calcifications, no carcinoma was detected. There was no difference in the size of the calcifications between benign and malignant disease. The incidence of calcifications in a palpable mass, however, was lower than that in occult cancers.[49] The selection of mammography vesus xeroradiography for breast evaluation is one of preference. Wolfe prefers xeroradiography,[50] believing that it provides greater resolution, which permits identification of smaller structures, especially tumor calcifications. All structures within the breast are recorded in good detail on one image, in contrast with conventional film mammography, in which proper exposure of the subaerolar area precludes visualization of the deeper structures. Finally, Wolfe notes that xeroradiograms are more easily interpreted without special means of viewing.[45] The authors also prefer xeroradiograms for patients with dense breasts, in the study of microcalcifications, for evaluation of lesions in the

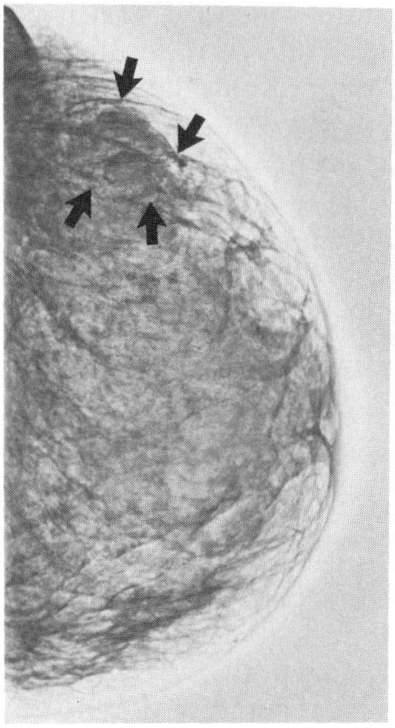

FIGURE 4–8. Xeromammogram demonstrating a malignancy in the upper outer quadrant of the right breast. There is asymmetry of the breast when compared with xeromammograms of the opposite breast. The mass has irregular, spiculated borders, contains suspicious calcifications, and is associated with venous dilatation and retraction of the skin.

posterior aspect or the periphery of the breast, and for performing specimen radiograms. Because any previous films may be helpful for comparison, the same technique (mammography or xeroradiography) should be used consistently, when possible.

Mammography, in addition to defining a palpable mass, may detect occult lesions elsewhere in the same breast or in the opposite breast. This is a further advantage of obtaining mammograms before the biopsy of a mass is performed. If another occult lesion is found it can be biopsied at the same time as the palpable mass, eliminating the need for two separate surgical procedures, as might be the case if the occult lesion were found on x-rays obtained only after biopsy of the palpable lesion. The authors routinely obtain a mammogram in all women over the age of 30 with a solid mass, to provide information both about the malignant characteristics of the mass and about the remaining tissue in the affected and the contralateral breasts. For women in the 20 to 30 year age group with a solid mass the authors obtain mammograms preoperatively if the patient is at high risk for breast cancer or if there is a strong suspicion of malignancy. Otherwise, a mammogram is obtained postoperatively if the mass is malignant. For cystic lesions in this age group, ultrasonography is useful in defining the mass and confirming complete resolution after aspiration (see later).

A mammogram obtained to evaluate a mass should be done to support, not to exclude, the diagnosis of malignancy. A negative mammogram should never be a substitute for cytologic or histologic evaluation of a palpable mass and should never prevent the adequate evaluation of a mass seen as suspicious on physical examination. This is one of the most common therapeutic errors in the management of breast masses, and one of the most disastrous.

TABLE 4–9. Ultrasound Mammography Descriptive Criteria of Breast Cancer

Descriptive Criteria	*Percentage of Breast Cancers with This Characteristic (%)*
SHAPE	
Round	27.0
Oval	15.0
Tubular	30.0
Lobulated	27.0
CONTOUR	
Smooth	27.0
Irregular	72.0
INTERNAL ECHOES	
Weak	72.0
Intermediate	12.0
Strong	4.0
None	10.0
BOUNDARY ECHOES	
Anterior	
Strong	27.0
Intermediate	56.0
Weak	16.0
Posterior	
Strong	4.0
Intermediate	6.0
Weak	35.0
Absent	55.0
ATTENUATION EFFECTS	
Great	60.0
Intermediate	30.0
Minimal	10.0

Source: Cole-Beuglet C, Soriano RZ, Kurtz AB, et al.: Ultrasound Analysis of 104 breast carcinomas classified according to histopathologic type. Radiology 147:191, 1983.

ULTRASONOGRAPHY OF BREAST MASSES

Ultrasonography has been used with increasing frequency to evaluate breast abnormalities. Ultrasound has the advantage of avoiding ionizing radiation and may be performed using either a hand-held transducer or whole-breast water baths. The diagnostic criteria for ultrasonographic evaluation of breast abnormalities are summarized in Table 4–9.[51–53] These breast changes are, in general, less subtle than those detected by mammography. As an imaging procedure, ultrasonography is most useful for distinguishing solid from cystic masses, detecting solid components within cysts (Fig. 4–9), and evaluating palpable masses not readily identified on mammography. It is also useful for evaluating palpable masses in women under 30 years of age (because of the density of the breast tissue) and for evaluating breast symptoms in adolescents, pregnant and post-partum women, and patients with inflammatory conditions of the breast.[53] Finally, it may be used to guide needle aspiration of cysts and to determine whether complete resolution has been achieved following aspiration of cysts.[52]

Ultrasound is less reliable than mammography when used either for detection and early diagnosis of breast cancer or for distinguishing benign from malignant lesions. Sickles and associates[55] reported that whereas mammography detected over 90 percent of

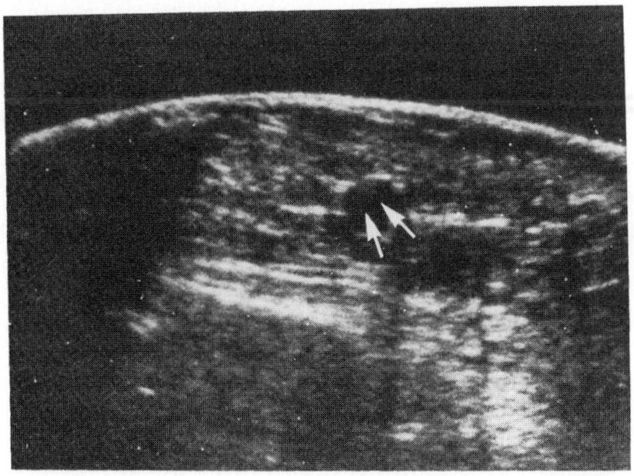

FIGURE 4–9. Breast ultrasonogram demonstrating a cystic papillary adenocarcinoma. The tumor mass is seen projecting into the cyst from the anterior cyst wall. (With permission from McSweeney MB, Murphy CH: Whole-breast sonography. Radiol Clin North Am 23:157, 1985.)

cancers of all categories, sonography detected only 48 percent of the cancers that had not yet spread to axillary lymph nodes, only 30 percent of the nonpalpable malignancies, and only 8 percent of the cancers less than 1 cm in diameter. Teixidor and Kazam[56] found that sonography correctly diagnosed 78.8 percent of proven cancers, versus 94 percent for mammography. Kobayashi and colleagues[57] reported the following diagnostic accuracy according to TNM tumor size: T_1, 76 percent; T_2, 90 percent; and T_3, 93 percent.[43] Jellins and colleagues[58] noted a sensitivity of 84 percent and 79 percent, respectively, for masses less than 2 cm or greater than 2 cm. Ultrasound is therefore not reliable for detecting occult malignancies or for detecting or evaluating microcalcifications of the breast.[59, 60] It is also viewed as less reliable for detecting masses deep to the nipple.[61] Ultrasound is therefore appropriate for distinguishing solid from cystic lesions, evaluating the results of aspiration of cystic lesions, and evaluating breast complaints in women for whom mammography is less reliable (see earlier). Ultrasonography should not be used to exclude the presence of occult lesions in the remaining breast tissue.

Breast Thermography

Thermography offers the same relative advantages as ultrasonography in that it is simple, nonhazardous, and noninvasive. It is based on the principle that inflammatory and neoplastic processes produce an increase in local temperature that can be detected at the skin surface. Thermography has been used extensively to screen asymptomatic patients for breast cancer and to evaluate patients with breast symptoms. When used to evaluate suspicious breast lesions, thermography has a true-positive rate of 72 to 85 percent, a false-positive rate of 6 to 14 percent, and a false-negative rate of 28 to 30 percent.[62–65] Thermography is more accurate for larger tumors and for those that are rapidly growing.[62, 66] Thermography may also be used to identify high-risk individuals: Amalric and colleagues[67] found that among patients with a persistently abnormal thermogram, 26 percent developed breast cancer within five years. However, because of its inability to diagnose smaller tumors, thermography is generally not considered to be a useful technique for breast evaluation. Isard and Ostrum[62] concluded, from a review of 4393 asymptomatic women, that thermography as an isolated procedure cannot diagnose breast cancer. Moskowitz and associates,[68] reviewing 42 patients with Stage I breast cancer, concluded that thermography cannot identify patients harboring early cancer, currently detectable by other means, in a general population of patients. Sterns and colleagues[65] do not recommend that an abnormal thermogram be used as an indication for mammography, and they concluded that thermography is a modality not sufficiently precise for use in routine breast examination. Finally, Johnsen and Burstam[45] feel there is no place for thermography in the diagnosis of breast symptoms. The authors support these conclusions and also the position of Kopans and associates[59] that thermography should be considered experimental, with no proven clinical efficacy.

Computerized Tomography of the Breast

The application of computerized tomography (CT scans) to the evaluation of breast masses has been well reviewed by Kopans and associates.[59] While offering the potential for increased resolution of breast masses, especially with the use of intravenous contrast material, computerized tomography has several disadvantages vis-à-vis conventional mammography. It delivers a higher dose of radiation (up to 1 rad) and necessitates irradiation of the entire chest. Breast tissue is evaluated in 1 cm slices; thus, smaller lesions such as microcalcifications can easily be missed. The overall resolution and delineation of structures are considerably poorer than with conventional mammography. The technique is also tedious and time consuming. Because of these limitations, CT scans of the breast offer few advantages over mammography and are not recommended as a standard procedure. Further refinements in the technique may increase its applicability.

Summary and Recommendations

Noninvasive studies may provide important information in the evaluation of breast symptoms. Noninvasive studies should be obtained prior to invasive procedures. Mammography and ultrasonography are the most useful of these studies. Ultrasonography is recommended for the evaluation of breast symptoms in women under 30 years of age, for pregnant or post-partum women, and for women with inflammatory conditions of the breast or with cystic lesions. Mammography should be performed preoperatively for all solid lesions in women over 30 years of age. For women 20 to 30 years of age, a mammogram should be obtained preoperatively in those at high risk for breast cancer or if there is a strong suspicion of malignancy. Mammography should be performed for cystic lesions in women over 30 if the patients are at increased risk for breast cancer, if the cysts do not completely resolve with aspiration, or if no previous mammograms have been obtained. In the last situation, the mammogram will serve for baseline screening purposes. Mammography is the only reliable method for detecting occult lesions in the breast. Biopsies should be performed on all suspicious lesions, regardless of the findings on noninvasive studies. Thermography and computerized tomography are not recommended either for screening purposes or for evaluation of breast symptoms. Their use should be restricted to investigational studies.

Invasive Studies for the Evaluation of a Breast Mass

The history, physical examination, and noninvasive studies are important for defining the clinical characteristics of the mass and of the remaining breast tissue. Invasive procedures, however, are necessary to establish the cause of breast abnormalities as well as the need for definitive treatment. Invasive diagnostic procedures used in the evaluation of breast lesions include needle aspiration of breast cysts, fine-needle aspiration to obtain material for cytologic analysis, percutaneous Tru-Cut or drill biopsies, and open biopsy, either incisional or excisional, to obtain material for histologic studies. These procedures differ primarily in the quantity of tissue and the manner in which it is obtained. The procedure selected will depend on the nature of the lesion being evaluated and the clinical setting.

Aspiration of Breast Masses and Cytologic Analysis

Technique. Fine-needle aspiration of breast masses may provide information regarding the cystic or solid nature of the mass and, especially in the case of solid masses, may provide material for cytologic examination. The aspiration of cystic and solid lesions will be considered separately. The technical aspects of performing aspiration, however, are the same for both lesions.[69–71] Fine-needle aspiration is commonly performed with an 18- to 22-gauge needle and a 10-ml syringe. For aspiration, a special syringe holder is available to facilitate obtaining cellular material (Fig. 4–10). After the overlying skin is cleansed, a 1-cm area of the skin is anesthetized. A variety of local anesthetics are available. The authors prefer 1 percent xylocaine without epinephrine. The needle is directed percutaneously into the mass. If a cystic lesion is encountered, the fluid is aspirated. If the fluid is to be analyzed (for blood or cytologic abnormalities), either the syringe is capped or the fluid is transferred to a clean glass screw-top tube. If a solid lesion is encountered, it is aspirated by rapid upward suction pressure on the syringe barrel, three or four times. The needle is moved to additional areas of the mass and the process repeated to obtain additional samples. The needle is then withdrawn, and the material is expressed onto a clean glass slide. The slide is immediately fixed in methyl alcohol, stained, and evaluated. Alternatively, the syringe with the aspirated material can be filled with saline and the contents transferred to a glass screw-top tube; appropriate analysis can then be done on the suspension or on a cell pellet. Except for an occasional small hematoma, there is no morbidity. The procedure takes five to ten minutes. There was initial concern that aspiration of a malignancy might seed the needle tract. Berg and Robbins[72] found, however, that long-term survival of patients diagnosed by aspiration biopsy is not different from that of nonaspirated control patients.

Aspiration of Cystic Breast Masses

When cystic breast masses are aspirated, one should note the character of the aspirate, whether the aspiration is followed by complete resolution of the mass, and whether the mass reaccumulates within a two- to three-week period. Aspiration of benign cysts will produce straw-colored or greenish-gray nonbloody fluid. In the case of a benign cyst, aspiration should result in complete resolution of the mass, without reaccumulation in a two- to three-week period. The diagnosis of benign cyst is supported by the finding of a correspnding cyst or dysplastic changes on mammography. Ultrasonography can also be used to verify complete resolution of the cyst. If these criteria are met (aspiration of clear or greenish-gray fluid with complete resolution of the mass), the patient should be reexamined in two to three weeks. If mammography has not been performed and the patient is over 30 years of age, mammography should be done for baseline and screening purposes. If the cyst has not reaccumulated, the diagnosis of benign breast disease is confirmed, and the patient can be followed with routine evaluations. Because the underlying mastopathy persists, the patient should be advised about the possibility of developing cysts at other locations in the future. Initial aspiration of cystic palpable masses is preferred to observation for the duration of a menstrual cycle. Properly performed aspiration should be associated with minimal discomfort or morbidity and should promptly confirm the diagnosis of benign breast disease, thus sparing the patient and the physcian further concern over the etiology of the mass.

A cystic breast mass should be excised to exclude the possibility of malignancy if aspiration of the mass does not result in complete resolution, if the cyst reaccumulates following a second aspiration in two or three weeks, or if the aspirate is bloody. The technical aspects of the excisional biopsy are the same as for solid masses (see later). For benign cysts, the authors excise the entire cyst wall to allow for a more thorough histologic examination and to prevent reaccumulation.

The role of cytologic analysis of cyst fluid remains unclear. Cystic carcinoma rarely occurs. Strawbridge and colleagues[73] reviewed 834 cyst aspirates and found 20 cases of carcinoma (2.2 percent), seven of which had bloody aspirates. Kline and associates,[74] reviewing 916 cyst aspirates, observed eight cases of carcinoma (0.9 percent), five of which had bloody or serosanguineous aspirates. Three additional series reported a total of 61 cases among 14,412 cyst aspirates, for an incidence of 0.4 percent.[75–77] The likelihood, therefore, of finding a carcinoma in a cystic lesion in which the aspirate is not bloody and there is complete resolution of the cyst is less than 1.0 percent. For this

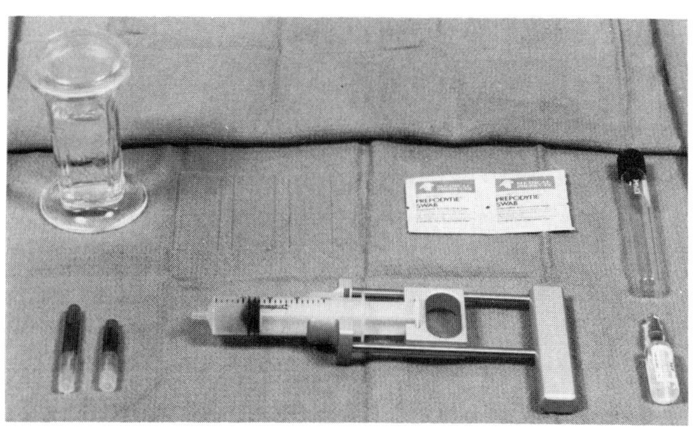

FIGURE 4–10. Equipment used for performing fine-needle aspiration of the breast. Included are a syringe and syringe holder, fine needle, slide holder containing fixative, screw-top tube to collect fluid, saline vial, and a Betadine swab for skin cleansing. The syringe holder allows a rapid suction motion on the syringe barrel, facilitating collection of cellular material from solid masses.

reason, the authors do not view cytologic analysis of cystic aspirates as a useful or productive procedure.

Aspiration of Solid Breast Masses

Aspiration cytology has been used extensively to diagnose solid breast masses. The results of aspiration cytology of palpable solid masses of the breast for eight series are summarized in Table 4–10. The rate of false-positive findings for aspiration cytology of solid masses ranges from 0 to 4 percent. False-positive cytologic findings may be artifactual on the basis of apocrine cell alterations or changes resulting from air-drying, or as a result of the histologic character of the underlying lesion. Histologic entities that have been associated with false-positive cytologic findings include intraductal papillomas, fibroadenoma, fibrocystic disease, gynecomastia,[74] fat necrosis, mastitis tuberculosa,[43] pseudolymphoma of the breast, and atypical lobular hyperplasia.[73, 74] The likelihood of a false-positive diagnosis can be reduced by proper preparation of the slide and increased experience of the cytologist. While a rate of false-positive findings of 1 percent represents a high degree of diagnostic accuracy, this error rate is unacceptable if the procedure represents the sole basis for determining definitive therapy for a breast mass. The use of aspiration cytology to recommend radical surgery for a breast mass must therefore be individualized from center to center. A large experience must be accumulated and a rate of false-positive findings of 0 percent must be demonstrated before aspiration cytology is used in place of histologic studies. As Kline has stated, "The greater the experience, the more rapidly specific diagnoses may be made. But it must be stressed that without a large volume of cases and at least one year's experience, definitive therapy should not follow aspiration biopsy."[74] If there is any question about the diagnosis from the aspirate, a biopsy of the mass should promptly be performed.

TABLE 4–10. Cytologic Analysis of Aspirates of Breast Masses

Series	*False-Negative Diagnoses (%)*	*False-Positive Diagnoses (%)*
Shabot et al.[46]	3.8	0.0
Frable[71]	7.0	2.0
Strawbridge et al.[73]	9.6	3.0
Kline et al.[74]	9.5	1.9
Thomas et al.[78]	6.0	4.0
Johnsen[79]	8.7	0.4
Zajicek[80]	1.8	—
Gardecki et al.[81]	7.9	0.0

The rate of false-negative findings for aspiration of solid masses ranges from 1.8 to 9.6 percent (Table 4–10). A false-negative diagnosis by this technique may occur for several reasons, including small tumor size, a significant fibrotic component, and absence of carcinoma cells in the aspirate. Kreuzer and Zajicek[82] noted that the incidence of false-negative reports for tumors less than 1 cm in diameter was 50 percent, resulting, in part, from the difficulty in localizing a small target with the needle. Fibrotic tissue was frequently found to yield few cells, which may be due to poor cellularity of the area explored by the needle or difficulty in detaching cells from the surrounding stroma by negative pressure created between needle and tissue. In cells with pronounced atypia, there may also be difficulty in distinguishing between fibroadenomas and atypical intraductal proliferation. Kline and colleagues[74] noted that 37 percent of infiltrating lobular carcinomas were diagnosed as negative, in contrast with 8 percent of the total number of infiltrating ductal carcinomas. This large percentage was probably due to the small, regular cells trapped in much of the connective tissue. A negative aspiration cytology, showing the absence either of cellular material or of malignant cells, should never be accepted as diagnostic of a benign lesion. All negative cytologic analyses of solid breast masses should be confirmed by histologic study of specimens. The use of a positive cytologic finding to plan definitive therapy will depend, as stated earlier, on the degree of confidence in the nature of the sample and on the expertise of the cytologist. Routine histologic biopsy should be performed on all suspicious breast lesions if there is any reason to question the results of the cytologic examination.

Procedures Providing Histologic Material of Breast Masses

Material from solid masses for histologic review or other studies may be obtained percutaneously with a Tru-Cut or drill needle or by an open incisional or excisional biopsy.

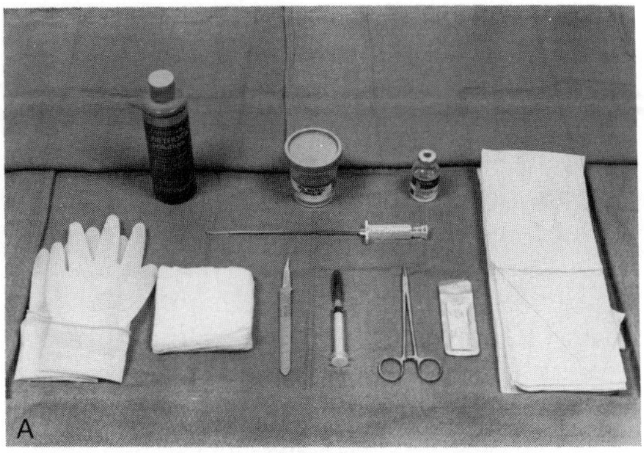

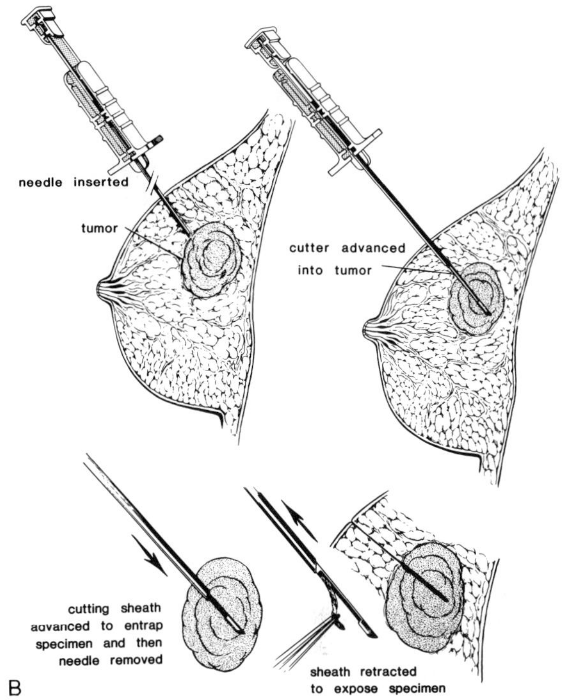

FIGURE 4–11. A, Equipment for performing Tru-Cut needle biopsy of the breast. Materials include local anesthetic with needle and syringe, antiseptic for skin cleansing, scalpel with No. 11 blade for skin puncture, Tru-Cut needle, formalin for handling of the specimen, and suture for skin closure. *B,* Technique for performing percutaneous biopsy of a breast mass with the Tru-Cut needle. (With permission from Donegan WL: General Considerations. *In*: Nora, PF (ed.): Operative Surgery: Principles and Techniques, 2nd ed. Philadelphia: Lea and Febiger, 1980.)

These procedures differ in both the quantity of material obtained and the requirements for the procedure. Selection of the procedure depends on the size and nature of the mass and the information desired from the specimen (e.g., histologic diagnosis and steroid receptor determination).

Tru-Cut Needle Biopsy. Material from a solid breast mass may be obtained percutaneously by a Tru-Cut needle biopsy.[35, 46, 83–85] The Tru-Cut needle provides for histologic review a core of tissue measuring approximately 0.2 by 1.0 to 2.0 cm (Fig. 4–11).[86] The tissue can be examined by either frozen or permanent section.[87] The procedure is performed under local anesthesia and is easily done in the office or an outpatient facility. It also has the advantage of avoiding incisional or excisional biopsy scars and does not compromise definitive treatment options, as can be the case following excisional biopsy of larger masses. The Tru-Cut needle biopsy may produce more ecchymotic and reactive tissue changes in the breast than does aspiration cytology; however, if only two or three cores are obtained these changes should be minimal. It is most easily performed on masses 2 cm or larger. "Targeting" smaller lesions may prove difficult. The Tru-Cut needle is generally inadequate when used to obtain material for steroid receptor determinations. At least 100 mg of tissue is necessary for reliable estrogen or progesterone receptor measurements. Because this information may be important for the management of patients, immediately or in the future, if a percutaneous biopsy establishes the diagnosis of malignancy, one should obtain adequate tissue for receptor determinations by an incisional or excisional biopsy, or on the tumor mass in the mastectomy specimen, at the time definitive treatment is instituted.

The rate of false-negative findings for the Tru-Cut needle biopsy from five series (totaling 711 patients) ranged from 12 to 33 percent (Table 4–11). The rate of false-positive findings, however, was 0 percent in all five series. The false-negative diagnosis of a malignancy by this technique is due mainly to

TABLE 4–11. Tru-Cut Needle Biopsy of Breast Masses

Series	*False-Negative Diagnoses (%)*	*False-Positive Diagnoses (%)*
Coates et al.[35]	12.0	0.0
Shabot et al.[46]	21.1	0.0
Davies et al.[83]	26	0.0
Elston et al.[84]	26.5	0.0
Roberts et al.[85]	33.0	0.0

inadequate material or tissue unrepresentative of the mass. This may occur with smaller masses (less than 2 cm); lesions with a significant desmoplastic component, which prevents penetration of the mass by the needle; or necrotic masses. Roberts and colleagues[85] noted that no tissue was obtained at biopsy in 5 percent of their cases. For masses less than 2 cm in diameter, adequate tissue was obtained in 36 percent of cases, compared with 88 percent of cases in which the mass was larger than 5 cm.

There have been no reports of false-positive diagnoses with Tru-Cut needle biopsies, and thus when the findings are positive, this technique can reliably and confidently be used to plan definitive therapy. This method should be used to establish the diagnosis of malignancy but *not* to exclude the diagnosis of malignancy. The high number of false-negative results confirms this. A negative diagnosis with a Tru-Cut biopsy of a suspicious mass, just as with aspiration cytology, should be followed with an incisional or excisional biopsy. Finally, Tru-Cut needle biopsy is much less reliable for defining the histologic type of benign lesions. Elston and associates[84] found that fibroadenoma was diagnosed with Tru-Cut biopsy in only 56 percent of cases, and the focal nature of mammary dysplasia was established in only a third of cases. For larger masses with a high index of suspicion on physical examination or mammography, the Tru-Cut needle biopsy is an excellent method for rapidly establishing the diagnosis. The limitations of the procedure, which relate predominantly to sample size, should be understood.

High-Speed Drill Biopsy. The high-speed drill biopsy is an additional technique by which material may be obtained percutaneously from solid breast masses for histologic examination.[88] It is a reliable technique with 93 to 95 percent accuracy and no false-positive diagnoses.[88, 89] Its diagnostic accuracy, like that of the Tru-Cut needle, is proportional to tumor size. High-speed drill biopsy may provide an advantage over Tru-Cut needle biopsy in that, because a high-speed drill is used, it can more readily penetrate fibrotic, acellular tumors. It requires, however, specialized equipment that is more difficult to use than the Tru-Cut needle. Tru-Cut needle biopsy is therefore preferred in the vast majority of patients in whom percutaneous material of solid breast masses is to be obtained for histologic analysis.

Incisional and Excisional Biopsies. Incisional and excisional biopsies have been the conventional means for establishing the diagnosis of solid breast masses. Both procedures are performed in the operating room and provide adequate tissue for diagnosis of breast masses and for steroid receptor determinations. These techniques remain the most definitive means for establishing the diagnosis of breast lesions, for determining malignant histologic subtypes, and for determining whether the malignancy is invasive or noninvasive. There are three major questions that are frequently considered in performing these biopsies: (1) whether they should be incisional or excisional, (2) whether they should be done under local or general anesthesia, and (3) whether they should be performed on an inpatient or outpatient basis.

INCISIONAL VERSUS EXCISIONAL BIOPSY. The primary objective of an incisional or excisional biopsy is to obtain tissue for diagnosis and to avoid sampling errors that may occur with breast and other tumors. The selection of an incisional or excisional biopsy will depend primarily on the size of the breast tumor and whether it appears clinically to be benign or malignant. For tumors smaller than 2 to 3 cm in diameter, these objectives can best be achieved by an excisional biopsy. If the tumor is benign, excisional biopsy will also constitute effective treatment and will avoid further concern over a persistent breast mass. If the tumor is malignant, an excisional biopsy will provide the maximum amount of tissue for diagnosis and steroid receptor determinations. If primary radiation therapy is to be the definitive treatment, an excisional biopsy may also make a subsequent excision unnecessary. In this case, if an incisional biopsy is done initially and the biopsy site must be reexplored one to two weeks later to remove remaining gross tumor, efforts to identify gross tumor in the presence of scarring, reactive changes, and hematoma may be difficult at best.

For solid tumors measuring 4 cm or larger, we initially perform a Tru-Cut needle biopsy. If this does not establish a malignancy, an incisional biopsy and frozen section are obtained. If the tumor is benign, a local excision can be performed at that time. Whether local excision is performed under local or general anesthesia will depend on several factors, which are discussed later. If a malignancy is confirmed, appropriate treatment is dis-

cussed with the patient (if treatment options have already been discussed, and mastectomy is selected, one may proceed with the procedure at the time of frozen section confirmation; see Chapter 8, NCI trial for radiation therapy for Stages I, and II breast cancer).

TECHNIQUE. Careful attention must be paid to the technical aspects of the biopsy procedure.[86, 90] The choice of anesthesia is discussed later. The patient is placed in the supine position and suitably prepared and draped. The margins of the mass are identified at the skin surface and noted with a marking pencil. In placing the incision, consideration should always be given to the possibility that the mass will prove malignant and a subsequent mastectomy will be necessary. The biopsy incision should not compromise the mastectomy incision. A periareolar incision along Langer's lines is frequently used (Fig. 4–12)[90]; however, for masses at the periphery of the breast for which there is a high index of suspicion, a radial incision is appropriate and can be more easily incorporated into the mastectomy incision. The biopsy incision should be extended 1 to 2 cm beyond the palpable limits of the mass. A larger incision not only may compromise a subsequent mastectomy but also may compromise the cosmetic benefit if primary radiation therapy is the selected treatment. After the skin incision, the authors prefer to use electrocautery for dissection of the subcutaneous tissues. The mass is identified, and if an incisional biopsy is to be performed, an adequate sample is obtained. Hemostasis is easily achieved on the surface of the remaining tissue with electrocautery or Gelfoam sterile sponges. If an excisional biopsy is to be performed, the authors prefer to excise the mass with a margin of 1 to 2 cm of normal tissue in all directions. There is no advantage in including a wide margin of tissue at this time, especially since the diagnosis has not been established. A wide margin not only may compromise the cosmetic result but provides little diagnostic or therapeutic benefit should the lesion prove to be benign. For lesions that subsequently prove malignant and that are to be treated with radiation therapy, it is also unclear whether "quadrantectomy" offers any advantage over local excision in reducing local recurrence (see the section on partial mastectomy in Chapter 5). Hemostasis is secured with cautery or absorbable sutures. The margins of the defect are approximated to provide a good cosmetic result, and the skin is closed with a running 4–0 or 5–0 subcuticular Vicryl suture and Steri-Strips. Wound drainage is not used. If biopsies are to be performed in previously irradiated breasts or on patients receiving adjuvant chemotherapy, the authors prefer to close the skin with interrupted 4–0 or 5–0 nylon or other nonabsorbable sutures.

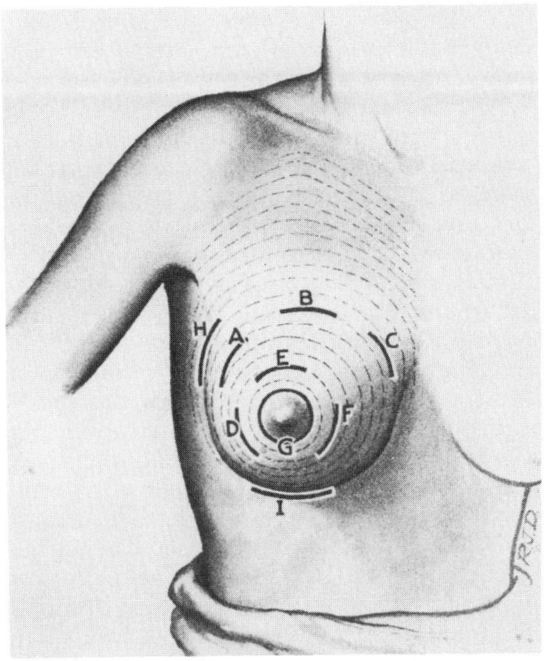

FIGURE 4–12. Langer's lines in the skin of the breast. Several options for placement of a circumareolar incision for a breast biopsy are illustrated. The incision should be along Langer's lines to provide the best cosmetic result. (With permission from Haagensen CD: Diseases of the Breast, 2nd ed. Philadelphia: W. B. Saunders Co., 1971.)

LOCAL VERSUS GENERAL ANESTHESIA. The selection of local or general anesthesia for breast biopsies will be determined by the size of the tumor, the compliance of the patient, and the nature of the definitive treatment contemplated if the lesion is malignant. Percutaneous biopsies, either aspiration cytology or Tru-Cut needle biopsies, can safely and comfortably be performed under local anesthesia. They produce minimal irritation of tissue and can be rapidly performed, and a wide variety of local anesthetics are available for effective anesthesia. These percutaneous biopsies are routinely performed as office procedures.

Incisional and excisional biopsies can also be performed safely under local anesthesia.

Breast biopsies performed under local anesthesia have several advantages over those done under general anesthesia.[27, 29, 30, 91–95] They avoid the risks of general anesthesia, relieve a good deal of the psychologic trauma to the patient, are easily performed and well tolerated, and reduce medical costs. Preliminary biopsy of malignant lesions using local anesthesia permits more efficient use of diagnostic procedures to stage the extent of the disease prior to treatment.[91] Patient concerns about breast biopsies under local anesthesia have included objections to the sounds of cutting instruments, duration of the procedure, inadequate analgesia, and subsequent delay in reporting the histologic diagnosis. These problems, however, can be easily avoided. A careful explanation to the patient as to the nature of the procedure will do much to relieve her concerns. Background music, as suggested by others, will diminish the sounds of the operative procedure.[92] The duration of the procedure, the need for retraction and hemostasis, and additional tissue trauma can be reduced by limiting excision under local anesthesia to masses of 3 cm or less. A wide variety of local anesthetics are available, and adequate infiltration of surrounding tissue should provide complete relief from discomfort. Some surgeons have objected to the use of local anesthesia because of concern that it distorts tissue planes and makes it more difficult to distinguish the tumor from normal tissue. The authors have not found this to be the case. The margins of the tumor can be easily discerned by palpation and inspection. The use of electrocautery for dissection reduces bleeding and facilitates visualization of the tissue planes. As with all other surgical procedures, biopsies under local anesthesia can most easily be performed by surgeons experienced in these techniques. Excision of a large mass by a junior house officer, with the patient under local anesthesia, may be unnecessarily traumatic for both the surgeon and the patient.

Frozen section review of the specimen may provide an immediate diagnosis.[96, 97] A definitive diagnosis can be established by frozen section in 80 to 95 percent of cases. Factors that make frozen section diagnosis difficult include inadequate sample size, small or occult breast lesions, and certain histologic patterns. The histologic patterns that frequently cause problems in frozen section diagnosis are listed in Table 4–12. For occult mammographic lesions that are localized preoperatively, the authors do not perform frozen section (see later). Agnantis and colleagues[98] reviewed frozen section diagnoses in 3451 breast biopsies. Twenty percent were deferred for permanent sections. Among those in which an immediate diagnosis was made, there were seven false-negative and one false-positive diagnosis. The latter was a case of juvenile papillomatosis misinterpreted as intraductal carcinoma. Thus, while frozen section is a valuable diagnostic tool, understanding its limitations may help to avoid unnecessary preparation for definitive procedures at the time of the biopsy and may allow optimum use of the specimen. The patient should be cautioned that a frozen section diagnosis is not always possible and that more careful study by the pathologist may be necessary. However, if the diagnosis can be established, the patient should be so informed; further delay only adds to the psychologic trauma.

TABLE 4–12. Histologic Patterns that Cause Problems during Frozen Section Diagnosis

All papillary lesions, including:
Atypical intraductal papilloma
Early intraductal carcinoma
Subareolar papillomatosis
Sclerosing adenosis with pseudoinfiltrative pattern
Florid adenosis and blunt duct adenosis
Atypical duct hyperplasia
Fat necrosis
Lobular carcinoma *in situ*

Source: Kagali VA: The role and limitations of frozen section diagnosis of a palpable mass in the breast. Surg Gyn Obstet 156:168, 1983.

OUTPATIENT VERSUS INPATIENT BREAST BIOPSY. Traditionally, breast masses were biopsied under general anesthesia, with preparations for immediate radical mastectomy if the mass proved malignant. This required hospitalization in addition to general anesthesia and deprived the patient of the opportunity to consider the diagnosis and alternative treatment options. In addition to the advantages of performing breast biopsies under local anesthesia discussed earlier, many data have been accumulated on the performance of these biopsies as outpatient procedures.[27, 29, 30, 91–99] These studies have shown that outpatient breast biopsies performed under local anesthesia have many advantages over inpatient biopsies done under general anesthesia:

1. Outpatient breast biopsy affords the patient the opportunity to discuss the diagnosis and treatment options with her physician. An understanding of the malignancy will aid in her psychologic adjustment, and the discussion of the advantages and disadvantages of alternative treatment regimens (e.g., mastectomy versus radiation therapy for early stage breast cancer) will help her to accept the treatment regimen selected.

2. A delay of one to three weeks between biopsy and institution of treatment does not have an adverse effect on prognosis.[31, 100–102] Bertario and colleagues[103] compared 57 patients who had an excisional biopsy done under local anesthesia, followed by an extended radical mastectomy an average of 25 days later, with 152 patients who underwent excisional biopsy performed under general anesthesia (the specimens of which were analyzed by frozen section) and then had immediate extended radical mastectomy. They found no difference in the ten-year actuarial survival between the two groups and concluded that a delay between biopsy and radical surgery of breast cancer is not an important prognostic factor. Hunt also supported the premise that delays up to several weeks seem to have no effect on ultimate prognosis.[92]

3. Outpatient breast biopsy will reduce hospital costs. In 1978, Walker and associates[91] estimated that inpatient hospital charges for biopsy of benign breast disease were 7.2 times higher than those for biopsy on an outpatient basis. In 1980, Doberneck[99] estimated that the use of local rather than general anesthesia reduced the cost of a breast biopsy by $694. In view of the increase in cost of hospital rooms, laboratory and x-ray studies, and anesthesia, this difference is probably greater today.

4. Outpatient breast biopsies can be performed safely with a negligible complication rate.[27, 29, 30, 91, 93, 94]

5. The risks of general anesthesia can be avoided.

6. The pathologist is allowed more time to evaluate the mass and adjacent tissue. This may be particularly important for *in situ*, intraductal, or microinvasive lesions.

The authors routinely perform essentially all breast biopsies as outpatient procedures under local anesthesia, including biopsies of both benign and malignant lesions as well as occult lesions that require preoperative radiographic localization. They reserve general anesthesia for complete excision of larger masses (4 to 5 cm), for bilateral breast biopsies, and for cases in which general anesthesia is requested by the patient. Outpatient breast biopsies done under local anesthesia are therefore suitable to the vast majority of breast lesions and, in the authors' experience, are most preferred by the patient.

EVALUATION OF THE PATIENT WITH NIPPLE DISCHARGE

The discharge of material from the nipple is uncommon, except in the post-partum state, and may be the first manifestation of a malignancy. Among all patients with breast symptoms, the incidence of nipple discharge ranges from 3 to 8 percent.[104–109] Nipple discharge may occur from either diffuse or localized changes within the breast. Diffuse changes usually accompany systemic physiologic alterations, including pregnancy, hormonal therapy, prolactin-secreting pituitary tumors, and certain drugs (chlorpromazine or oral contraceptives).[107–111] Discharge as a result of diffuse changes in the breast is usually nonspontaneous and bilateral, occurs from multiple ducts, and is clear to milky. This type of discharge should not be considered as a primary breast disorder, and treatment is directed at the underlying pathophysiologic stimulus.

Localized changes in the breast may result in focal changes in the intraductal epithelium, which are manifested by nipple discharge. The causes of nipple discharge and their frequency are listed in Table 4–13. Under these circumstances, the discharge is usually spontaneous, intermittent, and persistent and occurs from a single point at the nipple.[107–111] While a malignancy must clearly be excluded in a patient with unilateral nipple discharge, the majority of patients who have a nipple discharge have benign conditions. Among all patients with a nipple discharge, the discharge will be associated with a benign condition in 89 to 92 percent, and with a malignancy in 8 to 11 percent.[105–106] Conversely, 10 to 15 percent of patients with benign breast conditions and 2 to 3 percent with breast malignancy have associated spontaneous nipple discharge.[109–110] The discharge in patients with either a benign or a

TABLE 4–13. Character of Nipple Discharge from Different Breast Conditions*

Breast Condition	Type of Discharge				
	SEROUS	BLOOD-STAINED†	PURULENT	WATERY	GRUMOUS
Duct ectasia	36.4% (4.8–60.0%)	44.3% (21.4–71.3%)			73.8%
Infection			100.0%		
Intraductal papilloma	45.6% (42.0–49.1%)	72.0% (50.9–100%)		1.9%	
Fibrocystic disease	85.9% (71.7–100%)	36.9% (20.8–52.9%)	7.5%		
Cancer	23.0% (7.1–38.9%)	74.6% (57.1–100%)	14.3%	5.6%	
Lobular carcinoma *in situ*	12.5%	59.1% (55.6–62.5%)	12.5%		
Intraductal carcinoma	5.3%	78.9%	15.8%		

*Values expressed as mean and range (parentheses) for conditions for which more than one series reported findings.
†Includes grossly bloody or serosanguineous discharge, or discharge positive for blood by Hemoccult testing.
Source: Chaudary et al.,[104] Haagensen,[107] Leis and Pilnik,[108] Urban and Egeli,[110] and Rimsten et al.[112]

malignant lesion will contain blood in the majority of cases: 46 to 74 percent of discharges from benign lesions and 66 to 100 percent of discharges from malignancies will be positive for hemoglobin.[107, 109, 110] The strongest correlation between hemoglobin positivity and malignancy was noted by Chaudary and colleagues.[104] They performed microdochotomies on 270 patients with nipple discharge and no palpable breast abnormalities. In 16 cases, carcinomas were found (eight invasive and eight intraductal), all of which had hemoglobin-positive discharge. No instance of carcinoma was found among patients with hemoglobin-negative discharge. Age and the presence of an associated palpable mass are also important considerations. Copeland and Higgins[113] found that a serosanguineous or bloody discharge was usually benign in patients younger than 50 years of age but more often was due to cancer in older women.

The evaluation of a patient with a nipple discharge should begin with a complete history and physical examination. Possible systemic causes should be excluded, and the character and location of the discharge should be determined. Information acquired in the history may be adequate for these purposes; however, much more reliable information can usually be obtained if the physician observes the secretion. This allows more careful analysis of the discharge and permits the physician to identify the location of the duct in the nipple and, hence, the quadrant of the breast containing the pathologic changes. The discharge can usually be expressed from the nipple by palpation and mild pressure in the periareolar area. Each quadrant should be examined in turn and the location of the discharge noted. The discharge should be collected either on white gauze or on a glass slide and the character noted (milky, multicolored and sticky, purulent, watery, serous, serosanguineous, or bloody).[106] Examination by Hemostix and Wright's stain will reveal the presence of blood or purulent cells.

The usefulness of cytologic examination of nipple secretions remains unclear. The accuracy of cytologic diagnosis is dependent on the method of preparation of the smear and review by an experienced pathologist. Best results are obtained by applying a clear slide to the nipple area, followed by a lateral motion to smear the secretion. To avoid drying, the slide should be transferred immediately to a receptacle containing fixative. If the quantity of secretion is sufficient, it can be collected and placed in a glass tube containing saline. The cells are then separated and analyzed as for a smear. Among patients with a malignancy, the accuracy rate is 60 to 80 percent, with false-negative findings occurring in 12 to 35 percent of cases.[109, 114–120] Several groups have reported a false-positive rate (in patients with benign disease) of 3 to 4 percent.[109, 115, 121] Uei and colleagues[115] found that the presence of a spherical cell cluster with a smooth rim and the presence of blood in the smear increased the diagnostic accuracy of the procedure. Cytologic examination may support the diagnosis of malignancy, but definitive treatment should not be planned exclusively on the basis of these findings. Conversely, a negative cytologic examination should in no way exclude the diagnosis of breast cancer. Cytologic findings may thus be helpful but should be corroborated by more definitive procedures before treatment options are considered.

Mammography may further define the breast changes responsible for nipple discharge. Occult lesions, including carcinoma, as well as dysplastic changes, fat necrosis, and calcification associated with duct ectasia or fibrocystic disease may be recognized. The location of any abnormality should be correlated with the quadrant from which the discharge originates. Comparison with previous films may further suggest that the appearance of a new lesion and the discharge are temporally related.

The injection of mammary ducts with contrast material (galactography) in patients with nipple discharge has allowed the identification of ductal pathologic conditions in up to 70 percent of cases (Fig. 4–13).[120–126] The duct responsible for the discharge is identified and cannulated with a fine plastic catheter, and contrast material is injected. Using this technique, Taber and colleagues[121] identified intraductal papillomas in 38 percent of cases, mastopathy in 53 percent, and carcinoma in 9.4 percent. Nunnerly and Field[123] reviewed 21 cases and identified intraductal papillomas in six, duct ectasia in six, carcinoma in one, and proximal duct dilatation in one. While galactography may facilitate duct excision, it is time consuming and not readily available in many centers. Because the abnormality responsible for the discharge may not be in close proximity to the nipple, galactography is indicated in patients with negative mammograms and large breasts or other anatomic considerations that might make complete excision of the duct system difficult.

Patients who have single duct nipple discharge that is spontaneous, persistent, and intermittent and who have no associated abnormalities on physical examination or by mammography should have the duct system of that quadrant excised. The excision should include the duct from its terminus at the nipple to its proximal branching within the breast parenchyma. Occasionally, isolation of a single duct will not be possible either because of involvement of adjacent ducts, such as with duct ectasia, or because of a multifocal process such as papillomatosis. In these instances, the major duct system should be excised, through a circumareolar incision, with excision of a cone-shaped portion of tissue including the ducts, as described by Urban and Egeli.[110] Excision of the major duct system is also indicated for multiple duct or recurrent nipple discharge. The cosmetic results of this procedure should be quite good; however, excision of the major duct system precludes future nursing from that breast, which should be explained to the patient.

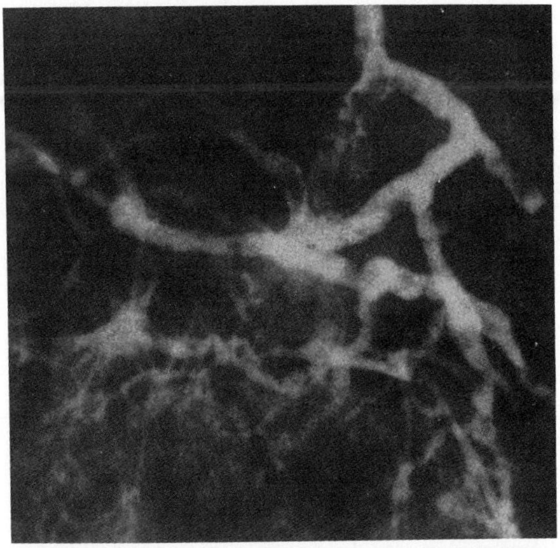

FIGURE 4–13. Breast galactogram. The ductal orifice is cannulated at the nipple and contrast material injected. Note extensive filling defects caused by papillomatosis. (With permission from Threatt B: Ductography. *In*: Bassett LW, Gold RH (eds.): Mammography, Thermography, and Ultrasonography in Breast Cancer Detection. New York: Grune & Stratton, 1982.)

The surgical approach to patients with nipple discharge and an occult lesion detected by mammography will depend primarily upon whether the quadrant in which the lesion is located is the same quadrant as that of the discharge. Occult lesions detected by mammography may be localized by a variety of techniques (see later). If the lesion is in the same quadrant as the discharge, it is appropriate to excise both the duct system of that quadrant and the lesion at the same time. Alternatively, one could excise only the occult lesion; however, if the discharge persisted, excision of the duct system would be required as a second procedure. If the lesion is not in the same quadrant and meets the criteria for excision, the lesion should be localized preoperatively and removed, along with the duct system from the quadrant responsible for the nipple discharge. The authors perform excision of the duct system under general anesthesia, especially if the entire duct system is to be removed. Frozen sections of the duct system or of occult abnormalities detected by mammography are not obtained because histologic sections of high quality are required for small lesions such as these.

EVALUATION OF OCCULT ABNORMALITIES DETECTED BY MAMMOGRAPHY

The increased use of mammography as a screening procedure in women has led to the detection of mammographic abnormalities that may not be associated with any symptoms or findings on physical examination (Fig. 4–14*A*). These abnormalities may take the form, in decreasing order of frequency, of a tumor mass, distortion of adjacent tissues (spiculation or retraction), calcifications, secondary abnormalities (skin thickening, skin or nipple retraction, or breast edema), or asymmetry.[128] Because these abnormalities may accompany either benign or malignant disease, their interpretation is not straightforward. The radiologic signs of breast cancer and their predictive value have been reviewed (Table 4–8). The concern for the surgeon (and the radiologist) is which of these abnormalities warrants biopsy. Just as with a palpable mass, histologic proof of the malignancy of an occult mammographic abnormality is required before definitive therapy is instituted. Schwartz and associates[129] have reviewed the mammographic findings for which biopsy is recommended. These are listed in Table 4–14. Any mammographic abnormality, however, should be reviewed with an experienced radiologist. The characteristics of malignancy may be subtle, and because an occult cancer in this stage has a high probability of cure, inappropriately recommending observation for a suspicious lesion must be avoided.

The accuracy of the radiographic signs will depend upon the character and the number of the signs present. Homer[130] has reviewed several large series of nonpalpable breast abnormalities that were biopsied. These series revealed that the rate of true-positive findings for nonpalpable breast abnormalities demonstrated by mammography is in the range of 20 to 30 percent. This is comparable to the true-positive biopsy rate for palpable breast lesions. Powell and colleagues[131] found that when calcifications were the only criteria used for biopsy, carcinoma was found in 17 percent of cases. Benign lesions that may be associated with calcifications on mammogram have been discussed previously (see Breast Mammography). The majority of occult mammographic abnormalities are therefore associated with benign disease. This incidence should not discourage an aggressive approach to occult mammographic changes. Detection of a malignancy at this stage represents the best opportunity for cure.

Localization and Biopsy

Occult lesions can be localized for biopsy purposes by a variety of techniques. All of these methods provide a means by which the surgeon can identify the occult lesion in the operating room, avoiding the need for a blind biopsy and the possibility of removing inappropriate or unnecessary tissue. In each of these procedures, under x-ray guidance a small-gauge needle is percutaneously placed into the area identified on the mammogram. Localization of a suspicious area for needle placement may be facilitated by use of compression grids.[132–135] The needle may be taped in place, serving as a track during the biopsy for identification of the lesion.[136–138] Alternatively, use of a needle with a barbed

TABLE 4–14. Mammographic Findings for Which Biopsy is Recommended

Breast calcifications suggestive of malignancy because of their size (less than 2 mm), shape (punctate, microlinear, or branching), distribution (clustered, grouped, or along ducts), or concentration (more than 5 calcifications per cm^3)
Stellate breast masses
Breast masses with ill-defined borders or nodular contours
Dominant, well-circumscribed, smooth masses that are significantly larger than any other mass in either breast
Areas of increased tissue density or distorted breast architecture

Source: Schwartz GF, Feif SA, Patchefsky AS: Clinicopathologic correlations and significance of clinically occult mammary lesions. Cancer 41:1147, 1978.

hook at the end, which secures it in place, avoids the problem of needle displacement during transport to the operating room.[132–134, 139–144] A third method, use of a nonabsorable dye to stain the tissue, has proved the most satisfactory in the authors' experience (Fig. 4–14*B*).[135, 145, 146] Opaque substances that have been used include a mixture of Lipiodol ultra fluid and Patent blue,[139] a suspension of carbon powder,[135] or methylene blue.[146] Following needle localization of the lesion, a drop of the localizing solution is injected through the needle; the stained tissue is then identified in the operating room and excised. Each of the localization methods has proved successful, and selection is a matter of preference for both the surgeon and the radiologist.

The technical aspects of excision of occult lesions are similar to those for other exci-

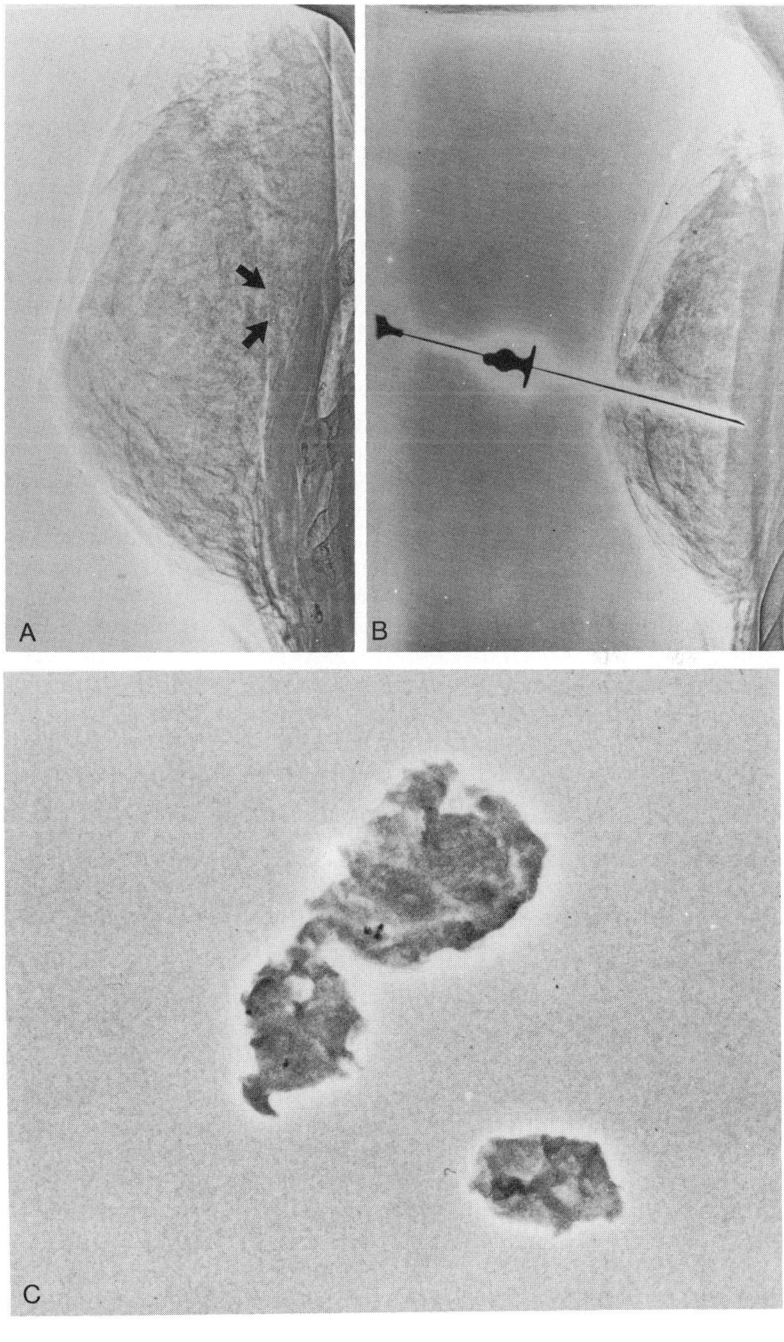

FIGURE 4–14. *A*, Xeromammogram revealing occult suspicious calcification in the outer middle quadrant of the right breast. *B*, Xeromammogram demonstrating needle localization of occult suspicious calcification depicted in *A*. *C*, Xeroradiogram of breast tissue specimen obtained following needle localization of occult suspicious calcification. The occult calcifications are contained within the specimen, confirming adequate excision. The occult calcifications were found, histologically, to be associated with intraductal carcinoma.

sional biopsies; however, several points should be emphasized. The needle should be placed in, or in close proximity to, the suspicious lesion. Inadequate placement can result in incomplete excision, with the potential need for a subsequent relocalization and excision. If the staining technique is used, not only the lesion but also the needle track should be stained out to the skin surface. This provides an easy landmark from which to begin the dissection, which is then carried down to the point of maximum staining representing the occult lesion. While occult lesions can be adequately stained with methylene blue, the diffusion capacity of this and other dyes through breast tissue is unpredictable. Excision of dye-localized lesions should be performed as soon after localization as possible to limit extension of the dye to adjacent tissues. Such extension would result in the unnecessary inclusion of additional tissue in the excision. The authors have found that methylene blue remains localized for at least two to three hours after injection.

The choice of local or general anesthesia for excision of occult lesions depends upon the condition of the individual patient. The technical aspects of the procedure, as mentioned, are quite similar to those of other excisional biopsies. There is little difference in the degree of tissue trauma or the requirement for local anesthesia. If specimen radiography is employed (see later), the duration of the procedure is lengthened by 15 to 30 minutes. With proper psychologic preparation of the patient, however, this is easily tolerated. The authors perform all excisions of localized lesions under local anesthesia, except in cases in which excision may be especially difficult and may require more than one specimen radiogram, when bilateral or multiple lesions are present, or when the patient's emotional status makes this inadvisable.

Specimen radiography is an indispensable adjunct to the excision of occult lesions.[147–151] Examination of the specimen by radiographs will ensure that the suspicious calcifications have been removed and will avoid the need for a postoperative mammogram to ascertain this (Fig. 4–14C). In addition, with reactive changes from the biopsy, a postoperative mammogram may be difficult to interpret, especially in the identification of small calcifications. Four to six weeks may be required before adequate films can be obtained. The authors routinely slice the specimen prior to specimen radiography. This facilitates identification of small calcifications and aids the pathologist in the selection of tissue for histologic sections. Frozen sections are not performed. As Gallager[147] has pointed out, to identify certain lesions (lobular carcinoma *in situ* or intraductal or microinvasive carcinoma), histologic sections of high quality are required, and a delay of two to three days for permanent sections will not have an adverse effect on response to treatment. Postoperative mammograms should not be considered a substitute for specimen radiography. If the lesion is not identified in the specimen radiogram, additional tissue can be excised at that time, avoiding the need for a repeat biopsy if only a postoperative mammogram is performed.

Specimen radiography is most useful for lesions that contain calcifications and is generally less reliable when used to identify noncalcified densities and lucencies in breast tissue.[148, 149] Pitzen and associates,[151] however, recently reported that resolution of noncalcified lesions is improved with xeroradiography of the specimen submersed in water. Precise localization with excision of at least 1 to 2 cm of surrounding tissue and careful palpation and inspection of adjacent tissue are the best means for ensuring complete excison of noncalcified lesions. Routine specimen radiography is not necessary for masses that are palpable preoperatively and that are completely excised. Multiple histologic sections of the mass can be prepared, and for specimens that are found to be benign, the probability of detecting an occult carcinoma by specimen radiography (to search for calcifications) is less than 1 percent.[147] For nonpalpable calcified lesions, however, specimen radiography is a very important, perhaps essential, adjunct to localization and excision.

BILATERAL BREAST CANCER AND BIOPSY OF THE OPPOSITE BREAST

Women who develop cancer in one breast are at increased risk for developing a malignancy in the opposite breast. The second malignancy may be synchronous or metachronous and invasive or noninvasive. The incidence of synchronous clinically apparent cancer in the second breast is approximately 0.81 percent (range 0.2 to 2.0 percent)[152, 153] and of metachronous clinically apparent breast cancer, 3.1 percent (range 1.0 to 6.5 per cent).[152–154] Eighty-eight to ninety-five percent of these second cancers will be of the invasive variety.[152–154] The annual risk of developing a metachronous second breast cancer is 0.65 per cent to 1.0 percent.[154, 155] Factors associated with the development of metachronous breast cancer include more advanced stage of the first primary tumor[152]; an initial tumor greater than 2 cm; an initial tumor associated with invasive cancer or proliferative fibrocystic disease, with nipple involvement, absent nodal sinus histiocytosis, or lobular carcinoma *in situ* in the vicinity of the dominant mass; an initial tumor of the lobular invasive or tubular type[154]; and multicentric primary lesions.[156] The effect on survival of developing a second breast cancer is not clear. Three studies have shown no significant difference in survival (10-year[152, 154] and 20-year[157]) between patients with unilateral and those with bilateral breast cancers,[152–154] whereas two other reports note a decreased survival rate among women with bilateral malignancies.[153, 155]

The incidence of occult contralateral breast cancer varies with the histologic character of the primary tumor. Among patients with lobular carcinoma *in situ* in one breast, approximately 23 to 42 percent will have noninvasive lesions in the opposite breast.[158–163] For intraductal carcinoma, the incidence of bilaterality is 4 to 6 percent[159, 161] (noninvasive breast cancer is discussed further in Chapter 10). These findings and the aforementioned risk for developing invasive carcinoma in the second breast in patients with unilateral invasive disease suggest that a contralateral breast biopsy would be a useful method for identifying patients at high risk for a second malignancy. Urban and colleagues[164] performed opposite breast biopsies in 954 patients. Of those with physical findings and mammography indicating carcinoma in the opposite breast, 71.0 percent had infiltrating cancers and 7.0 percent *in situ* carcinomas. Among those patients with indeterminate thickening of the opposite breast, 39.7 percent had infiltrating carcinomas and 60.3 percent had noninfiltrating lesions. Among patients with no clinical or radiologic abnormalities, 1.6 percent had infiltrating lesions and 6.4 percent had noninfiltrating lesions. Overall, 12.5 percent (of 954 patients) had carcinomas, of which 45 percent were infiltrating. If patients with positive findings on physical examination and mammography were excluded, 3.7 percent had infiltrating and 6.6 percent had noninfiltrating tumors, for a total of 10.3 percent. They concluded that contralateral breast biopsy at the time of mastectomy for a known cancer represents an additional method for the early detection of carcinoma in a very high-risk group.

Leis[165] performed random opposite breast biopsies in 321 patients, all of whom had no clinical or x-ray evidence of malignancy in that breast. Malignancy was found in 24 patients (7.5 percent), of which 10 (41.7 percent) were invasive and 14 (58.3 percent) were noninvasive. Wanebo and associates[153] performed contralateral biopsies in 52 patients with invasive breast cancer. Ten of these biopsies revealed malignancies: seven *in situ* lesions (four intraductal and three lobular carcinoma *in situ*) and three invasive malignancies. At least three of the ten patients had palpable lesions or suspicious mammograms of the opposite breast. The investigators concluded that contralateral biopsy provides the opportunity to reduce the risk of invasive cancer in that breast as well as to provide important diagnostic and prognostic information. Martin and colleagues,[156] however, noted a 2 percent incidence of carcinoma (all invasive) among 100 contralateral biopsies in clinically normal breasts. King and associates performed contralateral biopsies on 109 women with normal findings on physical examination and found one infiltrating carcinoma and four noninfiltrating lesions (two intraductal and two lobular carcinoma *in situ*). They concluded that these results did not justify the routine use of opposite breast biopsy as a diagnostic tool in patients with unilateral breast carcinoma and no abnormalities on physical examination or mammography. They rely, instead, on xeromammography for the selection of patients and the site of biopsy.

Summary and Conclusions

Women with unilateral breast cancer are at increased risk for developing a malignancy in the opposite breast. Clearly any clinically or radiographically suspicious areas, whether synchronous or metachronous, should be biopsied. The likelihood of finding a malignancy under these circumstances is high, and such detection provides the best opportunity for cure. Among patients with normal findings on clinical and radiologic examinations of the opposite breast, a blind biopsy of this breast will reveal a malignancy in approximately 10 percent of cases.[153, 165] Sixty to seventy percent of these malignancies will be noninfiltrating. Furthermore, based on the series of Wanebo and associates[153] and King and associates,[166] 43 to 50 percent of these noninfiltrating lesions will be lobular carcinoma *in situ*, for which continued observation is an appropriate treatment. Therefore, it can be estimated that among women with normal findings on examination of the opposite breast, up to 6 to 7 percent will be found to have intraductal or invasive carcinoma. This frequency does not in itself appear to justify routine biopsies of the normal breast in all women with unilateral breast cancer. Clearly, the patient group in the aforementioned studies (with normal evaluations but positive histologic findings on biopsy of the contralateral breast) needs to be better defined. An important task would be the correlation of these histologic findings in a retrospective (or, better, prospective) manner, with the factors outlined by Fisher and colleagues[154] that are associated with an increased risk for metachronous bilateral breast cancer. This might help to define guidelines for increasing the yield from biopsy of the normal contralateral breast. For the present, we agree with Fisher and colleagues[154] and King and associates[166] and recommend close observation of these patients by physical examination and mammography, reserving biopsy for any suspicious lesions that appear.

PREOPERATIVE EVALUATION OF THE BREAST CANCER PATIENT

Invasive breast cancer has the propensity for dissemination to a variety of organs and tissues. The distant sites most commonly affected in decreasing order of frequency are lung, bone, liver, and the adrenal.[20] Approximately 10 percent of all patients will have distant metastases at the time of presentation. Because the detection of distant metastases will obviously change both the stage assigned to the disease and the appropriate treatment options, it has been the practice to screen all patients at presentation with x-rays (skeletal and chest) and radionuclide scans. For patients with any of the grave signs of breast cancer and for patients with signs or symptoms of distant metastases, this is an appropriate policy. The probability of metastatic disease in this population is sufficient to justify these procedures, and it is important to clarify symptomatic areas that can be relieved by local treatment. In asymptomatic patients with early stage breast cancer (Stage I or Stage II), however, the extent to which a metastatic work-up should be pursued is less clear. The most extensive studies evaluating preoperative screening have been for those procedures used to detect lung, bone, and liver metastases. These will be discussed in the following sections.

Screening for Intrathoracic Metastases

Breast cancer may metastasize to pulmonary parenchyma, pleura, or mediastinal lymph nodes. Pulmonary parenchymal metastases may be either nodular or diffuse lymphangitic.[167] Nodular pulmonary metastases are the most common intrathoracic metastases; however, they are usually asymptomatic until they have reached a large size (Fig. 4–15). Lymphangitic metastases, although less common, are symptomatic much earlier in their developmental course (Fig. 4–16). They are often diffuse and may be associated with hemoptysis or shortness of breath. Pleural metastases are also often symptomatic and may be associated with chest pain, pleural effusions, or shortness of breath. Metastases to mediastinal lymph nodes are uncommon; however, they rarely may enlarge to the point of causing esophageal or superior vena caval obstruction. All of these abnormalities may be noted on a chest x-ray.

The incidence of pulmonary metastases in patients with Stage I or II breast cancer at presentation is low. Casey and associates[168] reviewed the chest x-rays of 1416 patients with breast cancer and found that 3 percent had a solitary nodule, either at the time of presentation or on follow-up. More impor-

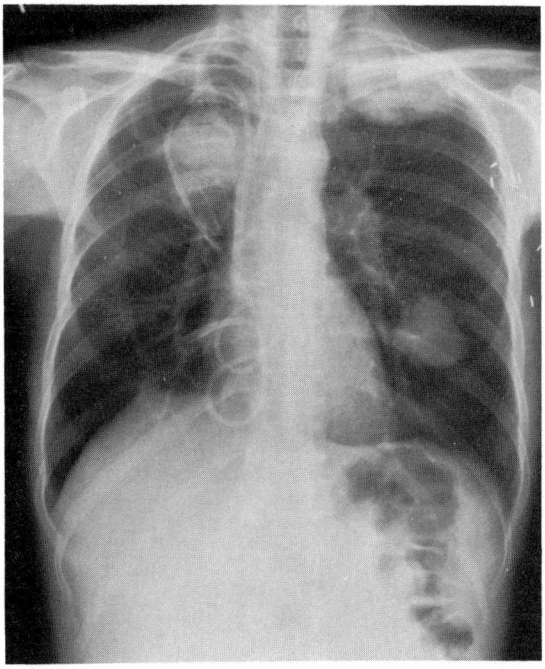

FIGURE 4–15. Chest x-ray demonstrating nodular type of pulmonary metastases from breast cancer.

tant, they found that whereas in 43 percent of these patients the solitary pulmonary nodule proved to be metastatic breast cancer, in 52 percent of patients the nodule proved to be a primary lung tumor. Cahan and colleagues[169] noted that among 78 breast cancer patients who had a solitary lesion on chest x-ray, 49 patients (63 percent) were found to have primary lung cancer. A *solitary* pulmonary nodule appearing in a patient with breast cancer, either past or present, is thus more likely to be a primary lung cancer than a metastasis from breast cancer.

While the likelihood of detecting metastatic disease on a chest x-ray in women with Stage I or II breast cancer at presentation is low, the chest x-ray remains a valuable technique for screening the patient for a variety of other thoracic disorders, including inflammatory and obstructive pulmonary problems, cardiomegaly, diaphragmatic disorders, bony abnormalities, and a second malignancy. The presence of any of these problems may have a significant effect on the treatment options selected, including both primary and adjuvant therapy. Because the vast majority of patients with early stage breast cancer will undergo a major surgical procedure (mastectomy or axillary lymph node dissection), a chest x-ray is indicated as part of the preoperative evaluation. However, the x-ray should also be carefully reviewed for the possibility of pulmonary or bony metastatic disease.

The sensitivity of the chest x-ray is such that a pulmonary nodule must be 1 to 2 cm in diameter before it can be visualized. More sensitive tests for evaluating the pulmonary parenchyma and thoracic structures include lung tomography, computerized tomography, and magnetic resonance imaging (MRI). However, these tests are more time consuming and costly and, in the case of the former two, deliver a substantially higher dose of radiation than does the chest x-ray. In view of the low incidence of pulmonary metastases in early stage breast cancer, these techniques are not indicated as routine screening procedures but should be used to further evaluate abnormalities found on chest x-ray.

The chest x-ray has been used routinely to follow patients for pulmonary metastases after definitive therapy for breast cancer. The chest x-ray, when abnormal, is a reliable means of evaluating patients for recurrent disease. Tesaro-Tess and colleagues[170] have reviewed the accuracy of the chest x-ray for

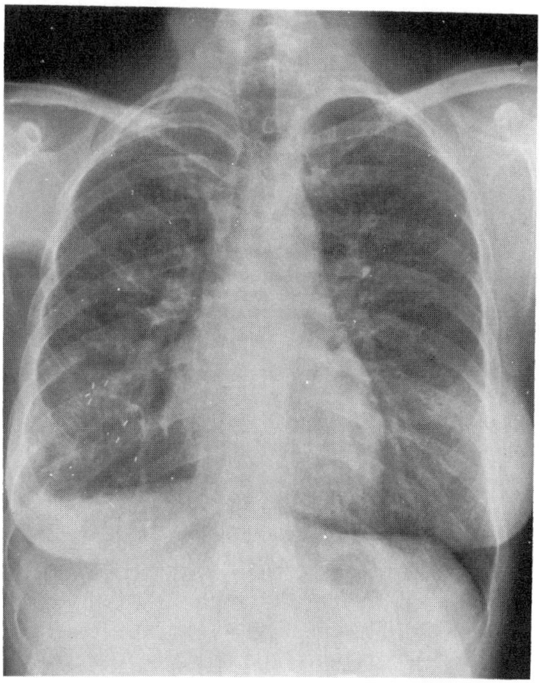

FIGURE 4–16. Chest x-ray demonstrating diffuse lymphangitic type of pulmonary metastases from breast cancer.

detecting pulmonary lesions as metastatic disease and found the accuracy of the chest x-ray to be 75 percent for parenchymal lung metastases, 84.6 percent for adenopathies, and 89.4 percent for pleural effusion. Among asymptomatic patients, however, the chest x-ray is usually unremarkable. Ciatto and Herd-Smith[171] evaluated the role of the chest x-ray in the follow-up of 1697 patients and found that its use resulted in the detection of only 39 cases of isolated thoracic metastases in asymptomatic patients. Chaudary and colleagues[172] evaluated serial chest x-rays in the follow-up of 241 patients with operable breast cancer. Pulmonary metastases were noted in 12 patients (5 percent), four of whom were symptomatic. Winchester and associates[33] found that among 87 patients with recurrent breast cancer, the recurrence was heralded by symptoms in 90 percent; in two of three asymptomatic patients, the recurrence was detected by routine chest x-ray. The chest x-ray in follow-up, as in preoperative, screening of the asymptomatic patient is useful for evaluation of the heart, lungs, and bony thorax but is unlikely to reveal asymptomatic metastatic disease. The chest x-ray should be included as a part of any yearly medical examination. Its more frequent use in breast cancer patients is indicated only by the presence of symptoms, for evaluation of previously detected abnormalities, or for following the response to therapy.

Screening for Skeletal Metastases

Bone represents the second most common site of distant metastatic disease in women with breast cancer. The pelvis and spine (in order of descending frequency, the lumbar, thoracic, and cervical) are the most common sites of osseous metastasis, followed by the ribs, femur, skull, and humerus.[173, 174] Metastases distal to the knee or elbow are uncommon. Bone metastases may be one of four types (in decreasing order of frequency): osteolytic, osteoblastic, intertrabecular, or mixed.[175] Osteolytic metastases are also the type most frequently seen on x-ray (Fig. 4–17). The osteoblastic type accounts for 5 to 10 percent of bone metastases (Fig. 4–18). Intertrabecular metastases, which constitute 15 to 20 percent of bone metastases, do not produce radiographic abnormalities.

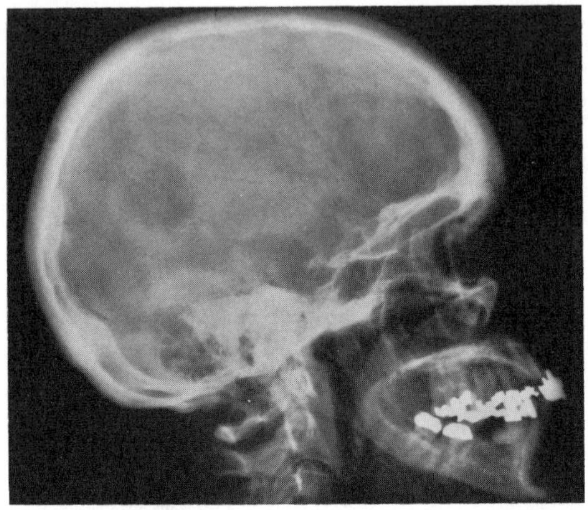

FIGURE 4–17. Skull x-ray demonstrating osteolytic type of metastases of the skull from breast cancer.

The two principal methods for screening for bone metastases have been plain-film skeletal x-rays and radionuclide bone scanning. Osseous metastases commonly are not demonstrable by radiologic examination until they are approximately 1 to 2 cm in diameter or until 50 to 75 percent of bone minerals have been lost.[176] For lesions of the spine, an even greater percentage of bone minerals

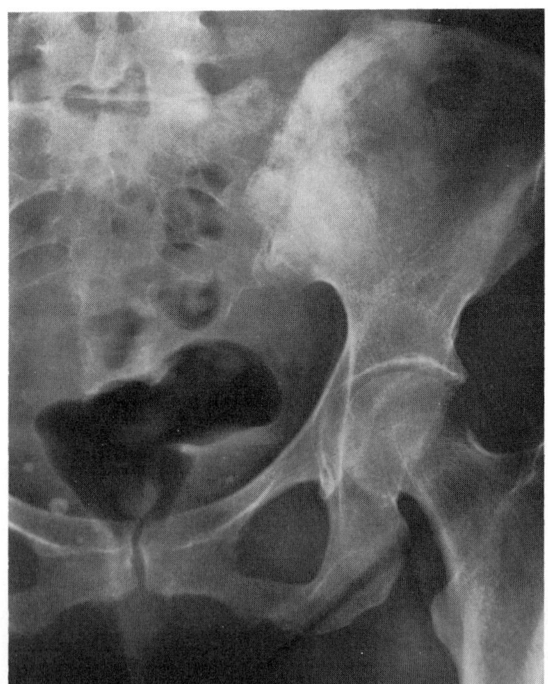

FIGURE 4–18. Pelvic x-ray demonstrating osteoblastic type of metastases of the ilium from breast cancer.

must be destroyed.[177] Furthermore, in less than half of patients with documented bone metastases at autopsy will these metastases be visualized by skeletal x-rays.[177] Thus, skeletal x-rays are not a sensitive means of detecting bone metastases from breast cancer. The usefulness of bone x-rays is principally in the evaluation of symptomatic areas or abnormalities noted on bone scan.

Bone scanning with technetium-99m is a more sensitive method for the detection of osseous metastases and has been used to evaluate patients with Stages I and II breast cancer, both preoperatively and in follow-up. The appearance of a bone lesion on a bone scintiscan will, in general, predate radiographic visualization by 2 to 18 months.[179] The average incidence of positive findings on bone scan is 1 to 4 percent for Stage I breast cancer, 5 to 7 percent for Stage II, and 14 to 25 percent for Stage III.[176, 180, 181] Lindholm and colleagues[180] found the following frequency of positive findings on bone scan according to clinical lymph node status: N_0, 5 percent; N_1, 15 percent; N_2, 30 percent; N_3, 63 percent. Other parameters with which positive findings on bone scan have shown a direct correlation include:

1. *Tumor size.* There is a direct correlation between the size of the primary tumor and the incidence of positive bone scans. Whereas no patients with tumors less than 1 cm in diameter had positive bone scans, 3 to 7 percent of patients with tumors of 2 to 5 cm and 13 to 45 percent of patients with tumors greater than 5 cm had positive bone scans.[176, 180]

2. *Grade of malignancy.* Lindholm and colleagues[180] noted that among patients with positive scans, 12.3 percent had low-grade tumors and 47.8 percent had high-grade tumors.

3. *Age.* Postmenopausal women have a higher frequency of positive findings on bone scan than do premenopausal women.[176, 180, 182] This increase with age, however, is also accompanied by an increased rate of positive findings resulting from benign disease. Benign lesions such as trauma, old fractures, infections, or degenerative joint disease may cause increased uptake of the isotope. It has been estimated that metastatic tumors may account for only 54 to 64 percent of the solitary lesions on abnormal bone scans, even in patients with proven extraosseous malignancies.[183, 184] Khandekar[185] estimated that the predictive value of a positive finding on bone scan in Stage I or II patients was only 23.5 percent. Rappaport and associates[186] followed 29 patients with unifocal lesions seen on bone scans for at least 18 months, and in only four patients did the lesions prove to be truly metastatic. Monypenny and colleagues[187] reviewed the initial bone scans in 685 patients with operable primary breast cancer. They found that 19 patients (2.8 percent) had positive findings on initial bone scan and negative findings on skeletal x-ray; only nine of these developed other evidence of metastatic disease after a mean follow-up period of 21 months.

4. *Symptomatic versus asymptomatic abnormalities.* Schaffer and Kalisher[188] followed 42 women with minimal or occult breast cancer for up to 48 months and found a 14 percent incidence of bone metastases; no patients who were asymptomatic had positive findings on bone scan. Schutte[189] found that 82 percent of patients without bone pain had negative findings on bone scan, whereas 63 percent of patients with pain had metastases and positive findings on bone scan. The bone scan, when findings are negative, is thus a reliable means of excluding bone metastases. Positive findings, however, must be interpreted in the context of the patient's age and history. Skeletal x-rays may be useful for further defining abnormalities noted on bone scan.

The bone scan has also been used in the follow-up of patients with operable breast cancer. Bishop and associates[190] evaluated 354 women with primary operable breast cancer with serial bone scans and found the incidence of positive findings on scans to be 4.3 percent at one year and 9.2 percent at two years. Monypenny and colleagues[187] reviewed serial bone scans in 510 patients after simple mastectomy. Fifty-one patients (10 percent) had scan conversion, of whom 37 developed clinical or radiologic confirmation of recurrent disease at a mean follow-up time of 13 months. Conversely, 12 of 45 patients with radiologically proven bone metastases had negative findings on scan. For this reason, these investigators did not consider routine bone scanning to be clinically useful as a follow-up procedure in patients with operable breast cancer. Arnstein and associates,[191] however, reviewed serial bone scans in 102 patients who underwent mastectomy and received adjuvant chemotherapy for breast carcinoma. All patients had negative findings on scan prior to chemotherapy. Scans of 23 patients (23 percent) showed a conversion to positive findings during follow-up at a mean interval of 29.5 months after surgery. At conversion, 5 of 21 patients had bone pain and none had an elevated alkaline phosphatase level. The investigators emphasized the importance of bone scanning in breast cancer patients who have received adjuvant chemotherapy, as the scan may be the only indicator of bone involvement. Coker and colleagues[192] reviewed serial bone scans in 57 patients with operable breast cancer. The initial rates of positive findings were 0 percent, 3 percent, and 0 percent for Stage I, II, and III, respectively. The corresponding conversion rates were 8 percent, 26 percent, and 60 percent, respectively, with an average follow-up of 34 months for each stage. They concluded that routine follow-up bone scan in Stage I patients is not warranted but is of value in the follow-up of high-risk patients, especially those with Stages II and III breast cancers and those with pathologically proven positive nodes.

SUMMARY AND CONCLUSIONS

Bone is a common site of metastasis following treatment failure in women with breast cancer. Bone metastases at the time of presentation in patients with Stage I or II breast cancer are uncommon. Preoperative bone scans need not be obtained routinely in patients with Stage I breast cancer but are indicated in patients with symptomatic bone lesions or an elevated alkaline phosphatase level that is specific for bone. Postoperatively and in follow-up, routine bone scans in Stage I patients are not necessary. Bone scans should be obtained in Stage II patients with positive lymph nodes, especially those with four or more positive nodes. These women are at increased risk for future systemic failure, and bone scans will serve both for baseline purposes and for evaluation of adjuvant chemotherapy regimens. It is therefore appropriate to obtain bone scans at yearly intervals in these patients. In Stage I or other Stage II (T_2N_0) patients, routine follow-up bone scans are not indicated. Any patient with breast cancer with either bone symptoms or an elevated alkaline phosphatase level should have a bone scan to evaluate these findings. A normal alkaline phosphatase level in the presence of bone pain, however, does not exclude the possibility of bone metastases. Among patients with positive findings on bone scan, 38 to 62 percent will have normal alkaline phosphatase levels.[178, 193] Patients with Stage III_a or III_b breast cancer should have a bone scan as part of their initial evaluation. The incidence of positive findings on bone scan in this group of patients ranges from 16 to 50 percent.[176, 178, 194–196] These should be repeated at yearly intervals, even in asymptomatic patients after therapy has been initiated, or as indicated by bone symptoms or an elevated alkaline phosphatase level. These patients are at significant risk for bone metastases throughout their lives. The evaluation and management of these patients is also discussed in Chapter 9.

Suspicious abnormalities on bone scans should be further evaluated with skeletal x-rays. This may further characterize the lesion and facilitates localization if a biopsy is indicated. CT scans or MRI usually do not provide additional useful information. If the suspicious lesion is visualized on x-ray and a biopsy is indicated, the biopsy can be performed either by percutaneous needle aspiration (to obtain material for cytologic examination) or by an open biopsy for histologic purposes. The authors prefer to attempt needle aspiration initially; this can be done under local anesthesia, using fluoroscopy to guide the needle. If this is unsuccessful, an open biopsy under general anesthesia can be performed. For lesions that are not visualized on plain-film x-rays, localization for biopsy purposes can be accomplished by placement of overlying radiopaque skin markers with the aid of the bone scan. Radiopaque markers are used if a needle aspiration under fluoroscopic guidance is to be performed. The technique of aspiration and processing of material for cytologic analysis is otherwise the same as for breast lesions (see earlier). A bone biopsy may require decalcification before histologic review can be performed.

Screening for Liver Metastases

The liver represents the third most common site of metastatic disease in breast cancer. Liver metastases are almost always nodular densities that remain asymptomatic until an advanced stage is reached, at which time pain, jaundice, or pruritus may be superimposed. The incidence, size, and extent of liver metastases will, of course, vary with the length of the interval from diagnosis of the breast cancer. The incidence of hepatic metastases in Stage I or II breast cancer at presentation is less than 5 percent (see later). Sears and associates[197] noted that among 84 patients with advanced or metastatic breast cancer who underwent exploratory laparotomy for major endocrine ablation, only six patients had liver metastases. At autopsy, approximately 60 percent of patients with metastatic breast cancer have disease in the liver.[18] Approximately 30 percent of liver metastases at autopsy, however, will be less than 2 cm in diameter.[198]

The screening procedures to detect hepatic metastases include the radioisotopic liver scan, computerized tomography with or without contrast enhancement, MRI, and blood chemistry biomarkers. Liver scanning to screen for space-occupying lesions is most frequently performed with a radiolabeled colloidal material, which is taken up by the reticuloendothelial system.[198] When used to detect metastatic breast cancer the liver scan has a rate of false-negative findings of approximately 19.1 percent (range 13 to 33 percent) and rate of a false-positive findings of 16.2 percent (range 9 to 31 percent).[199–207] False-negative diagnoses are due to limited resolution of the scan, restricted information from regions deep within the liver, and motion. False-positive findings are due predominantly to inflammatory conditions, benign tumors, or unusual anatomic variations. The liver scan, when used to evaluate patients with Stage I or II breast cancer at the time of presentation and in follow-up, has been found to be of little benefit. Nomura and colleagues[206] reviewed liver scans in 129 patients with TNM Stage I, II, or III breast cancer and found not one case of positive findings on scan. On follow-up of 2 to 36 months (mean, 17 months), no patient subsequently developed hepatic metastases. Sears and associates[197] evaluated liver scans in 100 patients and noted five cases of positive findings on scan, only one of which was subsequently proved to represent metastatic disease. Haid and colleagues[208] reviewed 66 patients with breast cancer and found only four who had focal defects on liver scan. Two of these four patients had normal hepatic enzyme levels and had prolonged disease-free survival. Weiner and Sachs[209] reviewed liver scans in 234 patients with primary breast cancer and found 11 scans to be abnormal; for eight of these patients the findings were subsequently proved to be falsely positive, as determined by surgical exploration, biopsy, or subsequent follow-up. Arnstein and associates[191] reviewed serial liver scans in 101 patients who underwent mastectomy and received adjuvant chemotherapy for breast cancer. All patients had negative findings on scan initially. Scan findings of 13 patients converted to positive at an average interval of 31.5 months after surgery. The liver scan was the first indicator of liver involvement in only 3 of 13 cases of conversion. In no case was the liver scan the first indication of metastatic disease. The investigators concluded that liver scans do not appear to be useful for screening patients without other evidence of metastatic liver involvement. Liver scans are thus indicated to evaluate either symptomatic patients or those patients with elevated liver-specific blood chemistries. CT scans similarly should be used only to evaluate abnormalities noted on liver scan. While CT scans are more sensitive procedures, they are costly and time consuming and are not indicated as routine screening procedures for breast cancer.

Liver metastases may be associated with abnormalities in plasma hepatic enzyme levels. These enzymes include alkaline phosphatase, LDH, SGOT, SGPT, 5′-nucleotidase, and γ-glutamyl transpeptidase. Alkaline phosphatase has been the enzyme studied most extensively and is the most useful as an indicator of hepatic metastases. The rate of true-positive findings for alkaline phosphatase levels used to detect hepatic metastases is approximately 78.1 percent (range 64 to 90 percent)[201–203, 207, 210–213]; the rate of false-positive findings is 30.6 percent (range 14 to 41 percent)[202, 203, 207, 210, 213]; and the rate of false-negative findings is 26.5 percent (range 11 to 41 percent).[202, 210] SGOT levels are elevated in 53 to 63 percent of patients with known metastatic liver cancer.[202, 210, 212] Coombes and colleagues[214] studied ten tumor markers in the serum or urine, as follow-up for patients with primary breast cancer. They found only three markers: Alkaline phosphatase, CEA, and γ-glutamyl transpeptidase levels were consistently abnormal prior to the development of detectable metastases in more than one patient. Castagna and associates[202] found that if results of only one of three tests (alkaline phosphatase, albumin, and SGOT) were abnormal, the likelihood of hepatic metastases was 40.7 percent but increased to 92.0 percent if results of all three tests were abnormal.

Liver scans and alkaline phosphatase determinations are of similar value when used as screening procedures for hepatic metastases. Combining these studies does not increase the sensitivity of either test. White and colleagues[210] reviewed liver scans and alkaline phosphatase determinations in 146 patients with breast cancer and found that radioisotopic liver scans are unlikely to provide additional useful information in the staging or follow-up of breast cancer patients in whom the alkaline phosphatase level remains normal. Smith and Williams[201] reviewed liver scans and alkaline phosphatase determinations in 296 patients and concluded that there was little evidence that the liver scan was more accurate than liver enzyme determinations in the diagnosis of hepatic space-occupying lesions. Jhingran and associates[213] noted that the liver scan was as accurate as a combination of scan and liver function tests in detecting hepatic involvement by metastases. The authors use the alkaline phosphatase level (and the CEA level; see later) as an initial screening test for detection of hepatic metastases. If the alkaline phosphatase level is elevated, it should be fractionated into isoenzymes, or a 5′-nucleotidase level should be obtained. If the 5′-nucleotidase level (or the CEA; see later) is elevated, the patient should be further evaluated with a liver scan or CT scan, or both.

Carcinoembryonic antigen (CEA) is a glycoprotein initially identified in association with colon carcinoma but subsequently found to be present in a variety of neoplasms of differing histogenesis, including breast cancer. In 1969, Thomson and associates[215] described a radioimmunoassay by which CEA antigen-antibody complexes could be detected in the plasma of individuals. Since that time plasma CEA levels have been widely used to evaluate patients with breast cancer. Lee[216] reviewed patients with early stage breast cancer and found 3 percent of those with Stage I and 6 percent of those with Stage II disease had elevated (greater than 5 ng/ml) CEA levels. Of those patients who developed recurrent disease, 48 percent had elevated CEA levels. Patients with chest wall recurrences rarely had abnormal CEA levels, whereas patients with visceral metastases had higher CEA levels. Similarly, Beatty and colleagues[217] found that only 15 percent of patients with localized breast cancer and 53 percent of patients with advanced disease had CEA levels greater than 5 ng/ml. The incidence of metastatic disease was 100 percent for patients with CEA levels greater than 25 ng/ml. For patients with localized disease, there was no correlation between CEA level and node positivity versus negativity.

The CEA level, when interpreted in conjunction with the liver scan, may increase the sensitivity of either test. McCartney and Hoffer[218] found that all patients with a CEA level greater than 9 ng/ml and positive findings on liver scan had liver metastases, whereas only 4 of 291 patients with negative findings on liver scan and CEA levels below 9 ng/ml were found to have liver metastases. Sugarbaker and associates[203] found CEA levels to have a rate of true-positive findings of 25 percent. When CEA levels were combined with liver scan, no false-positive findings were observed when results of both tests were abnormal. Plasma CEA levels are thus a useful screening test for patients with breast cancer. If the CEA level is elevated, determination of whether it represents hepatic metastatic disease can be confirmed with a liver scan. Coombes and colleagues[214] found that CEA, alkaline phosphatase, and γ-glutamyl transpeptidase determinations combined with findings of physical examination and chest x-ray were the best indices of the metastatic state in breast cancer patients, being collectively abnormal in 98 percent of patients at first presentation with metastases. They recommended screening patients postoperatively for metastases with these five tests; more detailed tests should be carried out only if results of one or more of these tests are abnormal.

In summary, patients with Stage I breast cancer can be effectively screened for hepatic metastases, both preoperatively and in follow-up, with a complete history and physical examination and alkaline phosphatase, γ-glutamyl transpeptidase, and CEA determinations. Any abnormalities detected in this manner can be further evaluated with a liver or CT scan. The incidence of hepatic metastases in Stage II patients at presentation is also low, and therefore these patients should have the same evaluation preoperatively as in Stage I patients. Postoperatively, a routine baseline liver scan is appropriate in patients with positive lymph nodes, especially those with four or more positive nodes. These patients are at increased risk for hepatic metastases at some point in their lives, and a baseline liver scan will be of value for comparative purposes. Subsequent liver scans should be obtained as indicated by findings on history and physical examination and blood chemistries. All patients with Stage III_a or III_b breast cancer should have a liver scan as part of their initial evaluation. Because many of these patients are now treated with combined-modality therapy, the scheduling of follow-up liver scans will be determined by their response to therapy, and by the findings on physical examination and serum and plasma chemistries.

Summary and Recommendations

Patients with Stage I or II breast cancer can be easily and effectively screened preoperatively for metastasis in lung, bone, or liver with a complete history and physical examination and blood chemistries (Table 4–15). Because the incidence of metastases to these sites in patients with Stage I or II breast cancer at presentation is low, negative findings on this evaluation do not need to be corroborated by radionuclide scans or tomography. Patients with abnormalities on any part of this evaluation should be further evaluated with bone or liver scans or full-lung or computerized tomography, as suggested by the abnormality. Postoperatively, patients with Stage II (T_1 or T_2/N_1) breast cancer should have a baseline bone and liver scan. Subsequent bone scans are recom-

TABLE 4–15. Suggested Follow-up Schedule for Patients with Stage I or II Breast Cancer

Procedures	Initial Examination Month	Year 1 (Monthly Intervals) 3	6	9	12	Year 2 (Monthly Intervals) 3	6	9	12	Year 3 (Monthly Intervals) 3	6	9	12	Subsequent Years (Monthly Intervals) 6	12
History															
Complete	X				X				X				X		X
Family	X														
Chest wall	X	X	X	X	X	X	X	X	X	X	X	X	X	X	X
Arm	X		X		X		X		X		X		X	X	X
Cough/dyspnea	X	X	X	X	X	X	X	X	X	X	X	X	X	X	X
Pain	X														
Pelvic/rectal symptoms	X				X				X				X		X
Breast self-examination	X	X	X	X	X	X	X	X	X	X	X	X	X	X	X
Physical examination															
Complete	X				X				X				X		X
Pulse, blood pressure, weight	X				X										
Breast/chest wall	X	X	X	X	X	X	X	X	X	X	X	X	X	X	X
Axillary, supraclavicular,	X	X	X	X	X	X	X	X	X	X	X	X	X	X	X
parasternal areas	X				X										
Arm	X				X										
Lung bases	X		X		X		X		X		X		X	X	X
Liver size	X				X				X				X		X
Pelvic and rectal	X				X				X				X		X
Diagnostic Studies	X														
CBC, platelets	X				X				X				X		X
Blood chemistries	X				X				X				X		X
Mammogram	X				X				X				X		X
Chest x-ray	X				X				X				X		X
Pap test	X				X				X				X		X
Occult blood in stool	X				X				X				X		X
Bone scan	X*				X†				X†				X†		X†
Liver scan	X*														

*Postoperatively in Stage II patients with histologically positive lymph nodes
†In follow-up in Stage II patients with histologically positive nodes
Adapted from Horton J: Follow-up of breast cancer patients. Cancer 53:790, 1984.

mended at yearly intervals. Routine liver scans are not recommended but should be obtained as indicated by findings on history and physical examination and blood chemistries.

All patients who have been treated for Stage I or II breast cancer should be followed at regular intervals with a complete history and physical examination. We recommend visits every three months during the first three years, every four to six months during the next two years, and at yearly intervals thereafter. Blood chemistries, including plasma alkaline phosphatase, CEA, and γ-glutamyl transpeptidase levels, should be determined at six-month intervals. A chest x-ray should also be obtained at yearly intervals, principally because it is an important part of a general medical examination (for evaluation of heart, mediastinum, lungs, and bony thorax) rather than because it represents a productive screening procedure for metastatic breast cancer. This schedule will allow effective follow-up of patients with breast cancer, without subjecting them to costly and time-consuming studies that are apt to be of little benefit.

REFERENCES

1. Fisher B, Wolmark N, Bauer M, et al.: The accuracy of clinical nodal staging and of limited axillary dissection as a determinant of histological nodal status in carcinoma of the breast. Surg Gynecol Obstet 152:765, 1981.
2. Beahrs OH, Myers MH (eds.): Manual for Staging of Cancer: American Joint Committee on Cancer, 2nd ed. Philadelphia: J.B. Lippincott Co., 1983, pp. 127–133.
3. Haagensen CD: Diseases of the Breast, 2nd ed. Philadelphia: W.B. Saunders Co., 1971, p. 630.
4. Windeyer BW: Cancer of the breast. Am J Roentgenol Radium Ther Nucl Med 62:345, 1949.
5. Beahrs OH, Myers MH (eds): Manual for Staging of Cancer: American Joint Committee on Cancer, 2nd ed. Philadelphia: J.B. Lippincott Co., 1983, pp. 127–133.
6. Donegan WL: Diagnosis: *In*: Donegan WL, Spratt JS (eds.): Cancer of the Breast, 2nd ed. Philadelphia: W.B. Saunders Co., 1979, p. 50.
7. Haagensen CD: Diseases of the Breast, 2nd ed. Philadelphia: W.B. Saunders Co., 1971, p. 630.
8. Henderson C, Canellos GP: Carcinoma of the breast: The past decade. N Engl J Med 302:17, 1980.
9. Vana J, Bedwani R, Mettlin C, et al.: Trends in diagnosis and management of breast cancer in the U.S.: From the surveys on the American College of Surgeons. Cancer 48:1043, 1981.
10. Haagensen CD: Diseases of the Breast, 2nd ed. Philadelphia: W.B. Saunders Co., 1971, p. 467.
11. Preece PE, Mansel RE, Bolton PM, et al.: Clinical syndromes of mastalgia. Lancet 2:670, 1976.
12. Haagensen CD: Diseases of the Breast, 2nd ed. Philadelphia: W.B. Saunders Co., 1971, p. 124.
13. Haagensen CD: Diseases of the Breast, 2nd ed. Philadelphia: W.B. Saunders Co., 1971, pp. 545–569.
14. Ashikari R, Park K, Huvos AG, et al.: Paget's disease of the breast. Cancer 26:680, 1970.
15. Satiani S, Powell RW, Mathews WH: Paget's disease of the male breast. Arch Surg 112:587, 1977.
16. Muir R: Further observations on Paget's disease of the nipple. J Pathol Bacteriol 49:299, 1939.
17. Haagensen CD: Diseases of the Breast, 2nd ed. Philadelphia: W.B. Saunders Co., 1971, p. 401.
18. Danforth DN, Jr., Findlay PA, McDonald HD, et al.: Complete axillary lymph node dissection for stage I, II carcinoma of the breast. J Clin Oncol 4:655, 1986.
19. Jessiman AG: The breast. *In* Warren R (ed.): Surgery. Philadelphia: W.B. Saunders Co., 1963, p. 720.
20. Haagensen CD: Diseases of the Breast, 2nd ed. Philadelphia: W.B. Saunders Co., 1971, p. 426.
21. Haagensen CD, Bodian C, Haagensen DE: Breast Carcinoma: Risk and Detection. Philadelphia: W.B. Saunders Co., 1981, pp. 460–472.
22. Goldstein DP, Miler V: Breast masses in adolescent females. Clin Pediatr 21:17, 1982.
23. Oberman HA: Breast lesions in the adolescent female. Pathol Annu 14:175, 1979.
24. Dewhurst J: Breast disorders in children and adolescents. Pediatr Clin North Am 28:287, 1981.
25. Turbey WJ, Buntain WL, Dudgeon DL: The surgical management of pediatric breast masses. Pediatrics 56:736, 1975.
26. Donegan WL: Diagnosis. *In* Donegan WL, Spratt JS (eds.): Cancer of the Breast, 2nd ed. Philadelphia: W.B. Saunders Co., 1979, p. 51.
27. Scher KS: Outpatient breast biopsies: A selective approach. Milit Med 144:823, 1979.
28. Haagensen CD: Diseases of the Breast, 2nd ed. Philadelphia: W.B. Saunders Co., 1971, p. 101.
29. Mitchell GW, Homer MJ: Outpatient breast biopsies on a gynecologic service. Am J Obstet Gynecol 144:127, 1982.
30. Baker RR: Outpatient breast biopsies. Ann Surg 185:543, 1977.
31. Abramson DJ: 857 breast biopsies as an outpatient procedure: Delayed mastectomy in 41 malignant cases. Ann Surg 163:478, 1966.
32. Love SM, Gelman RS, Silen W: Fibrocystic "disease" of the breast—a nondisease. N Engl J Med 307:1010, 1982.
33. Winchester DP, Sener S, Immerman S, et al.: A systematic approach to the evaluation and management of breast masses. Cancer 51:2535, 1983.
34. Kagali VA: The role and limitations of frozen section diagnosis of a palpable mass in the breast. Surg Gynecol Obstet 156:168, 1983.
35. Coates MR, Pilch YH, Benfield JR: Changing concepts in establishing the diagnosis of breast masses. Am J Surg 134:77, 1977.
36. Hermann RE, Esselstyn CB: Crile G, Jr., et al.: Results of conservative operations for breast cancer. Arch Surg 120:746, 1985.
37. Baker HL: The Breast Cancer Detection Demonstration Projects: Five-year summary report. CA 32:194, 1982.

38. Sickles EA, Klein DL, Goodsen WH, et al.: Mammography after needle aspiration of palpable breast masses. Am J Surg 145:395, 1983.
39. Moskowitz M: Minimal breast cancer redux. Radiol Clin North Am 21:93, 1983.
40. Sokol ES, Walker B, Terz JJ, et al.: Role of mammography with palpable breast lesions. Surgery 67:748, 1970.
41. Egan RL: Mammography: An aid to early diagnosis of breast carcinoma. JAMA 182:839, 1962.
42. Clark RL, Copeland MM, Egan RL, et al.: Reproducibility of the technique of mammography (Egan) for cancer of the breast. Am J Surg 109:127, 1965.
43. Kreuzer G, Boquoi E: Aspiration biopsy cytology, mammography, and clinical exploration: A modern setup in diagnosis of tumors of the breast. Acta Cytol 20:319, 1976.
44. Hahn P, Hallberg O, Schnürer LB: Combination of clinical examination, mammography, and aspiration cytology in the diagnosis of carcinoma of the breast (179 cases). Strahlentherapie 156:475, 1980.
45. Johnsen C, Bjurstam N: Diagnostic methods in breast cancer. World J Surg 1:290, 1977.
46. Shabot MM, Goldberg IM, Schick P, et al.: Aspiration cytology is superior to Tru-Cut needle biopsy in establishing the diagnosis of clinically suspicious breast masses. Ann Surg 196:122, 1982.
47. Robbins GF: Diagnosis of potentially curable breast carcinoma. *In*: Robbins GF (ed.): Breast Cancer Monography. New York: Memorial Hospital for Cancer and Allied Diseases, 1973, pp. 25–31.
48. Colbassani HJ, Feller WF, Cigtay OS, et al.: Mammographic and pathologic correlation of microcalcifications in disease of the breast. Surg Gynecol Obstet 155:689, 1982.
49. Frankl G, Ackerman M: Xeromammography and 1200 breast cancers. Radiol Clin North Am 21:81, 1983.
50. Wolfe JN: Xeroradiography of the breast. Springfield, IL: Charles C Thomas, Publisher, 1972, p. 5.
51. Kobayashi T: Gray-scale echography for breast cancer. Radiology 122:207, 1977.
52. Jellins J, Kossoff G, Reeve TS: Detection and classification of liquid-filled masses in the breast by gray-scale echography. Radiology 125:205, 1977.
53. Cole-Beuglet C, Soriano RZ, Kurtz AB, et al: Ultrasound analysis of 104 breast carcinomas classified according to histopathologic type. Radiology 147:91, 1983.
54. McSweeney MB, Murphy CH: Whole-breast sonography. Radiol Clin North Am 23:157, 1985.
55. Sickles EA, Filly RA, Callen PW: Breast cancer detection with sonography and mammography: Comparison using state-of-the-art equipment. AJR 140:843, 1983.
56. Teixidor HS, Kazam E: Combined mammographic-sonographic evaluation of breast masses. Am J Roentgenol 128:409, 1977.
57. Kobayashi T, Takatani O, Hattori H, et al: Differential diagnosis of breast tumors: The sensitivity graded method of ultrasonotomography and clinical evaluation of its diagnostic accuracy. Cancer 33:940, 1974.
58. Jellins J, Reeve TS, Croll J, et al.: Results of breast echographic examinations in Sydney, Australia: 1972–79. Semin Ultrasound 3:58, 1982.
59. Kopans DB, Meyer JE, Sadowski N: Breast imaging. N Engl J Med 310:960, 1984.
60. Rosner D: Ultrasonography in diagnosis and management of palpable breast masses. NY State J Med 81:1066, 1981.
61. Harper P, Kelly-Fry E: Ultrasound visualization of the breast. Radiology 137:465, 1980.
62. Isard HJ, Ostrum BJ: Breast thermography: The mammatherm. Radiol Clin North Am 12:167, 1977.
63. Amalric R, Brandone H, Robert F, et al.: Dynamic telethermography of 2200 breast cancers. Acta Thermogr 3:46, 1978.
64. Davison TW, Ewing KL, Fergason J, et al.: Detection of breast cancer by liquid crystal thermography. Cancer 29:1123, 1972.
65. Sterns EE, Curtis AC, Miller S, et al.: Thermography in breast cancer. Cancer 50:323, 1982.
66. Fournier VD, Kubli F, Klapp J, et al.: Infra-red thermography and breast cancer doubling time. Acta Thermogr 3:107, 1978.
67. Amalric R, Giraud D, Thomassin L, et al.: The persistently abnormal isolated thermogram: The highest known risk of cancer. Acta Thermogr 7:91, 1982.
68. Moskowitz M, Milbrath J, Gartside P, et al.: Lack of efficacy of thermography as a screening tool for minimal and stage I breast cancer. N Engl J Med 295:249, 1976.
69. Martin RE, Graham R: Office evaluation of breast tumors, with emphasis on needle aspiration therapy. Md State Med J 31:51, 1982.
70. Ulanow RM, Galblum L, Canter JW: Fine-needle aspiration in the diagnosis and management of solid breast lesions. Am J Surg 148:653, 1984.
71. Frable WJ: Thin-needle aspiration biopsy: A personal experience with 469 cases. Am J Clin Pathol 65:168, 1976.
72. Berg JW, Robbins GF: A late look at the safety of aspiration biopsy. Cancer 15:826, 1962.
73. Strawbridge HTG, Bassett AA, Foldes I: Role of cytology in management of lesions of the breast. Surg Gynecol Obstet 152:1, 1981.
74. Kline TS, Joshi LP, Neal HS: Fine-needle aspiration of the breast: Diagnosis and pitfalls: A review of 3545 cases. Cancer 44:1458, 1979.
75. Gatchell FG, Dockerty MB, Clagett OT: Intracystic carcinoma of the breast. Surg Gynecol Obstet 106:347, 1958.
76. Rosemond GP, Maier WP, Brobyn TJ: Needle aspiration of breast cysts. Surg Gynecol Obstet 128:351, 1969.
77. Tong D: The treatment of solitary cysts in the breast: A new technique. Br J Surg 56:885, 1969.
78. Thomas JM, Fitzharris BM, Redding WH, et al.: Clinical examination, mammography, and fine-needle aspiration cytology in diagnosis of breast tumors. Br Med J 2:1139, 1978.
79. Johnsen C: Diagnostic accuracy of clinical examination, mammography and aspiration biopsy, and the effect of combining these methods. Acta Chir Scand (Suppl) 454:56, 1975.
80. Zajicek J: Aspiration Biopsy Cytology. Basel, Switzerland: S Karger AG, 1974.
81. Gardecki TIM, Melcher DH, Hogbin BM, et al.: Aspiration cytology in the preoperative management of breast cancer. Lancet 2:790, 1980.
82. Kreuzer G, Zajicek J: Cytologic diagnosis of mammary tumors from aspiration biopsy smears III. Studies on 200 carcinomas with false-negative or doubtful cytologic reports. Acta Cytol 16:249, 1972.

83. Davies CJ, Elston CW, Cotton RE, et al: Preoperative diagnosis of carcinoma of the breast. Br J Surg 64:326, 1977.
84. Elston CW, Cotton RE, Davies CJ, et al.: A comparison of the use of the Tru-Cut needle and fine-needle aspiration cytology in the preoperative diagnosis of carcinoma of the breast. Histopathology 2:239, 1978.
85. Roberts JG, Preece PE, Bolton PM, et al.: The "Tru-Cut" biopsy in breast cancer. Clin Oncol 1:297, 1975.
86. Nora PF (ed.): Operative Surgery: Principles and Techniques, 2nd ed. Philadelphia: Lea & Febiger, 1980, pp. 177–183.
87. Gonzales E, Grafton WD, Morris DM, et al.: Diagnosing breast cancer using frozen sections from Tru-Cut needle biopsies. Ann Surg 202:696, 1985.
88. George WD, Burn JI: Drill biopsy in the diagnosis of breast cancer. Clin Oncol 1:291, 1975.
89. Sieinski W, Danska M: Usefulness of drill biopsy in the diagnosis of breast tumors. Cancer 38:2567, 1976.
90. Haagensen CD: Diseases of the Breast, 2nd ed. Philadelphia: W.B. Saunders Co., 1971, pp. 149–154.
91. Walker GM, Foster RS, McKegney CP, et al.: Breast biopsy: A comparison of outpatient and inpatient experience. Arch Surg 113:942, 1978.
92. Hunt TK, Cross RA: Breast biopsies on outpatients. Surg Gynecol Obstet 141:591, 1975.
93. Stein HD: Ambulatory breast biopsies: The patient's choice. Am Surg 48:221, 1982.
94. Lou MA, Mandal AK, Alexander JL: The pros and cons of outpatient breast biopsy. Arch Surg 111:668, 1976.
95. Scanlon EF: The case for and against two-step procedure for the surgical treatment of breast cancer. Cancer 53:677, 1984.
96. Kagali VA: The role and limitations of frozen section diagnosis of a palpable mass in the breast. Surg Gynecol Obstet 156:168, 1983.
97. Bauermeister DE: The role and limitations of frozen section and needle aspiration in breast cancer diagnosis. Cancer 40:947, 1980.
98. Agnantis NJ, Apostolikas N, Christodoulou I, et al.: The reliability of frozen section diagnosis in various breast lesions: A study based on 3451 biopsies. Recent Results Cancer Res 90:205, 1984.
99. Doberneck RC: Breast biopsy: A study of cost effectiveness. Ann Surg 192:152, 1980.
100. Pierce EH, Clagett OT, McDonald JR: Biopsy of the breast followed by delayed radical mastectomy. Surg Gynecol Obstet 103:559, 1956.
101. Jackson PP, Pitts HH: Biopsy with delayed radical mastectomy for carcinoma of the breast. Am J Surg 98:184, 1959.
102. Caffee HH, Benfield JR: Data favoring biopsy of the breast under local anesthesia. Surg Gynecol Obstet 140:88, 1975.
103. Bertario L, Reduzzi D, Piromalli D, et al.: Outpatient biopsy of breast cancer: Influence on survival. Ann Surg 201:64, 1985.
104. Chaudary MA, Millis RR, Davies GC, et al.: Nipple discharge: The diagnostic value of testing for occult blood. Ann Surg 196:651, 1982.
105. Geschickter CF (quoted by Hinckley PR): Nipple discharge. Ann Surg 113:301, 1941.
106. Donnelly BA: Nipple discharge: Its clinical and pathological significance. Ann Surg 181:342, 1950.
107. Haagensen CD: Diseases of the Breast, 2nd ed. Philadelphia: W.B. Saunders Co., 1971, pp. 102–103.
108. Leis HP, Pilnik S: Nipple discharge. Hosp Pract 6:29, 1970.
109. Leis HP, Pilnik S, Dursi J, et al.: Nipple discharge. Int Surg 58:162, 1973.
110. Urban JA, Egeli RA: Non-lactational nipple discharge. CA 28:130, 1978.
111. Rosemond GP, Maier WP: Nonlactational nipple discharge. Breast 1:23, 1975.
112. Rimsten A, Skoog V, Stenkvist B: On the significance of nipple discharge in the diagnosis of breast disease. Acta Chir Scand 142:513, 1976.
113. Copeland MM, Higgins CG: Significance of discharge from the nipple in nonpuerperal mammary conditions. Ann Surg 151:638, 1960.
114. Takeda T, Suzuki M, Sato Y, et al.: Cytologic studies of nipple discharges. Acta Cytol 26:35, 1980.
115. Uei Y, Watanabe Y, Hirota T, et al.: Cytologic diagnosis of breast carcinoma with nipple discharge: Special significance of the spherical cell cluster. Acta Cytol 24:522, 1980.
116. Muller JWT, In der Maur GAP: Pathological secretion of the breast. Diagn Imaging 51:62, 1982.
117. Papanicolaou NA: Pathological secretion of the breast. Panminerva Medica (Turin) 19:275, 1977.
118. Saphir O: Cytologic examination of breast secretion. Am J Clin Pathol 20:1001, 1950.
119. Barnes AB: Diagnosis and treatment of abnormal breast secretions. N Engl J Med 275:1184, 1966.
120. Kjellogren O: Cytologic diagnosis of cancer of the breast. Acta Cytol 8:216, 1964.
121. Taber L, Kadas I, Marton Z, et al.: The significance of mammography, galactography, and pneumocystography in detecting occult carcinomas of the breast. Surg Gynecol Obstet 137:965, 1973.
122. Taber L, Marton Z, Kadas I: Galactography in the examination of secretory breasts. Am J Surg 127:282, 1974.
123. Nunnerly HB, Field S: Mammary duct injection in patients with nipple discharge. Br J Radiol 45:717, 1972.
124. Funderburk WW, Syphax B: Evaluation of nipple discharge in benign and malignant conditions. Cancer 24:1290, 1969.
125. Bjorn-Hansen R: Contrast mammography. Br J Radiol 38:947, 1965.
126. Paulus D: Nipple discharge in relation to breast disease. Ninth Annual Seminar on Cancer of the Breast. Denver, Colorado, 1970.
127. Threatt B: Ductography. *In*: Bassett LW, Gold RH (eds.): Mammography, Thermography, and Ultrasonography in Breast Cancer Detection. New York: Grune & Stratton, 1982, pp. 109–119.
128. Lundgren B: Malignant features of breast tumors at radiography. Acta Radiol (Diagn) 19:623, 1978.
129. Schwartz GF, Feif SA, Patchefsky AS: Clinicopathologic correlations and significance of clinically occult mammary lesions. Cancer 41:1147, 1978.
130. Homer MJ: Nonpalpable breast abnormalities: A realistic view of the accuracy of mammography in detecting malignancies. Radiology 153:831, 1984.
131. Powell RW, McSweeney MB, Wilson CE: X-ray calcifications as the only basis for breast biopsy. Ann Surg 197:555, 1983.
132. Rasmussen OS, Seerup A: Preoperative radiographically guided wire marking of nonpalpable breast lesions. Acta Radiol (Diagn) 25:13, 1984.

133. Goldberg RP, Hall FM, Simon M: Preoperative localization of nonpalpable breast lesions using a wire marker and perforated mammographic grid. Radiology 146:833, 1983.
134. Blichert-Toft M, Dyreborg U, Bogh L, et al.: Nonpalpable breast lesions: Mammographic wire-guided biopsy and radiologic-histologic correlation. World J Surg 6:119, 1982.
135. Svane G: A stereotaxic technique for preoperative marking of nonpalpable breast lesions. Acta Radiol Diagn 24:145, 1983.
136. Peyester RG: Needle localization of nonpalpable lesions of the breast. Surg Gynecol Obstet 148:703, 1979.
137. Bigongiari LR, Fidler W, Skerker LB, et al.: Percutaneous needle localization of breast lesions prior to biopsy: Analysis of failures. Clin Radiol 28:419, 1977.
138. Libshitz HI, Feig SA, Fetouh S: Needle localization of nonpalpable breast lesions. Radiology 121:557, 1976.
139. Lefor AT, Numann PJ, Levinsohn EM: Needle localization of occult breast lesions. Am J Surg 148:270, 1984.
140. Homer MJ: Localization of nonpalpable breast lesions: Technical aspects and analysis of 80 cases. AJR 140:807, 1983.
141. Meyer JE, Kopans DB, Stomper PC, et al.: Occult breast abnormalities: Percutaneous preoperative needle localization. Radiology 150:335, 1984.
142. Frank HA, Hall FM, Steer ML: Preoperative localization of nonpalpable breast lesions demonstrated by mammography. N Engl J Med 295:259, 1976.
143. Hoehn JL, Hardacre JM, Swanson MK, et al.: Localization of occult breast lesions. Cancer 49:1142, 1982.
144. Chetty U, Kirkpatrick AE, Anderson TL, et al.: Localization and excision of occult breast lesions. Br J Surg 70:607, 1983.
145. Raininko R, Linna MI, Rasanen O: Preoperative localization of nonpalpable breast tumors. Acta Chir Scand 142:575, 1976.
146. Egan JF, Sayler CB, Goodman MJ: A technique for localizing occult breast lesions. CA 26:31, 1976.
147. Gallager HS: Breast specimen radiography: Obligatory, adjuvant and investigative. Am J Clin Pathol 64:749, 1975.
148. Bauermeister DE, Hall MH: Specimen radiography—a mandatory adjunct to mammography. Am J Clin Pathol 59:782, 1973.
149. Rosen PP, Snyder RE, Robbins G: Specimen radiography for nonpalpable breast lesions found by mammography: Procedures and results. Cancer 34:2028, 1974.
150. Prorok JJ, Trostle DR, Scarlato M, et al.: Excisional breast biopsy and roentgenographic examination for mammographically detected microcalcifications. Am J Surg 145:684, 1983.
151. Pitzen RH, Urdaneta LF, Al-Jurf AS, et al.: Specimen xeroradiography after needle localization and biopsy of noncalcified, nonpalpable breast lesions. Am Surg 51:50, 1985.
152. Haagensen CD: Diseases of the Breast, 2nd ed. Philadelphia: W.B. Saunders Co., 1971, p. 450.
153. Wanebo HJ, Senofsky GM, Fechner RE, et al.: Bilateral breast cancer: Risk reduction by contralateral biopsy. Ann Surg 201:667, 1985.
154. Fisher ER, Fisher B, Sass R, et al.: Pathologic findings from the National Surgical Adjuvant Breast Project (Protocol No. BO4). XI: Bilateral breast cancer. Cancer 54:3002, 1984.
155. Robbins GF, Berg SW: Bilateral primary breast cancers: A prospective clinico-pathological study. Cancer 17:1501, 1964.
156. Martin JK, van Heerden JA, Gaffey TA: Synchronous and metachronous carcinoma of the breast. Surgery 91:12, 1982.
157. Schell SR, Montague ED, Spanos WJ, et al.: Bilateral breast cancer in patients with initial stage I and II disease. Cancer 50:1191, 1982.
158. Newman W: In situ lobular carcinoma of the breast: Report of 26 women with 32 cancers. Ann Surg 157:591, 1963.
159. Ashikari R, Huvos AG, Snyder RE: Prospective study of noninfiltrating carcinoma of the breast. Cancer 39:435, 1977.
160. Snyder RE: Mammography and lobular carcinoma in situ. Surg Gynecol Obstet 22:255, 1966.
161. Urban JA: Biopsy of the "normal" breast in treating breast cancer. Surg Clin North Am 49:291, 1969.
162. Barnes JP: Bilateral lobular carcinoma in situ of the breast. Texas J Med 55:581, 1959.
163. Benfield JR, Jacobsen M, Wraner NE: In situ lobular carcinoma of the breast. Arch Surg 91:130, 1965.
164. Urban JA, Papachristou D, Taylor J: Bilateral breast cancer: Biopsy of the opposite breast. Cancer 40:1968, 1977.
165. Leis HP: Managing the remaining breast. Cancer 46:1026, 1980.
166. King RE, Terz JJ, Lawrence W: Experience with opposite breast biopsy in patients with operable breast cancer. Cancer 37:43, 1976.
167. Haagensen CD: Diseases of the Breast, 2nd ed. Philadelphia: W.B. Saunders Co., 1971, pp. 427–432.
168. Casey JJ, Stempel BG, Scanlon EF, et al.: The solitary pulmonary nodule in the patient with breast cancer. Surgery 96:801, 1984.
169. Cahan WG, Castro EB, Huvos AG: Primary breast and lung carcinoma in the same patient. J Thorac Cardiovasc Surg 68:546, 1974.
170. Tesaro-Tess JD, Valagussa P, Gardani G, et al.: Usefulness of chest and skeletal survey to assess the time of relapse in breast cancer. Tumori (Milan) 67:35, 1981.
171. Ciatto S, Herd-Smith A: The role of chest x-ray in follow-up of primary breast cancer. Tumori (Milan) 69:151, 1983.
172. Chaudary MA, Maisey MN, Shaw PJ, et al.: Sequential bone scans and chest radiographs in the postoperative management of early breast cancer. Br J Surg 70:517, 1983.
173. Staley CJ: Skeletal metastases in cancer of the breast. Surg Gynecol Obstet 102:683, 1956.
174. Sutherland CG, Decker FH, Cilley EI: Metastatic malignant lesions in bone. Am J Cancer 16:1457, 1932.
175. Haagensen CD: Diseases of the Breast, 2nd ed. Philadelphia: W.B. Saunders Co., 1971, pp. 433–436.
176. Lee YT: Bone scanning in patients with early breast cancer: Should it be a routine staging procedure? Cancer 47:486, 1981.
177. Bachman AL, Sproul EE: Correlation of radiographic and autopsy findings in suspected metastases in the spine. NY Acad Med Bull 31:146, 1955.

178. Baker R: Preoperative assessment of the patient with breast cancer. Surg Clin North Am 58:681, 1978.
179. O'Mara RE: Skeletal scanning in neoplastic disease. Cancer 37:480, 1976.
180. Lindholm A, Lundell L, Martenson B, et al.: Skeletal scintigraphy in the initial assessment of women with breast cancer. Acta Chir Scand 145:65, 1979.
181. Harbert JC: Efficacy of bone and liver scanning in malignant diseases: Facts and opinions. *In*: Freeman LM, Weissman HS (eds.): Nuclear Medicine Annual. New York: Raven Press, 1982, pp. 373–401.
182. Campbell DJ, Banks AJ, Oates GD: The value of preliminary bone scanning in staging and assessing the prognosis of breast cancer. Br J Surg 63:811, 1976.
183. Shirazi PH, Rayudu GV, Fordham EW: Review of solitary ^{18}F bone scan lesions. Radiology 112:369, 1974.
184. Corcoran RJ, Thrall JH, Kyle RW, et al.: Solitary abnormalities in bone scans of patients with extraosseous malignancies. Radiology 121:663, 1976.
185. Khandekar JD: Role of routine bone scans in operable breast cancer: An opposing viewpoint. Cancer Treat Rep 63:1241, 1979.
186. Rappaport AH, Hoffer PB, Genant HK: Unifocal bone findings by scintigraphy—clinical significance in patients with known primary cancer. West J Med 129:188, 1978.
187. Monypenny IJ, Grieve RJ, Howell A, et al.: The value of serial bone scanning in operable breast cancer. Br J Surg 71:466, 1984.
188. Schaffer DL, Kalisher L: Incidence of bone metastases in women with minimal and occult breast carcinoma. Radiology 124:675, 1977.
189. Schutte HE: The influence of bone pain on the results of bone scans. Cancer 44:2039, 1979.
190. Bishop HM, Blamey RW, Morris AH, et al.: Bone scanning: Its lack of value in the followup of patients with breast cancer. Br J Surg 66:752, 1979.
191. Arnstein NB, Harbert JC, Byrne PJ: Efficacy of bone and liver scanning in breast cancer patients treated with adjuvant chemotherapy. Cancer 54:2243, 1984.
192. Coker DD, Lambrecht RW, Kehn BD: The value of initial and followup bone scans in patients with operable breast cancer. Milit Med 145:492, 1980.
193. Cowan RJ, Young KA: Evaluation of serum alkaline phosphatase determinations in patients with positive bone scans. Cancer 32:887, 1973.
194. Gerber FH, Goodreau JJ, Kirchner PT, et al.: Efficacy of preoperative and postoperative bone scanning in the management of breast carcinoma. N Engl J Med 297:300, 1977.
195. Clark DG, Painter RW, Sziklas JJ: Indications for bone scans in preoperative evaluation of breast cancer. Am J Surg 135:667, 1978.
196. McNeil BJ, Pace PD, Gray EB, et al.: Preoperative and followup bone scans in patients with primary carcinoma of the breast. Surg Gynecol Obstet 147:745, 1978.
197. Sears HF, Gerber FH, Sturtz DL, et al.: Liver scan and carcinoma of the breast. Surg Gynecol Obstet 140:409, 1975.
198. Ozardo A, Picksen J: The topographic distribution of liver metastases in relation to surgical and isotope diagnosis. J Nucl Med 3:149, 1962.
199. Viamonte M, Schiff E: Diagnostic approach to hepatic neoplasms. JAMA 238:2191, 1977.
200. Lunia S, Parthasarathy KL, Bender MA: An evaluation of ^{99m}Tc sulfur colloid liver scintiscans and their usefulness in metastatic workup: A review of 1424 studies. J Nucl Med 16:62, 1975.
201. Smith LB, Williams RD: The relative diagnostic accuracy of liver radioactive isotope photoscanning. Arch Surg 96:693, 1968.
202. Castagna J, Benfield JR, Yamada H, et al.: The reliability of liver scans and function tests in detecting metastases. Surg Gynecol Obstet 134:463, 1972.
203. Sugarbaker PH, Beard JO, Drum DE: Detection of hepatic metastases from cancer of the breast. Am J Surg 133:531, 1977.
204. Ruiter DJ, Byck W, Pauwels EK, et al.: Correlation of scintigraphy with short interval autopsy in malignant focal liver disease: A study of 59 cases. Cancer 39:172, 1977.
205. Drum DE, Beard JM: Scintigraphic criteria for hepatic metastases from cancer of the colon and breast. J Nucl Med 17:677, 1976.
206. Nomura Y, Kondo H, Yamagata J, et al.: Evaluation of liver and bone scanning in patients with early breast cancer, based on results obtained from more advanced cancer patients. Eur J Cancer 14:1129, 1978.
207. Ferrier FL, Hatcher CR, Achord JL, et al.: The value of liver scanning for detection of metastatic cancer. Am Surg 35:112, 1969.
208. Haid M, Singh J, Nevinny HB: Liver scanning in newly diagnosed breast cancer. J Surg Oncol 13:265, 1980.
209. Weiner SN, Sachs SH: An assessment of routine liver scanning in patients with breast cancer. Arch Surg 113:126, 1978.
210. White DR, Maloney JJ, Muss HB, et al.: Serum alkaline phosphatase determination. Value in the staging of advanced breast cancer. JAMA 242:1147, 1979.
211. Stehlin JS, Hafstrom L, Greeff P: Experience with infusion and resection in cancer of the liver. Surg Gynecol Obstet 138:855, 1974.
212. Fenster L, Klatskin G: Manifestations of metastatic tumors of the liver. Am J Med 31:238, 1961.
213. Jhingran SG, Jordan L, Jahns MF, et al.: Liver scintigrams compared with alkaline phosphatase and BSP determinations in the detection of metastatic carcinoma. J Nucl Med 12:227, 1971.
214. Coombes RC, Powles TJ, Gazet JC, et al.: Screening for metastases in breast cancer: An assessment of biochemical and physical methods. Cancer 48:310, 1981.
215. Thomson DM, Krupey J, Freedman SO, et al.: The radioimmunoassay of circulating carcinoembryonic antigen of the human digestive system. Proc Natl Acad Sci 64:161, 1969.
216. Lee YT: Carcinoembryonic antigen as a monitor of recurrent breast cancer. J Surg Oncol 20:109, 1982.
217. Beatty JD, Romero C, Broan PW, et al.: Clinical value of carcinoembryonic antigen: Diagnosis, prognosis, and followup of patients with cancer. Arch Surg 114:563, 1979.
218. McCartney WH, Hoffer PB: Carcinoembryonic antigen assay in hepatic metastases detection. JAMA 236:1023, 1976.
219. Horton J: Follow-up of breast cancer patients. Cancer 53:790, 1984.

Surgical Treatment of Breast Cancer

DAVID N. DANFORTH, JR., M.D.
MARC E. LIPPMAN, M.D.

5

Surgery plays a major role in virtually all aspects of the diagnosis and treatment of breast cancer. Surgeons usually have patients referred to them for the evaluation of breast abnormalities and to obtain specimens from primary breast lesions for diagnostic purposes. A careful initial evaluation will define the abnormality and indicate which procedure should be used to obtain material for cytologic and histologic analyses. The initial evaluation will also indicate the appropriate diagnostic studies (radiographic and radionuclide examinations). For malignant lesions, this approach will result in accurate clinical staging. The diagnosis of breast abnormalities and the evaluation of the patient suspected of having breast cancer are discussed in detail in Chapter 4.

The present chapter is concerned with the surgical management of the patient with a breast malignancy. The surgical treatment of breast cancer includes removal of breast tissue, tissues adjacent to the malignancy, and the regional lymph nodes. Because of differing concepts of the biology of breast cancer and based on the anatomic relationships of the breast to adjacent tissue, many surgical procedures have been introduced for primary treatment. These include the Halsted radical mastectomy, the extended radical mastectomy, the superradical mastectomy, the modified radical mastectomy, the total (simple) mastectomy, and the partial (segmental) mastectomy. While all of these procedures remove the malignancy, they differ in the extent to which adjacent tissues are included in the resection. Most of these procedures have been evaluated extensively in retrospective series and have been compared with others in prospective randomized trials. These trials have clarified the relative merits of each procedure in terms of survival and local control rates and have added significantly to our understanding of the biology of breast cancer. The results of and the experience gained from each of these procedures, from both retrospective series and randomized trials, are discussed in this chapter.

The analysis of axillary lymph nodes is also an important part of the management of breast cancer patients. Information about the presence and number of axillary lymph node metastases is important for staging and prognostic purposes and for determining the need for adjuvant chemotherapy. The degree to which the axillary lymph nodes should be dissected (axillary sampling versus complete axillary dissection) to accurately obtain this information is controversial. The distribution of axillary lymph nodes and the pattern of spread of axillary metastases as well as the information provided by different types of axillary procedures are reviewed in the section on axillary lymph node dissection.

The procedures available for the treatment of breast cancer have been used predominantly for Stage I or Stage II breast cancer. Also, a reasonable amount of experience has been gained in the use of the Halsted radical mastectomy for treatment of locally advanced breast cancer (Stage III_a or III_b). This experience has defined the local characteristics of breast cancer (grave signs) that are associated with high local recurrence and poor survival rates. These findings emphasize the importance of accurate clinical staging of the patient at presentation, so that appropriate treatment may be selected. The results of treatment of locally advanced breast cancer with the Halsted radical mastectomy are discussed later; the results of treatment of this stage of breast cancer with combined-modality regimens are discussed in Chapter 9.

Finally, while many women with breast cancer will be cured by primary therapy, others will develop recurrent tumor. For these women, surgery may also play an important role. Biopsies of recurrent lesions, palliative mastectomies, or adrenalectomies or oophorectomies for hormone-dependent metastatic breast cancer may be indicated. The importance of surgery in the management of women with breast cancer is thus considerable, from clarification of an original breast complaint to primary treatment of a breast malignancy or effective palliation of advanced disease. An understanding of the surgical procedures available, their indications, and what they may achieve is thus essential for the effective management of these patients.

HISTORICAL ASPECTS

Breast cancer has been recognized since ancient times. The Edwin Smith papyrus from 3000 B.C. contains at least one description of carcinoma of the breast.[1] While cauterization was used to treat certain breast problems at the time, it is unclear whether these included breast malignancies. In the fifth century B.C., Hippocrates referred to malignancies that were either "deep-seated" or "hidden."[2] Hippocrates recognized the poor prognosis of these tumors and did not consider surgery to be beneficial: "It is better to give no treatment in cases of hidden cancer; treatment causes speedy death, but to omit treatment is to prolong life."[2] Theophilus, commenting on Hippocrates, remarked that "even if the disease is eradicated by cutting or burning, many untoward symptoms follow."[3] Throughout most of the pre-Christian era, the treatment of breast cancer was surveillance, with invocations for help from the gods. Breast amputation was used as punishment (Fig. 5–1); however breast surgery played little or no role as definitive treatment during this period.

The dawn of the Christian era witnessed the beginning of the surgical treatment of breast cancer. In the first century A.D., Leonides[4] described the operative technique of breast cancer as follows:

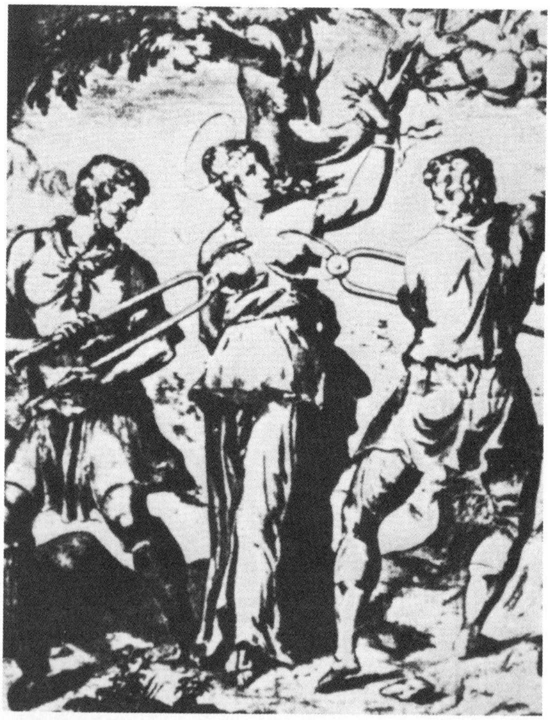

FIGURE 5–1. The Martyrdom of St. Agatha. (With permission from Degenshein GA, Ceccarelli F. The history of breast cancer: Early beginnings to Halsted. Breast 3:28, 1977.)

> I make the patient lie on her back. Then I make an incision into the sound part of the breast above the cancer and I apply cauteries until an eschar is produced that stops the bleeding. I then make another incision and cut into the deep of the breast and again sear the severed parts. This I repeat often, alternately cutting and burning in order to arrest the bleeding. For in this way the danger of hemorrhage is avoided. When the amputation is completed, I burn once again all parts until they are dry. The first cauterizations are made for the purpose of arresting hemorrhage. The rest, however, with the intention of eradicating all remnants of the disease. Often, however, I even completed the task without resorting to cautery, namely in such cases where an indurated tumor threatened to turn into a cancer in the breast. For in such a case an amputation up to the sound part suffices, since here no danger of hemorrhage is threatening.

Galen (born in 130 A.D.) proposed excision of breast cancer discovered at an early stage.[3] During the Middle Ages excision was used for smaller tumors. Hemostasis was achieved by compression, cautery, or suture ligatures. Locally advanced tumors were treated with diet, phlebotomy, and topical applicants. The mastectomy appears to have been introduced during the sixteenth century. The Spanish surgeon Arceo described an operation for removing the breast in 1574. In 1590, Cabrol recommended radical mastectomy with removal of the pectoral muscles for breast cancer, and the Italian Severinus practiced axillary dissection at the time of radical surgery. In the seventeenth century, Bidloo and Tabor developed specialized instruments for performing a mastectomy (Fig. 5–2). In 1844, Pancoast emphasized the importance of removing the breast and the involved axillary lymph nodes as a single procedure.[5]

During the latter part of the nineteenth century, surgeons further defined the surgical treatment of breast cancer. In 1867, Charles Moore emphasized the importance of not exposing the tumor during the procedure, of removing diseased axillary lymph glands, of removing all breast tissue in continuity with the axillary lymphatics, and of not dividing the intervening lymphatics.[6] Gross and Volkmann advocated removal of all breast tissue and the pectoral fascia, in conjunction with a complete axillary dissection for diseased lymph nodes. Kuster proposed, in addition, that a complete axillary dissection be performed in all patients, regardless of whether the lymph nodes were clinically positive.[7] The procedures proposed by these pioneering surgeons represent the prototype for the modified radical mastectomy used extensively in the twentieth century.

In 1894, William Halsted reported his experience with the radical treatment of breast cancer in 50 patients.[8] He removed all breast tissue, the pectoralis major muscle, and the axillary lymphatics. The pectoralis minor was divided but not removed. In his report of 1898, he described removal of the pectoralis minor as well.[9] This procedure became known as the classic Halsted radical mastectomy (Fig. 5–3). In this procedure, the breast tissue was removed first, followed by the

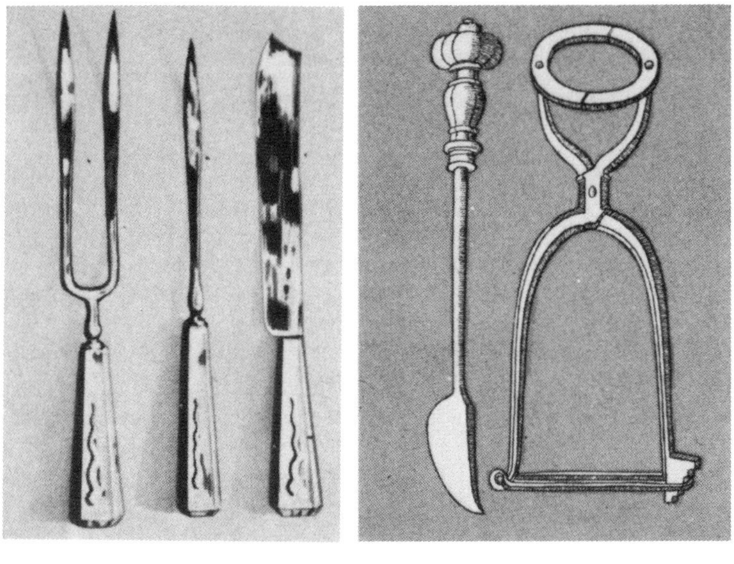

FIGURE 5–2. Mastectomy instruments used by Godefridus Bidloo (left). Compression instrument and knife used by Gerhard Tabor (right) (17th century). (With permission from Degenshein GA, Ceccarelli F. The history of breast cancer: Early beginnings to Halsted. Breast 3:28, 1977.)

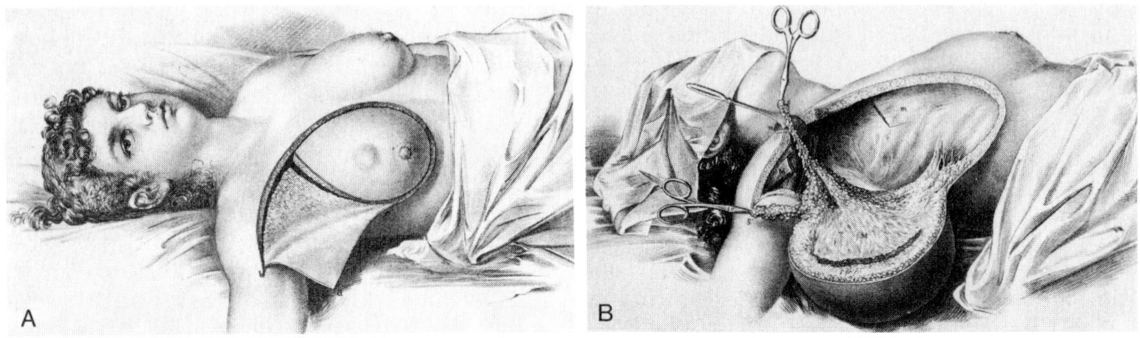

FIGURE 5–3. Halsted's radical mastectomy. *A*, Skin incisions, triangular flap of skin (*a*, *b*, *c*) and triangular flap of fat. *B*, Mastectomy demonstrating the pectoralis major muscle (*M*), pectoralis minor muscle (*m*), apex of infraclavicular fat below the subclavian vessels (*S*), and apex of fat above the vessels (*s*). (With permission from Halsted WS: The results of operations for the cure of cancer of the breast performed at the Johns Hopkins Hospital from June 1889 to January 1894. Johns Hopkins Hosp Bull 4:297, 1894.)

pectoral muscles, and then, beginning at the apex of the axilla, the axillary lymphatics. This procedure, although applied to all stages of breast cancer, represented a substantial improvement in both local control and survival rates over those of Halsted's predecessors. Whereas prior surgical treatment of breast cancer was associated wtih local recurrence rates of 60 to 82 percent and a three-year survival rate of 9 to 39 percent, Halsted reported a 6 percent local recurrence rate and three-year survival rate of 38 to 42 percent.[8, 11] In 1894, Meyer proposed an alternative method of performing the radical mastectomy.[12] In this procedure, the axillary lymphatics were dissected first, followed by the breast tissue and pectoral muscles. The extent of the surgical resection for the two procedures (Halsted and Meyer mastectomies) was the same; only the sequence of removing the tissues was different.

The radical mastectomy of both Halsted and Meyer was based on the premise that breast cancer spreads in an orderly manner, first to the regional lymphatics and then to distant sites. Removal of adjacent tissues and lymph nodes both improved local control and, by including the regional lymphatics, interrupted the spread to distant organs. This concept of dissemination was universally held until well into the twentieth century, when Crile as well as Fisher and colleagues established that the axillary dissection did not confer a survival benefit and was therapeutic only in that it prevented recurrent axillary disease.[13, 14]

Further experience with the radical mastectomy defined the extent of local breast cancer for which this procedure was effective. Whereas Halsted initially applied the radical mastectomy to all patients with breast cancer, in the 1940's Haagensen defined the disease characteristics that, when radical mastectomy alone was the therapy, were associated with high local recurrence and poor survival rates.[15] These characteristics are known as the grave signs of breast cancer (see Chapter 4). The presence of any of these signs is now considered evidence of inoperability. Haagensen also did much to establish the use of the staging classification in the treatment of breast cancer. His Columbia Clinical Classification was among the first to stage each patient according to the extent of disease at presentation (both local and distant) and to correlate local recurrence and long-term survival rates after radical mastectomy with this stage. An appreciation of the importance both of accurate staging and of the selection of therapy according to stage has been one of the most significant developments in the treatment of breast cancer in the twentieth century.

In 1948, Patey proposed that removal of the pectoralis major did not add to the value of surgical treatment with the radical mastectomy.[16] He described the modified radical mastectomy, in which all breast tissue was removed in conjunction with the pectoralis minor and the axillary contents, while preserving the pectoralis major. Both Auchincloss and Madden further modified this procedure by preserving both the pectoralis major and the pectoralis minor muscles.[17, 18] Subsequently, large retrospective series by many surgeons and two prospective randomized trials confirmed that local control and survival rates achieved with the modified radical mastectomy were comparable to those for the Halsted radical mastectomy.[19, 20] As a result of this experience, by 1982, 72.3 percent of all radical mastectomies were of the modified variety (Table 5–1).[21]

Halsted was also impressed with the frequency with which the internal mammary and supraclavicular lymph nodes were involved in breast cancer. This observation led him and Harvey Cushing to consider inclusion of these two areas in the radical mastectomy. In his address to the American Surgical Association, Halsted remarked, "Our present method of operating for the cure of breast cancer is even more radical than at the time of the writer's first publication on this subject. The supraclavicular region is almost invariably cleaned out. Hence it would appear that for the present, our rule should be to operate on the neck in every case."[19] Subsequently, Wangensteen,[22] Margottini,[23, 130] Dahl-Iversen,[24, 133] and Veronesi and Zingo[25] each reported on patients treated with supraclavicular node dissections (plus radical mastectomy) for breast cancer. However, there was never much enthusiasm for this procedure among the surgical community, and when it became clear that supraclavicular metastases represented disseminated disease, the procedure was abandoned.

With regard to mediastinal lymph node metastases, Halsted also remarked: "Dr. H. W. Cushing, my house surgeon, has in three instances cleaned out the anterior mediastinum on one side for recurrent cancer. It is likely, I think, that we shall see, in the near future, removal of the mediastinal contents at some of our primary operations."[9] Dissection of the mediastinal lymph nodes has since been used extensively in the treatment of operable breast cancer. Large retrospective series from several centers,[24–29, 130] and three prospective randomized trials have been conducted.[30, 33] Although enthusiasm for the procedure has diminished considerably, it is still applied in some centers on a limited basis for the treatment of breast cancer.

While some groups in the twentieth century were applying more extended procedures to the treatment of breast cancer, others were evaluating more conservative therapy options. Crile and others at the Cleveland Clinic were among the first proponents of total (simple) mastectomy and partial mastectomy as definitive treatment for breast cancer. The total mastectomy removed only the breast tissue, leaving the axillary lymph nodes intact.[34] This was associated with a significant axillary recurrence rate and also omitted important staging and prognostic information about axillary lymph node status. Nevertheless, the experience of this group and others,[13, 35–43, 145] including prospective randomized trials,[44–46] confirmed that the survival rate following total mastectomy was comparable with those for the more radical procedures.

The modified radical and total mastectomies, while providing an improved cosmetic result over the Halsted radical, were still accompanied by the psychological trauma of breast amputation. This encouraged the evaluation of more conservative procedures, in which the major portion of the breast tissue was preserved. Because it was clear even to Halsted's predecessors that partial mastectomy alone was followed by significant local recurrence rates, some form of adjuvant therapy for the remaining breast tissue was needed. Beginning with Keynes in the 1930's, many series and trials have demonstrated that breast conservation in conjunction with definitive postoperative radiation therapy for early stage breast cancer can result in survival and local control rates comparable to those for radical surgery, with a much superior cosmetic result. The long-term effects of the radiation as well as the socioeconomic impact on the individual of a postoperative course of radiation therapy are still under evaluation. Nevertheless, conservative treatment regimens have come to represent an accepted alternative in the therapy for early stage breast cancer. The extent to which these regimens will replace the modified radical mastectomy, which at present represents the dominant form of therapy, remains to be seen.

TABLE 5–1. Use of the Halsted Radical Mastectomy and Modified Radical Mastectomy by Year in the Treatment of Breast Cancer

Year	Radical Mastectomy (%)	Modified Radical Mastectomy (%)
1972	47.9	27.7
1976	25.5	51.9
1977	20.9	55.4
1981	3.4	72.3

Source: Report by The American College of Surgeons Commission on Cancer, Chicago, IL, October 22, 1982.

ANATOMIC CONSIDERATIONS

The breasts are paired organs on the anterior chest wall composed of a network of glands and ducts contained within fibrous and adipose tissue.[47–49] The basic subunit of glandular tissue is the alveolus. Clusters of alveoli form lobules, which, in turn, aggregate to form lobes. The alveoli empty into the lactiferous ducts. These ducts unite to form larger ducts, which correspond to one of the chief subdivisions of the breast. There are 15 to 20 major excretory ducts that converge and open into the nipple.[47] In addition to the major paired breast tissue, there may also be accessory breasts or nipples in 1 to 2 percent of subjects.[49] Accessory breast tissue is usually situated along the embryonic milk line between the axilla and the groin, most frequently in the axilla, and may consist of any combination of glandular tissue and nipple.[49]

Breast tissue extends from the second or third rib superiorly to the sixth or seventh costal margin inferiorly and from the lateral border of the sternum to beyond the anterior axillary fold (Fig. 5–4).[50] The peripheral boundaries of the breast tissue are neither well defined nor uniform and may extend superiorly to the brachial plexus and apex of the axilla, inferiorly to the epigastrium, laterally to the anterior border of the lattisimus dorsi, and medially to the midsternal line.[50, 51] The breast tissue is surrounded anteriorly by the superficial layer, and posteriorly by the deep layer, of the superficial fascia. Anteriorly, the superficial layer of the superficial fascia derives from the fibrous tissue of the tela subcutanea. The deep layer of the superficial fascia is adjacent to the pectoral fascia.[49]

The breast has a rich lymphatic network (Fig. 5–5). A dense areolar and nipple lymphatic network is continuous with the surrounding cutaneous lymphatics and also communicates with the deeper part of the central portion of the breast.[49] From the subareolar plexus there are usually two major trunks, one from the superior and one from the inferior portion, which drain into the axillary lymph nodes. The deep lymphatics, which originate in the interlobular and perilobular regions, either may converge into the subareolar plexus or may drain peripherally into one or more lymph node–bearing re-

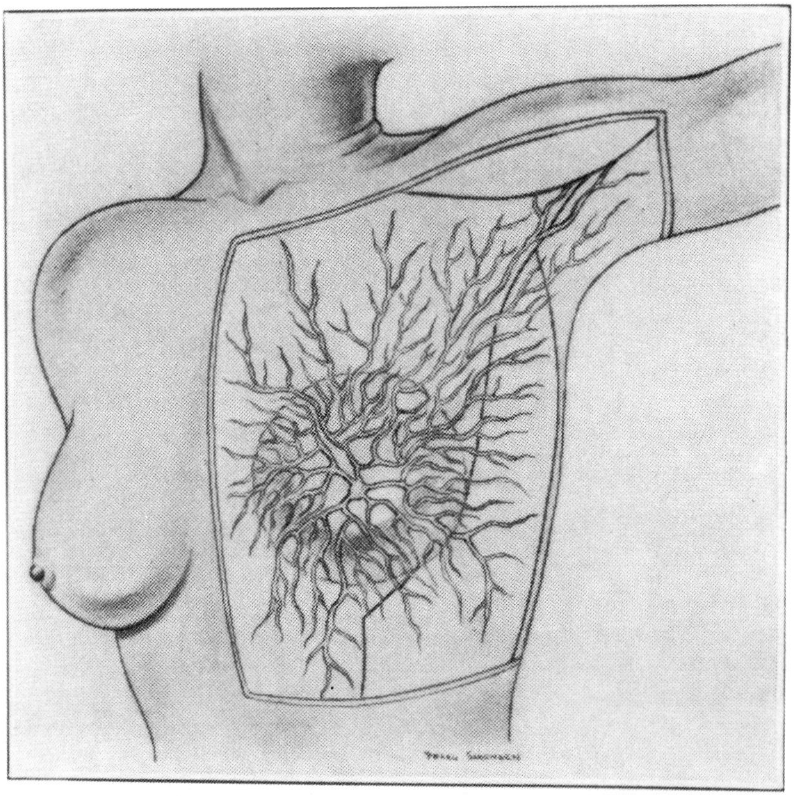

FIGURE 5–4. Diagram demonstrating the extent of breast tissue as determined from anatomic studies. (With permission from Hicken NF: Mastectomy: A clinical pathologic demonstrating why most mastectomies result in incomplete removal of the mammary gland. Arch Surg 40:6, 1940.)

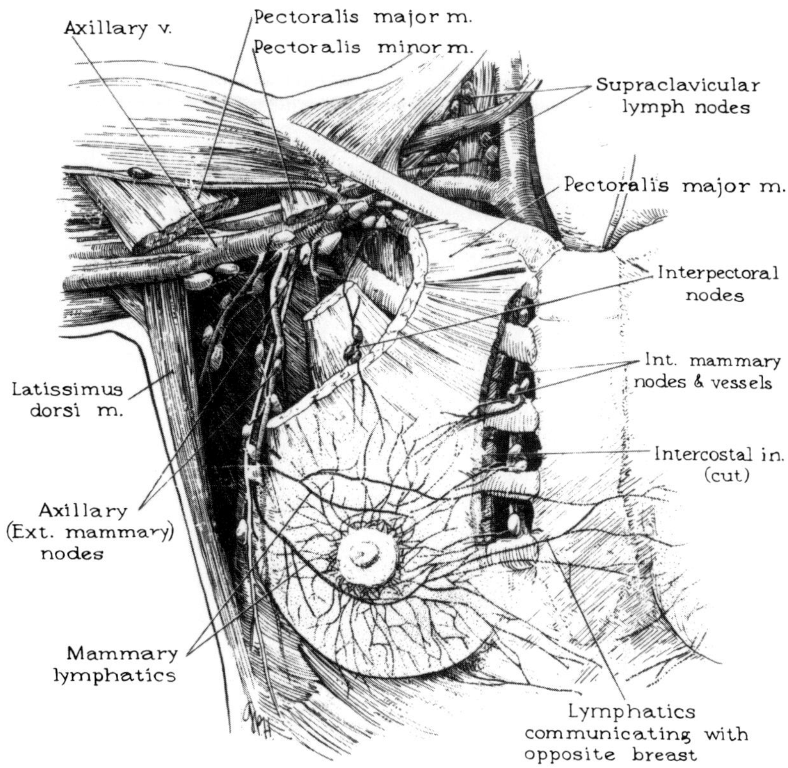

FIGURE 5–5. Lymphatic drainage of the breast and regional lymph node–bearing areas. (With permission from Sugarbaker ED: Thorax. *In:* An Atlas of Surgical Oncology, Vol. 1. Boca Raton, FL: CRC Press, 1983.)

gions. The latter include the axillary lymph nodes, the internal mammary lymph nodes, and the interpectoral lymph nodes. Vessels from the lateral portion of the breast usually drain into the axillary lymphatics, and vessels from the medial portion of the breast drain into the internal mammary lymph nodes located substernally along the internal mammary vessels. Lymphatics may also pass directly to the apical axillary (infraclavicular or subclavicular) nodes, some of which may penetrate the pectoral muscles in their course.

The axillary lymph nodes are contained in adipose tissue along and inferior to the axillary vein. The axillary space containing the axillary lymph nodes is bordered medially by the thoracic outlet, laterally by the latissimus dorsi muscle, posteriorly by the chest wall and subscapularis muscle, and superiorly by the axillary vein (Fig. 5–5). Inferiorly, the axillary tissue is continuous with the breast. The average number of axillary lymph nodes on each side in an individual is approximately 27.[53–56] Pickren noted that the number may range from 8 to 87 among individuals.[57] The axillary tissue is commonly divided anatomically according to its relationship to the pectoralis minor muscle (lateral, inferior, or medial).[58] These locations are referred to as the axillary levels (I, II, and III, respectively; Fig. 5–6). The distribution of axillary lymph nodes according to axillary level (I, II, or III) and its importance in the staging and prognosis of breast cancer are discussed later in the section on axillary lymph node dissection.

The internal mammary lymph nodes lie substernally upon the endothoracic fascia in the intercostal spaces. There are an average of three to five lymph nodes on either side of the sternum, located most frequently in the first, second, third, and fourth intercostal spaces.[59, 60] The importance of the internal mammary lymph nodes for diagnosis and treatment purposes is examined later in the section on extended radical mastectomy and in Chapter 4 in the discussion on biopsy of internal mammary lymph nodes.

The interpectoral, or Rotter's, lymph nodes lie on the inferior surface of the pectoralis major muscle, alojng the pectoral branch of the thoracoacromial artery. They are present in up to 95 percent of individuals, with an average of two to three lymph nodes per individual.[61, 62] While these nodes are com-

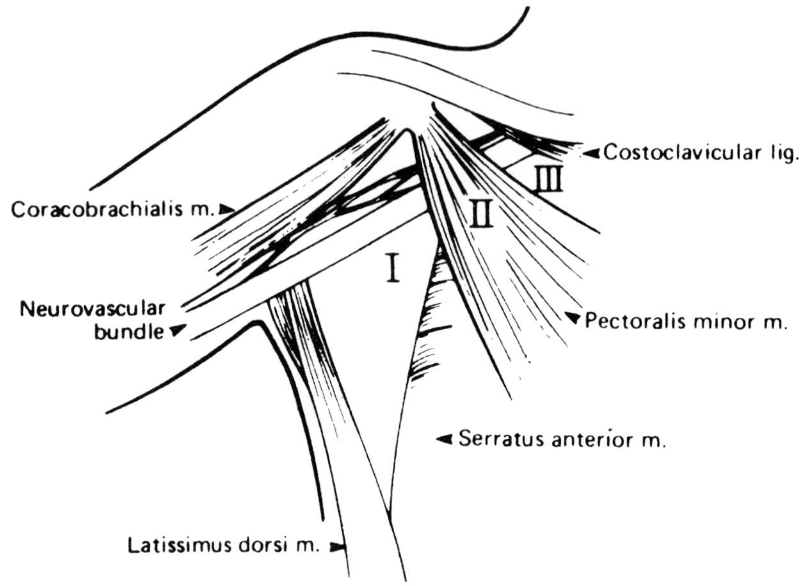

FIGURE 5–6. The anatomical levels (I, II, III) of the axillary contents, designated according to their relationship to the pectoralis minor muscle (see text for description). (With permission from deMoss EV, et al.: Complete axillary lymph node dissection before radiotherapy for primary breast cancer. *In*: Harris JR, Hellman S, Silen W (eds.): Conservative Management of Breast Cancer. Philadelphia: J. B. Lippincott, 1983.)

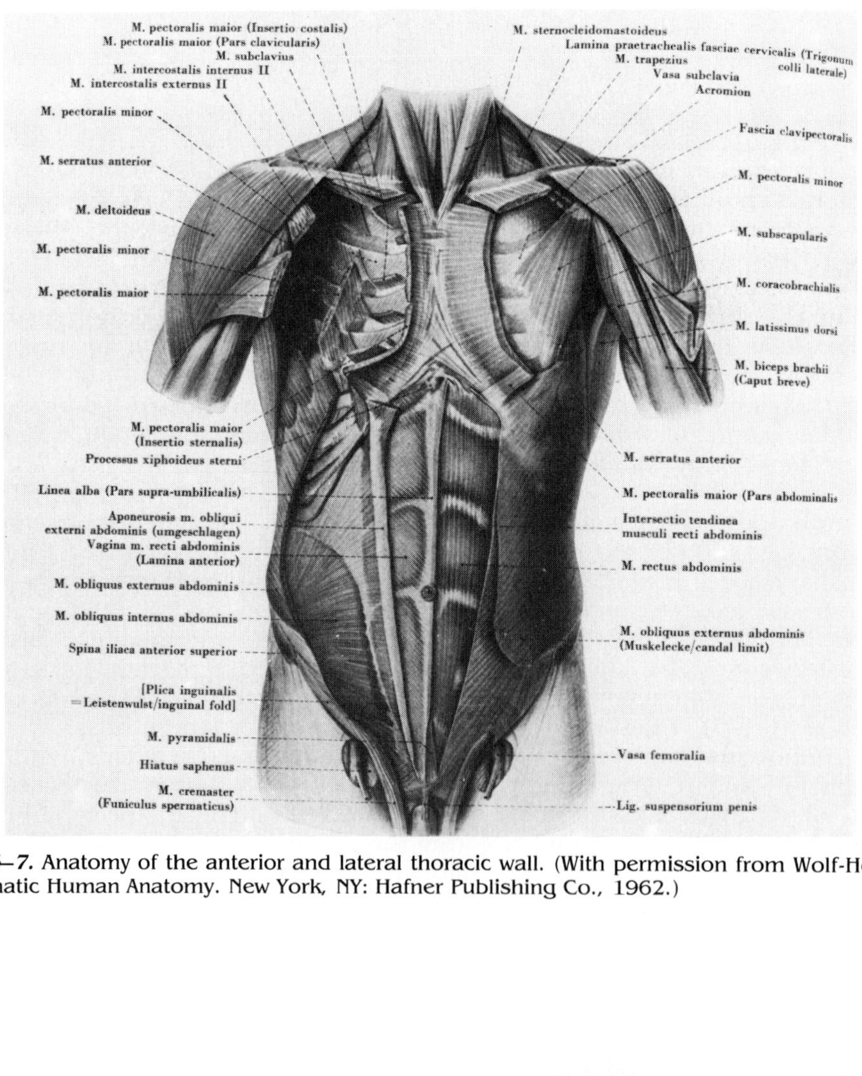

FIGURE 5–7. Anatomy of the anterior and lateral thoracic wall. (With permission from Wolf-Heidegger, G: Atlas of Systematic Human Anatomy. New York, NY: Hafner Publishing Co., 1962.)

monly included in the axillary dissection, they probably do not play a major role in the diagnosis and treatment of breast cancer. Cody and associates[61] found that 8.2 percent of patients with positive axillary nodes and 0.5 percent of node-negative patients had interpectoral lymph node metastases. Haagensen found interpectoral node metastases only in patients with positive axillary nodes.[49]

The posterior boundary of the breast is formed by the chest wall muscles, including the pectoralis major and minor muscles, the serratus anterior muscle, and the latissimus dorsi muscles (Fig. 5–7). Inferiorly, the breast may approach the superior aspect of the rectus abdominis muscle. The pectoralis major muscle originates on the clavicle, the sternum, and the costal cartilages of the second to the sixth ribs and inserts on the upper end of the humerus. The pectoralis major is supplied by the medial and lateral pectoral nerves and the thoracoacromial vessels. The medial pectoral nerve courses through the pectoralis minor muscle and supplies the lateral portion of the pectoralis major muscle (the anterior axillary fold). The pectoralis minor muscle originates on the outer surfaces of the third, fourth, and fifth ribs, near their costal cartilages, and inserts on the medial border and the upper surface of the coracoid process. The serratus anterior muscle arises from the upper eighth or ninth rib and inserts on the whole of the medial border of the scapula. It is supplied by the long thoracic nerve. The latissimus dorsi muscle arises from the spinous processes of the lower thoracic and lumbar vertebrae and sacrum and from the iliac crest. It has an attachment to the scapula and inserts on the humerus. The latissimus dorsi forms the posterior axillary fold and is supplied by the thoracodorsal vessels.

SURGICAL PROCEDURES FOR THE MANAGEMENT OF BREAST CANCER

The following surgical procedures are or have been used in the management of patients with breast cancer: (1) Halsted radical mastectomy, (2) extended radical mastectomy, (3) superradical mastectomy, (4) modified radical mastectomy, (5) total (simple) mastectomy, (6) partial mastectomy, (7) subcutaneous mastectomy, (8) axillary lymph node dissection, and (9) breast biopsy.

Halsted Radical Mastectomy

The standard radical mastectomy, as developed by Halsted and Meyer, removes all breast tissue and the pectoralis major and minor muscles in conjunction with a complete axillary dissection.[15, 63, 64] The Halsted and Meyer radical mastectomies differ in the sequence used to remove these tissues. The Halsted mastectomy removes the breast and pectoral muscles first, followed by the axillary dissection. The Meyer mastectomy dissects the axilla first, followed by removal of the breast and pectoral muscles. The final result is the same; however, the Meyer approach is rarely, if ever, used today. Both procedures are commonly performed through a vertical incision to facilitate detachment of the pectoralis major from the clavicle and the lower costal cartilages. A variety of other incisions have also been used (Fig. 5–8).[64, 183] All incisions incorporate the nipple and the biopsy site. The pectoralis major is completely removed from its attachments to the clavicle, sternum, costal cartilages, and humerus and the pectoralis minor from its attachments to ribs and the coracoid process. A complete axillary dissection is performed from the thoracic outlet medially, to the latissimus dorsi muscle laterally, and inferiorly to the junction of the long thoracic nerve and thoracodorsal vessels with their respective muscles. In the original descriptions of the procedure by Halsted and Meyer, both the long thoracic nerve and the thoracodorsal vessels were excised. Haagensen preserved the long thoracic nerve but removed the thoracodorsal vessels to the latissimus dorsi muscle. Today, both of these neuromuscular structures are commonly preserved to ensure scapular function and to maintain the function of the latissimus dorsi muscle so that it is available for future breast reconstruction. The original premise for excision of these structures was to allow for more complete axillary lymph node clearance. Both of these structures, however, can be easily and completely cleared of adjacent lymph node–bearing tissue and should be preserved, unless involved by tumor. The standard radical mastectomy also advocated wide excision of skin around the tumor and the biopsy site.

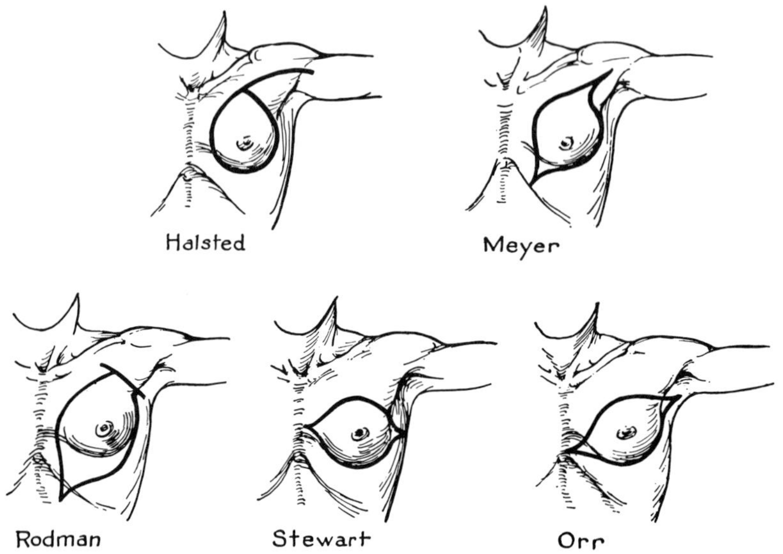

FIGURE 5–8. Skin incisions for mastectomy. The vertical incision of Meyer is commonly used for the Halsted radical mastectomy, and the transverse incisions of Stewart and Orr are commonly used for the modified radical or the total mastectomy. (With permission from Allen JG: The breast. *In*: Rhoades JE, et al. (eds.): Surgery: Principles and Practice, 4th ed. Philadelphia: J.B. Lippincott, 1970.)

A skin graft was commonly used to close the defect. This is rarely practiced today, both because adequate margins of skin can be obtained for smaller tumors and primary closure still achieved and because larger tumors, especially those with skin ulceration, edema, or other grave signs, are now considered inoperable and are treated initially with other forms of therapy. The significant cosmetic defect following the standard radical mastectomy is less easily repaired by reconstructive procedures than is that associated with the modified radical or total mastectomies. Postoperative drainage with Hemovac or Silastic catheters is routinely performed for the Halsted as well as other mastectomies.

Extended Radical Mastectomy

The extended radical mastectomy removes the internal mammary lymph nodes in conjunction with either a conventional Halsted or a modified radical mastectomy. The distribution of internal mammary nodes has been discussed previously (see discussion on anatomic considerations). The skin incision incorporates the nipple and biopsy site as with other radical mastectomies and may be either vertical or transverse, depending upon whether the pectoralis major is removed. The radical mastectomy portion of the procedure removes all breast tissue in conjunction with an axillary dissection. The pectoralis major or pectoralis minor muscle may also be included.[68] The mediastinal lymph node dissection can be performed in a discontinuous manner,[65] as a monobloc dissection with removal of the internal mammary lymph node chain extrapleurally[23] or as an *en bloc* procedure with removal of the bony chest wall, which contains the internal mammary lymph nodes.[66, 67] The chest wall defect may be reinforced with Marlex mesh, fascia lata, or other materials. The skin is usually closed primarily.

Superradical Mastectomy

The superradical mastectomy goes beyond the Halsted radical mastectomy to include removal of all breast tissue and both pectoral muscles and dissection of the axillary, internal mammary, and supraclavicular lymph nodes. The supraclavicular nodes can be removed either in a discontinuous manner,[65] with resection of the first rib,[22] or as an *en bloc* resection, with removal of the clavicle, the medial portion of the first and second ribs, and the corresponding half of the sternum.[25] Because it has become clear that the presence of supraclavicular lymph node metastases represents advanced disease (variously Stage III_b or Stage IV, depending on the classification scheme), the superradical mastectomy is no longer used in the treatment of breast cancer.

Modified Radical Mastectomy

There are two types of modified radical mastectomy, that described by Patey[16, 69] and that described by both Auchincloss[17] and

Madden.[18] The Patey modified radical mastectomy alters the Halsted radical mastectomy by preserving the pectoralis major muscle. All breast tissue and the fascia of the pectoralis major are removed as well as the pectoralis minor in conjunction with a complete axillary lymph node dissection. The Auchincloss and the Madden modified radical mastectomies remove all breast tissue and the axillary lymph nodes; however, they preserve both the pectoralis major and the pectoralis minor muscles. The fascia of the pectoralis major may or may not be removed in these latter two procedures. The modified radical mastectomy is commonly performed through a transverse incision that incorporates the nipple and the biopsy site. The breast tissue and pectoral fascia can be easily dissected off the pectoralis major through this incision, and good exposure of the axilla is obtained. Complete removal of the pectoralis minor (in the Patey modified radical) is accompanied by loss of the medial pectoral nerve, which courses through this muscle and which supplies the lateral border of the pectoralis major muscle. Because the Auchincloss and the Madden mastectomies preserve the pectoralis minor muscle, access to the apex of the axilla is restricted and the axillary dissection performed is usually less complete than that in the Patey modified radical mastectomy. Axillary dissection for the Auchincloss and the Madden procedures usually removes Levels I and II lymph nodes, leaving Level III intact (see the following discussion on axillary lymph node dissection). The pectoralis minor muscle may be divided and retracted while the apex is dissected and then reapproximated to its tendinous insertion. In all modified radical mastectomies, the long thoracic nerve and the thoracodorsal vessels are preserved. The skin incision is closed primarily, skin grafts are rarely needed, and the wound is drained postoperatively with suction catheters.

Total (Simple) Mastectomy

The total mastectomy removes all of the breast tissue.[70] Both the pectoralis major and the pectoralis minor muscles are preserved, and there is no axillary lymph node dissection. A transverse incision is used and includes the nipple and the biopsy site. Dissection of the skin flaps is performed in the same manner as for the radical mastectomy. Postoperative catheter drainage is routinely employed.

Partial Mastectomy

The term partial mastectomy refers to procedures in which only a portion of the breast tissue containing the malignancy is removed. The major portion of the breast tissue as well as the nipple and both pectoral muscles is left intact. More descriptive terms for the partial mastectomy may be used to describe the quantity of tissue removed, including quadrantectomy, segmentectomy, lumpectomy, tylectomy, and local excision. *Quadrantectomy* involves radical removal of the entire quadrant of the breast containing the primary carcinoma.[71] The overlying skin and the fascia of the pectoralis major muscle are removed, together with the breast tissue. *Segmentectomy* involves resection of the tumor with removal of enough normal tissue to ensure that the specimen margins are free of tumor. Removal of pectoral fascia or overlying skin is not required.[72] *Local excision, lumpectomy,* and *tylectomy* are synonymous and refer to removal of gross tumor only, with a margin of 0.5 to 1 cm of adjacent normal tissue.[73] No attempt is made to achieve negative margins. This procedure is the same as an excisional biopsy of a breast mass. Microscopically, positive margins will be present at the excision site in 30 to 35 percent of patients.[73]

Subcutaneous Mastectomy

The subcutaneous mastectomy removes only the major portion of the breast tissue, preserving the nipple, both pectoral muscles, and the axillary lymph nodes.[74] The procedure may be performed through either a periareolar or an inframammary incision. The skin is subcutaneously dissected off the underlying breast tissue, leaving a skin flap 4 to 8 mm in thickness. Immediate reconstruction is frequently performed. Subcutaneous mastectomy is commonly performed for lobular carcinoma *in situ* (but not intraductal carcinoma), severe fibrocystic disease, or gynecomastia. It should not be used for the treatment of invasive breast carcinoma. The role of this procedure is discussed further in Chapter 14.

Axillary Lymph Node Dissection

This procedure refers to the removal of lymph nodes from the axilla and is commonly performed to obtain nodes for staging and prognostic purposes and to prevent axillary recurrence of tumor. Axillary dissection is an integral part of radical mastectomies. Total and partial mastectomies, by definition, do not disturb the axillary contents. However, an axillary lymph node dissection is commonly performed in conjunction with a total or a partial mastectomy, for staging and prognostic purposes. When local excision or segmental resection is used, the axillary dissection is performed in a discontinuous manner, through a separate axillary incision. When quadrantectomy is performed, the axillary dissection can be continuous (for upper outer quadrant tumors) or discontinuous (for medial lesions).[71]

The anatomic distribution of axillary lymph nodes according to axillary level (I, II, III) is covered later in the discussion on axillary lymph node dissection. The procedures available for removing axillary lymph nodes include the complete axillary lymph node dissection, partial axillary dissection, axillary lymph node sampling, and local excision of clinically involved lymph nodes. All of these procedures may be performed either in conjunction with a mastectomy or as a single discontinuous procedure (such as when partial mastectomy is used). When performed as a single discontinuous procedure, an S-shaped or transverse axillary incision is used.[52, 174] A complete axillary dissection removes all lymph nodes (Levels I, II, III) from the thoracic outlet laterally, with skeletonization of the axillary vein (Fig. 5–6). The pectoralis minor muscle is either removed or divided and reapproximated, to provide exposure of the apex of the axilla. The dissection is carried laterally to the junction of the axillary vein with the latissimus dorsi muscle and inferiorly to the junction of the thoracodorsal vessels with the latissimus dorsi muscle and the long thoracic nerve with the serratus anterior muscle. Both of these vessels and nerves are preserved. One to 2 cm of the tail of the breast is usually included in the specimen. Postoperative axillary drainage is used routinely for all types of axillary dissection. Perioperative antibiotics are not administered.

A partial axillary dissection removes adipose tissue containing lymph nodes lateral and inferior to the pectoralis minor muscle (Levels I and II).[72, 157] The apex of the axilla is not dissected, and the pectoralis minor is preserved. This procedure removes 70 to 80 percent of the axillary contents. The technical aspects and the lateral and inferior extent of the dissection are otherwise the same as for a complete axillary dissection.

An axillary sampling removes only lymph nodes lateral to the lateral border of the pectoralis minor muscle (Level I).[75] This may be done with or without skeletonization of the axillary vein. Less than 40 percent of the axillary lymph nodes are removed by this procedure.

Excision of axillary lymph nodes refers to the local excision of one to two lymph nodes that are usually adjacent to the tail of the breast (pectoral node biopsy).[45] No attempt is made to formally dissect the axilla. A frozen section may be performed on these nodes, and if findings are positive, an axillary dissection should follow.[76] Local excision of involved lymph nodes is not usually done as a single procedure, but rather is done at the time of total mastectomy. Postoperative axillary drainage is used routinely for all types of axillary dissection. Perioperative antibiotics are not given.

Breast Biopsy

The breast biopsy obtains material from a breast abnormality for diagnostic purposes. Procedures for securing specimens include fine-needle aspiration for cytologic analysis, Tru-Cut needle biopsy or high-speed drill biopsy for histologic analysis, and incisional or excisional biopsies for histologic and steroid receptor analyses. The selection of a particular procedure depends upon the nature of the lesion being evaluated and the facilities available. Each of these procedures is discussed in Chapter 4.

PRINCIPLES OF BREAST CANCER SURGERY

The effective treatment of breast cancer requires a complete history and physical examination and accurate clinical staging of each patient. This will define the extent of the malignancy and will indicate what treatment will provide the best opportunity for local control and cure. The primary tumor and regional lymph node–bearing areas, the skin, and the remaining breast tissue should be carefully examined. An accurate measurement of the tumor is especially important. Tumors 5 cm or less in diameter (Stage I or II) may be effectively treated with radical surgery. Partial mastectomy with postoperative radiation therapy has been shown to be effective for tumors 4 cm or less in diameter but not for larger lesions, according to one study with modest follow-up.[72] Tumors larger than 5 cm in diameter (Stage III_a or III_b) are not effectively managed with either radical surgery or radiation therapy alone (such treatment results in high local recurrence and poor survival rates). These tumors are more appropriately managed with combined-modality regimens (see the following discussion on locally advanced breast cancer).

The local extent of the tumor should be carefully determined. Any of the grave signs of breast cancer should be noted, since these are categorical evidence of inoperability and require combined-modality therapy. The grave signs of breast cancer include extensive edema of the skin over the breast, satellite nodules, inflammatory carcinoma, parasternal tumor, supraclavicular metastases, arm edema, skin ulceration, fixation of the tumor to the chest wall, and fixation of axillary lymph nodes to each other and to the deep structures of the axilla (see Table 5–31 and the Columbia Clinical Classification in Chapter 4). Skin changes caused by inflammatory carcinoma or satellite nodules may be quite subtle and do not necessarily occur in the skin directly overlying the mass. Biopsies should be performed on any suspicious skin areas, using a skin punch.

The mobility of the breast mass should be determined. Loss of mobility of a tumor may result from fixation to pectoral fascia or muscle or to the chest wall (ribs, intercostal muscles, or serratus anterior muscle). The distinction between fixation to pectoral fascia or muscle or to the chest wall must be made on clinical grounds and can be assessed by noting the relative mobility of the lesion. Masses that are fixed to the chest wall are completely immobile and, as has often been stated, "The patient will move with the mass." Tumors involving only pectoral tissue, however, have some relative mobility. Fixation to pectoral fascia does not alter the stage of the breast cancer as defined by the TNM Classification. Fixation to the chest wall, however, represents locally advanced disease (Stage III_b). While Stage I and Stage II tumors that are fixed to pectoral fascia or pectoralis major muscle may be effectively treated with radical mastectomy, these characteristics may preclude radiation therapy as primary treatment. This is because of the difficulty in implantation of the fascia or muscle with radioactive needles (used to provide a radiation boost to the tumor site). Similarly, multifocal tumors are also not considered suitable for primary radiation therapy.

Breast cancer is often a multicentric disease. If a radical surgical procedure is to be effective in preventing local recurrence, all breast tissue must be removed. The incidence of multicentricity for invasive carcinoma ranges, among several series, from 7 to 37 percent.[78] Gallagher, after a careful review of these series, concluded that 30 percent is a minimum estimate of the incidence of multicentricity in the average group of patients with operable breast cancer.[78] As pointed out previously (see the discussion on technical aspects), the breast tissue is surrounded anteriorly by the superficial fascia. During formation of skin flaps, dissection should be done superficial to this layer. This will leave 2 to 3 mm of fat and areolar tissue on the skin flaps, which will have a network of small vessels but no large ones.[63] Similarly, the posterior dissection should remove the fascia from the anterior surface of the pectoralis major muscle. When only a partial mastectomy is performed, there will be recurrence in the breast. On the average, one fourth of patients will have microscopic tumor in the biopsy site or multicentric tumor foci in the remaining breast tissue (see the following discussion on partial mastectomy).

Treatment of the nipple-areola complex is an important part of radical surgery for breast cancer. The mammary ducts, as noted, converge and terminate in the nipple. For invasive ductal carcinoma, there is thus the potential for disease of the nipple either by contiguous involvement or by multicentric tumor. Histologic analysis of the nipple from mastectomy specimens has revealed an 8 to 31 percent incidence of carcinoma.[79–82, 189] At least three cases have also been reported in which carcinoma developed in a nipple autotransplanted to the thigh for future breast reconstruction.[83–85] The nipple-areola complex should therefore be included in the skin incision and excised with the breast tissue in a radical or total mastectomy. Because the ducts terminate in the nipple and not in the areola, it is not necessary to include a wide margin of skin around the areola, unless a periareolar incision was used for the biopsy.

Since breast cancer frequently metastasizes to axillary lymph nodes, these nodes are routinely removed to obtain information for staging and prognostic purposes. In addition, removal of axillary lymph nodes will prevent axillary recurrence in patients with clinically negative lymph nodes and will prevent progression of the disease in patients with clinically positive nodes. The thoracoacromial vessels supplying the pectoralis major muscle should be preserved during the axillary dissection if a Halsted radical mastectomy is not being performed. These vessels course along the inferior-superior aspect of the muscle. One of the major advantages of the modified radical and the total mastectomies is the cosmetic benefit of preserving the pectoralis major muscle. This benefit will be lost if the thoracoacromial vessels are injured, resulting in atrophy of the muscle. The thoracodorsal vessels and, especially, the long thoracic nerve should be preserved during dissection of the axillary lymph nodes. Both these structures can be easily cleared of adjacent tissue, and their preservation will prevent loss of function of the muscles they innervate. The latissimus dorsi muscle, in addition, may be needed for future breast reconstruction.

The axillary vein should represent the superior limit of the axillary dissection. There are no lymph nodes superior to the vein in the region of the brachial plexus. The axillary dissection should include lymph node–bearing tissue inferior to the axillary vein and medial to the latissimus dorsi muscle. The degree to which the axilla should be dissected (partial versus complete) is covered in the discussion on axillary lymph node dissection.

The principles of multiple synchronous biopsies should be observed. Occasionally, a patient will present with more than one lesion upon which biopsies are to be performed during a single procedure. Patients may have multiple lesions in the same breast, bilateral breast lesions, or a single breast lesion with, simultaneously, a soft-tissue nodule elsewhere on the body. If a biopsy is to be performed on more than one lesion during the same procedure, it is essential that malignant cells from the initial biopsy do not contaminate the second site. Strict adherence to the principles of cancer surgery must therefore be observed. When possible, a biopsy should be performed on the least suspicious lesion first (an exception to this would be the random opposite breast biopsy in patients with a proven malignancy in one breast). Following completion of the initial biopsy and closure of the skin, the field should be covered. Gloves and gown should be changed, a new set of instruments used, and the second biopsy site appropriately prepared and draped. The importance of this approach cannot be overemphasized. If a biopsy site for a benign lesion in some other region of the body is contaminated with invasive breast cancer cells from a preceding biopsy, this contaminated area will require definitive treatment, just as for any invasive malignancy. If a segmental breast excision is to be done in conjunction with an axillary dissection, the axillary dissection should be done first, to avoid contaminating the axilla with cells from the biopsy site. The sequence of multiple biopsies and their details should be clearly stated in the operative site for the benefit of others involved in the care of the patient.

RESULTS OF THE SURGICAL TREATMENT OF BREAST CANCER

The results of treatment of operable breast cancer with each type of mastectomy are discussed in the following section. For each type of procedure, the experience from retrospective series is considered first, followed by a discussion of prospective randomized trials comparing that particular procedure with others. The survival and local control rates and the complications are considered for each procedure. The role of the axillary lymph node dissection and the role of surgery for locally advanced breast cancer are considered in separate sections. Before beginning the discussion of treatment results, the reader should review the discussions in Chapter 4 on the staging classifications of breast cancer. There are three major classifications used to stage patients and to report treatment results: the TNM Classification, the Columbia Clinical Classification, and the Manchester Classification. These classifications differ somewhat in the characteristics assigned to each stage. An understanding of these classifications will clarify both the results of each series or trial and the recommendations of the participating authors.

Halsted Radical Mastectomy

The Halsted radical mastectomy (HRM) was introduced approximately 100 years ago by William Halsted for the treatment of breast cancer. Its development and the rationale for its use are examined in the preceding discussion on the historical aspects of the surgical treatment of breast cancer. This procedure represented the standard form of treatment for breast cancer until the 1970's, when it was replaced by more conservative procedures, especially the modified radical mastectomy. Because of the long history of use of the Halsted radical mastectomy, a considerable amount of experience has been gained regarding its curative potential, the patterns of recurrence following its use, and its complications. This experience is found in many large retrospective series, the most prominent of which is Haagensen's series of over 1000 radical mastectomies, which were followed for 47 years,[86] and in several prospective randomized trials comparing the Halsted radical mastectomy with other forms of therapy. Knowledge of the findings of these studies is important for defining the operability of breast cancer and for evaluating the effectiveness of alternative treatment regimens.

Before discussing treatment results, a comment should be made about survival in untreated breast cancer. In a classic study, Bloom and colleagues[87] reviewed the clinical records of 356 patients with untreated breast cancer admitted to the Middlesex Hospital between 1805 and 1933. Histologic documentation of the breast cancer was available for 250 patients. The survival curves for these 250 patients are reproduced in Figure 5–9. The median period of survival for untreated breast cancer is 2.7 years; 18 percent of patients survived for 5 years, and 10 percent for 10 years. It was against this background that the Halsted radical mastectomy was introduced as treatment of breast cancer.

SURVIVAL RATES

The survival rates, according to tumor stage, following radical mastectomy from nine series are summarized in Table 5–2. The mean ten-year survival rate among these series for Stage I and Stage A patients is 65 percent and for Stage II/Stage B patients, 43 percent. This represented a considerable im-

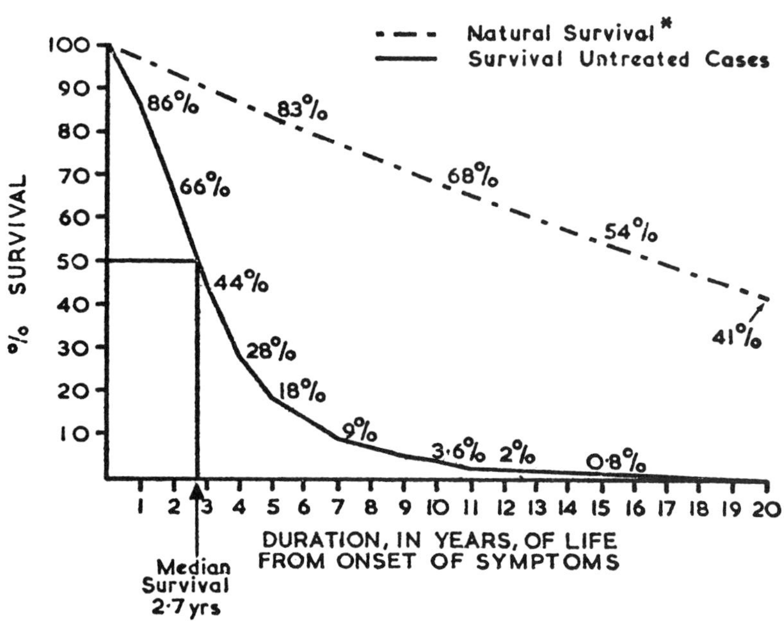

FIGURE 5–9. Survival of patients with untreated breast cancer, based on 250 cases evaluated at the Middlesex Hospital, 1805–1933. (With permission from Bloom HJG, Richardson WW, Harries EJ: Natural history of untreated breast cancer (1805–1933). Br Med J, July 28, 1962, pp. 213–221.)

TABLE 5–2. Survival Rates for Halsted Radical Mastectomy, Retrospective Series

Series	*5-Year Survival Rate (%)*	*10-Year Survival Rate (%)*
Ariel[91]		
Stage I*	81.7	60.3
II	63.7	47.2
III	31.1	17.4
Baker et al.[95]		
Stage I*	85.0	
II	83.0	
III	48.0	
Ferguson et al.[94]		
Stage I*	84.0	76.0
II	52.0	44.0
III	29.0	17.0
Haimov et al.[97]		
Stage I*	70.1	55.5
II	61.4	33.2
III	18.0	12.0
Lee and Lambley[96]		
Stage I†		53.0
II		29.0
Anglem and Leber[90]		
Stage A‡		67.0
B		60.0
C		20.0
D		0.0
Butcher[92]		
Stage A‡	76.0	56.0
B	48.0	30.0
C	48.0	31.0
D	11.0	0.0
Donegan[93]		
Stage A‡	77.0	70.0
B	57.0	43.0
C	52.0	30.0
D	22.0	7.0
Haagensen and Cooley[88]		
Stage A‡	82.5	77.0
B	59.0	45.0
C	38.0	25.0
D	20.0	18.0

*TNM Classification
†Manchester Classification
‡Columbia Clinical Classification

provement over both no treatment and the methods used by Halsted's predecessors. Long-term survival following the Halsted radical mastectomy has been reviewed for four series (Figs. 5–10 and 5–11; Table 5–3). Robbins and Berg[98] found that survival rates for Grades I and II ductal cancer continued to decline at 30 years, whereas those with Grades III and IV cancer remained constant after 20 years. Haagensen's and Ariel's data suggest that survival rates diminish for up to 35 years.[86, 91] Duncan and Kerr found that patients with lesions less than 2 cm in diameter, but not with larger lesions, had a higher death rate 20 years after primary treatment than did an age-matched normal population.[99] While five- and 10-year survival rates may be adequate for comparing the relative effectiveness of two procedures,[46] longer follow-up is required to establish the curativeness of any procedure for the treatment of operable breast cancer.

Table 5–4 summarizes survival rates according to the number of axillary lymph node metastases following treatment with the Halsted radical mastectomy. The results are grouped according to the number of positive nodes (0, 1–3, or ≥4) because of significant differences in survival according to these criteria. The presence of any axillary lymph node metastases is a poor prognostic sign. Among node-positive patients, those with three or fewer lymph node metastases have a significantly better prognosis than patients with four or more positive nodes. In addition, data suggest that the prognosis for patients with micrometastases (less than 2 mm in diameter) in axillary nodes may be better than for patients with macrometastases. Huvos and associates[191] found that the eight-year survival rate for patients with micrometastases of Level I only (94 percent) was as good as that for patients with no metastases at all (82 percent). The survival rate among patients with micrometastases of Level III (59 percent) was comparable with that of patients with macrometastases of Level I (62 percent). Attiyeh and colleagues[102] also found that the presence of micrometastases in axillary nodes was not associated with a worse prognosis than that for patients with no lymph node metastases. This iden-

TABLE 5–3. Long-Term Survival after Halsted Radical Mastectomy for Patients with Stage A and Stage B Breast Cancer, Haagensen's Personal Series

Interval After Surgery (Years)	*Cumulative Proportion of Patients Surviving Breast Carcinoma to End of Interval (%)*	
	STAGE A	STAGE B
0–10	82	51
11–15	79	45
16–20	76	36
21–25	73	36
26–30	67	—
31–35	63	—

Adapted from: Haagensen CD, Bodian C: A personal experience with Halsted's radical mastectomy. Ann Surg 199:143, 1984.

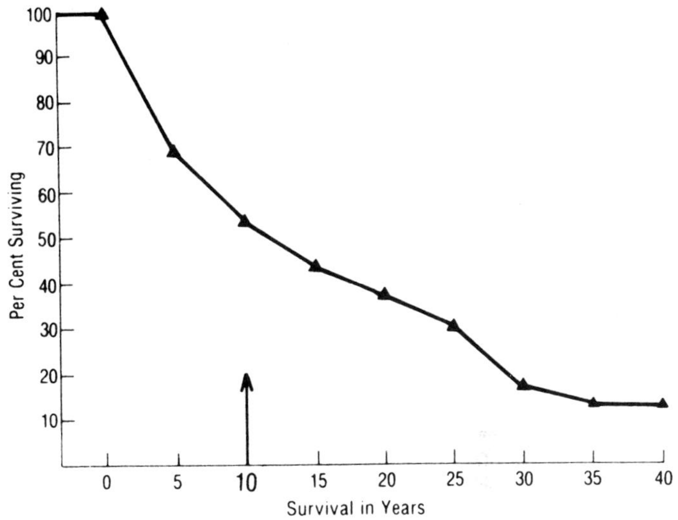

FIGURE 5–10. Overall survival curve for 1178 cases (all stages) of breast carcinoma treated with the Halsted radical mastectomy. (With permission from Ariel IM: Results of 1178 patients with breast cancer treated by radical mastectomy and postoperative radiation where metastases to axillary lymph nodes occurred. J Surg Oncol 12:137, 1979.)

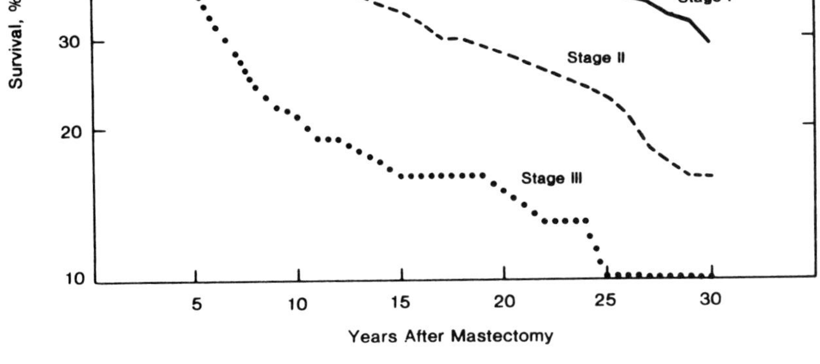

FIGURE 5–11. Comparison of expected and overall survival rates for patients with TNM Stage I, II, or III breast cancer treated with the Halsted radical mastectomy. (With permission from Ferguson DJ, et al.: Staging of breast cancer and survival rates. An assessment based on 50 years of experience with radical mastectomy. JAMA 248: 1337, 1982.)

TABLE 5–4. Survival Rates According to Axillary Node Status after Halsted Radical Mastectomy

Node Status	Haagensen†[89] Series STAGE A	Haagensen†[89] Series STAGE B	Robinson*[100] Series	Ferguson†[94] Series	Fisher†[101] Series	Ariel†[91] Series
Negative	78.0	66.0	86.0	72.0	64.9	60.3
1–3	70.7	44.0	73.0	52.0	37.5	53.9
≥4	—	—	57.0	—	13.4	23.7
4–6	—	—	—	41.0	—	—
>6	—	—	—	10–25	—	—
4–7	42.9	35.7	—	—	—	—
≥8	18.8	15.6	—	—	—	—

*Five-year survival rates (%)
†Ten-year survival rates (%)

tification of subgroups of patients with positive axillary nodes emphasizes the importance of the axillary dissection for staging and prognostic purposes. All patients treated with the Halsted radical mastectomy have a complete axillary dissection. While lesser procedures (e.g., axillary sampling) may establish node positivity, they are thought to be inadequate for accurately quantitating the number of positive nodes (see the following discussion on axillary lymph node dissection).

The ten-year survival rate according to primary tumor size among patients treated with the Halsted radical mastectomy is summarized in Table 5–5. The survival rate progressively decreases with the increasing size of smaller tumors; however, this correlation diminishes for larger lesions (greater than 4 cm). This observation has been made by others.[89] A similar phenomenon has been noted for the incidence of axillary metastases according to tumor size (see following discussion and Table 5–28).[103] The explanation for this correlation is not known. The influence of location of the primary tumor on survival rate is controversial. A worse prognosis has been reported for tumors in the central or medial areas than for outer quadrant tumors.[104] This was not confirmed, however, in the NSABP-B04 trial, in which there was no difference in survival rates between inner and outer quadrant tumors.[105]

TABLE 5–5. Survival According to Size of Primary Tumor in Patients with Breast Cancer Treated with Halsted Radical Mastectomy

Size of Tumor (cm)	No. of Patients	5-Year Survival Rate (%)	10-Year Survival Rate (%)
1 or less	90	77.7	67.9
2	239	74.1	57.1
3	222	65.2	52.8
4	112	63.4	40.3
5	74	59.4	42.9
6	41	46.3	35.1
7	24	44.7	44.7
8	11	54.5	44.6
9 or more	22	27.3	10.9

Adapted from Ariel IM: Results of 1178 patients with breast cancer treated by radical mastectomy and postoperative irradiation where metastases of axillary lymph nodes occurred. J Surg Oncol 12:137, 1979.

LOCAL RECURRENCE

The areas at risk for local recurrence following the Halsted radical mastectomy include the axilla, chest wall, parasternal region, and supraclavicular region. The local recurrence rates among six series evaluating the Halsted radical mastectomy for operable breast cancer are summarized in Tables 5–6 and 5–7. The size and local extent of the primary tumor as well as axillary lymph node metastases are the major determinants of local recurrence. In these series, the overall recurrence rate among axillary node–negative patients ranged from 2.1 to 11.0 percent (average 5.6 percent) and among axillary node–positive patients, from 18 to 48 percent. The highest local recurrence rates have been noted for locally advanced breast cancer (Stages III_a and III_b; see following discussion and Table 5–31).

The Halsted radical mastectomy includes a complete axillary dissection, and therefore the axillary recurrence rate should be low when this procedure is used for operable breast cancer. Axillary recurrence rates ranged from 0 to 5.5 percent (Table 5–6). Haagensen noted no axillary recurrences among Stage A or Stage B node-negative patients and an incidence of 0.2 percent among node-positive patients.[106] Postoperative radiation therapy was rarely adminis-

TABLE 5–6. Locoregional Recurrence after Halsted Radical Mastectomy

Site	Haagensen*§106 Series STAGE A	Haagensen*§106 Series STAGE B	Valagussa*§[107] Series	Donegan‡[108] Series	Fisher†§[46] Series	Ferguson§[94] Series	Veronesi and Valagussa[32] Series
Chest wall	2.7/21.7	1.7/42.2			4.4/7.2		1.7/5.5
Axilla	0.0/0.0	0.0/0.2			1.4/1.0		0.0/5.5
Parasternal area	2.2/5.7	2.7/5.1			0.0/0.0	1.5	1.1/5.5
Supraclavicular area					1.1/5.8	3.0	2.3/8.9
Chest wall/supra-clavicular area			6.0/17.0				
Chest wall, axilla						5.8	
Operative field							
Negative nodes				11.0	2.1		
1–2 positive nodes				21.0			
1–3 positive nodes				—	4.5		
3–4 positive nodes				38.0			
Four or more positive nodes				40.0–52.0	12.5		

*Axillary lymph node pathologically negative or positive
†Axillary lymph node clinically negative or positive
‡Five-year local recurrence rates (%)
§Ten-year local recurrence rates (%)

tered to the chest wall or to the axilla in these node-negative patients. Unless there is extracapsular extension of a metastasis or transection of tumor-bearing lymphatics, the complete axillary dissection should effectively prevent axillary recurrence.

The incidence of chest wall recurrence ranges from 1.7 percent, in lymph node–negative patients, to 42 percent, in lymph node–positive patients (Table 5–6). Among all patients in Haagensen's series, only 15 percent received postoperative radiation therapy, and these were predominantly patients with extensive axillary nodal involvement.[106] Chest wall recurrence is thought to represent implantation of tumor cells at the time of surgery. This emphasizes the importance of including an adequate margin of skin around the tumor (or the biopsy) site and incorporating the nipple in the incision. Skin flaps should be carefully formed, dissecting the skin from the subcutaneous tissue superficial to the superficial fascia. Because chest wall recurrence rates are even higher for locally advanced tumors, these tumors are now considered inoperable (see following discussion).

The parasternal and supraclavicular lymph nodes are not in the operative field and, therefore, should probably not be considered treatment failures. An accurate assessment of parasternal recurrence after the Halsted radical mastectomy is difficult because the lymph nodes are located substernally and must grow to a reasonable size before a parasternal mass is detected and because many patients with inner quadrant tumors or positive axillary nodes received postoperative internal mammary irradiation. The incidence of clinically apparent parasternal recurrence, however, is usually low, averaging less than 6 percent.[59, 110] The incidence of supraclavicular recurrence ranges from 1.0 to

TABLE 5–7. Incidence of Local Recurrence According to Tumor Size after Treatment with Halsted Radical Mastectomy

Tumor Size (cm)	Local Recurrence Rate (%)
<2	3.0
2–3	24.0
3–4	23.0
4–5	24.0
5–6	31.0
6–7	29.0
7–8	28.0
8–9	29.0
9–10	28.0
>10	41.0

Adapted from Donegan WL: Primary treatment options and end results. *In*: Donegan WL, Spratt JS (eds.): Cancer of the Breast, 2nd ed. Philadelphia: W.B. Saunders Co., 1979, p. 262.

TABLE 5–8. Survival Rates of Patients with Locoregional Recurrence after Radical or Modified Radical Mastectomy

Series	5-Year Survival Rate (%)	10-Year Survival Rate (%)	15-Year Survival Rate (%)
Chu et al.[184]	21.0	5.0	—
Donegan et al.[111]	3.9	—	—
Bedwinek et al.[185]	36.0	—	—
Zimmerman et al.[186]	3.0	—	—
Gilliland et al.[187]	18.0	5.0	—
Ferguson et al.[94]	—	—	6.0
Haagensen[106]	12.0	—	—

Adapted from Wilson RE: Surgical management of locally advanced and recurrent breast cancer. Cancer 53:752, 1984.

18 percent (Table 5–6). Approximately one fourth of all local recurrences are in the supraclavicular area.[134]

Local recurrence at any of these sites is a very poor prognostic sign (Table 5–8). Donegan and colleagues[111] noted that, of those patients treated with radical mastectomy who developed a local recurrence, 46 percent died within one year, and only 4 percent survived five years. In Haagensen's series of 135 patients, 30 percent of patients with local recurrence died within one year and 12 percent survived for five years.[106] Ferguson and associates[94] found that only 3 of 51 patients with local recurrence survived more than 20 years without further recurrence, and one of these died of carcinoma at 37 years. Local recurrence in a site that was previously operated on is thus a manifestation of systemic failure. The site of local recurrence (chest wall versus node), however, does not appear to influence survival.[188] These observations stress the need for effective systemic adjuvant therapy in women with breast cancer.

Locally Advanced Breast Cancer

Locally advanced breast cancer includes all Stages III_a and III_b and Stages C and D tumors. In this grouping are all tumors with any of the grave signs of breast cancer. The management of these patients is examined in the following discussion on locally advanced breast cancer and in Chapter 9. It should be pointed out at this time that treatment of locally advanced tumors with the Halsted radical mastectomy alone is ineffective. The 10-year survival rate for Stages III_a and III_b and Stages C and D breast cancer ranges from 0 to 30 percent (Table 5–2), with locoregional recurrences occurring in up to 60 percent of patients (see Table 5–31). The characterization of the grave signs by Haagensen did much to define the operability of breast cancer. The presence of any of these signs precludes the use of the radical mastectomy for curative purposes. These findings also emphasize the importance of accurate clinical staging of the patient at presentation. Detection of inflammatory changes, chest wall fixation, fixed axillary nodes, or other evidence of locally advanced disease not only will spare the patient ineffective radical surgery but also will direct her toward more appropriate and effective treatment from the outset.

Operative Complications

The potential complications following the Halsted radical mastectomy include operative mortality, skin-flap necrosis, seroma formation, arm edema, and wound infection. The incidences of these complications for several series are summarized in Table 5–9. The operative mortality ranged from 0.0 percent to 1.5 percent.[88, 96, 114, 117] Lee and Lambley noted five deaths among 403 patients, with the cause of death including pulmonary embolus in three patients, shock in one patient, and cerebrovascular accident in one patient.[96] With appropriate selection of patients, adequate preoperative preparation, careful operative technique, and early ambulation, the operative mortality from this procedure (as well as from all mastectomies) should be negligible.

Skin-flap necrosis is a frequent and important complication of the Halsted radical mastectomy. The incidence among the four series totaling 1692 patients ranged from 15 to 61 percent (Table 5–9). The largest series (1323 patients) noted an incidence of 36.1 percent. This included partial- and full-thickness skin loss. Factors that are associated with an increased incidence of skin-flap necrosis include increased duration of the surgical procedure, the presence of postoperative serum collections, and vertical rather than transverse incisions.[114, 118] Jolly and Viar[115] reported that skin-flap necrosis occurred in 61 percent of cases in which a vertical incision was used, but in only 17 percent of cases in which a transverse incision was used. The incidence

TABLE 5–9. Postoperative Complications of Mastectomy for Breast Cancer

Complication	Incidence (%)			
	Extended Radical Mastectomy	Standard Radical Mastectomy	Modified Radical Mastectomy	Total Mastectomy
Skin flap necrosis[113–116, 131, 146]				
Mean incidence	24.7 ± 1.2	31.2 ± 11.0	21.4 ± 6.4	9.3 ± 3.5
Range	23.0–26.3	14.5–61.0	7.1–33.0	4.0–16.0
Wound infection[113–116, 146]				
Mean incidence	21.1	10.6 ± 2.7	6.2 ± 1.0	4.7 ± 1.5
Range	(21.1)	5.6–15.0	5.2–7.1	2.0–7.2
Seroma[113–116, 131, 146]				
Mean incidence	31.8 ± 20.9	10.6 ± 2.7	11.5 ± 4.4	18.3 ± 6.7
Range	11.0–52.6	5.6–15.0	7.1–16.0	8.0–30.9
Arm edema[35, 113–116, 131, 146]				
Mean incidence	23.2 ± 13.7	19.9 ± 9.9	8.2 ± 6.3	4.7 ± 2.6
Range	9.5–36.8	2.9–42.0	0.0–27.0	0.0–9.1

of skin-flap necrosis is reduced by increased experience of the operating surgeon and by closure with a split-thickness skin graft rather than by primary closure (skin grafting, however, is rarely used today because the criteria for operability have excluded large tumors as well as those with ulcerations, an inflammatory component, or other grave signs).[114] Krohn and colleagues[190] compared 45 patients undergoing radical mastectomy who had wide skin excision, without ultrathin skin flaps, and autogenous skin grafts with 45 patients treated with radical mastectomy with less wide skin excision, without ultrathin skin flaps but closed primarily. They found that the five- and ten-year survival and local recurrence rates were comparable between the two groups but that wound complications, hospital stays, and subsequent lymphedema were significantly greater in the series with thinner skin flaps. The investigators recommended that the routine use of ultrathin skin flaps be abandoned as treatment of breast cancer.

Skin-flap necrosis occurs more frequently in the upper than in the lower flap. This, presumably, is because the lower flap maintains a richer blood supply from the superior epigastric vessels. Inadvertent separation of the skin from the subcutaneous tissue at the edge of the skin flap will impair viability. Closure of the skin under tension should be avoided. The intraoperative use of fluorescein dye may also help reduce the incidence of skin-flap necrosis in radical mastectomy by allowing detection and excision of nonviable tissue. Myers and associates[119] reported primary healing without any significant wound problems in 90 percent of patients with tissue shown to be viable by this technique.

Seroma formation is a common complication of the Halsted radical mastectomy as well as other mastectomies. In Say and Donegan's series of 1323 radical mastectomies, 41.2 percent of patients developed a seroma postoperatively.[114] This complication is due to persistent drainage from transected lymphatics and other small vessels in the axilla and on the surface of the chest wall. Adherence of the skin flaps to the chest wall facilitates closure of these vessels. For this reason, suction catheters are used routinely to drain the operative field. Morris[120] reported on a controlled trial in which after radical mastectomy, wound healing occurred more rapidly (with a reduction in the incidence of wound infection, breakdown, and necrosis) with suction catheter drainage than with dependent drainage. The authors prefer Hemovac catheters to soft Silastic (Jackson-Pratt) catheters because more effective suction drainage is achieved with the former. Hemovac catheters are left in place until drainage is reduced to 20 ml in a 24-hour period, whichever occurs first. Catheter drainage is usually not required for longer than six to seven days. There appears to be little added benefit in leaving catheters in place for longer than two weeks; beyond this time, they often become associated with chronic, low-grade inflammation of adjacent tissues. Soft Silastic catheters left in place for extended periods of time may also adhere to adjacent tissues. Becker and colleagues[121] reported two cases in which Jackson-Pratt catheters, left in place for two to three weeks, broke beneath the skin surface when they were removed; in both cases, an operative procedure was required to remove the retained fragment. Other methods of promoting skin-flap adherence, such as wrapping the chest with elastic bandages, have largely been abandoned both because their effectiveness has not been proved and because of discomfort to the patient.

Seroma formation is easily treated with percutaneous needle aspiration. Aspiration will eliminate the space under the skin and facilitate adherence of the skin flaps to the underlying chest wall. Repeated aspiration may be necessary. Persistent seromas may be treated with tetracycline, a sclerosing agent. Sitzmann and associates[122] found that instillation of 2 gm of tetracycline in 100 ml of normal saline into postoperative seromas after evacuation enhanced resolution of the seromas without complication. Open drainage of persistent seromas is not recommended because this may introduce infection and/or result in chronic sinus formation.

Postoperative physical rehabilitation also has an important effect on catheter drainage. Lotze and colleagues[123] found that when patients began range of motion exercises on the first postoperative day, there was more total wound drainage and more days of drainage than if physical therapy was started on postoperative day seven. A carefully outlined physical therapy program plays an important role in the management of these patients (see also Chapter 16).

The incidence of arm edema following the Halsted radical mastectomy is difficult to quantitate because the literature is not consistent regarding the criteria used to establish the presence of this complication. The incidence among four series (Table 5–9) ranged from 30 to 42 percent. Britton and Nelson[124] reviewed the incidence among 14 series between 1908 and 1960 and noted a range of 7 to 63 percent.[224] They analyzed 114 cases of postmastectomy edema. Recurrent cancer was an infrequent cause of arm edema. Radiodermatitis, late fibrosis in the axilla resulting from radiation or surgery, and anatomic or functional obstruction of the axillary vein were considered to be major factors contributing to postmastectomy edema. Halsted also recognized the importance of infection as a contributing factor. He noted, "For many years I have entertained the view that although blocking of the lymphatics and occasionally also of the veins was the underlying factor, infection played a conspicuous part in the determination of the amount of swelling and the time of its manifestation."[125] Postoperative axillary radiation after radical mastectomy has also been shown to significantly increase the incidence and severity of arm edema.[124, 126] Britton and Nelson concluded that control of existing infection, instruction in skin care, restoration of shoulder function, pneumatic compression to eliminate pitting edema, and wearing of a precision-fitted elastic sheath were effective in controlling edema in about 90 percent of the patients.[124] Because of the increased risk of arm edema with postoperative (or subsequent) wound infection, the patient who has undergone a complete axillary dissection should not have blood drawn or blood pressure taken or receive any intravenous infusions in that arm. Any cuts or inflammatory reactions in that arm should receive careful and prompt attention. This applies to any patient undergoing a complete axillary dissection, whether it is part of a radical mastectomy or not. The complication of arm edema and its management is also considered in Chapter 16.

The incidence of postoperative wound infection following the Halsted radical mastectomy ranged from 6 to 15 percent (Table 5–9). However, the criteria for designating a wound infection (abscess formation, purulent drainage versus skin inflammation) or use of antibiotics are often not clearly defined in the literature. Certain factors, including seroma formation, skin-flap necrosis, and prolonged catheter drainage, are considered to contribute to the incidence of this complication.[116, 118] Say and Donegan[114] reported that postoperative irradiation increased the postoperative wound infection rate from 15.0 to 28.3 percent. Many of these contributing factors can obviously be eliminated by careful surgical technique. Perioperative antibiotics, however, have not been shown to significantly reduce the postoperative wound infection rate after radical mastectomy.[127]

Extended Radical Mastectomy

The extended radical mastectomy (ERM), as the name implies, extends either the Halsted or the modified radical mastectomy to include the internal mammary lymph nodes. The concept of the extended radical mastectomy is not new, having been proposed by Halsted and Harvey Cushing in the 1890's (see discussion on historical aspects). Since that time, a large number of retrospective studies and three prospective randomized trials have evaluated the role of this procedure in the treatment of operable breast cancer. The technical aspects of the procedure have been reviewed previously (see the discussion on surgical procedures for the management of breast cancer). While there are different methods for removing the internal mammary lymph nodes (*en bloc* resection, monobloc extrapleural dissection, and discontinuous dissection), the results are thought to be comparable. *En bloc* resection is used most commonly. The extended radical mastectomy is based on the premise that removal of diseased internal mammary nodes would prevent local recurrence, would provide important prognostic and staging information, and would remove a source of tumor cells that could otherwise seed distant sites.

The incidence of internal mammary lymph node metastases correlates with the location of the primary tumor and the presence or absence of axillary node metastases (Table 5–10). Internal mammary node metastases are more frequent with inner quadrant tumors. The highest incidence of internal mammary node involvement is among patients with inner quadrant lesions and positive axillary nodes. Interestingly, Handley found that among this subset of patients, the incidence of internal mammary node involvement was greater for lower inner quadrant than for upper inner quadrant tumors.[128] Nevertheless, it can thus be appreciated that without an internal mammary node dissection, a portion (2 to 14 percent) of patients with negative axillary nodes would be understaged and deprived of the potential benefits of adjuvant chemotherapy, whereas 22 to 59 percent of patients with positive axillary nodes would have residual disease in the internal mammary nodes. These and other factors discussed later encouraged the use of the extended radical mastectomy.

The survival rates for seven retrospective series including 1609 patients treated with the extended radical mastectomy are presented in Table 5–11. The results of most of these trials were presented in terms of the positivity and negativity of the axillary (Ax) and internal mammary (IM) nodes, whereas Margottini and colleagues[130] expressed their data according to the stage. In three of the series, *en bloc* resections of the IM nodes were performed,[26–28] and in three series extrapleural dissections were performed.[24, 25, 29, 130] The results for the two techniques, however, are comparable, and the superiority of one method of dissection over the other has not been clearly established. Postoperative radiation therapy was used in the series of Dahl-Iversen (48 percent of patients)[24] and of Urban (33 percent of patients)[28] and among all node-positive patients in Margottini's series.[130] Adjuvant chemotherapy was not used in any of the series. The mean five-year survival according to nodal status for these series is as follows: Ax−/IM−, 85.3 percent; Ax+/IM−, 60.2 percent; A−/IM+, 44.1 percent; and A+/IM+, 54.9 percent. Most of the authors have concluded from their respective series that the extended radical mastectomy improves the survival rate; however, there is disagreement as to which patient group benefits the most from this procedure.

Sugarbaker concluded that patients with combined Ax and IM metastases were responsible for most of the increased survival rate.[26] He recommended that the procedure be used for all patients with operable breast cancer unless there were medical contraindications (clinical pulmonary disease, cardiac disease, or advanced age). Urban noted that optimum results were obtained when the

TABLE 5–10. Incidence of Internal Mammary Lymph Node Metastases*

Location of Primary Tumor	*Incidence (Mean ± SEM) (%)*	*Range (%)*
Outer quadrant		
Negative axillary lymph nodes	4.1 ± 0.4	2.4–4.8
Positive axillary lymph nodes	30.0 ± 4.9	21.5–42.0
Inner quadrant		
Negative axillary lymph nodes	11.8 ± 0.9	9.0–14.3
Positive axillary lymph nodes	49.1 ± 2.9	43.2–59.2

*References 28, 29, 65, 128, and 129

TABLE 5–11. Survival Rates for Extended Radical Mastectomy, Retrospective Series

Series	5-Year Survival Rate (%)	10-Year Survival Rate (%)
Caceres[27]		
Ax −/IM −	84.6	66.6
Ax +/IM −	51.7	31.0
Ax −/IM +	55.5	—
Ax +/IM +	23.9	9.0
Dahl-Iversen and Tobiassen[24]		
Stage A	55.0	
B	50.0	
C	66.0	
D	0.0	
Livingston and Arlen[29]		
Ax −/IM −	89.0	82.0
Ax +/IM −	61.0	54.0
Ax −/IM +	60.0	38.0
Ax +/IM +	50.0	17.0
Sugarbaker[26]		
Ax −/IM −	86.0	
Ax +/IM −	70.0	
Ax −/IM +	14.0	
Ax +/IM +	51.0	
Urban[28]		
Ax −/IM −	87.0	74.7
Ax +/IM −	69.0	50.0
Ax −/IM +	67.0	55.0
Ax +/IM +	50.0	23.0
Veronesi and Zingo[25]		
Ax −/IM −	80.0	67.1
Ax +/IM −	49.4	28.7
Ax −/IM +	24.2	9.5
Ax +/IM +	(100.0)	(50.0)
Margottini et al.[130]		
Stage I	80.4	40.8
II	59.5	31.8
III	29.7	10.0

procedure was applied to proven Stage I cases with clear axillary nodes.[28] He recommended the procedure for Stage I and early Stage II inner quadrant infiltrating tumors. Veronesi and Zingo considered the procedure beneficial for patients with IM metastases but not for patients with combined axillary and internal mammary metastases.[25] Livingston and Arlen[29] compared their series with Haagensen's series of standard radical mastectomies by chi-square analysis and concluded that the extended radical was superior ($p < 0.01$). No details of the analysis were provided, and no statement was made as to which patient group(s) was responsible for the improved survival rate. In a retrospective manner, Margottini and colleagues[130] compared the results of the extended radical mastectomy with those of the Halsted radical at their institution and concluded that the extended radical mastectomy can achieve a much better five-year cure rate for cancers of the inner quadrant of the breast than can the standard operation. Caceres, however, compared in a nonrandomized manner patients who underwent extended radical mastectomy with those who underwent Halsted radical.[27] The two groups were comparable according to a variety of parameters, and all patients were treated at the same institution by the same group of surgeons. Caceres concluded that there was no statistically significant difference in five- or ten-year survival rates between the groups undergoing the two procedures, regardless of the distribution of axillary or internal mammary metastases.

Local Recurrence

The areas at risk for local recurrence following extended radical mastectomy include the axilla, chest wall, parasternal region, and supraclavicular region. The recurrence rates for these areas are summarized in Table 5–12. This summary includes findings from both retrospective series and prospective randomized trials (which are discussed later). The overall local recurrence rate ranged from 5.3 percent to 21.6 percent (average, 10.8 percent). The highest local recurrence rate was noted in patients with positive axillary and internal mammary lymph nodes (16.7 percent)[29] Because dissection of the axillary and parasternal lymph nodes is included in the extended radical mastectomy, local recurrence in these areas is infrequent. Livingston and Arlen[29] and Meier and associates[33] noted no recurrences in the axilla or the parasternal region, and Veronese and Valagussa[32] found an incidence of 0.3 percent in these two areas. This is to be compared with a parasternal recurrence rate of 4 to 6 percent for the Halsted radical mastectomy.[59, 110] The local recurrence rates in the chest wall and supraclavicular areas following the extended radical mastectomy are comparable to that of the Halsted radical mastectomy (see also the Halsted radical mastectomy, Table 5–6). However, for either procedure, recurrences are higher in patients with positive axillary nodes than in those with negative nodes.

Postoperative Complications

The operative mortality rate for the extended mastectomy ranges from 0.1 to 1.5 percent and is generally less than 1.0 percent.[26–29, 32] The incidences of other postoperative complications for the extended radical mastectomy are summarized in Table 5–9. The incidences of skin-flap necrosis and arm edema in the extended radical mastectomy are comparable with those in the Halsted radical mastectomy. The incidence of wound infection and seroma formation may be higher for the extended radical mastectomy. Morbidity that can be directly attributed to the internal mammary node dissection is not well defined, nor is it clear whether extrapleural dissection or *en bloc* resection of the nodes is preferable. Livingston and Arlen[29] considered the extended extrapleural radical mastectomy to be an uncomplicated procedure, with no mortality and few postoperative complications. Meier and colleagues[33] noted that the duration of the surgery was approximately one hour longer and the average number of blood units required was greater for the extended radical than for the standard radical mastectomy but reported no difference in the postoperative complication rate. Donegan and associates[131] concluded that the operative mortality and morbidity after the three procedures (standard, modified, and extended radical mastectomies) were similar when all three were performed by skilled surgeons. The technique used for closure of the chest wall defect will vary according to the preference of the surgeon. Urban prefers use of a fascia lata graft. The skin is closed primarily.

It is very difficult to come to definitive conclusions about the superiority of the extended radical mastectomy over the Halsted radical based solely on the retrospective experience, especially when small differences are involved. Retrospective trials are subject to variability in patient selection, treatment modalities, method of follow-up, data analysis, and method of reporting observations. The retrospective experience and the observations were, however, sufficient to justify prospective randomized trials comparing the extended radical with the Halsted radical mastectomy. These trials have been conducted and are discussed in the following section.

Prospective Randomized Trials

Three prospective randomized trials have been conducted comparing the extended radical with the Halsted radical mastectomy. These are presented chronologically.

International Cooperative Trial, 1963–1968.[30, 31] Patients with tumors less than 7 cm in diameter (clinically N_0 or N_1) were randomized to receive either Halsted radical mastectomy (HRM, 746 patients) or Halsted radical plus internal mammary node dissection (HRM plus IMND, 697 patients). There were five participating centers. No adjuvant radiation therapy or chemotherapy was administered. There have been two reports, the first for five-year results (1976) and the second for ten-year results (1983). There were no significant differences in either overall or disease-free survival rates between the two groups at five years and at ten years (Fig. 5–12). The locoregional recurrence rate at ten years was higher for the HRM (24 percent) than for HRM plus IMND (14 percent). This difference was statistically significant ($p < 0.05$); however, recurrences were mainly noted in patients who developed metastases and thus did not have an impact on survival.

At the time of the five-year report (1976), there was felt to be a significant improvement in the survival rate among patients with inner

TABLE 5–12. Locoregional Recurrence after Extended Radical Mastectomy

Site	*Livingston and Arlen[29] Series*	*Urban[28] Series*	*Veronesi and Valagussa†[32] Series*	*Meier[33] Series*	*Lacour†[30, 31] Series*	*Caceres†[27] Series*
Operative field						
Overall	7.7	7.5		5.3	14.0	9.8
Axillary nodes negative		0.8				
Axillary and internal mammary nodes positive	16.7					
Axilla	0.0		0.3	0.0		
Parasternal area	0.0		0.3	0.0		
Supraclavicular area			10.5	4.8		

*Five-year recurrence rates (%)
†Ten-year recurrence rates (%)

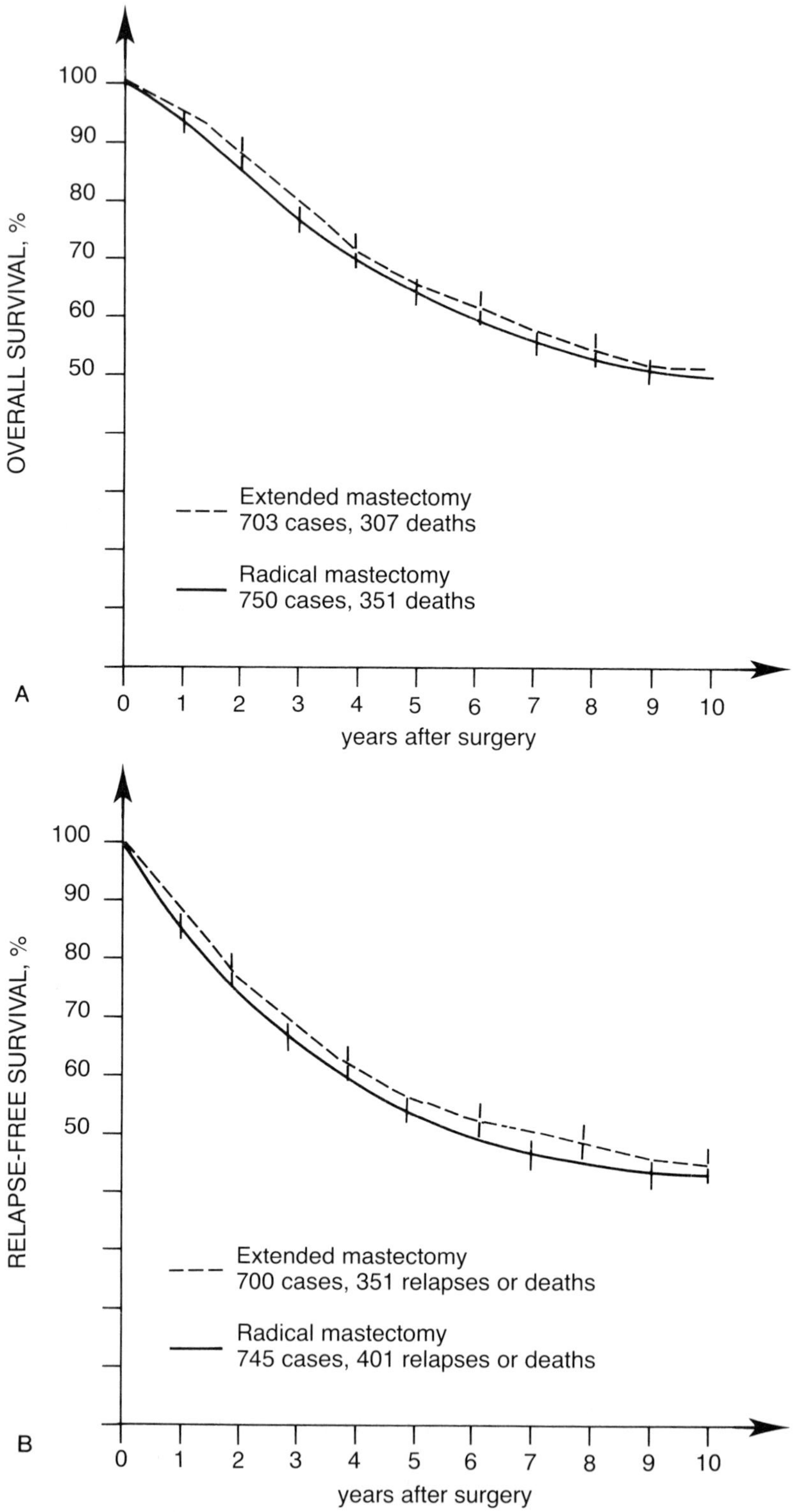

FIGURE 5–12. International cooperative randomized trial comparing the Halsted radical mastectomy with the extended radical mastectomy for patients with T_{1-3}/N_0 or N_1 breast cancer. *A,* ten-year overall survival curves by treatment. *B,* ten-year relapse-free survival curves by treatment. (With permission from Lacour J, et al.: Radical mastectomy vs. radical mastectomy plus internal mammary dissection. Cancer 51:1941, 1983.)

or medial T_1 or T_2 tumors with positive axillary lymph nodes treated with HRM plus IMND versus HRM alone (HRM plus IMND, 71 percent; HRM, 52 percent; $p < 0.01$). There was no significant difference for outer quadrant tumors or for inner or medial quadrant tumors without axillary involvement. However, at the time of the ten-year report and following a reanalysis of data, the survival difference in this subgroup was no longer considered significant because of center-to-center variability in the nodal status of the patients (see later). The investigators concluded that except for a reduction in locoregional recurrence rate with the extended radical, which was not accompanied by a survival benefit, this trial failed to demonstrate the superiority of the extended radical mastecomy over the Halsted radical mastectomy.

CRITIQUE. Upon completion of entry subjects into the trial, there was a slight excess of Halsted operations (51 percent versus 49 percent for HRM plus IMND) and a greater percentage of patients over the age of 50 years in the Halsted group. These differences appear minor and should not have a significant impact on the results. One center had 25 percent of its patients lost to follow-up and thus was excluded from the analysis. All analyses were based on 1443 patients from the remaining four centers. There was also a disparity in distribution of patients according to nodal status. The incidence of axillary node positivity varied from 53 percent to 62 percent and the incidence of internal mammary node positivity varied from 14 to 29 percent among the four centers. The ten-year survival rate for lymph node–positive patients varied from 15 to 44 percent. The reasons for this variability as well as detailed analyses of survival by center for three of the final four participating centers are not given (see NCI [Milan] trial, discussed later).[32] It is stated that two of the centers performed *en bloc* removal of the internal mammary nodes and two performed extrapleural dissections. The results of this trial support the conclusion that the extended radical mastectomy, when applied to all patients with Stage I or II breast cancer, provides no significant benefit over the Halsted radical. The original proposal by Veronesi and Zingo[25] and Urban[28] that the procedure is of benefit for inner quadrant lesions with negative axillary nodes is not substantiated. Whether those patients with positive axillary and internal mammary nodes benefit from this procedure (as proposed by Sugarbaker[26]) remains unresolved, based on this trial.

National Cancer Institute (Milan), 1964–1968.[32] This is a detailed analysis of the Milan contribution to the International Cooperative Trial discussed earlier. Patients with TNM T_1, T_2, T_{3a}, N_0, and N_1 tumors were randomized to receive Halsted radical mastectomy (HRM, 374 patients) or Halsted radical mastectomy plus internal mammary node dissection (HRM plus IMND, 342 patients). An *en bloc* dissection was used for the node dissection. There was no postoperative adjuvant radiation therapy. Follow-up is at ten years.

There was no significant difference in the ten-year overall or disease-free survival rates between the two treatment groups (Table 5–13). No significant difference was noted between the two groups when they were analyzed according to nodal status or location of the primary tumor. No significant difference was noted in the locoregional recurrence rate at ten years between HR and HR plus IMND for the operative field, homolateral axilla, or homolateral supraclavicular region (Table 5–14). The parasternal recurrence rate was slightly higher with HRM (3.7 percent) than with HRM plus IMND (0.3 percent), although this apparently was not statistically significant. The investigators concluded that their findings do not support the usefulness of internal mammary node dissection for either all patients or any subset of patients with breast cancer. In addition, because only 2.3 percent of patients with negative axillary nodes had positive internal mammary nodes, the investigators do not support the IMND for staging purposes.

CRITIQUE. This was a well-controlled, single-institution randomized trial. The two treatment groups were comparable according to tumor size, age, menopausal status, location of primary tumor, and axillary nodal status. All patients who underwent extended radical mastectomy receive an *en bloc* resection of the internal mammary nodes. There was no adjuvant radiation therapy or chemotherapy. The results confirm that the extended radical, when applied to all patients with Stage I or II breast cancer, offers no significant advantage over the Halsted radical mastectomy. This trial also argues against the proposal that the extended radical mastectomy is of benefit for patients with inner

TABLE 5–13. Disease-Free and Overall Ten-Year Survival: NCI (Milan) Prospective Randomized Trial Comparing Halsted Radical Mastectomy with Extended Radical Mastectomy

Survival	Halsted Radical Mastectomy No. of Patients	%	Extended Radical Mastectomy No. of Patients	%
Disease-Free				
Total	374	49.7	342	47.3
N −	174	75.8	161	72.1
N +	200	27.0	181	25.4
Overall				
Total	374	60.7	342	57.0
N −	174	80.4	161	79.5
N +	200	43.2	181	38.1

Source: Veronesi U, Valagussa P: Inefficacy of internal mammary node dissection in breast cancer surgery. Cancer 47:170, 1981.

quadrant tumors and negative axillary lymph nodes. The only subgroup in this category that showed a survival benefit (overall or disease-free, five- or ten-year) was that of patients with T_3 lesions (Table 5–15). A total of only 16 patients (2.2 percent of total population) had inner quadrant T_3 lesions with negative axillary nodes. This represents a very small percentage of all patients who may benefit from the extended radical mastectomy. In addition, there is increasing evidence that all T_3 lesions should now be treated with combined-modality therapy (see later).

University of Chicago, 1973–1985.[33] One hundred twenty-three women with TNM clinical Stage I or II breast cancer were randomized to receive Halsted radical mastectomy (HRM, 62 patients) or extended radical mastectomy (ERM, 61 patients). All patients in the ERM group received an *en bloc* resection of the internal mammary nodes. No postoperative radiation therapy was given. Adjuvant chemotherapy was administered to 24.5 percent of the HRM patients and 36.4 percent of the ERM patients. Follow-up was at five years for all patients. The investigators found no significant differences between the two treatment groups in overall five-year survival rates, either for all patients or for any subgroup according to tumor location, including central-medial tumors (Fig. 5–13). The local recurrence rate for all patients was 5.3 percent, with no significant differences between the two treatment groups. The investigators conducted a separate analysis in which 11 patients from the total trial population were excluded (two patients because of protocol violations, two patients with intraductal carcinoma, and seven patients in whom the operative procedure was not performed by the same surgeon, in contrast with the remaining 112 patients). Among these 112 patients, they found no significant difference between the two groups in overall five-year survival but noted a trend favoring survival with ERM for central-medial lesions (HRM, 88 percent; ERM, 66 percent; $p < 0.6$).

CRITIQUE. There were several differences in the patient population between the two treatment arms. The unequal distribution according to adjuvant chemotherapy has been mentioned. In addition, the ERM group included patients with more favorable prognostic factors: There were fewer premenopausal patients, more patients with nonductal invasive carcinoma, fewer patients with vascular invasion, fewer patients with more

TABLE 5–14. Overall Locoregional Recurrence Rate for Halsted Radical Mastectomy and Extended Radical Mastectomy: NCI (Milan) Prospective Randomized Trial

Site	Halsted Radical Mastectomy 5-Year (%)	10-Year (%)	Extended Radical Mastectomy 5-Year (%)	10-Year (%)
Operative field	7.2	8.3	6.4	8.2
Parasternal region	3.7	3.7	0.3	0.3
Homolateral axilla	0.3	0.3	0.3	0.3
Homolateral supraclavicular region	8.0	8.0	8.8	10.5

Source: Veronesi U, Valagussa P: Inefficacy of internal mammary node dissection in breast cancer surgery. Cancer 47:170, 1981.

TABLE 5–15. Overall Survival Rate Related to Extent and Location of Primary Tumor and to Axillary Lymph Node Involvement: NCI (Milan) Prospective Randomized Trial Comparing Halsted Radical with Extended Radical Mastectomy

	Halsted Radical Mastectomy		*Extended Radical Mastectomy*	
Patient Category	5-YEAR (%)	10-YEAR (%)	5-YEAR (%)	10-YEAR (%)
T_1–T_2 lateral	76.9	63.3	70.8	60.8
N −	93.6	85.0	81.4	77.9
N +	63.2	45.7	61.1	45.3
T_1–T_2 medial	70.2	62.2	71.0	57.0
N −	81.5	78.9	92.6	80.2
N +	57.7	45.8	51.6	37.9
T_3 lateral	70.8	60.8	35.3	29.4
N −	91.7	91.7	75.0	75.0
N +	50.0	25.0	23.1	7.7
T_3 medial	47.4	36.1	61.9	43.3
N −	60.0	60.0	100.0	84.7
N +	42.9	28.6	30.8	15.1

Source: Veronesi U, Valagussa P: Inefficacy of internal mammary node dissection in breast cancer surgery. Cancer 47:170, 1981.

than 4 positive axillary nodes, more patients with estrogen receptor–positive tumors, and a smaller average primary tumor diameter. When analyzed separately, the difference in tumor diameter was significant ($p < 0.05$). The difference in vascular invasion, nodal status, pathologic stage, and ERM status was not significant. Nevertheless, while statistically significant differences for individual prognostic factors were not seen, the potential cumulative effect of these factors in one group is not clear. With several prognostic factors tending to favor one group (ERM), one is reluctant to conclude that the trend toward a survival benefit (for central-medial lesions) is based solely on the procedure itself. It is also not clear why the exclusion of 11 patients made such a difference in survival for central-medial lesions (14 percent difference, $p < 0.14$ when the 11 patients were included, versus a 22 percent difference, $p < 0.06$ when the patients were excluded). With the exclusion, 35 patients are present in each arm for this subgroup. Larger numbers of patients, with a balance according to prognostic factors, are needed to make definitive conclusions about the role of the ERM for central-medial lesions. It is noted,

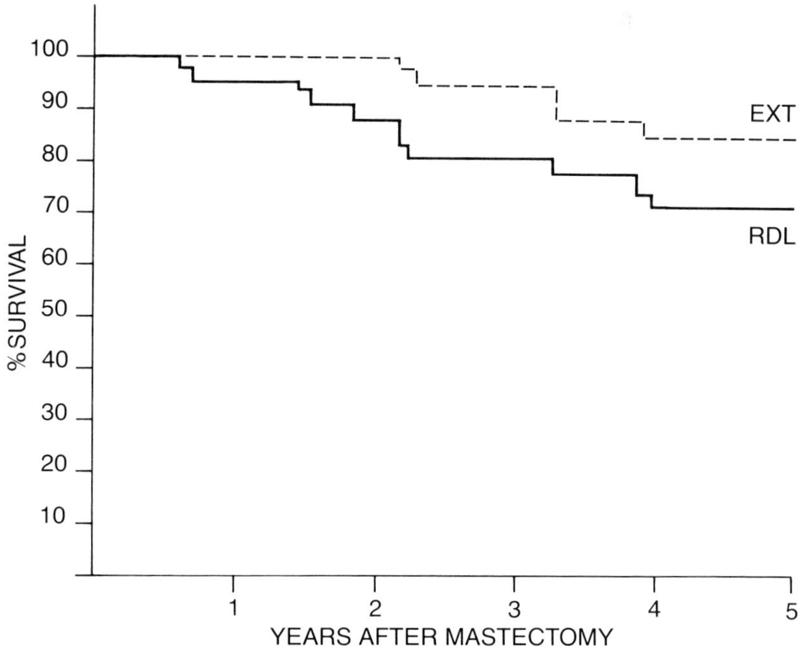

FIGURE 5–13. University of Chicago randomized trial comparing the Halsted radical mastectomy (RDL) with the extended radical mastectomy (EXT) for patients with TNM Stage I or II breast cancer. Overall survival curves by treatment. (With permission from Meier P, Ferguson DJ, Karrison T: A controlled trial of extended radical mastectomy. Cancer 55:880, 1985.)

however, that the authors no longer recommend the ERM for lateral tumors.

Summary and Consensus

In summary, retrospective series using the extended radical mastectomy for the treatment of operable breast cancer suggested a survival benefit of this procedure over the Halsted radical. This survival benefit was principally for inner quadrant lesions, although there was disagreement as to whether this benefit occurred in patients with internal mammary lymph node metastases alone or in patients with combined internal mammary and axillary metastases. None of these series suggested a survival benefit for patients without any lymph node metastases. The retrospective series also suggested that by identifying patients with internal mammary node metastases only (without axillary metastases), there was a staging and prognostic benefit to the extended radical mastectomy. These series showed that the extended radical could be performed with negligible operative mortality and with a morbidity that is comparable to or slightly higher than that for the Halsted radical mastectomy.

Prospective randomized trials from several centers comparing the Halsted radical mastectomy with the extended radical mastectomy all failed to show any survival benefit among all patients with Stage I or II breast cancer. Among subgroups of patients, there was no additional benefit for patients with lateral lesions when treated with the extended radical mastectomy. Two trials (Lacour and colleagues[30, 31] and Meier and associates[33]) suggested a possible survival benefit of the extended radical for central-medial lesions, although in one, this was not statistically significant,[33] and in the other, it was significant only if variability in lymph node status within the treatment groups was disregarded.[30, 31] Therefore, at this time it cannot be unequivocally concluded that the ERM confers a definite survival advantage over the Halsted radical mastectomy for any subgroup of patients with Stage I or II breast cancer.

The internal mammary node dissection for staging and prognostic purposes may be beneficial in identifying patients with positive internal mammary and negative axillary lymph nodes. The incidence of internal mammary metastases (and negative axillary nodes), as noted, ranges from 2 to 14 percent and is associated with a worse prognosis. Because adjuvant chemotherapy is being considered for axillary node–negative patients, information about internal mammary lymph node status would be important for evaluation of this treatment. Internal mammary node dissection (or biopsy) would most appropriately be applied to patients with inner quadrant lesions and clinical negative axillary nodes. More information is needed about the role of chemotherapy in the treatment of axillary node–negative patients before internal mammary node dissection or biopsy can be recommended as a routine procedure in these patients.

Superradical Mastectomy

The superradical mastectomy extends the Halsted radical to include the supraclavicular and internal mammary lymph nodes. This procedure was originally proposed by Halsted. In 1898, he reported on 67 cases in which the supraclavicular fossa had been dissected.[9] He found nodal involvement in this region in 23 cases (36 percent). He concluded that "our rule should be to operate on the neck in every case." This recommendation was not adopted by other surgeons until the 1940's and 1950's when the procedure was revived by a few groups, most notably Wagensteen,[22] Margottini,[23, 130] Dahl-Iversen,[24, 65, 133] and Veronesi and Zingo.[25] Wagensteen and colleagues[22] removed the first rib and divided the sternocleidomastoid and strap muscles and the sternum.[22] The sternum was reapproximated after the internal mammary nodes were dissected. Dahl-Iversen and Tobiassen[24] performed a discontinuous dissection, first removing the supraclavicular nodes through a separate neck incision, followed by closure and then the mastectomy and internal mammary node dissection. Margottini performed the supraclavicular node dissection as a second stage in patients with axillary and internal mammary node metastases.[23] Veronesi and Zingo[25] performed an *en bloc* resection, removing the clavicle, the first and second ribs, and the corresponding half of the sternum.[25]

The incidence of supraclavicular metastases alone (without axillary or internal mammary metastases) among these series ranged from 2 to 6 percent.[22, 65] The incidence of

TABLE 5–16. Five-Year Survival Rates According to Stage for Superradical Mastectomy: Dahl-Iversen–Tobiassen Series of 366 Patients

Stage	*No. of Patients*	*5-Year Survival Rate (%)*
A	277	77.0
B	61	48.0
C	20	50.0
D	8	37.7

Source: Dahl-Iversen E, Tobiassen T: Radical mastectomy with parasternal and supraclavicular dissection for mammary carcinoma. Ann Surg 157:170, 1963.

supraclavicular metastases with involvement of axillary or parasternal lymph nodes ranged from 17 to 43 percent.[22, 23, 25, 65] The highest incidence (43 percent) was noted by Veronesi and Zingo,[25] who applied the superradical mastectomy to patients with massive invasion of axillary nodes or palpable supraclavicular nodes. Haagensen performed supraclavicular node biopsies on patients with breast cancer and found a 2 percent incidence of supraclavicular involvement alone and a 17 percent incidence with internal mammary node involvement.[134]

The five-year survival rates for Dahl-Iversen and Tobiassen's series of 366 patients is presented in Table 5–16.[24] Among patients with supraclavicular metastases, they noted a five-year survival rate of 17 percent. They concluded that "removal of the parasternal and supraclavicular lymph nodes has not improved the recurrence rate."[65] Wangensteen and colleagues[22] noted a five-year survival rate of 17 percent among all patients treated with the superradical mastectomy and concluded that it was unlikely that the overall survival with this procedure would be greater than that obtained by the conventional operation (Halsted radical). Margottini, however, reported a 14 percent improvement in survival rate over the Halsted radical.[23]

The operative mortality for two series evaluating the superradical mastectomy was 1 percent.[22, 24] The morbidity attributable to the supraclavicular node dissection was minimal when this was done as a discontinuous procedure or in a second stage.[23, 65] The morbidity of the *en bloc* resection of supraclavicular and internal mammary nodes used by Veronese and Zingo was not described.[25]

The superradical mastectomy was never adopted to any degree by the surgical community. While the procedure did provide information about the incidence of supraclavicular metastases in breast cancer, it became clear the surgical treatment of the supraclavicular area provided no therapeutic benefit to these patients. The experience with this procedure simply reaffirmed the concept that supraclavicular metastases represented advanced disease and required other forms of treatment. Accordingly, the procedure is no longer used.

Modified Radical Mastectomy

The modified radical mastectomy (MRM) was introduced because of a concern among surgeons that the Halsted radical mastectomy resulted in a significant cosmetic deficit and because of the suggestion that survival and local control rates could be just as effectively achieved with less radical procedures. The classic modified radical mastectomy, as described by Patey, removes all breast tissue, the pectoralis minor, and all axillary tissue, preserving the pectoralis major muscle.[16] A further modification of this procedure was introduced by Auchincloss[17] and Madden.[18] In these latter two procedures, all breast tissue and essentially the lateral 80 percent of the axillary tissue are removed, preserving both pectoral muscles. The terms Auchincloss and Madden mastectomies are used interchangeably in the literature with the term total mastectomy with axillary dissection and are synonymous. The degree to which the axillary contents can be dissected with and without removing the pectoralis minor muscle is examined later in the discussion on axillary lymph node dissection. Although the concept of the modified radical mastectomy was introduced by Moore in 1867, it was not until the 1960's and 1970's that the procedure was used by a large number of surgeons. During this time, its popularity increased dramatically, and by the 1980's, the modified radical became the standard procedure for the radical treatment of breast cancer. As of 1981, 72.3 percent of all radical mastectomies were of the modified radical variety and only 3.4 percent were of the Halsted radical type (Table 5–1). Because of this trend, a large experience has accumulated from both retrospective series and prospective randomized trials defining the curative potential, the ability to achieve local control, and the associated complications of the modified radical mastectomy.

TABLE 5–17. Survival Rates for Modified Radical Mastectomy, Retrospective Series

Series	5-Year Survival Rate (%)	10-Year Survival Rate (%)
Baker et al.[95]		
Stage I*	90.0	
II	73.0	
III	45.0	
Hermann and Steiger[135]		
Stages I and II†	71.0	46.0
Leis[138]		
Stage I† (T_1, T_2, T_3/N_0)		72.2
Stage II (T_1, T_2, T_3/N_1)		40.2
Madden et al.[137]		
Stage I*	73.4§	
II	52.0	
III	50.0	
Robinson et al.[100]		
Stages I, II, and III*	78.0	
Handley[139]		
Stage A‡	83.0	79.0
B	72.0	48.0
C	51.1	46.0
Delarue et al.[136]		
All stages*	51.0	
Meyer et al.[140]		
All stages	74.0	43.0

*TNM Classification
†Manchester Classification
‡Columbia Clinical Classification
§Three- to 13-year follow-up

The five- and ten-year survival rates according to stage and node status for eight retrospective series evaluating the modified radical mastectomy are summarized in Tables 5–17 and 5–18. Among these series, a Patey mastectomy with removal of the pectoralis minor muscle was employed by Handley[139] and by Leis.[138] An Auchincloss-Madden modified radical mastectomy with preservation of the pectoralis minor was performed by Robinson,[100] Hermann and Steiger,[135] Delarue,[136] and Madden.[137] While comparisons between procedures using retrospective series alone are impossible to accomplish reliably, these series suggest that the survival rates according to both stage and node status for the modified radical mastectomy are comparable to those for the Halsted radical mastectomy (Tables 5–2 and 5–4). In addition, these series suggest that the survival rates for the Auchincloss-Madden mastectomy are comparable to those for the Patey mastectomy. In the latter procedure, the apical axillary tissue is removed, whereas in the former this tissue is preserved. It has been shown that the axillary dissection does not confer a survival benefit (see the following discussions on total mastectomy and on axillary lymph node dissection). Therefore, one would not expect a difference in survival between these two procedures.

The incidence of locoregional recurrence following modified radical mastectomy is summarized in Table 5–19. In Handley's series, radiation therapy was used for patients with positive axillary or internal mammary nodes (41 percent of patients).[139] Radiation therapy was used in 12 percent of patients in Baker's series[95] and not at all in those of Delarue[136] and Madden.[137] Because the modified radical mastectomy preserves the pectoralis major (and in some cases the pectoralis minor), one might expect the modified radical to have higher chest wall and, perhaps, axillary recurrence rates than those of the Halsted radical mastectomy. (The internal mammary and supraclavicular nodes are not disturbed in either procedure.) Handley, among his first 200 patients, noted only one local recurrence in the axilla and no instance of recurrence in the pectoralis major muscle.[141] Delarue and colleagues observed no local or regional recurrences in patients with Stage I disease.[136] Madden and associates reported no local recurrences at ten years in the pectoral muscles.[137] Baker found no significant difference in local recurrence rates between the modified radical and the Halsted

TABLE 5–18. Survival Rates According to Axillary Lymph Node Status after Modified Radical Mastectomy

Axillary Lymph Node Status	Madden*[137] Series	Handley†[139] Series	Robinson*[100] Series
Negative	81.6	90.0	84.0
Any positive nodes	32.4	67.0	—
1–3	—	—	73.0
≥4	—	—	55.0

*Five-year survival rates (%)
†Ten-year survival rates (%)

radical mastectomies for Stage I and II disease but a statistically higher incidence for Stage III disease (HRM, 8 percent; MRM, 39 percent).[95] Thus, the local recurrence rates in the operative field are not substantially different from those of the standard radical mastectomy, despite the fact that the pectoralis major muscle and the accompanying intrapectoral lymph node chain were not removed in any of these patients and neither excision of the pectoralis minor nor a complete axillary dissection was performed in many. These observations support the view that removal of the pectoralis major muscle is not essential to achieving good local control in Stage I or II and Stage A or B breast cancers (both the modified radical mastectomy and the Halsted radical are inadequate alone for achieving local control in Stage III and Stage C or D tumors; see following discussion on locally advanced breast cancer). In all of these series, the nipple and an adequate margin of skin around the biopsy site were removed. In all but one series (Hermann and Steiger[135]) the skin flaps were thin, leaving, at most, occasional islands of fat to promote vascularity of the skin. Handley made his skin flaps up to one fifth of an inch thick in stout patients but considerably thinner in less well-developed patients. In all series, the fascia was removed from the pectoralis major muscle. These principles of breast cancer surgery appear to be adequate for providing local control in patients with operable (Stage I or II) breast cancer.

The postoperative complications following modified radical mastectomy are summarized in Table 5–9. The operative mortality was negligible and was zero in four series (356 patients).[113, 114, 136, 141] The exact incidence of each of the remaining four major complications (skin-flap necrosis, seroma formation, arm edema, and wound infection) is variable. In general, however, the incidence of these complications is comparable or even less than that for the Halsted radical mastectomy. Feigenberg and associates[142] compared the incidence of postoperative complications follow-

TABLE 5–19. Locoregional Recurrence After Modified Radical Mastectomy

Site	*Delarue**[136] Series	*Madden*†[137] Series	*Leis*‡[138] Series	*Handley*‡[139] Series	*Baker**[95] Series	*Maddox**[20] Series
Operative field						
Stage I	0.0		5.0		13.1	9.3
I and II	12.5		13.8			
II					9.0	7.1
III					38.7	20.0
I, II, and III		10.0				
Negative axillary nodes				5.0		
Positive axillary nodes				27.0		
Chest wall						
Stage A				10.0		
B				22.6		
C				63.6		
I					13.1	
II			0.8		9.0	
III					22.5	
Axilla						
Stage A				1.8		
B				0.1		
C				9.1		
I					1.0	
II					4.5	
III					22.5	
Parasternal area						
Stage A				1.8		
B				3.0		
C				9.1		

*Five-year recurrence rates (%)
†Three- to 13-year recurrence rates (%)
‡Ten-year recurrence rates (%)
For staging classifications, see Table 5–20.

ing the modified radical mastectomy with those of the Halsted radical. They found that for the modified radical, there were considerably fewer immediate postoperative complications (seroma formation, wound infection, and skin-flap necrosis) and a significantly lower incidence of late complications (limb edema and recurrent infection) than for the Halsted radical mastectomy. Leis[138] considered the modified radical to be associated with an increased percentage of better arm and shoulder function and a decreased percentage of significant arm edema as compared with the Halsted radical mastectomy. Dunphy[143] considered the modified radical mastectomy to be associated with improved wound healing, less blood loss, and a decidedly superior cosmetic result compared with the Halsted radical. This probably reflects the more frequent use of the transverse incision, preservation of the pectoralis major muscle (and, in some cases, the pectoralis minor), reduced frequency of complete axillary dissection, and shorter operative time for the modified radical mastectomy. The factors contributing to each of these complications are reviewed in detail in the earlier discussion on postoperative complications following the Halsted radical mastectomy.

Prospective Randomized Trials

The retrospective analysis of a large experience with the modified radical mastectomy thus suggested that this procedure could achieve survival rates and local control comparable to the Halsted radical mastectomy, with perhaps fewer complications, and with a clear cosmetic advantage. The comparability of these two procedures has been further tested in two prospectively randomized trials. These are discussed chronologically.

Manchester Trial, Manchester, England, 1969–1976.[19] Patients with TNM T_1 or T_2/N_0 or N_1 tumors were prospectively randomized to receive Halsted radical (HRM, 278 patients) or modified radical mastectomies (MRM, 256 patients). Surgical procedures were performed by six participating surgeons. No adjuvant radiation or chemotherapy was given. Results were reported according to whether tumors were pathologically Stage I or II under respective clinical Stage I or II headings; hence, a range is given for each category. The median follow-up period is five years.

The investigators found no significant difference in five-year overall or disease-free survival between the two groups undergoing the procedures for either Stage I or Stage II tumors (Fig. 5–14). The five-year local recurrence rates (skin flap, chest wall or axilla) for Stage I patients and for Stage II patients were also comparable between the two treatment arms (Table 5–20). The investigators concluded that the Halsted radical mastectomy confers no measurable advantage over the modified radical mastectomy in terms of rate of total survival, local recurrence, distant metastases, or disease-free survival.

Critique. There were eight protocol violations (patients receiving surgical procedures other than those assigned to them). Among clinical Stage II patients, the Halsted radical group was, on the average, three years older than the modified radical group. The two groups were otherwise comparable. The local recurrence rates (skin flap, chest wall, and ipsilateral axilla) among pathologic Stage II patients (average 39 percent) were high. The number of positive nodes per patient is not stated, but unless virtually all of the Stage II patients had four or more positive nodes, these recurrence rates would be higher than those reported by other groups. The technical

TABLE 5–20. Local Recurrence Rates in Manchester Trial: Prospective Randomized Comparison of Halsted Radical Mastectomy with Modified Radical Mastectomy

Patient Category	*5-Year Local Recurrence Rate (%)*
All Cases	
Radical	25.0
Modified radical	21.0
Clinical Stage I	
Pathologic Stage I	
Radical	15.0
Modified radical	10.0
Pathologic Stage II	
Radical	43.0
Modified radical	26.0
Clinical Stage II	
Pathologic Stage I	
Radical	9.0
Modified radical	12.0
Pathologic Stage II	
Radical	41.0
Modified radical	44.0

Adapted from Turner L, Bell WGT, Hartley RC, et al.: Radical versus modified radical mastectomy for breast cancer. Ann R Coll Surg Engl 63:239, 1981.

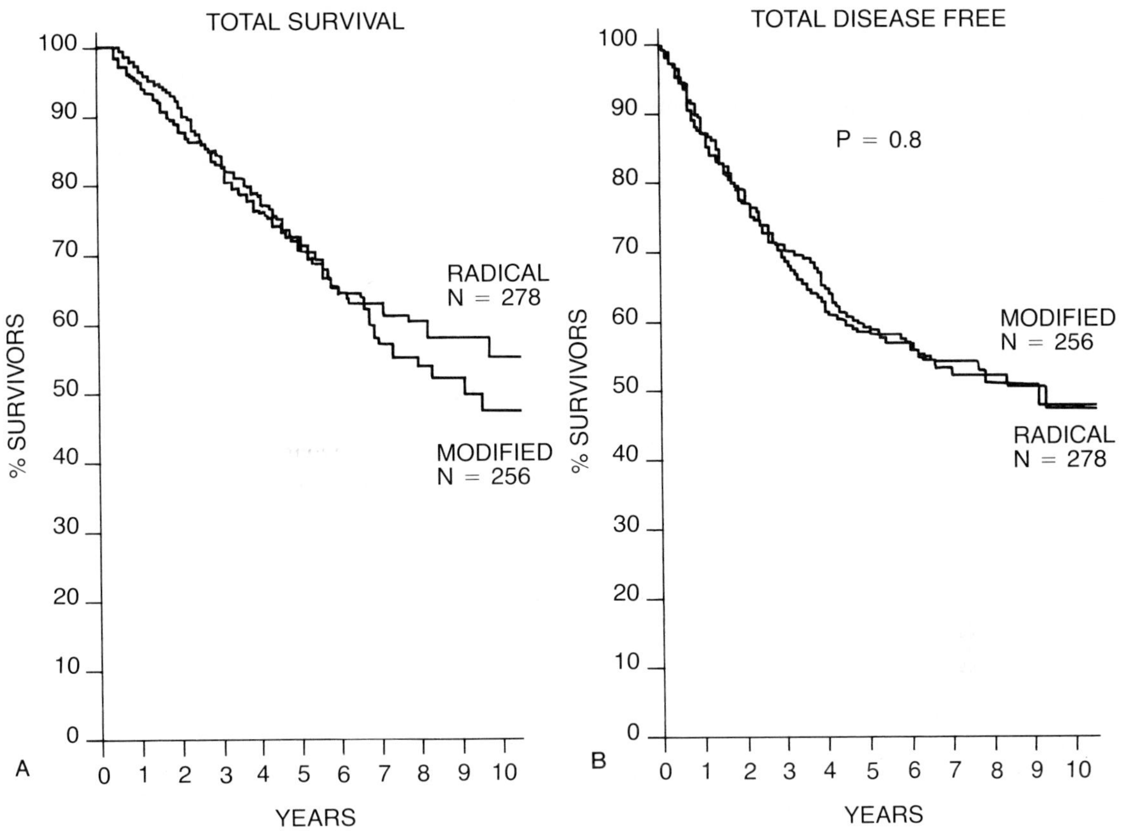

FIGURE 5–14. Manchester randomized trial comparing the Halsted radical mastectomy with the modified radical mastectomy for patients with Stage I or II breast cancer. *A,* ten-year total survival curves by treatment. *B,* ten-year total disease-free survival curves by treatment. (With permission from Turner L, et al.: Radical versus modified radical mastectomy for breast cancer. Ann R Coll Surg Engl 63:239, 1981.)

details of the procedure and the degree to which they might contribute to the high recurrence rate are not specified for either the Halsted radical or the modified radical groups. Without this information, one cannot exclude the possibility that the five-year local recurrence and disease-free survival rates could be improved in one or both treatment groups. The trial supports the comparability of the two procedures, but it needs to be shown that the procedures were optimally applied to patients at high risk for recurrence.

University of Alabama, W. Maddox, 1975–1978.[20] Patients with TNM T_{1a}, T_{2a}, and T_{3a}/N_0 or N_1 tumors were randomized to receive Halsted radical mastectomy (HRM, 136 patients) or modified radical mastectomy (MRM, 175 patients). A prerandomization scheme was used (the participating surgeon knew the selected treatment when discussing the protocol with the patient). Axillary node–positive patients were in turn randomized to receive either CMF (cyclophosphamide, methotrexate, and fluorouracil) or melphalan. Ninety-one surgeons from the state of Alabama participated. There was no postoperative radiation therapy. The median follow-up period was 65 months. The investigators found no statistically significant differences in five-year overall or disease-free survival rates between the two treatment groups (Fig. 5–15). There were no significant differences in local recurrence rates (Table 5–21). There was a trend, however, favoring HRM in each of these three categories.

CRITIQUE. This is a well-conducted trial under the direction of a single institution. The use of a prerandomization scheme probably accounted for the greater number of patients in the modified radical arm. The two arms are, however, well balanced according to age, race, menopausal status, clinical and pathologic stage, node status, and adjuvant chemotherapy. The number of patients rejecting the study and their distribution is not given. The number of patients in each arm

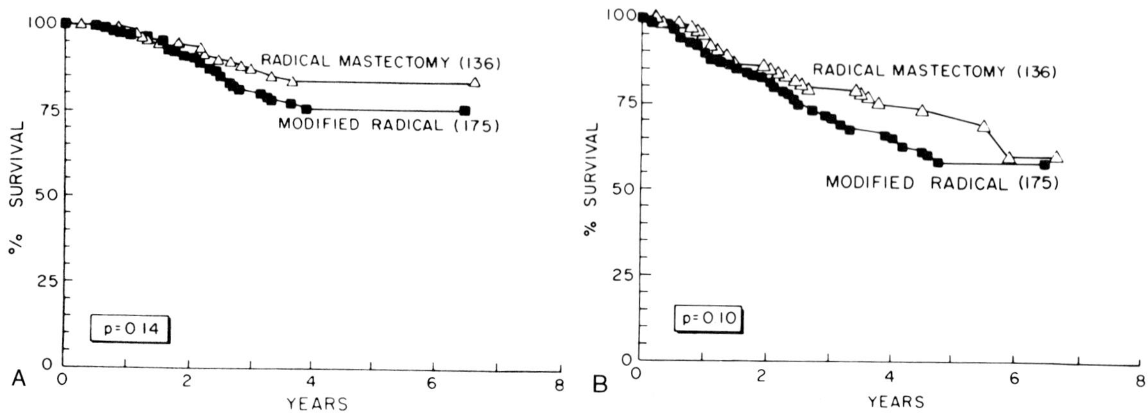

FIGURE 5–15. University of Alabama randomized trial comparing the Halsted radical mastectomy with the modified radical mastectomy for patients with TNM Stage I, II, or III breast cancer. *A*, Disease-free survival by treatment. *B*, Overall survival by treatment. (With permission from Maddox WA, et al.: A randomized prospective trial of radical (Halsted) mastectomy versus modified radical mastectomy in 311 breast cancer patients. Ann Surg 198:207, 1983.)

required to demonstrate a significant difference as well as the alpha and beta error is also not given. While there was a trend toward higher local recurrence rates in the modified radical group, this was predominantly among Stage III patients. Recurrence rates among Stages I and II patients were comparable. The survival curves comparing the two procedures are presented for all patients rather than according to stage. Thus, if Stage III is eliminated from the curves, it is entirely possible the survival rates for the two treatments would be even more comparable and would not tend to favor the Halsted radical mastectomy. This is particularly important in view of evidence suggesting that combined-modality therapy is more appropriate for Stage III patients (see following discussion on locally advanced breast cancer). This trial, however, supports the premise that the modified radical mastectomy is as effective as the Halsted radical in terms of survival and local control rates in the treatment of operable breast cancer.

TABLE 5–21. Local Recurrence Rates in University of Alabama Trial: Prospective Randomized Comparison of Halsted Radical Mastectomy with Modified Radical Mastectomy

	5-Year Local Recurrence Rate (%)	
Stage	Halsted Radical Mastectomy	Modified Radical Mastectomy
I	9.3	5.4
II	7.1	3.6
III	20.0	6.3

Adapted from Maddox WA, Carpenter JT, Laws HL, et al: A randomized prospective trial of radical (Halsted) mastectomy versus modified radical mastectomy in 311 breast cancer patients. Ann Surg 198:207, 1983.

Summary and Consensus

There are two types of modified radical mastectomy, the Patey type and the Auchincloss-Madden type. In the former, the pectoralis minor is removed and a complete axillary dissection is performed. In the latter, the pectoralis minor is preserved and the major portion (80 percent) of the axillary contents are removed, leaving the apical axillary tissue intact. Retrospective series evaluating these two types of modified radical mastectomy suggest that they are equivalent in terms of survival and local recurrence rates and morbidity. Study of the apical axillary tissue may yield information regarding lymph node metastases that is important for staging and prognostic purposes in a small number of patients (see following discussion on axillary lymph node dissection). Retrospective series suggested that the survival and local control rates achieved with the modified radical mastectomy are comparable with those for the Halsted radical but that the former procedure yields better cosmetic results and a reduced incidence of postoperative complications. Two prospective randomized trials have confirmed that the overall and disease-free survival rates following treatment with the modified radical mastectomy are not significantly different from those of the Halsted radical. The local recurrence rates for operable breast cancer in one of these trials (University of Alabama)[20] were comparable for these two procedures and with those reported previously for retrospective series. In the other trial (Manchester),[19] the local recurrence rates were high for Stage II patients following treatment with either procedure (Halsted or modified radical mastectomy). Based on both retrospective series and prospective randomized trials, it seems clear that the Halsted radical offers no advantage in terms of survival and local control rates and, certainly, cosmetic results over the modified radical mastectomy. The NIH Consensus Development Conference, in its review of the experience with the Halsted radical versus the modified radical mastectomy, concluded that the total mastectomy with axillary dissection (synonymous with Auchincloss-Madden modified radical mastectomy) is a satisfactory alternative to the Halsted radical mastectomy for women with clinical Stage I and Stage II disease.[144] While no prospective randomized trial has been conducted comparing the modified radical mastectomy with the extended radical, available information suggests that these two procedures are also comparable in terms of survival and local control rates. It is the authors' position that the modified radical mastectomy is the procedure of choice when radical surgery is used for the treatment of operable breast cancer. Finally, the authors prefer the Patey mastectomy over the Auchincloss-Madden mastectomy. Removal of the pectoralis minor muscle is easily performed and is well tolerated. The Patey modified radical mastectomy may provide additional information for staging and prognostic purposes by including the apical axillary tissue in the axillary dissection and can more effectively prevent local progression of disease in patients with clinically positive nodes.

Total Mastectomy

The total mastectomy (TM) for the treatment of operable breast cancer represents a further modification of the radical mastectomy in that it preserves both pectoralis major and pectoralis minor muscles and omits dissection of the axillary lymph nodes; only the breast tissue is removed. Total mastectomy is synonymous with simple mastectomy. It is based on the premise that breast cancer is a systemic disease from the outset. Surgical procedures directed at the breast and regional lymph nodes are methods for achieving local control and therefore should not influence survival. If this is true, the total mastectomy should provide the same cure rates, with reduced cosmetic deformity, as do the more radical procedures. In addition, it has been proposed (without validation) that intact axillary lymph nodes are immunologically competent and may possess inherent tumoricidal activity. By leaving these lymph nodes intact, one would not disturb the host-tumor defense mechanism.

Information about the effectiveness of the total mastectomy in the treatment of breast cancer comes from both retrospective series and randomized trials. Some of the randomized trials compare total mastectomy alone with more radical procedures, while others evaluate total mastectomy with or without postoperative radiation therapy. Adjuvant radiation therapy (and the respective trials) is considered in detail in Chapter 8; however, information regarding total mastectomy alone from these trials will be included in the following discussion.

The survival rates for nine series evaluating the total mastectomy alone as definite treatment for breast cancer are summarized in Table 5–22. The clinical staging system is used (by necessity) in all of these series. The average five-year survival rate among these series for clinical Stage I tumors is 73.9 percent (range 55.7 to 83.0 percent) and for clinical Stage II tumors, 51.9 percent (range 33.7 to 72.0 percent). The problems of using retrospective series to compare two procedures notwithstanding, these survival results are, in general, comparable to those achieved with the radical mastectomy.

The local recurrence rates for the series evaluating total mastectomy alone are summarized in Table 5–23. Postoperative radiation therapy was not administered to any of these patients. The operative field recurrence rates in the series of Crile[13] and Williams[35] refer to the chest wall, parasternal, and supraclavicular regions. Turnbull and associates[43] performed axillary lymph node biopsy at the time of total mastectomy; recurrences for all sites are reported overall as well as according to results of the node biopsy. The recurrence rates in Table 5–23 appear similar to those for the radical mastectomy; however, the absence of information about axillary node status makes any comparisons difficult. The technical aspects

TABLE 5–22. Survival Rates from Retrospective Series for Total Mastectomy

Series	5-Year Survival Rate (%)	10-Year Survival Rate (%)
Cleveland Clinic[13, 34, 153]§		
Stage I	78.0	60.0 (42.0)†
II	53.0	37.0 (37.0)†
Stage I and II	72.0	45.0 (27.5)†
Baum and Coyle[42]‡		
Stage I	83.0*	
II	64.0*	
Den Besten and Ziffren[145]		
Negative axillary nodes	55.7	
Positive axillary nodes	33.7	
Devitt[37, 38]§		
Stage II	52.0	50.0
Lythgoe et al. (Manchester regional study)[40, 41]‡		
Stage I	69.0	55.0
Kyle et al. (CRC trial)[39]§		
Stage I	78.0	
II	72.0	
Turnbull et al.[43]‡		
Stage I and II*	78.0*	
Williams et al.[35]§		
Stage I	77.0	33.0
Shimkin et al.[36]		
All stages	51.0	31.0

*Three-year survival (%)
†Figures in parentheses, 15-year survival (%)
‡TNM Classification
§Manchester Classification

of skin flap formation and removal of breast tissue and pectoral fascia should be the same for both the total and radical mastectomies. The parasternal and supraclavicular regions are not dissected in either procedure. Because the axilla is not dissected with the total mastectomy, recurrences in this area are considered separately later.

The total mastectomy does not remove any axillary node tissue, and patients treated with this procedure should be at significant risk for axillary recurrences. The axillary recurrence rate after total mastectomy for clinical Stage I patients ranges from 17 to 37 percent (Table 5–24). Crile[34] reported a recurrence rate of 30 percent, with palpable axillary

TABLE 5–23. Locoregional Recurrences after Total Mastectomy

Series	Operative Field	Chest Wall/Scar	Supraclavicular Area	Supraclavicular Parasternal Area	Parasternal Area
Crille*[13]	5.6				
Williams et al.*[35]	16.0				
Lythgoe et al. (Manchester regional study)*[40, 41]	20.0	15.0			
Fisher et al. (NSABP-B06)*[46]		7.6	3.0		0.0
Kyle et al. (CRC trial)†[39]		8.0	2.1		
Forrest et al. (Cardiff trial)†[147] (5 yr.)	5.3			3.0	
Turnbull et al.‡[43]	15.0/43.0‖				
Capetown trial§[44, 45]		13.7			

*Ten-year recurrence rates
†Five-year recurrence rates
‡Two- to four-year recurrence rates
§One- to two-year recurrence rates
‖Patients with clinically negative and positive axillary nodes

TABLE 5–24. Axillary Recurrences Among Clinically Node-Negative Patients Treated with Total Mastectomy

Series	Follow-up Period (yr)	Recurrence Rate (%)
Lythgoe et al. (Manchester regional study)[41]	10	37.0
Fisher et al. (NSABP-B06)[46]	10	17.8
Forrest et al. (Cardiff trial)[147]	10	16.0
Crile[34]	6	30.0
Kyle et al. (CRC trial)[39]	5	17.1
Baum and Coyle[42]	1	20.8

nodes appearing on the average of 22 months after mastecomy (range, 1 month to 6 years) Baum and Coyle[42] noted a recurrence rate of 21 percent with a median follow-up time of 7.5 months. In the NSABP-B04 trial (see later) the recurrence rate was 17.8 percent, with the median interval to recurrence being 14.7 months.[46] One can therefore expect that approximately one fourth of patients with clinically negative axillae treated with total mastectomy alone will develop an axillary recurrence within two years. Crile[13] observed, however, that the survival among patients undergoing a delayed axillary dissection (at the time of the axillary recurrence) was not different from that of clinically node-negative patients undergoing an axillary dissection initially (prophylactically). These findings were confirmed in the NSABP-B04 trial (see later).[14] For Stage II patients, Baum and Coyle[42] reported that 48 percent of patients with clinically palpable axillary nodes had progression of their disease within eight months.

The analysis of axillary lymph nodes is important for staging and prognostic purposes and for the selection of adjuvant chemotherapy. These concepts are examined in the discussion on axillary lymph node dissection. Because the total mastecomy does not remove any axillary lymph nodes, this information is not available. This disadvantage and the fact that many women will require a second procedure (delayed axillary dissection) for axillary recurrence represent the two major objections to the total mastectomy.

The postoperative complications following total mastectomy are summarized in Table 5–9. While incidences of the complications of this procedure are generally lower than those for the radical procedures, skin-flap necrosis and seroma still frequently occur. The factors contributing to these complications are covered in the preceding discussion on Halsted radical mastectomy. The transverse incision is used routinely for the total mastectomy. The formation of skin flaps and the excision of breast tissue are the same as for the modified radical mastectomy. Suction wound drainage is used routinely. Bourke and associates[146] compared, in a randomized manner, suction wound drainage with corrugated drainage following total mastectomy. They found that suction drainage was associated with a reduced requirement for wound dressing changes and a reduced duration of postoperative drainage. The total mastectomy is thus a well-tolerated operation and, if properly performed, should have a low associated morbidity.

Prospective Randomized Trials

The findings of several series suggested that survival rates for operable breast cancer comparable to those with the radical mastectomy could be achieved with the total mastectomy. Because the total mastectomy was associated with less morbidity than was the radical mastectomy and provided a superior cosmetic result, there was much enthusiasm for using the total mastectomy for operable breast cancer. Prospective randomized trials were needed to establish comparable survival benefits and to define further the role of this procedure. Three such trials have been conducted, all of which include at least one group undergoing treatment with total mastectomy alone that is compared with a group undergoing radical mastectomy. These trials are discussed later. The role of postoperative radiation therapy following total mastectomy and the respective trials are discussed in Chapter 8.

Capetown Trial, 1968–1971.[44] This is a single-institution, prospective randomized trial in which patients with TNM T_1 or T_2/N_0 or N_1 tumors were randomized to receive Halsted radical mastectomy (HRM, 44 patients) or simple mastectomy (SM, 51 patients). Simple mastectomy involved removal of breast tissue for Stage I tumors or removal of breast tissue and enlarged axillary lymph nodes but without formal block lymph node dissection for Stage II tumors. Postoperative radiation therapy or chemotherapy was not given in either arm of the trial. The median follow-up time is not stated; however, the findings were reported in 1972. The overall survival (HRM, 93.2 percent; SM, 92.2 percent) and the distant disease-free survival (HRM, 81.8 percent; SM, 82.4 percent) rates within this interval were comparable between the two groups. A significant difference was noted, however, in the incidence of local recurrence (axillary or skin flap). The local recurrence rate in the simple mastectomy group was 23.5 percent (9.8 percent with enlarged lymph node recurrences and 13.7 percent with skin flap recurrences). In all five patients with axillary recurrences, the nodal recurrences were inoperable. In contrast, there was one skin flap recurrence and no axillary recurrences in the radical mastectomy group. Because of the high local recurrence rate in the simple mastectomy arm and the severe discrepancy between the two treatment modalities, the investigators elected to terminate the trial after three years. They concluded that simple mastectomy without postoperative radiation therapy should not be performed for operable breast cancer and that patients with operable breast cancer should be treated with radical mastectomy or any other form of mastectomy that includes axillary node dissection with postoperative radiation therapy.

CRITIQUE. The duration of this trial is short and the number of patients small. In addition, information regarding distribution according to stage between the two procedures as well as the number of node-positive patients in the radical mastectomy group is not given. These factors do not permit any meaningful evaluation of survival rates between the two procedures. It is stated that, among the five total mastectomy patients who developed axillary recurrence, the distribution according to stage was as follows: T_2N_0, two patients; T_1N_1, one patient; and T_2N_1, two patients. All of these patients therefore had TNM Stage II disease. The high rate of skin flap recurrence among the TM group (13.7 percent) is also of concern. The fact that the skin flap recurrence rate in the Halsted radical group was only 2.3 percent suggests either that there was an uneven distribution according to stage between the two arms or that the same technical principles of skin flap formation and excision of breast tissue were not equally applied to the two groups. The trial does, however, confirm the high rate of axillary recurrence that can be expected when the total mastectomy is used to treat operable breast cancer.

Cardiff–St. Mary's Trial, 1967–1973.[45, 147] This is a prospective randomized trial conducted at University Hospital, Cardiff, Wales, and St. Mary's Hospital, London. Patients with TNM T_1, T_2/N_0, N_1/M_0 were randomized to receive modified radical mastectomy (MRM, 97 patients) or total mastectomy with pectoral node biopsy (TM, 103 patients). The proposed treatment regimen, however, resulted in four treatment groups. If pectoral node biopsy (or the axillary dissection in the MRM group) revealed histologically positive lymph nodes, the patient received full-course postoperative radiation therapy (XRT). The distribution according to treatment groups was as follows: TM alone (75 patients), TM plus XRT (49 patients), MRM (79 patients), and MRM plus XRT (40 patients). No adjuvant chemotherapy was given. The duration of follow-up is to the date of the 1982 publication, or approximately ten years. The survival curves (which, unfortunately, are reported for all SM patients versus all MRM patients) show no significant difference in overall ten-year survival rates between the two treatment groups (Fig. 5–16). The axillary recurrence rate among patients treated with total mastectomy alone was 16 percent, versus 1 percent for MRM alone. The investigators also noted a significantly higher incidence of arm swelling (46 percent versus 15 percent) and restricted arm elevation (25 percent versus 0 percent) in the MRM group than in the TM group. Among the modified radical mastectomy group receiving postoperative radiation therapy, the radiation fields included the axilla.

CRITIQUE. This trial supports the premise that survival rates for Stage I or II breast cancer treated with total mastectomy are comparable with those for radical mastectomy, while the axillary recurrence rates are higher following total mastectomy. This trial, however, suffers from small numbers of patients and several problems in data analysis. The number of patients entered for each stage and the survival curves according to stage and for each individual treatment are not given. The average number of axillary nodes per patient removed in the total mastectomy group is not given. This information would be particularly useful because 39.3 percent of all TM patients were found to

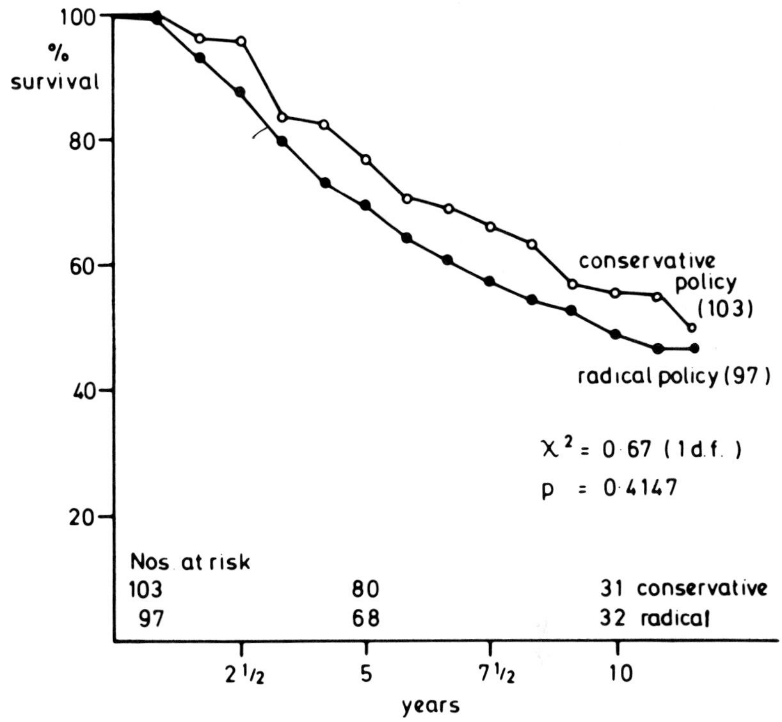

FIGURE 5–16. Cardiff randomized trial comparing the Halsted radical mastectomy (radical policy) with total mastectomy and pectoral node biopsy (conservative policy) for patients with TNM Stage I or II breast cancer. (With permission from Forrest APM, et al.: Simple mastectomy and axillary node sampling (pectoral node biopsy) in the management of primary breast cancer. Ann Surg 196:371, 1982.)

have positive axillary nodes (and received adjuvant radiation therapy). This incidence is higher than that among the MRM group (33.6 percent), members of which underwent a complete axillary dissection. This suggests either that there was an uneven distribution of patients according to stage between the conservative and radical treatment arms or that considerably more than a "pectoral node biopsy" for lymph node analysis was done in the TM group. Also, it is not clear, from a statistical standpoint, why this trial (which had four treatment groups and stratification into 24 subgroups) was closed after only 243 patients were entered. This number appears to be too small to allow conclusive statistical analysis. Finally, full-course axillary radiation therapy as was administered to the patients undergoing complete axillary dissection has been shown by others to be unnecessary, and in this trial was associated with a 58 percent incidence of arm edema of more than 2 cm and a 67 percent incidence of restricted arm motion. In summary, the trial results generally support the premise that total mastectomy can achieve survival rates for Stages I and II breast cancer comparable with those of radical mastectomy but do not allow definitive conclusions for the large number of subgroups.

NSABP-B04, 1971–1974.[14, 46, 104] This is a prospective randomized trial conducted at 34 participating United States and Canadian institutions. Patients with T_1, T_2/N_0, N_1 or with T_3/N_0 tumors were entered into the study. Patients with clinically negative axillary nodes were randomized to one of three treatment regimens: Halsted radical mastectomy (HR), total mastectomy alone (TM), or total mastectomy and regional irradiation (TM + XRT). Patients with clinically positive axillary nodes were randomized to receive either Halsted radical mastectomy or total mastectomy and regional irradiation. No adjuvant chemotherapy was given. Follow-up is at ten years.

Among the clinically node-negative patients, there was no significant difference at ten years in disease-free or overall survival rates between HR, TM + XRT, or TM (Fig. 5–17). The regional recurrence rates (axillary, supraclavicular, internal mammary, or subclavicular areas) are summarized in Table 5–25. There were no significant differences in regional recurrence rates between TM and HR. The regional recurrence rate included a 17.8 percent axillary node recurrence rate among the TM group. The median time from mastectomy to axillary dissection in this latter group was 14.7 months (range 3 to 113

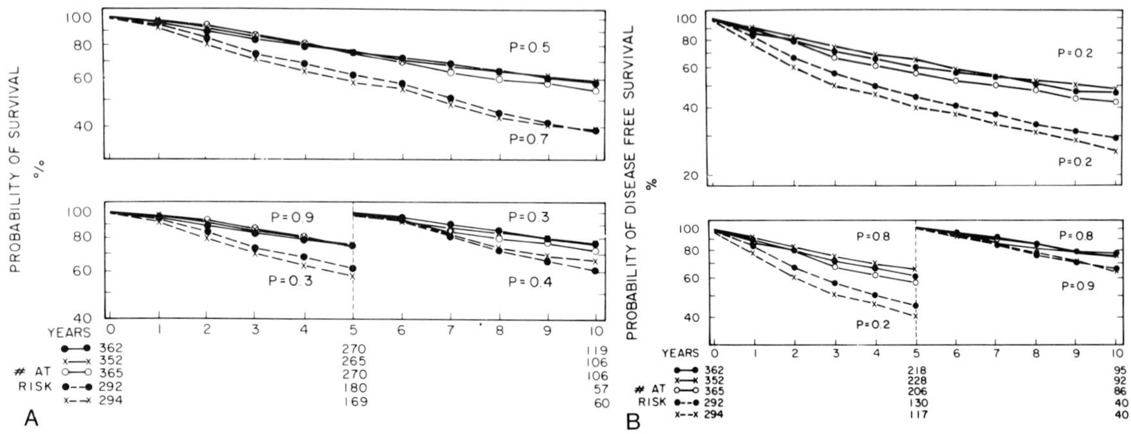

FIGURE 5–17. NSABP B-04 randomized trial comparing Halsted radical mastectomy (solid circle) and total mastectomy and radiation (×) or total mastectomy (open circle) for patients with TNM Stage I or II breast cancer (solid line, node-negative patients; broken line, node-positive patients). *A, Top,* Survival through ten years. *Bottom left,* Survival during the first five years. *Bottom right,* Survival during the second five years for patients alive at the end of the fifth year. *B, Top,* Survival free of disease through ten years. *Bottom left,* Survival free of disease during the first five years. *Bottom right,* Survival free of disease during the second five years for patients free of disease at the end of the fifth year. (With permission from Fisher B, et al.: Ten year results of a randomized clinical trial comparing radical mastectomy and total mastectomy with or without radiation. N Engl J Med 312:674, 1985.)

months). Seventy-nine percent of recurrences occurred within the first two years. The axillary recurrence rate after delayed axillary dissection was 11 percent. There were no significant differences, however, in survival rates between this group (delayed axillary dissection) and those who presented with histologically positive nodes and who underwent TM + XRT or HR. It was also noted by the investigators that while the axillary recurrence rate in the TM group was 17.8 percent, the projected incidence of positive axillary nodes (based on the HR group) was 40 percent. The reason that, among these patients, an additional 22.2 percent did not develop axillary recurrences is unknown. The investigators concluded that axillary dissection in conjunction with total mastectomy is useful for disease-staging purposes and is therapeutic only in that it reduces the possibility of subsequent regional recurrences. Axillary dissection does not alter the incidence of systemic recurrence or of patient survival. The investigators further concluded that, among clinically node-negative patients, there is no significant difference in disease-

TABLE 5–25. Local and Regional Recurrence Rates at Ten Years in NSABP-B04 Randomized Trial Comparing Halsted Radical Mastectomy, Total Mastectomy, and Total Mastectomy plus Radiotherapy

Site	*Recurrence Rate (%), Patients with Clinically Negative Axillary Nodes*			*Recurrence Rate (%), Patients with Clinically Positive Axillary Nodes*	
	HR	TM	TM + XRT	HR	TM + XRT
Local					
Chest wall	3.0	5.2	0.9	5.8	0.7
Scar	0.8	1.6	0.3	0.3	0.3
Both	0.6	0.8	0.0	1.0	0.7
Regional					
Axilla	1.4	1.1	3.1	7.5	11.9
Supraclavicular area	1.1	3.0	0.3	5.8	0.0
Internal mammary area	0.0	0.0	0.0	0.0	0.0
Subclavicular area	0.0	0.0	0.0	0.0	0.0
More than one site	0.0	0.0	0.0	0.7	0.0

Source: Fisher B, Redmond C, Fisher ER, et al.: Ten-year results of a randomized clinical trial comparing radical mastectomy and total mastectomy with or without radiation. N Engl J Med 312:674, 1985.

free, distant disease–free, or overall survival rates among patients without clinical evidence of axillary node involvement who were treated by the three regimens.

Among the clinically node-positive patients, there were no significant differences in disease-free or overall survival rates at ten years between HRM or TM + XRT. The ipsilateral axillary node recurrence rate was higher for the TM + XRT group (11.9 percent versus 1.0 percent for HRM); however, supraclavicular node recurrences were higher in the radical mastectomy group (5.8 percent versus 0.0 percent for TM + XRT). The investigators concluded that among clinically node-positive patients, there was no significant difference in disease-free, distant disease–free, or overall survival rates between the two treatment regimens (this aspect of the trial is discussed further in Chapter 8).

For all patients, the investigators concluded that the location of the tumor in the breast does not influence the prognosis and does not provide justification for varying local and regional therapy. There was no difference in survival for medial versus lateral primary tumors, among either clinically node-negative or node-positive patients.[105] Despite the beneficial effect of radiation therapy for local and regional disease control, survival rate was not improved.

CRITIQUE. This is a well-conducted prospective randomized trial evaluating a large number of subjects with long-term (ten-year) follow-up. Major treatment violations were present in 14.6 percent of patients, with the majority of violations being radiation therapy variations. To what degree this influenced the higher axillary recurrence rate in the TM + XRT group is not clear; the study did demonstrate that adjuvant radiation therapy had no impact on survival. Center-to-center variability is also apparent in the number of lymph nodes included in the TM group, which ranged from none to more than ten nodes. This has been shown (by the investigators) to influence the axillary recurrence rate. Among clinically node-negative patients, if no lymph nodes were removed, the axillary recurrence rate was 22 percent, in contrast with no recurrences if six to 10 lymph nodes were removed.[14] The trial, however, is considered to represent a valid comparison between the two treatment groups.

The principal issue regarding this trial is how the results are to be interpreted. The trial demonstrated that for operable breast cancer, total mastectomy without radiation therapy (for patients with clinically negative lymph nodes) or with radiation therapy (for patients with clinically positive nodes) is as effective as Halsted radical mastectomy in terms of curative potential. While the pectoralis major and minor muscles clearly do not need to be removed to cure breast cancer, at face value the trial also suggests that there is no need to perform an axillary dissection in patients who present with clinically negative nodes. This needs to be clarified. A prophylactic axillary dissection will not alter survival rates but will prevent axillary recurrence in 22 percent of these patients and thus spare them the need for a second operation. An axillary lymph node dissection does provide important information about lymph node status for staging and prognostic purposes (see discussion on axillary lymph node dissection). For these reasons, an axillary lymph node dissection is considered an essential part of the management of all patients with operable breast cancer. While radical surgery to the extent of a Halsted mastectomy is not necessary to provide effective treatment for these patients, neither should a total mastectomy without axillary lymph node dissection be considered optimum management. It is important to note that in the subsequent NSABP trial (B06), all patients received at least a complete dissection of Levels I and II, in conjunction with either a total mastectomy or a segmentectomy with primary breast irradiation, confirming that the investigators agree to the importance of the axillary procedure.

SUMMARY AND CONSENSUS

Retrospective series suggested that the total mastectomy could achieve survival rates comparable to those of the Halsted radical mastectomy, with an improved cosmetic result and reduced postoperative morbidity. Because axillary tissue is not dissected with the total mastectomy, axillary recurrence rates in the untreated axilla were substantial with this procedure, more so among patients with clinically positive lymph nodes. Among clinically node-negative patients undergoing total mastectomy alone, one fourth will subsequently require an axillary dissection for recurrent axillary disease. Approximately one half of clinically node-positive patients will have progression of their axillary disease if an axillary dissection is not performed. It has been shown, however, that among clinically node-negative patients, a delayed axillary dissection (at the time of axillary recurrence) is not associated with a worse prognosis than if the axillary dissection were to be done at the time of the mastectomy. For clinically node-positive patients, a delay in the axillary dissection may result in unresectable axillary disease. The total mastectomy is well tolerated, with fewer postoperative complications and a superior cosmetic result, compared with the radical mastectomy.

Prospective randomized trials have confirmed that survival rates among clinically node-negative patients treated with total mastectomy alone are not significantly different from those of the Halsted radical. While the axillary recurrence rate is higher following total mastectomy, a delayed axillary dissection is associated with the same long-term survival as when the axillary dissection is done initially. Apparently, axillary lymph node metastases are not, in themselves, sources of distant metastatic disease but are simply indicators of an increased risk for future systemic failure. All patients with an axillary recurrence should undergo a complete axillary dissection (including the apical tissue) whether the recurrence appears in a patient who previously had clinical negative nodes, or whether it represents progression of disease in clinically node-positive patients.

The axillary dissection provides important information about axillary lymph node metastases for staging and prognostic purposes. This information is currently essential for decisions regarding the use of adjuvant chemotherapy and for evaluating adjuvant treatment regimens. An axillary lymph node dissection should therefore be considered an essential component in the management of all patients with operable cancer. The NIH Consensus Development Conference, evaluating the experience with the Halsted radical versus the total mastectomy, concluded that axillary dissection has become a procedure necessary for staging purposes, regardless of the debate on its therapeutic benefit.[144] While long-term survival rates with the total mastectomy are comparable with those of the radical mastectomy, the total mastectomy alone disregards the importance of the axillary lymph node dissection and thus should not be considered to represent optimum management of these patients.

Partial Mastectomy

Partial mastectomy refers to the excision of a malignancy and adjacent breast tissue, leaving the major portion of the breast as well as the pectoral muscles and axillary lymph nodes intact. The terms quadrantectomy, segmental mastectomy (segmentectomy), and local excision are also included in this category. The terms as they have been discussed in clinical trials are defined at the beginning of this chapter.

Partial mastectomy was introduced for the treatment of Stages I and II breast cancer for two reasons. There was continued concern about the disfigurement resulting from total mastectomy as well as an appreciation that local control could be achieved by methods other than total breast removal without compromising long-term survival. The principal method of obtaining local control following partial mastectomy has been with postoperative adjuvant radiation therapy. A large experience with this approach has been accumulated over the past 50 years. The technical aspects of adjuvant treatment with radiation therapy and the results from retrospective series and prospective randomized trials are discussed in detail in Chapter 8. It is clear from this discussion that conservative treatment of Stage I tumors and Stage II tumors $\leq$ 4 cm in diameter with partial mastectomy and postoperative radiation therapy can achieve local control and survival rates equivalent to those for total or radical mastectomy alone. A smaller but significant experience has also been acquired with partial mastectomy alone, without adjuvant therapy, in the treatment of early stage breast cancer. This experience will be discussed in the following section.

The two principal questions that must be asked of partial mastectomy in the treatment of breast cancer are "What is the recurrence rate in the breast?" and "Will treatment of these recurrences result in the same long-term survival as would be observed if mastectomy were performed at the time of presentation?" The recurrence rates within the breast following partial mastectomy for seven series are summarized in Table 5–26. The

TABLE 5–26. Incidence of Breast Recurrence after Partial Mastectomy

Series	5-Year Recurrence Rate (%)	10-Year Recurrence Rate (%)	15-Year Recurrence Rate (%)
Clark et al. (Princess Margaret)[148]	24.8	26.5	
Montgomery et al.[149]	33.0		
Freeman et al.[150]			
T_1 tumors	16.0		
T_2 tumors	47.0		
Targart[151]	37.0		
Lagios et al.[152]			
Overall	28.0		
Negative margins	13.0		
Positive margins	71.0		
Cleveland Clinic[153–156]	11.0	15.0	16.0
Fisher et al. (NSABP-B06)[72]			
Negative axillary nodes	27.9		
Positive axillary nodes	36.2		
T_1 tumors	26.0		
T_2 tumors	30.0		

mean overall breast recurrence rate within five years was 27.5 ± 3.8 percent. The findings of Clarke[148] and Hermann[153] suggest that the majority of these recurrences arise within the first year, with fewer subsequent recurrences. Freeman and associates[150] found that the median time to failure was 12.5 to 15 months. Tagart[151] found that the average time to relapse was 25 months. The vast majority of breast recurrences after partial mastectomy will appear in the biopsy site. Among patients with breast recurrences, the mean recurrence rate outside the biopsy site was 4.3 percent (range 0 to 7.3 percent).[148, 150, 151, 155] Recurrences at the biopsy site are thought to represent positive margins or cells implanted at the time of surgery, although multicentric tumor at the margins may occur. It can be seen from Table 5–26 that the incidence of local breast recurrence is increased in patients with T_2 versus T_1 tumors,[72, 150] positive margins,[152] and positive axillary nodes.[72] The highest recurrence rates (71 percent) were noted for patients with positive margins.[152] Freeman and associates[150] also noted the recurrence rates to be higher following local excision than with wide resection. Breast recurrences following partial mastectomy in the aforementioned series were treated most often with total mastectomy. The results for alternative forms of treatment (reexcision with or without radiation therapy) are not well defined, in terms of either survival or cosmetic result.

The survival rates for two retrospective series and the NSABP-B06 prospective randomized trial evaluating partial mastectomy are summarized in Table 5–27. The NSABP-B06 trial (which is discussed in Chapter 8) included one category in which 390 patients with T_1 or T_2 tumors 4 cm or less in diameter were treated with segmental resection to achieve negative margins and with axillary lymph node dissection.[72] No postoperative radiation therapy was given if negative margins in the breast were obtained. The average

TABLE 5–27. Survival Rates for Partial Mastectomy

Series	5-Year Survival Rate (%)	10-Year Survival Rate (%)	15-Year Survival Rate (%)
Cleveland Clinic[153]			
Stage I	80.0	58.8	51.1
II			
Clark et al. (Princess Margaret)[148]	80.0	70.0	
Fisher et al. (NSABP-B06)[72]			
Disease-free	68.1/54.8*		
Distant disease–free	72.8/63.8		
Overall	90.7/73.8		

*Patients with negative and positive axillary nodes

follow-up time was 39 months. Among patients with clinically negative axillary nodes, the recurrence rate in the ipsilateral breast was 27.9 percent, and among patients with clincially positive axillary nodes, 36.2 percent. All of these patients were treated with total mastectomy for their recurrences. The overall and disease-free survival rates among this group of patients were not significantly different from those of patients of comparable nodal status treated initially with total mastectomy or segmental mastectomy with radiation therapy (Fig. 5–18).

The five-year actuarial survival rates for Stages I and II tumors for all series in Table 5–27 are comparable to those of the radical mastectomy. The ten-year survival rate for the Princess Margaret series is similarly comparable;[148] however, the findings for the Cleveland Clinic[153] are lower than those for the Halsted radical mastectomy reported by Haagensen for both Stages I/A and II/B tumors at both 10 and 15 years (see Table 5–2). The average follow-up period for the NSABP trial was only 39 months.[72] These findings would suggest that, at least in terms of five-year survival, breast recurrences after partial mastectomy do not have an impact on survival. Breast recurrences can be effectively treated with total mastectomy without altering prognosis. Therefore, breast recurrences do not appear to be sources of distant metastases or to be associated with an increased systemic failure rate. Long-term survival rates (10 and 15 years) following treatment for Stages I and II tumors with partial mastectomy, however, need to be defined.

Regional recurrence rates, excluding breast recurrences, following partial mastectomy are comparable with those following radical mastectomy.[72, 148, 153] That is, recurrence rates in the internal mammary or supraclavicular regions, in a previously dissected axilla, or in the chest wall following total mastectomy for breast recurrence are not different from those among patients undergoing modified radical mastectomy. Nonbreast regional recurrences carry the same poor prognosis following partial mastectomy as they do after definitive surgical procedures (see previous discussion on local recurrence and the Halsted radical mastectomy). Axillary recurrences in a previously undissected axilla, however, are not associated with a worse prognosis when treated with a delayed axillary dissection. This was discussed earlier under total mastectomy.

The size of the primary tumor to which partial mastectomy should be applied and the technical aspects of the procedure are not well defined. The procedure should achieve a good cosmetic result and reduce as much as possible the risk of breast recurrence. Postoperative radiation therapy can significantly reduce the local recurrence rate after partial mastectomy (see Chapter 8). Based upon the available experience, patients with primary tumors greater than 4 cm in diameter and patients for whom positive margins cannot be obtained should not be considered candidates for partial mastectomy alone. With regard to technical aspects, in the Milan

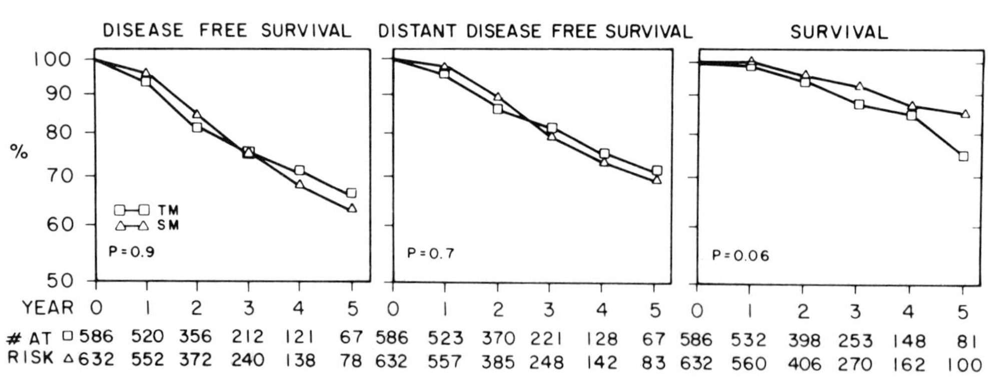

FIGURE 5–18. NSABP B-06 randomized trial comparing total mastectomy (TM) with segmental mastectomy alone (SM) for patients with TNM Stage I or II (T < 4 cm) breast cancer. Disease-free survival, distant disease–free survival, and overall survival by treatment. (With permission from Fisher B: Five year results of a randomized clinical trial comparing total mastectomy and segmental mastectomy with or without radiation in the treatment of breast cancer. N Engl J Med 312:665, 1985.)

trial, which evaluated only patients with T_1 tumors, a quadrantectomy with removal of overlying skin and adjacent pectoral fascia was performed.[71] Approximately 30 percent of women considered the cosmetic result to be unsatisfactory. In the NSABP trial (B06), segmental resection of breast tissue was performed to achieve negative margins.[72] Skin and pectoral fascia were not removed. Results from a cosmetic standpoint have not been reported. It is apparently not necessary to include pectoral fascia or overlying skin in the excision. If postoperative radiation therapy is used, a much more limited resection may be possible. In an ongoing NCI (USA) trial, patients with T_1, T_2/N_0, N_1 tumors undergo local excision to remove gross disease only; positive margins are present in 35 percent of patients. Local recurrence rates (with postoperative radiation therapy) are 2 percent with a median follow-up period of 2.5 years.[73]

Summary and Consensus

Retrospective series suggested that the partial mastectomy could achieve five-year survival rates comparable with those for the radical mastectomy, with reduced morbidity and a clearly improved cosmetic result. At least one series (Cleveland Clinic),[153] however, suggested that long-term survival rates (10 and 15 years) with the partial mastectomy may be inferior to those for the radical mastectomy. Local recurrence within the breast appears in approximately 28 percent of cases; however, when these recurrences are treated with total mastectomy, the five-year survival rate is comparable with that for patients undergoing total mastectomy initially. There has been only one prospective randomized trial in which patients with T_1 or T_2 tumors (less than 4 cm in diameter) were treated with partial (segmental) mastectomy and axillary lymph node dissection alone, without further treatment to the breast (NSABP-B06[72]; see also Chapter 8). Patients with positive margins at the time of segmental mastectomy, as well as those with recurrences in the breast, underwent total mastectomy. Approximately 36 percent of all patients assigned to segmental mastectomy (without radiation therapy) underwent total mastectomy. This trial confirmed that recurrence rates in the breast following segmental mastectomy were high: 23.5 percent in patients with negative axillary lymph nodes and 36.2 percent in lymph node–positive patients. When these recurrences were treated with total mastectomy, the five-year survival rate was not significantly different from that for patients undergoing either segmental mastectomy with postoperative radiation therapy or total mastectomy as primary treatment. The follow-up period for this study was short, and the report from the Cleveland Clinic that long-term survival following partial mastectomy alone may be inferior to that for radical mastectomy is of concern. In addition, none of these reports addresses the fact that up to a third of women treated with this procedure are left with concern over local recurrence and the potential for a subsequent mastectomy.

It is established that postoperative radiation therapy can prevent local recurrence in the breast and, hence, the need for a subsequent mastectomy in the overwhelming majority of women undergoing conservative breast surgery. Radiation therapy can be delivered with an excellent cosmetic result and negligible morbidity. For these reasons, partial mastectomy alone with axillary dissection does not appear to represent optimum treatment for Stages I and II breast cancer. Partial mastectomy alone, without axillary dissection, has no role in the treatment of these patients. Before partial mastectomy alone with axillary dissection (without radiation) can be recommended, it must be demonstrated from prospective randomized trials that long-term survival rates after this treatment are equivalent to those for either radical surgery or conservative surgery with postoperative radiation therapy and that concern among women about the possibility of a subsequent mastectomy is not significant.

Axillary Lymph Node Dissection

The axillary lymphatics represent the principal site of regional metastases from breast cancer. The incidence of axillary lymph node metastases varies directly according to the size of the primary tumor. The incidence ranges from approximately 20 percent for tumors less than 1 cm in diameter to 60 percent for lesions greater than 5 cm (Table 5–28). The location of the primary tumor is also an important factor. Axillary metastases are found more often from outer quadrant tumors than from inner quadrant tumors

TABLE 5–28. Incidence of Axillary Metastases According to Primary Tumor Size, Haagensen's Personal Series

Primary Tumor Size (cm)	*No. of Patients*	*Incidence of Axillary Metastases (%)*
No palpable tumor	26	19.2
Less than 1	22	22.7
1.0–1.9	119	24.2
2.0–2.9	223	30.5
3.0–3.9	180	46.7
4.0–4.9	147	46.3
5.0–5.9	101	60.4
6.0–7.9	77	51.9
8.0 or larger	27	51.9
Total	922	40.6

Source: Haagensen CD: Diseases of the Breast, 2nd ed. Philadelphia: W. B. Saunders Co., 1971, p. 401.

(Fig. 5–19). The presence and number of axillary lymph node metastases are important factors in determining prognosis. The five-year survival rate for patients with no axillary involvement following radical surgery is approximately 82.5 percent, as opposed to 50.0 percent if one to three nodes are involved, and 21.1 percent for four or more positive nodes.[158] In addition, the nature of the axillary involvement is important. Patients with lymph nodes fixed to each other or to adjacent structures are considered to have locally advanced (Stage III_a) breast cancer and are therefore inoperable.

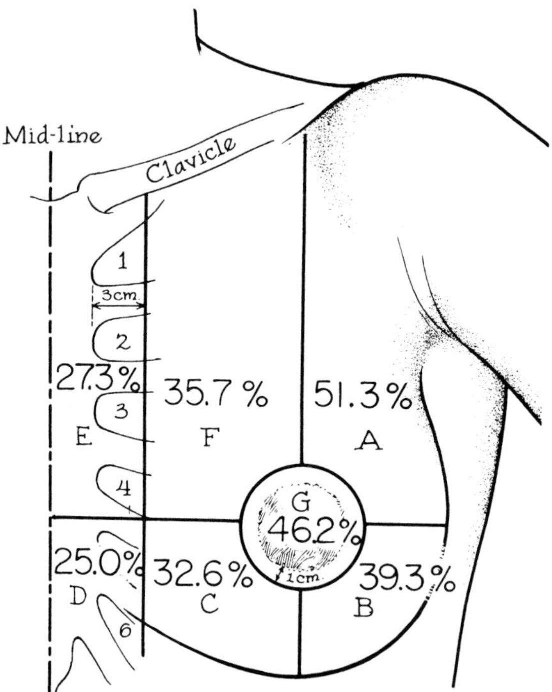

FIGURE 5–19. The frequency of axillary lymph node metastases according to location of carcinoma in the breast. (From Haagensen CD: Diseases of the Breast, 2nd ed. Philadelphia: W. B. Saunders Co., 1971.)

The status of the axillary lymph nodes can be determined either clinically or pathologically. The clinical evaluation of lymph node status, however, is frequently inaccurate (Table 5–29). Among patients with clinically negative axillae, approximately 29 percent will have axillary metastases on histologic review.[14] Conversely, among patients with clinically palpable lymph nodes thought to be positive, on the average 38 pecent will not have lymph node metastases on histologic review.[14] Clinical examination also provides no information about the number of positive lymph nodes in node-positive patients. This information is important for identifying subgroups of patients (one to three versus four or more positive nodes) at risk for recurrent tumor and for evaluating the effectiveness of adjuvant chemotherapy regimens. Axillary dissection and pathologic analysis of lymph nodes are thus necessary and important parts of the management of patients with Stages I and II breast cancer. Clinical staging, however, should be performed in all patients. This not only will identify locally advanced disease but also may influence the extent of the axillary dissection among clinically node-positive patients (see later).

The axillary contents are divided anatomically into three levels (Fig. 5–6). Level I represents the tissue between the latissimus dorsi muscle and the lateral border of the pectoralis minor muscle. Level II is that axillary tissue between and inferior to the lateral and medial borders of the pectoralis minor muscle. Level III is that tissue between the medial border of the pectoralis minor and Halsted's ligament, or the apex of the axilla. There are, on the average, 27 lymph nodes in the axilla (range 6 to 80).[53–57] This range is due both to patient-to-patient variation and to the techniques used by the pathologist to isolate lymph nodes from the axillary specimen. Level I contains approximately 38 percent of the total number of nodes; Level II, 38 percent; and Level III, 24 percent.[53, 56, 159, 160] The level of axillary involvement with lymph node metastases has been correlated with prognosis. The three-year survival for patients with positive lymph nodes at Level I only is 87.0 percent, in contrast with 75.0

TABLE 5–29. Accuracy of Clinical Examination in Determining Axillary Node Status

Axillary Node Status and Series	*No. of Patients*	*Pathologically Negative (%)*	*Pathologically Positive (%)*
Clinically negative axilla			
Cutler[177]	881	62	38
Haagensen[178]	724	69	31
Wallace and Champion[179]	119	74	26
Roberts et al.[180]	62	79	21
Johnsen[181]	36	67	33
National Surgical Adjuvant Breast and Bowel Project, 1981[14]	355	61	39
Danforth et al.[53]	109	63	37
Clinically positive axilla			
Cutler[177]	461	37	63
Haagensen[178]	198	25	75
Atkins et al.[182]	81	25	75
Wallace and Champion[179]	55	55	45
Roberts et al.[180]	50	50	50
Johnsen[181]	94	36	64
National Surgical Adjuvant Breast and Bowel Project, 1981[14]	286	27	73
Danforth et al.[53]	27	7	93

Adapted from Fisher B, Wolmark N, Bauer M, et al.: The accuracy of clinical nodal staging and of limited axillary dissection as a determinant of histological nodal status in carcinoma of the breast. Surg Gynecol Obstet 152:765, 1981.

percent for Level II involvement and 36.1 percent if node metastases are present at Level III.[159]

Procedures used for removing lymph nodes from the axilla for purposes of histologic analysis include complete axillary dissection, partial axillary dissection, axillary sampling, and isolated axillary lymph node excision. The technical aspects of these procedures are defined at the beginning of this chapter (see the discussion on surgical procedures for the management of breast cancer). A complete axillary dissection (which includes Levels I, II, and III) will remove approximately 25 nodes; a partial axillary dissection (Levels I and II), approximately 20 nodes; an axillary sampling (at or below Level I), 10 nodes; and isolated lymph node excision, 1 to 5 nodes. Each of these procedures can be performed either in conjunction with a mastectomy or as a separate procedure through a single axillary incision. If a complete axillary dissection is to be done, it is most easily accomplished by removing the pectoralis minor muscle. The authors have found, among complete axillary dissection specimens, no difference either in the total number of lymph nodes removed or in the number of lymph nodes per level between specimens obtained as part of the Patey modified radical mastectomy and those obtained during a separate procedure.[53]

The selection of a particular type of axillary dissection must be based not only on the number of lymph nodes to be removed but also on an understanding of the distribution according to axillary level of lymph node metastases from breast cancer. The two major issues are what type of dissection is necessary to establish lymph node positivity or negativity and what is necessary to distinguish subgroups of patients with positive nodes (one to three versus four or more positive nodes). Several groups have examined, among lymph node–positive patients, the distribution of lymph node metastases according to axillary level.[53–56, 160] In all of these series, a complete axillary dissection was performed, the specimen divided into levels (I, II, and III), and the number of metastases at each level determined. Table 5–30 summarizes the findings of these series in terms of the percentage of the total number of metastases at each level or combinations thereof. It can be seen that in three series, 25.0 to 29.0 percent of all lymph node–positive patients had metastases only to Levels II and III, with Level I being negative.[53, 55, 160] This represents the incidence of "skip" metastases to the higher axillary levels with breast cancer. Between 25.0 and 29.0 percent of lymph node–positive patients would thus be inaccurately staged as being lymph node negative if only Level I were analyzed. Two

TABLE 5–30. Incidence of Axillary "Skip" Metastases from Breast Cancer*

	Incidence (%)				
	PIGOTT[55] SERIES	SMITH[160] SERIES	BOOVA[56] SERIES	ROSEN[54] SERIES	DANFORTH[53] SERIES
Skip metastases	25.0	27.0	8.9	2.5	29.2

*Incidence of axillary metastases to only Levels II or III or both, with Level I being negative.

series, however, reported an incidence of only 2 to 11 percent of skip metastases.[54, 56] This discrepancy in the incidence of skip metastases among these series appears to be due to technical differences in the manner in which the axillary specimens were divided and analyzed according to levels. In the series that report a low incidence of skip metastases to Levels II or III, it appears that the specimens were processed in a manner such that Level II tissue was included in Level I for analysis.[53] This would account for the disparity in the distribution of metastases between these two series and the remaining three series. It is the authors' conclusion that skip metastases from breast cancer to the higher axillary levels are a real phenomenon and occur in 25 to 29 percent of node-positive patients. The failure to identify this in all series is due to a discrepancy in the way the axillary specimens were analyzed.[53]

Removal of axillary Levels I and II is also necessary to accurately quantitate the number of positive lymph nodes in patients wtih breast cancer. In the authors' series of 65 patients with axillary metastases, 19 percent of lymph node–positive patients would have been identified as having one to three positive nodes if only Level I were dissected but more than four positive nodes if the upper axillary levels were included in the dissection.[53] This information is important both for identifying subgroups of node-positive patients and for evaluating the effectiveness of adjuvant chemotherapy regimens. An axillary sampling, which removes approximately ten or fewer lymph nodes, is inadequate both for determining node positivity or negativity and for accurately quantitating the number of positive nodes.

The inclusion of Level III in the axillary dissection may be beneficial in a select number of patients. On the average, 3 percent of lymph node–positive patients will have metastases only to Level III (without metastases to Level I or II).[53–56, 160] In the authors' series, in addition, 3 percent of patients would have been converted from three or fewer to four or more positive nodes by the addition of Level III.[53] Thus, for staging and prognostic purposes, information contained in Level III will benefit only a small number of patients.

The axillary dissection is of therapeutic benefit in that it will prevent axillary recurrence or progression of axillary disease, but it will not have an impact upon survival rate. In the previous discussion on total mastectomy, it was pointed out that among clinically node-negative patients, if an axillary dissection is not performed, 17 to 37 percent of patients will develop recurrent axillary disease.[34, 39, 41, 42, 44, 45] If a delayed axillary dissection is done at that time, the survival rate is no different from that of an axillary dissection done at the time of presentation.[153] Therefore, axillary metastases are not, in themselves, sources of distant metastases. Fisher and colleagues[14] demonstrated that if more than six lymph nodes are removed from clinically node-negative patients, the subsequent axillary recurrence rate is zero. Among clinically node-positive patients, however, if an axillary dissection is not performed initially, 48 percent will have progression of their axillary disease and, in many, the disease will become unresectable.[42] Therefore, for clinically node-negative patients, the authors recommend dissection of at least Levels I and II. This will provide accurate information for staging and prognostic purposes and will effectively prevent axillary recurrence. Among clinically node-positive patients, Levels I and II should also be dissected for the same reasons. The apex of the axilla should be carefully examined, and if palpable nodes are identified, they should be dissected as well. The premise that leaving clinically positive lymph nodes intact in the axilla is of some immunologic benefit to the host has never been substantiated. Gross residual disease may progress and become unresectable. Patients with unresectable axillary disease, with attendant pain and venous obstruction, are among the most difficult to manage.

The potential morbidity of the axillary dissection procedures includes arm and breast edema, seroma formation, and neurovascular injury. Arm edema following complete axillary dissection has been discussed previously (see the discussion on the Halsted radical mastectomy and postoperative complications). The incidence and severity of arm edema do not appear to differ according to whether the axillary dissection is done as a single procedure or whether it is combined with a mastectomy.

The authors reviewed the incidence of arm edema following a complete axillary dissection along with postoperative breast radiation therapy compared with that following modified radical mastectomy and found no significant differences.[161] Removal of the axillary lymph nodes and lymphatics is the principal cause of arm edema. The addition of breast tissue and the pectoralis major or minor muscles does not appear to add significantly to the incidence, except perhaps by affecting range of motion of the shoulder. Postoperative radiation therapy or axillary infection will, however, significantly increase the incidence of arm edema.[124, 126] For this reason, axillary radiation therapy is now rarely given after a complete axillary dissection. Any evidence of skin inflammation in the shoulder, the arm, or the chest wall should be promptly treated. The guidelines for following patients after a complete axillary dissection are reviewed in the previous discussion on arm edema and the Halsted radical mastectomy. Finally, the incidence of arm edema after lesser axillary procedures has not been as extensively reviewed but should, however, be lower than that following the complete axillary dissection. Rose and associates[75] found that the incidence of mild arm edema when axillary sampling was combined with postoperative radiation therapy was 5 percent, and of moderate arm edema, 2 percent. The incidence of breast edema following breast irradiation has been found to correlate with the degree of axillary dissection. Clarke and colleagues[162] found that the incidence of breast edema following complete axillary dissection was 79 percent, as opposed to 25 percent after axillary sampling and 6 percent if there was no axillary surgery.

Seroma formation is a frequent complication of axillary dissection. Lotze and colleagues[123] reported a 23 percent incidence, and the authors observed a 21 percent incidence among 86 patients undergoing axillary dissection as a single procedure.[123] Table 5–10 shows that this incidence is comparable with that for the total and modified radical mastectomies. The role of the chest wall component in seroma formation following the modified radical mastectomy is thus unclear. Adherence of the skin flaps to the chest wall should minimize this complication. Following a complete axillary dissection as a single procedure, the axillary skin flaps will adhere to the lateral chest wall; however, a space between the pectoralis major and the chest wall frequently persists. Unsealed transected lymphatics and the raw surface area of the excised pectoralis minor muscle probably contribute to seroma formation. Liberal use of Hemoclips at the time of surgery (for division of lymphatics) and postoperative catheter (Hemovac) suction drainage may reduce the incidence of this complication. The role of postoperative rehabilitation therapy remains unclear. Lotze and colleagues also found that the incidence of postoperative seroma formation was the same regardless of whether rehabilitation therapy was started on the first or seventh day postoperatively.[123] The problem of postoperative seroma formation is also considered in the discussion on the Halsted radical mastectomy.

Injury to the axillary vein, thoracodorsal vessels, and long thoracic nerve may occur during axillary procedures, although with careful surgical technique, these problems should be easily avoided. Lotze and colleagues[123] reported a 30 percent incidence of transient serratus anterior dysfunction and a 5 percent incidence of latissimus dorsi dysfunction following complete axillary dissection. This neuropraxia probably occurs during clearing of these structures of adjacent lymph node–bearing tissue; however, the practice of "tweaking" the long thoracic nerve to elicit serratus contracture (for purposes of identification) almost certainly contributes to the problem. This practice should be condemned. The long thoracic nerve can be easily identified throughout its course and easily separated from adjacent tissue. Removal of the pectoralis minor is usually accompanied by division of the medial pectoral nerve supplying the lateral border of the pectoralis major muscle. Loss of this portion of the muscle may result in a less prominent anterior axillary fold. Injury to the axillary vein has been reported during axillary sampling procedures. Rose and associates reviewed 176 patients undergoing axillary sampling and postoperative radiation therapy. They noted vascular complications in four patients.[75] These included axillary vein thrombosis (one patient), venous swelling (two patients), and superficial phlebitis (one patient). Carabell and colleagues[163] reported an 8 percent incidence of axillary vein thrombosis following axillary node sampling.

SUMMARY AND CONCLUSIONS

The analysis of axillary lymph nodes for both the presence and the number of lymph node metastases is an essential part of the management of patients with Stages I and II breast cancer. Such analysis provides important staging and prognostic information and identifies subgroups of patients for the selection and evaluation of adjuvant chemotherapy regimens. An axillary dissection of at least Levels I and II is the minimal procedure that should be performed to reliably obtain this information. Dissection of Level III (apex of the axilla) may provide additional information in a small number of patients. A complete axillary dissection including Level III should be performed in clinically node-positive patients to prevent local progression of disease. Axillary sampling or lesser procedures are not recommended in the management of patients with Stages I and II breast cancer. They are inadequate for staging and prognostic purposes and depend upon postoperative radiation therapy to prevent progression of axillary disease in clinically node-positive patients. In clinically node-negative patients, the axillary dissection will prevent recurrent disease but does not confer a survival advantage. An axillary dissection can be easily and safely performed with a low incidence of long-term complications.

LOCALLY ADVANCED BREAST CANCER

Locally advanced breast cancer refers to all TNM Stage III tumors. At the time that Halsted introduced the radical mastectomy, no distinction was made between Stages I, II, and III breast cancer and the radical mastectomy was applied uniformly to all patients with localized disease. In 1943, Haagensen[15] reviewed his experience with the use of the radical mastectomy for locally advanced tumors and defined the characteristics of breast cancer that, when the disease was treated with surgery alone, were associated with high local recurrence rates and a poor prognosis. Haagensen placed these characteristics in one of two groups for staging and prognostic purposes: the five grave signs of advanced breast cancer (Stage C of the CCC) and the characteristics of more advanced breast cancer (Stage D of the CCC). These signs of advanced breast cancer are listed in Table 5–31. Any sign from either of these two groups is considered evidence of inoperability. The five-year survival and local recurrence rates observed when patients with grave signs of breast cancer are treated with radical mastectomy are also given in Table 5–31. It can be seen that, with the presence

TABLE 5–31. Local Recurrence Rates and Five-Year Survival Among Patients with Stage C or Stage D Breast Cancer after Treatment with Halsted Radical Mastectomy

Stage of Breast Cancer	*Local Recurrence Rate (%)*	*5-Year Survival Rate (%)*
STAGE C (GRAVE SIGNS)		
Edema of the skin involving less than ⅓ of the breast	32.0	22.7
Skin ulceration	14.3	35.7
Solid fixation of tumor to chest wall	40.0	5.0
Massive involvement of axillary lymph nodes	12.5	37.5
Fixation of axillary lymph nodes	12.5	12.5
STAGE D		
A combination of any two or more grave signs listed in Stage C	30.8–58.3	0.0–5.3
Edema of the skin involving more than ⅓ of the breast	60.8	0.0
Satellite skin nodules	57.1	0.0
Inflammatory carcinoma	60.0	0.0
Clinically involved supraclavicular or parasternal lymph nodes	56.2	0.0
Edema of the arm	41.4	0.0

Adapted from Haagensen CD: Diseases of the Breast, 2nd ed. Philadelphia: W. B. Saunders Co., 1971, pp. 662–630.

of any one of the grave signs alone, five-year survival rates of less than 40 percent and local recurrence rates of up to 40 percent are observed following radical mastectomy. With more advanced disease, higher local recurrence rates and fewer five-year survivors are noted. These findings have been confirmed by others. Among four series totaling 99 cases of inflammatory cancer, there were two reported five-year survivors following radical mastectomy.[164] Petrek and colleagues reviewed 38 patients with ulcerating breast cancer treated with a variety of regimens and observed a 19 percent three-year survival rate.[165]

Several points should be emphasized regarding the locally advanced nature of Stage III tumors. First, the majority of the criteria for diagnosing Stage III tumors are clinical characteristics. This stresses the importance of a careful physical examination and accurate clinical staging at the time of presentation. Fixation to the chest wall should be distinguished from fixation to pectoral fascia or muscle (the latter does not represent Stage III disease). Fixed or matted axillary nodes, skin edema or inflammation, satellite nodules, and arm edema can all be readily detected by physical examination. The diagnosis of inflammatory cancer requires skin inflammation that is not the result of direct skin extension by the tumor and/or histologic evidence of tumor in the subdermal lymphatics. The inflammatory components of these tumors may be quite subtle and at some distance from the primary tumor. A skin punch biopsy of the inflammatory area will establish the diagnosis. Second, there is a subset of Stage III tumors that should be distinguished from the remainder of the locally advanced tumors. These are the 5- to 6-cm tumors with clinically negative axilla and no associated grave signs, or the $T_3/N_0/M_0$ (or $T_2/N_0/M_0$ by the new TNM classification) tumors. These tumors may respond adequately to radical surgery alone. Haagensen[89] reported a 66 percent ten-year survival with radical mastectomy for these lesions. (Clearly, there is still room for improvement in the treatment of these Stage III tumors, and it is appropriate to treat these patients under investigational studies evaluating combined-modality therapy). In this regard, the findings of Arnold and Lesnick are of interest.[166] They reviewed 228 patients with Stage III breast cancer treated with radical mastectomy. The five-year survival rate for T_3/N_0 patients was 77 percent and for T_4/N_0, 65 percent. These two groups represented 14 percent of all Stage III patients. The characteristics establishing the T_4 classification were not given. While there may be subsets of patients within Stage III with a more favorable prognosis, until these patients are better defined and confirmed by others, all T_3 lesions (or T_4 by the old TNM classification) are best considered not appropriate candidates for surgery and/or for radiation therapy.

The role of radiation therapy in the treatment of Stage III lesions, both as definitive therapy and as an adjunct to surgery, is discussed in Chapters 6 and 8. In general, the ability of radiation therapy to achieve local control is comparable with that of surgery alone. Valagussa and associates[167] evaluated three combined-modality regimens in the treatment of patients with T_{3b} to T_4 tumors: chemotherapy (doxorubicin and vincristine), followed by surgery (Halsted or modified radical mastectomy) or radiation therapy and (in two groups) additional chemotherapy (Fig. 5–20). While the investigators found that additional chemotherapy was associated with improved freedom from progression as well as overall survival rates, they discerned no significant differences according to whether surgery or radiation therapy was used to achieve local control. Townsend and colleagues[168] reported on 55 patients with TNM Stage III or IV disease treated by preoperative radiation therapy followed by total mastectomy. With a median follow-up time of 12 to 26 months, the investigators noted a local recurrence rate of 4 percent. Copeland[169] also reported on the treatment of 353 patients with grave signs of breast cancer who received total mastectomy and Level I axillary dissection followed by postoperative radiation therapy. A ten-year local recurrence rate of 6 to 14 percent was observed. Balawadjer and associates[176] treated 108 patients with Stage III breast cancer with either radiation therapy alone or radiation therapy in combination with surgery or chemotherapy or both. The results of their series are summarized in Table 5–32. Local control was most effectively achieved by chemotherapy followed by radiation therapy and surgery; however, there were no significant differences in five-year survival rate among any of the treatment regimens.[176]

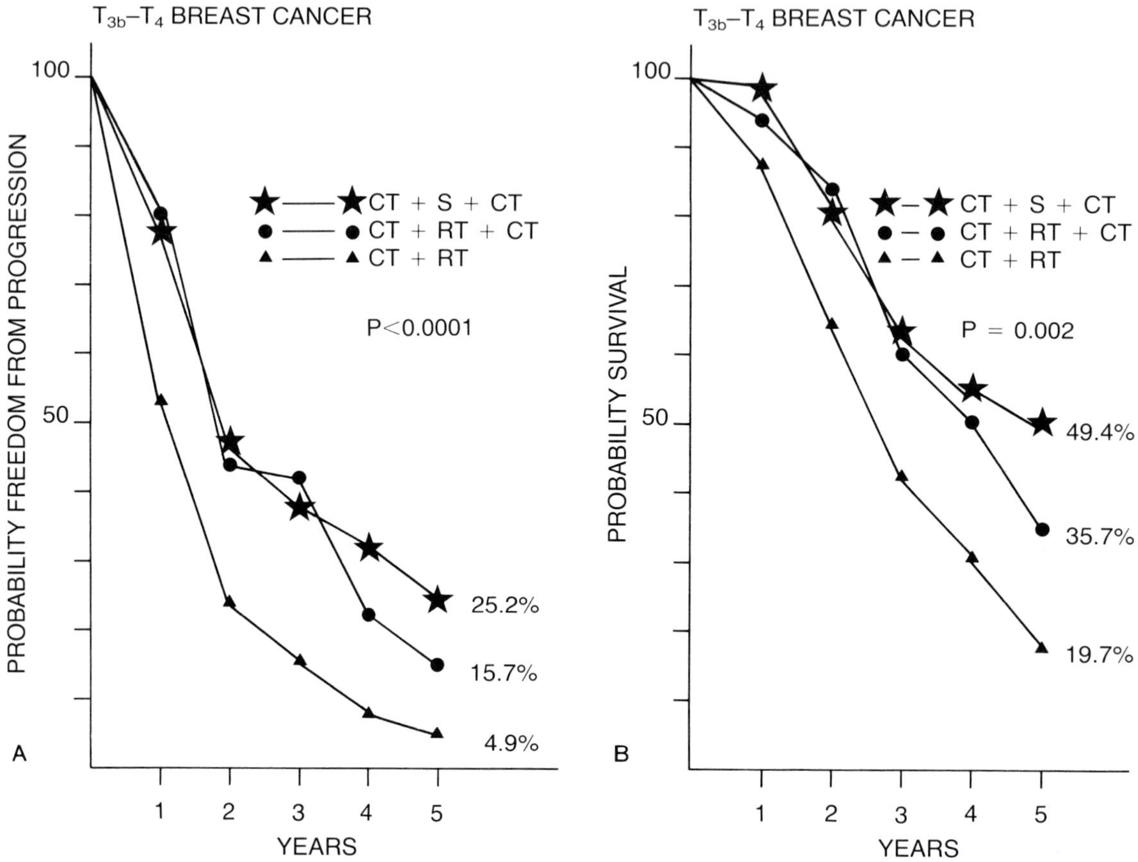

FIGURE 5–20. Treatment with combined-modality regimens of patients with T_{3b} or T_4 breast cancer. Probability of freedom from progression (*A*) and overall survival (*B*), according to treatment (CT, chemotherapy; RT, radiation therapy; S, surgery). (With permission from Valagussa P, et al.: T3b-T4 breast cancers: Factors affecting results in combined modality treatments. Clinical Experimental Metastases 1:191, 1983.)

The most promising therapy for locally advanced breast cancer appears to be combined-modality regimens using chemotherapy initially, followed by surgery or radiation therapy or both (to consolidate local control) and, then, by maintenance chemotherapy. The details of these regimens and the results are discussed in Chapter 9. With this approach, Perloff and Lesnick[170] reported a median survival of 40 months among 29 patients with inflammatory carcinoma. Hortobagyi and colleagues[171] observed that among 52 patients with T_3, T_4/N_2, N_3/M_0 tumors, 94 percent were rendered free of clinically detectable disease at a median follow-up time of 60 months; 40 percent of patients remained

TABLE 5–32. Treatment of Stage III Breast Cancer with Combined-Modality Therapy. Actuarial Results at Five Years for Local Control

		Actuarial Five-Year Results (%)		
Treatment Group	*No. of Patients*	Local Control Rate	Rate of Freedom from Metastases	Survival Rate
C→ R→ S	30	88 ± 8	36 ± 9	38 ± 10
C→ R	23	54 ± 14	41 ± 12	46 ± 12
R→ S	17	55 ± 22	21 ± 12	44 ± 14
R	38	38 ± 10	14 ± 7	38 ± 10

With permission from Balawajder I, Antich PP, Boland J, et al.: An analysis of the role of radiotherapy alone and in combination with chemotherapy and surgery in the management of advanced breast cancer. Cancer 51:574, 1983.

disease-free off all therapy. Sorace and colleagues[172] reported that among 26 patients with Stage III breast cancer, 96 percent achieved an objective response and 78 percent of these patients were rendered disease-free by the combined-modality approach.

Thus, surgery may play an important role as part of combined-modality regimens for locally advanced breast cancer.[171–173] Surgical procedures in this context are performed to remove gross disease in the breast and axillary lymph nodes remaining after initial chemotherapy. Eradication of gross disease will facilitate subsequent chemotherapy and radiation therapy and will provide the most effective means of local control. The recommended surgical procedure for these patients has not been defined. For patients with a residual breast mass, the authors have performed a total mastectomy. There has been no reported experience with local excision of the mass under these circumstances. In addition, because of the associated inflammatory reaction from the chemotherapy, the margins of the tumor mass may be ill defined. If palpable axillary nodes are present, the authors perform an axillary dissection. The extent of the dissection should be determined at the time of surgery. If involved nodes are limited to Level I, only this portion needs to be removed. However, if grossly involved lymph nodes extend to the apex of the axilla, a complete axillary dissection should be done to provide more effective local control.

The timing of the surgical procedure is important. The authors prefer to perform the procedure approximately three weeks after the last cycle of cytoxic chemotherapy. This allows recovery from the myelosuppression of cytotoxic drugs without prolonging the interval between chemotherapy treatments. At the time of the mastectomy, the skin flaps must be carefully dissected. The nipple and biopsy site are included in the skin incision. Thick flaps are made because the procedure is designed to remove only areas of gross disease. Because of the recent cytotoxic chemotherapy, wound healing may be diminished. With careful surgical technique, skin-flap necrosis in the postoperative period can be avoided. This complication is particularly significant in these patients, as it may delay for up to several weeks resumption of chemotherapy and treatment with adjuvant radiation therapy while wound healing occurs. Nonabsorbable sutures are used to close the skin and are left in place for ten days. Perioperative antibiotics are not given.

In summary, while surgery as primary therapy is no longer considered appropriate for locally advanced (Stage III) breast cancer, surgery continues to play an important role in the management of these patients. Careful surgical technique must be practiced to allow these patients to derive maximum benefit from combined-modality regimens.

REFERENCES

1. Breasted JH: The Edwin Smith Papyrus. Chicago: University of Chicago Press, 1930.
2. De Moulin D: A Short History of Breast Cancer. Boston: Martinus Nijhoff Publishers, 1983, p. 2.
3. Degenshein GA, Ceccarelli F: The history of breast cancer surgery: Early beginnings to Halsted. Breast 3:28, 1977.
4. De Moulin D: A Short History of Breast Cancer. Boston: Martinus Nijhoff Publishers, 1983, pp. 5–6.
5. Pancoast J: Treatise on Operative Surgery. Philadelphia: Carey and Hart, 1844, p. 269. *In*: Robbins GF: The Breast. Austin, TX: Silvergirl, Inc., 1984, pp. 50–53.
6. Moore CH: On the influence of inadequate operations on the theory of cancer. Royal Med Chir Soc 1:245, 1867. *In*: Robbins GF: The Breast. Austin, TX: Silvergirl, Inc., 1984, pp. 58–64.
7. Madden JL: Modified radical mastectomy. Ann Surg 5:624, 1972.
8. Halsted WS: The results of operations for the cure of cancer of the breast performed at the Johns Hopkins Hospital from June 1889 to January 1894. Johns Hopkins Bulletin 4:297, 1894.
9. Halsted WS: A clinical and histological study of certain adenocarcinoma of the breast; and a brief consideration of the superclavicular operation and of results of the operations for cancer of the breast from 1889–1898 at the Johns Hopkins Hospital. Ann Surg 28:557, 1898.
10. Donegan WL: Mastectomy in the primary management of invasive mammary carcinoma. Adv Surg 6:1, 1972.
11. Halsted WS: The results of radical operations for cure of carcinoma of the breast. Ann Surg 46:1, 1907.
12. Meyer W: An improved method of the radical operation for carcinoma of the breast. Med Rec 46:746, 1894.
13. Crile G, Jr.: Results of conservative treatment of breast cancer at ten and 15 years. Ann Surg 181:26, 1975.
14. Fisher B, Wolmar, N, Bauer M, et al.: The accuracy of clinical nodal staging and of limited axillary dissection as a determinant of histological nodal status in carcinoma of the breast. Surg Gynecol Obstet 152:765, 1981.
15. Haagensen CD, Stout AP: Carcinoma of the breast. Criteria of operability. Ann Surg 118:1032, 1943.
16. Patey DH, Dyson WH: The prognosis of carcinoma

of the breast in relation to the type of operation performed. Br J Cancer 2:7, 1948.
17. Auchincloss H: Significance of location and number of axillary metastases in carcinoma of the breast: A justification for a conservative operation. Ann Surg 158:36, 1963.
18. Madden JL: Modified radical mastectomy. Surg Gynecol Obstet 121:1221, 1965.
19. Turner L, Bell WGT, Hartley RC, et al.: Radical versus modified radical mastectomy for breast cancer. Ann R Coll Surg Engl 63:239, 1981.
20. Maddox WA, Carpenter JT, Laws HL, et al.: A randomized prospective trial of radical (Halsted) mastectomy versus modified radical mastectomy in 311 breast cancer patients. Ann Surg 198:207, 1983.
21. Report by The American College of Surgeons Commission on Cancer, Chicago, IL, October 22, 1982.
22. Wangensteen OH, Lewis FJ, Arhelger SW: The extended or superradical mastectomy for carcinoma of the breast. A justification for a conservative operation. Surg Clin North Am 36:1051, 1956.
23. Margottini M: Arguments in favor of superradical operations for carcinoma of the breast. Acta Unio Internat Contra Cancrum 15:1037, 1958.
24. Dahl-Iversen E, Tobiassen T: Radical mastectomy with parasternal and supraclavicular dissection for mammary carcinoma. Ann Surg 157:170, 1963.
25. Veronesi U, Zingo L: Extended mastectomy for cancer of the breast. Cancer 20:677, 1967.
26. Sugarbaker ED: Extended radical mastectomy: Its superiority in the treatment of breast cancer. JAMA 187:96, 1964.
27. Caceres E: An evaluation of radical mastectomy and extended radical mastectomy for cancer of the breast. Surg Gynecol Obstet 125:337, 1967.
28. Urban JA: The role of superradical operations for breast cancer. Proc Natl Cancer Conf 6:145, 1970.
29. Livingston SF, Arlen M: The extended extrapleural radical mastectomy: Its role in the treatment of carcinoma of the breast. Ann Surg 179:260, 1974.
30. Lacour J, Bucalossi P, Caceres E, et al.: Radical mastectomy versus radical mastectomy plus internal mammary dissection: Five-year results of an international cooperative study. Cancer 37:206, 1976.
31. Lacour J, Le M, Caceres E, et al: Radical mastectomy versus radical mastectomy plus internal mammary dissection: Ten-year results of an international cooperative trial in breast cancer. Cancer 51:1941, 1983.
32. Veronesi U, Valagussa P: Inefficacy of internal mammary node dissection in breast cancer surgery. Cancer 47:170, 1981.
33. Meier P, Ferguson DJ, Karrison T: A controlled trial of extended radical mastectomy. Cancer 55:880, 1985.
34. Crile G, Jr.: Results of simplified treatment of breast cancer. Surg Gynecol Obstet 118:517, 1964.
35. Williams IG, Murley RS, Curwen MP: Carcinoma of the female breast: Conservative and radical surgery. Br Med J 2:788, 1953.
36. Shimkin MB, Koppel M, Connelly RR, et al.: Simple and radical mastectomy for breast cancer: A reanalysis of Smith and Meyer's report from Rockford, Illinois. J Natl Cancer Inst 27:1197, 1961.
37. Devitt JE: The influence of conservative and radical surgery on the survival of patients with breast cancer. Can Med Assoc J 87:906, 1962.
38. Devitt JE: The significance of regional lymph node metastases in breast carcinoma. Can Med Assoc J 92:289, 1965.
39. Kyle J, Norman JN, Carr J, et al.: Management of early cancer of the breast: Report of an international multicenter trial supported by the Cancer Research Campaign. Br Med J 1:1035, 1976.
40. Lythgoe JP, Leck I, Swindell R: Manchester regional breast study: Preliminary results. Lancet 1:744, 1978.
41. Lythgoe JP, Palmer MK: Manchester regional breast study—5- and 10-year results. Br J Surg 69:693, 1982.
42. Baum M, Coyle PJ: Simple mastectomy for early breast cancer and the behavior of the untreated axillary nodes. Bull Cancer 64:603, 1977.
43. Turnbull AR, Turner DT, Chant ADB, et al: Treatment of early breast cancer. Lancet 2:7, 1978.
44. Helman P, Bennett MB, Louw JH, et al.: Interim report on trial of treatment for operable breast cancer. S Afr Med J 46:1374, 1972.
45. Forrest APM, Stewart HJ, Roberts MM, et al.: Simple mastectomy and axillary node sampling (pectoral node biopsy) in the management of primary breast cancer. Ann Surg 196:371, 1982.
46. Fisher B, Redmond C, Fisher ER, et al.: Ten-year results of a randomized clinical trial comparing radical mastectomy and total mastectomy with or without radiation. N Engl J Med 312:674, 1985.
47. Goss CM (ed.): Gray's Anatomy of the Human Body. Philadelphia: Lea & Febiger, 1966, pp. 1330–1334.
48. Woodburne RT: Essentials of Human Anatomy. New York: Oxford University Press, 1965, p. 72.
49. Haagensen CD: Diseases of the Breast, 2nd ed. Philadelphia: W.B. Saunders Co., 1971, p. 403.
50. Hollinshead WH: Anatomy for Surgeons: The Thorax, Abdomen, and Pelvis. New York: Paul B. Hoeber, Inc., 1956, Vol. 2, pp. 10–16.
51. Hicken NF: Mastectomy: A clinical pathologic study demonstrating why most mastectomies result in incomplete removal of the mammary gland. Arch Surg 40:6, 1940.
52. de Moss EV, Lichter AS, Lippman ME, et al.: Complete axillary lymph node dissection before radiotherapy for primary breast cancer. *In*: Harris JR, Hellman S, Silen W (ed.): Conservative Management of Breast Cancer: New Surgical and Radiotherapeutic Techniques. Philadelphia: J.B. Lippincott, 1983, pp. 163–182.
53. Danforth DN, Jr., Findlay PA, McDonald HD, et al.: Complete axillary lymph node dissection for Stage I, II carcinoma of the breast. J Clin Oncol 4:655, 1986.
54. Rosen PP, Lesser ML, Kinne DW, et al.: Discontinuous or "skip" metastases in breast cancer. Ann Surg 197:276, 1983.
53. Pigott J, Nichols R, Maddox WA, et al: Metastasis to the upper levels of the axillary lymph nodes in carcinoma of the breast and its implications for nodal sampling procedures. Surg Gynecol Obstet 158:255, 1984.
56. Boova RS, Bonanni R, Rosato FE: Patterns of axillary nodal involvement in breast cancer. Ann Surg 196:642, 1982.
57. Haagensen CD: Diseases of the Breast, 2nd ed. Philadelphia: W.B. Saunders Co., 1971, p. 38.
58. Friedell GH, Gallagher HS, Hartmann WH, et al.:

Standardized management of breast specimens. Am J Clin Pathol 60:789, 1973.
59. Smithers DW, Rigby-Jones P: Clinical evidence of parasternal lymph node involvement in neoplastic disease. Acta Radiol (Suppl) 188:235, 1959.
60. Urban JA: Clinical experience and results of excision of the internal mammary lymph node chain in primary operable breast cancer. Cancer 12:14, 1959.
61. Cody HS, Egeli RA, Urban JA: Rotter's node metastases. Ann Surg 199:266, 1984.
62. Netter FH: Ciba Collection of Medical Illustrations. Summit, NJ: Ciba Pharmaceutical Co., 1979, Vol. 7, p. 6.
63. Haagensen CD: Diseases of the Breast, 2nd ed. Philadelphia: W.B. Saunders Co., 1971, pp. 674–704.
64. Madden JL: Atlas of Technics in Surgery, 2nd ed. New York: Appleton-Century-Crofts, 1964, pp. 134–147.
65. Dahl-Iversen E: Extended Radical Operation for Mammary Carcinoma. Proceedings of the Third National Cancer Conference, Philadelphia: J.B. Lippincott, 1956, pp. 148–156.
66. Sugarbaker ED: An Atlas of Surgical Oncology. Boca Raton, FL: CRC Press, 1983, Vol. 1, pp. 141–158.
67. Beattie EJ, Economou SG: An Atlas of Advanced Surgical Techniques. Philadelphia: W.B. Saunders Co., 1968, pp. 88–103.
68. Handley RS, Patey DH, Hand BH: Excision of the internal mammary chain in radical mastectomy: Results in 57 cases. Lancet 1:457, 1956.
69. Kinne DW, DeCosse JJ: Modified radical mastectomy for carcinoma of the breast: How I do it. Am Surg 48:543, 1982.
70. Nora PF: Operative Surgery: Principles and Techniques. Philadelphia: Lea & Febiger, 1972, pp. 182–187.
71. Veronesi U, Saccozzi R, Del Vecchio M, et al.: Comparing radical mastectomy with quadrantectomy, axillary dissection, and radiotherapy in patients with small cancers of the breast. N Engl J Med 305:6, 1981.
72. Fisher B, Bauer M, Margolese R, et al.: Five-year results of a randomized clinical trial comparing total mastectomy and segmental mastectomy with or without radiation in the treatment of breast cancer. N Engl J Med 312:665, 1985.
73. Findlay PA, Lippman ME, Danforth DN, Jr., et al.: Mastectomy vs. radiotherapy as treatment for stage I, II breast cancer: A prospective randomized trial at the National Cancer Institute. World J Surg 9:671, 1985.
74. Shons AR, Press BHJ: Subcutaneous mastectomy: Indications, technique, and applications. Arch Surg 118:844, 1983.
75. Rose CM, Botnick LE, Weinstein M, et al.: Axillary sampling in the definitive treatment of breast cancer by radiation therapy and lumpectomy. Int J Radiat Oncol Biol Phys 9:339, 1983.
76. Esselstyn CB, Jr., Hermann RE, Crile G, Jr., et al.: The results of selective conservative treatment in breast cancer: A five- to ten-year follow-up. Bull Soc Int Chir 6:513, 1975.
77. Haagensen CD: Diseases of the Breast, 2nd ed. Philadelphia: W.B. Saunders Co., 1971, pp. 629–634.
78. Gallagher HS: Multicentricity in breast cancer. *In* Harris JR, Hellman S, Silen W (eds.): Conservative Management of Breast Cancer. Philadelphia: J.B. Lippincott, 1983, pp. 117–122.
79. Parry RG, Cochran TC, Jr., Wolfert FG: When is there nipple involvement in carcinoma of the breast? Surg Gynecol Obstet 59:535, 1977.
80. Smith J, Payne WS, Carney JA: Involvement of the nipple and areola in carcinoma of the breast. Surg Gynecol Obstet 143:546, 1976.
81. Lagios MD, Gates EA, Westdahl PR, et al: A guide to the frequency of nipple involvement in breast cancer. A study of 149 consecutive mastectomies using a serial subgross and correlated radiographic technique. Am J Surg 138:135, 1979.
82. Morimoto T, Komaki K, Inui K, et al.: Involvement of nipple and areola in early breast cancer. Cancer 55:2459, 1985.
83. Allison AB, Howorth MB: Carcinoma in a nipple preserved by heterotopic auto-transplantation. N Engl J Med 298:1132, 1978.
84. Khandekar JD: Carcinoma in a heterotopically autotransplanted nipple. Cancer 43:2502, 1979.
85. Rose JH: Carcinoma in a transplanted nipple. Arch Surg 115:1131, 1980.
86. Haagensen CD, Bodian C: A personal experience with Halsted's radical mastectomy. Ann Surg 199:143, 1984.
87. Bloom HJG, Richardson WW, Harries EJ: Natural history of untreated breast cancer (1805–1933). Br Med J 5299:213, 1962.
88. Haagensen CD, Cooley E: Radical mastectomy for mammary carcinoma. Ann Surg 157:166, 1963.
89. Haagensen CD: Diseases of the Breast, 2nd ed. Philadelphia: W.B. Saunders Co., 1971, pp. 647–658.
90. Anglem TJ, Leber RE: Characteristics of ten-year survivors after radical mastectomy. Am J Surg 121:363, 1971.
91. Ariel IM: Results of 1178 patients with breast cancer treated by radical mastectomy and postoperative irradiation where metastases to axillary lymph nodes occurred. J Surg Oncol 12:137, 1979.
92. Butcher HR: Radical mastectomy for mammary carcinoma. Ann Surg 170:883, 1969.
93. Donegan WL: Primary treatment options and end results. *In* Donegan WL, Spratt JS (eds.): Cancer of the Breast, 2nd ed. Philadelphia: W.B. Saunders Co., 1979.
94. Ferguson DJ, Meier P, Karrison T, et al.: Staging of breast cancer and survival rates. An assessment based on 50 years of experience with radical mastectomy. JAMA 248:1337, 1982.
95. Baker RR, Montague ACW, Childs JN: A comparison of modified radical mastectomy to radical mastectomy in the treatment of operable breast carcinoma. Ann Surg 189:553, 1979.
96. Lee RO, Lambley DG: Radical mastectomy in the treatment of breast cancer: A followup study over 10 and 15 years. Br J Surg 58:138, 1971.
97. Haimov H, Kark AE, Lesnick GJ: Carcinoma of the breast: Thirty years experience with radical mastectomy. Am J Surg 115:341, 1968.
98. Robbins GF, Berg J: Curability of patients with invasive breast carcinoma based on a 30-year study. World J Surg 1:284, 1977.
99. Duncan W, Kerr GR: The curability of breast cancer. Br Med J 2:781, 1976.

100. Robinson GN, Van Heerden JA, Payne WS, et al.: The primary surgical treatment of carcinoma of the breast: A changing trend toward modified radical mastectomy. Mayo Clin Proc 51:433, 1976.
101. Fisher B, Slack N, Katrych D, et al.: Ten-year follow-up of results of patients with carcinoma of the breast in a cooperative clinical trial evaluating surgical adjuvant chemotherapy. Surg Gynecol Obstet 140:528, 1975.
102. Attiyeh FF, Jensen M, Huvos AG, et al.: Axillary micrometastases and macrometastases in carcinoma of the breast. Surg Gynecol Obstet 144:839, 1977.
103. Haagensen CD: Diseases of the Breast, 2nd ed. Philadelphia: W.B. Saunders Co., 1971, p. 400–401.
104. Leis HP, Jr.: Diagnosis and Treatment of Breast Lesions. Flushing, NY: Medical Examination Pub. Co., 1970, p. 126.
105. Fisher B, Wolmark N, Redmond C, et al.: Findings from NSABP Protocol No. B-04: Comparison of radical mastectomy with alternative treatments. II. The clinical and biological significance of medial-central breast cancers. Cancer 48:1863, 1981.
106. Haagensen CD: Diseases of the Breast, 2nd ed. Philadelphia: W.B. Saunders Co., 1971, pp. 706–710.
107. Valagussa P, Bonadonna G, Veronesi U: Patterns of relapse and survival following radical mastectomy: Analysis of 716 consecutive cases. Cancer 41:1170, 1978.
108. Donegan WL: Primary treatment options and end results. *In* Donegan WL, Spratt JS (eds.): Cancer of the Breast, 2nd ed. Philadelphia: W.B. Saunders Co., 1979, p. 242.
109. Fisher B, Slack NH, Cavanaugh PJ, et al.: Postoperative radiotherapy in the treatment of breast cancer: Results of the NSABP clinical trial. Ann Surg 172:711, 1970
110. Haagensen CD: Diseases of the Breast, 2nd ed. Philadelphia: W.B. Saunders Co., 1971, p. 415.
111. Donegan WL, Perez-Mesa CM, Watson FR: A biostatistical study of locally recurrent breast carcinoma. Surg Gynecol Obstet 122:529, 1966.
112. Haagensen CD: Diseases of the Breast, 2nd ed. Philadelphia: W.B. Saunders Co., 1971, pp. 622–629.
113. Budd DC, Cochran RC, Sturtz DL, et al.: Surgical morbidity after mastectomy operations. Am J Surg 135:218, 1978.
114. Say CC, Donegan WL: A biostatistical evaluation of complications from mastectomy. Surg Gynecol Obstet 138:370, 1974.
115. Jolly PC, Viar W: Reduction of morbidity after radical mastectomy. Am Surg 47:377, 1981.
116. Zintel HA, Nay HR: Postoperative complications of radical mastectomy. Surg Clin North Am 44:313, 1964.
117. Gray EB, Anglem TJ: Radical mastectomy for carcinoma of the breast. N Engl J Med 261:1310, 1959.
118. Aitken DR, Minton JP: Complications associated with mastectomy. Surg Clin North Am 63:1331, 1983.
119. Myers MB, Brock D, Cohn I, Jr.: Prevention of skin slough after radical mastectomy by use of a vital dye to delineate devascularized skin. Ann Surg 173:920, 1971.
120. Morris AM: A control trial of closed wound suction: Drainage in radical mastectomy. Br J Surg 60:357, 1973.
121. Becker C, Sener SF, Scanlon E: Complications of drainage system for modified radical mastectomy. Arch Surg 117:859, 1982.
122. Sitzmann JV, Dufresne C, Zuidema GD: The use of sclerotherapy for treatment of postmastectomy wound seromas. Surgery 93:345, 1983.
123. Lotze MT, Duncan MA, Gerber LH, et al.: Early vs. delayed shoulder motion following axillary dissection. Ann Surg 193:288, 1981.
124. Britton RC, Nelson PA: Causes and treatment of postmastectomy lymphedema of the arm. JAMA 180:95, 1962.
125. Halsted WS: The swelling of the arm after operations for cancer of the breast—elephantiasis chirurgica—its cause and prevention. Johns Hopkins Hosp Bull 32:309, 1921.
126. Brismar B, Ljungdahl I: Postoperative lymphedema after treatment of breast cancer. Acta Chir Scand 149:687, 1983.
127. Chodak GW, Plaut ME: Use of systemic antibiotics for prophylaxis in surgery. Arch Surg 112:326, 1977.
128. Handley RS: Carcinoma of the breast. Ann R Coll Surg Engl 57:59, 1975.
129. Caceres E: Incidence of metastases in the internal mammary chain in operable carcinoma of the breast and 5-year results. Acta Unio Int Contra Cancrum 19:1566, 1963.
130. Margottini M, Jacobelli G, Cau M: The end results of enlarged radical mastectomy. Acta Unio Int Contra Cancrum 19:1555, 1963.
131. Donegan WL, Sugarbaker ED, Handley RS, et al.: The management of primary operable breast cancer: A comparison of time-mortality factors after standard, extended, and modified radical mastectomy. Proceedings of the Sixth National Cancer Conference, Philadelphia: J.B. Lippincott, 1968, pp. 135–143.
132. Urban JA: Extended radical mastectomy for breast cancer. Am J Surg 106:399, 1963.
133. Dahl-Iversen E, Tobiassen T: Radical mastectomy with parasternal and supraclavicular dissection for mammary carcinoma. Ann Surg 170:889, 1969.
134. Haagensen CD: Diseases of the Breast, 2nd ed. Philadelphia: W.B. Saunders Co., 1971, pp. 412–413.
135. Hermann RE, Steiger E: Modified radical mastectomy. Surg Clin North Am 58:743, 1978.
136. Delarue NC, Anderson WD, Starr J: Modified radical mastectomy in the individualized treatment of breast carcinoma. Surg Gynecol Obstet 1969 129:79, 1969.
137. Madden JL, Kasndalaft S, Bourque R: Modified radical mastectomy. Ann Surg 175:624, 1972.
138. Leis HP, Jr.: Modified radical mastectomy: Definition and role in breast cancer surgery. Int Surg 65:211, 1980.
139. Handley RS: The conservative radical mastectomy of Patey: 10-year results in 425 patients. Breast 2:16, 1976.
140. Meyer AC, Smith SS, Potter M: Carcinoma of the breast: A clinical study. Arch Surg 113:364, 1978.
141. Handley RS: The technic and results of conservative radical mastectomy (Patey's operation). Prog Clin Cancer 1:462, 1965.
142. Feigenberg Z, Zer M, Dintsman M: Comparison of

postoperative complications following radical and modified radical mastectomy. World J Surg 1:207, 1977.
143. Dunphy JE: Modified radical mastectomy. Cancer 28:1624, 1971.
144. Moxley JH, Allegra JC, Henney J, et al.: Treatment of primary breast cancer: Summary of the National Institutes of Health Consensus Development Conference. JAMA 244:797, 1980.
145. Den Besten L, Ziffren SE: Simple and radical mastectomy. Arch Surg 90:755, 1965.
146. Bourke JB, Balfour TW, Hardcastle JD, et al.: A comparison between suction and corrugated drainage after simple mastectomy: A report of a controlled trial. Br J Surg 63:67, 1976.
147. Forrest APM, Roberts MM, Preece RP, et al.: The Cardiff–St. Mary trial. Br J Surg 61:766, 1974.
148. Clark RM, Wilkinson RH, Mahoney LJ, et al.: Breast cancer: A 21-year experience with conservative surgery and radiation. Int J Radiat Oncol Biol Phys 8:967, 1982.
149. Montgomery ACA, Greening WP, Levene AL: Clinical study of recurrence rate and survival time of patients with carcinoma of the breast treated by biopsy excision without any other therapy. J R Soc Med 71:339, 1978.
150. Freeman CR, Belliveau NJ, Kim TH, et al.: Limited surgery with or without radiotherapy for early breast carcinoma. J Can Assoc Radiol 32:125, 1981.
151. Tagart REB: Partial mastectomy for breast cancer. Br Med J 2:1268, 1978.
152. Lagios MD, Richards VE, Rose MR, et al.: Segmental mastectomy without radiotherapy: Short-term follow-up. Cancer 52:2173, 1983.
153. Hermann RE, Esselstyne CB, Jr., Crile G, Jr., et al.: Results of conservative operations for breast cancer. Arch Surg 120:746, 1985.
154. Crile G, Jr.: Treatment of breast cancer by local excision. Am J Surg 109:400, 1965.
155. Crile G, Jr., Hoerr SO: Results of treatment of carcinoma of the breast by local excision. Surg Gynecol Obstet 132:780, 1971.
156. Crile G, Jr.: The case for local excision of breast cancer in selected cases. Lancet 1:549, 1972.
157. Cady B: Total mastectomy and partial axillary dissection. Surg Clin North Am 53:313, 1973.
158. Henderson C, Canellos GP: Carcinoma of the breast: The past decade. N Engl J Med 302:17, 1980.
159. Berg JW: The significance of axillary node levels in the study of breast carcinoma. Cancer, 8:776, 1955.
160. Smith JA, Gamez-Araujo J, Gallagher H, et al.: Carcinoma of the breast: Analysis of total lymph node involvement versus level of metastases. Cancer, 39:527, 1977.
161. Wood C, Gerber L, Findlay P, et al.: Prospective assessment of functional outcome in breast cancer patients undergoing mastectomy vs. radiotherapy in a randomized trial. Proceedings, American Society of Clinical Oncology Annual Meeting, Houston, Texas, May 19–21, 1985, Abstract No. C-393.
162. Clarke D, Martinez A, Cox RS, et al.: Breast edema following staging axillary node dissection in patients with breast carcinoma treated by radical radiotherapy. Cancer, 49:2295, 1982.
163. Carabell SC, Richter MP, Bryan JH, et al.: Radiation therapy as an alternative to mastectomy for breast cancer—the role of axillary sampling. Int J Radiat Oncol Biol Phys, 7 (Suppl 1):31, 1981.
164. Camp E: Inflammatory carcinoma of the breast: The case for conservatism. Am J Surg, 131:583, 1976.
165. Petrek JA, Glenn PD, Cramer AR: Ulcerated breast cancer: Patients and outcome. Am. Surg 49:187, 1983.
166. Arnold DJ, Lesnick GJ: Survival following mastectomy for Stage III breast cancer. Am J Surg, 137:362, 1979.
167. Valagussa P, Zambetti M, Pignami P, et al.: T_{3b}–T_4 breast cancers: Factors affecting results in combined modality treatments. Clin Exp Metastasis 1:191, 1983.
168. Townsend CM, Abston S, Fish JC: Surgical adjuvant treatment of locally advanced breast cancer. Ann Surg, 201:604, 1985.
169. Ibid, p. 609, see discussion by EM Copeland.
170. Perloff M, Lesnick GJ: Chemotherapy before and after mastectomy in Stage III breast cancer. Arch Surg, 117:879, 1982.
171. Hortobagyi GN, Blumenschein GR, Spanos W, et al.: Multimodal treatment of locally advanced breast cancer. Cancer, 51:763, 1983.
172. Sorace RA, Lippman ME, Bagley CS, et al.: Effective combined modality treatment for locally advanced breast cancer using primary induction chemotherapy with hormonal synchronization followed by radiation therapy with or without debulking surgery. World J Surg, 9:775, 1985.
173. Hagelberg RS, Jolly PC, Anderson RP: Role of surgery in the treatment of inflammatory breast carcinoma. Am J Surg 148:125, 1984.
174. Chretien PB, Ketcham AS, Hoye RC, et al.: Axillary dissection with preservation of the pectoralis major muscle. Ann Surg 173:554, 1971.
175. Wilson RE: Surgical management of locally advanced and recurrent breast cancer. Cancer 53:752, 1984.
176. Balawajder I, Antich PP, Boland J: An analysis of the role of radiotherapy alone and in combination with chemotherapy and surgery in the management of advanced breast cancer. Cancer 51:574, 1983.
177. Cutler SJ: The prognosis of treated breast cancer. *In*: Forrest APM (ed.): Prognostic Factors in Breast Cancer, Proceedings of the First Tenovus Symposium. Edinburgh: E. Livingston, Ltd. 1967, pp. 20–31.
178. Haagensen CD: Diseases of the Breast, 2nd ed. Philadelphia: W.B. Saunders Co., 1971, p. 631.
179. Wallace IWJ, Champion HR: Axillary nodes in breast cancer. Lancet, 29:217, 1972.
180. Roberts MR, Forrest APM, Blumgart LH, et al.: Simple versus radical mastectomy. Lancet, 19:1073, 1973.
181. Johnsen C: Breast disease. Acta Chir Scand (Suppl), 454:1, 1975.
182. Atkins H, Hayward JL, Klugman DJ, et al.: Treatment of early breast cancer: A report after 10 years of a clinical trial. Br Med J 2:243, 1972.
183. Jessiman AG: The Breast. *In*: Warren R (ed.): Surgery. Philadelphia: W.B. Saunders Co., 1963.
184. Chu FCH, Lin F-J, Kim JH, et al.: Locally recurrent carcinoma of the breast: Results of radiation therapy. Cancer 37:2677, 1976.

185. Bedwinek JM, Lee J, Fineberg B, et al.: Prognostic indicators in patients with isolated locoregional recurrence in breast cancer. Cancer 47:2232, 1981.
186. Zimmerman KW, Montague ED, Fletcher GH: Frequency, anatomical distribution and management of local recurrence after definitive therapy for breast cancer. Cancer 19:67, 1966.
187. Gilliland MD, Barton RM, Copeland EM, III: The implications of local recurrence of breast cancer as the first site of therapeutic failure. Ann Surg 197:284, 1983.
188. Bedwinek JM, Lee J., Fineberg B, et al.: Prognostic indicators in patients with isolated local-regional recurrence of breast cancer. Cancer 47:2232, 1981.
189. Quinn RH, Barlow JF: Involvement of the nipple and areola by carcinoma of the breast. Arch Surg 116:1139, 1981.
190. Krohn IT, Cooper DR, Basett JG: Radical mastectomy: Thick vs. thin skin flaps. Arch Surg 117:760, 1982.
191. Huvos AG, Hutter RV, Berg JW: Significance of axillary macrometastases and micrometastases in mammary cancer. Ann Surg 173:44, 1971.

Radiation Therapy as Definitive Treatment of Breast Cancer

PEGGIE A. FINDLAY, M.D.

6

The application of radiation therapy as primary curative treatment for patients with carcinoma of the breast in many ways parallels the evolution of clinical radiation oncology. In the early years of the century, use of low-energy equipment and a rapidly administered dose did not produce a very satisfactory outcome. In the 1920's and the 1930's, Keynes[1] in England and Baclesse[2] in France developed clinical treatment techniques that were capable of achieving permanent local tumor control with acceptable effects on normal tissue. Later, advances in physics and equipment led to the development of improved treatment techniques. Over the last decade, there has been considerable critical evaluation of treatment results, integration of local and systemic therapy, and the initiation of a number of controlled clinical trials.

Like surgery, radiation therapy is a local treatment modality, and also like surgery, the objective of therapy is to eradicate all cancer in the treated area, ensuring no recurrence. In addition, this objective should be achieved with maintenance of a cosmetically intact breast. If these two goals can be attained simultaneously, the ultimate result should be a substantial reduction in the physical and psychologic morbidity of treatment and an improvement in the patient's quality of life. It is to be hoped that by reducing women's fear of potentially disfiguring surgery, they will be encouraged to seek medical attention for breast cancer at an earlier, and hence potentially more curable, stage of the disease.

For many years, the recommended treatment for locoregional breast cancer was *en bloc* surgical resection of all involved and potentially contaminated tissues using the radical mastectomy (which in recent years has been supplanted by the modified radical mastectomy). This treatment approach was predicated on the concept, largely espoused by surgeons such as Handley and Halsted, that breast cancer was primarily a local disease that spread to other areas of the body in a contiguous, centrifugal fashion, moving from the breast to the rest of the body through the lymphatic system and along fascial planes.

Although it undoubtedly occurs, I am not sure that I have observed from breast cancer, metastasis which seemed definitely to have been conveyed by way of the blood vessels; and my views as to the dissemination of carcinoma of the breast accord . . . fully with Handley's . . . . We believe with Handley that cancer of the breast in spreading centrifugally preserves, in the main, continuity with the original growth . . . the dissemination probably takes place by way of the lymphatics—not by the blood vessels—and the disease holds together without important interruptions. It permeates to the bone rather than metastasizes to it and, by the lymphatics, along fascial planes. There is then a definite . . . quite uninterrupted connection between the original focus and all the outlying deposits of cancer. It must be our endeavor to trace more definitely the roots traveled in the metastasis to bone, particularly to the humerus, for it is even possible in case of involvement of this bone, that amputation of the shoulder joint plus a proper removal of the soft parts might irradicate the disease. So, too, it is conceivable that, ultimately, when our knowledge of the lymphatics traversed in cases of femur involvement becomes sufficiently exact, amputation at the hip joint may seem indicated.[3]

In the late 1930's, this concept was called into question, while emphasis shifted to an embolic spread of the disease. This is the view that predominates today. As expressed by Bernard Fisher,[4] "In most patients, by the time a breast cancer becomes clinically discernible it is already systemically disseminated." Fisher believes that regional lymph nodes are "indicators rather than instigators of distant disease" and, thus, variations in locoregional treatment are unlikely to affect patient survival rates. Some have doubted the curability of any patient with breast cancer, suggesting that the disease is always systemic and, therefore, every patient would eventually manifest disease recurrence that would prove fatal, if long enough follow-up were possible.

The truth probably lies somewhere between these opposing points of view. Rutqvist and Wallgren[5] identified 458 women aged 40 or younger at the time of diagnosis of breast cancer, in whom the likelihood of mortality from other causes would presumably be minimal. The minimum follow-up period was 20 years, with a maximum of 51 years. At 40 years from diagnosis, actuarial survival for patients with negative axillary nodes was 53 percent and for patients with positive axillary nodes, 19 percent. Although only a few patients remained at risk after 40 years from diagnosis, no breast cancer deaths were observed after that time. Actuarial survival of this population is shown in Figure 6–1. These data suggest strongly that there is a cured group of patients.

Roth and Bayat[6] conducted an autopsy study of patients with a history of breast cancer. Every patient with metastatic disease was found to have chest wall disease as well, generally not clinically apparent. Histologically, the chest wall disease appeared to be the result of direct extension and infiltration by the primary tumor, as opposed to hematogenous metastasis. Although this observation is consistent with several hypotheses, one of which is that these findings are mainly an indication of biologically aggressive cancer, an optimistic interpretation would be that complete eradication of the primary tumor is important in achieving a cure.

To call the radiotherapeutic management of locoregional breast cancer "conservative" is something of a misnomer. Such treatment is conservative only in that it aims to preserve a cosmetically intact breast. The goal of therapy is to eradicate all tumor cells in the treated region and ensure no recurrence, that is, in a very real sense to perform the equivalent of a "radical mastectomy," without surgical resection.

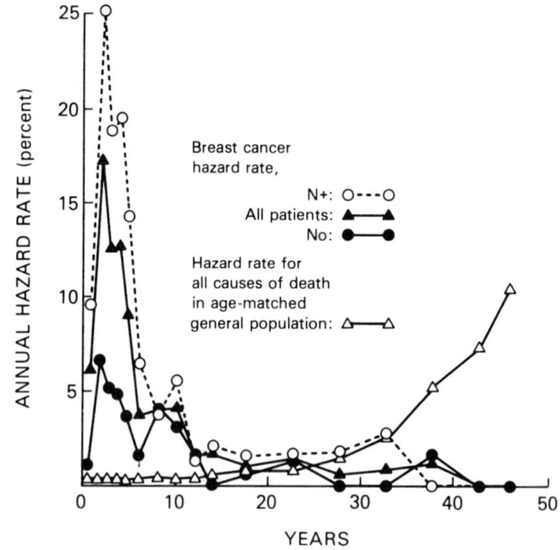

FIGURE 6–1. Long-term survival of young breast cancer patients. Annual breast cancer hazard rates of patients grouped by histologic status of axillary nodes and of all patients. Annual hazard rates for all causes of death in age-matched populations. (With permission from Rutqvist LE, Wallgren A: Long-term survival of 458 young breast cancer patients. Cancer 55:658, 1985.)

A truly meaningful assessment of breast cancer treatment must evaluate a number of factors. Survival rate is only one of several important end points. Local tumor control in the treated region, acute and chronic effects on normal tissue, the ability to integrate effectively local and systemic therapy, and the psychologic impact of treatment are all issues that should be considered.

EARLY RADIATION THERAPY EXPERIENCES

Geoffrey Keynes and Interstitial Radium

In the first two decades of the century, radiation therapy was used sporadically in the treatment of breast cancer, generally as a palliative measure in patients with inoperable disease and occasionally as definitive therapy in severely debilitated patients or those in whom local recurrences appeared after radical surgery. Only primitive external radiation equipment was available. In 1922, at St. Bartholomew's Hospital Geoffrey Keynes[7] began an investigation of treatment of carcinoma of the breast with radium needles, a venture suggested by G.E. Gask. Because the quantity of available radium was limited, Keynes decided to distribute it in platinum needles, which could be implanted directly into tissue. In order to reduce the damage to normal tissues, small amounts of radium were used in each needle and the time of administration of radiation was prolonged. From 1922 to 1924, seven patients were treated for recurrent chest wall disease after surgery. Six of the seven died within a short time; one was alive and well eight years after treatment. The experience with these patients demonstrated that nodules of recurrent tumor could be eradicated with radium, and Keynes decided to attempt treatment of primary tumors in the same way. From 1924 to 1927, he treated 50 patients with very advanced or inoperable tumors. Results in this group were so encouraging (6 of the 50 were alive ten years after treatment, and in many patients local tumor control and alleviation of symptoms were achieved) that he subsequently applied his treatment to patients with operable primary tumors.

Keynes's fully developed technique is illustrated in Figure 6–2. The entire breast area was treated, as were the axillary, supraclavicular, and internal mammary nodes. Although initially no surgery other than biopsy was performed, in later years he did incorporate local removal of large tumors. Needles were usually inserted with the patient under general anesthesia, were left in place for a period of about seven days, and were then removed with or without local anesthesia. Examples of the appearances of the breast before and after radium-needle treatment are shown in Figure 6–3.

In 1937, Keynes[8] published the survival rates of his treatment, with patients divided into three groups: Group I, disease clinically confined to the breast; Group II, disease clinically confined to the breast and axilla; and Group III, advanced or inoperable disease. By that time, he had treated a total of 325 patients, 250 of whom had been followed for a minimum of three years. For purposes of comparison, he included survival rates obtained from the University College Hospital for a similar number of patients treated with surgery alone. These results are shown

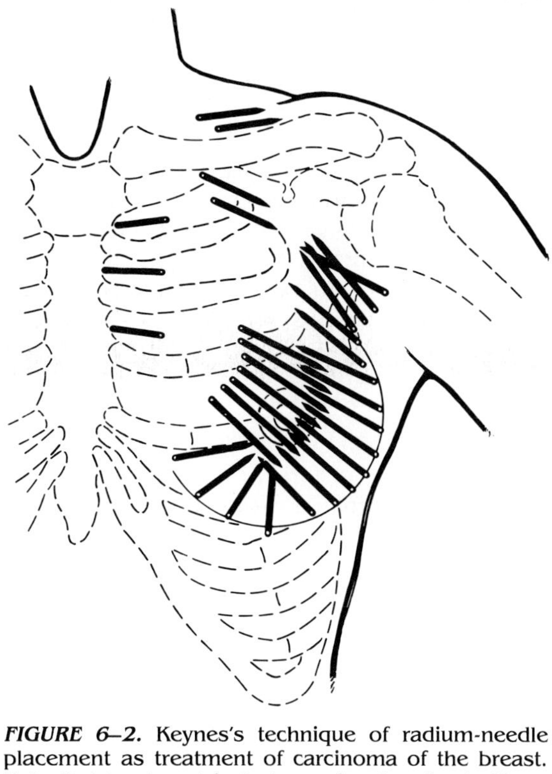

FIGURE 6–2. Keynes's technique of radium-needle placement as treatment of carcinoma of the breast. Note that treatment includes regional nodes (axillary, infraclavicular, supraclavicular, and internal mammary) in addition to the entire breast. (With permission from Keynes G: Conservative treatment of cancer of the breast. Br Med J, 1937, pp. 643–647.)

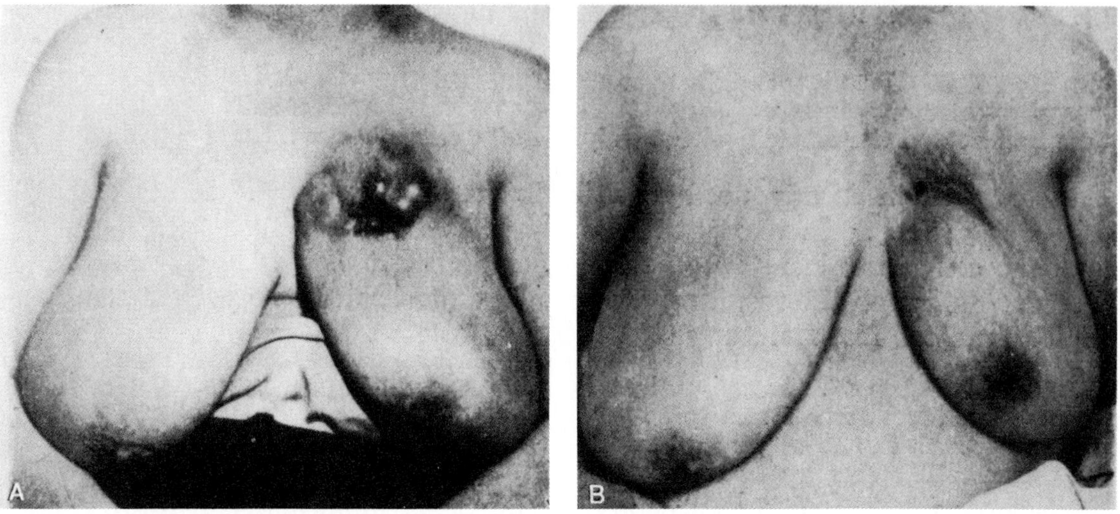

FIGURE 6–3. Cosmetic outcome of Keynes's radium-needle treatment. *A,* Pretreatment photograph. *B,* Sixteen months after treatment. (With permission from Keynes G: Conservative treatment of cancer of the breast. Br Med J, 1937, pp. 643–647.)

in Table 6–1. Certainly, the results of radium-needle treatment compare favorably with those of surgery. It should be noted that the surgical patients in Group I had *histologically* negative axillary nodes, whereas the Group I patients treated with radium needles had only *clinically* negative nodes. Despite publication of these results as well as lectures throughout Great Britain, Africa, and Canada and in New York City, Keynes's work was not favorably received. In 1939, with the coming of World War II, he was appointed as senior consultant to the Royal Air Force. His duties took him away from London, and the system of follow-up of his private patients irretrievably collapsed. Furthermore, the danger of enemy bombings during the war largely prevented the use of radium needles. In the late 1940's, Keynes abandoned further work in the treatment of breast cancer and turned his attention to the treatment of myasthenia gravis.[9]

TABLE 6–1. Results of Radium-Needle Treatment Compared with Results of Surgery

Group	3-Year Survival Rate (%)		5-Year Survival Rate (%)	
	RADIUM	SURGERY	RADIUM	SURGERY
I*	83.5	79.2	71.4	69.1
II†	51.2	52.3	29.3	30.5
III‡	31.4	—	23.6	—

*Disease clinically confined to the breast (85 radium patients).
†Disease clinically confined to the breast and axilla (91 radium patients).
‡Advanced or inoperable disease (74 radium patients)
Data from Keynes G: Conservative treatment of cancer of the breast. Br Med J, 1937, pp 643–647.

During this time, a few physicians, influenced by Keynes's reports, also applied radium to patients with breast cancer. In 1929, Roy Ward of the Radium Institute, London, published the results of radium treatment in 633 patients with primary inoperable or recurrent breast cancer.[10] For this group of patients, he claimed a 22 percent three-year and a 12 percent five-year survival rate and an improved quality of life, with healed ulcerations, pain relief, and reduced lymphedema in the majority of patients. Ward remarked on the radioresponsiveness of tumors, as related to their histologic type, with anaplastic or highly cellular tumors responding more rapidly than the scirrhous variety. He correlated some failures of radiation therapy with inadequate radiation dosage.

In 1930, G. Lenthal Cheatle,[11] a surgeon at King's College Hospital, London, published an account of his treatment philosophy and method, again similar to those of Keynes. Cheatle emphasized the importance of treating the entire breast to a sufficient dose and suggested that a lower dose over a longer period of time might be a technical improvement. He also suggested exploration of the use of external as well as interstitial radiation, stating that, "the final treatment by radiation will emerge as experience is gained by the use of external radiation alone, interstitial radiation alone, and by the combined use of external radiation and interstitial radiation."

External Beam Radiation Therapy—Baclesse, Mustakallio, and Peters

Over the next several decades, the use of radium needles as definitive management of breast cancer virtually disappeared. Physicians in a few centers maintained an interest in curative radiation management of the disease but applied external radiation rather than interstitial needles. A landmark paper was published in 1949 by François Baclesse of the Foundation Curie in Paris.[2] This paper describes the outcome of treatment in 130 patients with advanced breast cancer who received external radiation therapy. Patients were treated using a 180-kVp (orthovoltage) machine with a 1-mm copper filter, a source-to-skin distance (SSD) of 60 cm, and an intensity of 20 roentgen per minute. The average number of treatment fields per patient was six to seven, as is illustrated in Figure 6–4, and overlapping of fields was avoided. Two fields, and rarely three, were treated daily. Instead of giving the entire dose in one or a few treatments, Baclesse developed a technique of fractionation, administering small daily doses over a prolonged period to a greater total dose. Total dose increased directly with overall treatment time. He analyzed his results in terms of dose administered, treatment time, and clinical characterizations of the primary tumor. His results (Table 6–2) showed that higher doses given over protracted periods are more effective in obtaining tumor control than are lower rapidly administered doses and that even in this extremely unfavorable group of patients, permanent local tumor control can be achieved (Table 6–3). Baclesse noted complications in the "skin, subcutaneous tissues, muscles and nerves, bones (fractures), lungs, and heart," which varied according to dose and fields and which he ascribed to "obvious mistakes" and to high doses.

Beginning in the 1940's, Sakari Mustakallio[12] in Helsinki, Finland, began to treat patients with clinical Stage I breast cancer with conservative therapy. Clinical Stage I included cases in which the primary tumor was not fixed to the chest wall, had no satellite skin nodules or "striking" edema, and had clinically negative regional nodes. Tumor size was not considered. Treatment consisted of either local excision of the tumor or a segmental resection followed by postoperative irradiation. (Interestingly, Mustakallio remarks, "In the early days I often

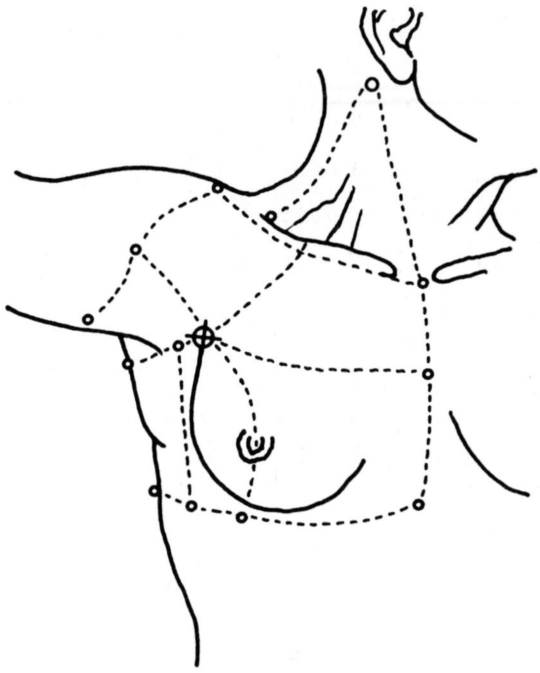

FIGURE 6–4. Orthovoltage treatment fields utilized by Baclesse. (With permission from Baclesse F: Roentgen therapy as the sole method of treatment of cancer of the breast. Am J Roentgenol Radium Ther Nucl Med 62:311, 1949.)

TABLE 6–2. Clinical Disappearance of Tumor at Least One Year after Treatment Compared with Breast Tumor Dose

*Dose**	*Patients Treated†*	*Patients with Tumor Control*	*Percentage (%)*
4100	4	3	75
4500–5000	15	2	13
6000–6800	31	21	68
7000–8000	32	22	69
9000	18	13	72
>9000	17	14	82

*Tumor dose evaluated at center of breast.

†Five cases with inflammatory carcinoma are included. Thirteen cases with distant metastasis or bilateral tumors are excluded.

Data from Baclesse F: Roentgen therapy as the sole method of treatment of cancer of the breast. Am J Roentgenol Radium Ther Nucl Med 62:311, 1949.

TABLE 6–3. Treatment Results by Clinical Stage of Primary Tumor

Characteristics of Primary Tumor	*No. of Patients*	*1 Year Clinically Well*	*3 Years Clinically Well*
4–6 cm; movable; ± skin/nipple involvement	33	27	22
>6 cm, ± fixation; ± skin invasion/edema/peau d'orange; ± skin nodules	42	25	8
Ulcerated tumor	28	15	7
Extensive; fixed; ± ulceration	9	7	2
Inflammatory	5	1	0
Distant metastases; extension to opposite breast	13	4	2
All patients	130	79	41

Data from Baclesse F: Roentgen therapy as the sole method of treatment of cancer of the breast. Am J Roentgenol Radium Ther Nucl Med 62:311, 1949.

removed the tumor myself.") Radiation therapy was administered with orthovoltage equipment of 180 to 250 kVp, with a 0.5-mm copper filter and an SSD of 40 to 50 cm. Five separate fields were used in the treatment of patients. The dose to each field was 2100 R to the skin, delivered in six doses of 350 R per dose. This regimen often produced a "fairly pronounced" skin reaction in the axilla and breast. An illustration of the treatment fields is provided in Figure 6–5. Seven hundred and two patients were followed for a minimum of five years. Mean age at diagnosis was 54 years (103 patients were aged 70 or older, and 20 patients were aged 80 or older). All deaths in the series were attributed to breast cancer. The absolute survival rate of the entire group was 79 percent at five years and 60 percent at ten years. The relative survival rate (observed survival divided by the estimated survival from the Finnish life tables) was 87 percent at five years and 72 percent at ten years. Comments on complications are absent. The description regarding cosmesis is "The normal shape of the breast is usually preserved." One hundred and two of the 418 patients surviving for ten or more years developed locoregional recurrences. Unfortunately, no breakdown of the site of local recurrence was provided.

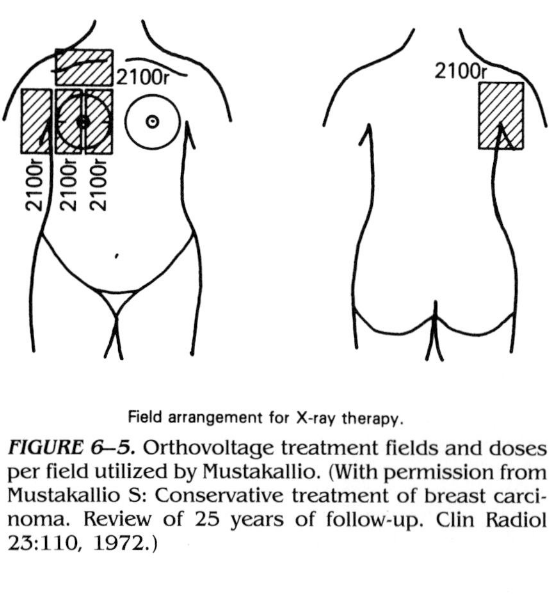

Field arrangement for X-ray therapy.

FIGURE 6–5. Orthovoltage treatment fields and doses per field utilized by Mustakallio. (With permission from Mustakallio S: Conservative treatment of breast carcinoma. Review of 25 years of follow-up. Clin Radiol 23:110, 1972.)

This paper is notable in a number of respects. Despite the inaccuracies of clinical staging in the assessment of axillary lymph node involvement and the lack of information on tumor size, the survival rates are quite good and appear to be comparable with those of radical surgery series. The radiation therapy was unsophisticated, the administered doses were relatively low, and homogeneity of dose distribution throughout the breast was lacking (each breast tangent field received a total of 2100 rad to the skin; therefore, the dose to the breast itself must have varied with individual patient size and configuration). Although at ten years nearly 25 percent of surviving patients had developed a locoregional recurrence, most locoregional recurrences appeared four years or longer after treatment, which suggests at least a delay in tumor growth in the treated area. Interestingly, there was no difference in the ten-year relative survival rate between the patients who developed local recurrence and either the entire group or those patients who did not develop local recurrence. The implication is that salvage therapy for local recurrence may be effective.

In 1975, M. Vera Peters[13] published a study done at the Princess Margaret Hospital in Toronto. She analyzed 217 patients with clinical Stage I breast cancer (T_1 to T_2, N_0, M_0) who had been treated with local excision of the primary tumor and radiation therapy from 1939 to 1969. All patients with these characteristics who were treated at the Princess Margaret Hospital during these years were included. Each patient was matched according to age, lump size, and year of treatment with a patient treated with radical or modified radical mastectomy and postoperative irradiation. The reasons given for the selection of patients for excision and radiation therapy included patient refusal of mastectomy as well as the surgeon's concern about infectious complications. A large proportion of this patient group were women whose advanced age and significant medical illnesses made them poor surgical candidates. In an attempt to eliminate a possible bias in treatment outcome due to associated medical illnesses, Peters analyzed survival data in two ways: (1) including all 217 excision and irradiation patients and their matched controls and (2) excluding all pairs of which either woman had died of a cause other than breast cancer in the first ten years after treatment. Pairs eliminated in this fashion numbered 72, leaving a study population of 145. Survival rates to 30 years are depicted in Figure 6–6*A* for the entire set of 217 pairs and in Figure 6–6*B* for the subpopulation of 145 pairs. Ten mastectomy patients developed a local recurrence, and all subsequently developed distant metastasis; 23 excision plus irradiation patients developed a local recurrence, of whom ten developed distant metastases but 13 remained free of disease for a subsequent 5 to 30 years following reexcision or mastectomy. Of note, the incidence of histologically positive nodes in the mastectomy patients was only 24 percent, a lower than expected percentage, implying a relatively favorable set of patients undergoing that treatment.

Peters expanded her analysis in a paper published in 1977.[14] Patients were included who had been seen from 1939 to 1972 with clinical T_1 to T_2, N_0, M_0 breast cancer. Patients undergoing excision (ranging from excisional biopsy to quadrantectomy) with or without postoperative radiation therapy were matched with patients undergoing mastectomy with or without postoperative radiation therapy. Patients were again matched according to age, size of the primary tumor, and year treated. Each excision patient was matched with three controls undergoing mastectomy only, and each excision plus irradiation patient was matched with three controls undergoing mastectomy with radiation therapy. A set of patients was eliminated from analysis if any patient of the set, regardless of her breast cancer treatment, died of intercurrent disease less than ten years after undergoing breast cancer therapy. Two hundred and three cases (19 excision and 184 excision plus irradiation) were compared with 609 controls (57 mastectomy and 552 mastectomy plus irradiation). Survival and

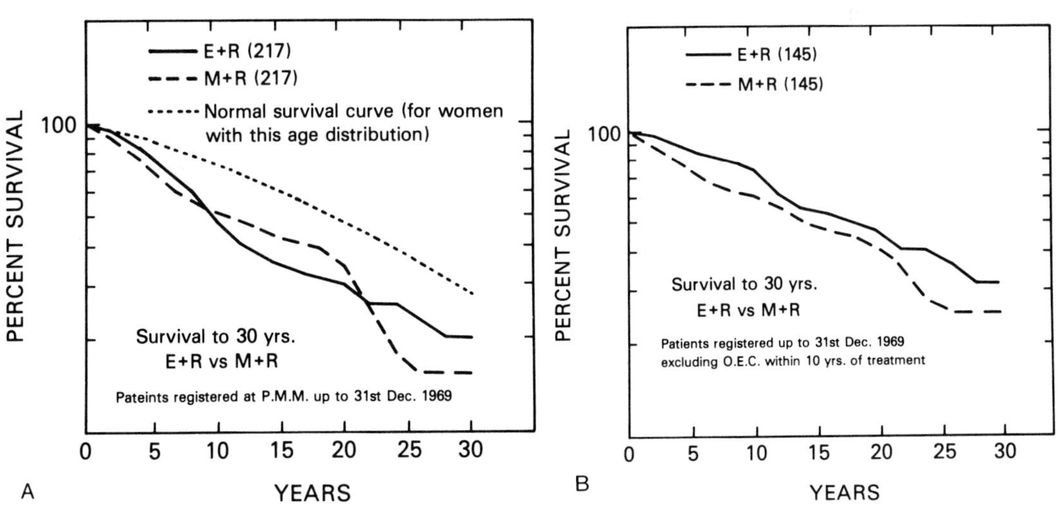

FIGURE 6–6. Survival of patients at the Princess Margaret Hospital. Each patient treated with excision and irradiation is matched with one patient treated with mastectomy and irradiation. *A*, Survival of all patients. *B*, Survival of patients, excluding pairs of patients with a member dying of causes other than breast cancer. (With permission from Peters MV: Cutting the "Gordian Knot" in early breast cancer. Ann R Coll Physicians Surg Can 8:186, 1975.)

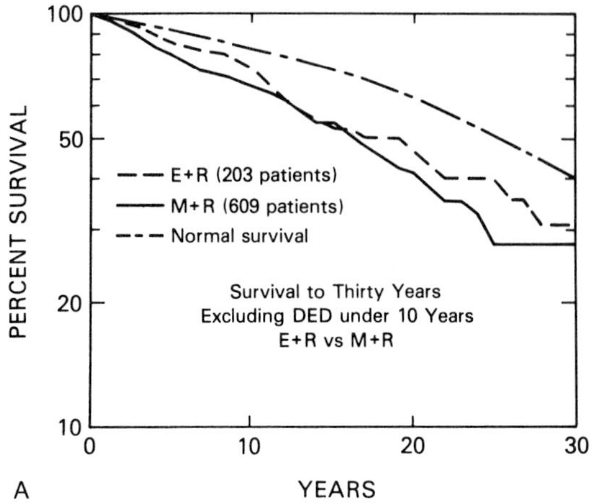

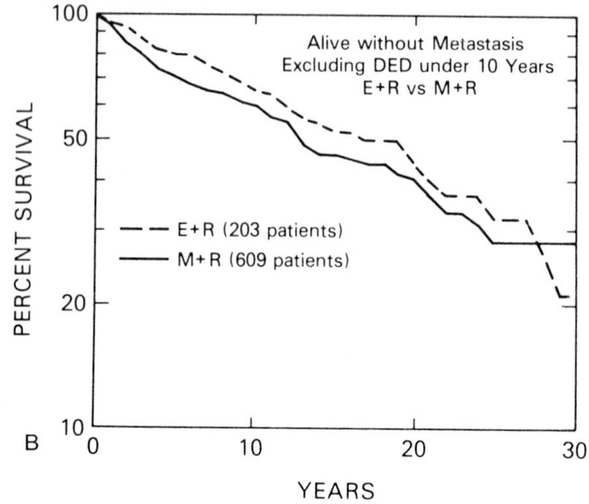

FIGURE 6–7. Survival of patients at the Princess Margaret Hospital. Each excision and irradiation patient is matched with three mastectomy and irradiation patients. *A,* Survival (normal survival for an age-matched population shown for comparison.) *B,* Survival without metastasis. Patients dying of causes other than breast cancer are excluded. (With permission from Peters MV: Wedge resection with or without radiation in early cancer. Int J Radiat Oncol Biol Phys 2:1151, 1977.)

disease-free survival rates are shown in Figure 6–7. Of interest, 17 excision patients developed breast cancer in the breast residuum and underwent reexcision or mastectomy. Seven of the 17 developed distant metastases, but 10 of 17 remained disease free after salvage treatment for five years or more. There was no difference in survival rate when the two groups were analyzed according to patient age or size of the primary tumor. (In T_2 patients, the survival rate to 20 years was consistently higher in the excision plus irradiation group, although this difference did not achieve statistical significance.) Although not a prospectively randomized study, analysis of potentially important prognostic indicators (tumor size, patient age, and infiltrating versus noninfiltrating histologic type) failed to reveal any significant difference between the two study groups, and patient numbers seemed to be sufficient so that unknown factors would be unlikely to bias the outcome.

RADIATION THERAPY IN THE ERA OF MEGAVOLTAGE EQUIPMENT—SINGLE-INSTITUTION EXPERIENCES

Since modern megavoltage equipment has become available, results from, initially, a number of French and Canadian institutions and, more recently, United States institutions have been reported on the outcome of more than 8000 patients with locoregional breast cancer treated with comprehensive radiation therapy without mastectomy. The following representative reports (Table 6–4) are discussed.

The French Experience—Institute Curie, Creteil, and Marseilles Cancer Institute

Calle and colleagues[15] have reported on the ten-year results in 606 patients treated from 1960 to 1971 at the Institute Curie. Patients were considered for treatment if the primary tumor was 7 cm or less in diameter, was not fixed to the chest wall, and was without peau d'orange, skin infiltration, or ulceration and if the axillary nodes were clinically negative or positive but movable (Fig. 6–8). If the tumor was larger than 3 cm in diameter or if the nodes were clinically positive, excision of the tumor was not performed. The ten-year absolute disease-free survival rate in patients undergoing lumpectomy and irradiation was 78 percent; 90 percent of these patients had their breasts preserved. Cosmetic results were excellent to good (no or minimal radiation fibrosis or skin telangiectasia) in 66 percent, good to fair (fibrosis or telangiectasia or both involving less than one third of the

TABLE 6–4. Results of Treatment of Locoregional Breast Cancer with Radiation Therapy Without Mastectomy

Institution	Clinical Stage	No. of Patients	Minimum Follow-up Time	5-Year Survival NED (%)	10-Year Survival NED (%)
Curie[15]	T_1N_0	87	10 years		84
	$T_2 \leq 3$ cm, N_0	56			68
	$T_2 > 3$ cm, N_0	178			66
	T_2N_1	89			42
	$T_3 \leq 7$ cm, N_0	95			39
	$T_3 \leq 7$ cm, N_1	101			25
Creteil[16]	T_1	99	5 years	84	65
	(N_0)	(95)			
	($N_1 < 2$ cm)	(4)			
	T_2	235		75	64
	(N_0)	(207)			
	($N_1 < 2$ cm)	(28)			
	$T_3 < 7$ cm	74		65	45
	(N_0)	(48)			
	($N_1 < 2$ cm)	(26)			
Marseilles[18]	T_1–T_2 N_0	895	5 years	79	72
	(*T_1N_0)	(309)		(92)	(81)
	(*T_2N_0)	(259)		(82)	(71)
	T_1–T_2 N_1	851		67	51
	(*T_1N_1)	(79)		(82)	(79)
	(*T_2N_1)	(133)		(74)	(61)
	$T_3 \leq 8$ cm, N_0–N_1	435		44	32
Princess Margaret Hospital[19]	All partial mastectomy and irradiation, N_0	800	5 years (median)	79†	62
	T_{IS}	10	(2 to 20 years)		
	T_1	249			
	T_2	149			
	T_3	6			
	T_4	10			
	Multifocal	6			
	Bilateral	7			
	T_x	363			
JCRT[21]	I (T_1N_0)	89	3.6 years (median) (2.7 to 13 years)	93†	(85‡)
	II	166		84†	(75‡)
	(T_1N_1)	(20)			
	(T_2N_0)	(105)			
	(T_2N_1)	(41)			
M. D. Anderson Hospital[22]	I (T_1N_0)	134	3 years	85	78
	II (T_1N_1, T_1–T_2, N_0)	157		78	73
Univ. of PA[23]	I, II	196	2 years		
	(T_1 path N_0)			86§	
	(T_1 path N_1, T_2 path N_0–N_1)			69§	
Yale[24]	I (T_1N_0)	110	3 years (3 to 23 years)	88	
	II	69		66	
	(T_2N_0)	(57)			
	(T_1–T_2, N_1)	(12)			

*Tumor excision prior to radiation.
†Actuarial overall.
‡Actuarial freedom from distant relapse.
§Four-year actuarial survival.

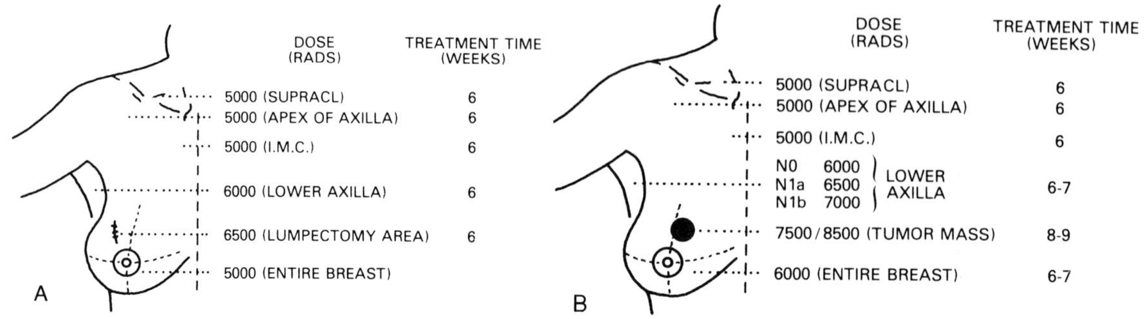

FIGURE 6–8. Treatment fields and doses used at the Institute Curie. *A,* Radiation doses given to patients treated with lumpectomy followed by radiation therapy. *B,* Radical radiation therapy alone (without lumpectomy). (With permission from Calle R, Pilleron JP, Schlienger P, et al.: Conservative management of operable breast cancer: Ten years experience at the Foundation Curie. Cancer 42:2047, 1978.)

breast, without significant distortion) in 29 percent, and poor (fibrosis or telangiectasia or both involving more than half of the circumference of the breast) in 4 percent. One of the 111 patients had a significant irradiation complication (brachial nerve paralysis). Of the 463 patients treated exclusively with irradiation, absolute disease-free survival at ten years was 47 percent. Fifty-three of these patients had breasts preserved. Cosmesis was excellent to good in 41 percent, good to fair in 44 percent, and poor in 15 percent. Six patients had severe radiation sequelae (unspecified). At a minimum follow-up time of ten years, 20 of 143 patients (14 percent) treated with lumpectomy with irradiation had developed locally recurrent disease (18, in the breast, and 2, in the axilla). Eighteen of the 20 underwent salvage surgery; 13 of these 18 were alive without evidence of disease at a minimum of four years following salvage treatment.

Between 1961 and 1982, more than 900 patients were treated with radiation therapy at Creteil.[16, 17] Four hundred and eight of these patients have been followed for a minimum of five years, and 126 patients, for a minimum of ten years. Patients in the treatment schema had single primary breast tumors up to 7 cm in diameter, clinically negative axillary nodes or positive nodes less than 2 cm in diameter, and no evidence of distant metastasis. The treatment schema is shown in Figure 6–9. Five- and ten-year disease-free survival rates for T_1 tumors were 84 percent and 65 percent; for T_2 tumors, 75 percent and 64 percent; and for limited T_3 tumors, 65 percent and 45 percent, respectively. Cosmesis was "very good" (no or very minimal sequelae) in 87 percent of T_1, 54 percent of T_2, and 40 percent of T_3 lesions; "quite good" (obvious sequelae but preferable to mastectomy) in 12 percent of T_1, 39 percent of T_2, and 45 percent of T_3 lesions; and poor (initial surgery would have been preferable) in 1 percent of T_1, 7 percent of T_2, and 15 percent of T_3 lesions. Complications of therapy included pain in the breast or chest wall in 5 percent, mild limitation of shoulder movement in 5 to 10 percent, arm edema in 5 percent, and radiation-induced breast necrosis in one case.

From 1960 to 1981, 3786 patients with operable breast cancer underwent breast-conserving therapy at the Marseilles Cancer Institute.[18] Two thousand two hundred sixteen were followed for a minimum of five years, and 704, for a minimum of ten years. Patients included had tumors up to 8 cm in diameter (T_1, T_2, and limited T_3), clinically negative or positive but movable axillary nodes (N_0, N_1),

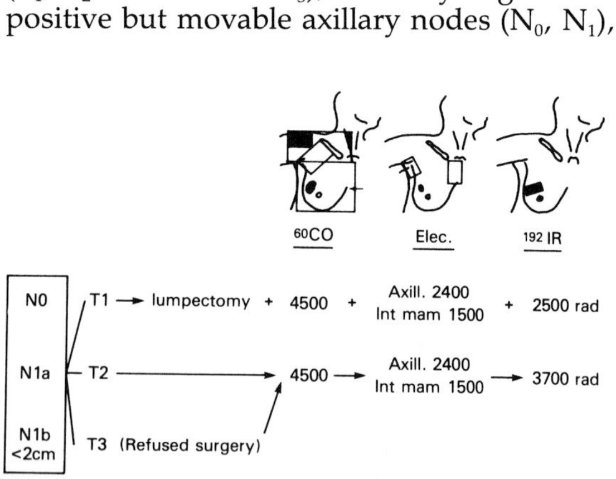

FIGURE 6–9. Treatment schema used at Creteil according to clinical stage. (With permission from Pierquin B: Conservative treatment for carcinoma of the breast: Experience of Creteil. *In* Harris JR, Hellman S, Silen W (eds.): Conservative Management of Breast Cancer. Philadelphia: J. B. Lippincott, 1983.)

and no distant metastasis. The treatment schema was predicated upon clinical stage (Table 6–5). Tumors less than 5 cm in diameter with no or minimal adenopathy and no clinical signs of rapid growth were excised prior to radiation therapy. Before 1970, this was done as a simple excision, but since that time, the group utilized wedge resection that included the tumor with a margin of normal tissue. Subsequent to 1975, this tumor excision was accompanied by a limited dissection of the lower and middle axillary nodes. All other tumors received irradiation alone without prior tumor excision. The breast and axilla were treated with a cesium unit or cobalt 60 with a dose of 5000 to 6000 rad over five weeks, and internal mammary and supraclavicular nodes were treated to a dose of 4000 to 5000 rad over five weeks. The tumor bed was boosted to a total of 7500 rad in patients who had had prior excision and 8000 rad in those without prior excision. Positive axillae were boosted to a total dose of 7000 rad. A minority of patients received a short course of perioperative chemotherapy, and selected premenopausal patients with adverse prognostic indicators underwent prophylactic oophorectomy. Five- and 10-year survival rates for T_1 to T_2, N_0 patients were 79 percent and 72 percent; for T_1 to T_2, N_1 patients, 67 percent and 51 percent; and for limited T_3, N_0 to N_1 patients, 44 percent and 32 percent, respectively. Eight percent of patients undergoing limited surgery prior to breast irradiation had locoregional failures at ten years in the breast only; 4 percent, in the breast and axilla; and 2 percent, in the axilla only. The ten-year locoregional failure rate for patients without prior tumor excision was 38 percent. Among the 704 patients followed for ten years, 227 had locoregional persistence or recurrence, especially those with T_3 tumors treated with radiation therapy alone. One fifth of these recurrences were inoperable because of either extensive local disease or distant metastasis. Salvage surgery was performed on 179 patients; an additional 56 patients had a surgical procedure with negative pathologic findings for cancer. The five-year survival rate after salvage treatment for histologically positive locoregional recurrence was 5 percent. Complications included extensive fibrosis (5 percent), mild arm edema (5 percent), severe arm edema (1 percent), shoulder stiffness (1 percent), and brachial plexus injury (1 percent).

TABLE 6–5. Marseilles Cancer Institute Treatment Schema

STAGE OF DISEASE	PROCEDURE
Surgery	
T_1–T_2, N_0, M_0 rapid growth, M_0	Tumor excision Limited axillary dissection (after 1975)
All other T/N, M_0	Incisional or needle biopsy of primary tumor
Radiation	
Breast and axilla	5000–6000 rad/5 weeks
Internal mammary nodes	4000–5000 rad/5 weeks
Supraclavicular nodes	4000–5000 rad/5 weeks
Axilla, boost to	7000 rad (positive nodes only)
Tumor bed, boost to	7500 rad (prior excision) 8000 rad (no prior excision)

Data from Amalric R, Santamaria F, Robert F, et al.: Conservative therapy of operable breast cancer—results at five, ten, and fifteen years in 2216 consecutive cases. *In*: Harris JR, Hellman S, Silen W (eds.): Conservative Management of Breast Cancer. New Surgical and Radiotherapeutic Techniques. Philadelphia: J. B. Lippincott, 1983.

The North American Experience—Princess Margaret Hospital, Harvard, M.D. Anderson Memorial Hospital, University of Pennsylvania, and Yale

Clark[19] has reported on the treatment of 800 patients referred to the Princess Margaret Hospital between January 1958 and March 1980. All patients had undergone partial mastectomy, ranging from excisional biopsy to segmental resection, and had clinically negative axillae. Radiation therapy was administered with cobalt 60; the dose was 4000 rad in 16 fractions over three weeks. Thirty-four percent of patients underwent a 500-rad boost to the primary site with cobalt 60 or orthovoltage. The various treatment fields utilized in the patient population are tabulated in Table 6–6. Patients who received excision without postoperative irradiation tended to have smaller tumors (T_1) than did the population as a whole. The breast relapse rate was affected by the volume irradiated; axillary relapse was small in all groups. The actuarial survival rate of the entire group was 79 percent at five years and 52 percent at 10 years. When the survival rate was analyzed

TABLE 6–6. Princess Margaret Hospital—Treatment Groups by Volume Irradiated

None	177 (22%)
Breast only	252 (32%)
Breast and all regional nodes	248 (31%)
Breast and limited regional nodes	105 (13%)
Some nodes ± breast	18 (2%)

Data from Clark RM: Alternatives to mastectomy—The Princess Margaret Hospital experience. *In*: Harris JR, Hellman S, Silen W (eds.): Conservative Management of Breast Cancer. New Surgical and Radiotherapeutic Techniques. Philadelphia: J. B. Lippincott, 1983.

with regard to presence and site of relapse, there was a definite decrement in survival with relapse in the breast only (Fig. 6–10). This effect was seen only after five years of follow-up. This observation is consistent with the hypothesis that local control in the primary site is important for patient survival and suggests that initial treatment should aim to achieve complete tumor eradication. Although no details are given, Clark reports that overall cosmetic results were usually excellent and that there were no major complications.

Increasing numbers of women in the United States have undergone primary irradiation as management for breast cancer. Initial reports from this country included small numbers of patients. In 1977, physicians from four institutions (Yale, Harvard, Hahnemann, and Jefferson) reported on the results in 150 patients pooled from these institutions.[20] All patients had invasive carcinoma, clinical Stages I and II. One hundred and forty-five patients underwent excisional biopsy, and five had needle biopsy of the primary tumor only. Patients had been referred for radiation therapy for various reasons, initially because of medical contraindications to surgery, but later because of patient refusal to undergo mastectomy. Irradiation techniques were similar in the four institutions and were based on guidelines outlined by Fletcher. Only megavoltage equipment was used (cobalt 60, 4-MeV, and 6-MeV linear accelerators). The entire breast and lymph node–draining areas were encompassed in the treated volume. Breast and ipsilateral internal mammary lymph nodes were covered in tangential fields, and the supraclavicular and axillary nodes were treated in a direct *en face* field, sometimes supplemented by irradiation of a posterior axillary field. Occasionally, because of individual anatomy, a separate internal mam-

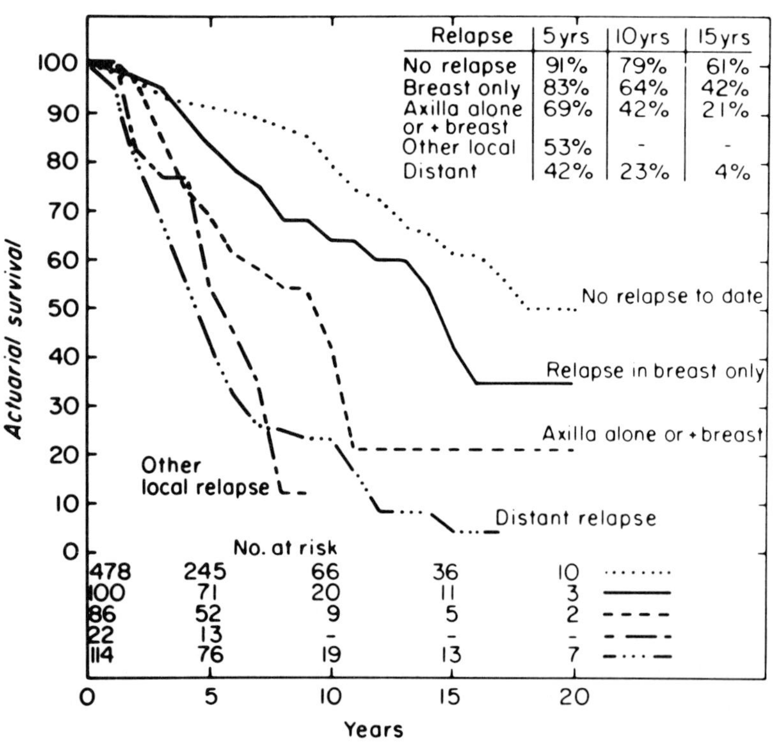

FIGURE 6–10. Comparison of survival based on diagnosis of patients with no relapse, with relapse in breast only, with relapse in axilla alone or with breast, with other local relapse, and with distant relapse in Princess Margaret Hospital series. No relapse versus breast relapse p = 0.042; breast relapse versus axillary relapse p = 0.012. (With permission from Clark RM: Alternatives to mastectomy—The Princess Margaret Hospital experience. *In*: Harris JR, Hellman S, Silen W (eds.): Conservative Management of Breast Cancer. Philadelphia: J. B. Lippincott, 1983.)

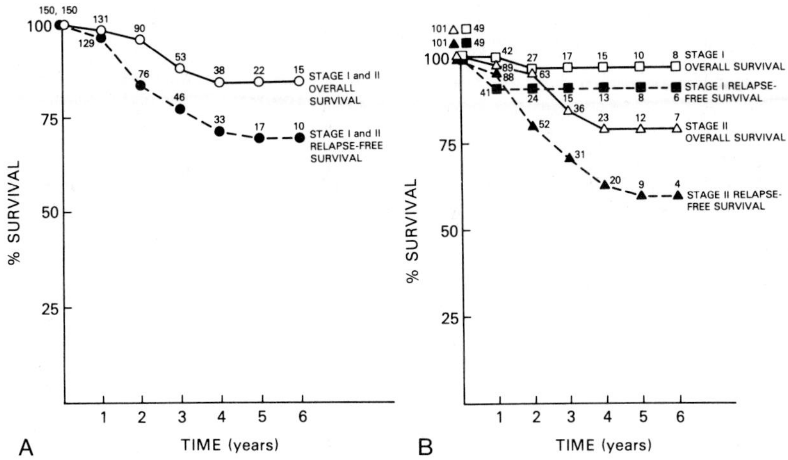

FIGURE 6–11. Cumulative overall survival and relapse-free survival of patients treated with breast-conserving radiation therapy. *A,* All patients combined. *B,* Patients separated by clinical stage. (With permission from Prosnitz LR, et al.: Radiation therapy as initial treatment for early stage cancer of the breast without mastectomy. Cancer 39:917, 1977.)

mary field matched to the tangents was employed to cover these lymph nodes. The breast and node areas received a total dose of 4400 to 5000 rad, generally at a rate of 1000 rad per week. In some patients, the excisional biopsy site was given an additional 1000 to 2000 rad by either continued external beam therapy or an interstitial implant. Clinically involved lymph nodes in the axilla were boosted with an external beam. Actuarial survival and relapse-free survival rates by stage are shown in Figure 6–11. Ten patients developed a recurrence of tumor within the irradiated volume, five of whom then underwent mastectomy. Complications included non–steroid-requiring pneumonitis (2 percent), rib fracture (2 percent), arm edema (less than 1 percent), skin ulceration (less than 1 percent), and pleural effusion (less than 1 percent). The cosmetic appearance was reported to be "quite satisfactory," although the investigators comment that overweight women with large, pendulous breasts tended to have a less satisfactory cosmetic result.

In the years following, larger numbers of patients were treated in these and other United States institutions, and reports from those most active in this type of treatment are summarized later. Selection of patients tended to follow the same pattern, that is, patients treated in the earlier years generally came for radiation therapy because of medical contraindications to surgery, while patients treated in the later years had refused mastectomy. Most recently, patients have chosen this treatment after it had been offered initially as an alternative to breast amputation.

At the Harvard Joint Center for Radiation Therapy between 1968 and 1978, 255 women with clinical Stages I and II breast cancer underwent primary radiation therapy.[21] The median follow-up time for the group was 44 months. Eleven patients had bilateral breast cancer; therefore, a total of 266 breasts were treated. In 22 cases, needle or incisional biopsy was performed, and in the remainder, at least an excisional biopsy was performed. Radiation therapy was given with a 4-MeV linear accelerator. The breast and ipsilateral internal mammary nodes were irradiated in opposed tangential fields, and the axillary and supraclavicular nodes were treated using a direct *en face* anterior field occasionally supplemented with a posterior axillary boost field. Treatment was given at a rate of 900 to 1000 rad per week, in five-week treatments, to a total of 4400 to 5000 rad. Some patients received an additional boost to the tumor bed of 1500 to 2500 rad with implant or external beam, particularly when the margins of resection were felt to be close. The actuarial five-year survival rate was 93 percent for Stage I and 84 percent for Stage II patients; the five-year actuarial distant disease–free survival rate was 85 percent for Stage I and 75 percent for Stage II; and the five-year actuarial probability of local control was 97 percent for Stage I and 87 percent for Stage II. These results are shown graphically in Figure 6–12. Major complications developed in 2 percent of patients (arm edema, three patients; arm weakness, one; radiation pericarditis, one; soft-tissue necrosis, one; and acute leukemia, one); and transient or mild complications appeared in 12 percent of patients (rib fractures, fourteen patients; arm

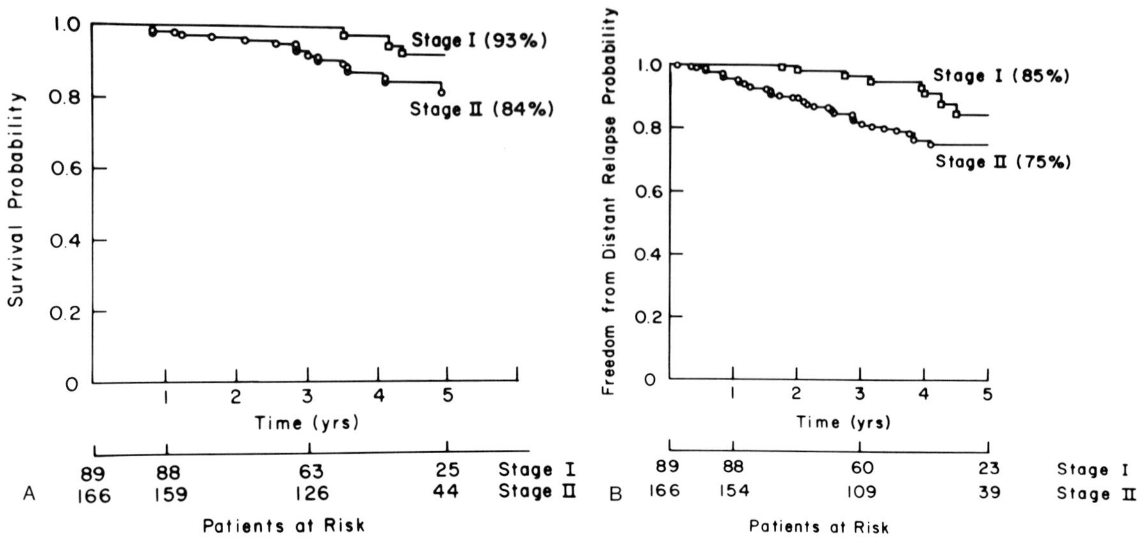

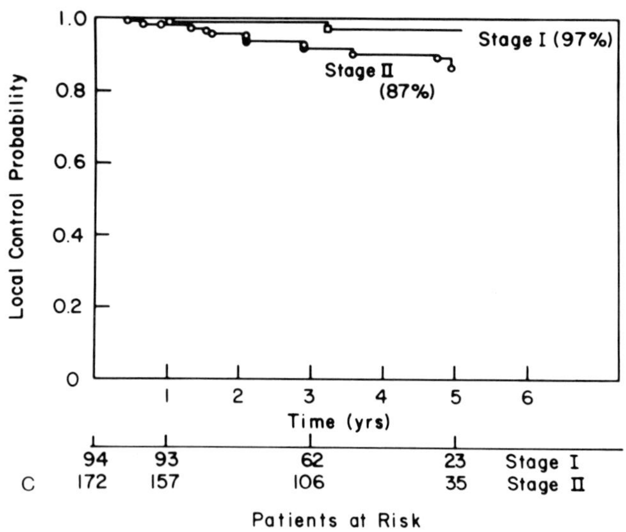

FIGURE 6–12. Patients treated at the Joint Center for Radiation Therapy. *A,* Actuarial survival. *B,* Actuarial distant disease–free survival. C, Local recurrence. (With permission from Harris JR, Hellman S: The results of primary radiation therapy for early breast cancer at the Joint Center for Radiation Therapy. *In*: Harris JR, Hellman S, Silen W (eds.): Conservative Management of Breast Cancer. Philadelphia: J. B. Lippincott, 1983.)

edema, ten; radiation pneumonitis, five; and paresthesia, one).

Montague[22] has reported on results of conservative surgery and radiation therapy in 345 patients treated at the M. D. Anderson Memorial Hospital between 1955 and 1980. Prior to 1974, conservative surgery consisted of gross tumor excision only. Since that time, the treatment policy has been excision of the primary tumor with a rim of normal tissue ("segmental mastectomy") and dissection of the lateral axilla. This surgery was followed by irradiation of the breast and node-draining regions. Using cobalt 60, the breast was irradiated in opposing tangential fields; the axillary supraclavicular nodes, in a direct *en face* field and a supplemental posterior axillary field; and the ipsilateral internal mammary nodes, in a straight-on field using a mixture of photons and electrons. The total dose to these regions was 4500 to 5000 rad at a rate of 1000 rad per week. The tumor was boosted with an additional 1000 rad over five days using electrons or with 1500 to 2000 rad (in patients with unknown or positive margins of resection) with an interstitial implant. Actuarial disease-free survival rates at five and ten years were 85 percent and 78 percent, respectively, in Stage I and 78 percent and 73 percent, respectively, in Stage II. These disease-free survival rates, when retrospectively compared with those of patients undergoing radical or modified radical mastectomy alone at the same institution, appear to be comparable (Table 6–7), although selection bias could be influencing these results. Eighteen patients developed local recurrences, 16 patients, in the breast alone, and

TABLE 6–7. Disease-Free Survival: Mastectomy versus Radiation Therapy for Breast Cancer (M. D. Anderson Memorial Hospital)

Stage	Radiation* No. of Patients	Radiation* 5-Year Survival	Radiation* 10-Year Survival	Mastectomy No. of Patients	Mastectomy 5-Year Survival	Mastectomy 10-Year Survival
I (T_1, N_0)	134	85%	78%	224	88%	80%
II (T_1, N_1, T_2, N_0–N_1)	157	78%	73%	370	77%	65%

*Prior to 1974, all radiation patients had only clinical evaluation of the axilla.

Data from Montague ED: Conservative surgery and radiation therapy in the treatment of operable breast cancer. Cancer 53:700, 1984.

2 patients, in the breast and axilla. Complications included symptomatic pneumonitis in 7 percent, rib fracture in 1.5 percent, severe matchline fibrosis in 14 percent, brachial plexopathy in 1 percent, arm edema in 7 percent, and breast edema in 22 percent. Cosmesis was reported to be "good" in about 75 percent of patients at five years.

The University of Pennsylvania group has reported on 196 patients treated with excisional biopsy, axillary dissection, and radiation therapy from 1977 to 1982.[23] One hundred and fourteen had T_1, and 82 had T_2 tumors; lymph nodes were histologically negative in 143 patients and histologically positive in 53 patients. The median follow-up time was 24 months. Radiation therapy consisted of megavoltage irradiation to 4600 to 5000 rad to the breast and draining lymph nodes over 4.5 to 5 weeks, with a boost to the primary site of 1500 to 2000 rad with electrons or an interstitial implant. Patients with histologically negative nodes had only the breast irradiated. Forty-six of 53 patients with histologically positive nodes received adjuvant chemotherapy. The four-year actuarial disease-free survival rate in pathologic Stage I patients (T_1, pathologic N_0) was 86 percent, and in pathologic Stage II patients (T_1, pathologic N_1; T_2 pathologic N_0 or N_1) was 69 percent. The four-year actuarial locoregional recurrence rate was five percent. Complications included arm edema (6 percent), symptomatic pneumonitis (1 percent), rib fracture (1 percent), pericarditis (1 percent), and pleural effusion (1 percent). Cosmetic outcome was judged to be good to excellent in 90 percent of the patients treated.

From 1960 to 1980, 179 patients with clinical Stage I or II breast cancer were treated at Yale University.[24] Excisional biopsy was performed on all but five patients; 20 patients also underwent surgical staging of the axilla. Radiation was administered with a 6-MV linear accelerator. The breast was treated in opposed tangential fields; node-draining areas (axillary, supraclavicular, and ipsilateral internal mammary nodes) were treated in separate anterior *en face* fields. The breast and nodal regions received 4500 to 5000 rad over 4.5 to 5 weeks. Following this, a boost of 1500 to 2000 rad was given to the primary tumor area with either electrons or an iridium-192 implant. The actuarial disease-free survival of 110 Stage I patients was 88 percent and of 69 Stage II patients was 66 percent. Local recurrence was seen in 15 patients (8 percent). Complications included radiation pneumonitis in five patients, pericarditis in one patient, arm edema in two patients, limitation of arm motion in two patients, and brachial plexopathy in one patient. Cosmesis was evaluated in 161 patients and was judged to be good to excellent in 90 percent.

Reports such as these describing the treatment of operable breast cancer with radiation therapy provide evidence that modern techniques of limited surgery and comprehensive irradiation can offer patients a sound alternative to mastectomy. However, the inherent difficulty with all retrospective series is the issue of patient selection. For example, inclusion of patients with favorable disease (who are genetically predisposed to fare well in the tumor-host interaction) can lead to erroneous conclusions regarding the effectiveness of a given treatment. Thus, randomized prospective trials have been necessary to evaluate alternative therapies as rigorously as possible.

PROSPECTIVE RANDOMIZED STUDIES

A number of studies are now available that compare the efficacy of treatments incorporating breast amputation with therapy that conserves the breast.

Guy's Hospital Trials

Since 1960, two randomized prospective trials have been conducted at Guy's Hospital in London.[25] The first study (Guy's I) was conducted between 1961 and 1971. Patients aged 50 and over with operable breast cancer (T_1 to T_{3a}, N_0 to N_1, M_0) were eligible and were randomly treated with either wide local excision or radical mastectomy, both followed with radiation therapy. The surgical procedure for wide excision patients was removal of the lump and 3 cm of surrounding clinically normal breast tissue in all directions; no axillary surgery was permitted. Mastectomy patients underwent complete breast removal with full axillary clearance, including removal of the pectoralis minor muscle and that part of the pectoralis major muscle beneath the primary tumor. Radiation therapy consisted of treatment of the axilla and supraclavicular and ipsilateral internal mammary nodes in all patients, using a 300 kVp orthovoltage unit and administering a total dose of 2500 to 2700 rad, even to those patients with clinically positive axillae. Mastectomy patients received this dose over a period of 18 days, and wide excision patients, over a period of 12 days. The wide excision patients also received breast irradiation with a 6-MV linear accelerator delivering 3500 to 3800 rad over three weeks, with bolus used to eliminate skin sparing of the megavoltage machine. This schema is outlined in Figure 6–13. Three hundred and seventy-six patients were entered into this trial.

Between 1971 and 1975, a second study was performed. In this series, only patients with clinically negative axillae were included, but patients of any age were eligible. The treatments compared were exactly the same as those administered in the first trial (Fig. 6–13). Two hundred and fifty-two patients were entered in the second study. Local recurrence was defined as the development of tumor within an area bounded by the midline medially, the clavicle superiorly, the posterior axillary line laterally, and the costal margin inferiorly. Recurrences in the ipsilateral supraclavicular fossa (in the skin or subcutaneous tissues, lymph nodes, or retained breast in wide excision patients) were considered to be local, whether the recurrence appeared alone or as a part of disseminated disease. Published results of the first trial with a minimum follow-up time of 11 years and of the second trial with a minimum follow-up time of seven years are available.

Results from the Guy's I trial have been analyzed according to clinical node status. For patients with Stage I disease (clinically negative nodes), overall survival, local recurrence, and distant recurrence are shown in Figure 6–14. In these patients, there is no difference between the two treatments in terms of either survival or distant disease–free survival rates, although the incidence of local recurrence in patients undergoing wide excision was high. Survival, distant disease–free survival, and local recurrence rates for patients with clinically positive nodes are shown in Figure 6–15. In this group, there is a statistically significant difference in both survival and local recurrence rates, but contrary to what one would expect, there is no difference in distant recurrence rates between the two treatments. Results in patients from the second series, all of whom had clinically negative nodes, in terms of survival, local recurrence, and distant recurrence rates are shown in Figure 6–16. These results demonstrate a statistically significant

Schema: Guy's Hospital Randomized Trials

<u>Guy's I</u>

T_{1-3}, N_{0-1}, M_0
Age ≥ 50 y.

<u>Guy's II</u>

T_{1-3}, N_0, M_0
Any Age

RANDOMIZE

Radical Mastectomy + Nodal Radiation
2500-2700r/18d
300 KVP

Wide Excision + Breast Irradiation + Nodal Irradiation
(Tumor + 3cm) 3500-3800r/3 wk 2500-2700r/12d
6 MV/Bolus 300 KVP

FIGURE 6–13. Schema—Guy's Hospital randomized trials.

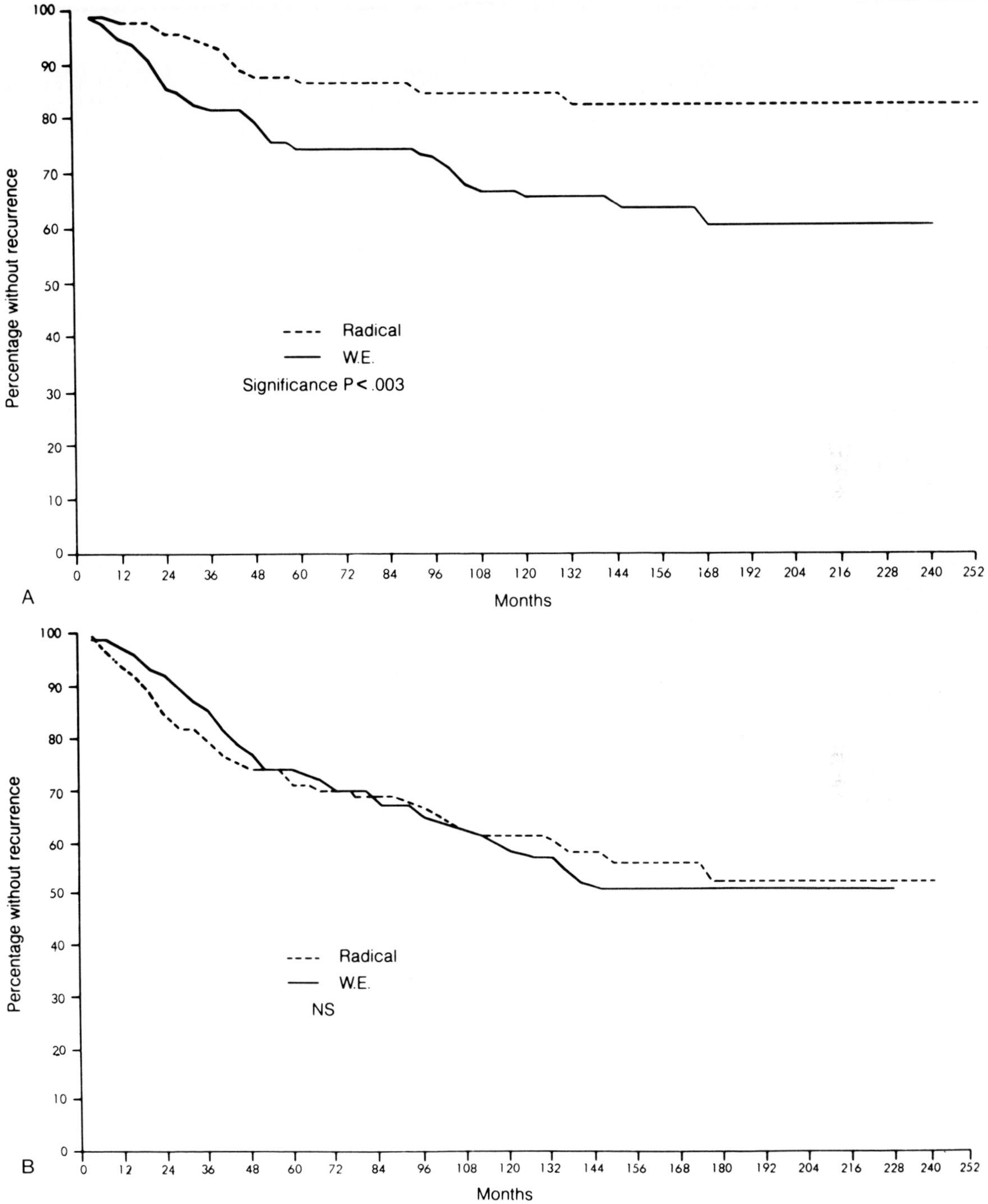

FIGURE 6–14. Guy's Hospital Trial I, Stage I patients—wide excision versus radical mastectomy. *A,* Local recurrence. *B,* Distant recurrence.

Illustration continued on following page

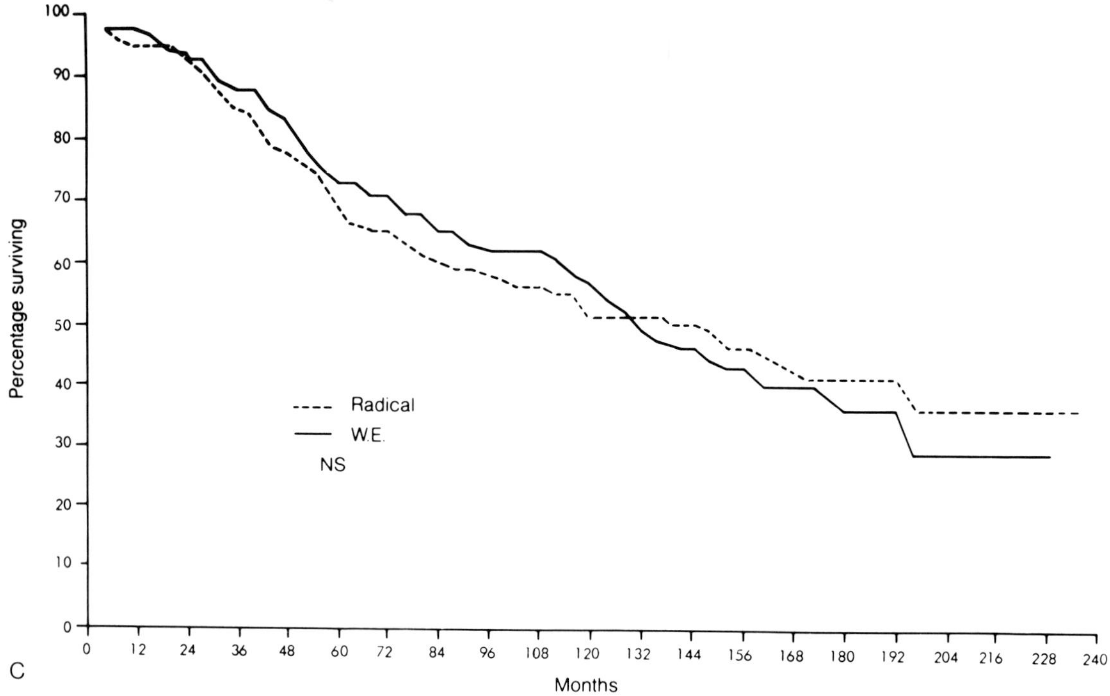

FIGURE 6–14 Continued. *C,* Survival. (With permission from Hayward J: The Guy's Hospital trials on breast conservation. *In*: Harris JR, Hellman S, Silen W (eds.): Conservative Management of Breast Cancer. Philadelphia: J. B. Lippincott, 1983.)

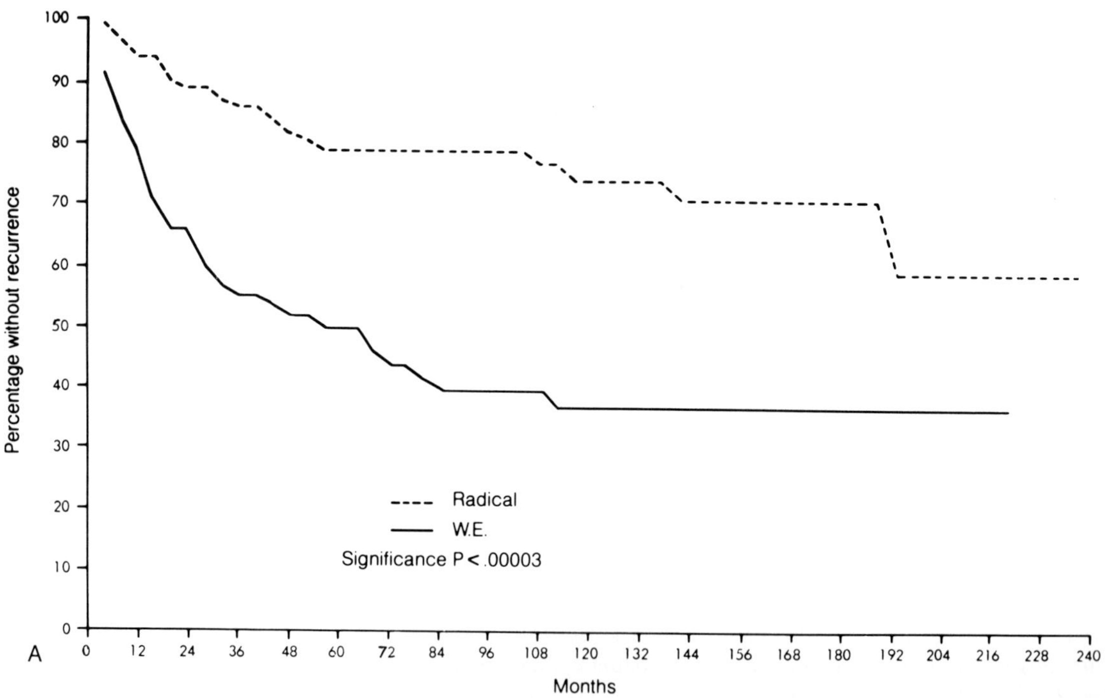

FIGURE 6–15. Guy's Hospital Trial I, Stage II patients—wide excision versus radical mastectomy. *A,* Local recurrence.

Illustration continued on opposite page

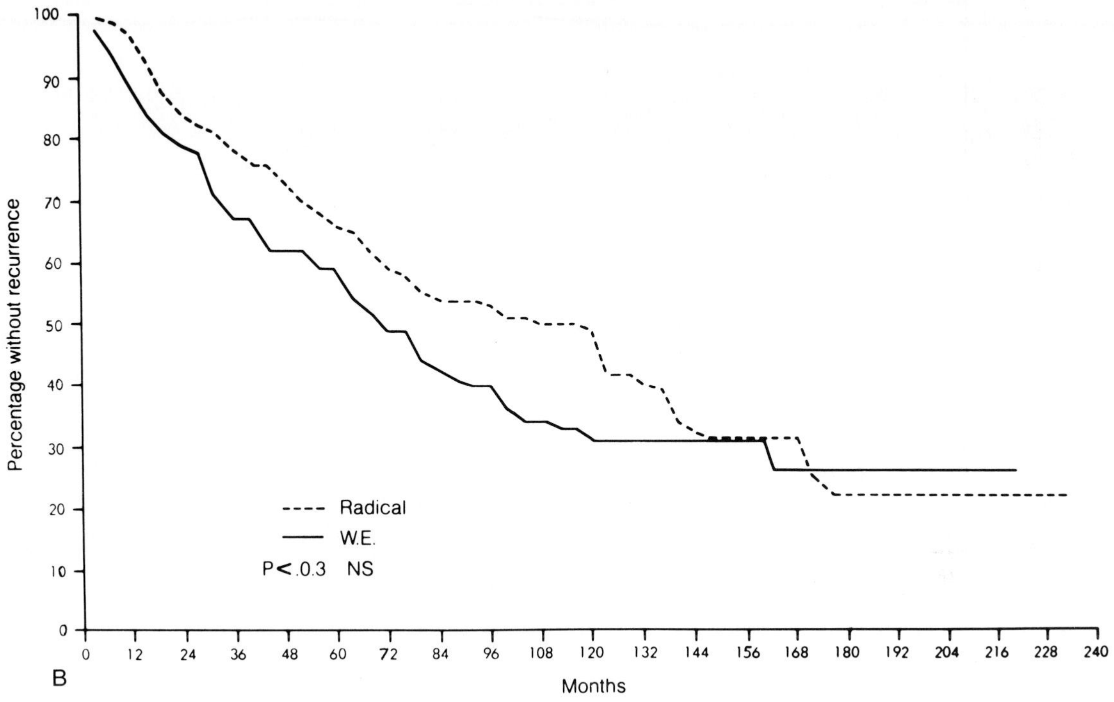

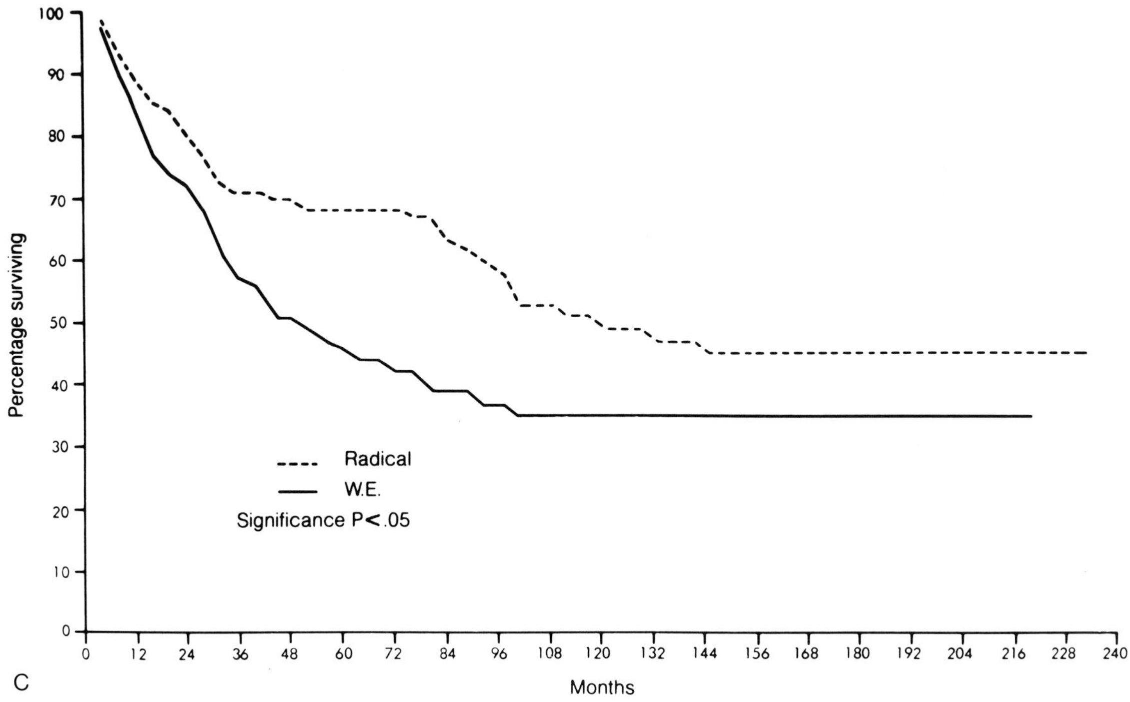

FIGURE 6–15 *Continued. B,* Distant recurrence. *C,* Survival. (With permission from Hayward J: The Guy's Hospital trials on breast conservation. *In*: Harris JR, Hellman S, Silen W (eds.): Conservative Management of Breast Cancer. Philadelphia: J. B. Lippincott, 1983.)

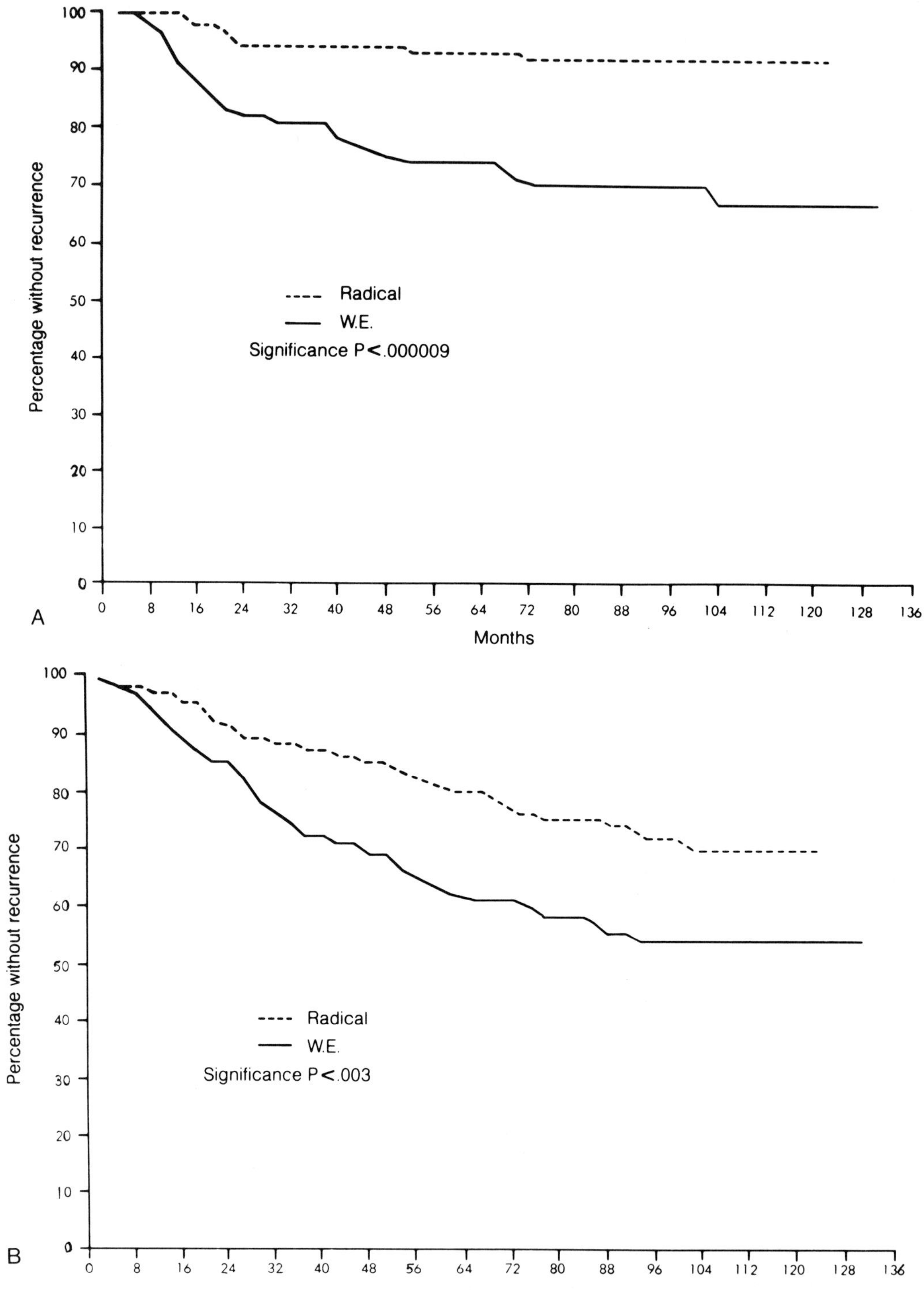

FIGURE 6–16. Guy's Hospital Trial II, Stage I patients—wide excision versus radical mastectomy. *A,* Local recurrence. *B,* Distant recurrence.

Illustration continued on opposite page

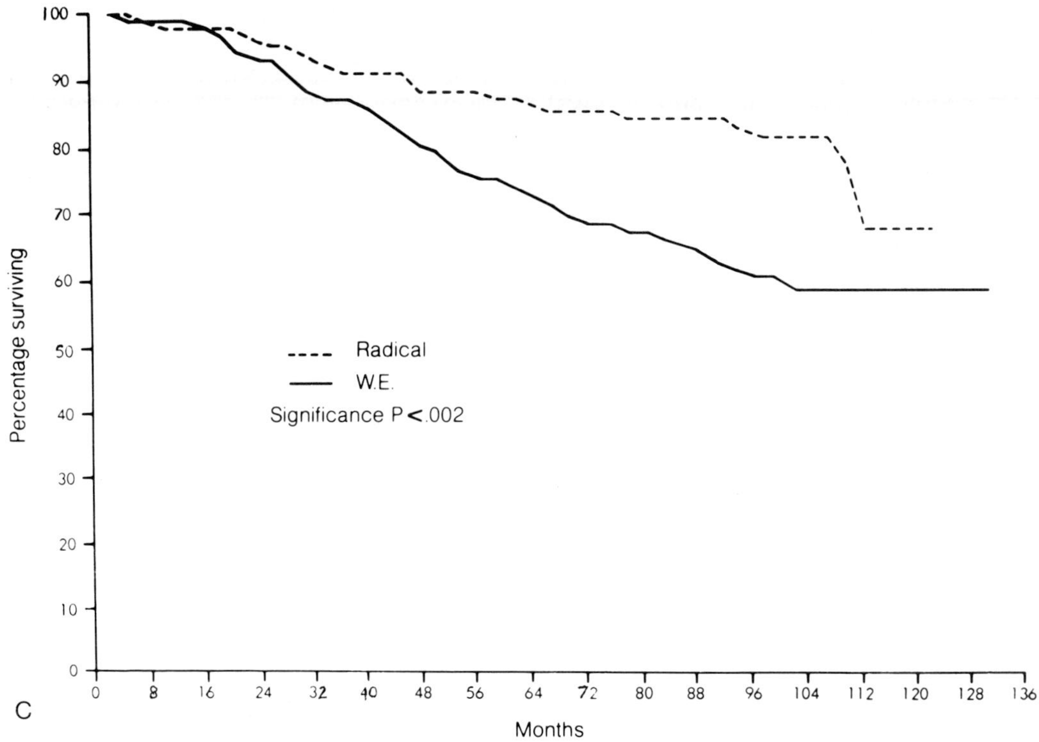

C

FIGURE 6–16 Continued. C, Survival. (With permission from Hayward J: The Guy's Hospital trials on breast conservation. *In*: Harris JR, Hellman S, Silen W (eds.): Conservative Management of Breast Cancer. Philadelphia: J. B. Lippincott, 1983.)

difference between the treatment groups in terms of all three parameters. Sites of local recurrence for patients in both series are described in detail in Table 6–8.

The issues involved in the analysis of these trials are complicated and confusing. The design of these trials has been criticized strongly: By modern standards, the doses of radiation administered are inadequate, particularly to the axilla. This is reflected in the high incidence of axillary recurrence in the N_0 patients. The doses of radiation administered to the breast were also inadequate. If local disease control is important in patients who have not yet developed micrometastatic disease, increased local control failure should be reflected in a higher rate of distant disease and, ultimately, in a decreased survival rate. If one examines the local and distant disease curves and the survival curves for Guy's II study, this hypothesis appears to be borne out. However, in the Guy's I study, although patients treated with wide excision had a higher rate of local recurrence than did patients treated with radical mastectomy, there was no difference in distant recurrence rates between the two treatment groups for either Stage I or Stage II patients and no treatment-related difference in survival rates for Stage I patients. Surprisingly, in Stage II patients, despite the *lack* of difference in distant disease recurrence rates between the treatment groups, there *is* a statistically significant difference in survival rates! When one compares local recurrence, distant recurrence, and survival rates for Stage I patients undergoing

TABLE 6–8. Sites of Local Recurrence According to Clinical Node Status (Guy's Hospital Trials)

	Guy's Trial I			*Guy's Trial II*
	N_0	N_1	ALL	N_0
Total patients treated	121	63	184	122
Node recurrence	22	14	36 (20%)	14 (12%)
Ax	20	13	33	13
Sc	2	1	3	1
Breast recurrence	5	7	12 (12%)	5 (15%)
Skin recurrence	5	11	16	13

Data from Hayward J: The Guy's Hospital trials on breast conservation. *In*: Harris JR, Hellman S, Silen W (eds.): Conservative Management of Breast Cancer. New Surgical and Radiotherapeutic Techniques. Philadelphia: J. B. Lippincott, 1983.

wide excision in each trial (Fig. 6–17), as expected, there is no detectable difference. On the other hand, when one compares local recurrence, distant recurrence, and survival rates for patients treated with radical mastectomy in the two trials (Fig. 6–18), there is a trend (not statistically significant), in both local and distant recurrence rates, for the

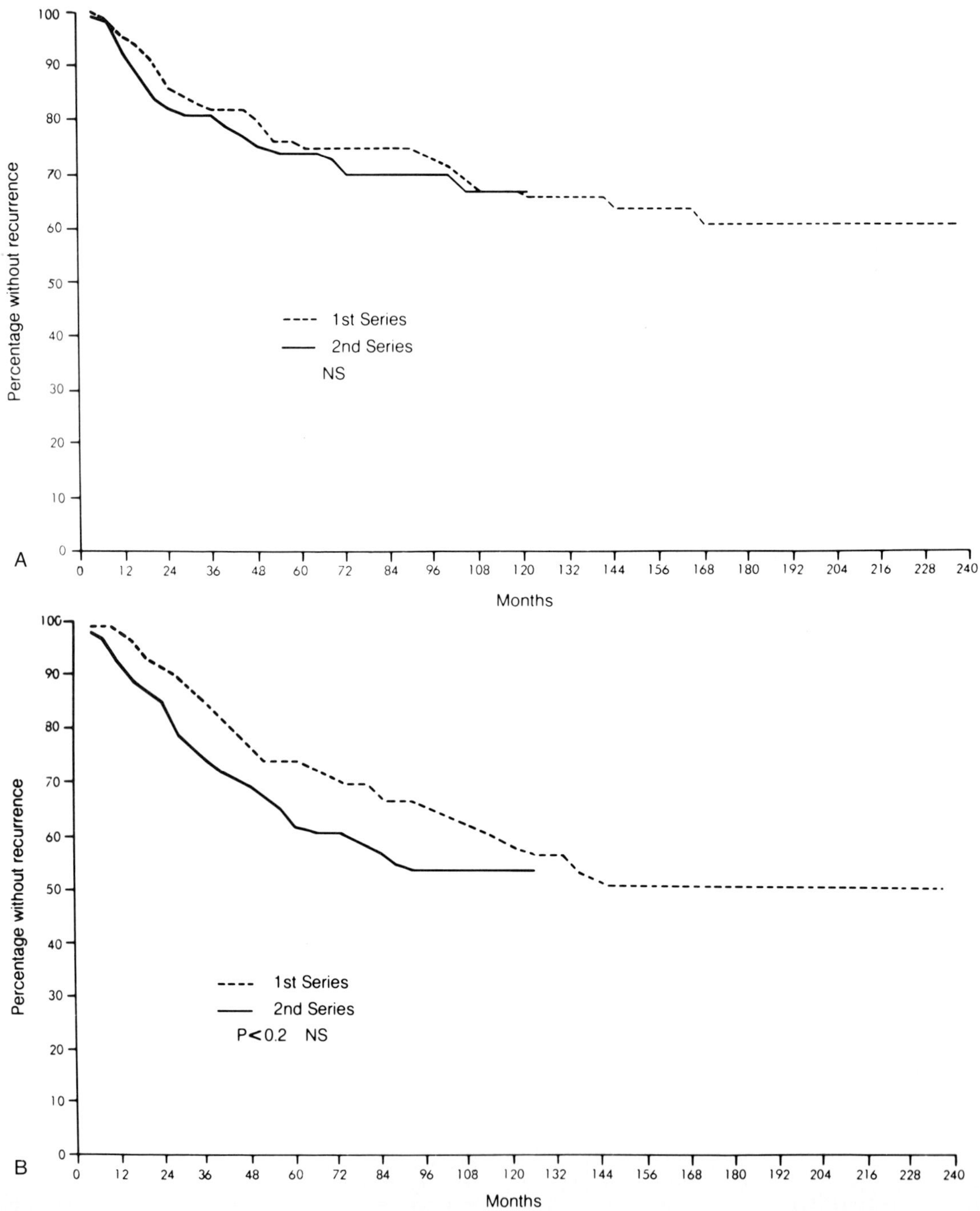

FIGURE 6–17. Guy's Hospital, Stage I patients treated with wide excision. Trial I versus Trial II. *A,* Local recurrence. *B,* Distant recurrence.

Illustration continued on opposite page

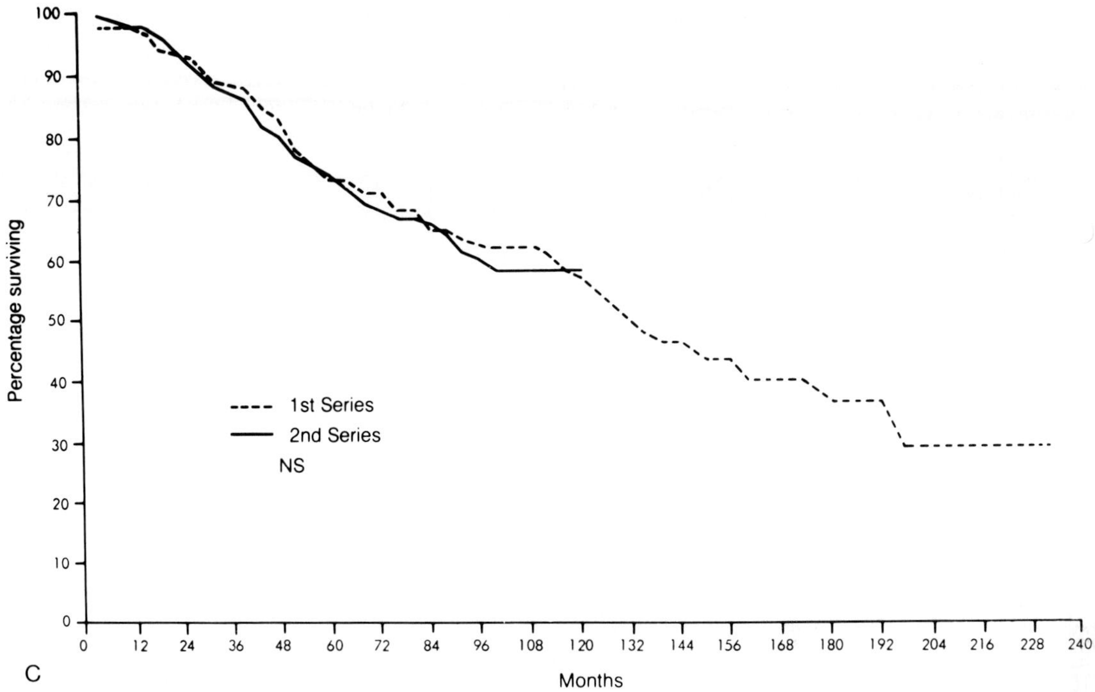

FIGURE 6–17 Continued. C, Survival. (With permission from Hayward J: The Guy's Hospital trials on breast conservation. *In*: Harris JR, Hellman S, Silen W (eds.): Conservative Management of Breast Cancer. Philadelphia: J. B. Lippincott, 1983.)

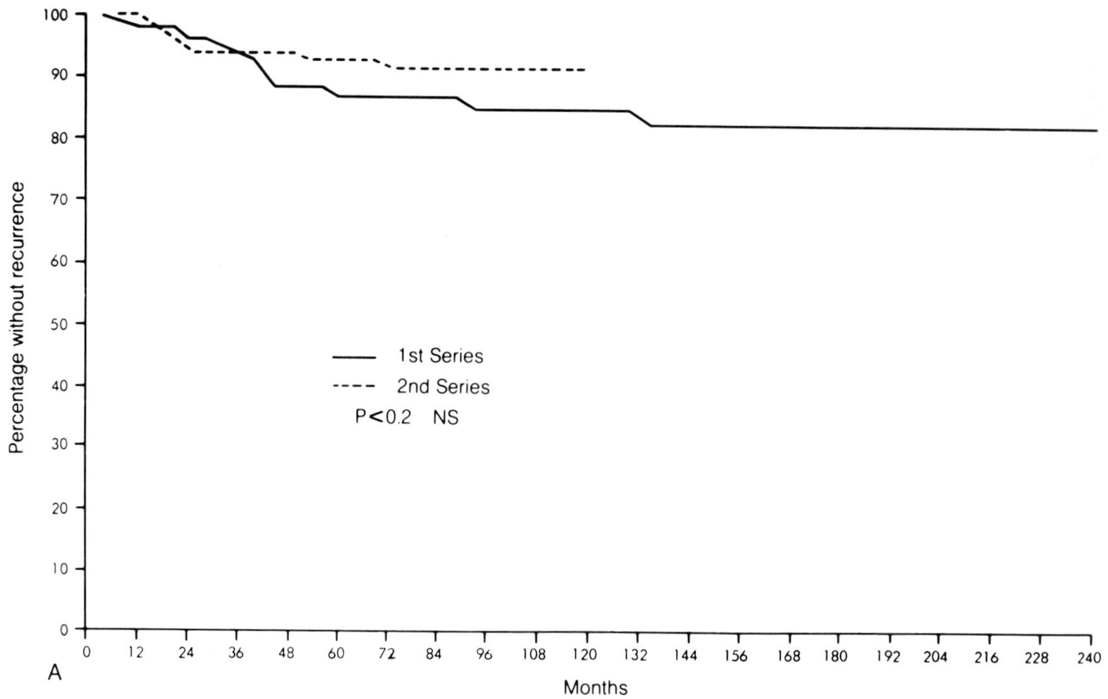

FIGURE 6–18. Guy's Hospital, Stage I patients treated with radical mastectomy. Trial I versus Trial II. *A,* Local recurrence.

Illustration continued on following page

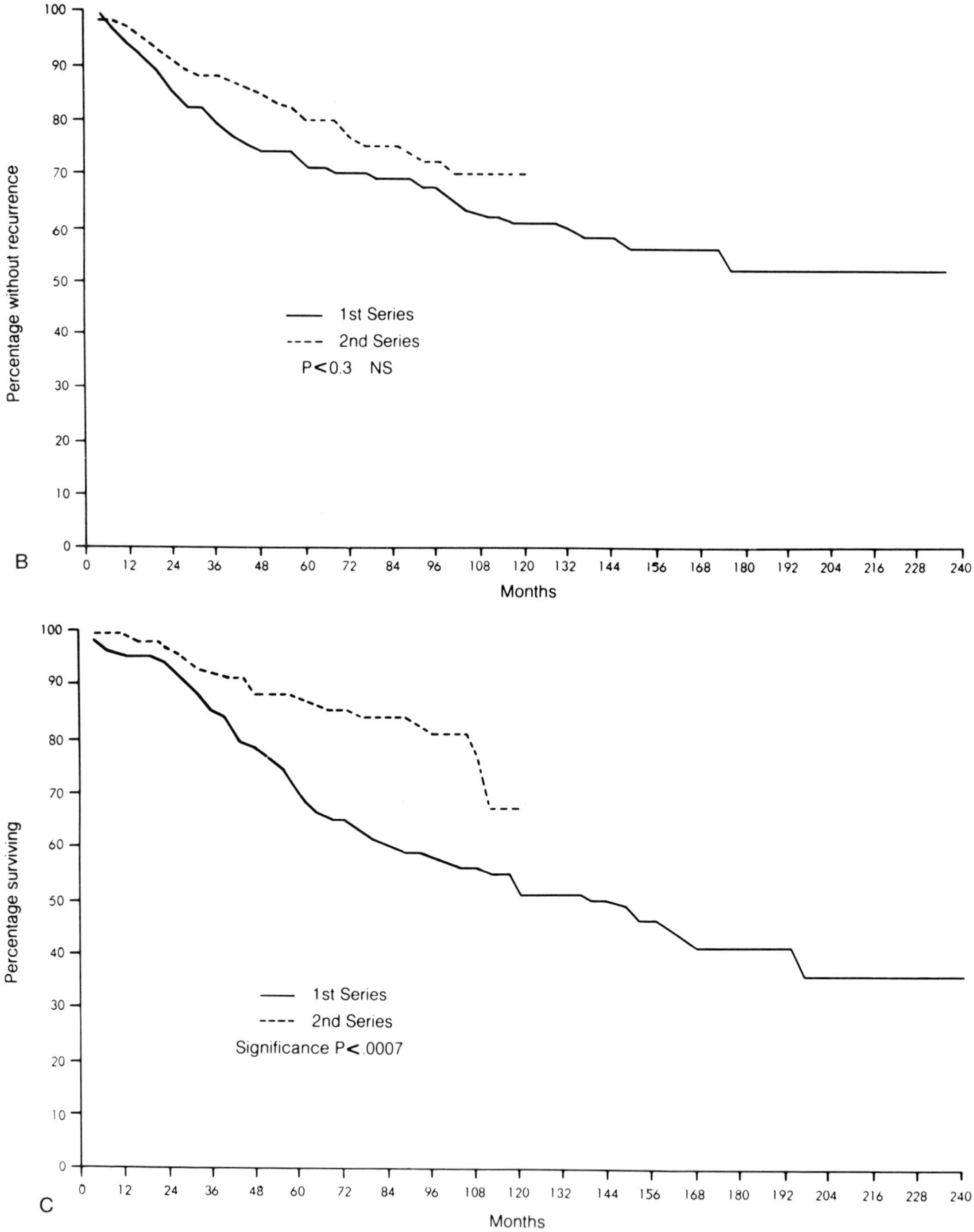

***FIGURE 6–18** Continued. B,* Distant recurrence. C, Survival. (With permission from Hayward J: The Guy's Hospital trials on breast conservation. *In*: Harris JR, Hellman S, Silen W (eds.): Conservative Management of Breast Cancer. Philadelphia: J. B. Lippincott, 1983.)

mastectomy patients in the second series to do better. Furthermore, there is a statistically significant increase in the survival rate of mastectomy patients in the second series.

What conclusions can be made from these two trials in which the evidence is conflicting? Unquestionably, the doses of radiation administered were inadequate, and therefore, it can be argued reasonably that these trials cannot shed light on the comparative efficacy of irradiation versus surgery. It can be further argued that these data do support the notions that local control is important and that inadequate treatment of local disease may adversely affect both disease control and survival, despite the results in patients with Stage II disease treated in the first trial. In those patients, there was a definite increase in local recurrence rates in wide excision patients as well as a small, but significant decrement in the survival rate. On the other hand, since distant disease recurrence rates were the same in both groups, why did these patients die? A final possibility is that there was a difference in the patient populations making up the treated groups. Histologically positive nodes were found in 25 percent and 31 percent of N_0 patients in the first and second series, respectively. Both figures are lower than the expected incidence of node positivity in clinically N_0 patients with T_1 to T_3 primary tumors. Unfortunately, information on the histologic node status of the N_0 patients treated with wide excision cannot be determined.

Probably the most conservative conclusion to be derived from these studies is that wide excision patients clearly had inferior local tumor control when compared with mastectomy patients. Since it is conceivable that poor local control may adversely affect overall survival, techniques to maximize initial local tumor sterilization should be utilized.

National Cancer Institute of Milan

From 1973 to 1980, the National Cancer Institute of Milan (Italy) conducted a randomized prospective trial comparing radical mastectomy with *QU*adrantectomy, *A*xillary node dissection, and *R*adiation *T*herapy (QUART technique) for patients with clinical Stage I (T_1, N_0) infiltrating breast cancer (Fig. 6–19).[26, 27] Surgery consisted of the classic Halsted radical mastectomy during the first five years of the trial; in the last two years, the procedure was modified, with the extent of surgery slightly reduced to preserve a large portion of the pectoralis major muscle. The conservative treatment (QUART) consisted of quadrantectomy, that is, radical removal of the entire quadrant of the breast containing the primary cancer, as well as a complete axillary dissection. The pectoralis minor muscle was removed to facilitate excision of the nodes up to the apex of the axilla. With primary tumors located in the upper quadrants, these two surgical procedures were carried out *en bloc*; with lower quadrant lesions, the quadrantectomy and axillary dissections were carried out through separate incisions. Radiation therapy was administered to the entire breast using cobalt 60 or a 6-MV linear accelerator to a dose of 5000 rad over five weeks. A cone-down boost of 1000 rad to the skin surrounding the scar and underlying breast was delivered with orthovoltage radiation therapy. Until the end of 1975, node-positive patients in both groups were randomly selected to receive or not receive adjuvant node irradiation to the supraclavicular and ipsilateral internal mammary nodes consisting of 4000 to 4500 rad over four to five weeks. In 1976, this policy was discontinued. Beginning in 1976, all patients with positive axillary lymph nodes were treated with 12 cycles of chemotherapy

Schema: Milan

Clinical Stage T_1, N_0 — RANDOMIZE

- Halsted Radical Mastectomy
- QUadrantectomy + Axillary Dissection + Radiation Therapy

FIGURE 6–19. Cancer Institute of Milan treatment schema.

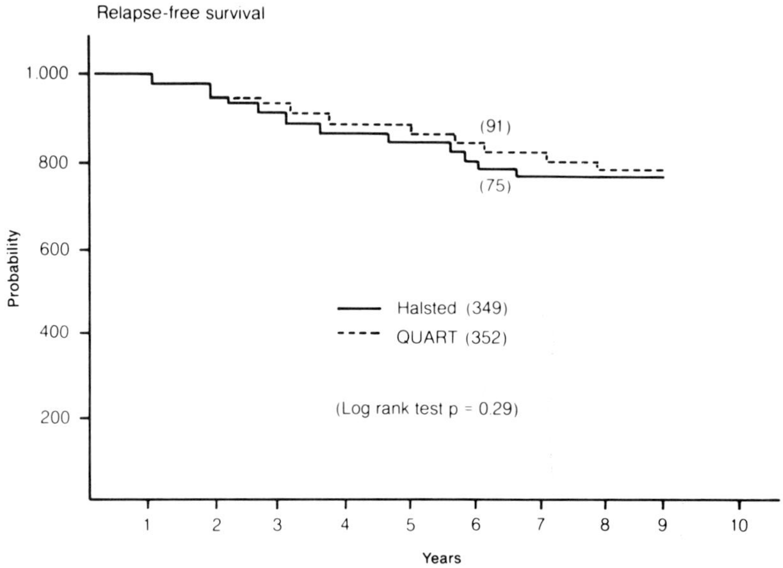

FIGURE 6–20. Cancer Institute of Milan. Actuarial disease-free survival in patients treated with Halsted radical mastectomy or with quadrantectomy, axillary dissection, and radiation therapy (QUART). (With permission from Veronesi U, et al.: Results of quadrantectomy, axillary dissection, and radiotherapy (QUART) in T1N0 patients. *In*: Harris JR, Hellman S, Silen W (eds.): Conservative Management of Breast Cancer. Philadelphia: J. B. Lippincott, 1983.)

consisting of CMF, as previously described by Bonadonna.

A total of 701 evaluable patients were entered into the study; 349 received mastectomy (295, Halsted radical mastectomy, and 54, modified radical mastectomy), and 352 were treated with QUART. The patient groups were entirely comparable in terms of age, menopausal status, tumor size, pathologic node positivity, and number of positive lymph nodes. Relapse-free and overall survival rates for the entire group according to treatment regimen (Figs. 6–20 and 6–21) demonstrate no significant difference between the two treatments. When analyzed in terms of node-positive and node-negative patients, there was again no difference in relapse-free survival in patients with histologically negative axillary nodes (Fig. 6–22). Interestingly, there was a statistically significant difference in actuarial disease-free survival in patients with histologically positive axillary nodes, favoring the radiation group (Fig. 6–23).

Sites of first disease recurrence are listed in Table 6–9. Local recurrences were seen in four mastectomy patients and one QUART patient. Ipsilateral "second primary tumors"

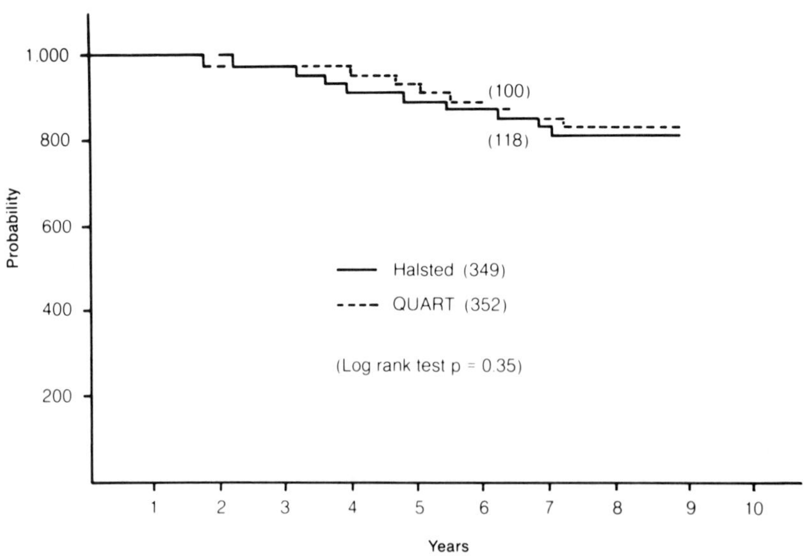

FIGURE 6–21. Cancer Institute of Milan. Actuarial overall survival in patients treated with Halsted radical mastectomy or with quadrantectomy, axillary dissection, and radiation therapy (QUART). (With permission from Veronesi U, et al.: Results of quadrantectomy, axillary dissection, and radiotherapy (QUART) in T1N0 patients. *In*: Harris JR, Hellman S, Silen W (eds.): Conservative Management of Breast Cancer. Philadelphia: J. B. Lippincott, 1983.)

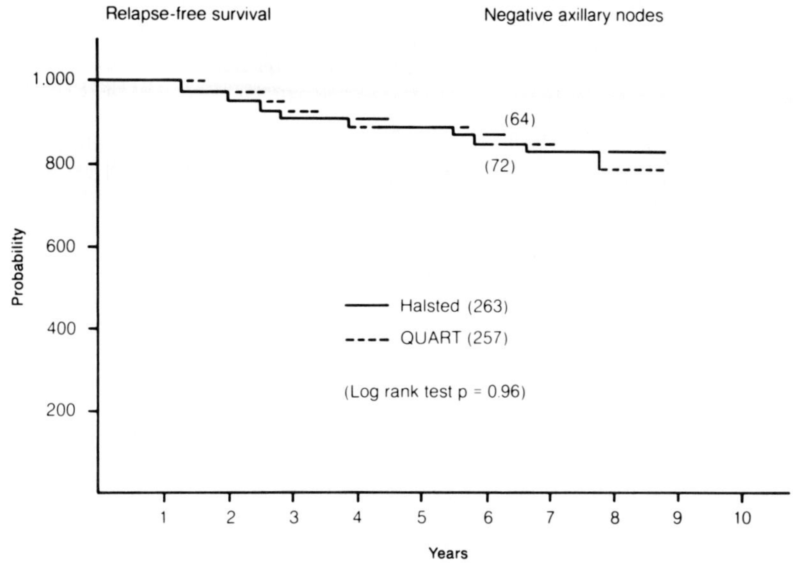

FIGURE 6–22. Cancer Institute of Milan. Actuarial disease-free survival in node-negative patients treated with Halsted radical mastectomy or with quadrantectomy, axillary dissection, and radiation therapy (QUART). (With permission from Veronesi U, et al.: Results of quadrantectomy, axillary dissection, and radiotherapy (QUART) in T1N0 patients. *In*: Harris JR, Hellman S, Silen W (eds.): Conservative Management of Breast Cancer. Philadelphia: J. B. Lippincott, 1983.)

were seen in an additional seven QUART patients. The distinction between local recurrence and second primary tumor in a breast treated with limited surgery and radiation therapy can be difficult. This distinction depends heavily on issues such as pathology of the two tumors as well as location of the two tumors within the breast, particularly with regard to their proximity to each other. Contralateral breast cancers occurred in 8 mastectomy and 12 QUART patients.

It is difficult to overestimate the importance of this trial. It compares in a scientifically meticulous fashion, two local treatment strategies, both designed to maximize initial local disease control. The study demonstrates unequivocally that a surgical procedure that conserves the breast, combined with adequate radiation therapy, does not compromise survival, when compared with a radical surgical procedure incorporating complete breast amputation. It cannot be concluded

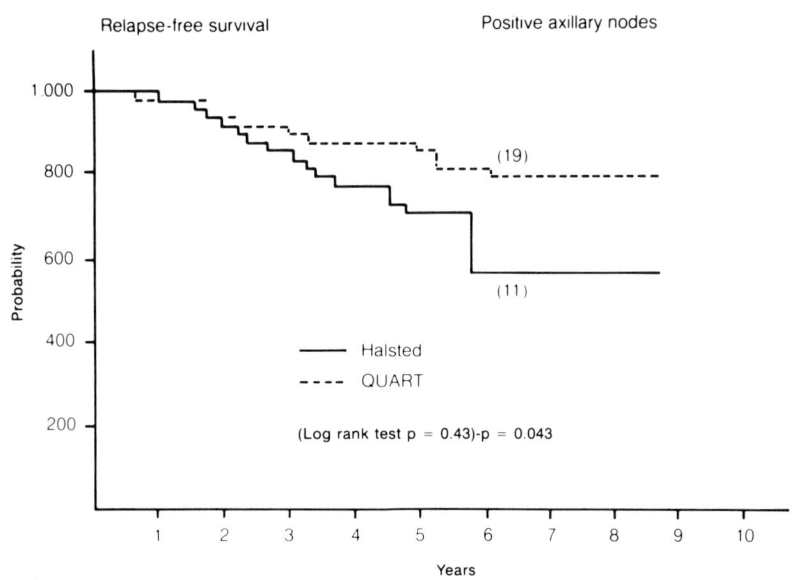

FIGURE 6–23. Cancer Institute of Milan. Actuarial disease-free survival in node-positive patients treated with Halsted radical mastectomy or with quadrantectomy, axillary dissection, and radiation therapy (QUART). (With permission from Veronesi U, et al.: Results of quadrantectomy, axillary dissection, and radiotherapy (QUART) in T1N0 patients. *In*: Harris JR, Hellman S, Silen W (eds.): Conservative Management of Breast Cancer. Philadelphia: J. B. Lippincott, 1983.)

TABLE 6–9. Sites of First Recurrence after Radical Mastectomy versus QUART

	RM	*QUART*
Local recurrence	4	1
Second primary breast cancer	8	19
Ipsilateral	0	7
Contralateral	8	12
Distant metastasis	44	33

Data from Veronesi U, Del Vecchio M, Greco M, et al.: Results of quadrantectomy, axillary dissection, and radiotherapy (QUART) in T1N0 patients. *In*: Harris JR, Hellman S, Silen W (eds.): Conservative Management of Breast Cancer. New Surgical and Radiotherapeutic Techniques. Philadelphia: J. B. Lippincott, 1983.

from this study that all local treatments are equivalent for all patients with early or operable breast cancer; the treatments that were compared in this study were quite specific, and the study was limited to the subset of patients with clinical Stage I (T_1, N_0) disease. Nonetheless, the implications raised are extremely important. Based on the results of this trial, the Halsted radical mastectomy has been abandoned and the QUART technique embraced as the standard treatment for patients with clinical Stage I breast cancer at the National Cancer Institute of Milan.

Institute Gustav-Roussy

In 1984, results of a randomized prospective trial conducted at the Institute Gustav-Roussy between 1972 and 1979 were reported.[28] Patients were eligible for this study if they were 70 years of age or younger and had unilateral breast cancer with primary tumors that were 2 cm or smaller on mammography and that were confirmed to be 2 cm or smaller pathologically ("pathologic" T_1), with N_0 to N_1, and M_0 (Fig. 6–24). The patients were randomly selected to receive either total mastectomy or tumorectomy (removal of the primary cancer with 2 cm of surrounding tissue) followed by radiation therapy. All patients underwent a low axillary dissection with identification, at the time of surgery, of at least seven lymph nodes. If any lymph node was found to contain tumor, a complete axillary dissection was performed. (For patients with pathologically positive axillary nodes, a second randomized selection was carried out for comprehensive node irradiation versus no radiation.) Radiation therapy was delivered with a cobalt 60 unit. The dose consisted of 4500 rad to the locoregional area in 18 fractions over four weeks, with a boost of 1500 rad in six fractions applied to the tumor bed. In patients with pathologically negative low axillary nodes, only the breast was irradiated. This is shown diagrammatically in Figure 6–25. One hundred seventy-nine patients entered the study; 88 underwent mastectomy, and 91, tumorectomy with irradiation. The two groups were comparable in terms of age, tumor size, tumor location, and number of histologically positive axillary nodes. The five-year actuarial disease-free survival rates (Fig. 6–26) show no significant treatment-related difference. The local recurrence rate at five years (site unspecified) was 5 percent in tumorectomy and 12 percent in mastectomy patients. Cosmesis in the tumorectomy patients was judged to be excellent in 32 percent, good in 60 percent, and poor in 8 percent of patients. Complications varied with the treatment received. One hundred eighteen patients had negative axillary nodes, 59 of whom received tumorectomy, and 59, mastectomy. One tumorectomy patient developed pneumonitis, and two mastectomy patients developed arm lymphedema with functional impairment (both had undergone complete axillary dissection, contrary to protocol design). Seventy-two patients had positive axillary nodes. Fifty-eight of these patients were part of the randomized trial comparing mastectomy with tumorec-

Schema: Institute Gustav-Roussy

T Pathologic 1, N_{0-1}, M_0 Age < 70y.	R A N D O M I Z E	Mastectomy + Low Axillary Dissection Tumorectomy + Low Axillary Dissection (Tumor Excision + 2cm Normal Breast)

FIGURE 6–24. Institute Gustav-Roussy treatment schema. (With permission from Sarrazin D, et al.: Conservative treatment versus mastectomy in breast cancer tumors with macroscopic diameter of 20 millimeters or less. Cancer 53:1209, 1984.)

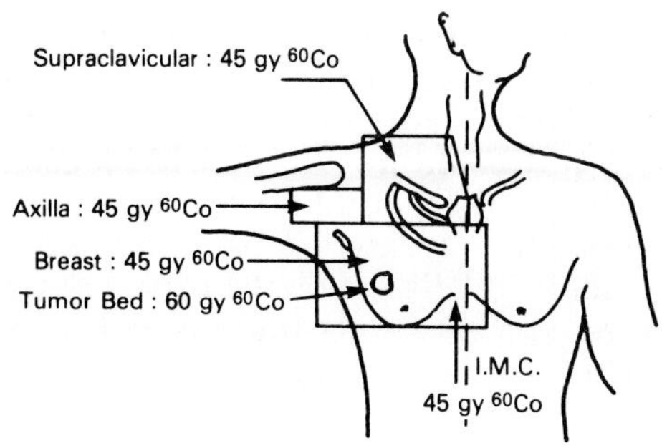

Technique of irradiation: target volumes and doses.

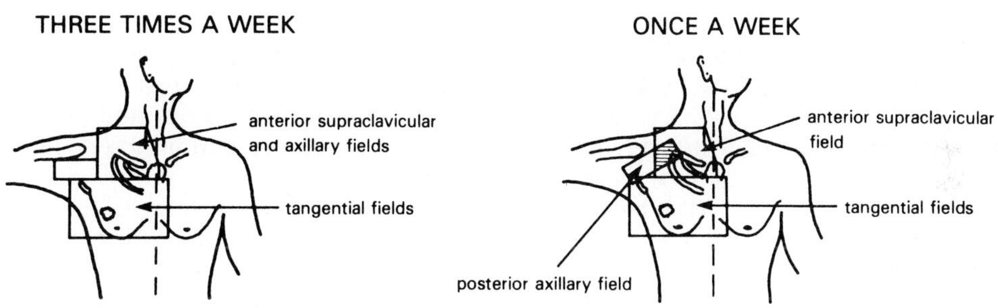

FIGURE 6–25. Institute Gustav-Roussy. Technique of irradiation. Target volumes, doses, and fields. (With permission from Sarrazin D, et al.: Conservative treatment versus mastectomy in breast cancer tumors with macroscopic diameter of 20 millimeters or less. Cancer 53:1209, 1984.)

tomy, and 14 patients who were not part of this study but who had undergone tumorectomy and radiation therapy were also included. Forty-one of these 72 patients had been randomly selected to receive node radiation therapy, and 31 were randomly selected to receive no node radiation therapy. All these patients had full axillary node dissection. Three of 31 patients without node radiation therapy developed arm edema. No other complications are reported for this group. Five of 41 patients with node irradiation developed edema, and one of these subsequently developed angiosarcoma. In addition, one patient developed brachial plexopathy, one, pneumonitis, and three, shoulder periarthritis.

This trial differs somewhat from the aforementioned Milan study. The patient population was again restricted to those with small (T_1) primary tumors, although it did allow inclusion of patients with clinically positive axillary lymph nodes. The treatments com-

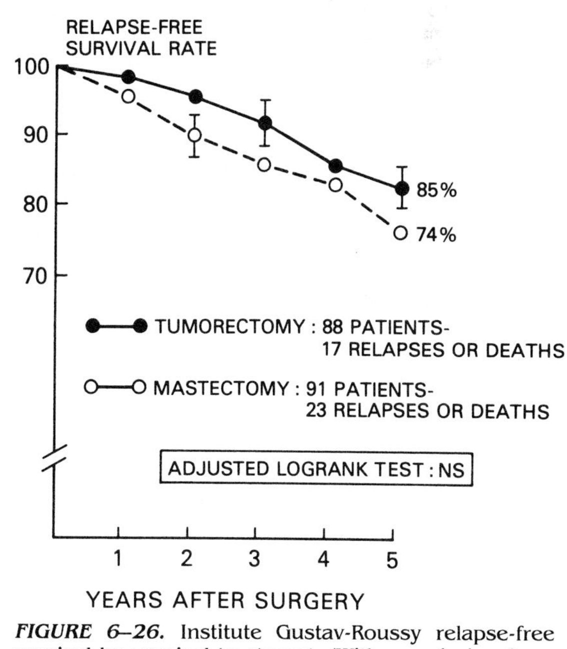

FIGURE 6–26. Institute Gustav-Roussy relapse-free survival by surgical treatment. (With permission from Sarrazin D, et al. Cancer 53:1209, 1984.)

pared in this study, in both the surgery and the radiation therapy groups, were more limited. Mastectomy patients had the entire breast removed, but the pectoralis major and the pectoralis minor muscles were left intact, and axillary surgery was limited, except in the case of histologically positive low axillary nodes. Likewise, the surgery performed in patients undergoing primary radiation therapy was more strictly limited to include only the identified gross tumor mass with a moderate margin of normal surrounding tissue. Although including a larger number of patients in the trial would have increased the reliability of the study outcome, the study does demonstrate that in this subset of patients with early breast cancer, limited surgery with comprehensive irradiation appears as effective as breast amputation in terms of five-year disease-free and overall survival rates.

Local recurrence appears to be at least comparable, and in fact, at five years the tumorectomy patients were faring better than the mastectomy patients. It should be pointed out that a 12 percent local recurrence rate for patients with T_1 tumors undergoing mastectomy is rather high. Overall, 35 percent of the patients included in this study had histologically positive lymph nodes, which is a rather high percentage of this patient population as well.

National Surgical Adjuvant Breast Project B-06

The NSABP has recently published results of a randomized prospective trial conducted from 1976 to 1984.[29] The patients had unilateral breast cancer 4 cm or less in diameter, which was movable in relation to the skin, underlying muscle, and chest wall, with no clinical evidence of skin involvement. In addition, the breast had to be of sufficient size, and the tumor located such that tumor resection would leave a cosmetically acceptable breast. Lymph nodes could be clinically negative or positive but movable (N_0 to N_1), but there could be no evidence of distant metastasis. Patients were randomly assigned to three different breast treatments: total mastectomy, in which the entire breast and pectoral fascia were removed; segmental mastectomy, in which the tumor was removed with free margins of resection; or segmental mastectomy with postoperative radiation therapy consisting of 5000 rad in 25 fractions of 200 rad per day, with tangential fields to the entire breast with megavoltage equipment. In addition to undergoing treatment to the breast, all patients underwent axillary node dissection. This was not performed *en bloc* in patients undergoing segmental mastectomy. Patients undergoing segmental mastectomy, in whom it was impossible to obtain a microscopically free margin at surgery or in whom postoperative pathologic examination detected a positive margin, received total mastectomy. Radiation boosts to the tumor bed were not employed. All patients with one or more positive lymph nodes received adjuvant chemotherapy consisting of L-phenylalanine mustard and 5-fluorouracil.

Local failure was defined as recurrence of tumor in the chest wall or operative scar; regional failure was defined as tumor recurrence in internal mammary, axillary, or ipsilateral supraclavicular lymph nodes; and distant metastasis was defined as disease in any other site. In patients undergoing segmental mastectomy alone or segmental mastectomy with radiation therapy, appearance of tumor in the residual breast parenchyma was *NOT classified as local failure* and was *NOT scored as disease recurrence*. These patients were classified as having a *cosmetic failure ONLY* and were treated with a total mastectomy.

In the early years of the study, patient accrual was quite slow. This was attributed to the psychologic difficulty of randomization between surgical procedures. Thus a prerandomization scheme was adopted whereby patients considered eligible for the study were randomized initially; once the assigned treatment had been determined, the physician then presented the study and the assigned treatment to the patient. The use of prerandomization risked the introduction of bias into the treatment results because of patient refusal of assigned treatment. However, only 8 percent of patients refused their assigned treatment, and this did not affect the statistical outcome of the study.

A total of 2163 patients were entered into the study. Of these, 320 (15 percent) were considered unevaluable, leaving 1843 patients who were analyzed for end results. Patients were considered unevaluable if they refused all protocol participation (41 patients), had noninvasive tumors (32), had other confounding medical conditions (40), refused assigned treatment (174), had insufficient follow-up at the time of analysis (24), or had no pathologic test results available at time of analysis (9). Overall, 8 percent of patients refused study treatment. There was a tendency for more patients to refuse assigned mastectomy (78 of 713, or 10 percent, as opposed to segmental mastectomy (41 of 719, or 6 percent) or segmental mastectomy with irradiation (55 of 731, or 8 percent). The mean time on study was 39 months, with a range of 5 to 99 months at the time of analysis; the estimated median time on the study is somewhat shorter, about 30 months.

Of patients undergoing segmental mastectomy, approximately 10 percent had total mastectomy because of the presence of positive margins. The risk of undergoing total mastectomy because of positive margins was increased by the presence of positive nodes (15 percent of patients with positive nodes and 7 percent of patients with negative nodes had positive margins) and by extensive nodal involvement (33 percent of patients with more than ten positive nodes also had positive margins). Additionally, the presence of positive margins seemed to be related to tumor size: 7 percent of patients with primary tumors up to 2 cm and 13 percent of patients with primary tumors from 2.1 to 4 cm had positive margins.

The NSABP analyzed results of all patients entered into the study and of only evaluable patients. Although specific data are not provided, no differences were noted between these two analyses, and thus results are reported only for the 1843 evaluable patients. When total mastectomy was compared with segmental mastectomy or when total mastectomy was compared with segmental mastectomy with radiation therapy, no significant difference was apparent in terms of overall survival, disease-free survival (see aforementioned definition), or distant disease–free survival rates, either for the groups as a whole (Fig. 6–27) or when examined by subgroups according to pathologic status of axillary nodes (Table 6–10). When segmental mastectomy patients were compared with segmental mastectomy plus radiation therapy patients, patients with positive margins were *eliminated* from the analysis. In these analyzed patients, no significant differences in distant disease–free survival or survival rates were detected.

With regard to local failure in segmental mastectomy patients, five-year projections indicated that 28 percent of patients not receiving radiation therapy as opposed to 8 percent of patients receiving radiation therapy would develop recurrent disease in this site (Fig. 6–27). This difference was even

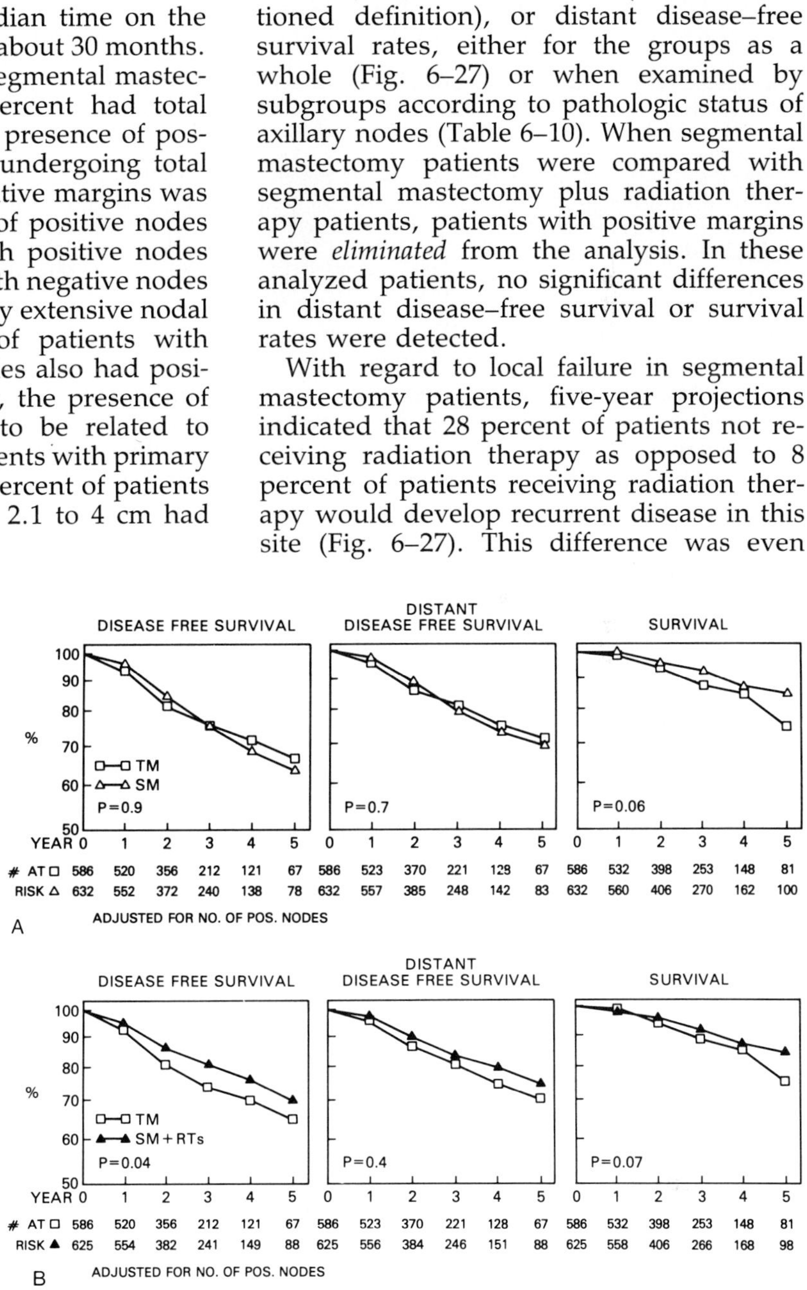

FIGURE 6–27. NSABP B-06 trial. Treatment outcome: disease-free survival, distant disease–free survival, survival. *A*, Total mastectomy versus segmental mastectomy. *B*, Total mastectomy versus segmental mastectomy and irradiation. (With permission from Fisher B, et al.: Five-year results of a randomized clinical trial comparing total mastectomy and segmental mastectomy with or without radiation in the treatment of breast cancer. N Engl J Med 312:665, 1985.)

TABLE 6–10. Comparison of Total Mastectomy versus Segmental Mastectomy and versus Segmental Mastectomy Plus Breast Irradiation According to Node Status of Patients—Life-Table Estimates of End Results Five Years after Operation

	Negative Nodes			*Positive Nodes*		
End Results	TM** (362 Patients)	SM (390 Patients)	SM + RTX (396 Patients)	TM (224 Patients)	SM (242 Patients)	SM + RTX (229 Patients)
Disease–free survival	71.9* ±3.5	68.1 ±3.5 0.7†	81.4 ±2.9 0.1	57.9 ±5.3	54.8 ±5.7 0.4‡	57.5 ±5.4 0.6
Distant disease–free survival	81.3 ±3.0	72.8 ±3.4 0.2	85.3 ±2.6 0.2	58.6 ±5.6	63.8 ±5.7 0.2	61.3 ±5.4 1.0
Overall survival	81.7 ±3.9	90.7 ±2.4 0.05	91.6 ±2.1 0.09	66.4 ±5.3	73.8 ±5.3 0.3	75.2 ±4.5 0.4

*% ± SE.
**TM = total mastectomy; SM = segmental mastectomy; RTX = radiation.
†p value versus TM.
‡p value versus TM; adjusted for number of positive nodes (1–3, 4–9, 10 or more)
With permission from Fisher B, Bauer M, Margolese R, et al.: Five-year results of a randomized clinical trial comparing total mastectomy and segmental mastectomy with or without radiation in the treatment of breast cancer. N Engl J Med 312:665, 1985.

more striking in patients with positive axillary nodes and was highly statistically significant. Node-positive patients receiving radiation had only a 2 percent incidence of breast recurrence, as opposed to a 36 percent incidence in node-positive patients not receiving radiation therapy. This observation suggested that adjuvant chemotherapy may be additive to irradiation in reducing disease recurrence in the breast after segmental mastectomy.

This study differs from the aforementioned Italian and French studies in terms of patient selection (patients with tumors 4 cm or smaller and with clinically negative or positive but movable nodes) as well as the extent of surgical resection (requirement was for pathologically negative margins in the resection specimen). Since relatively few patients, approximately 15 percent of the study group, have been followed for five years, the confidence intervals on projected treatment outcome at five years are somewhat broad. Nonetheless, the study does demonstrate that at least for this subset of patients with early breast cancer, procedures involving less than breast amputation do not appear to compromise overall survival.

Certainly, the definition of local recurrence that is used by the NSABP is unconventional. It will be very important to see what happens to the segmental mastectomy groups with and without radiation therapy over time, particularly in node-negative patients. Such a comparison will provide important information on the significance of initial local tumor control. It is conceivable that in node-positive patients who are known to be at extremely high risk for distant micrometastatic disease, local treatment, no matter how effective in eliminating disease in the treated area, will not have a detectable impact on overall survival. On the other hand, in patients with only local disease, initial therapy to maximize eradication of local tumor cells may well prove to be important in terms of ultimate cure. Information to be gained from following these patients over the long term will therefore be invaluable.

National Cancer Institute

At the National Cancer Institute in Bethesda, Maryland, the author and colleagues are engaged in an ongoing prospective randomized trial.[30] This study began in 1979 and compares surgical management consisting of total mastectomy and complete axillary node dissection followed by optional breast reconstruction with comprehensive radiation therapy consisting of gross tumor excision, complete axillary node dissection, and locoregional external beam radiation therapy of 4680 rad over five and a half weeks, combined with a 1500 to 2000 rad boost to

TABLE 6–11. Randomized Trials in Early Breast Cancer: Surgery versus Radiation Therapy

Institution	Stage	Control	Investigation
Milan[26]	T_1, N_0	Radical mastectomy	Quadrantectomy; axillary dissection; 5000 rad/5 wk breast only + 1000 rad scar boost
Gustav-Roussy[28]	T_1, N_0–N_1	Mastectomy, low axillary dissection	Tumor excision + 2 cm surrounding tissue; low axillary dissection; 4500 rad breast + nodes; 1500 rad tumor bed boost
NSABP[29] (B-06)	T < 4 cm, N_0–N_1	Mastectomy, axillary dissection	Sequential mastectomy with negative margins; axillary dissection ± 5000 rad breast only
NCI[30]	T_1–T_2, N_0–N_1	Mastectomy, complete axillary dissection	Tumor excision; complete axillary dissection; 4600 rad breast + nodes; 1500 rad tumor bed boost

the tumor bed generally with interstitial iridium. Patients are eligible if they have a solitary primary breast cancer that is clinical Stage T_1 to T_2, N_0 to N_1, M_0 and have no prior history of malignancy. All patients with pathologically demonstrated axillary node metastases receive adjuvant chemotherapy consisting of doxorubicin (40 mg/m^2, IV, day 1) and cyclophosphamide (200 mg/m^2, PO, days 3 to 6) with escalation to maximally tolerated doses. Initially, chemotherapy was given in 11 cycles of four weeks per cycle, with the first cycle being given within 7 to 10 days of surgery and the second cycle delayed for seven weeks to allow for an administration of radiation therapy. Currently, we administer nine cycles of therapy on a three-week basis without interruption, although doxorubicin is withheld during the third cycle. In addition, patients over 50 years of age with positive lymph nodes receive tamoxifen, 40 mg PO q.d. until relapse, upon the completion of adjuvant chemotherapy. This study differs in several respects from those cited earlier. All patients with Stages I and II breast cancer are eligible, including those with primary tumors up to 5 cm in diameter. In the irradiation patients, we require only gross tumor excision, without microscopically disease-free margins of resection. This excision is complemented by a radiation boost to the tumor bed. This treatment policy is founded on the beliefs that gross tumor excision facilitates radiation therapy but that wide excision is therapeutically unnecessary when coupled with a radiation boost and is likely to lead to surgically induced breast deformity. As of July 1, 1985, 194 patients had entered the study. The median follow-up time of 34 months is too short a period from which to make definitive treatment-related conclusions, although survival and disease-free survival rates are very similar in the two groups. In addition to the determination of treatment-related survival outcome, we are investigating prospectively numerous other aspects of the impact of these two therapies, especially in terms of cosmetic and functional outcomes and the psychologic and psychosocial impact of treatment.

LOCAL RECURRENCE

Definitions and Background

Analysis of the results of any local treatment of breast cancer mandates an examination of the issue of tumor control in the treated area as well as overall survival. In this context, definitions are important. Since the breast that is managed radiotherapeutically (including the nipple-areola complex and the overlying skin) is not removed, it is at risk for recurrence of cancer, which is termed *local recurrence*. Local recurrence may take two forms. The first is a true recurrence of the original tumor, which would be expected to be in the vicinity of the original tumor bed and to be of a histologic appearance similar if not identical to the original primary tumor. The second form of local recurrence in the breast would be the emergence of another independent primary cancer. This cancer may arise at a location remote from the original tumor bed and may be of a histologic appearance that may or may not be identical to the original primary tumor.

TABLE 6–12. Residual Cancer in Mastectomy Specimens

Pathologic Tumor Size	*No. of Patients*	*Patients without Tumor Foci*	*Patients with Tumor Foci*	*Distance from Reference Tumor* ≤ 2 CM	≥ 2 CM
≤ 2 cm	130	53 (41%)	77 (59%)	22	55
≤ 4 cm	264	101 (38%)	163 (62%)	54	109
≤ 5 cm	182	105 (37%)	177 (63%)	56	121

With permission from Holland R, Veling SHJ, Mravunac M, et al.: Histologic multifocality of Tis, T1–2 breast carcinomas. Implications for clinical trials of breast-conserving surgery. Cancer 56:979, 1985.

Regional recurrence is disease appearing in the ipsilateral lymph node–draining regions, including the axillary, internal mammary, infraclavicular, and supraclavicular lymph nodes.

From a number of pathologic studies, including serial sectioning of whole-organ mastectomy specimens, it is clear that breast cancer is a multicentric condition in a significant proportion of patients. Generally, this proportion has been estimated to be approximately 30 percent of early breast cancer patients, but estimates vary with the definition applied and the pathologic technique used. In 1985, Holland and associates[31] published the analysis of consecutive mastectomy specimens from patients who would be suitable, on clinical grounds, for breast-conserving therapy. In this study, chilled mastectomy specimens were microscopically sectioned at approximately 5-mm intervals, with tissue blocks taken of all grossly and radiologically suspicious areas, in addition to random samples of normal-appearing tissue. Pathologic findings were then diagrammed for each specimen. Results of this study are summarized in Table 6–12. In approximately 40 percent of patients with tumors 5 cm or less in diameter, no other focus of cancer was detected in the breast. However, in the remaining 60 percent, additional foci of either invasive or noninvasive cancer were identified in regions adjacent to or remote from the identified primary tumors. Of interest, the proportion of patients with multicentric disease and the location of these multicentric foci (that is, adjacent to or remote from the identified primary tumor) did not vary with primary tumor size. Of the tumor foci located farther than 2 cm from the primary tumor, approximately 25 percent were invasive cancer and about 75 percent were noninvasive cancer. Although the biologic significance of these multicentric sites of tumor is not completely known, a few series are available on the treatment of highly selected and, presumably, favorable breast cancer with limited surgery only.[32–34] These studies are summarized in Table 6–13. The breast cancer recurrence rate in patients so treated is approximately 30 percent, which is consistent with the aforementioned pathologic findings. This subject is discussed in Chapter 10.

Technical and Biologic Factors Influencing Local Control

A number of factors may influence the likelihood of local tumor control. These include technical factors of treatment such as extent of surgery, radiation dose, and irradiation technique as well as biologic factors including tumor size and histologic patterns.

Excision of the Primary Tumor

Probably the most important technical determinant of local tumor control is complete gross excision of the primary tumor. Review of the data from a number of series, summarized in Table 6–14, reveals that local recurrence appears in approximately one third of patients who have less than total gross excision of the primary tumor, whereas this incidence is generally reduced to less than 10 percent in patients who have at least a total gross excision. At this time, available data are insufficient to draw firm conclusions regarding the necessity for microscopically disease-free margins or inclusion of a rim of normal-appearing breast parenchyma around the identified primary tumor. At the National Cancer Institute, the policy is to require only gross tumor excision, without regard for the presence of microscopic tumor deposits at the resection margins, in the belief that limited excision will reduce breast deformity. However, these limited excisions are accompanied by a boost dose to the tumor bed to

TABLE 6–13. Breast Recurrence after Tumor Excision

	No. of Patients	*Stage*	*Follow-up*	*Surgery*	*Local Recurrence*
Royal Marsden[32]	26	T_1, N_0	19–74 months	Quadrantectomy; axillary dissection	15%
Newmarket[33]	44	T_1–T_2, N_0–N_1	36–72 months	Mass + 2 cm surrounding tissue ± axillary dissection	37%
Princess Margaret Hospital[19]	154	T_1–T_2*	5–25 years	Partial mastectomy	26%
NSABP B-06[29]	565	$T \leq 4$ cm, N_0–N_1	5–99 months	Segmental mastectomy (negative margins); axillary dissection	28%
UCSF[34]	43		6–48 months	Mass + 2 cm surrounding tissue axillary dissection	19%

*122 T_1–T_2, 34 TX, 8 T_3–T_4.

eliminate the potentially higher concentration of microscopic tumor deposits in this area. Three of 96 patients treated in the NCI early breast cancer study have developed local tumor recurrence, for a five-year actuarial local recurrence rate of 9 percent. This compares favorably with the five-year actuarial local recurrence rate of 7 percent from the Joint Center for Radiation Therapy,[35] whose treatment policy regarding the extent of excision of the primary tmor has also been total gross tumor excision without the requirement for negative margins. The NSABP, in protocol B-06, required pathologically free margins and gave *no* boost dose of radiation. Their rate of breast tumor recurrence was 7.7 percent.[29] With attention to detail, a careful excision can be performed that can preserve cosmesis and lead to maximum local control.[38]

Radiation Dose

Radiation dose also appears to be a factor, but it is essential to examine this parameter in conjunction with removal of gross disease. As illustrated in Table 6–15, the local tumor control rate appears to be greater than 90 percent in patients receiving at least 6000 rad to the tumor bed when the primary tumor has been completely excised. Not surprisingly, with less than total gross excision, much higher radiation doses are necessary, and even with very high doses, the risk of local tumor recurrence is approximately one third. It has been the policy in France that patients with larger tumors (3 cm or more in diameter) are treated with radiation therapy without gross tumor excision. This was predicated on the notion that removal of tumors of this size would induce significant breast deformity. At Marseilles, radiation therapy, including tumor bed boosts, is administered exclusively with external radiation, whereas at Creteil, the boost to the tumor is delivered using an interstitial implant. Although the total tumor doses prescribed in these two institutions are similar, it should be remembered that with an implant the dose prescribed is a minimum dose and a substantial portion of the implanted volume receives a significantly higher dose. The ten-year local failure rates for T_2 and T_3 tumors treated at Marseilles are 35 percent and 39 percent, respectively.[18] At Creteil, the corresponding figures are 7 percent and 15 percent.[16] These

TABLE 6–14. Local Recurrence versus Extent of Excision

Institution	*Stage*	*Follow-up*	*No. of Patients*	*Less Than Complete Excision*	*No. of Patients*	*Complete Excision and Beyond*
JCRT[35]	I–II	52 months (median)	24	35%	342	7%
Curie[15]	I–III	5 + years	122	57%	67	15%
MGH[36]	I–II	5–28 years	18	39%	128	10%
Marseilles[18]	I–III	10 years minimum	303	34%	286	11%
Creteil[37]	I–III	5 + years	309	9%	99	3%

TABLE 6–15. Local Control versus Radiation Dose

Institution	No. of Patients	Surgery	Radiation Dose	Local Recurrence (%)
JCRT[39]	89	GTE	<6000 *rad	7†
	144	GTE	6000–6999 *rad	4†
	109	GTE	>7000 *rad	1†
Curie[40]	43	GTE	<7000 rad	19
	24	GTE	>7000 rad	8
	31	None	≤1950 ret‡	77
	47	None	1950–2150 ret	64
	44	None	>2150 ret	36
MGH[36]	7	<GTE	TDF <70§	71
	11	<GTE	TDF ≥70	18
	37	GTE	TDF <70	14
	73	GTE	TDF ≥70	8 (2 geographic misses)
	10	>GTE	TDF <70	10
	14	>GTE	TDF ≥70	7

*GTE, gross tumor excision.

†Recurrence of disease in tumor bed. Excludes patients with marginal recurrence (4% overall, not related to dose or volume of boost) or recurrence elsewhere in the breast (1% overall).

‡By the NSD formula, 1943 ret is equivalent to 7000 rad and 2128 ret is equivalent to 8000 rad of conventionally fractionated radiation.

§TDF 70 is thought to be equivalent to 4500 rad of conventionally fractionated radiation.

data, although not conclusive, are certainly consistent with the notion that total dose is an important determinant of local control.

Tumor Size

The size of the primary tumor appears not to predict local recurrence, provided that gross disease has been completely excised.[17, 35] This is consistent with the pathologic findings in mastectomy specimens discussed earlier.

Tumor Histologic Types

Specific histologic subtypes of invasive carcinoma (e.g., invasive ductal, lobular, or medullary carcinoma) have not been found to be important in determining subsequent local recurrence. Since the majority of breast cancers are infiltrating ductal carcinoma, substantial numbers of patients would be necessary for a meaningful assessment of the influence of histologic subtypes on local recurrence. In Clark's analysis of 800 patients treated at the Princess Margaret Hospital,[19] no influence of histologic status on local recurrence was detected. Schnitt and associates[41] from the Joint Center for Radiation Therapy (JCRT) reviewed pathologic features in 255 patients undergoing primary radiation therapy. Two hundred thirty-one cases were available for complete pathologic review. Of these, the majority of tumors (76 percent) were predominantly of the infiltrating ductal type. Eighteen patients developed local recurrence, pathologic material of which was available for review in 17. Fifteen of the 17 local failures (88 percent) had infiltrating ductal cancer as the most aggressive histologic condition in the primary tumor, one patient had infiltrating lobular carcinoma, and one had an adenoid cystic carcinoma.

Axillary Node Status

Interestingly enough, the presence of histologically positive axillary lymph nodes has not been found to correlate with increased risk of breast recurrence.[17, 41, 23]

Extensive Intraductal Carcinoma

The JCRT group have retrospectively analyzed the histopathologic features in their series of patients undergoing primary breast irradiation, with particular attention to those who subsequently suffered local recurrence.[41] In the analysis, they included only patients with infiltrating ductal carcinoma who had had excisional biopsy prior to radiation therapy, a total of 356 patients. Extensive intraductal carcinoma was defined as a moderate or marked intraductal component within the confines of the infiltrating tumor *and* intraductal carcinoma in the adjacent breast tissue. When extensive intraductal carcinoma was found in the excision specimen, there was a five-year actuarial risk of local recurrence of 24 percent in 133 patients, in contrast with a 2 percent risk in patients without these features. Of the 29 local recurrences in patients with extensive intraductal involvement, 25 were at a site consistent with recurrence of the primary tumor. Of the five local recurrences in patients without extensive intraductal carcinoma, two were considered true recurrences and three were located elsewhere in the breast. Based on these observations, the investigators speculate that extensive intraductal disease both within and adjacent to the primary tumor indicates a more extensive volume of cancer in the breast than the disease that is clinically detectable and is therefore less likely to be eradicated with moderate, well-tolerated doses of radiation. Since the treatment policy during the study period included gross excision of the primary tumor without regard for microscopic involvement of the resection margins, the investigators recommend that patients with extensive intraductal involvement and unknown or uncertain resection margins undergo reexcision of the tumor bed prior to radiation therapy. Despite the increased incidence of local failure in this patient subgroup, the five-year actuarial risk of distant disease was not affected (20 percent and 21 percent in patients with and without extensive intraductal cancer, respectively).

Time Course of Local Recurrence

The time course of local recurrence following radiation therapy in patients undergoing at least gross tumor excision has been examined in a combined group of patients from the Joint Center for Radiation Therapy, the Marseilles Cancer Institute, the Institute Curie, and the Princess Margaret Hospital.[42] One hundred fifty-two patients with early breast cancer who were followed for a minimum of 15 years were analyzed. All patients had at least tumor excision preceding radiation therapy; no axillary surgery was performed. In this group, local recurrence appeared at a fairly constant rate, approximately 2 percent per year, over the first 14 years after treatment. Of the 35 local recurrences in these 158 breast cancers studied, 16 were in the breast alone; 3, in the axilla alone; 7, in both breast and axilla; and 9, in an unspecified location. Thirty of these patients underwent secondary salvage treatment in the hope of cure. Their actuarial disease-free survival was 58 percent at five years and 50 percent at ten years. These data suggest that the time course of local recurrence following primary irradiation is different from that following mastectomy, in which most local recurrences cluster within the first three years after treatment. This is potentially very important in planning the follow-up of patients receiving radiation therapy as a primary treatment.

As mentioned earlier, recurrence of tumor in the breast may appear either in the vicinity of the original primary tumor or at a distant separate focus in the breast. Whether breast recurrence represents failure to control the original primary tumor or emergence of a second tumor can be difficult, if not impossible, to resolve. In the Milan trial, nine QUART patients developed breast recurrence.[26, 27] In three patients, this was considered to be recurrence of the original tumor, and in the remaining six, it was viewed as a second primary tumor in the ipsilateral breast. These second primary tumors appeared two to five years after the original treatment. An analysis of patients from the JCRT[25] related site of recurrence (i.e., in the region of the original tumor bed versus distant sites in the breast) to time of recurrence after treatment. This study revealed that recurrences in the tumor bed tend to happen within the first few years of treatment, whereas recurrences elsewhere in the treated breast tend to arise after five years.

Treatment and Prognosis of Local Recurrence

Data are now beginning to accumulate concerning treatment and prognosis of local recurrence following primary radiation therapy. Information from a combined group of patients from Harvard, the Marseilles Cancer Institute, The Institute Curie, and the Princess Margaret Hospital with a minimum of 15 years of follow-up indicates that the five-year actuarial survival rate after salvage treatment for locoregional recurrence is approximately 50 percent.[42] Data from Toronto also support this conclusion.[19] It is apparent that the prognosis of patients with local recurrence following primary radiation therapy differs dramatically from that of patients with local recurrence following radical surgery in that local recurrence following radiation therapy is not necessarily a harbinger of systemic disease. Salvage therapy after local recurrence may be curative in a significant proportion of patients, although this percentage has not been determined with absolute certainty. Results from the NSABP B-06 trial[29] indicate that early in a patient's disease course, recurrence in the breast does not impair survival in a statistically significant manner. However, results from very long follow-up of patients at the Princess Margaret Hospital[19] (Fig. 6–10) suggest that recurrence in the breast alone may have an adverse effect. Clearly, until more information is available, initial therapy should be planned to maximize local control. Salvage treatment for most patients with locoregional recurrence has been mastectomy. When mastectomy has followed modern radiation therapy, the surgery does not seem to be plagued with excessive complications. Interestingly, salvage was apparently achieved in a number of patients treated with lesser surgical procedures such as wide re-excision, sometimes in conjunction with a local radiation implant.

COMPLICATIONS

Complications of treatment vary somewhat with the treatment technique, including extent of the surgical procedures performed in the breast and the axilla, total radiation dose, dose fractionation, field arrangement, and methods of boost. Table 6–16 summarizes reported complications from a number of institutions using modern equipment and techniques. Pneumonitis, when it occurs in this setting, is usually manifested clinically as a dry cough that may appear toward the end of external beam therapy or within the first several months after treatment. The vast majority of patients with this complication have not required either steroids or hospitalization. Rib fractures occur in a variable proportion of patients and are frequently asymptomatic, being detected on a routine follow-up chest x-ray or bone scan. Virtually all rib fractures heal spontaneously with conservative management. Severe breast fibrosis and soft-tissue necrosis are unusual when the total dose to the entire breast is limited to 5000 rad or less and no bolus is used. However, even with the best technique, a very rare patient will manifest severe breast fibrosis without obvious cause. Brachial plexopathy and limitation of arm motion occur infrequently, and clinical impairment is usually mild. Myositis and chest wall pain vary in incidence and are usually transient. Symptoms generally respond well to anti-inflammatory agents. Pericarditis is a rare occurrence, as is pleural effusion. The incidences of breast and arm edema vary both with radiation technique and, probably more importantly, with the extent of axillary surgery. Clearly, the incidence of arm edema is increased when complete axillary dissection is combined with axillary irradiation. The re-

TABLE 6–16. Complications of Primary Radiation Therapy

Complication	*MDAH*[44]	*JCRT*[21]	*Yale*[24]	*Palo Alto*[43]	*Univ. of PA*[23]	*NCI*
Pneumonitis	7%	3%	3%	2%	1%	0%
Rib fracture	2%	5%			1%	8%
Severe breast fibrosis	4%			3%		0%
Soft-tissue necrosis	<1%	<1%				0%
Brachial plexopathy	1%	1%	<1%	2%	0%	0%
Limited arm mobility	1%					0%*
Arm edema	7%	5%	1%	6%	6%	18%†
Pericarditis		<1%	<1%		1%	0%
Breast edema	22%			38%		
Myositis				6%		9%
Leukemia		1 patient				

*All patients have at least functional range of motion.

†All patients receive upper extremity measurements before treatment at three locations on the arm. Measurements are repeated prospectively after treatment. If at any time any one measurement increases by 2 cm, a prophylactic Jobst stocking is prescribed. This figure represents patients with Jobst stocking prescriptions.

ported incidence of edema varies with the methods of assessment and is lower in series relying on subjective observation and higher in series using prospective objective measurements.

Induction of Second Tumors

One of the concerns regarding the use of radiation therapy as a primary treatment modality for patients with breast cancer is the issue of tumor induction. It is well established that ionizing radiation is a carcinogen, and this is a legitimate concern. In this regard, attention has been focused on two specific neoplasms, acute leukemia and a second primary breast cancer.

The relationship between radiation exposure and the development of leukemia, particularly acute myelogenous leukemia and its histologic subtypes, has been studied in several populations, most notably the survivors of the atomic bombs,[45] radiologists,[46] patients undergoing radiation therapy for alkylosing spondylitis,[47] and patients treated with irradiation for benign pelvic conditions.[48, 49] The exposures of these populations are similar in three important respects. First, the persons in these populations had a relatively long life expectancy after exposure, thus allowing for the expression of a late leukemogenic effect. Second, significant proportions of the active bone marrow were exposed (i.e., the whole body in the atomic bomb survivors and radiologists; the sternum, spine, and pelvis in those with alkylosing spondylitis; and the pelvis in patients with benign pelvic disorders). Third, the exposures involved relatively low doses of radiation. In the radiation treatment of locoregional breast cancer, very little active bone marrow is irradiated and the doses employed are higher and thus more likely to inhibit or to eliminate the proliferative capacity of marrow stem cells than to induce somatic mutations. Leukemia induction as a result of this therapy is unlikely.

An association between breast cancer and acute leukemia has been noted by Rosner, Carey, and Zarrabi,[50] who reviewed 24 of their own and 54 reported cases of breast cancer with acute leukemia. Eight of these patients had synchronous diagnosis of acute leukemia and breast cancers, while the remaining 70 developed leukemia subsequent to the diagnosis of breast cancer. The median interval from the diagnosis of breast cancer to the diagnosis of acute leukemia for patients with metachronous tumors was five years. No causal relationship to therapy for breast cancer could be demonstrated.

Curtis and associates[51] have recently analyzed SEER (*S*urveillance, *E*pidemiology, and *E*nd *R*esults Program) data with respect to leukemia risk associated with the first course of cancer treatment (Table 6–17). The first course of cancer treatment was considered to be therapy begun within the first four months after diagnosis. Information was obtained from the SEER program abstracts of hospital records. Fifty-nine thousand one hundred fifteen registered breast cancer patients were analyzed. The relative risk of leukemia during the third to seventh year following initial breast cancer therapy was calculated to be 1.3 for surgery alone, 3.2 for surgery with irradiation, and 8.9 for surgery and chemotherapy. Unfortunately, there was no documentation of treatment actually received and no information at all on therapy of any kind recommended or given subsequent to initial therapy. With such uncertainty in the data base, no substantive conclusions from the study are possible.

In 1985, the NSABP reported their experiences of the incidence of leukemia in breast

TABLE 6–17. Breast Cancer Initial Therapy and Leukemia Risk

No. of Patients	*Treatment*	*Relative Risk in Years 3–7 after Diagnosis*
59,115 Registered breast cancer patients		
39,416	Surgery	1.3
10,854	RT, no chemo	3.2
6040	Chemo	8.9
2805	None/other	0
29,656 Localized disease		
25,485	Surgery	1.0
3187	RT, no chemo	1.1
447	Chemo	0
540	None/other	0
22,380 Regional disease		
12,040	Surgery	2.4
6194	RT, no chemo	4.9
3755	Chemo	13.2
391	None/other	0

Data from Curtis RE, Hankey BF, Myers MH, et al.: Risk of leukemia associated with the first course of cancer treatment: An analysis of the Surveillance, Epidemiology, and End Results Program experience. JNCI 72:531, 1984.

TABLE 6–18. Cumulative Risk Rate of Occurrence of Leukemia (L) or Myeloproliferative Syndrome (MPS): NSABP Trials B-04 to B-10

Assigned Therapy	No. of Patients	No. of Occurrences L	No. of Occurrences MPS	Average Annual Occurrence Rate per 100 Patients	Cumulative Risk Rate per 100 Patients 4-Year	Cumulative Risk Rate per 100 Patients 8-Year
Operation						
Alone	2068	3	0	0.028	0.05	0.27
Plus breast irradiation	470	1	0	0.081	0.42	0.42
Plus regional irradiation	646	5	0	0.109	0.17	1.02
Plus chemotherapy	5299	27	7	0.153	0.44	1.68

Data from Fisher B, Rockette H, Fisher E, et al.: Leukemia in breast cancer patients following adjuvant chemotherapy or postoperative radiation: The NSABP experience. J Clin Oncol 3:1640, 1985.

cancer patients following adjuvant chemotherapy or postoperative irradiation.[52] Eight thousand four hundred eighty-three women who participated in seven trials (B-04 through B-10) were evaluated. Forty-three patients were judged to have a blood dyscrasia; 36 of 8483 (0.4 percent) were classified as having leukemia and 7 of 8483 (0.1 percent), myeloproliferative syndrome. Of the 2068 patients treated with operation alone, three (0.1 percent) had leukemia. Of the 1116 patients receiving postoperative irradiation, six (0.5 percent) had leukemia; 1 of 470 (0.2 percent) patients treated with irradiation only to the breast and 5 of 646 (0.8 percent) patients treated with irradiation to the chest wall and lymph node–draining areas developed leukemia. After adjuvant chemotherapy, 34 occurrences appeared in 5299 patients (0.6 percent); 27 were leukemia (0.5 percent) and seven were myeloproliferative syndrome (0.1 percent). The cumulative risk rates are shown in Table 6–18. The relative risk is shown in Table 6–19, both for all leukemias and for acute myelocytic leukemia as related to initial treatment. Two of the cases of leukemia seen in irradiated patients were chronic lymphocytic leukemia, a cell type not associated with radiation exposure. Although the NSABP data indicate that there may be an increased incidence of leukemia associated with irradiation, the risk appears to be small.

Probably a more important concern is the issue of induction of breast cancer, especially in the parenchyma of the contralateral breast. It is well established that the risk of developing a contralateral breast cancer is greater in women undergoing mastectomy for invasive breast cancer than in the normal population. This risk has been estimated to be 1 percent per year.[53] Since radiation has been shown to be capable of inducing breast cancer[45, 54, 55] and since the opposite breast receives some amount of radiation from treatment, this is a subject that warrants close scrutiny and continued follow-up.

Breast cancer incidence among the survivors of the Hiroshima and Nagasaki atomic bombs, related to estimated dose and age at exposure, is demonstrated in graphic form in Figure 6–28.[56] From these data, breast cancer risk appears to increase directly with dose and is highest in persons exposed at younger ages. Dose estimates in these graphs are based on the 1965 exposure estimates. Although revision of the dose estimates for

TABLE 6–19. Observed (O) and Expected (E) Incidence of Leukemia and Relative Risk (RR) by Initial Treatment (NSABP Trials B-04 through B-10)

Leukemias	Surgery Only No. at Risk	O	E	RR	Surgery Plus Radiation Therapy No. at Risk	O	E	RR	Surgery Plus Chemotherapy No. at Risk	O	E	RR
All L	2068	3	1.94	1.5	1,116	6	0.99	6.1*	5299	27	2.45	11.0†
AML only		2	0.78	2.6		4	0.39	10.3†		26	1.08	24.0†

*$p < 0.05$.
†$p < 0.01$.
Data from Fisher B, Rockette H, Fisher E, et al.: Leukemia in breast cancer patients following adjuvant chemotherapy or postoperative radiation: The NSABP experience. J Clin Oncol 3:1640, 1985.

exposed persons is currently in progress, such revision is unlikely to result in any substantial change in these risk estimates.

In the earlier years of the twentieth century, an accepted treatment for tuberculosis was induction of lung collapse by iatrogenic pneumothorax (and, rarely, pneumoperitoneum). This treatment was administered under fluoroscopic guidance. An increased incidence of breast cancer has been noted in women so exposed to these diagnostic x-rays. Boice and Monson[57] analyzed patients from two Massachusetts tuberculosis sanatoria, an exposed group of 1047 women treated with pneumothorax who had multiple fluoroscopies, and a comparison group of 717 women with tuberculosis treated with other therapy. Demographics of the two

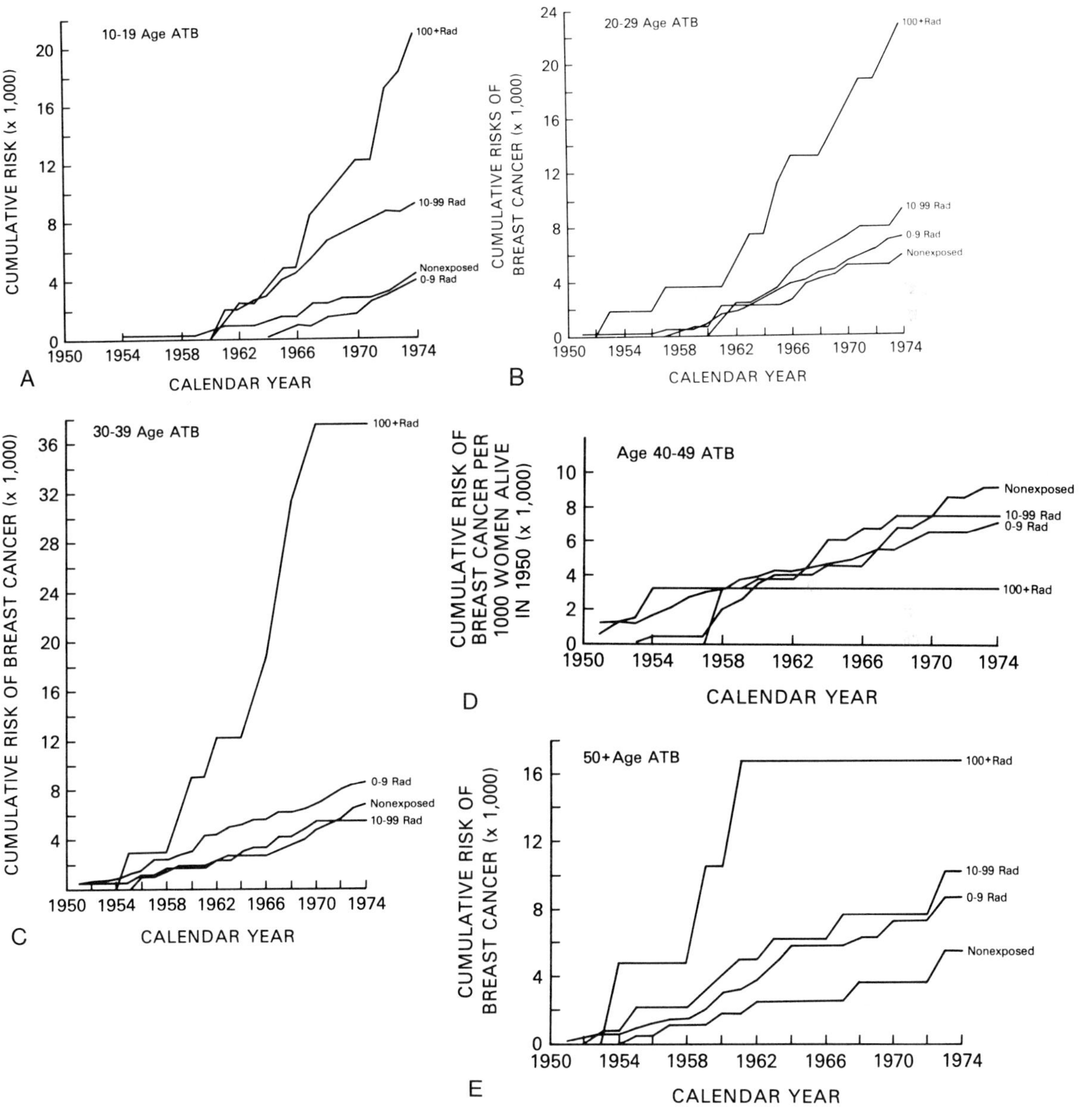

FIGURE 6–28. Cumulative probability of development of breast cancer in women exposed to the atomic bombs at Hiroshima and Nagasaki over calendar time by radiation dose class. *A*, Ten to 19 years old at time of the bomb (ATB). *B*, Twenty to 29 years old ATB. *C*, Thirty to 39 years old ATB. *D*, Forty to 49 years old ATB. *E*, Fifty years old or more ATB. (With permission from Tokunaga M, et al.: Malignant breast tumors among atomic bomb survivors, Hiroshima and Nagasaki, 1950–74. J Natl Cancer Inst 62:1347, 1979.)

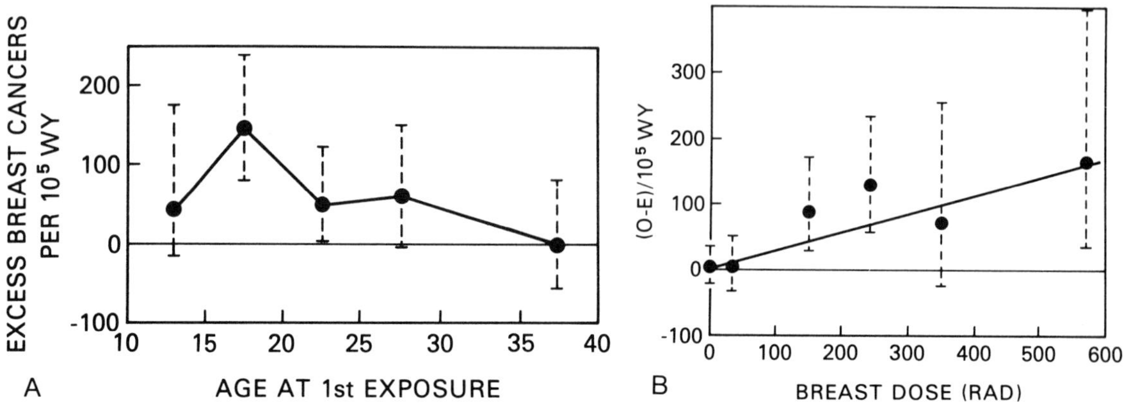

FIGURE 6–29. Excess breast cancer in women exposed to multiple chest fluoroscopies per 100,000 WY at risk; 80 percent confidence limits are presented. *A*, By age at first exposure. *B*, By estimated average dose to breast. Best fitting least-squares line presented (O-E, Observed-expected). (With permission from Boice JD, Manson RR: Breast cancer in women after repeated fluoroscopic examinations of the chest. J Natl Cancer Inst 59:823, 1977.)

groups were comparable, except for the severity of tuberculosis (which was worse in the fluoroscopically treated patients) and, of course, the therapy administered. Breast cancer risk factors, including family history, previous benign breast disease, and parity, were equivalent between the two groups. Six percent of the identified patient population could not be traced. The ratio of observed to expected cases in the exposed persons was 1.76, in contrast with an O/E ratio in the nonexposed patients of 1.06. Risk was related to age at exposure (Fig. 6–29*A*) and was highest in patients exposed before the age of 30. Incidences also appeared to be directly related to the estimated dose received, as shown in Figure 6–29*B*. There was no correlation with the side of the pneumothorax and the breast developing cancer. (Standard practice involved scanning both lungs, using fully opened shutters; thus both breasts were exposed.) Interestingly, the excessive breast-cancer risk was apparent only after 15 years of observation.

Information is available from the M. D. Anderson Memorial Hospital comparing the incidence of contralateral breast cancer in patients with early stage breast cancer treated with surgery alone versus surgery with postoperative irradiation.[44] Data are shown in Table 6–20. Although the techniques used for postoperative radiation therapy after mastectomy were somewhat variable, they are very similar to the techniques used in the treatment of the intact breast. The scatter dose to the opposite breast would be expected to be virtually equivalent. As can be seen from examination of these data, an excessive incidence of contralateral breast cancer in irradiated patients has not been detected.

In summary, theoretic concern remains about the induction of contralateral breast cancer in patients treated with comprehensive radiation therapy. This risk, if real, is probably too small to detect, except in the follow-up of enormous numbers of patients. The median age of breast cancer patients is 50, and even the theoretic risk in this patient population would be minute. It is perhaps of more concern in very young patients, particularly those younger than 30 at diagnosis, since their theoretic risk is higher and their life expectancy may allow for expression of breast cancer induction.

TABLE 6–20. Consecutive Bilateral Breast Cancer: Incidence Correlated with Treatment of the First Breast (M.D. Anderson Hospital)

Treatment	*Patients Developing Second Breast Cancer* Number	%	
Surgery only	30/409	7.3	
Peripheral lymphatic XRT	27/553	4.9	57/1673 (3.4%)
Peripheral lymphatic XRT and electron beam to chest wall	7/321	2.2	
Chest wall tangents	23/799	2.9	

Data from Montague ED, Schell SR, Romsdahl MM, et al.: Conservation surgery and irradiation in clinically favorable breast cancer. *In*: Harris JR, Hellman S, Silen W (eds.): Conservative Management of Breast Cancer. New Surgical and Radiotherapeutic Techniques. Philadelphia: J. B. Lippincott, 1983.

COSMESIS

Cosmesis is one of the most important areas, as well as the most difficult area to evaluate, in the primary radiation therapy of locoregional breast cancer. It is axiomatic that the advantage of radiation therapy over surgery is that the former can preserve a cosmetically intact breast. Several observer-based cosmesis scales have been employed to evaluate treatment outcome and to identify factors that may contribute to achieving excellent cosmesis. Two of the most widely used are shown in Table 6–21.[58] Like all subjective measurements, assessments may be quite variable from observer to observer. Assessments do not evaluate individual factors affecting cosmetic outcome but do document that modern techniques produce a "good" cosmetic outcome in the majority of patients treated. At the National Cancer Institute, in addition to a global cosmesis assessment, the author and colleagues attempt to evaluate the independent contributions of several factors. They have noted, as have others,[59] that patients tend to judge cosmetic outcome more favorably than medical observers. Factors influencing cosmesis are related to surgical techniques, radiation techniques, and patient anatomy.

There is unanimous agreement among investigators in this field that the extent of surgical resection of the primary tumor had profound influence on ultimate cosmesis.[58, 59] Although optimum local control requires total excision of gross tumor, the extent of resection beyond the gross tumor is a matter of considerable controversy. The greater the volume of tissue removed, the greater the risk of a tissue defect resulting in irreparable breast deformity, especially in patients with small breasts. In any patient, removal of excessive tissue results in distortion of breast contour and retraction of the nipple. To avoid these problems, at the National Cancer Institute the author and colleagues recommend conservative excision consisting of resection of the primary tumor and only a small, 1- to 2-cm rim of surrounding normal-appearing breast parenchyma. If there is any uncertainty concerning the possibility of residual gross tumor, the policy is to reexcise the tumor bed. The author and colleagues at the NCI believe that it is not necessary to obtain *microscopically* disease-free margins of resection, particularly since they routinely employ a radiation boost to the primary site. However, a careful preplanned excision can usually obtain pathologically free margins.[38] If extensive intraductal cancer is found in the specimen, a re-excision is recommended. Generally, the extent of excision of the primary tumor and the administration of a radiation boost to the tumor bed are complementary. When the primary tumor has been excised completely and all resection margins are free of microscopic disease (e.g., following wedge resection or quadrantectomy), a local boost of radiation is probably not necessary.[29] With more limited resections of the primary tumor, the conservative approach would include some sort of local radiation boost.

The surgical incision should be planned so that the scar is unobtrusive and does not distort breast projection or contour. The NSABP, as part of protocol B-06, has made recommendations for placement of tumorectomy incisions, shown in Figure 6–30. In planning boost treatment, it is helpful for the pathologist to ink the specimen margins and for the surgeon to place radiopaque clips at

TABLE 6–21. Two Observer-Based Cosmesis Scales Employed by Volunteers to Evaluate Photographs of Patients Treated for Breast Cancer

Scale A	*Scale B*
0 = Treated breast nearly identical to untreated breast	0 = Appearance of treated breast almost identical in size and configuration to opposite breast; no breast deformity from fibrosis or biopsy; no skin changes
1 = Treated breast slightly different from untreated breast	1 = Retraction and/or skin changes involving less than ¼ of breast
2 = Treated breast clearly different from untreated breast, but not seriously distorted	2 = Retraction and/or skin changes involving ¼ to ½ of breast
3 = Treated breast seriously distorted	3 = Deformity involving over ½ of breast

With permission from Pezner RD, Lipsett JA, Vora NL, et al.: Limited usefulness of observer-based cosmesis scales employed to evaluate patients treated conservatively for breast cancer. Int J Radiat Oncol Biol Phys 11:1117, 1985.

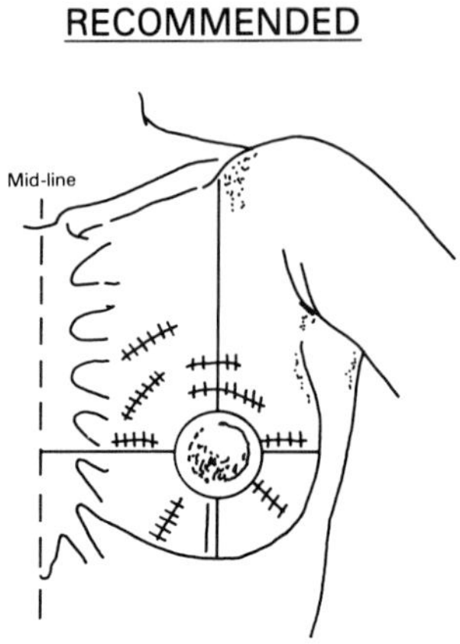

FIGURE 6–30. NSABP recommendations for placement of incisions for tumor excision. Curvilinear incisions are appropriate in all locations. (Used with permission of B. Fisher.)

the deep, superficial, and lateral margins of resection.

Surgery of the axilla also has a significant impact on breast cosmesis. The incidence of both breast and arm edema appears to be directly related to the extent of axillary dissection.[43, 60, 61] Axillary nodes can be divided anatomically into three levels, using the pectoralis minor muscle as a landmark: Level I nodes are lateral to the lateral border of the pectoralis minor muscle; Level 2 nodes are located deep to the pectoralis minor muscle; and Level 3 nodes are medial to the medial border of the pectoralis minor muscle. A complete axillary node dissection involves removal of all three node levels. Not surprisingly, more extensive removal of axillary nodes, presumably because of more extensive disruption of lymphatic channels, is accompanied by a greater incidence of edema. Additionally, to ensure complete removal of Level 3 nodes, the pectoralis minor muscle must be either removed or divided and reapproximated. When this is done, the medial pectoral nerve, which traverses the pectoralis minor muscle and innervates the lateral border of the pectoralis major muscle, must be removed. The consequent denervation atrophy of the lateral portion of the pectoralis major frequently causes noticeable asymmetry, although in the experience at the National Cancer Institute, this does not lead to impairment of arm mobility or strength. With any extent of axillary surgery, the axillary incision should be separate from the lumpectomy incision. A single incision leads to superolateral breast retraction, with undesirable distortion of breast contour.

Several anatomic features have been identified as important. Most investigators have noted that patients with large pendulous breasts frequently have a worse cosmetic outcome than do patients with smaller breasts.[58, 59] This has not been definitely correlated with dose inhomogeneities throughout the treatment volume, and the cause of this effect is unknown. A large tumor-to-breast ratio has also been associated with poorer cosmetic results.[59] Tumors in a central location, particularly in the subareolar area, may also have an inferior cosmetic outcome, since their complete excision may require removal of the nipple. However, the appearance of the natural breast following removal of the nipple or areola, or both, is cosmetically superior to breast reconstruction, and subareolar primary tumors may be successfully treated with excision plus radiation.

Numerous components of radiation technique have also been identified as influencing cosmesis. Not surprisingly, the total dose administered to the entire breast is critical in this regard,[59, 62] with the incidence of undesirable fibrosis and retraction rising sharply between total doses of 5000 and 6000 rad to the whole breast with conventional fractionation. Use of bolus is unnecessary for local tumor control, leads to undesirable pigmentary changes and telangiectasia, and should not be used. Overlap of fields, especially between the tangential and *en face* axillary supraclavicular fields, leads to severe match line fibrosis in as many as 14 percent of patients and more modest degrees of fibrosis in an even larger percentage.[43] Various techniques can eliminate this problem. Tissue compensators such as wedges are a standard part of modern treatment techniques to ensure dose homogeneity. At the National Cancer Institute, the author and associates have found that lung density corrections incorporated into the treatment plan have affected the beam modifiers used, and this correction is taken into account in all patients. For an in-depth discussion of radiation techniques, the reader is referred to Chapter 7.

Boost to the tumor bed can be applied with several techniques. Interstitial implant has been most commonly employed; electron beam boost is also frequently used; and orthovoltage or megavoltage cone-down treatment field can also be applied. One boost technique has not been shown to be definitely superior to another in terms of cosmetic outcome, and the choice between the

TABLE 6–22. Effect of Adjuvant Chemotherapy on Cosmesis

	RT Only		RT + Chemo	
Institution	No. of Patients	Good to Excellent	No. of Patients	Good to Excellent
Penn[63]	19	89%	27	81%
JCRT[64]	37	92%	40	67%
NCI	24	80%	16	70%
Palo Alto[60]	73	88%	37	73%

various methods of applying the boost is largely a matter of individual style. With careful attention to technique, the available methods are probably equivalent.

At the Joint Center for Radiation Therapy, for example, use of interstitial therapy did not significantly contribute to breast fibrosis and retraction.[59] This seems to be consistent with the general experience, although some investigators prefer to use electrons.[60] At the NCI, an interstitial boost is favored when there is probable microscopic residuum in the tumor bed and when the tumor has been located fairly deep to the surface. Larger interstitial implants involving several planes of needles predictably lead to more breast fibrosis than do smaller implants, undoubtedly because of a larger dose to a larger volume. Use of plastic spacers between the skin surface and the metal-stabilizing button decreases scatter dose from the button to the skin. For unknown reasons, the skin scars from the guide needles tend to be more prominent at the sites of needle entrance than at those of exit. Thus, with an upper outer quadrant lesion, it is recommended that the needles be placed from the side to the median plane, to avoid entrance-point scars in the neckline region.

If electrons are used, lower energies to treat more superficial lesions have been shown to give better cosmetic results.[60] The dose administered with electrons should be given using conventional rather than accelerated fractionation to avoid a localized area of subcutaneous fibrosis and skin telangiectasia. At the NCI, electrons are preferred when the tumor has been removed from an area with very little breast parenchyma, such as the very medial portions of the breast and the upper inner quadrant, and in areas directly over the ribs. Implants in these circumstances have been associated with rib fractures and myositis resulting from less breast tissue to attenuate dose to these structures.

Adjuvant chemotherapy in several standard regimens has been associated with a decrement in cosmetic outcome, although this has generally been from a decrease in the percentage of patients in the excellent cosmetic category, with their reassignment to a good cosmetic category (Table 6–22).[63, 64] Cosmesis has been observed to stabilize at two to three years after completion of therapy,[63] except in patients undergoing adjuvant chemotherapy, for whom cosmetic change seems to continue for a longer, but as yet undefined, period of time.

INTEGRATION WITH ADJUVANT CHEMOTHERAPY

The major change in the therapy of early breast cancer has been the administration of adjuvant chemotherapy, initiated in the 1970's. There are a number of important issues regarding the combination of chemotherapy with comprehensive radiation therapy. The first question that arises is whether adequate drug doses can be delivered. Bonadonna and Valagussa,[66] in a retrospective analysis, demonstrated that the effectiveness of adjuvant CMF chemotherapy was dependent upon the percentage of the drug dose delivered. Although these conclusions are controversial,[67] it is important to determine what effect, if any, primary radiation therapy has on the ability to deliver a drug.

The University of Pennsylvania group has reported on the tolerance of cyclic CMF or CMFP in 31 patients receiving primary radiation therapy.[68] Instead of decreasing drug dosage for hematopoietic toxicity, drug cycles were delayed. No significant difference was detected in the median time for completion of chemotherapy in irradiated patients versus mastectomy patients treated at the same hospital. Thirty-four of 40 patients treated with adjuvant CMF at the Joint Center for Radiation Therapy were able to receive greater than 85 percent of their prescribed drug dose.[69] No significant delay in overall treatment time was noted. Increased severity of acute skin reactions was observed in these patients, who received concurrent irradiation and chemotherapy, and there was also a suggestion of an increased incidence of clinically apparent radiation pneumonitis.

At the National Cancer Institute, adjuvant chemotherapy is administered to all node-positive patients and consists of doxorubicin, 40 mg/m^2 IV on day 1, and cyclophosphamide, 150 mg/m^2 PO on days 3 through 6. It should be noted that cyclophosphamide doses are escalated to achieve targeted myelosuppression. This practice ensures that each patient receives the maximally tolerated dose rather than an arbitrary, preset dose. When the author and colleagues at the NCI analyzed their initial cohort of patients, they noted that the total white blood count was persistently lower in irradiated patients but that this was due to lymphopenia in these women. Therefore, to avoid inappropriate drug dose reduction, they adjust the chemotherapy dosages on the basis of total granulocyte count. In their most recent analysis of 652 chemotherapy cycles (343 in mastectomy patients and 309 in irradiation patients), the median percentage dose of cyclophosphamide was 114 percent for mastectomy patients and 100 percent for irradiation patients; for doxorubicin, mastectomy patients received a median of 99 percent and irradiation patients, 97 percent, of their predicted dose.

In contrast with these reports are the findings of the group from the Stanford University Medical Center and the Palo Alto Medical Foundation. In a retrospective analysis of 42 patients undergoing either primary or postoperative irradiation compared with 42 similar patients undergoing surgery alone, the group observed that the irradiated patients received lower doses of adjuvant CMF.[70] There are several possible explanations for this observed discrepancy. Radiation is a potent lympholytic agent, and even after local radiation, lymphocyte counts may be affected for variable periods of time. Granulocyte counts are affected to a much lesser degree. Dosage modifications of chemotherapy based on total white blood count may result in inappropriate dosage reductions. Also, a major difference exists between the radiation therapy technique used at Stanford and Palo Alto and those a employed at the other institutions. Although all of these reported patients had regional lymph nodes included in the treated volume, the internal mammary nodes of the patients treated by the Stanford and Palo Alto group were irradiated with a direct *en face* internal mammary field rather than being incorporated in the breast tangents, as was done at the other institutions. Myelosuppression may be due to irradiation of the thoracic vertebral bodies with the exit dose from this field. Additionally, with use of this direct internal mammary field, virtually all the circulating blood volume is irradiated as it passes through the heart and great vessels, and the pool of circulating stem cells may be reduced as a result.

Most important, in the randomized prospective trials conducted at the National Cancer Institute in Milan[26] and the NSABP B-06 trial,[29] in which patients with positive nodes, regardless of local therapy, received adjuvant chemotherapy, no adverse effect on disease recurrence or survival rate was noted in patients undergoing irradiation. It should be noted that in these two trials, irradiated patients received therapy to the chest wall with tangential fields only. From this evidence, it is safe to conclude that primary radiation therapy can be effectively combined with aggressive adjuvant chemotherapy. It would seem prudent to avoid as much as possible the use of irradiation techniques that incorporate the thoracic vertebral bodies and mediastinal contents in the treated volume as well as to base modifications of drug dosage on total granulocyte count rather than total white blood count.

The optimal timing of irradiation and chemotherapy has not been determined. There is a suggestion from at least one study that the benefit seen from adjuvant chemotherapy is greatest when chemotherapy is given close to the time of initial surgery.[71] Additionally, although the optimal number of chemotherapy cycles is not certain, information from Milan suggests strongly that the initial cycles of chemotherapy are the most important.[72] Thus, to delay initiation of chemotherapy while local therapy is being administered may lead to a compromise in the effectiveness of systemic treatment. On the other hand, there is concern over the possibility of disease recurrence within the breast during a prolonged initial period of chemotherapy, and thus, to delay initiation of irradiation may lead to a decrease in local control. Specialists in the field are beginning to develop strategies that address both these concerns.

At the National Cancer Institute, the author and colleagues have recently modified their treatment schema to incorporate chemotherapy in the perioperative period as well as to initiate prompt irradiation. Axillary node dissection is followed in approximately one week by the first of 9 three-week cycles of doxorubicin and cyclophosphamide. Patients undergo an iridium implant to the tumor bed between Cycles 1 and 2, preceding external radiation therapy. During external beam radiation therapy, begun after Cycle 2 of chemotherapy, a third cycle of drug is started, consisting of cyclophosphamide alone. The remainder of the chemotherapy cycles consist of both drugs given in three-week cycles.

GUIDELINES FOR PATIENT TREATMENT

A number of characteristics of both the patient and the tumor should be considered in the evaluation and treatment of any individual. *Tumor size* per se, as discussed earlier, is not an important consideration, provided that the entire gross tumor mass is excised. The NCI usually recommends that patients with more than one clinically detectable tumor undergo mastectomy with breast reconstruction, since the surgical deformity induced by multiple tumor removals may severely compromise cosmetic outcome and because a better result may be obtained with complete breast reconstruction. Similarly, patients with a large tumor-to-breast ratio may also be better served with mastectomy and breast reconstruction, again because of problems with surgically induced breast deformity. Patients with large pendulous breasts may develop more retraction and fibrosis after treatment than do patients with smaller breasts, and the former patients are technically more difficult to treat. On the other hand, breast reconstruction after mastectomy is also more difficult in these patients. Some radiotherapists prefer not to treat patients with tumors in a subareolar location, since tumor excision usually requires removal of the nipple, which certainly compromises cosmesis. Nonetheless, an individual patient may find the cosmetic deficit from nipple removal preferable to breast amputation and reconstruction, and artistically applied tattooing or nipple-areola reconstruction can correct much of the defect.

It is essential that patients undergo bilateral mammography prior to initiation of radiation therapy. The identification of diffuse, suspicious-looking breast microcalcifications is a relative contraindication to primary radiation therapy, since this finding may indicate substantial amounts of tumor diffusely infiltrating breast parenchyma. One would expect a higher incidence of local failure with primary radiation therapy in the presence of this finding, although this has not been demonstrated conclusively. If a patient with these characteristics strongly desires breast conservation therapy, this can be considered, with mastectomy reserved for salvage treatment of local failure. In such circumstances, it is important that the patient be aware of her potential increased risk for local recurrence, be instructed in good breast self-examination techniques, and be available for close follow-up. Furthermore, if microcalcifications are left behind prior to radiation treatment, the usefulness of this roentgenographic sign for follow-up purposes is negated. It is difficult, if not impossible, to count whether there are more or fewer punctate microcalcifications on serial mammograms, and thus, one of the most sensitive indicators of recurrence is rendered useless. The breast should be cleared of all suspicious microcalcifications prior to treatment. If this is not possible, mastectomy is preferable.

Other characteristics of a more general nature are also important. Primary radiation therapy requires daily outpatient visits for treatment for five to six weeks, and a short hospital stay if an iridium implant is performed, all of which may be unacceptably inconvenient for a particular individual. Psychologically, some patients prefer the physical certainty of surgical removal. Age of the patient is not generally a major consideration. Many older patients prefer to undergo breast-conserving therapy when offered this option. In very young patients, particularly those under the age of 25, a careful explanation of risks versus benefits is especially important.

Management of the Axilla

The decision of how to manage the axilla should be based on the importance of several factors in the individual patient and a careful balance of the risks and benefits of various procedures. Treatment options are extraordinarily diverse and include surgery, ranging from complete axillary node dissection to limited node sampling or biopsy; radiation therapy to the axilla; combinations of radiation therapy and surgery; and no axillary intervention at all. Obviously, the toxicities of treatment are as variable as the treatment methods, and these toxicities must be weighed against the advantages of the various options. This is particularly true in the case of the clinically negative axilla.

Therapy directed at the axilla performs several functions. For many years, heated arguments raged concerning the necessity of treating effectively all of the regional lymph nodes, since such prophylactic treatment was thought to improve patient survival. Randomized prospective trials have failed to demonstrate a survival benefit from prophylactic node treatment in any subgroup of early breast cancer patients. Veronesi,[73] from the Tumor Institute of Milan, published results of a trial comparing patients treated with radical mastectomy (which included *en bloc* axillary node dissection) versus extended radical mastectomy (which, in addition to *en bloc* axillary node dissection, also included *en bloc* resection of the ipsilateral internal mammary lymph nodes), which failed to show a benefit from treatment of the internal mammary lymph nodes. The NSABP B-04 study randomly selected patients with clinically negative axillae to receive, in addition to total mastectomy, axillary node dissection, axillary node irradiation, or no axillary node treatment.[74] At ten years, there was no difference in survival rate between these groups. This is not the place for a detailed discussion of this issue, but such evidence indicates that prophylactic node treatment is unlikely to have a significant impact on patient survival rates. Even if survival is unlikely to be affected by node treatment, uncontrolled tumor growth in the axilla, with consequent arm edema, pain, and brachial plexopathy, is to be scrupulously avoided. Likewise, undesirable consequences of treatment, especially treatment administered prophylactically, must be minimized.

Patients with clinically positive axillary lymph nodes require treatment to achieve local tumor control. Although radiation therapy can be used in this circumstance, the presence of gross axillary nodal disease requires high doses, and permanent tumor control in these circumstances is not a certainty. Therefore, with a clinically positive axilla, the NCI recommends that patients undergo complete axillary node dissection. Following such surgery, postoperative irradiation of the axilla should be avoided, except in the very rare circumstance of extension of the tumor outside the capsule of the lymph nodes and into the axillary fat and the presence of an extremely high number (20 or more) of positive axillary nodes. A small field that is limited to the ipsilateral supraclavicular triangle can be added after full axillary node dissection, without increase in treatment-related morbidity, and will decrease the incidence of tumor recurrence in this site. The information obtained from pathologic examination of the removed lymph nodes can be used for determination of patient prognosis and of administration of appropriate systemic therapy.

The issues in the patient with a clinically negative axilla become much more complex. If the pathologic status of the axillary lymph nodes will determine systemic treatment, intervention to determine this status is necessary. The only available method of determination is pathologic examination. Options for various procedures are shown in Table 6–23. If it is essential to identify with absolute certainty a patient's pathologic node status, a complete axillary dissection encompassing axillary node Levels I, II, and III is necessary. A more limited axillary dissection, involving removal of Levels I and II, will not identify the very small group of patients with early breast cancer who have skip metastases to Level III lymph nodes, with negative lymph nodes at Levels I and II. The complete axillary dissection specimens of 136 patients from the NCI early breast cancer study have been analyzed by axillary node level. Sixty-five patients had pathologically positive lymph nodes, but only two patients had pathologically positive lymph nodes at Level III concurrent with negative nodes at Levels I and II. These data indicate that removal of Levels I and II lymph nodes provides an accurate pathologic assessment of axillary lymph nodes and is incorrect in less than 2 percent (2 of 136) of patients (Table 6–24).[75] Since this procedure does not require removal of the medial pectoral nerve, it probably results in a lesser incidence of arm edema, while obtaining virtually the same information as a complete axillary dissection. In most situations, it is the treatment of choice. Axillary

TABLE 6–23. Management Options for Clinically Negative Axilla

Treatment	*Advantages*	*Disadvantages*
None	No treatment-related morbidity May require subsequent therapy for regional tumor control (approximately 20% of patients)	Cannot determine pathologic node status
Complete axillary dissection (Levels I, II, and III)	Most accurate method to assess pathologic node status (Levels I, II, and III) Effective local tumor control, without need for postoperative radiation therapy, except in rare circumstances	Increased risk (10 to 20%) of arm and/or breast edema Removal of medial pectoral nerve leads to denervation of lateral border of pectoralis major muscle and obvious asymmetry Axillary anesthesia, usually permanent Tissue removal leads to cosmetic defect Requires postoperative physical therapy to assure functional range of motion
Limited axillary dissection (Levels I and II)	Does not require removal of medial pectoral nerve A lesser incidence of arm/breast edema than with complete dissection Less cosmetic deformity than with complete dissection	Will not identify patients with skip metastases to Level III lymph nodes In patients with positive nodes, may not identify all patients with 4 or more positive lymph nodes If nodes are positive, axillary radiation therapy is usually recommended for local tumor control but may increase the incidence of arm and breast edema.
Axillary node biopsy	Little or no treatment-related morbidity	Unable to identify reliably patients with positive nodes (approximately 15 to 30% false-negative rate)
Radiation therapy	Effective permanent control of regional disease Avoids surgical deformity Less arm/breast edema than with surgical dissection (approximately 4%) Does not require posttreatment physical therapy for functional range of motion, except in very rare circumstances	Unable to determine pathologic node status Technically difficult treatment (matching fields with breast tangents)

TABLE 6–24. Axillary Node Positivity by Node Level

Level(s) with Positive Nodes	*All Patients (n = 136)*			*Clinical N_0 (n = 109)*	*Clinical N_1 (n = 27)*
I only	20			15	5
I and II	13	46 (I only through I, II, and III)		6	7
I and III	1			0	1
I, II, and III	12		63 (I only through II and III)	5	7
II only	14			13	1
II and III	3			1	2
III only	2			1	1
Total all levels	65			41	25

Data from Danforth DN, Jr., Findlay PA, McDonald HD, et al.: Complete axillary node dissection for stages I–II carcinoma of the breast. J Clin Oncol 4:655, 1986.

node biopsy or limited node samplings will lead to false-negative results in an estimated 15 to 30 percent of patients depending on other clinical characteristics. Radiation therapy to the clinically negative axilla is capable of achieving excellent permanent tumor control,[74] with a low incidence of treatment-related morbidity (brachial plexopathy, less than 1 percent; arm edema, approximately 4 percent; radiation pneumonitis, approximately 2 percent).[35, 75–77] Match line fibrosis can be virtually eliminated with use of appropriate matching techniques. The disadvantage of using radiation therapy in this circumstance is that pathologic node status is undetermined. As stated, if determination of pathologic node status is not important for determination of systemic therapy, radiation therapy is a viable treatment option in an individual patient. Treatment of the breast alone without axillary surgery or irradiation is also an alternative, but patients have about a 20 percent risk of needing subsequent axillary treatment for control of later-appearing clinically positive nodes.[74]

PATIENT FOLLOW-UP AFTER PRIMARY IRRADIATION

Physical Examination

The principles of examination of the treated breast are virtually identical with those of the standard breast examination. Since certain breast changes are expected to evolve over time, it is extremely important that examination be performed in a consistent manner and that findings be documented in the patient record. Diagrams are very helpful, in addition to written descriptions.

In the region of the tumor bed, changes related to surgical excision of the primary tumor are common. If the breast tissue has not been approximated, there may be a defect in this area from lack of tissue. Occasionally, tissue adjacent to this defect may feel firm by comparison, leading to the false impression of a mass. Induration in the excision site is not unusual and is attributed to a combination of surgical scarring and localized radiation-related change from a boost dose, especially if the boost has been delivered with an interstitial implant.

Changes in the breast parenchyma are usually fairly subtle. With modern techniques, it is rare to see breast fibrosis and retraction. The texture of the treated breast may be somewhat firmer than that of the untreated breast, particularly in large-breasted women. Cystic changes are often improved. Especially if the patient has undergone a complete axillary dissection, some amount of breast edema may be present. This usually appears about four to six months after treatment and may improve slowly over ensuing months. Again, this finding is more common in large-breasted women.

In the skin, subtle pigmentary changes can sometimes be seen, both hyperpigmentation and depigmentation, particularly in the areola and nipple. Peau d'orange, especially in the dependent portions of the breast, frequently appears. As is the case with parenchymal breast edema, onset is usually about four to six months after treatment. Telangiectasias may appear in the region of the tumor bed after one or two years, particularly if interstitial sources were positioned too close to the skin. Similar changes can be seen in the skin following an electron boost, especially if accelerated fractionation was used. In this situation, the skin changes tend to be outlined by the boundaries of the electron field.

Unfortunately, some patients will develop recurrent tumor in the treated breast. The physical findings in such circumstances will be virtually identical with those seen in patients not having received previous radiation treatment.[78] With the presence of a new, enlarging, or changing mass either in the original tumor bed or elsewhere in the breast, mammographic examination and biopsy as appropriate are recommended.

Mammography

The mammographic appearance of the treated breast, like the results of physical examination, can be confusing, particularly in the area of the primary site.[79, 80] Obviously, changes in the physical aspect of the breast over time (for example, the occurrence of peau d'orange) are reflected in the mammographic appearance. Virtually all patients will have obvious distortion in the region of the tumor bed, related to both the surgical excision and the use of a radiation boost. Importantly, this distortion remains very stable over time, which distinguishes it from recurrent tumor. Generally, no marked changes that are noticeable in the breast parenchyma itself can be attributed to radiation.

Calcium deposition in the breast does change after treatment and generally can be fitted into one of three categories.[81] The first is disappearance of fine calcifications in the first several months and up to a year following treatment. This has been postulated to reflect eradication of residual microscopic or noninvasive disease or to signify improvement in fibrocystic mammopathy. The second category is the appearance of coarse calcifications, usually in the area of the tumor bed. These are especially likely to appear if an interstitial implant has been employed as a boost. These large, coarse calcifications are treatment related and should not cause alarm. The third category of calcium deposition is the appearance of new clustered microcalcifications. These are very suggestive of malignancy and should prompt biopsy.

REFERENCES

1. Keynes G: The treatment of primary carcinoma of the breast with radium. Acta Radiol 10:393, 1929.
2. Baclesse F: Roentgen therapy as the sole method of treatment of cancer of the breast. Am J Roentgenol Radium Ther Nucl Med 62:311, 1949.
3. Halsted WS: The results of radical operations for the cure of carcinoma of the breast. Ann Surg 46:1, 1907.
4. Fisher B: Surgical adjuvant therapy for breast cancer. Cancer 30:1556, 1972.
5. Rutqvist LE, Wallgren A: Long-term survival of 458 young breast cancer patients. Cancer 55:658, 1985.
6. Roth D, Bayat H: The role of residual tumor in the chest wall in the late dissemination of mammary cancer. Ann Surg 168:887, 1968.
7. Keynes G: The radium treatment of carcinoma of the breast. Br J Surg 19:415, 1932.
8. Keynes G: Conservative treatment of cancer of the breast. Br Med J, 1937, pp. 643–647.
9. Keynes G: Breast cancer: A case for conservation. (Letter to the editor) Br Med J 282:1392, 1981.
10. Ward R: Inoperable carcinoma of the breast treated with radium. Br Med J, 1929, pp. 242–244.
11. Cheatle GL: A lecture on treatment of mammary carcinoma by radiation. Br Med J, 1930, pp. 807–811.
12. Mustakallio S: Conservative treatment of breast carcinoma—review of 25 years of follow-up. Clin Radiol 23:110, 1972.
13. Peters MV: Cutting the "Gordian Knot" in early breast cancer. Ann R Coll Phys Surg Can 8:186, 1975.
14. Peters MV: Wedge resection with or without radiation in early breast cancer. Int J Radiat Oncol Biol Phys 2:1151, 1977.
15. Calle R, Vilcoq JR, Pilleron JP, et al.: Conservative treatment of operable breast carcinoma by irradiation with or without limited surgery—10-year results. *In:* Harris JR, Hellman S, Silen W (eds.): Conservative Management of Breast Cancer. New Surgical and Radiotherapeutic Techniques. Philadelphia: J.B. Lippincott, 1983, pp. 3–9.
16. Pierquin B: Conservative treatment for carcinoma of the breast: Experience of Creteil—ten-year results. *In:* Harris JR, Hellman S, Silen W (eds.): Conservative Management of Breast Cancer. New Surgical and Radiotherapeutic Techniques. Philadelphia: J.B. Lippincott, 1983, pp. 11–14.
17. Pierquin B, Owens R, Maylin C, et al.: Radical radiation therapy of breast cancer. Int J Radiat Oncol Biol Phys 6:17, 1980.
18. Amalric RE, Santamaria F, Robert F, et al.: Conservative therapy of operable breast cancer—results at five, ten, and fifteen years in 2216 consecutive cases. *In:* Harris JR, Hellman S, Silen W (eds.): Conservative Management of Breast Cancer. New Surgical and Radiotherapeutic Techniques. Philadelphia: J.B. Lippincott, 1983, pp. 15–21.
19. Clark RM: Alternatives to mastectomy—The Princess Margaret Hospital experience. *In:* Harris JR, Hellman S, Silen W (eds.): Conservative Management of Breast Cancer. New Surgical and Radiotherapeutic Techniques. Philadelphia: J.B. Lippincott, 1983, pp. 35–46.
20. Prosnitz LR, Goldenberg IS, Packard RA, et al.: Radiation therapy as initial treatment for early stage cancer of the breast without mastectomy. Cancer 39:917, 1977.
21. Harris JR, Hellman S: The results of primary radiation therapy for early breast cancer at the Joint Center for Radiation Therapy. *In:* Harris JR, Hellman S, Silen W (eds.): Conservative Management of Breast Cancer. New Surgical and Radiotherapeutic Techniques. Philadelphia: J.B. Lippincott, 1983, pp. 47–52.
22. Montague ED: Conservative surgery and radiation therapy in the treatment of operable breast cancer. Cancer 53:700, 1984.
23. Danoff BF, Goodman RL: Excisional biopsy, axillary node dissection and definitive radiotherapy for stage I and II breast cancer. (Abstract) Int J Radiat Oncol Biol Phys 9:113, 1983.
24. Prosnitz LR, Goldenberg IS, Weshler Z, et al.: Radiotherapy instead of mastectomy for breast cancer—the Yale experience. *In:* Harris JR, Hellman S, Silen W (eds.): Conservative Management of Breast Cancer. New Surgical and Radiotherapeutic Techniques. Philadelphia: J.B. Lippincott, 1983, pp. 61–70.
25. Hayward J: The Guy's Hospital trials on breast conservation. *In:* Harris JR, Hellman S, Silen W (eds.): Conservative Management of Breast Cancer. New Surgical and Radiotherapeutic Techniques. Philadelphia: J.B. Lippincott, 1983, pp. 77–90.
26. Veronesi U, Saccozzi R, Del Vecchio M, et al.: Comparing radical mastectomy with quadrantectomy, axillary dissection, and radiotherapy in patients with small cancers of the breast. N Engl J Med 305:6, 1981.
27. Veronesi U, Del Vecchio M, Greco M, et al.: Results of quadrantectomy, axillary dissection, and radiotherapy (QUART) in T1N0 patients. *In:* Harris JR, Hellman S, Silen W (eds.): Conservative Management of Breast Cancer. New Surgical and Radio-

therapeutic Techniques. Philadelphia: J.B. Lippincott, 1983, pp. 91–99.
28. Sarrazin D, Le M, Rouesse J, et al.: Conservative treatment versus mastectomy in breast cancer tumors with macroscopic diameter of 20 millimeters or less. Cancer 53:1209, 1984.
29. Fisher B, Bauer M, Margolese R, et al.: Five-year results of a randomized clinical trial comparing total mastectomy and segmental mastectomy with or without radiation in the treatment of breast cancer. N Engl J Med 312:665, 1985.
30. Findlay PA, Lippman ME, Danforth D, Jr., et al.: Mastectomy vs. radiotherapy as treatment for stage I–II breast cancer: A prospective randomized trial at the National Cancer Institute. World J Surg 9:671, 1985.
31. Holland R, Veling SHJ, Mravunac M, et al.: Histologic multifocality of Tis, T1–2 breast carcinomas. Implications for clinical trials of breast-conserving surgery. Cancer 56:979, 1985.
32. Greening WP, Montgomery AC, Gowing NF: Report on pilot study of treatment of breast cancer by quadrantic excision with an axillary dissection and no other therapy. J R Soc Med 71:261, 1978.
33. Tagart REB: Partial mastectomy for breast cancer. Br Med J 2:1268, 1978.
34. Lagios MD, Richards VE, Rose MR, et al.: Segmental mastectomy without radiotherapy: Short-term follow-up. Cancer 52:2173, 1983.
35. Recht A, Silver B, Schnitt S, et al.: Breast relapse following primary radiation therapy for early breast cancer. I. Classification, frequency, and salvage. Int J Radiat Oncol Biol Phys 11:1271, 1985.
36. Chu AM, Cope O, Russo R, et al.: Patterns of locoregional recurrence and results in stages I and II breast cancer treated by irradiation following limited surgery, an update. Am J Clin Oncol 7:221, 1984.
37. Pierquin B, Otmezguine Y, Lobo PA: Conservative management of breast carcinoma: The Creteil experience. Acta Radiol (Oncol) 22:101, 1983.
38. Fisher B: Reappraisal of breast biopsy prompted by the use of lumpectomy. JAMA 253:24, 1985.
39. Harris JR, Connolly JL, Schnitt SJ, et al.: Clinical-pathologic study of early breast cancer treated by primary radiation therapy. J Clin Oncol 1:184, 1983.
40. Bataini JP, Picco C, Martin M, et al.: Relation between time-dose and local control of operable breast cancer treated by tumorectomy and radical radiotherapy or by radical radiotherapy alone. Cancer 42:2059, 1978.
41. Schnitt SJ, Connolly JL, Harris JR, et al: Pathologic prediction of early local recurrence in stage I and II breast cancer treated by primary radiation therapy. Cancer 53:1049, 1984.
42. Harris JR, Recht A, Amalric R, et al.: Time course and prognosis of local recurrence following primary radiation therapy for early breast cancer. J Clin Oncol 2:37, 1984.
43. Ray GR, Fish VJ, Lee RH, et al.: Biopsy and definitive radiation therapy in stages I and II carcinoma of the female breast. Int J Radiat Oncol Biol Phys 9:23, 1983.
44. Montague ED, Schell SR, Romsdahl MM, et al.: Conservation surgery and irradiation in clinically favorable breast cancer. *In:* Harris JR, Hellman S, Silen W (eds.): Conservative Management of Breast Cancer. New Surgical and Radiotherapeutic Techniques. Philadelphia: J.B. Lippincott, 1983, pp. 53–60.
45. Beebe GW, Kato H, Land CE: Studies of the mortality of A-bomb survivors. Radiat Res 75:138, 1978.
46. March HC: Leukemia in radiologists, ten years later. Am J Med Sci 242:137, 1961.
47. Court-Brown WM, Doll R: Mortality from cancer and other causes after radiotherapy for ankylosing spondylitis. Br Med J 2:1327, 1965.
48. Doll R, Smith PG: The long-term effects of x-irradiation in patients treated for metropathia haemmorrhagica. Br J Radiol 41:362, 1968.
49. Smith PG: Leukemia and other cancers following radiation treatment of pelvic disease. Cancer 39:1901, 1977.
50. Rosner F, Carey RW, Zarrabi MH: Breast cancer and acute leukemia: Report of 24 cases and review of the literature. Am J Hematol 4:151, 1978.
51. Curtis RE, Hankey BF, Myers MH, et al.: Risk of leukemia associated with the first course of cancer treatment: An analysis of the Surveillance, Epidemiology, and End Results Program experience. J Natl Cancer Inst 72:531, 1984.
52. Fisher B, Rockette H, Fisher E, et al.: Leukemia in breast cancer patients following adjuvant chemotherapy or postoperative radiation: The NSABP experience. J Clin Oncol 3:1640, 1985.
53. McCredie JA, Inch WR, Alderson M: Consecutive primary carcinomas of the breast. Cancer 35:1472, 1975.
54. Shore RE, Hempelmann LH, Kowaluk E, et al.: Breast neoplasms in women treated with x-rays for acute postpartum mastitis. J Natl Cancer Inst 59:813, 1977.
55. Baral E, Larsson LE, Mattsson B: Breast cancer following irradiation of the breast. Cancer 40:2905, 1977.
56. Tokunaga M, Norman JE, Jr., Asano M, et al.: Malignant breast tumors among atomic bomb survivors, Hiroshima and Nagasaki, 1950–74. J Natl Cancer Inst 62:1347, 1979.
57. Boice JD, Monson RR: Breast cancer in women after repeated fluoroscopic examinations of the chest. J Natl Cancer Inst 59:823, 1977.
58. Pezner RD, Lipsett JA, Vora NL, et al.: Limited usefulness of observer-based cosmesis scales employed to evaluate patients treated conservatively for breast cancer. Int J Radiat Oncol Biol Phys 11:1117, 1985.
59. Harris JR, Levene MB, Svensson G, et al.: Analysis of cosmetic results following primary radiation therapy for stages I and II carcinoma of the breast. Int J Radiat Oncol Biol Phys 5:257, 1979.
60. Ray GR, Fish VJ: Biopsy and definitive radiation therapy in stage I and II adenocarcinoma of the female breast: Analysis of cosmesis and the role of electron beam supplementation. Int J Radiat Oncol Biol Phys 9:813, 1983.
61. Rose CM, Botnick LE, Weinstein M, et al.: Axillary sampling in the definitive treatment of breast cancer by radiation therapy and lumpectomy. Int J Radiat Oncol Biol Phys 9:339, 1983.
62. Spanos WJ, Montague ED, Fletcher GH: Late complications of radiation only for advanced breast cancer. Int J Radiat Oncol Biol Phys 6:1473, 1980.
63. Danoff BF, Goodman RL, Glick JH, et al.: The effect of adjuvant chemotherapy on cosmesis and complications in patients with breast cancer treated by definitive irradiation. Int J Radiat Oncol Biol Phys 9:1625, 1983.
64. Beadle GF, Come S, Henderson IC, et al.: The effect

of adjuvant chemotherapy on the cosmetic results after primary radiation treatment for early stage breast cancer. Int J Radiat Oncol Biol Phys 10:2131, 1984.

65. Pierquin B, Baillet F, Wilson JF: Radiation therapy in the management of primary breast cancer. Am J Roentgenol 127:645, 1976.
66. Bonadonna G, Valagussa P: Dose-response effect of adjuvant chemotherapy in breast cancer. N Engl J Med 304:10, 1981.
67. Redmond C, Fisher B, Wieand HS: The methodologic dilemma in retrospectively correlating the amount of chemotherapy received in adjuvant therapy protocols with disease-free survival. Cancer Treat Rep 67:519, 1983.
68. Glick JH, Danoff BF, Haller DG, et al.: Adjuvant chemotherapy in patients undergoing definitive irradiation for primary breast cancer—The University of Pennsylvania experience. *In:* Harris JR, Hellman S, Silen W (eds.): Conservative Management of Breast Cancer. New Surgical and Radiotherapeutic Techniques. Philadelphia: J.B. Lippincott, 1983, pp. 311–320.
69. Botnick LE, Come S, Rose CM, et al.: Primary breast irradiation and concomitant adjuvant chemotherapy. *In:* Harris JR, Hellman S, Silen W (eds.): Conservative Management of Breast Cancer. New Surgical and Radiotherapeutic Techniques. Philadelphia: J.B. Lippincott, 1983, pp. 321–328.
70. Levine JF, Coleman CN, Cox RS, et al.: The effect of postoperative and primary radiation therapy on delivered dose of adjuvant cyclophosphamide, methotrexate and 5-fluorouracil (CMF) chemotherapy in breast cancer. Cancer 53:237, 1984.
71. Nissen-Meyer R: One short chemotherapy course in primary breast cancer: 12-Year follow-up in series 1 of the Scandinavian Adjuvant Chemotherapy Study Group. *In:* Jones SE, Salmon SE (eds.): Adjuvant Therapy of Cancer II. New York: Grune & Stratton, 1979, pp. 207–213.
72. Tancini G, Bonadonna G, Valagussa P, et al.: Adjuvant CMF in breast cancer: Comparative 5-year results of 12 vs. 6 cycles. J Clin Oncol 1:2, 1983.
73. Veronesi U, Valagussa P: Inefficacy of internal mammary nodes dissection in breast cancer surgery. Cancer 47:170, 1981.
74. Fisher B, Redmond C, Fisher E, et al.: Ten-year results of a randomized clinical trial comparing radical mastectomy and total mastectomy with or without radiation. N Engl J Med 312:674, 1985.
75. Danforth DN, Jr., Findlay PA, McDonald HD, et al.: Complete axillary node dissection for stage I–II carcinoma of the breast. J Clin Oncol 4:655, 1986.
76. Amalric R, Santamaria F, Robert F, et al.: Radiation therapy with or without primary limited surgery for operable breast cancer: A 20-year experience at the Marseilles Cancer Institute. Cancer 49:30, 1982.
77. Calle R, Pilleron JP, Schlienger P, et al.: Conservative management of operable breast cancer: Ten years experience at the Foundation Curie. Cancer 42:2045, 1978.
78. Schnitt SJ, Connolly JL, Recht A, et al.: Breast relapse following primary radiation therapy for early breast cancer. II. Detection, pathologic features, and prognostic significance. Int J Radiat Oncol Biol Phys 11:1277, 1985.
79. Bloomer WD, Berenberg AL, Waissman BN: Mammography of the definitively irradiated breast. Radiology 118:425, 1976.
80. Paulus DD, Libschitz HL, Montague ED: Malignant masses in the therapeutically irradiated breast. AJR 135:789, 1980.
81. Libschitz HI, Montague ED, Paulus DD: Calcifications and the therapeutically irradiated breast. AJR 128:1021, 1977.

Technical Aspects of the Treatment of Breast Cancer with Radiation Therapy

ALLEN S. LICHTER, M.D.

Radiation therapy can be used in a variety of ways in the treatment of breast cancer (Table 7–1). Radiation therapy is commonly employed to treat metastatic breast cancer, most frequently in bone or the central nervous system.[1] Techniques for treatment of bone or brain metastases are the same for virtually all metastatic cancers, regardless of their tissue of origin, and will not be discussed here. Unique to radiation therapy for breast cancer is the necessity of treating the intact breast, either preoperatively (to permit or improve surgical therapy) or following local excision of a breast tumor (as definitive treatment). Another unique application of radiation therapy in breast cancer management is the treatment of the postmastectomy chest wall. It is these latter two techniques that will be discussed in detail in this chapter. Technical advances in the quality of radiation therapy equipment, including linear accelerators, simulators, treatment planning computers, and CT scanners, have made the treatment of the intact breast or chest wall a technically demanding and challenging exercise for the radiation therapist.

RADIATION THERAPY FOR THE INTACT BREAST

Areas at Risk

In the treatment of the intact breast, the breast itself and the three major nodal areas—axillary, supraclavicular, and internal mammary—compose the areas at risk. However, the necessity or desirability of treating some or all of the regional nodal areas remains controversial. It is generally acknowledged that axillary recurrence following a full axillary dissection is an uncommon event, occurring in 1 percent or less of axillae at risk.[2] Therefore,

7

TABLE 7–1. Role of Radiation Therapy in Breast Cancer

Preoperative—usually borderline or inoperable tumors
Postoperative
Definitive
Palliative

if a full axillary dissection has been performed, there is no need to irradiate this region, unless gross tumor has been left behind or tumor has spread beyond the confines of the nodes into axillary fat. A more difficult decision concerns the need to irradiate the axilla in patients who have had only an axillary "sampling." In a recent NSABP study, there were no axillary recurrences following surgery alone if more than six nodes were removed from the axilla as part of a total mastectomy.[2] Similarly, data from the University of Pennsylvania support the contention that radiation can be safely omitted following an axillary operation that is less than a full dissection.[3] The best available data suggest that the use of a Level I and a Level II axillary dissection will accurately determine nodal status in the vast majority of cases and eliminate the need for radiation treatment to the axilla.

The supraclavicular nodes are generally treated only if the axilla is positive.[4] When the axilla is negative, recurrence in the supraclavicular nodes is rare. With axillary node positivity, the incidence of recurrence in the supraclavicular fossa at some time during the patient's illness approaches 25 percent[4] and can be reduced to less than 5 percent through the use of radiation to that area.

Treatment of the internal mammary lymph nodes is also somewhat controversial. The incidence of biopsy-proven internal mammary lymph node involvement is directly related to the location of the primary tumor and to the status of the axillary lymph nodes.[5] When the tumor is laterally located and the axilla is negative, the frequency of internal mammary involvement is approximately 5 percent, and such patients can have the internal mammary lymph node region safely excluded from the treatment volume. However, the incidence of internal mammary positivity jumps to approximately 20 percent for inner quadrant tumors with a negative axilla or outer quadrant tumors with a positive axilla. Internal mammary node involvement increases to 40 percent in women whose tumors are located in the inner quadrant and who have positive axillary lymph nodes. The aforementioned considerations formed the basis of the guidelines for areas at risk for irradiation of the intact breast presented in Figure 7–1.[6] These guidelines are dependent upon a good axillary dissection that captures lymph nodes at Levels I and II at a minimum. With a low axillary sampling obtaining only a few lymph nodes, axillary involvement may be missed in 10 to 20 percent of patients,[7, 8] making these guidelines difficult to employ.

REGIONS TREATED IN PRIMARY BREAST IRRADIATION

QUADRANT OF PRIMARY	HISTOLOGY OF NODES FOLLOWING AXILLARY DISSECTION	
	NEGATIVE	POSITIVE
LATERAL	BREAST ONLY	BREAST PLUS INTERNAL MAMMARY AND SUPRACLAVICULAR NODES
MEDIAL	BREAST PLUS INTERNAL MAMMARY NODES	BREAST PLUS INTERNAL MAMMARY AND SUPRACLAVICULAR NODES

FIGURE 7–1. Regions to be treated in primary breast irradiation.

Goals of Radiation Therapy

Obviously, the primary goal of irradiation of the intact breast is to sterilize all tumor cells within the treatment volume. Equally important is the ability to reliably accomplish this task with a minimum of complications and maximum preservation of cosmesis. Thus, the goals listed in Table 7–2 come into play. First, as in all radiation therapy that is to be taken to high curative doses, the irradiation should be as homogeneous as possible. The maximum tumor dose should be kept within 10 percent of the target volume dose to ensure a minimum of long-term com-

TABLE 7–2. Goals of Treatment in Definitive Breast Irradiation

Deliver homogeneous dose to target volume (± 5%)
Treat minimum amount of lung
Spare mediastinum
Treat internal mammary nodes
Avoid overlap or underlap of adjacent fields
Achieve easily reproducible, rapid setup

plications. As will be pointed out in the section on CT scanning, failure to appreciate the importance of lung density in radiation therapy treatment planning makes achieving the goal of 10 percent maximum dose extremely difficult. The need for homogeneous irradiation also implies that irradiation of the intact breast be done in a customized manner for each patient. Contours should be obtained and isodose curves plotted for each individual case.

A second goal of treatment is to spare normal uninvolved tissue as much as possible. The two major areas to be spared in irradiation of the intact breast are the underlying lung and the mediastinum. No firm guideline can be given as to the amount of lung that should or should not be included in a breast treatment plan. Clearly, enough lung must be included to encompass the underlying chest wall. In most tangential treatment plans, approximately 20 percent of the lung is taken to full dose.[9] In the author's experience, this is safe and complication free.

Third, the mediastinum should be spared whenever possible. This is especially important for patients who are to receive adjuvant chemotherapy. While evidence is circumstantial, those institutions that irradiate the mediastinum directly with *en face* internal mammary fields have considerably more difficulty in achieving full chemotherapy dosages,[10] as compared with those institutions that spare the mediastinum with the use of tangential fields.[11, 12, 13] Patients who receive chemotherapy and radiation therapy have been shown to lose circulating stem cells.[14] This loss is proportional to the amount of blood flow through the field of radiation. Since the mediastinal irradiation treats the aorta and vena cava, it delivers dosage to the maximum amount of blood flow possible. Thus, it is understandable that direct irradiation of the mediastinum may result in a patient who is less tolerant of chemotherapy and has a slower white count recovery following a cycle of chemotherapy.

A fourth goal is to deliver reliable dosage to the internal mammary lymph nodes when it is desired to treat such nodes. While the most precise way of dosing these nodes is to treat them directly with a photon field, such a technique delivers the maximum amount of radiation into the mediastinum and thus represents a substantial trade-off in terms of increasing the volume of normal tissue irradiated. Methods to treat the internal mammary lymph nodes without treating the mediastinum will be described later in this chapter.

A fifth goal is to avoid areas of overlap between adjacent sets of fields. Overlap between fields increases dose inhomogeneity and can lead to scarring, fibrosis, and cosmetic distortion.[15] A variety of techniques exist to prevent field overlap and will be described. Lastly, any treatment technique should be easy to set up and easy to reproduce. The patient will be treated 25 to 30 times. Reproducibility of the setup from day to day is critically important. It is also extremely uncomfortable for a patient to lie on the treatment couch for long periods of time while technologists carry out a complicated 30 to 40 minute set up. Ideally, any breast technique should take no more than 20 minutes to execute.

TECHNIQUES OF IRRADIATION OF THE INTACT BREAST

Tangential Breast Fields

All irradiation of the intact breast is done with tangentially directed fields that treat the breast and a portion of underlying lung, as illustrated in Figure 7–2. Two major types of field configurations are employed. In Figure 7–2*A*, only tangential fields are utilized. In order to treat the internal mammary nodes, the entrance point of the medial tangent can be brought across the midline, enlarging the treatment volume to encompass the internal mammary lymph node region. The internal mammary nodes, by definition, are situated along the internal mammary artery and vein. Those two blood vessels are located superior to the pleura and lateral to the sternum.[5] Therefore, if one includes the point where the pleura intersects the sternum, one must have the internal mammary lymph nodes within the treatment field. The notion that the internal mammary lymph nodes lie 3 cm lateral and 3 cm deep to a point along the midline of the patient[16] should be discarded. With modern CT scanning or ultrasound, it is rather easy to identify this pleural-sternal junction and to customize a patient's treatment accordingly.[17] It should also be noted that several authors have reported results

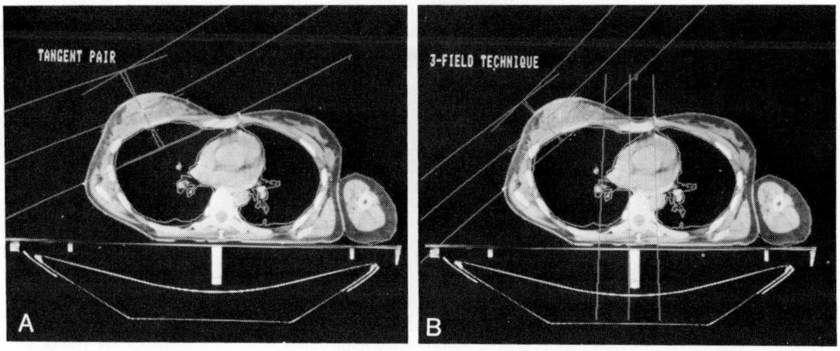

FIGURE 7–2. *A,* Primary breast cancer treatment, using tangential fields. The medial field entrance point is brought 2 to 3 cm beyond the midline, to allow the region of the internal mammary lymph nodes to be included in the high-dose treatment volume. *B,* A three-field approach for the same treatment volume, using a separate internal mammary field. Notice the wedge-shaped area where the internal mammary field joins the tangential field, which receives little treatment from irradiation of either tangential or internal mammary fields.

from internal mammary lymphoscintigraphy in which nodal structures have been imaged at significant distances from the anatomic internal mammary artery and vein. Nodes deep to the sternum itself and nodes extremely laterally placed on the chest wall have been noted.[18, 19] However, internal mammary lymphoscintigraphy is performed through an injection in the rectus sheath of the subcostal chest wall. While these aberrant lymph nodes apparently participate in the drainage from that distant space, it has never been shown that such lymph nodes participate in the lymphatic drainage of the breast itself. Histologic information concerning internal mammary node involvement is based solely on biopsy of nodes that are found along the internal mammary artery and vein in the intercostal spaces. Thus, it is the opinion of this author that treatment should be directed at those anatomically described nodes. To perform a lymphoscintigram and to place an unusually shaped field on a patient in order to encompass lymph nodes that lie in "left field" is, up to this point, an exercise that has not been proved worthwhile either by pathologic confirmation of nodal involvement or by outcome parameters.

The second method to treat the breast has its field configuration illustrated in Figure 7–2*B*. Here a direct internal mammary field is applied, usually having a medial border at the midline and extending a width of 5 cm. The tangentially directed breast fields match the internal mammary field edge.[4] There are two major drawbacks to this field configuration. First, as previously mentioned, this technique directs a great deal of radiation into the mediastinum and may interfere with chemotherapy tolerance. Second, the technique leaves a cold wedge-shaped area of tissue between the field junction points on the skin and the underlying pleura. In thin patients this wedge is quite small, whereas in larger patients a considerable volume of breast tissue may go untreated.[17] For these two reasons, a technique that uses a separate direct internal mammary field is not generally recommended for treating the intact breast. Such a technique may be more suitable for treatment of the postmastectomy chest wall.

The volume encompassed by tangential breast fields is illustrated in Figure 7–3. When the fields are to include the internal mammary nodes, the medial border of the medial tangent is placed 2 to 3 cm beyond the

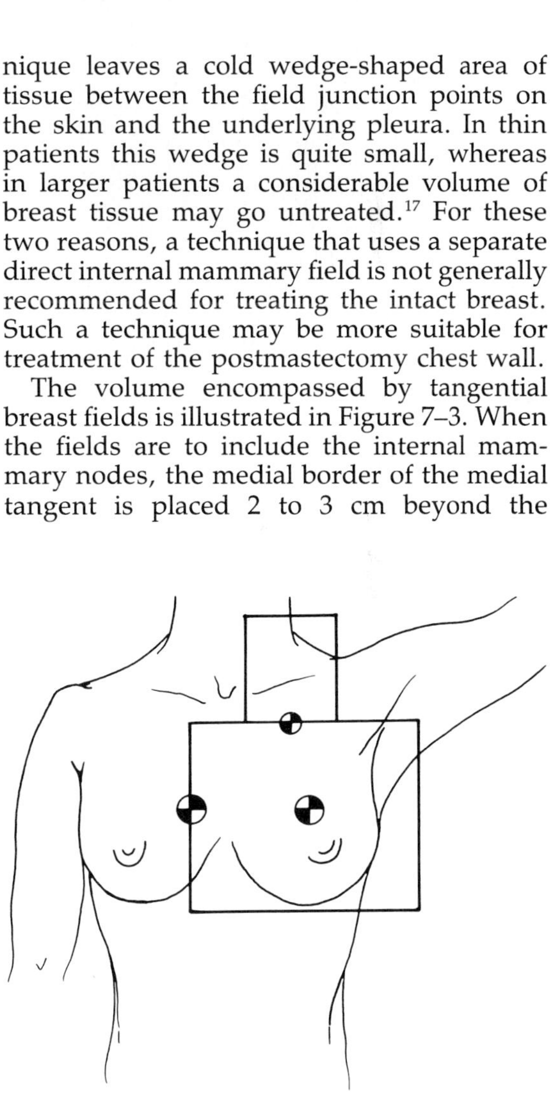

FIGURE 7–3. Volume encompassed by the breast cancer fields. Irradiation of the tangential fields treats the entire breast and internal mammary lymph node area. A small supraclavicular field encompasses the supraclavicular nodes and the apex of the axilla.

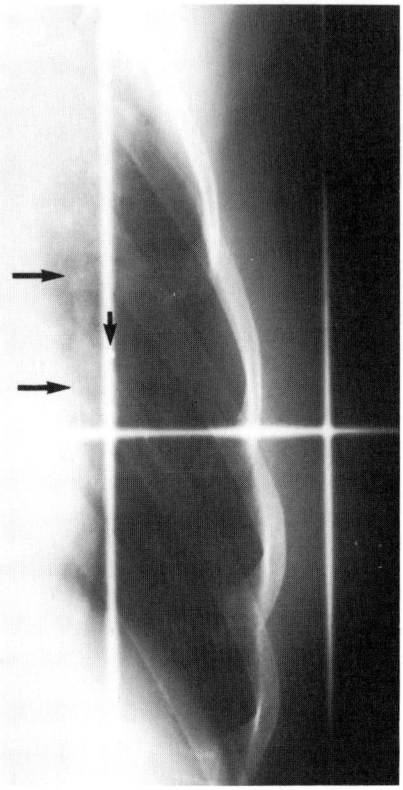

FIGURE 7–4. Simulator film for a tangential breast field. Note that the deep edge of the field bisects the sternum (large arrows). A BB dot (small arrow) is placed on the entrance for the complementary tangential field. The field edge intersects this BB, indicating that the deep edges of the field have been made coplanar.

midline. The superior border is positioned beyond palpable breast tissue, usually up to the base of the clavicle. The inferior border extends below the inframammary fold. The lateral tangent encompasses the same volume and is placed on the lateral chest wall below all palpable breast tissue.[20] The simulator film that treats this volume is shown in Figure 7–4. Because the internal mammary nodes are included in this patient's volume, the deep edge of the tangential fields bisects the sternum. This gives an immediate visual clue at the time of simulation that the treatment borders are deep enough to subtend the internal mammary node region.

Setting the Tangential Fields

In the opinion of the author, the setup is made much easier to put together and to reproduce if the tangential fields are positioned isocentrically. This almost demands a 100-cm isocentric distance because shorter distances such as 80 cm bring the head of the treatment machine too close to the patient and to the treatment couch, making an isocentric setup difficult, if not impossible. The technique for performing the isocentric setup has been described in detail[21] and is modified from the method developed by Svensson and colleagues at the Joint Center for Radiation Therapy in Boston.[22, 23] The setup begins with the patient lying flat on the simulator couch, with the arm carefully immobilized in an abducted position to move it away from the breast. The immobilization device that has been developed at the National Cancer Institute to perform this task is shown in Figure 7–5. The patient rests her head against a plastic piece, adjusted so that she rests on the board each day in the same position. The elbow is supported well up in the air, as this is a more comfortable position for patients than is having the elbow on the same level as the treatment couch, especially in the case of patients who have had recent axillary surgery. The position of the elbow in space is controlled by several adjustable parts of the arm board so that the patient can be

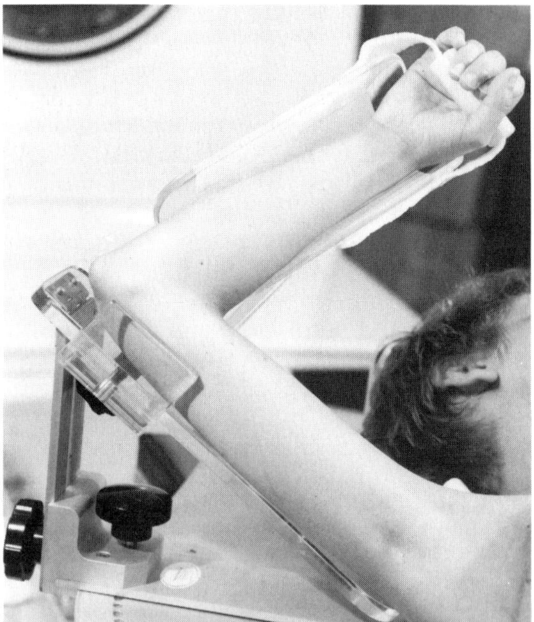

FIGURE 7–5. An adjustable arm board to position the patient precisely for each treatment. All angles and heights of this board are adjustable for patient comfort.

placed in exactly the same position each day. The arm board is adjustable from patient to patient. Occasionally, for a patient with very pendulous breasts, a tilt board must be utilized to prevent the breast from riding up too close to the clavicle. In such cases, the adjustable arm board is bolted on to the tilt board, and the setup proceeds in a standard fashion.

Once the patient is comfortably positioned with the arm board, the field borders are outlined on her skin. A breast bridge is then utilized, as illustrated in Figure 7–6. The measuring points of the bridge are placed at the edge of the medial and lateral tangential fields in the central axis of the beam. Once accurately positioned, three measurements are obtained. First, the angle from the horizontal that connects the medial and lateral entrance points is read from the inclinometer scale. This device easily gives accuracy to plus or minus one degree. Second, a scale on the bridge is read to note the separation between the two tangential field entrance points. Finally, a third scale on the bridge allows one to note the width of the field that will be necessary to produce approximately 2 cm of excess field size beyond the nipple.

Using these three measured parameters, one can calculate the location of the isocenter necessary to produce the appropriate field arrangement. This is illustrated in Figure 7–7. The geometry of the breast setup is standard from patient to patient. Using the point along the central ray where the medial tangent intersects the skin as a reference point, one can calculate the depth below this point that should be set as the isocentric treatment depth and the lateral shift of the treatment couch that would place the isocenter in the appropriate position within the breast. The gantry can then be rotated to the calculated medial and lateral treatment angles. A simple computer program will calculate these functions and is reproduced in Figure 7–8. To perform the setup, one first sets the isocenter to the calculated depth below the reference point. Since the setup is very sensitive to changes in this isocentric depth, the optical distance indicator of the machine is simply not accurate enough. The author uses the front pointer to set this isocentric distance to

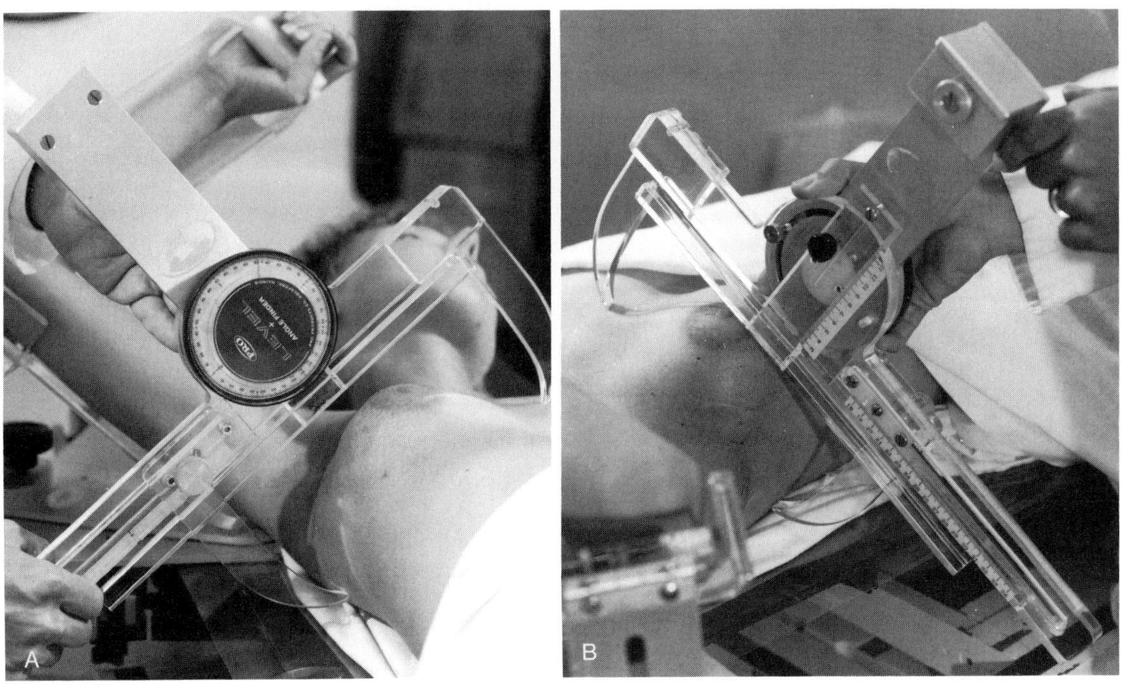

FIGURE 7–6. A, A front view of the breast bridge. When the caliper points are placed on the entrance and exit marks for the medial and lateral tangential fields, the inclinometer gives the angle that connects these two points. *B,* Back view of the breast bridge. The two centimeter scales indicate the separation between the caliper points and the width of the field necessary to clear the surface of the breast by a 1 to 2 cm margin.

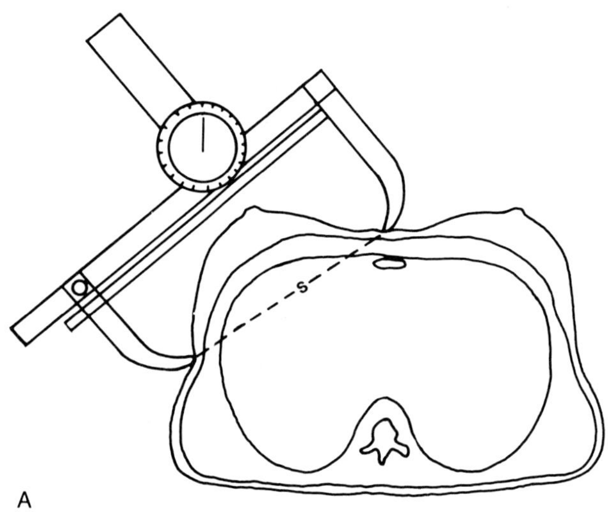

A

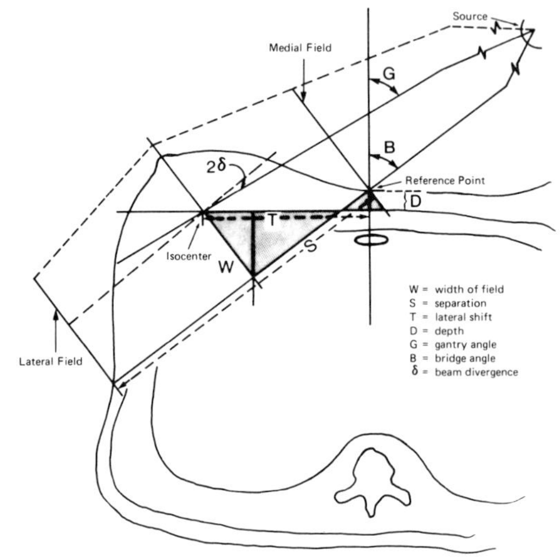

B

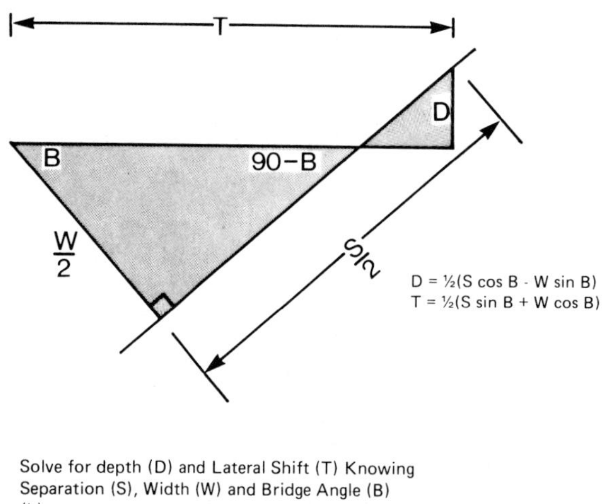

C

FIGURE 7–7. A, A schematic drawing of the breast bridge in place. The distance between the caliper points indicates the separation(s). The inclinometer measures the bridge angle. The width of the field is read off a scale on the back of the breast bridge (not illustrated). *B,* A detailed drawing of the known parameters (separation, field width, and bridge angle) and the calculated measurements needed to perform the setup (set-up depth, table shift, and gantry angle). The darkened triangles contain the variables. *C,* A blowup of the shaded triangles from *B*. The depth and the table shift can be solved by using the equations noted. The gantry angle is simply the breast bridge angle plus the beam divergence.

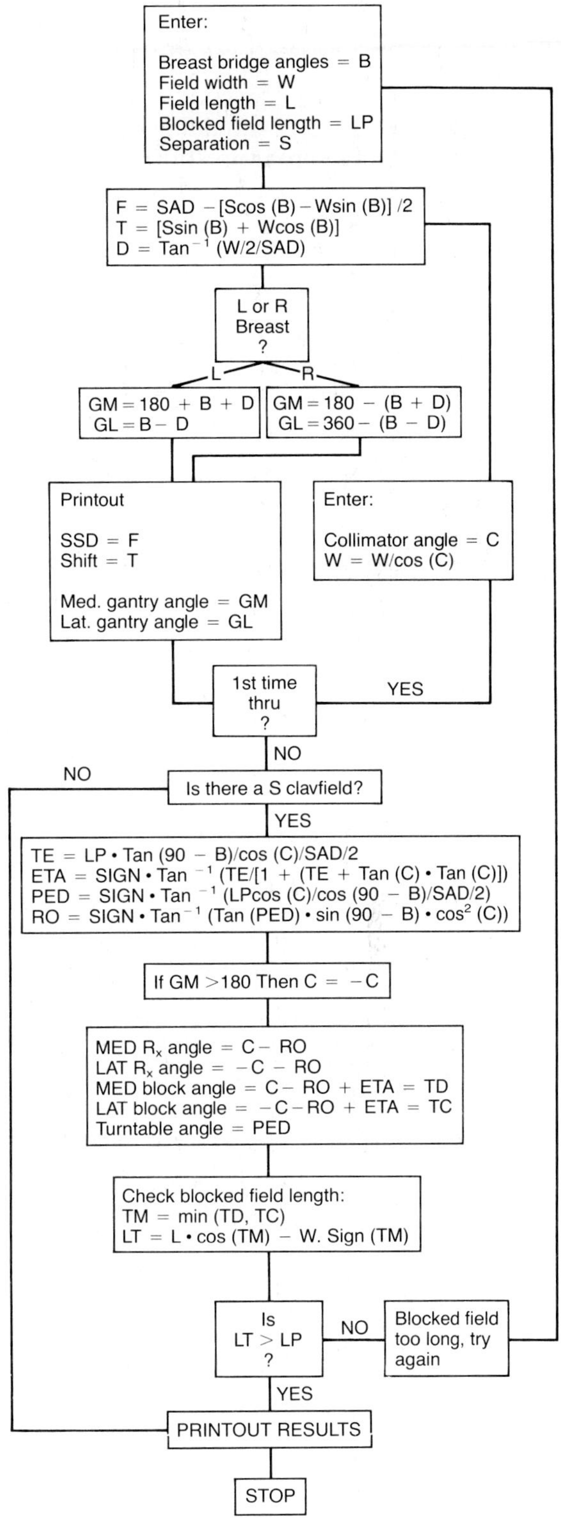

FIGURE 7–8. A schematic drawing of the computer program to solve the equations for the breast setup.

accuracies within 1 mm (Fig. 7–9). The table is then shifted laterally the calculated distance, and the gantry is rotated to the medial or lateral gantry angle to perform the treatment. If the setup is correct, the edge of the medial tangential field will exactly intersect the reference point. It should be noted that with the computer program shown in Figure 7–8, the two tangential beams are actually angled a few degrees beyond 180 and are opposed so that the deep edges of the beams are coplanar and extra divergence is directed into space and not into the underlying lung (Figure 7–7*B*). In such cases, a wire placed on the lateral tangential field edge should exactly line up with the medial tangential field edge on the simulator film (Fig. 7–4). In all cases, the collimator is rotated several degrees so that the field parallels the chest wall. In those patient who are raised up on a tilt board, such collimator rotation is required to a lesser degree or is not necessary at all.

The Supraclavicular Axillary Field and Field Matching

The supraclavicular field is utilized whenever there is axillary lymph node positivity as noted in Figure 7–1. This field is generally quite small, its medial border being placed along the edge of the spine and its lateral border encompassing the apex of the axilla (beyond where the first rib crosses the clavicle). Inferiorly, it matches the tangential breast fields, and superiorly, it comes up to the edge of the supraclavicular skin (Fig. 7–10). The field is made twice as long as necessary, and its central ray is placed at the match line that joins the tangents and the supraclavicular port. The inferior half of the field is then blocked so that the supraclavicular field is prevented from diverging into the tangential breast fields (Fig. 7–11). The entire field is angled 10 degrees medially so that the divergence is directed laterally, away from the spine. If the need ever arises to treat the cervical spine for a bony metastasis, this area will not have received any significant dosage. As stated previously, there is little need to treat the entire axilla once it has been dissected. However, in cases in which

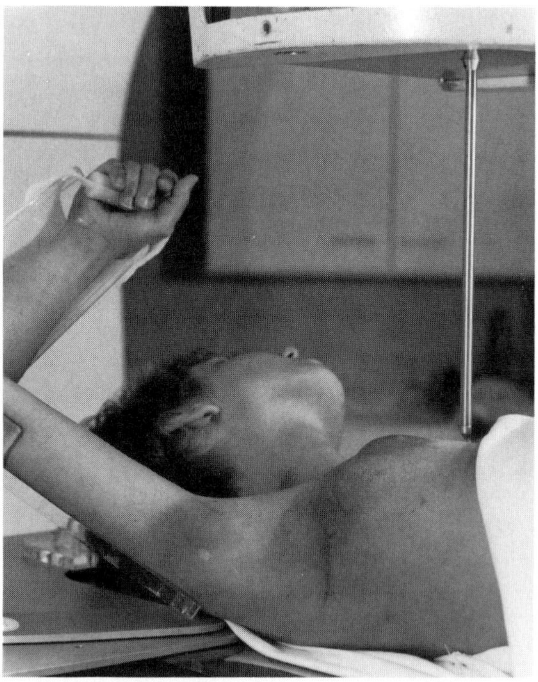

FIGURE 7–9. The front pointer on the accelerator is used to set carefully the treatment distance.

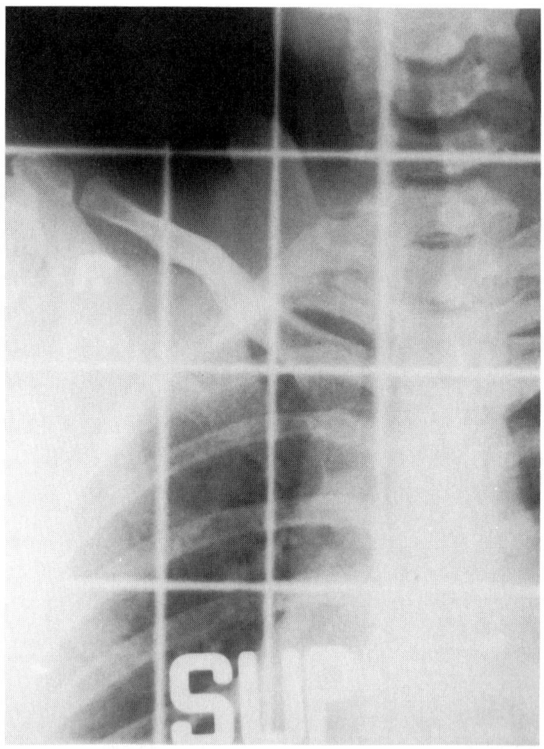

FIGURE 7–10. The supraclavicular port. The inferior half of this port is blocked out to avoid divergence into the tangential fields. The field is used after a full axillary dissection. It is designed to treat only the supraclavicular nodes and the apex of the axilla. If the axilla has not been dissected, the field is extended laterally to encompass the entire axillary content.

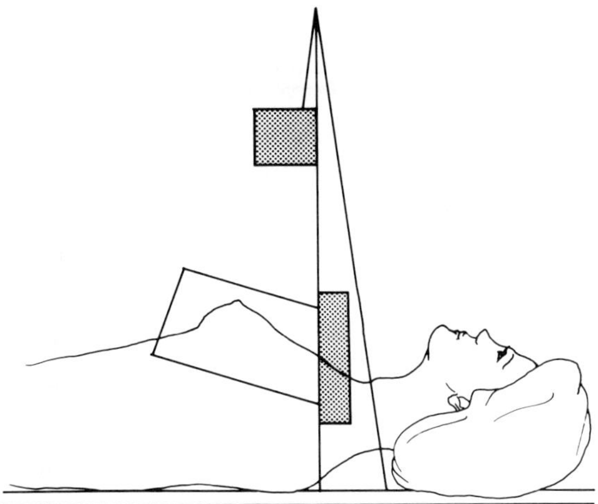

FIGURE 7–11. A schematic drawing of the relationship of the tangential fields to the supraclavicular field. The supraclavicular half-block prevents the supraclavicular field from diverging into the tangential field.

axillary treatment is necessary, the supraclavicular field is simply extended laterally to just beyond the head of the humerus. The humerus is then shielded with a carefully placed block. The posterior aspect of the axilla can be boosted in standard fashion with a small, posteriorly placed axillary field.

Matching the supraclavicular axillary field to the tangential breast fields without causing an area of underdose that could lead to recurrence or an area of overdose that could lead to match line fibrosis[15] has been the subject of a number of papers. A variety of techniques have been described, including treating the patient with a single isocenter with both the supraclavicular and the tangential fields half blocked to eliminate divergence.[24] Others have eliminated overlap through the use of a gravity-oriented hanging block,[22, 23] a rotatable half-beam block,[25] or the device on the simulator that allows one to cut a custom-shaped, field-matching block.[26] While all these techniques remedy the major problems with field overlap at the match line, they have the disadvantage of requiring special devices to be fabricated and mounted on the head of the simulator and the head of the treatment machine.

For a technique that is closely related to the aforementioned, a detailed account describes how an extremely accurate match line can be created using a straight block mounted with a wing nut to a standard tray that is slid into the tray holder of a standard collimator assembly.[21] A common theme in most of the literature delineating techniques of breast setup is their apparent complexity. This is due to the fact that it is difficult to describe a problem involving sophisticated three-dimensional geometry with simple words and pictures. The author has not encountered a single person who has, by simply reading a description of one of these complex breast setups, been able to use the technique in the clinic. However, the majority of breast setups are easy to comprehend if one simply sees them being carried out. Therefore, anyone wishing to change his breast setup to a different technique would be well advised to travel to one or two centers where these techniques are being employed and simply to observe several setups. In the author's opinion, this is worth hours and hours of studying journal articles and trying to decipher pictures. Nonetheless, it is important to document the techniques used for breast irradiation so that interested workers may refer back to them as necessary. Some of the basic features of the technique for field matching that is employed at the National Cancer Institute are described later to emphasize certain basic principles.

Setting the Supraclavicular Field

Again it should be emphasized that the foundation of accurate and reproducible breast cancer irradiation is an immobilization device that places the patient in exactly the same position each day. A device for accomplishing this critical task is illustrated in Figure 7–5. If it is determined that the patient needs a supraclavicular field, the simulation is done slightly differently from the procedure previously described for setting up the tangent fields alone. First, a match line is drawn on the patient's skin, indicating where the tangential breast fields will join the supraclavicular field. This is often at the level of the clavicular base. The tangential fields are then set up with at least 4 cm of overlap superiorly into the tangential field, allowing room for a block to be placed in the tangential field to define the match line. This match line block is necessary for two reasons (Table 7–3). First, and most obvious, the match line block must make the top edge of the tangential field parallel with the supraclavicular field after the collimator has been rotated to parallel the chest wall (Fig. 7–11). In most pa-

TABLE 7–3. Function of Match Line Block

Make superior edge of tangential field parallel the supraclavicular field after collimator rotation
Correct trapezoid effect

tients, a collimator twist of 10 to 20 degrees is necessary. Thus, the match line block is placed in the field at an angle corresponding to the chest wall inclination in order to make the superior aspect of the tangential field parallel to the supraclavicular field. However, there is a second and more subtle reason to include this match line block. This problem has been referred to as the trapezoid effect.[23] Simply stated, an oblique field that strikes a plane that is perpendicular to the couch surface and parallel to its long axis will describe a trapezoid and not a rectangle (Fig. 7–12). Thus, the top edge of the tangential field will appear not as straight vertical within the patient but as angled and therefore will need to be corrected with the insertion of the match line block. Even elevating the patient on a tilt board to eliminate collimator rotation does not correct this small error introduced by the trapezoid effect. A simple computer program can calculate the magnitude of the trapezoid effect and allow one to insert the match line block in such a way as to take this effect into account.[21] Of course, a gravity block is always vertical in its orientation and automatically adjusts for the trapezoid effect.[22, 23]

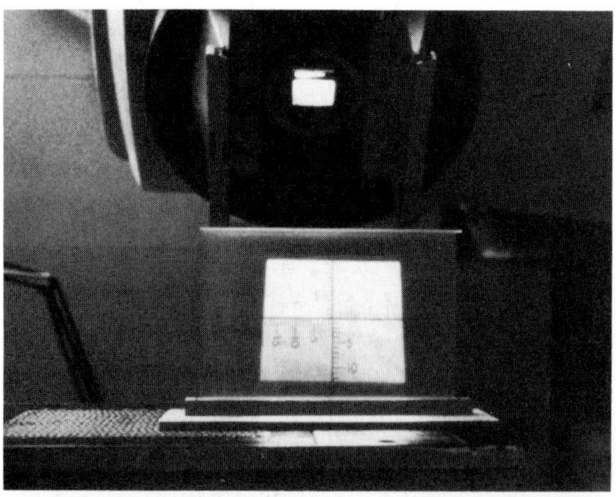

FIGURE 7–12. A rectangular field is photographed as the rays strike a vertical plane in a tangential manner. Notice that the field is no longer rectangular, but, actually, trapezoidal, as a result of beam divergence effects.

Once the match line block has been placed so that the top of the tangential field parallels the supraclavicular field, eliminating the effect of collimator rotation and the trapezoid effect, the tangential field will accurately match the supraclavicular field at the surface and at all depths. However, one must still correct the divergence of the tangential breast fields into the supraclavicular field. The easiest correction to make is to angle the couch pedestal several degrees to make the superior aspect of the tangential field parallel with the supraclavicular field as illustrated in Figure 7–13. Typically, the amount of pedestal angulation required is four to five degrees and can be easily calculated. However, once the pedestal is angled by several degrees, the medial and lateral tangents will no longer exactly match one another, since the pedestal is angled in opposite directions for each of these fields. The solution to this small but potentially significant problem is made utilizing a small adjustment to the match line block and collimator angle as described in detail elsewhere.[21]

A final key element in the setup is the ability to visualize the light field as being accurately located to define a precise match line for both tangential fields and the supraclavicular field. For this purpose, marks placed on the patient's skin are inadequate. There is no guarantee that a mark placed on the patient's skin will be parallel to the central axis of the machine. If the skin mark is angled, defining a precise match line will be impossible. Additionally, it is impossible to see the light field from a lateral tangential beam fall on the patient's anterior chest wall because the tissues of the lateral chest shield the light field from shining onto the anterior chest wall. To visualize the match line, the author has adopted a device first used by

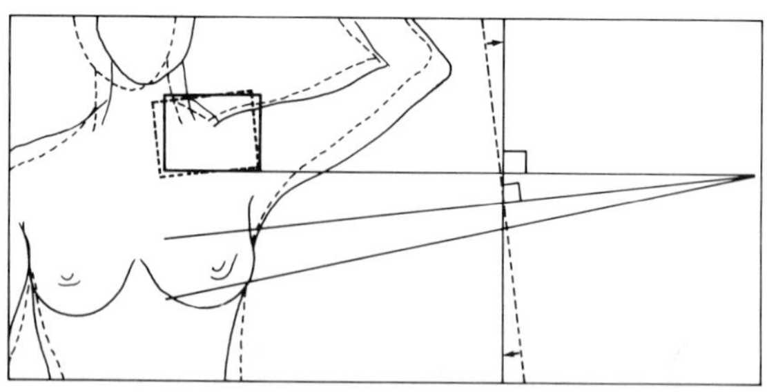

FIGURE 7–13. Rotation of the couch pedestal prevents the tangential field from diverging into the supraclavicular field.

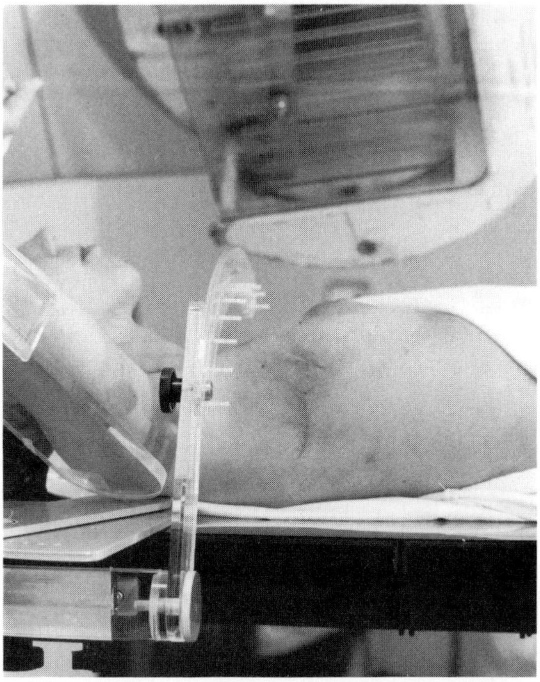

FIGURE 7–14. The "protractor" device, mounted on the edge of the treatment couch. The device is placed over the match line, and both the tangential and the supraclavicular fields are matched to the red scored lines that bisect each of the rods protruding from the protractor. In the collimator tray, the straight block that forms the superior match line can be seen.

Svensson and colleagues[22, 23] called a protractor (Fig. 7–14). This simple device is a gently curved piece of plastic in which a series of rods have been embedded. The rods are each scored with a small red line, and the device is mounted so that it is perpendicular to the side rail of the couch. A mounting device on the couch side rail itself can be used to attach this protractor for clinical use. The light fields from the breast tangents can be clearly seen to fall upon the rods extending from the protractor, thus assuring that the match line passes across the patient in a manner parallel to the central axis of the beam. The position of the table can be adjusted slightly, either with the couch pedestal or with small movements in the craniocaudal direction, to make this light field strike each rod at exactly the red scored mark. Both tangential fields are adjusted in this manner, and the supraclavicular axillary field is half blocked so that its central axis also falls on the red scored marks, ensuring that all three fields meet in exactly the same plane. Since the geometry of the setup guarantees that the three fields' edges are truly vertical, matching the fields at the red marks scored on the rods guarantees that the fields will match accurately at all depths within the patient. Another advantage of the protractor is that it is unlikely to be placed in exactly the same spot over the patient each day. This variation of 1 or 2 mm from day to day produces a natural "feathering" of the match line, smoothing out the dose in this match region. Additional details of the setup can be found in Reference 21.

TREATMENT PLANNING AND DOSIMETRY IN PRIMARY BREAST CANCER THERAPY

Once the patient simulation has been done, an external contour is obtained through the central ray and at levels 1 to 2 cm from the superior and inferior field edges. Until recently, most breast cancer dosimetry was performed using this contour as though it contained only unit density material. Thus, all breast cancer dosimetry used wedge filters to compensate for the slope of the breast, and plans with apparent dose homogeneity were created (Fig. 7–15). The ability to visualize anatomy by utilizing CT scans has had a great impact on breast cancer dosimetry.[17, 27, 28] A CT scan of the breast dramatically displays all the relevant anatomy necessary

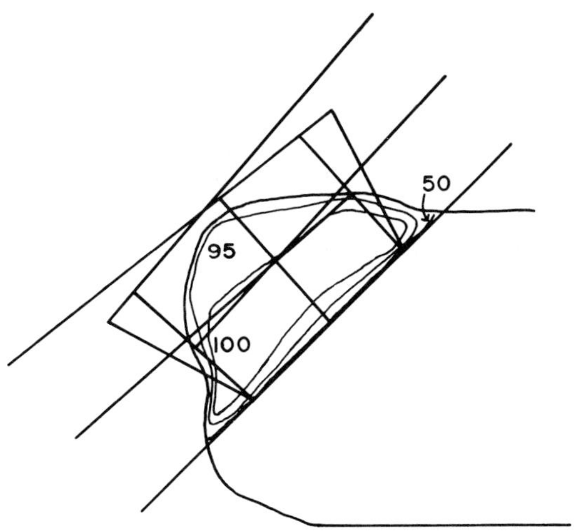

FIGURE 7–15. A treatment plan for breast cancer, using an external contour only. Two tangential fields with wedge filters create a uniform dose distribution.

for accurate treatment planning (Fig. 7–16). However, having the CT scan in no way eliminates the need for an accurate external contour, taken at the time of simulation. Since the CT scan is done at a separate session, on a different machine, and with a different type of couch surface, small changes in patient position can distort the shape of the CT image. Thus, it is always critical to compare the CT contour with the standard contour and to make any adjustments necessary to compensate for problems with the CT scanning process.

The manner in which CT scans are used for breast cancer treatment planning is illustrated in Figure 7–17. The CT scan is transferred to the treatment planning computer and is brought up on the video monitor (Fig. 7–17*A*). The markers on the surface of the patient correspond to the field edges of the medial and lateral tangents, as determined by the previous simulation; they are placed on the skin using thin angiography catheters. The treatment fields are then brought up on the screen and superimposed on the CT scan. The isocenter inside the breast is found by measuring the SSD and the table shift, using the cursor on the treatment planning computer in exactly the same manner as that in which the patient will be set up on the treatment machine. These distances have been determined from the equations illustrated in Figure 7–7 and utilizing the program presented in Figure 7–8. The field of appropriate length and width is placed at this isocenter and rotated to duplicate the appropriate gantry angle. If setup has been properly executed and the CT scan has been carefully obtained, this field will enter through the medial angiography catheter and exit through the lateral angiography catheter. A similar technique is used to position the lateral field (Fig. 7–17*B*). Dosimetry is then performed incorporating a correction for lung density.[29] The resultant dose distribution is displayed in Figure 7–17*C*. Notice that no wedge filters appear in this plan. This is because the reduced density of the lung, typically 0.2 relative to unit density soft tissue,[30] has virtually negated the need for wedge compensation. In our experience, 15-degree wedges are the most that are needed to achieve a uniform dose distribution. Without compensating for lung density, wedge filters are considerably overused in breast cancer treatment planning.

The ability to reduce or to eliminate wedge filters in breast cancer treatment planning carries with it an important benefit. In a recent study by Fraass and colleagues,[31] it

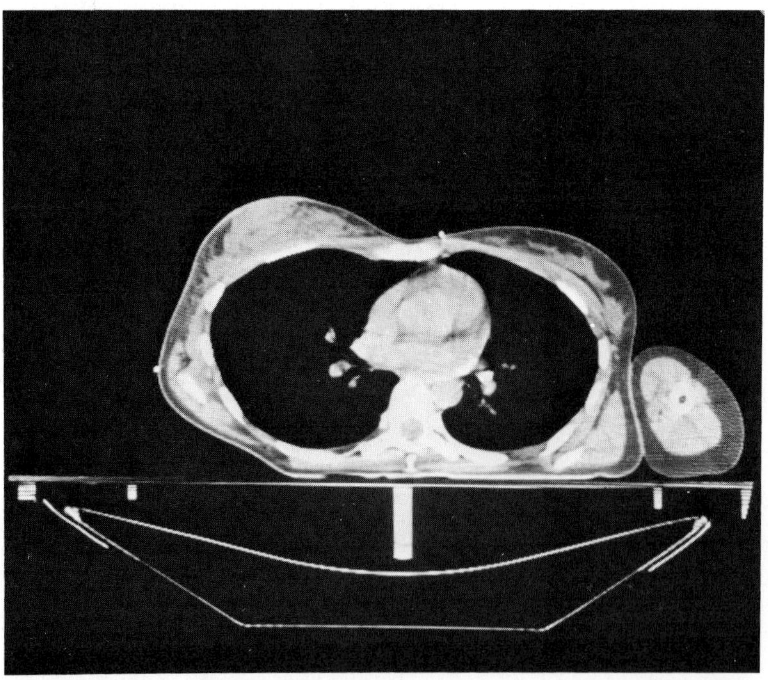

FIGURE 7–16. A CT scan of the breast, suitable for treatment planning. The patient has been scanned on a flat couch with the arm over the head, to duplicate the treatment position. Small opaque angiography catheters mark the entrance and exit points for the medial and lateral tangential fields.

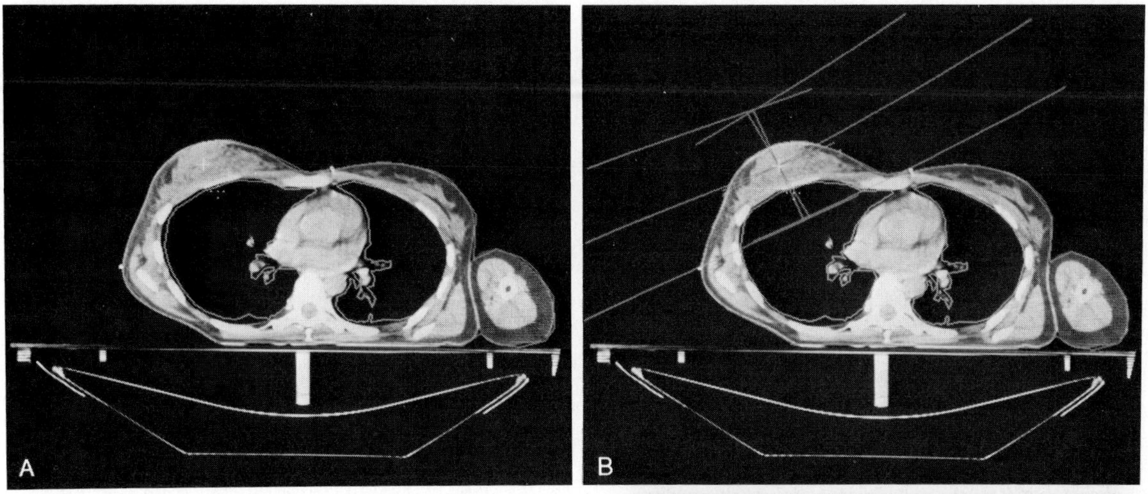

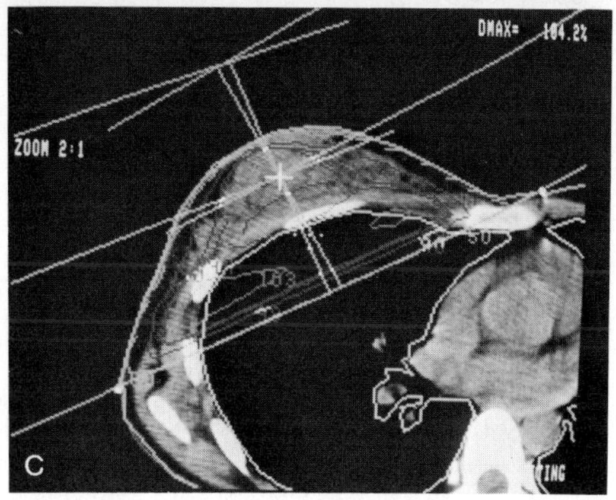

FIGURE 7–17. A, The CT scan in Figure 7–16 has been brought up on the video monitor of the treatment planning computer. The external contour and internal outline of the lungs have been added. *B,* The treatment fields have been placed. *C,* The dose distribution is plotted.

was found that dose scattered to the opposite breast is related to a number of factors listed in Table 7–4. The use of a half-beam block, or "beam splitter," in the tangential fields, even if such a block is six half-value layers thick, yields a direct transmission dose of over 1.5 percent. If the block is five half-value layers thick, a relatively standard block thickness, the transmitted dose is over 3 percent. This would account for an additional 75 to 150 rad scattered to the entire contralateral breast for a prescribed dose of 5000 rad to the ipsilateral breast. Therefore, the use of half-beam blocks in the tangential breast fields is not recommended. Another factor that significantly contributes to the dose deposited into the contralateral breast is the use of wedge filters. Not only is there low-energy scatter radiation that comes off the wedge itself (wedge scatter), but since the wedge attenuates the beam and requires the treatment machine to be on longer to provide the prescribed dose, the standard leakage radiation from the head of the machine also increases. The influence of the wedge is most pronounced for wedges placed in the medial tangential field. This is because the wedge filter placed in the lateral tangent has its low-energy wedge scatter filtered by the body, and it is absorbed before it can reach the contralateral breast. Of course, wedge scatter from the medially placed wedge encounters the contralateral breast directly.

TABLE 7–4. Factors that Contribute to Dose to the Contralateral Breast

Factors
Wedge in medial field
Use of "beam splitter" in tangents
Non-coplanar deep field edges

Thus, two conclusions can be drawn from the wedge data presented by Fraass.[31] First, the use of wedges should be minimized when possible, a task that is easy to accomplish if a correction for lung density is applied to breast cancer treatment plans. Such correction automatically decreases the necessity for the wedge in the treatment field and produces better dose homogeneity. Second, when a wedge filter is necessary, it should be used in the lateral field and not in the medial field. It has been found that such a shift of wedges to emphasize the lateral field does not dramatically alter dosimetry.[31] For example, if a pair of 15-degree wedges yields a well-balanced treatment plan, putting a single 30-degree wedge in the lateral field and leaving the medial field open and simply changing the weighting of the fields slightly produce a virtually identical isodose distribution.

Future Directions in Treatment Planning for the Intact Breast

With the use of modern simulators, CT scanning, and computerized dosimetry employing density corrections, the treatment of the intact breast has become far more sophisticated than ever before. However, there is still room for development.

All the CT-based treatment plans shown in this chapter have been two-dimensional representations of dosimetry using a single CT slice. While the author and others routinely look at dose distributions on planes superior and inferior to the central axis of the beam, this limited analysis can only hint at the complexities of the dose distribution in this irregularly shaped volume. Graphics tools for computerized display of three-dimensional anatomy as well as calculational algorithms for computation of three-dimensional dose distribution have become available. Since a multiple set of CT slices contains a series of two-dimensional representations of a three-dimensional volume, integration of those CT scans can create a three-dimensional picture. Drs. Daniel McShan and Benedick Fraass of the Department of Radiation Therapy, University of Michigan, have created the displays in Figure 7–18. These show the reconstructed body surface with treatment fields (Fig. 7–18*A*); a cut-away revealing underlying structures on transverse, sagittal, and coronal CT images simultaneously (Fig. 7–18*B*); a dose distribution on these planes (Fig. 7–18C); and a highlighted dose display for the 105 to 120 percent isodose volumes (Fig. 7–18*D*). The region of the electron beam boost is contained in the high-dose volume, but notice also areas of excessive dose at the extreme top and bottom of the breast. It is hoped that additional research into three-dimensional dose display will enhance the ability to visualize treatment volumes and to adjust them for optimal benefit and minimal complications.

Energy of the Beam to Treat the Intact Breast

In most centers, the intact breast has been treated with either 4- or 6-MV photons from 100 cm isocentric linear accelerators. To use machines with shorter isocentric distances makes performing an isocentric setup for breast treatment virtually impossible. A low-energy accelerator has been favored because measurements and clinical experience have suggested that the surface dose from a 4-MV[32] or a 6-MV linear accelerator gives appropriate levels of skin sparing for good cosmesis while still treating the superficial layers of the breast.

There has been a concern that using an accelerator of higher energy would be inappropriate for the intact breast because of an excessive skin-sparing effect. However, one frequently encounters patients with a large separation between medial and lateral tangents in whom a lower-energy beam, especially a 4-MV or ^{60}Co, will yield a poor isodose distribution with significant hot spots in the plan (Fig. 7–19*A*). The quality of the dose distribution is greatly improved by using 10-MV x-rays (Fig. 7–19*B*). The depth-dose characteristics of 4-, 6-, and 10-MV photons are displayed in Figure 7–20. With a plastic tray in the collimator assembly, the 10-MV doses are virtually identical to that of the 6-MV beam. Thus, the author believes that it is safe to treat the intact breast with x-rays from a 10-MV linear accelerator when necessary, provided that a tray is placed in the beam to add some additional dose to the surface.

Boost to the Tumor Bed

Most treatment centers that have a large volume of primary breast cancer patients undergoing irradiation deliver a boost dose to the tumor bed. Evidence in the literature indicates that local recurrence rates decrease

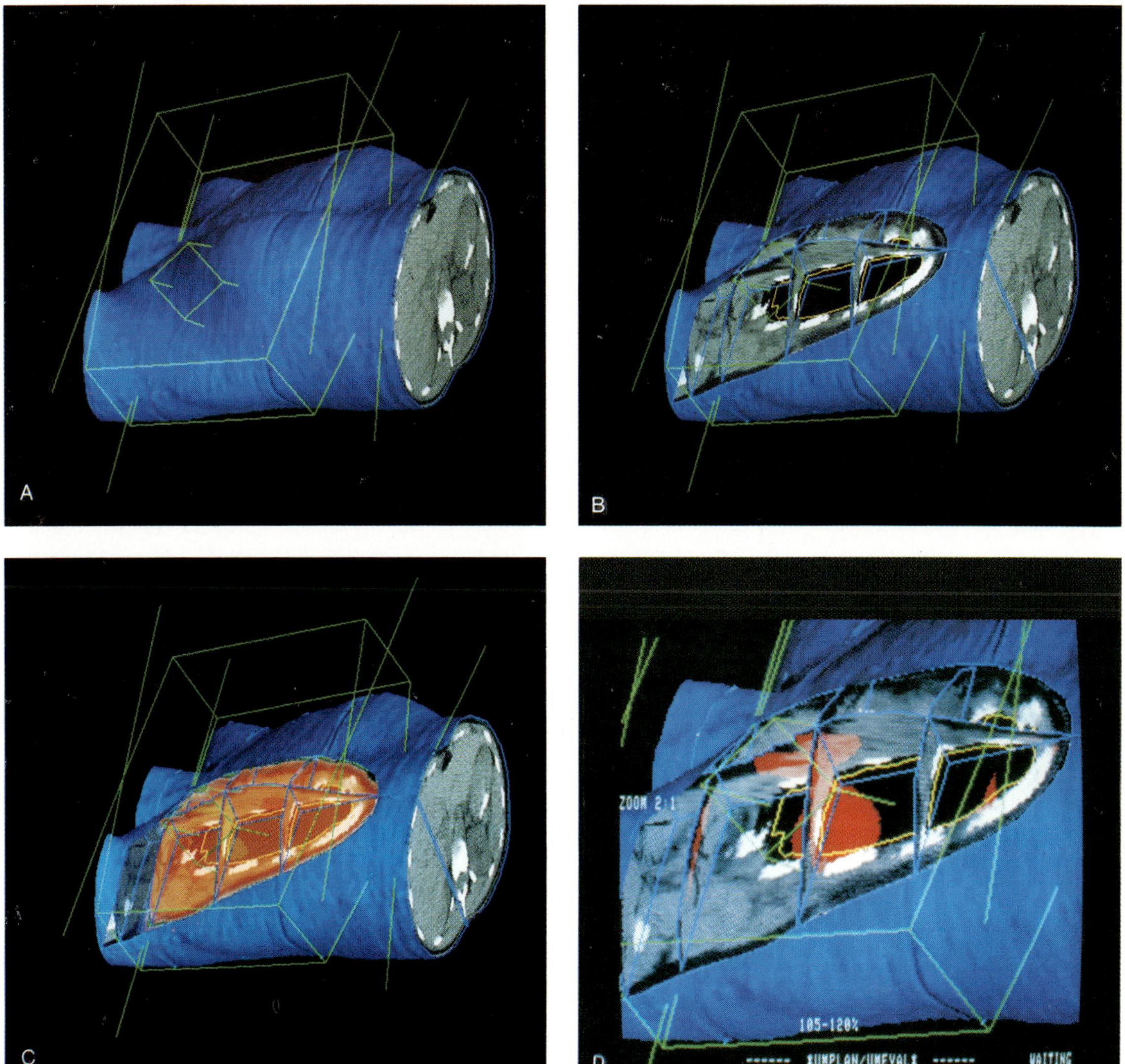

FIGURE 7–18. *A,* The body surface of a patient has been reconstructed using multiple CT slices. The two large rectangles indicate the medial and lateral tangential fields that are treating the right breast. The small square that looks like a coffee table indicates the small electron beam field that will boost the site of the primary tumor. *B,* Some of the surface has been cut away leaving behind one sagittal, one coronal, and three transverse CT slices. *C,* A dose distribution superimposed on this cutaway volume. The darker area underneath the electron beam boost is the high-dose boost volume. *D,* A dose display highlighting the 105 to 120 percent isodose volumes. The boost field contains this area of extra dose. Notice also that the thin areas of the breast in the upper and lower portions of the field also contain areas of extra dose.

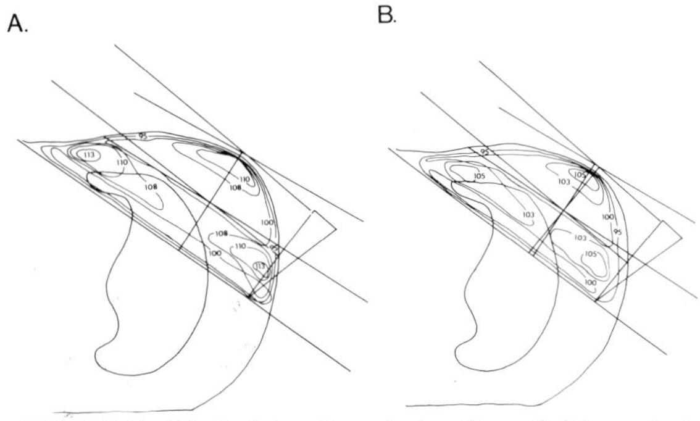

FIGURE 7–19. A, A treatment plan for a full-breasted patient, using a 4-MV beam. Notice the dose inhomogeneity up to 110 percent. *B,* The same treatment plan with 10-MV photons. The dose distribution is much more uniform.

when the local tumor bed is treated with such a boost.[33] In a recent study published by the NSABP,[34] no boost dose was given and the local recurrence rate at three years was 7.7 percent. The authors of the NSABP report argue that this indicates that boost doses of radiation are not indicated in every case. While this is likely to be true, it should be remembered that all patients in the NSABP trial had their tumor excised with pathologically free margins on the initial excision. Any patient with a positive margin was withdrawn from the study, and no reexcisions of microscopic residual tumor were allowed. Under those circumstances, whole-breast irradiation without a boost has produced the recurrence rates previously cited. With a median follow-up of only three years, it is likely that this 7.7 percent figure will increase somewhat. In most clinical situations, surgical excision with pathologically free margins is not demanded in every case. Furthermore, reexcision of a tumor whose complete removal is in doubt is allowed and encouraged. Under these circumstances, when the amount of residual disease may be greater than was the case in the NSABP trial, a boost dose is warranted. The two methods for boosting the tumor bed are an interstitial iridium implant or an electron beam.

Methodology to perform an implant of the breast has been carefully described in the literature.[35, 36] The first matter that must be decided upon is exactly where in the breast to place the implant needles. If the patient has been examined by the radiation oncologist prior to local tumor excision, such a

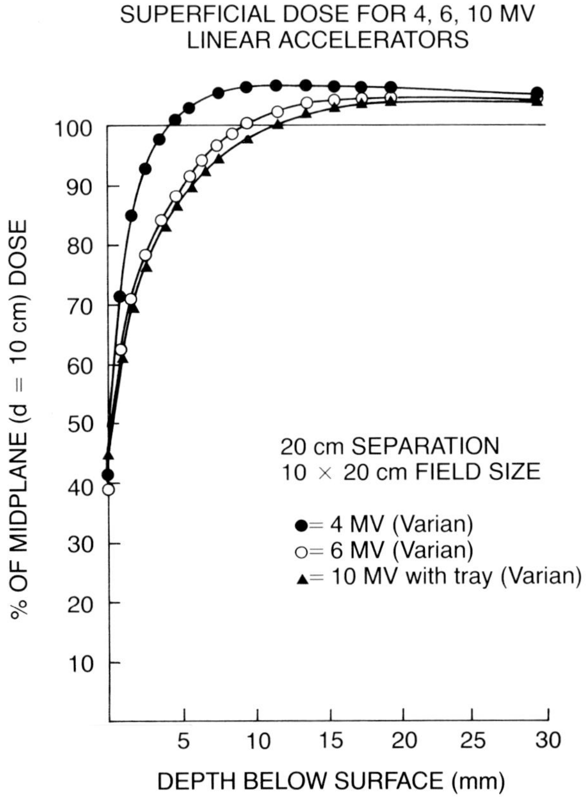

FIGURE 7–20. Surface dose characteristics from a 4-, 6-, and 10-MV accelerator. Although the 4-MV accelerator has a higher surface dose, the buildup regions for the 6- and 10-MV machines are virtually identical.

decision is greatly facilitated. After the findings of physical examination and mammography are noted, determining the proper location of the implant should be relatively straightforward. However, in many cases the patient is seen in the radiation therapy department after the tumor has been removed. At times the scar from local tumor excision has been placed directly over the tumor, which helps define the tumor bed. On many other occasions, however, the scar is circumareolar, and defining the exact location of the tumor bed is not straightforward. Under those circumstances, one must carefully read the surgeon's preoperative examination and discuss the tumor location with the surgeon. The patient is also helpful in pointing out the area of the breast where the tumor was palpable. Mammography, both before and after excision, can also help define the tumor bed. Finally, surgeons should be reminded to leave a metallic clip in the deep margin of the tumor bed when possible.[37]

When implanting the breast, the author commonly uses a two-plane implant and covers virtually the entire quadrant in which the tumor mass was located. A single-plane implant irradiates such a small amount of tissue that it is difficult to be certain that the volume of interest is being treated. Breast implants are performed under local anesthesia, with the help of intravenous diazepam and intravenous narcotic analgesics. The entire procedure takes approximately 30 minutes and is well tolerated by the vast majority of patients. The author always loads the implant with inert gold seeds and films the implant on the simulator for individual dosimetric computation. In doing a two-plane implant, a seed strength of 0.35 milligram radium equivalent is customary. The spacing between adjacent needles is 1.2 cm, and the spacing between planes is 1.5 cm. If these rules are followed, an isodose line of 35 to 45 rad per hour smoothly covers the entire implant bed. A dose between 1500 and 2000 rad is delivered, and this takes anywhere from 40 to 45 hours.

Whenever a two-plane implant is feasible, it is preferable to use that type of boost. However, when the amount of tissue receiving the implant is small and a two-plane implant is not possible, boosting the tumor bed with an electron beam is desirable. In patients who have tumors located in the periphery of the breast (such as high near the clavicle, medially along the sternum, laterally near the chest wall, or near the inframammary fold) the electron beam is preferred. The location of the tumor bed is carefully mapped out, and the angle of approach for the electron beam and its desired depth of penetration can be determined from CT scans, as described by Solin.[37] A 1600 rad boost delivered in eight fractions has been employed.

Total Dose for Primary Breast Cancer Treatment

In general, an analysis of treatment results has indicated that doses above 6000 rad produce local control following local tumor excision in over 95 percent of cases.[33] The author attempts to achieve a dose somewhere between 6200 and 6500 rad to the tumor bed. This dose is arrived at by delivering 4500 to 5000 rad to the entire breast in five to five and one half weeks, followed by a boost dose between 1500 and 2000 rad.

TREATMENT OF THE POSTMASTECTOMY CHEST WALL

When radiation is required after mastectomy, the treatment techniques are similar to those of the intact breast. One can employ two tangential fields brought slightly beyond midline to encompass the internal mammary node chain as well as the chest wall. These two fields are matched with a direct supraclavicular field, utilizing the same match line technique previously described. A bolus is used on the chest wall on alternate days to bring up the skin dose, since the skin is an organ at risk following mastectomy. This is in direct contrast with the treatment of the intact breast when the skin is at low risk and bolus is not indicated.

The postmastectomy chest wall can also be treated with electrons, as described in the literature by the group from M.D. Anderson Hospital.[38, 39] The electron beam can be employed to treat just the chest wall or can be used for both the chest wall and the adjacent nodal areas. Because the chest wall is a curving surface, it is often necessary to angle the chest wall electron field so that it falls perpendicular to the center of the curve of the chest. This often means that the chest wall field is angled into adjacent internal mammary fields, producing an overlap. Careful attention must be paid to this match line to avoid excessive dosage. Treatment of the chest wall with full-course electrons often produces a moist desquamation, which is quite uncomfortable. Therefore, the author prefers to treat the postmastectomy chest wall with photons whenever possible. However, a great deal of experience has been gained with electron beam therapy of the chest wall, and it clearly represents a useful treatment option.

REFERENCES

1. Montague ED, Delclos L: Palliative radiotherapy in the management of metastatic disease. *In:* Fletcher GH (ed.): Textbook of Radiotherapy. Philadelphia: Lea & Febiger, 1980, pp. 943–948.
2. Fisher B, Wolmark N, Baner M, et al.: The accuracy of clinical nodal staging and of limited axillary dissection as a determinant of histologic nodal status in carcinoma of the breast. Surg Gynecol Obstet 152:765, 1981.
3. Danoff BF, Goodman RL, Edelstein S, et al.: Results of omission of peripheral lymphatic irradiation in patients with clinical stage I and II breast cancer and histologically negative axillary nodes undergoing conservative surgery and radiation. (Abstract) Intl J Radiat Oncol Biol Phys (Suppl 2) 10:107, 1984.
4. Fletcher GH, Montague ED, Tapley N, et al.: Radiotherapy in the management of nondisseminated breast cancer. *In:* Fletcher GH (ed.): Textbook of Radiotherapy. Philadelphia: Lea & Febiger, 1980, pp. 527–579.
5. Haagensen CD: Lymphatics of the breast. *In:* Haagensen CD, Feind CR, Herter FP, et al. (eds.): The Lymphatics in Cancer. Philadelphia: W.B. Saunders Co., 1972, pp. 319–327.
6. Montague ED, Gutierrez AE, Barker JL, et al.: Conservation surgery and irradiation for the treatment of favorable breast cancer. Cancer 43:1058, 1979.
7. Pigott J, Nicholas R, Maddox WA, et al.: Metastases to the upper levels of the axillary nodes in carcinoma of the breast and its implications for nodal sampling procedures. Surg Gynecol Obstet 158:255, 1984.
8. Davies GC, Millis RR, Hayward JL: Assessment of axillary lymph node status. Ann Surg 192:148, 1980.
9. Roberson PL, Lichter AS, Bodner A, et al.: Dose to lung in primary breast irradiation. Intl J Radiat Oncol Biol Phys 9:97, 1982.
10. Levine JF, Coleman CN, Cox RS, et al.: The effect of postoperative and primary radiation therapy on delivered dose of adjuvant cyclophosphamide, methotrexate, and 5-fluorouracil (CMF) chemotherapy in breast cancer. Cancer 53:237, 1984.
11. Lippman ME, Lichter AS, Edwards BK, et al.: The impact of primary irradiation treatment of localized breast cancer on the ability to administer systemic adjuvant chemotherapy. J Clin Oncol 2:21, 1984.
12. Glick JH, Danoff BF, Haller DG, et al.: Adjuvant chemotherapy in patients undergoing definitive irradiation therapy for primary breast cancer. *In:* Harris JR, Hellman S, Silen W (eds.): Conservative Management of Breast Cancer. Philadelphia: J.B. Lippincott, 1983, pp. 311–320.
13. Botnick LE, Come S, Rose CM, et al.: Primary breast irradiation and concomitant adjuvant irradiation. *In:* Harris JR, Hellman S, Silen W (eds.): Conservative Management of Breast Cancer. Philadelphia: J.B. Lippincott, 1983, pp. 321–328.
14. Abrams RA, Lichter AS, Bromer JD, et al.: The hematopoietic toxicity of regional radiation therapy—correlations for combined modality therapy with systemic chemotherapy. Cancer 55:1429, 1985.
15. Harris JR, Levene MB, Svensson G, et al.: Analysis of cosmetic results following primary radiation for stages I and II carcinoma of the breast. Intl J Radiat Oncol Biol Phys 5:257, 1979.
16. Fletcher GH, Montague ED: Does adequate irradiation of the internal mammary chain and supraclavicular nodes improve survival rates? Intl J Radiat Oncol Biol Phys 4:481, 1978.
17. Lichter AS, Fraass BA, Fredrickson HA, et al.: Computed tomography in treatment planning: Primary breast cancer. *In:* Ling CC, Rogers CC, Morton RJ (eds.): Computed Tomography in Radiation Therapy. New York: Raven Press, 1983, pp. 99–107.
18. Rose CM, Kaplan WP, Marck A, et al.: Parasternal lymphoscintigraphy: Implication for the treatment planning of internal mammary lymph nodes in breast cancer. Intl J Radiat Oncol Biol Phys 5:1849, 1979.
19. Collier BD, Palmer DW, Wilson JF, et al.: Internal mammary lymphoscintigraphy in patients with breast cancer—correlation with computed tomography and impact on radiation therapy planning. Radiology 147:845, 1983.
20. Lichter AS, Padikal TN: Treatment planning in primary breast cancer. *In:* Bleehen NM, Glatstein E, Haybittle JL (eds.): Radiation Therapy Planning. New York: Marcel Dekker, 1983, pp. 639–661.
21. Lichter AS, Fraass BA, van de Geijn J, et al.: A technique for field matching in primary breast irradiation. Intl J Radiat Oncol Biol Phys 9:263, 1983.
22. Svensson GK, Bjärngard BE, Lawson RD, et al.: A modified three-field technique for breast treatment. Intl J Radiat Oncol Biol Phys 6:689, 1980.
23. Svensson GK, Chin LM, Siddon RL, et al.: Breast treatment techniques at the Joint Center for Radiation Therapy. *In:* Harris JR, Hellman S, Silen W (eds.): Conservative Management of Breast Cancer. Philadelphia: J.B. Lippincott, 1983, pp. 239–255.
24. Podgorsak EB, Gosselin M, Pla M, et al.: A simple isocentric technique for irradiation of the breast, chest wall, and peripheral lymphatics. Br J Radiol 57:57, 1984.
25. Siddon RL, Tonnesen GL, Svensson GK: Three-field technique for breast treatment using a rotatable half-beam block. Intl J Radiat Oncol Biol Phys 7:1473, 1981.
26. Siddon RL, Buck BA, Harris JR, et al.: Three-field technique for breast irradiation using tangential field cancer blocks. Intl J Radiat Oncol Biol Phys 9:583, 1983.
27. Lichter AS: Application of computerized tomography in radiotherapy treatment planning. *In:* Phillips TL, Pistenmaa DA (eds.): Radiation Oncology Annual. New York: Raven Press, 1984, pp. 179–203.

28. Glatstein E, Lichter AS, Fraass BA, et al.: The imaging revolution and radiation oncology: Use of CT, ultrasound and NMR for localization, treatment planning, and treatment delivery. Intl J Radiat Oncol Biol Phys 11:299, 1985.
29. Van de Geijn J: EXTDOS 71, revised and expanded version. The program for treatment planning in external beam therapy. Comput Programs Biomed 2:169, 1972.
30. Van Dyk L, Keane TJ, Rider WD: Lung density as measured by computerized tomography: Implications for radiotherapy. Intl J Radiat Oncol Biol Phys 8:1363, 1982.
31. Fraass BA, Roberson PL, Lichter AS: Dose to the contralateral breast due to primary breast irradiation. Intl J Radiat Oncol Biol Phys 11:485, 1985.
32. Svensson GK, Bjärngard BE, Chen GTY, et al.: Superficial doses in treatment of breast with tangential fields using 4MV x-rays. Intl J Radiat Oncol Biol Phys 2:705, 1977.
33. Harris JR, Beadle GF, Hellman S: Clinical studies on the use of radiation therapy as primary treatment of early breast cancer. Cancer 52:705, 1984.
34. Fisher B, Bauer M, Margolese R, et al.: Five-year results of a randomized clinical trial comparing total mastectomy and segmental mastectomy with or without radiation in the treatment of breast cancer. N Engl J Med 312:665, 1985.
35. Levene MB: Interstitial therapy of breast cancer. Intl J Radiat Oncol Biol Phys 2:1157, 1977.
36. Martinez A, Goffinet D: Irradiation with external beam and interstitial radioactive implant as primary treatment for early carcinoma of the breast. Surg Gynecol Obstet 152:285, 1981.
37. Solin LJ, Danoff BF, Schwartz GF, et al.: A practical technique for the localization of the tumor volume in definitive irradiation of the breast. Intl J Radiat Oncol Biol Phys 11:1215, 1985.
38. Tapley ND: Radiation therapy with the electron beam. Semin Oncol 8:49, 1981.
39. Montague ED, Tapley ND, Spanos WJ: Treatment techniques depending on tumor extent in cancer of the breast. *In:* Levitt SH, Tapley NV (eds.): Technological Basis of Radiation Therapy: Practical Clinical Applications. Philadelphia: Lea & Febiger, 1984, pp. 228–243.

Radiation Therapy as an Adjuvant to Surgery in the Treatment of Operable Breast Cancer

ALLEN S. LICHTER, M.D.
PEGGIE A. FINDLAY, M.D.

Certainly, no topic is more controversial in primary breast cancer therapy than the indications for and the effectiveness of adjuvant irradiation. Since the discovery of roentgen rays in the late 1890's, surgeons and radiation therapists have debated and researched these issues extensively. At least 20 clinical trials have been performed. It is a matter of considerable frustration to clinicians who treat breast cancer that despite the large number of clinical trials and the voluminous literature published on this topic, a general consensus as to the appropriate use of adjuvant irradiation has yet to be reached. This chapter will present an objective review of literature concerning adjuvant irradiation and will make recommendations about its use.

HISTORICAL BACKGROUND

The last decade of the nineteenth century witnessed a number of developments that had a profound impact on the treatment of breast cancer. In 1894, both Halsted[1] and Meyer[2] described operations for the *en bloc* removal of the breast, axillary contents, and pectoral musculature, forming the basis for radical surgery in the treatment of breast cancer. While there is uncertainty concerning the overall impact on survival that resulted from the introduction of the radical mastectomy, it is clear that the incidence of local recurrence was dramatically reduced.[3] In 1895, Roentgen announced the discovery of the x-ray, and as early as 1896, Gocht in Hamburg, Germany, applied the newly discovered rays to the treatment of two patients with advanced breast cancer. Relief of local pain was accomplished in both cases, although the patients died within a few weeks.[4] In the

8

United States, Grubbe in Chicago also reported irradiating advanced breast cancer before the turn of the century.[4]

The fact that the newly discovered x-rays could effect a response in advanced breast cancer was quickly seized upon by the contemporary surgical community. In the early 1900's, most surgeons were still operating on patients with locally advanced lesions. In a review of cases from the Mayo Clinic, Harrington reported that between 60 and 70 percent of their operable cases had pathologically involved lymph nodes.[5] Because of the relatively advanced nature of the cases and the fact that basic criteria for operability had yet to be defined, local persistence or local recurrence of breast cancer following operation was a common event. Radiation therapy was the only available modality that could address the problem of local recurrence and also could produce responses in patients with massive tumors, rendering them eligible for surgical therapy. One of the earliest practitioners of radiation therapy in the treatment of carcinoma of the breast was Pfahler in Philadelphia. In a series of papers,[6–10] Pfahler describes over 1000 cases of breast cancer treated between 1902 and 1928. The patients were treated for a variety of indications. Some received both preoperative and postoperative treatment, some just postoperative treatment; almost half the patients were treated solely for recurrence or metastasis, while another large group had primary inoperable cancer and were treated with radiation alone. A group of patients with small primary operable cancers was treated by radiation alone, representing the first reported group treated without benefit of radical surgical extirpation. It is interesting that 41 of the 50 patients (82 percent) treated in this breast-conserving manner were alive and "well" five years after treatment. Histologic confirmation was not obtained for any of these patients, and it is likely that some of them had benign disease.

Pfahler's reports were quite typical of the radiation papers published during the early 1900's. These reports were based on a varied assortment of patients and contained little indication as to how patients were selected for treatment. Not only were the technical aspects of irradiation ignored, but adherence to a uniform protocol was felt to be a hindrance to good radiation therapy results. As Pfahler stated, "We have no standard technique for all cases and until we can make cancer develop and distribute itself in some standard manner, no standard technique can be developed. Every case must be treated according to the individual indications."[9] Despite the poor equipment and the uncertainty regarding proper dosage, treatment responses were seen. Eleven percent of Pfahler's patients with inoperable cancers had their cancers made operable (20 of 178). Eighty-seven percent (43 of 49) of his patients with negative lymph nodes were well five years after surgery plus irradiation, and 58 percent (57 of 98) of patients who had had positive lymph nodes removed at the time of mastectomy survived five years. Pfahler reviewed the contemporary literature and concluded that results from postoperative irradiation were superior to those from surgery alone (Table 8–1). He strongly endorsed the use of irradiation as an adjuvant to surgery in the treatment of breast cancer and thought that all patients should receive such therapy.

Most reports of the time do not extend as far back as 1902 but rather begin their case accrual in the period from 1915 to 1918. This is because the Coolidge x-ray tube was invented in 1914 and allowed for a significant increase in x-ray voltage and an increase in tissue penetration.[11] A series of papers published in the late 1920's and throughout the 1930's reported on patients treated with this

TABLE 8–1. Comparative Survival in Breast Cancer Surgery With and Without Radiation Therapy

	No. of Series	*No. of Patients*	*Alive 5 Years* Stage II	All Operated Cases
Surgery alone	6	3021	27.9%	35.0%
Surgery and postoperative irradiation	11	1828	39.6%	46.8%

With permission from Pfahler GE: The treatment of carcinoma of the breast—Caldwell Lecture, 1937. Am J Roentgenol 39:1, 1938.

"modern" equipment. Virtually all of these papers reach a strong positive conclusion concerning the application of radiation therapy in the treatment of primary breast cancer. These statements are made despite the fact that there were no statistical analyses applied to the data, enormous selection bias, and certainly nothing even resembling a clinical trial. Lee,[12] Evans and Leucutia,[13] Portman,[14] and Adair[15] all proposed the value of irradiation. The report of Adair is typical of the type of papers published at the time and deserves careful scrutiny.

In February 1943, Adair published a review of cases seen at Memorial Hospital from 1920 through 1936.[15] A total of 1996 operable cases were seen, of which 613 were excluded from the analysis because of no pathologic confirmation of malignancy or because of death due to intercurrent disease. There were 194 patients treated with surgery alone, 669 treated with preoperative irradiation and surgery (many receiving postoperative radiation as well), and 338 patients treated with surgery followed by irradiation. There were also 182 patients treated with radiation therapy alone.

The survival rates of all of these groups were analyzed on the basis of whether they had positive or negative axillary lymph nodes (Table 8–2). The major conclusions from this paper were:

1. Preoperative irradiation was ineffective in improving survival beyond what could be achieved with surgery alone or with postoperative irradiation. For six years, all patients received preoperative therapy, following biopsy proof of cancer with aspiration cytology. The results of this form of treatment were no better than those of surgery alone or surgery plus postoperative irradiation.

2. As regards postoperative irradiation, Adair concludes that it is valuable, even though the survival rate of the irradiation group is identical with that of the group that had surgery alone. He ascribes the good results of surgery alone to "careful selection" of patients, but even when patients are stratified by nodal status, there is no difference in survival rate between the patients who were irradiated and those who were not. Adair comments on this situation as follows: "If we possessed a group of unselected cases treated by surgery alone, which we do not, we could tell how much irradiation adds; but we *already know* it to be of such great value that it is now too late to start to obtain an unselected group to be treated only by surgery."

3. A small group of patients were treated with biopsy plus radiation alone. Although the survival rate was low in these patients (44 of 182, or 24.2 percent), it does show that radiation is an effective agent against breast cancer.

Adair laments the "unfortunate turn of events" that has seen some people turn away from radical mastectomy to simple mastectomy. However, his results do not give any indication that such a move is undesirable. He reports a total of 99 patients treated with simple mastectomy, usually in conjunction with preoperative or postoperative irradiation. The overall five-year survival rate in

TABLE 8–2. Results of Surgery With and Without Radiation Therapy at Memorial Hospital

	Axilla Negative or ?		*Axilla Positive*	
	No. of Patients	5-Year Survival (%)	No. of Patients	5-Year Survival (%)
Surgery Alone				
Radical mastectomy	98	74	74	47
Simple mastectomy	14	71	—	—
Local excision	7	86	1	100
Preoperative XRT				
Radical mastectomy	245	68	337	35
Simple mastectomy	53	53	1	100
Local excision	28	68	5	0
Postoperative XRT				
Radical mastectomy	100	74	117	42
Simple mastectomy	30	73	1	0
Local excision	30	70	—	—
Radiation Only	180	24	2	0

With permission from Adair FE: The role of surgery and irradiation in cancer of the breast. JAMA 121:553, 1943.

these patients was 65 percent, which is slightly lower than that of patients treated with more radical surgery, but the former were patients selected because of poor general condition and older age. Intriguing results are also presented for local excision alone. Seventy-one patients were treated, with an overall survival rate near 70 percent. Most of these patients were treated with preoperative or postoperative irradiation, although there were seven patients treated with excision alone, of whom six survived beyond five years. Adair still claims that simple mastectomy or local excision is an inferior treatment and states, "It is up to the protagonist of this procedure to produce a series of cases as good as that produced by the combination of radical surgery and irradiation. We shall await with great anticipation a comprehensive report of a series of cases, statistically acceptable, so treated." However, since the majority of breast cancer patients were treated by surgeons whose philosophy of treatment paralleled that of the Memorial Hospital group, no such series were available for comparison, and it would take more than two decades for such a trial to begin. Even then, it was the British medical community that would launch this effort, not physicians in the United States.

In contrast with Adair's report, numerous negative reports concerning irradiation were appearing at the same time. The paper by Harrington[5] reported on 1859 patients treated with mastectomy from 1910 to 1923 at the Mayo Clinic. Slightly over half (1092 patients) of the entire group had postoperative radiation therapy; many were irradiated at other institutions. The five- and ten-year survival rates for patients treated with and without postoperative irradiation and stratified for axillary nodal status were similar. There is no mention of the type of radiation that patients received or the dosage or method of application. Similarly, there is no discussion of selection factors, such as number of positive lymph nodes or tumor size, that might have influenced the outcome. In 1929, Greenough[16] reported for the committee on x-ray treatment of the American College of Surgeons. They examined 774 records of breast cancer patients treated from 1918 through 1920. Five hundred thirty-six of these records were evaluable, and 408 of these had treatment for primary breast cancer. The five-year survival rate in operable cases was 28 percent, and the investigators report that there was no difference in outcome according to whether adjuvant irradiation was or was not given. Again, there was no mention of x-ray technique or criteria for selection of patients.

Adding to the confusion as to whether radiation therapy contributed to survival after mastectomy was the plethora of x-ray techniques used. While tangential techniques for the chest wall were employed relatively early by Pfahler,[10] most therapists used a technique that cross-fired radiation into the mediastinum via numerous direct chest wall fields. The paper by Pendergrass and Hodes[17] is illustrative of these multiple-field techniques. Between 20 and 40 fields were used (Fig. 8–1); over the years, this was reduced to 10 or 12 fields. Five to six hundred roentgens were given daily to numerous small

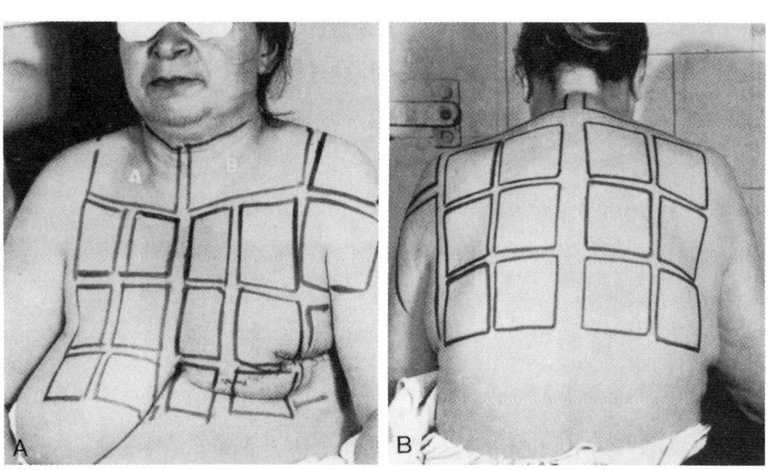

FIGURE 8–1. Field configurations for postoperative chest wall and lymph node irradiation in the 1920's. To compensate for the very low energy of the x-rays and the ill-defined nature of the regions at risk, multiple beams were cross-fired into the chest wall, lymph nodes, and mediastinum through anterior and posterior fields. (With permission from Pendergrass EP, Hodes PG: Some observations on carcinoma of the breast. Am J Roentgenol 39:397, 1938.)

portals or two to four of the large portals. When each field had received one treatment, the series was stopped and then repeated at two- to three-month intervals. Similar techniques were used by Evans and Leucutia[13] and also by Lee and Herendeen.[18] In this fashion, a series of treatments could extend over six to ten months and in some patients would extend over many years. It was not until the 1940's[11] and in some cases until the 1950's[19] that a continuous course of irradiation was routinely employed.

As the decade of the 1940's approached, sorting out a generally accepted treatment for carcinoma of the breast became impossible. Most authors acknowledged that very early cases could be cured with operation alone and that very advanced cases required a combination of surgery and irradiation. However, a vast middle ground of patients remained for whom there was no established therapeutic plan. As early as 1938, Pendergrass and Hodes, radiologists at the University of Pennsylvania, wrote, "It seems that the time is propitious for some large organization, representing radiologists and surgeons, to inaugurate one or several of the acceptable methods for treatment of cancer of the breast. In this manner, if careful records are kept, a sufficiently large number of patients treated by several methods could be accumulated in a few years for subjection to a critical analysis. If we carry on as we have been doing in the past, there will continue to be marked divergence of opinion because of the small groups of patients being reported by each individual, with the result that little progress will be made."[17] Eleven years later the first such clinical trial would take place.

THE ERA OF CLINICAL TRIALS—POSTOPERATIVE IRRADIATION

Since 1949, a major part of the knowledge concerning the treatment of primary breast cancer has come through analysis of prospective randomized trials. A detailed consideration of clinical trial development, methodology, and analysis is found in Chapter 19. Clinicians around the world have understood the potential biases concerning patient selection that make it impossible to compare consecutive series of patients treated at one hospital during different time periods or treated concurrently at different hospitals. While it is tempting to compare large series of patients treated by different methods (and one can find such comparisons as that of the M.D. Anderson Hospital[20] contrasting their treatment results with a reported outcome from the National Surgical Adjuvant Breast Project (NSABP)[21]), the information gained from this practice is limited and potentially misleading.

Two types of clinical trials have emerged over the years. In the trials of *radical* therapy, two treatments whose aim is the comprehensive therapy of the breast and locoregional lymph nodes are compared. Examples of these types of trials include (1) radical mastectomy versus radical mastectomy plus irradiation, (2) radical mastectomy versus simple mastectomy plus irradiation, and (3) extended radical mastectomy versus simple mastectomy plus irradiation.

In many respects, the Guy's Hospital trial,[22] as well as the Milan trial[23] and the NSABP B-06 trial[24] comparing radical or modified radical mastectomy against excision plus lymph node dissection (not done in the Guy's Hospital trial) plus radiation, is also an example of a radical therapy trial. Since one of the treatment arms in these trials did not use mastectomy, the results of these three studies are discussed in Chapter 6.

The other area of clinical investigation is the trial of *conservative* therapy. In this type of study, a comprehensive radical treatment is compared with a less aggressive treatment. Such conservative treatments avoid treatment of the axillary lymph nodes. Examples of these types of trials include (1) radical mastectomy versus simple mastectomy and (2) simple mastectomy plus irradiation versus simple mastectomy.

A recently completed trial by the NSABP (trial B-06)[24] also included a conservative treatment arm, which involved wide local excision of the breast lump with axillary dissection and no treatment to the remaining breast tissue. Again, this trial is discussed in Chapter 6.

The purpose of the numerous clinical trials was to demonstrate, if possible, the best treatment for breast cancer. Failing to identify a "best" treatment, the researchers running the trials sought to advance a less morbid form of treatment if it was equivalent, with respect to local control and survival rates, to a more aggressive one. At least 16 trials involving postoperative radiation therapy have been reported in the literature in the last three decades. In spite of these efforts, considerable controversy still exists concerning the proper role of postoperative radiation therapy in the treatment of operable breast cancer. Some of the reasons that clinical trials have yet to resolve the issue of postoperative radiation therapy are contained in a provocative paper by Bross and Blumenson.[25] Using predictive mathematical models based on the reported survival rates of breast cancer patients, these investigators conclude that any clinical trial in breast cancer is probably treating three groups of patients:

1. Patients with localized disease, in whom virtually all adequate local treatments will produce a "cure."
2. Patients who present with occult metastatic disease and who will succumb to their disease process. In this group, no variation in local therapy will produce a difference in outcome.
3. Patients with locoregional disease without distant metastases. It is in this group that a change in the philosophy of management of the locoregional tumor may produce a change in the survival rate. This subset of patients, if it even exists at all, is so small that even fairly important differences in outcome are diluted by the overall group.

Based on their mathematical models, Bross and Blumenson conclude that even clinical trials randomizing 10,000 patients would have a great deal of difficulty in showing any difference between one form of local therapy versus another. Since the largest clinical trials have randomized approximately 2500 patients, it is not surprising that there has not yet been a "positive" trial in the primary treatment of breast cancer; that is, all primary treatment programs tested have shown essentially equivalent overall survival rates.

The fact that the design of primary breast cancer clinical trials and the biologic aspects of this disease almost guarantee that each treatment arm will produce nonstatistically different overall results has a more insidious side. Such trials allow all participants and all practitioners to leave the trial with their preconceived views intact. As Bross and Blumenson point out, physicians who favor one approach (e.g., a conservative approach) can argue that trial after trial has shown that the conservative alternative is equivalent to the radical one. They can point out that whatever true difference may exist between the two treatments, this difference is likely to be small and relatively inconsequential. Thus, advocates of the conservative approach may feel that their treatment philosophy has been vindicated. On the other hand, physicians who favor a more radical approach may still cling to this treatment, arguing that the study design was flawed, that too few patients were randomized, and that no study so designed could be expected to show an advantage for radical treatment. Thus, the overall design of the trial is called unfair and these physicians continue to practice radical therapy. In the words of Bross and Blumenson, "Neither participant would be compelled by these hypothetical 'facts' to alter the position that he had taken prior to the study." In the recent literature, the types of critiques that Bross and Blumenson predicted would appear concerning breast cancer clinical trials have indeed been published.[26–29] Because of the problems inherent in the design of clinical trials and because of finite limitations on the number of patients that can be randomized in a clinical trial, the oncology community may never be able to reach a consensus concerning the value of postoperative radiation therapy in the management of primary breast cancer. Baum[30] recently used these same types of arguments concerning clinical trial evaluation for adjuvant chemotherapy.

Analysis of Clinical Trials Testing Radical Forms of Treatment

THE MANCHESTER TRIAL

This study, directed by Ralston Paterson of the Christie Hospital and the Holt Radium Institute in Manchester, England, was the first breast cancer clinical trial performed. It was begun in January 1949 and concluded patient accrual with 1461 cases in June 1955. The study design and outcome have been published on several occasions.[31–35] Patients were allocated at random to treatment with radical mastectomy alone or radical mastectomy followed by postoperative irradiation. The group that underwent surgery alone received radiation at the first sign of local or regional failure. This has led the investigators to emphasize that this trial represented a comparison of "immediate" versus "delayed" irradiation and not a trial of irradiation versus no irradiation.

The patients were irradiated using two completely different techniques. From 1949 to mid-1952, the "quadrate technique" was used; from mid-1952 to mid-1955, the "peripheral technique" was practiced. These two techniques are almost mirror images of one another; that is, while the quadrate technique irradiated the operative bed and virtually ignored the lymph nodes, the peripheral technique treated the nodes, leaving the chest wall untreated. With the quadrate technique, three oblique tangential fields covered the area of the chest wall (Fig. 8–2), while a fourth field extending from the back into the axilla was employed to supplement whatever dose entered the axilla through the tangential fields. The supraclavicular triangle was not irradiated. The overall treatment time was three weeks, and the dosage was between 3500 and 4000 R. It is not indicated whether this dose was given to a tumor volume or was an applied dose, but it is likely the latter. The peripheral technique consisted of a pair of opposed fields, usually 10 × 20 cm, directed anteriorly and posteriorly over the supraclavicular fossa and axilla. These fields were matched to a single anterior field, 6 × 12 cm, covering the homolateral side of the parasternal area (Fig. 8–3). The treatment

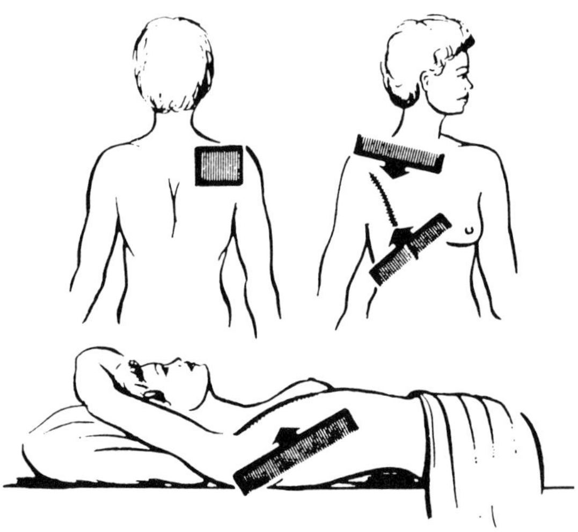

FIGURE 8–2. The quadrate technique, used in the first Manchester trial. Irradiation of three oblique fields treated the chest wall while irradiation of a fourth posterior field supplemented the axillary dose. (With permission from Eason EC: Postoperative radiotherapy in breast cancer. *In*: Forrest AP [ed.]: Prognostic Factors in Breast Cancer. Baltimore: Williams & Wilkins, 1968.)

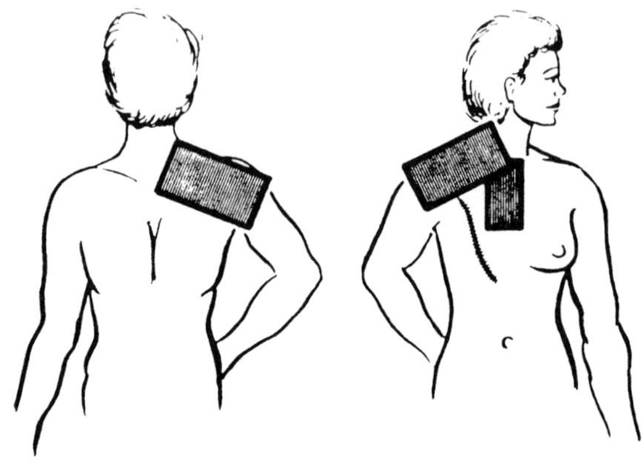

FIGURE 8–3. The peripheral technique, used in the Manchester trial. Irradiation of one posterior and two anterior fields treated the peripheral lymph nodes, leaving the chest wall untreated. (With permission from Eason EC: Postoperative radiotherapy in breast cancer. *In*: Forrest AP [ed.]: Prognostic Factors in Breast Cancer. Baltimore: Williams & Wilkins, 1968.)

time was three weeks, the opposed fields receiving 3250 R at midplane, while the applied dose to the parasternal field was 4250 R over three weeks. Both techniques used a 250-KV machine with a half-value level of 1.5 mm of copper, and both routinely produced moist desquamation and, in many cases, left permanent skin changes. A total of 723 patients were treated during the quadrate era and 741 during the peripheral technique period.

The results of the study showed no significant difference in survival rate for the overall study population. Similarly, there was no difference in survival rate when the total patient population was stratified according to axillary nodal status, although in the axilla-negative group, the unirradiated patients did slightly better (Fig. 8–4). There was no significant difference between the quadrate technique and the peripheral technique. It should be noted that watched patients in the peripheral series (1952 to 1955) did somewhat better than watched patients in the quadrate series (1949 to 1952). However, these differences were not statistically different.

A significant part of the analysis involved local recurrence (Table 8–3). Overall, 19 percent of the treated patients developed local recurrence versus 32 percent of the watched patients. However, once the treated patients had local failure, it was very difficult to control their disease and over two thirds of the patients manifesting a chest wall failure died with active disease at this site, which

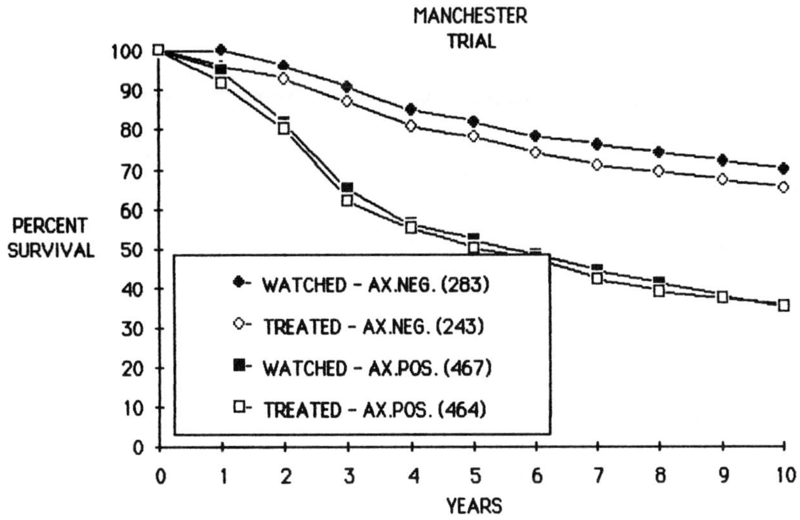

FIGURE 8–4. Results from the first Manchester trial, 1949 to 1955. No significant differences between groups were seen. (From Eason EC: Postoperative radiotherapy in breast cancer. *In* Forrest AP [ed.]: Prognostic Factors in Breast Cancer. Baltimore: Williams & Wilkins, 1968.)

represented 14 percent of the treated patients. In the watched group, half the patients who exhibited local failure had their local disease controlled until death with irradiation delivered at the time of recurrence. Thus, 16 percent of the watched patients died with active local tumor. In summary, this trial showed that postoperative irradiation did not have an impact on overall survival rate, and while the frequency of initial local recurrence was reduced by irradiation, there was little effect on the overall number of patients dying with uncontrolled chest wall disease.

Criticisms of this trial are centered in two major areas. Despite the large number of patients involved, patient selection could have influenced the outcome. Patients were randomized by odd or even date of birth, allowing the investigators to know which treatment a patient would receive prior to randomization. Thus, some patients with certain disease characteristics could have been systematically excluded from one arm of the trial or systematically overrepresented in the alternate arm. Since in the reports of this trial there is no mention of tumor size or number of nodes involved, one cannot be sure that these prognostic factors were evenly divided between the groups. The other criticism concerns the techniques of irradiation in this trial.[46] The quadrate technique was not designed to treat the internal mammary lymph nodes and gave a very uncertain dose to the axilla. The peripheral technique did not treat the chest wall at all and may have given a lower than intended dose to the upper internal mammary lymph nodes. Supporting this contention is the rather high local failure rate (19 percent) in irradiated patients followed to ten years. However, considering the time period of this trial and keeping in mind that 250-kV machines were the only machines available, the study employed treatment that was current. While one explanation for the failure to show that radiation therapy improves survival and ultimate local control may be that the radiation was inadequately delivered,[46] an equally plausible explanation is that postoperative irradiation does not influence the outcome in primary operable breast cancer.

TABLE 8–3. Incidence of Locoregional Failure and Ultimate Locoregional Control—The Manchester Trial

		Local Failure		*Local Disease Uncontrolled*	
Clinical Stage	*No. of Cases*	TREATED	OBSERVED	TREATED	OBSERVED
I	527	9.5%	16.0%	5.0%	7.5%
II	934	25.0%	41.5%	18.5%	21.0%
Total	1461	19.0%	32.0%	14.0%	16.0%

With permission from Eason EC: Post-operative radiotherapy in breast cancer. *In*: Forrest AF (ed.): Prognostic Factors in Breast Cancer. Baltimore: Williams & Wilkins, 1968.

THE TRIAL BY BRINKLEY AND HAYBITTLE (ADDENBROOKE'S HOSPITAL, CAMBRIDGE)

A review of cases seen at Addenbrooke's Hospital from 1947 to 1950 indicated that patients with Stage II breast cancer treated with simple mastectomy plus postoperative irradiation had a better survival rate than did patients treated with radical mastectomy and postoperative irradiation. However, since this was a retrospective review and patient selection could have introduced bias into the results, it was felt appropriate to perform a prospective clinical trial.[36, 37] The study began in October 1958 and ended in May 1965. It was confined to patients with tumor of any size at the primary site with clinically positive, mobile axillary nodes. Surgical treatment was either standard radical mastectomy or "modified" simple mastectomy, which was defined as removal of the entire breast without taking pectoral musculature, although accessible axillary glands could be removed. Radiation therapy was started three to four weeks after surgery. Two 30 × 10 cm tangential fields were used in an effort to treat the entire chest wall, the axilla, the supraclavicular fossa, and the internal mammary node regions. A minimum tumor dose of 3250 rad was delivered in 18 days, using 250-kV x-rays with bolus.

Patient entry into this trial was rather slow and over the seven years of the trial, only 204 patients were randomized. Overall, there was no significant difference in the survival or disease-free survival rates between the two treatment groups (Fig. 8–5), although with this relatively small sampling, a moderately sized difference could have been missed. The Addenbrooke study confirmed that the morbidity of the radical operation was greater than that of the simple operation.

The investigators point out that in 1965 the findings of Kaae and Johansen showed the results of simple mastectomy plus irradiation to be the equivalent of those of extended radical mastectomy. Based on those reported findings, the fact that there was no difference between the two groups, and the added morbidity of radical mastectomy, the investigators elected to discontinue patient entry.

It is difficult to place a great deal of confidence in the conclusions of this trial. The patient numbers are quite small, and subset analyses in which 20 to 25 patients are being compared in each arm are quite hazardous. The x-ray therapy technique used in this trial is rather obscure, since it is difficult to imagine how the chest wall and all regional lymph nodes could be included in a single pair of tangential x-ray fields. Nonetheless, this trial gave British surgeons and radiotherapists the confidence to use simple mastectomy plus postoperative irradiation as a standard treatment arm in subsequent trials. This particular study directly led to the Cancer Research Campaign trial of simple mastectomy plus postoperative irradiation versus simple mastectomy alone, which will be discussed later.

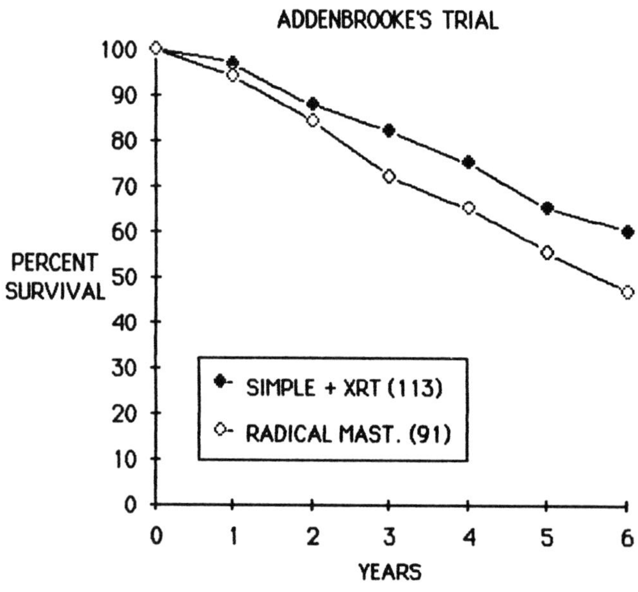

FIGURE 8–5. Results from the Addenbrooke trial, 1958 to 1965. No significant differences between groups were seen. (From Brinkley D, Haybittle JL: Treatment of stage two cancer of the female breast. Lancet 2:1086, 1971.)

NSABP Protocol No. 2

This study began in 1961 and terminated in mid-1968.[38] The complex schema of this trial differed for pre- and postmenopausal patients. While all patients received radical mastectomy, premenopausal patients were randomized to the following postsurgical treatments: 50 percent to radiation therapy; 25 percent to a placebo drug; and 25 percent to three days of postoperative thiotepa. Postmenopausal patients could be randomized in the same fashion, or at the discretion of the institution, node-positive postmenopausal patients could be randomized according to the premenopausal schema, while node-negative postmenopausal patients would receive no radiation therapy and would be evenly divided to receive either thiotepa or 5-FU. In May 1967, there was another change in the premenopausal category, and the placebo group was eliminated. Premenopausal patients were then randomized, with two thirds receiving radiation and one third receiving thiotepa. Node-positive postmenopausal patients were treated similarly.

While this study was in progress, another NSABP clinical trial (Protocol No. 3) was being carried out.[39] Following radical mastectomy, half the patients were treated with bilateral oophorectomy, while the other half received either thiotepa or a placebo. Analysis of the outcome of Protocol No. 3 premenopausal patients treated with thiotepa or a placebo showed that their results were similar to the results in the identical treatment arm of Protocol No. 2 (control arm). Therefore, the investigators chose to add 133 patients from Protocol No. 3 into the control arm of Protocol No. 2. According to the researchers, "Their inclusion enhances the reliability of the data in certain subsets of patients whose numbers are otherwise too small for valid interpretation."

A total of 1882 patients were randomized, and 779 (41.4 percent) were withdrawn, leaving 1103 patients suitable for analysis. Of those analyzed, 470 received radiation therapy, 316 received thiotepa, and 317 received a placebo. The researchers claim that careful analysis of the excluded patients did not introduce any bias into the results of the study.

The radiation therapy technique involved dosages from 3500 rad over three weeks to 4500 rad over five weeks to the peripheral nodes. The chest wall was not irradiated. Seventy-five percent of the patients received supervoltage radiation, while the other 25 percent received orthovoltage radiation with an energy of no less than 200 kV.

The results of this study showed that radiation therapy decreased local and regional failures in virtually all subsets of patients. This decrease was most marked for regional disease recurrence in the lymph nodes but was also true for local disease recurrence in the chest wall, even though the chest wall was not irradiated. However, there was no difference in overall recurrence or survival rates between the irradiated and the nonirradiated patients (Fig. 8–6).

A number of flaws are inherent in this trial. First, it is not widely appreciated that the results reported by the NSABP are crude recurrence and survival figures, not actuarial survival figures. Thus, while the investigators imply that the results are based on 1103 patients eligible for analysis, at the time of the report only 415 patients had been followed for five years or more, and the five-year results are based on an analysis of these 415 patients only. No analysis of all 1103 patients has, to our knowledge, been presented. Second, the method of randomization that allowed so many treatment exclusions can also be criticized. Not only were 41 percent of the patients deemed ineligible (in part because of insufficient information for follow-up), but these exclusions were not randomly distributed. This fact along with the complex randomization schema created an unequal distribution of the patients among the three arms of the study. Third, it is unacceptable statistical practice to include the results of control patients who were treated in another study simply because they matched the outcome of patients treated in Protocol No. 2. Such a statement implies that if these other control patients had an outcome that differed from that of the patients in Protocol No. 2, they would not have been included. This "padding" of the control population with an additional 133 patients whose outcome lives up to a preconceived expectation damages the credibility of the study. Finally, there was no monitoring of radiation therapy quality control in this study. Each radiation department was allowed to set up its radiation fields according to its best judgment, and no monitoring was done to see that the correct dosage of radiation was delivered to the proper targets.

In spite of the fact that this study showed

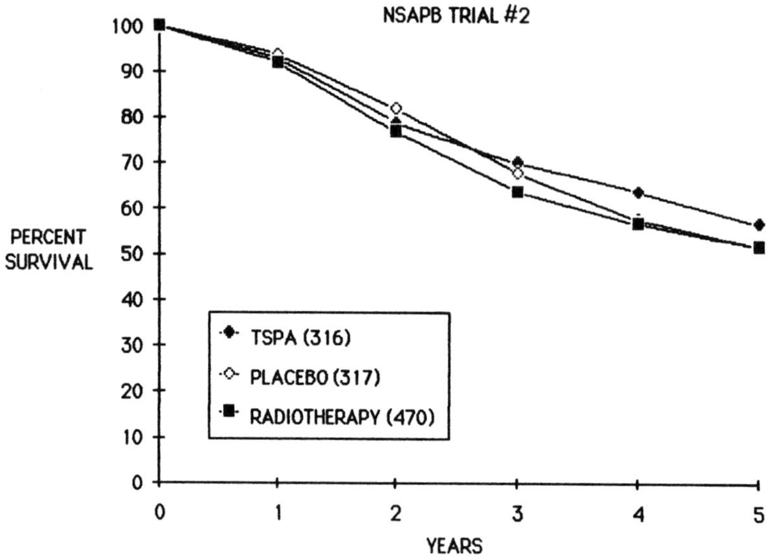

FIGURE 8–6. Results from NSABP trial no. 2, 1961 to 1968. No significant differences among groups were seen. (From Fisher B, Slack NH, Cavanaugh PJ, et al.: Postoperative radiotherapy in the treatment of cancer—results of the NSABP trial. Ann Surg 172:711, 1970.)

no advantage for radiation therapy, Harris and Hellman[40] have suggested that modest increases in disease-free survival rates for node-positive patients may be related to the improved locoregional control produced by the radiation. Examination of Tables 5 and 6 of the NSABP publication[38] shows that the percentage of improvement in the disease-free survival rate seen in irradiated patients was identicial with the improvement in the locoregional control rate produced by the radiation (Table 8–4). Among patients with no positive nodes or one to three positive nodes, the irradiated patients showed a 3 percent improvement in the disease-free survival rate and a 3 percent lowering in the rate of locoregional recurrence. Among patients with four or more positive nodes, the irradiated patients enjoyed a 10 percent increase in the disease-free survival rate, which corresponded exactly to their 10 percent lower incidence of locoregional failure. Harris and Hellman imply that the group of patients who could expect improved survival with postoperative irradiation is small, can be identified, and has been demonstrated by the NSABP study, but this group is simply not large enough to show statistical advantage. However, it should be remembered that while disease-free survival rates for certain subsets of patients were improved with radiation therapy, the overall survival rate was not affected and the subset analysis included rather small groups of patients. For example, in the group with four or more positive nodes who were followed for at least five years, 48 patients who received radiation therapy are compared with 59 patients who received a placebo or thiotepa. These 117 patients come from a population of 1103 randomized into the study.

It is reasonable to conclude that NSABP Prococol No. 2 contained too many design flaws to be considered the definitive trial as

TABLE 8–4. Relapse-Free Survival and Locoregional Recurrences—NSABP Protocol No. 2

	Axillary Node Status		
	Negative Nodes (%)	1–3 Positive Nodes (%)	4 or More Positive (%)
Relapse-free Survival			
Irradiation	78.6	49.1	28.4
Control	76.0	47.8	18.0
Locoregional Recurrence			
Irradiation	0	0	1.5
Control	2.1	4.5	12.5

With permission from Harris JR, Hellman S: Local and regional management of carcinoma of the breast. *In*: Carter S, Glatstein E, Livingston R (eds.): Principles of Cancer Treatment. New York: McGraw-Hill, 1982.

to the efficacy of postoperative radiation therapy. It is to the credit of the NSABP that two very similar treatment arms were included in a more modern trial (NSABP Protocol B-04) and that all the major design flaws from Protocol No. 2 were corrected in the later trial. The results of that trial will be discussed later in this chapter.

The Copenhagen Trial

From November 1951 until November 1957, Kaae and Johansen conducted a clinical trial comparing simple mastectomy plus postoperative irradiation versus extended radical mastectomy.[41–43] All patients who were seen at the Radium Center in Copenhagen and who were living in Copenhagen were randomized into the trial; however, only about three out of four patients actually received protocol therapy. Many randomized patients turned out to be ineligible for surgery because of the advanced stage of their disease or because of inoperability. For example, in the simple mastectomy plus postoperative irradiation group, 331 patients were randomized, 288 were operable, and 219 actually received the treatment. In the extended radical mastectomy group, 206 patients received the treatment. The results of the study are based on the outcome of these 425 patients. It should also be pointed out (as mentioned by Kaae and Johnansen and emphasized by Anglem and Leber[44]) that 25 patients out of the 206 assigned to the extended radical mastectomy arm as "operable" never actually received the extended radical mastectomy because at the time of surgery they were found to be technically inoperable. These patients are reported in the series of extended radical mastectomy because the researchers felt that similar exclusions could not be made in the simple mastectomy plus irradiation arm and that to exclude these poor prognosis patients from analysis would have introduced bias into the study.

Extended radical mastectomy was performed by the Dahl-Iversen method. This included a classic radical mastectomy plus a dissection of the internal mammary and supraclavicular area. The internal mammary node dissection was not performed *en bloc* but rather represented a local excision of this lymph node–bearing region. The simple mastectomy was followed by radiation delivered according to McWhirter's method.[45] The axilla and supraclavicular areas were treated via two opposing fields, and the chest wall was treated via tangential fields. The medial tangent was placed along the contralateral sternal border to include the internal mammary lymph nodes within the tangential fields, and bolus was used on all fields. The axillary-supraclavicular fields were treated with 400-kV photons, and the tangential fields were treated with 250-kV photons, with between 4200 and 4500 rad applied over three weeks. The central midaxillary dose varied from 3800 to 4000 rad.

Overall, there were no differences in survival or disease-free survival rates for the total group or any subset, regardless of treatment option (Fig. 8–7). In the patients with more advanced disease (excluding Stage I), there were fewer locoregional recurrences in the irradiated group versus the extended radical mastectomy group.

The following criticisms were leveled at this study. The patients were assigned to treatment by odd or even case numbers. This could allow an introduction of bias into the study through the selection of patients. However, the investigators maintain that all patients were randomized, which would seem to address this potential problem. The conclusions are based on relatively small numbers of patients: A total of 400 patients actually received the assigned therapies. However, this number is certainly large enough to rule out missing substantial differences that might exist between the two groups. Clinical Stage II and clinical Stage III patients were analyzed together, and thus, it is impossible to ascertain whether these two treatments were equivalent for patients with Stage II cancer only. Anglem and Leber[44] speculate about the quality of the surgical therapy. They point out that 12 percent of the patients in the extended radical mastectomy group could not receive the operation even after all supposedly inoperable patients were screened out. This 12 percent rate of inoperability seemed quite high to them. Anglem and Leber also point out that the Dahl-Iversen method (which is to simply locally excise internal mammary lymph nodes versus resecting them *en bloc*) has been implicated in promoting the dissemination of breast cancer, an argument that has never been proved. The x-ray therapy technique can also be criticized. One of the variables in the trial concerned the therapy of the internal

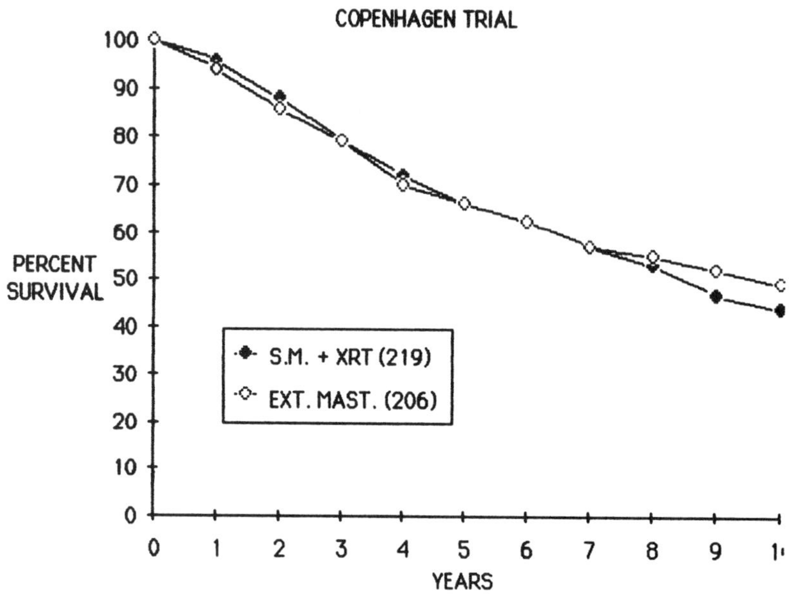

FIGURE 8–7. Results from the Copenhagen trial, 1951 to 1957. No significant differences between groups were seen. (From Kaae S, Johansen H: Simple mastectomy followed by irradiation offers survival comparable to radical procedures. Int J Radiat Oncol Biol Phys 2:1163, 1977.)

mammary lymph nodes. In the surgical group, these nodes were resected, whereas in the irradiation group, they were supposed to receive x-ray treatment. It is doubtful that tangential fields brought to the edge of the contralateral sternum and treated with 250-kV photons reliably irradiated the intramammary lymph nodes to full dose in most patients.[46]

THE NORWEGIAN TRIAL

In 1964, Høst and Brennhovd at the Norwegian Radium Hospital began a trial evaluating postoperative radiation therapy.[47–49] Patients who had undergone a Halsted radical mastectomy and were referred for irradiation were randomized to receive or not to receive such treatment, while all patients received ovarian irradiation of 650 to 900 R. The chest wall and nodal radiation differed in two periods of the study. From 1964 through 1967, 546 patients had their treatment delivered with 200-kV orthovoltage radiation. The radiation fields covered the internal mammary lymph node chain, axilla, supraclavicular fossa, and chest wall. The supraclavicular fossa was irradiated with a direct field delivering a surface dose of 3600 R. The remainder of the targets were irradiated in tangential fields with a surface dose of 2500 to 3100 R. A lateral field was used to boost the axilla, with an additional 1800 R delivered to the skin. The overall treatment time was four weeks. The investigators state that measurement in a phantom revealed a rapid falling off of dose, especially in the tangential fields, because of the amount of radiation that was directed into the air and because of the corresponding lack of tissue to scatter radiation back into the field. They note a very inhomogeneous dose distribution, with target exposures ranging from 1800 to 3600 R.

From 1968 to 1972, the remainder of the patients were irradiated with ^{60}Co. Direct fields covered the apex of the axilla, the supraclavicular region, and the internal mammary chains, while the chest wall was not irradiated at all. A dose of 5000 rad over four weeks was delivered at a 3 cm depth.

In 1977, the results from both the orthovoltage and the megavoltage series were reported.[48] For patients with negative lymph nodes, there was no difference in survival or recurrence rates between those who were irradiated and those who were not. However, in Stage II disease, there was a suggestion of an improved survival rate for the patients irradiated with ^{60}Co as compared with either the controls or the orthovoltage irradiation group. This improvement occurred solely in patients with medial quadrant tumors but was not quite statistically significant ($p = 0.075$). However, there was a statistically significant improvement in the disease-free survival rate for cobalt-treated patients ($p < 0.05$).

There are numerous criticisms of this 1977 analysis. Probably the most serious one is that the results of the cobalt-treated patients are not compared with those of the controls of the same four-year period, but rather with the results of all controls in the entire eight-year study. This means not only that the median follow-up time was considerably longer in the control group but also that statistical tests would be performed on a larger group of patients, allowing statistical significance to be reached when none may actually have existed. The series also employed no stratification for menopausal status and used ovarian irradiation in each patient. An unequal distribution with regard to menopausal status could have influenced the results. Finally, the results for the entire series are so outstanding that one wonders about their comparability with those of other treatment series. For example, the five-year survival rate in Stage II disease (positive lymph nodes) is quoted as 86 percent for the cobalt-irradiated group. The M.D. Anderson Hospital quotes a five-year survival rate of 67 percent[20] for a similar group of patients. This 86 percent survival rate is so high that one cannot help but think that careful patient selection has entered into the treatment of these patients.[50]

The statistical criticisms of the trial have been answered in a subsequent report from Høst, published in 1982.[49] In this report, the cobalt-treated patients were compared with the control subjects who were randomized and treated concurrently. When such an analysis was done in Stage II disease, there was no statistically significant improvement in the 95 cobalt-irradiated patients over the 92 concurrent controls (Fig. 8–8), and the disease-free survival rate was no longer statistically different. Patients irradiated during the cobalt era for *medial* quadrant tumors had five- and ten-year survival rates of 79 and 62 percent, respectively, compared with 55 and 45 percent for the corresponding controls. However, this difference was not statistically significant. As it now stands, this trial must be regarded as a negative study.

The Southeast Scotland Trial

By 1964, the surgeons of Edinburgh and the southeastern region of Scotland had over 20 years of experience in treating breast cancer with simple mastectomy plus postoperative irradiation. This policy had come under substantial criticism from surgeons who favored more radical surgical procedures, and the surgeons and radiotherapists of the region began a clinical trial to test radical mastectomy against simple mastectomy plus postoperative radiation.[51–53] Eligible patients had to be between 35 and 69 years of age

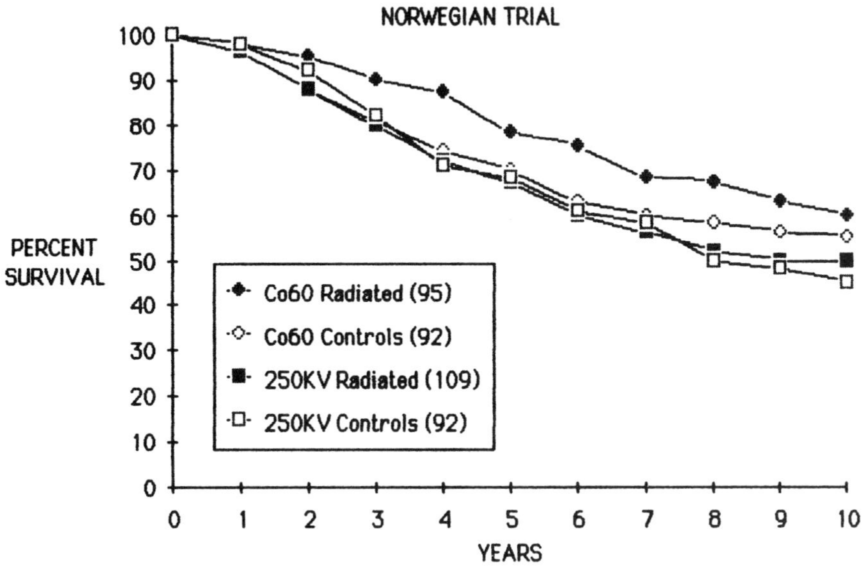

FIGURE 8–8. Results from the Norwegian trial, 1964 to 1982. No significant differences among groups were seen. (From Host H: Postoperative radiotherapy in breast cancer. Experientia [Suppl] 41:580, 1982.)

and had to have clinical Stage I or II or operable Stage III cancer. A negative chest x-ray and pelvic x-ray constituted the systemic work-up. The irradiation technique used 2-MV x-rays and treated the axilla and supraclavicular fossa in opposed fields, while treating the chest wall and internal mammary lymph nodes in tangential fields. The axilla and supraclavicular fossa received 4250 rad in 10 fractions on alternate days over four weeks, while the chest wall received an applied dose of 4500 rad with the same fractionation. All patients between 35 and 60 years of age had either oophorectomy or ovarian irradiation. A total of 1099 patients were randomized through 1971. Since the randomization was done prior to any surgical procedure, 512 patients were immediately withdrawn from the study because the breast tumor turned out to be histologically benign. Eighty-nine additional cases were withdrawn for a variety of other reasons. For example, 31 patients did not receive oophorectomy, 20 patients had noninvasive carcinoma or a sarcoma, 17 patients were too old or had a previous carcinoma, and 11 patients had an axillary dissection when they should have had a simple mastectomy alone. These exclusions left 256 patients in the radical mastectomy group and 242 patients in the simple mastectomy plus irradiation group.

Results showed that the number of recurrences was the same in both groups, with 107 treatment failures in patients undergoing simple mastectomy and 105 failures in patients treated with radical mastectomy. Although more patients in the simple mastectomy plus irradiation group had recurrence in the axilla, more patients in the radical mastectomy group exhibited recurrence in the supraclavicular nodes. In all, 30 patients in each group had recurrence in regional lymph nodes. The overall survival rate was statistically better in the group treated with radical mastectomy versus the simple mastectomy group (Fig. 8–9). This difference in outcome, interestingly enough, occurred entirely in the group with clinical Stage I disease. The survival rates in Stage II and Stage III disease were identical between the two groups. Another factor accounting for the difference in survival rate was a prolonged survival from the time of first recurrence in the radical mastectomy group.

This is the only randomized clinical trial that has shown a superiority of one treatment over another in terms of the overall survival rate. While it would be easy to criticize this

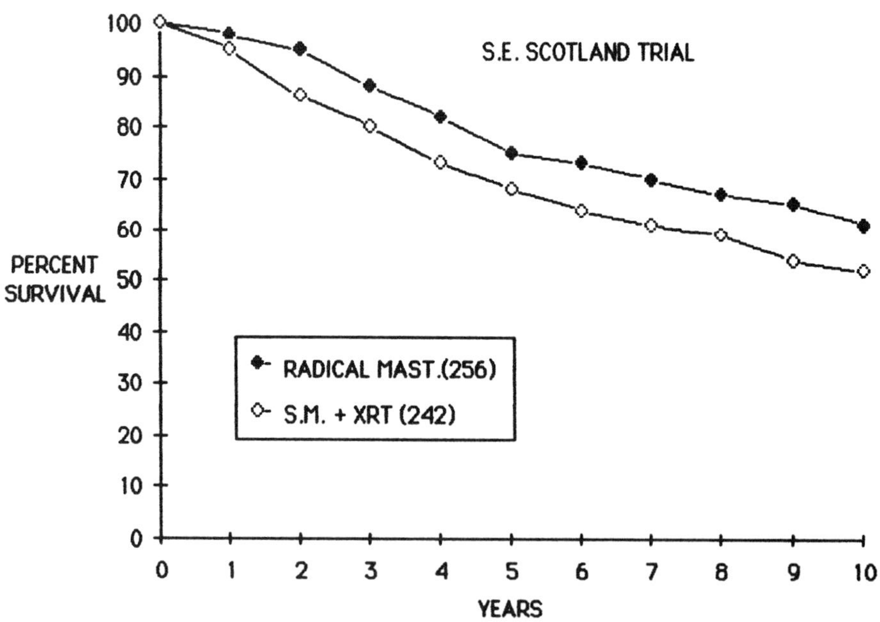

FIGURE 8–9. Results of the southeast Scotland trial, 1964 to 1971. A statistically significant advantage for the radical mastectomy group was seen. (From Langlands AO, Prescott JR, Hamilton T: A clinical trial in the management of operable cancer of the breast. Br J Surg 67:170, 1980.)

trial because of the withdrawal of slightly more than half of the patients who were randomized, the fact that randomization was done before biopsy justifies the vast majority of the exclusions. The patients who went through with the treatment did turn out to be a fairly well-balanced group. There was a slightly greater number of premenopausal patients in the radical mastectomy group (29 percent versus 26 percent), and since oophorectomy was performed on all patients, this may have added a slight advantage to the radical mastectomy group. It is also rather unusual that the superiority of radical mastectomy was seen only in clinically node-negative patients. A closer look at the survival curves broken down by stage indicates a very adverse outcome in clinical Stage I patients treated with simple mastectomy and irradiation, with a five-year survival rate of barely 70 percent, compared with 85 percent for radical mastectomy patients. There were twice as many noncancer deaths in the Stage I simple mastectomy group, as compared with the Stage I radical mastectomy group (12 versus 6).

The Villejuif Trial

In 1963, an international group of European hospitals initiated a cooperative study to investigate the benefits of dissection of the internal mammary lymph node chain. Over the next decade, 1580 cases were randomized to radical mastectomy versus extended radical mastectomy. The results from the study[54] showed no benefit from the removal of the internal mammary lymph nodes. However, one subset of patients, those with T_1 or T_2 tumors in the medial quadrants and with histologically positive axillary lymph nodes, did exhibit a survival advantage with internal mammary lymph node dissection. No patients in this study received radiation.

Tubiana and Sarrazin[55] employed a matching process to compare patients they treated in Villejuif, France, as part of the international cooperative trial with patients receiving postoperative irradiation and treated at the same hospital during the same period. A total of 431 patients were divided into four groups, radical mastectomy or extended radical mastectomy with or without postoperative irradiation. Radiation therapy (machine and energy not specified) delivered 4500 rad to the internal mammary node chain, supraclavicular lymph nodes, axilla, and chest wall.

Results showed that the patients who underwent extended radical mastectomy had no change in their relapse, disease-free survival, or overall survival rates with the addition of postoperative radiation therapy. However, the survival rate of patients who were treated with radical mastectomy significantly improved with postoperative radiation therapy, especially for those with tumors of the medial quadrants (Fig. 8–10). In this

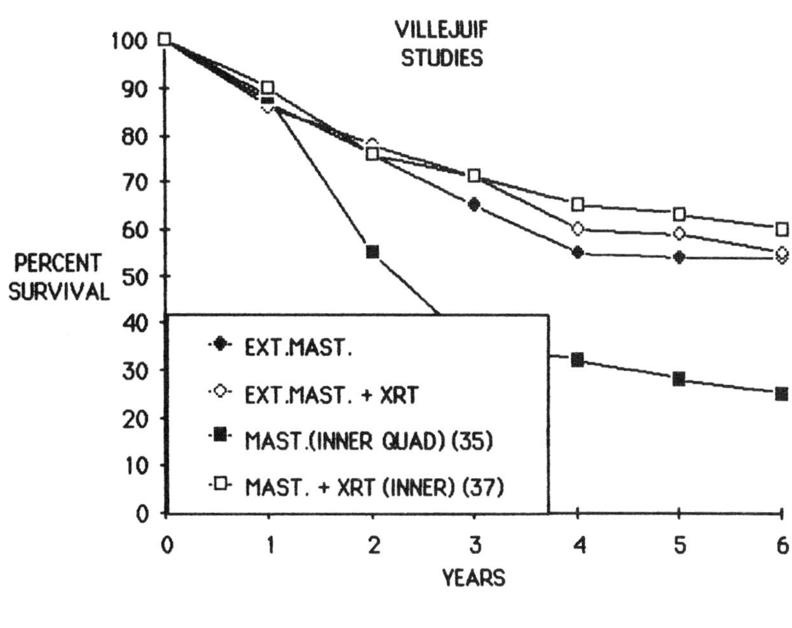

FIGURE 8–10. Results from the Villejuif study. Patients with inner-quadrant tumors, who had no treatment to internal mammary lymph nodes, had a significantly lower survival rate compared with that of patients who had their lymph nodes treated with irradiation or with surgery. (From Tubiana M, Sarrazin D: A reappraisal of radiotherapy in the treatment of operable breast cancer. The new light of the internal mammary chain roll. Eur J Cancer [Suppl] 1:243, 1980.)

comparison, the survival rate of patients treated with radical mastectomy plus dissection of the internal mammary lymph nodes also was significantly better than that of patients treated with radical mastectomy alone. The conclusion of this matched analysis is that treatment of the internal mammary lymph nodes does make a difference in patients with T_1, T_2, and early T_3 tumors with positive axillary lymph nodes, especially if the tumors are located in the medial half of the breast. The investigators further conclude that radiotherapeutic treatment of the internal mammary lymph nodes is the equivalent of surgical treatment.

Although this paper appeared in 1980 and stated that the study "shall be published in detail," no further reports concerning this trial have been put forward, to our knowledge. Details of how the radiation was administered and especially how the patients were selected for this nonrandomized trial are lacking. Until full publication of the trial, the results must be interpreted with caution.

The Hammersmith Trial

In 1965, the departments of surgery, radiation therapy, radiology, and pathology at Hammersmith Hospital began a clinical trial comparing total mastectomy plus postoperative radiation therapy versus radical Halsted mastectomy plus postoperative radiation therapy.[56]

The radiation therapy in both groups included treatment to the regional lymph nodes. However, in the patients who underwent total mastectomy, the chest wall and entire axilla were treated, while in the patients who received radical mastectomy, the chest wall was not irradiated, and only the apex of the axilla was treated. Details of the radiation were not given. All premenopausal patients and all postmenopausal patients within ten years of their menopause had a prophylactic oophorectomy. A total of 195 patients were randomized, and patient entry was closed in mid-1970. The eligibility criteria included clinical Stages I and II cancers and also resectable Stage III tumors.

Analysis of the results showed that local recurrence appeared in 10 percent of the group treated with radical mastectomy plus nodal irradiation versus 11 percent of the group who had total mastectomy with comprehensive postoperative irradiation. Morbidity was essentially the same between both groups: The simple mastectomy group had a higher incidence of shoulder stiffness, while the radical mastectomy group had a higher incidence of arm edema. The survival rates for the groups at five years were no different, with 65 percent of the simple mastectomy group and 70 percent of the radical mastectomy group remaining alive (Fig. 8–11).

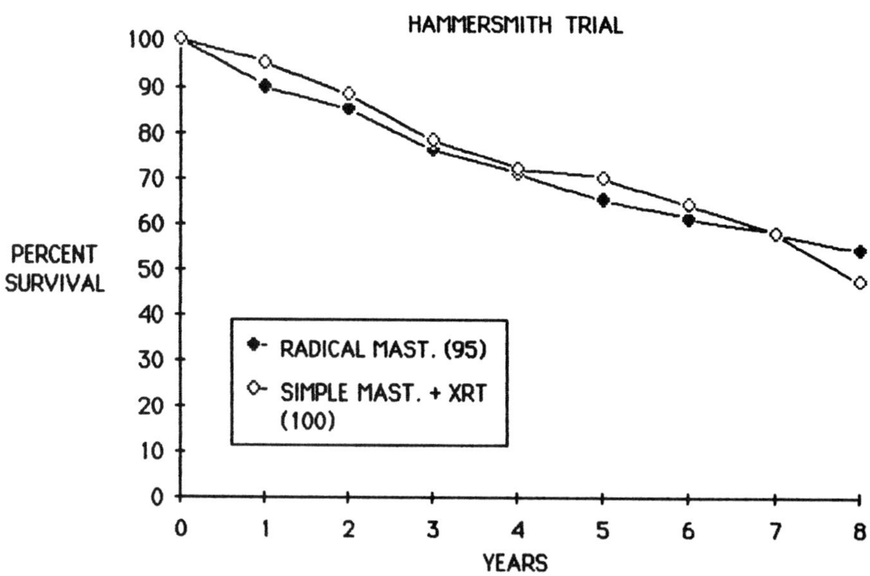

FIGURE 8–11. Results from the Hammersmith trial, 1965 to 1970. No statistically significant differences between groups were seen. (From Burn JI: Early breast cancer; the Hammersmith trial. Br J Surg 61:762, 1974.)

The major problems with this trial are the small number of patients randomized and the fact that 38 of the 195 patients had T_3 N_1 cancers. Thirty-one of these 38 (80 percent) had treatment failure. With such a high percentage of failures in this group, any differences between treatment outcome in early stage patients may have been obscured by the overwhelming number of failures in the more advanced stage patients.

DISCUSSION

These eight trials comparing radical forms of treatment have, in general, demonstrated a decreased rate of locoregional recurrences for patients receiving radiation. However, the majority of the data suggest no increase (or decrease) in the overall survival rate of patients receiving postoperative irradiation. While some trials used radiation techniques that could not be considered ideal,[46] trials with improved technical treatment also failed to show better results for the study population as a whole.

Whether larger numbers of patients randomized into clinical trials would be necessary to show an advantage for irradiation is a matter of speculation.[25, 26] These trials of radical therapy have also demonstrated that whether axillary or internal mammary nodes are treated with surgery or with irradiation, the ultimate outcome is identical. Since simple mastectomy plus irradiation appears to have less morbidity than does radical mastectomy, in patients for whom lymph node information is not critical, simple mastectomy plus postoperative irradiation is a treatment alternative.

Specific attention should be directed to the medial quadrant lesion in axilla-positive patients. For this small group of patients, treatment of the internal mammary node chain with either surgery[54] or irradiation[47, 55] may yield improved survival rates. However, since many axilla-positive patients receive chemotherapy or hormonal therapy, it is difficult to comment with certainty on the benefit of irradiation of node-positive patients with medial quadrant tumors who are receiving systemic therapy. This subgroup is the only one in which an improved survival rate following irradiation has been suggested. The remainder of the results from the eight trials analyzed fail to support the routine use of postoperative irradiation for any other subset of patients who have primary operable breast cancer without signs of locally advanced disease, such as a positive surgical margin, involvement of skin lymphatics, extracapsular nodal spread, or numerous positive axillary nodes.

Analysis of Trials Testing Conservative Forms of Treatment

CANCER RESEARCH CAMPAIGN (KING'S/CAMBRIDGE TRIAL)

This trial, begun in 1970, was the first trial to test a purely conservative treatment approach. At that time in England, simple mastectomy with postoperative irradiation was the most commonly used method for treating carcinoma of the breast, based on the work of McWhirter.[45] However, there was a great deal of concern at the time that irradiating the lymph nodes in the axilla would decrease immunity and adversely affect the host-tumor relationship, actually producing a decrease in survival rate.[57] Therefore, it was decided to test simple mastectomy plus postoperative irradiation against simple mastectomy alone. The working group that formulated the trial performed a careful statistical analysis before beginning the study.[58] They decided that the detection of a 7 percent difference would be important and that in order to have a 90 percent chance of finding such a difference, if it really existed, 2000 patients would be needed in the trial. The protocol treated women less than 70 years of age with tumors that were T_1 or T_2, N_0 or N_1. All patients had a simple mastectomy, and following this operation, patients were randomized by the physicians in their own treatment center to either receive or not receive irradiation. This postoperative randomization might have been a flaw, as surgeons could have refused to randomize some patients based on operative findings. However, the study was able to accrue over 2000 patients between May 1970 and April 1975.[59, 60]

The standards for radiation treatment were written rather broadly.[61] Orthovoltage or supervoltage could be used, and the dosage could be delivered in three fractions or five fractions per week. For the three fractions per week treatment, the dose range was 2850 rad over three weeks to 4050 rad over six weeks. For the five times per week schedule, the dose range was 3250 rad over three weeks to 4600 rad over six weeks. These doses were to be multiplied by a factor of 1.1 for supervoltage.

There were 2268 evaluable patients entered in the study and 336 nonevaluable patients. The breakdown was 1152 in the observation arm and 1116 in the x-ray therapy arm and was weighted toward patients with negative lymph nodes, as a number of centers (80 hospitals participated) had elected to treat only Stage I disease. No statistical differences in survival or distant recurrence rates were seen (Fig. 8–12), but there was a significant advantage in terms of local control in favor of the irradiated group. The axilla was the most common site of recurrence or persistence of disease. Of 158 recurrences in the observation group, 110 were in the axilla. Interestingly enough, of the 1152 patients who entered that arm of the trial, it would have been predicted that 370 would have had positive lymph nodes. However, only 110, less than one third, actually needed treatment to the axilla. This was the first indication that not all patients with microscopically positive axillary nodes would manifest a clinical axillary recurrence if nodes went untreated, a point later emphasized by the NSABP. Of the 110 patients who had recurrence in the axilla, 75 were alive after being treated for their axillary enlargement, indicating that *en bloc* removal of axillary nodes was not necessary to produce good survival rates in node-positive patients, a point confirmed in a later trial of the NSABP.

In 1980, this group performed a thoughtful analysis of the pitfalls of designing a multicenter clinical trial.[62] They point out that most of the inevaluable patients were those patients who were randomized "out of order," compared with the master randomization list that was held at the central office. Since randomization was performed in each hospital, it was not clear whether the out of order randomization represented a treatment selection bias of the physicians involved or whether it was in fact an innocent mistake. They conclude that randomization for a multi-institution trial should always be done centrally and should not be done by each individual center.

A detailed analysis of the pathologic findings, of this trial was performed.[63] This analysis showed that local recurrence rates increased with tumor size for the observation group but not for the irradiation group. Since increasing tumor size was associated with increasing tumor grade, the same observation was made for tumor grade. Therefore, while radiation therapy decreased local recurrence rates, this effect was most prominent in patients with large, high-grade tumors. They also found that in 27 percent of their cases (418 of the 1562 analyzed) lymph nodes were found, despite the fact that only a simple mastectomy was to be performed. In 179 patients, the nodes were negative, and freedom from local recurrence was seen in 81.2 percent of the observation patients and 92.3 percent of the irradiated patients. In 220

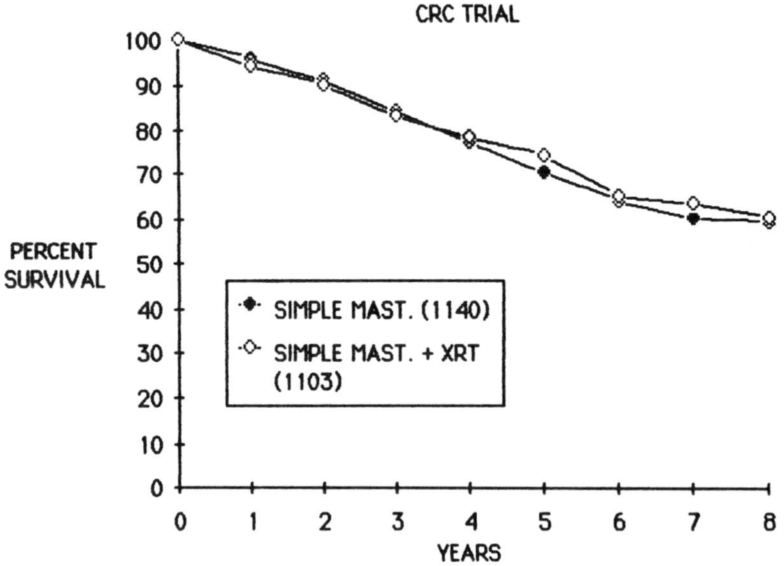

FIGURE 8–12. Cancer Research Campaign (King's/Cambridge trial), 1970 to 1975. No statistically significant differences between groups were seen. (From Cancer Research Campaign Working Party: Cancer Research Campaign [King's/Cambridge] trial for early breast cancer—a detailed update at the tenth year. Lancet 2:55, 1980.)

cases, the nodes were positive. Freedom from local recurrence was seen in only 58.9 percent of the observation patients but 88.2 percent of the irradiated patients.

The most recent report of this trial analyzed the radiation doses in some detail.[61] The investigators emphasize that the design of the actual fields was left completely up to the local radiotherapist. Although it was suggested to irradiate the chest wall and all regional lymph nodes, no quality control was used to make sure this was actually done. The ideal time-dose fractionation was 1320 to 1510 ret (a ret is a unit of radiation that incorporates total dose, fraction size, and total time. Five thousand rad in 25 fractions over five weeks is 1520 ret). In fact, only two thirds of the patients actually received this dose. Twenty-three percent of the patients received a lesser dose, and 10 percent of the patients received more. There was no difference in outcome whether the patient was treated three or five times per week. Similarly, there was no change in outcome relative to orthovoltage or supervoltage radiation. There was improvement in survival rates as higher doses of radiation were employed. The p value was 0.07 for this finding, and of course, since this study was not randomized to test different doses, there is always the possibility that patients who were irradiated with higher doses might have been healthier patients who displayed better tolerance of their treatment. However, the suggestion that higher doses produced better results is made by these data.

In summary, the CRC trial showed that while local treatment failure increased in women who did not have a formal axillary dissection and had no radiation to the axilla, no difference in survival resulted from these locoregional failures. Conversely, the trial failed to find any evidence that radiation therapy was detrimental. In patients with simple mastectomy alone, high rates of locoregional recurrence were seen with larger tumors, higher histologic grade, and positive axillary nodes in the breast specimen, indicating that postoperative irradiation might be selectively restricted to these subsets of patients.

The Cardiff and Edinburgh Trials

Since examination of simple mastectomy specimens often reveals the presence of nodes in the axillary tail and pectoral region, as noted in the CRC trial discussed earlier, Forrest and colleagues decided to test whether one could avoid giving radiation to those women in whom these nodes were negative or absent and give irradiation only to women who had histologically positive nodes.[64–66] This technique of simple mastectomy and pectoral node biopsy was randomly compared against modified radical mastectomy, with node-positive patients receiving radiation and node-negative patients being watched. The study population included T_1, T_2, N_0 and N_1 patients, and the study ran from 1967 to 1973, with 243 patients randomized according to the 1974 report.[64] For patients who had a simple mastectomy with positive pectoral lymph nodes, 4000 rad was given in ten fractions every other day for three weeks to the axilla only. In patients who had modified radical mastectomy with positive axillary nodes, the radiation was 3500 to 4000 rad, given in the same fraction scheme, but delivered comprehensively to regional nodes and the chest wall. Only about 80 percent of the simple mastectomy specimens contained any lymph nodes.

In this small group of patients, the chance of finding positive lymph nodes in either clinical Stage I or II patients appeared the same in the radical mastectomy arm as it was in the simple mastectomy arm, suggesting that the number of nodes removed was not critical in determining axillary positivity. However, 6 of 75 (8 percent) simple mastectomy patients with negative or absent pectoral nodes and no postoperative radiation had recurrence in the axilla. This is the false-negative rate from simple mastectomy alone in this trial.[64] Local recurrences were fewer in the modified radical mastectomy group (12 of 119, or 10 percent) versus the simple mastectomy group (22 of 124, or 18 percent). Morbidity was clearly less with simple mastectomy approaches, especially for measurement of arm edema and arm motion (Table 8–5).

When this trial was republished six[65] and eight years[66] later, only 200 patients were evaluated. No reference was made to the other 43 patients mentioned in the earlier report. No difference in survival rate was seen between the two groups (Fig. 8–13). There was also no difference in distant recurrence rate. However, interesting observations were made regarding local recurrence in patients with negative nodes. By trial de-

TABLE 8–5. Arm Complications by Treatment Type—The Cardiff Trial

Treatment (No. of Patients)	*Edema* (%)*	*Decreased Motion (%)*
CONSERVATIVE		
Simple Mastectomy (26)	15	0
Simple Mastectomy + XRT (19)	37	37
RADICAL		
Radical Mastectomy (28)	46	25
Radical Mastectomy + XRT (12)	58	67

*More than 2.0 cm difference from baseline arm circumference.

With permission from Forrest APM, Roberts MM, Preece P, et al: The Cardiff–St. Mary's trial. Br J Surg 61:766, 1974.

sign, if a simple mastectomy was performed and the sampled nodes were negative, radiation was withheld. The local recurrence rate in the axilla in such patients had now increased to 19 percent from the 8 percent reported previously. This recurrence figure is very similar to that reported from the NSABP Protocol B-04, in which no node sampling of the axilla was attempted.[67] It would thus appear that withholding treatment to the axilla based on an examination of the low pectoral nodes is no more accurate than withholding it based on clinical examination. In patients with positive nodes, those who had a simple mastectomy and irradiation to the axilla had a 28 percent recurrence rate in the chest wall but only a 3 percent recurrence rate in the axilla.

Survival rates with simple mastectomy or modified radical mastectomy were seen to be identical, and since the morbidity was less with simply mastectomy, this operation became the surgical standard in two new trials called Edinburgh Trial I and Edinburgh Trial II. All patients were treated with simple mastectomy and pectoral node biopsy. If they had negative nodes, they were randomized to no further treatment or x-ray therapy to the chest wall and the regional nodes (Trial I). Those patients with positive nodes were randomized to comprehensive irradiation or the same irradiation plus a year of 5-FU as a single agent (700 mg/M^2 IV every four weeks for one year) (Trial II). These trials accrued patients from 1974 to 1979, with 342 patients randomized in Trial I and 286 patients randomized in Trial II.[66] Early analysis of results from Trial I once again showed that in patients with negative pectoral nodes, a simple mastectomy alone produced an axillary recurrence rate of 16 percent, which was reduced to 5 percent with radiation treatment.

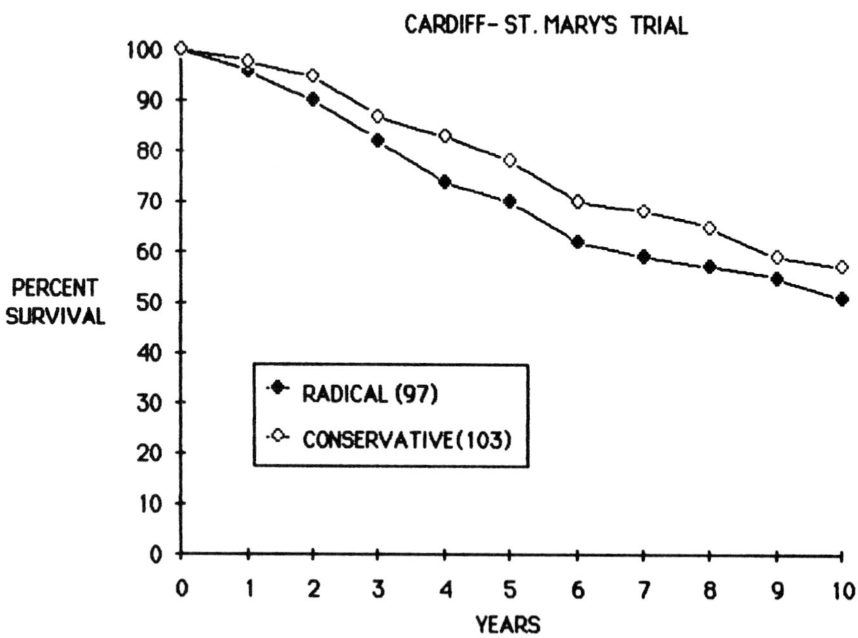

FIGURE 8–13. Results from the Cardiff–St. Mary's trial, 1967 to 1973. No statistically significant differences between groups were seen. (From Forrest APM, Stewart JH, Roberts MM, et al.: Simple mastectomy in axillary node sampling [pectoral node biopsy] in the management of primary breast cancer. Am J Surg 196:371, 1982.)

However, this study was flawed in that over one third of the patients had no nodes found in the simple mastectomy specimen. These node-absent patients experienced a local recurrence rate of 41 percent (24 of 59) when no radiation was given. Even in the group who were randomized to receive radiation, there was a 19 percent locoregional recurrence rate (11 of 57) when no lymph nodes were found. However, a recurrence in the axilla alone was not detrimental to overall survival. No data have been published concerning results from Trial II, the chemotherapy study.

A third trial was started in 1980. In Trial III, half of the patients are again treated with a simple mastectomy and pectoral node biopsy. Patients with negative nodes are watched, and patients' positive nodes are irradiated comprehensively. In contrast with Trials I and II, this study is being performed in a single institution where the techniques for obtaining pectoral node biopsies are more defined. The investigators state that nodes have been identified in 100 percent of patients.[66] The other group of patients are receiving modified radical mastectomy, and no radiation is being given regardless of nodal status. Since it has already been shown that the results of simple mastectomy with postoperative irradiation are equivalent to those of a modified radical mastectomy, the only thing that this study is likely to demonstrate is the identification of a group of patients with negative nodes following simple mastectomy who can be watched. However, that policy in two previous trials has lead to a 15 to 20 percent axillary failure rate that necessitated treatment. It is difficult to understand how the results of Trial III will influence therapy in the future.

The Southampton Trial

In 1973, the surgery and radiation therapy departments of Southampton University Hospital began a conservative breast cancer trial. Patients less than 70 years of age and presenting with clinical Stages I and II breast cancer were treated with a simple mastectomy and axillary lymph node biopsy.[68] Randomization took place postoperatively, one half of the patients receiving no further treatment, while the other half received radiation to the chest wall, internal mammary nodes, axillary nodes, and supraclavicular nodes. Radiation therapy was carried out on a cobalt unit, delivering 4600 rad in 20 fractions over four weeks to the chest wall and internal mammary lymph nodes, using tangential fields, while an anterior field treated the axilla and supraclavicular nodes with an applied dose of 5550 rad over four and one-half weeks. A supplemental posterior axillary boost was used to bring the midplane axillary dose to 4500 rad.

One hundred fifty patients were entered,[68] and 125 of those have been followed for at least three years. In the simple mastectomy only group, 28 percent of the patients had local recurrence, versus 9 percent in the group who had simple mastectomy plus postoperative irradiation. In the surgery only group, 58 percent of the patients were without evidence of disease at the time of the report, versus 72 percent in the postoperative radiation therapy trial. These figures are not statistically different (Fig. 8–14). There were no conclusions drawn from this small clinical trial. Radiation therapy was successful in reducing the rate of local treatment failures, and certainly there was no suggestion that postoperative radiation therapy adversely affected survival rate. What is puzzling is why the investigators discontinued their research with such a small number of patients enrolled. Possibly, other similar trials such as the Cancer Research Campaign Trial or the Manchester Trial were felt to have addressed this issue sufficiently.

The Manchester Regional Breast Study

Continuing in the footsteps of Patterson and Russell, the surgeons and radiotherapists at the Royal Marsden Hospital, Christie Hospital, and Holt Radium Institute in Manchester began another primary breast cancer study in 1970. Patients with T_1 and T_2 cancer with negative lymph nodes (clinical Stage I) were randomized to receive simple mastectomy or simple mastectomy plus postoperative irradiation. Patients with a similar tumor stage but with clinically positive nodes (Stage II) were randomized to receive modified radical mastectomy or simple mastectomy plus postoperative radiation therapy. From March 1970 until October 1975, 1020 cases were accrued,[69, 70] with 711 patients having clinical Stage I cancer and 309 patients having clinical Stage II cancer. Metastatic work-up included only a chest x-ray, and all

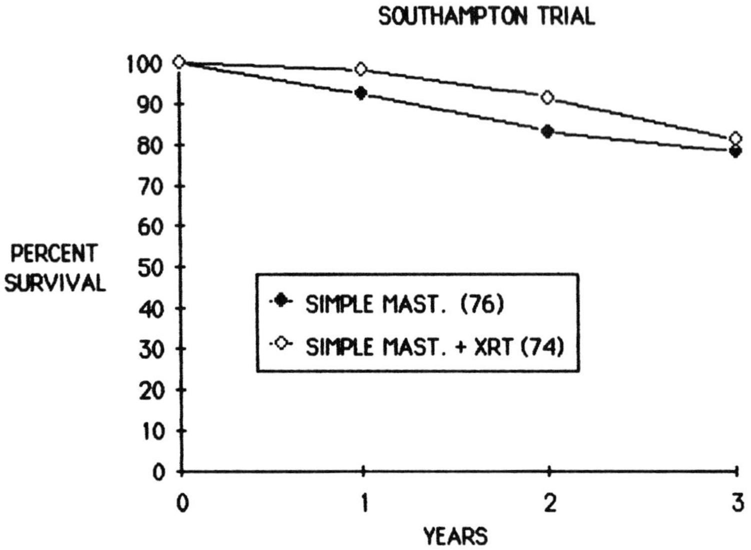

FIGURE 8–14. Results from the Southampton trial, begun in 1973. No statistically significant differences between groups were seen. (From Turnbull AR, Chant ADB, Buchanan RB: Treatment of early breast cancer. Lancet 2:7, 1978.)

patients who were premenopausal or less than three years postmenopausal had ovarian irradiation. The local radiation therapy involved two techniques, somewhat similar to the original Manchester trials.[32, 33] The quadrate technique included three fields that were tangentially directed to the chest wall. These fields were treated with 300-kV photons and were designed to treat the chest wall, internal mammary nodes, and axilla. There was also a separate field to the supraclavicular fossa and a posterior field directed to the apex of the axilla. The total estimated dose was 3700 rad over three weeks. The "peripheral plus tangent pair" technique used a single L-shaped 4-MV field directed at the internal mammary nodes, supraclavicular nodes, and axilla; a 4000 rad dose was applied over three weeks. The chest wall was then treated with a pair of tangential fields, using 300-kv photons with a midplane dose of 3000 rad over three weeks.

Results of the trial showed that between 12 and 13 percent of the patients did not

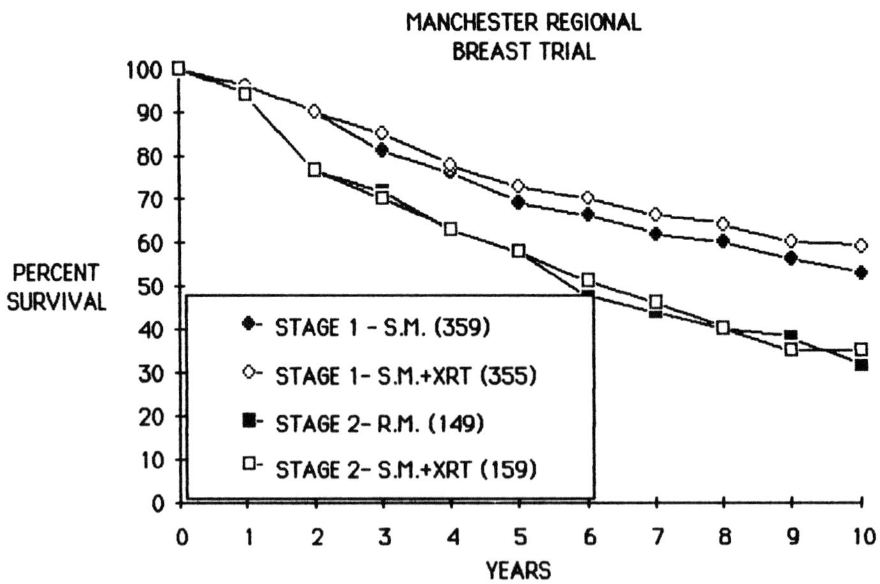

FIGURE 8–15. Results from the second Manchester trial, 1970 to 1975. No statistically significant differences among groups were seen. (From Lythgoe JP, Palmer MK: Manchester regional breast study—five- and ten-year results. Br J Surg 69:693, 1982.)

TABLE 8–6. Survival and Disease-Free Survival Rates

Clinical Stage	Treatment	No. of Patients	Survival (%) 5-YEAR	Survival (%) 10-YEAR	Disease-Free Suvival (%) 5-YEAR	Disease-Free Suvival (%) 10-YEAR
I	Simple mastectomy	359	69	55	49	36
	Simple mastectomy + XRT	355	74	62	65	52
			p = 0.2		p = 0.0001	
II	Radical mastectomy	149	57	35	38	19
	Radical mastectomy + XRT	159	55	31	39	28
			p = 0.9		p = 0.56	

With permission from Lythgoe JP, Palmer MK: Manchester regional breast study—five and ten year results. Br J Surg 69:693, 1982.

receive the protocol treatment.[69, 70] This was mainly due to patients receiving or not receiving the assigned radiation therapy or to patients refusing the ovarian irradiation. However, results are analyzed with all patients included in their original groups. For clinical Stage I patients, there was a highly statistically significant improvement in the disease-free survival rate in patients who were irradiated. This was due to a reduced incidence of chest wall and axillary failures. However, survival after recurrence was better for the patients treated with simple mastectomy alone, and thus, the overall survival rate was not statistically different (Fig. 8–15). At five and ten years, 74 and 62 percent of the irradiated patients were alive, versus 69 and 55 percent of those in the surgery alone group (Table 8–6).

In clinical Stage II patients, there was no difference in local recurrence, disease-free survival, or overall survival rates according to whether radiation was or was not given (Fig. 8–15 and Table 8–6). However, it should be noted that for Stage II cases, there was a very high rate of recurrence in the chest wall and axilla (Table 8–7). In patients treated with modified radical mastectomy, 34 percent had recurrence in the chest wall, while patients treated with simple mastectomy and radiation therapy had a 23 percent failure rate in the chest wall. The figures for axillary recurrences are also disturbingly high. Thus, there is a cause for concern as to the quality of both the modified radical mastectomy and the postoperative radiation therapy. A rate of treatment failure in the axilla that is greater than 1 to 2 percent following radical mastectomy is quite unusual. Similarly, a high rate of failure in the chest wall following radiation therapy is also rather unusual. The large percentage of failure in the chest wall cannot be explained by the use of the peripheral radiation technique, as formerly practiced in Manchester,[32, 33] because a pair of tangential fields was added to the nodal irradiation. However, the chest wall received only 3000 rad, which is probably too low a dose to reliably sterilize microscopic disease.[71]

Other criticisms of this trial should be noted. The published reports do not state how the randomization was performed. There is no comparison of the two radiation techniques in terms of outcome, even though these techniques are different in design. Additionally, the only staging test for entry into this trial was a chest x-ray. This fact indicates that some patients in the trial probably had metastases that would have been detected with a more thorough staging work-up. Nonetheless, these shortcomings and biases are likely evenly distributed in both arms of the trial.

The study conclusion that there is no sta-

TABLE 8–7. Percentage of Patients Free of Recurrence According to Site

Clinical Stage	Treatment	Chest Wall 5-YEAR	Chest Wall 10-YEAR	Axilla 5-YEAR	Axilla 10-YEAR	Supraclavicular Region 5-YEAR	Supraclavicular Region 10-YEAR
I	SM	84	80	67	63	89	85
	SM + XRT	94	91	84	81	92	89
II	RM	66	64	76	71	80	77
	RM + XRT	77	63	75	72	87	86

With permission from Lythgoe JP, Palmer MK: Manchester regional breast study—five and ten year results. Br J Surg 69:693, 1982.

tistically significant difference between the two treatment approaches as employed in this study has recently been criticized by Hughes,[72] who points out that at five years and at ten years there is a 16 percent disease-free survival advantage for patients treated with postoperative irradiation versus patients treated with surgery alone ($p < 0.0001$) (Table 8–6). He argues that since there are so many more disease-free patients in the irradiated group, it is likely that the survival rate will ultimately be affected as the study proceeds to 15 years. He further concludes that this study shows that treatment of clinical Stage I cancer with simple mastectomy alone is inadequate therapy. This trial bears watching as subsequent reports are published.

NSABP Protocol B-04

In 1971, the NSABP began comparing the value of radical mastectomy against that of alternative treatments, some of which involved radiation therapy. The schema (Fig. 8–16) allocated patients with clinically negative lymph nodes to one of three treatment arms, radical mastectomy, total mastectomy plus postoperative radiation, or total mastectomy alone. Patients with clinically node-positive cancer were allocated either to radical mastectomy or to total mastectomy plus postoperative radiation therapy.

Radiation therapy was directed at the regional lymph nodes and the chest wall. The internal mammary and supraclavicular nodes received 4500 rad over five weeks, while the chest wall received 5000 rad in 25 treatments over five weeks with tangentially directed fields. A clinically negative axilla was treated with 5000 rad over five weeks, with an anterior field supplemented by a posterior axillary boost field. Clinically positive axillae were treated with an additional 1000 to 2000 rad boost through the posterior portal. This is the only multicenter trial in breast cancer to conduct detailed quality control of the radiation therapy. Not only was each institution reviewed to make sure that its radiation therapy practices conformed to the standards of the trial, but each radiation machine used in the trial was measured to verify calibration, depth-dose characteristics, and other dosimetry parameters. Additionally, each case treated was reviewed by a radiotherapist and radiation physicist, with a copy of the patient's daily treatment record, a contour drawing of the patient's chest wall, copies of the dosimetry calculations and isodose printouts, and the radiation therapy portal films, to make sure that doses received were within 5 percent of the intended dose. Permissible dosages for the trial were as follows: supraclavicular nodes, 4300 to 5000 rad; internal mammary nodes, 4300 to 5250 rad; chest wall, 4700 to 5500 rad; negative axilla, 4700 to 5800 rad; and positive axilla, greater than 5800 rad. Using these criteria, 82 percent of clinically node-negative patients were treated without variation from protocol standards and 71 percent of node-positive patients were treated without variation.

Results from the study[67, 73–76] show no difference in the disease-free survival or overall survival rates for any of the treatment arms (Fig. 8–17). It should be noted that a failure in the axilla in a patient randomized to total mastectomy and no irradiation was treated with an axillary dissection at the time of that failure. However, that patient was *not* considered to have had a treatment failure for purposes of the disease-free survival rate. Overall, 17.8 percent of women who had clinically negative nodes and were treated with total mastectomy alone required subse-

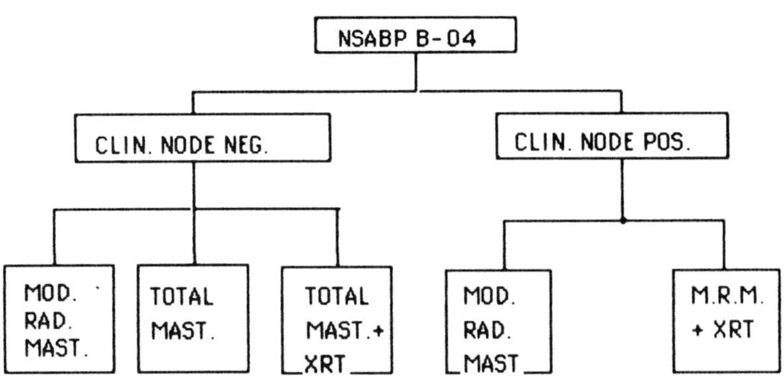

Figure 8–16. The randomization schema from NSABP Protocol B-04.

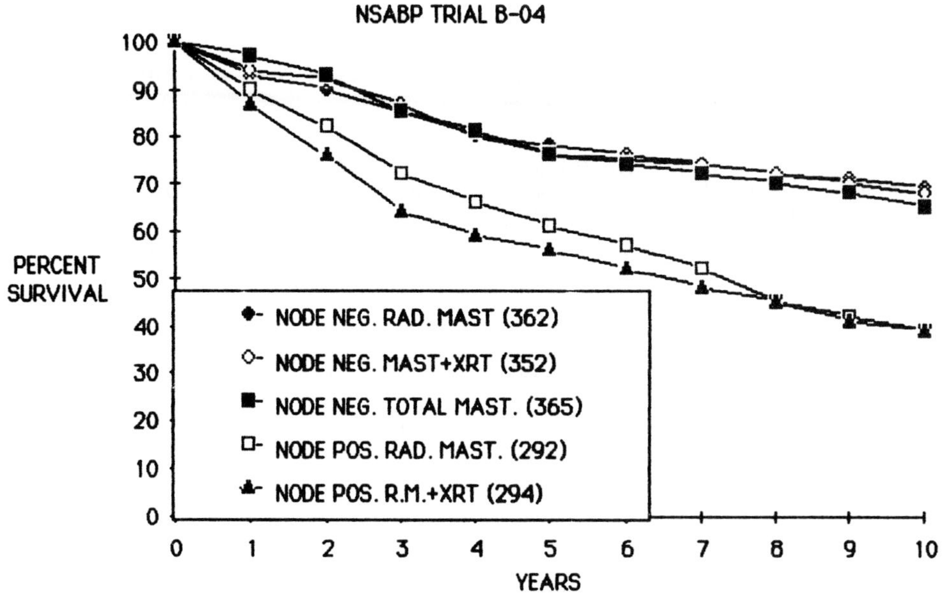

Figure 8–17. Results from NSABP trial B-04, 1971 to 1974. No statistically significant differences between groups were seen. (From Fisher B, Redmond C, Fisher E, et al.: Ten-year results of a randomized clinical trial comparing radical mastectomy and total mastectomy with or without radiation. N Engl J Med 312:674, 1985.)

quent axillary dissection for a clinically detectable node treatment failure.[74] Such a failure apparently had no influence on the overall survival rate, consistent with the British Cancer Research Campaign Trial.[59–61] Since 39 percent of women in the clinically node-negative group had positive nodes when undergoing radical mastectomy, it is concluded that fewer than half the women with pathologically positive lymph nodes will subsequently clinically manifest a lymph node treatment failure if those nodes are left untreated. However, this 17.8 percent figure is slightly misleading. In the performance of the total mastectomy, 129 of 365 (35 percent) patients so treated had lymph nodes removed.[75] In those patients who had any lymph nodes removed, only 7.8 percent subsequently required axillary dissection, and in the 49 patients who had more than six nodes removed, none later required axillary dissection. This contrasts with the 21.2 percent nodal treatment failure rate in the 236 women whose total mastectomy specimen did not contain any lymphatic tissue. Thus, it is likely that somewhat over half the women who have positive lymph nodes left untreated at initial surgery will subsequently require axillary dissection (Table 8–8).

Some of the criticisms leveled at the first NSABP trial (Protocol No. 2)[38] testing postoperative irradiation were (1) poor quality

TABLE 8–8. Axillary Failure Related to Number of Nodes Removed—NSABP B-04

	Axillary Failure after Simple Mastectomy			*Axillary Failure After Radical Mastectomy*		
No. of Nodes Removed	No. of Patients	No.	Percentage	No. of Patients	No.	Percentage
None	236	50	21.2	2	0	0.0
1–5	83	10	7.8	11	0	0.0
6–10	23	0	0.0	54	4	7.4
11 or more	26	0	0.0	290	1	0.3
Total	365	60	16.4*	357	5	1.4

*Total number of axillary failures have increased to 17.8 percent in a more recent update.[74]

With permission from Fisher B, Wolmark N, Bauer M, et al.: The accuracy of clinical nodal staging and of limited axillary dissection as a determinant of histologic nodal status in carcinoma of the breast. Surg Gynecol Obstet 152:765, 1981.

control of the irradiation, (2) inadequate radiation dosage, and (3) a large percentage of patients withdrawn from the study. The NSABP has made a major effort in Trial B-04 to avoid those problems. In a detailed analysis of radiation dosage,[76] they showed that while 53 percent of the irradiated patients in this trial had some degree of variation from the protocol treatment, 77 percent of the radiation fields received dose that was within the range acceptable to the protocol and only 6.7 percent of all sites received an unacceptable major variation in radiation. When analyzed separately, patients who had minor or major variations in radiation dosage did not have failure experiences or survival experiences that were statistically different from the group of patients who had no treatment variation. This fact, coupled with the knowledge that the overwhelming majority of fields were treated correctly, effectively eliminates the criticism that failure to show a survival advantage for radiation therapy in this study was based on poor radiation therapy compliance. It does show that radiation therapy can substitute for axillary dissection, so that women treated with total mastectomy plus irradiation have an outcome similar to that of patients treated with standard radical mastectomy. This study also supports the hypothesis that variations in local treatment of breast cancer, at least as it relates to lymph node management and postoperative irradiation, are unlikely to produce substantial variations in the survival rate.

Discussion

Trials of conservative therapy have shown that removal of axillary nodes in clinically node-negative patients can be avoided without affecting the survival rate. Without doubt, patients whose nodes are removed or whose nodes and chest wall are irradiated postoperatively have considerably fewer relapses and a higher disease-free survival rate, compared with patients treated with simple mastectomy alone. However, no increase in the overall survival rate was seen at least to ten years. This outcome supports the concept that axillary nodal metastases are indications of distant spread but are unlikely to be the instigators of that spread, since leaving some occultly node-positive patients untreated to their axilla does not alter their outcome. Critics of these studies emphasize that differences in the overall survival rate between irradiated and nonirradiated patients may emerge after 15 years of follow-up. Validation of this hypothesis obviously must await later analysis.

Modern treatment techniques employing adjuvant chemohormonal therapy demand accurate knowledge of the status of axillary lymph nodes. Thus, the concept that the axilla may be left alone during primary therapy has been largely relegated to an academic point; few breast cancer centers would forgo the prognostic information contributed by axillary node histology. Whether pectoral node biopsy can substitute for axillary dissection remains to be seen. The false-negative rate from this procedure appears to be high, in the range of 15 to 20 percent.

PREOPERATIVE IRRADIATION

The use of preoperative irradiation has largely been confined to patients with borderline operable or frankly inoperable tumors. In a significant percentage of patients, these large tumors can be rendered technically operable.[77, 78] However, research into the usefulness of preoperative irradiation for patients who have primary operable breast cancer has been modest. This is due, in part, to negative published experiences. Adair and colleagues at Memorial Hospital performed a rather extensive investigation of this technique in the 1930's and failed to show a survival advantage over standard surgery plus postoperative irradiation in a nonrandomized series.[15] Montague and Fletcher at the M.D. Anderson Hospital have treated 442 patients with preoperative irradiation.[79] The overall results from that treatment are not substantially different from those of patients given postoperative irradiation. Granted, some negative selection bias might have gone into the preoperative series, and thus, one may theorize that had they been treated with surgery and postoperative radiation, their treatment outcome might have been worse. Nonetheless, it would appear that the results of preoperative irradiation from retrospective series are no different than those of postoperative irradiation.

A recent trial from Stockholm[80–84] thoroughly tested the concept of preoperative irradiation. Women less than 71 years of age with operable breast cancer diagnosed by fine-needle aspiration cytology were eligible for the three-arm randomization. A total of 960 patients were randomized: 316 received preoperative radiation therapy, followed by modified radical mastectomy; 323 received postoperative radiation therapy; and 321 received surgery alone.

The radiation therapy was designed to treat the internal mammary and axillary lymph nodes as well as the breast and chest wall to a dose of 4500 rad over five weeks. During the first two years of the study, both sides of the internal mammary node chain were treated. However, in order to diminish the amount of lung in the treatment portal, this practice was discontinued, and only the ipsilateral internal mammary lymph nodes were irradiated. It should be noted that preoperative radiation therapy was given through tangential ^{60}Co portals, and the internal mammary lymph nodes were included within the tangential portals by extending the medial tangent entrance point across the midline. Postoperative irradiation, by contrast, was delivered with 12.5-MeV electrons aimed directly at the chest wall and the internal mammary lymph nodes. In one publication,[83] the study investigators indicated that there may have been an underdosage in the region of the internal mammary lymph nodes from this electron beam technique, such that in some patients, the dosage to the internal mammary nodes would be 60 to 70 per cent of that intended.

Preoperative irradiation was effective in sterilizing disease in axillary lymph nodes. Microscopically involved axillary nodes were found in 38 per cent of patients treated with surgery as initial therapy, but in only 20 percent of patients who were treated with preoperative irradiation. Both preoperative and postoperative irradiation had a dramatic effect in reducing local and regional recurrences (Table 8–9). However, there was no major difference in the number of distant recurrences among the three treatment groups. While earlier reports of this trial suggested an improved survival rate for patients treated with preoperative irradiation, longer follow-up has shown that this survival advantage has not persisted (Fig. 8–18). Comparing the ratio of mortality rates for irradiated patients with that for surgery only controls, no statistically significant difference is seen (Table 8–10). Also in the earlier reports, statistically significant differences were noted for the subset of patients who had medial quadrant tumors. While a survival advantage still persists for irradiated subjects with inner quadrant tumors, with longer follow-up the difference in mortality rates no longer has statistical significance (Table 8–10). Conclusions from this well-controlled and carefully conducted clinical trial are that radiation therapy, given either preoperatively or postoperatively, dramatically decreases the incidence of local and regional failures. However, the advantage in overall survival for irradiated patients as a whole and for the subset of irradiated patients who had medially located tumors does not reach statistical significance. Preoperative irradiation reduced the incidence of detectable axillary lymph node involvement by nearly half. In an era when adjuvant chemotherapy or adjuvant hormonal therapy or both, is to be applied in node-positive patients, such a decrease in the ability to detect patients with axillary lymph node involvement makes preoperative irradiation an inappropriate form of therapy in primary operable breast cancer.

NONRANDOMIZED STUDIES OF ADJUVANT POSTOPERATIVE IRRADIATION

There have been numerous single-institution reports concerning the use of adjuvant irradiation. The most prolific investigators in

TABLE 8–9. Recurrences by Site and Treatment—The Stockholm Trial

Treatment	*No. of Patients*	*Locoregional Failures*	*Distant Failures*	*All Failures*
Preoperative XRT	316	25	100	104
Postoperative XRT	323	23	94	96
Surgery only	321	83	110	135

With permission from Wallgren A, Glas U, Strender LE, et al.: Adjunctive therapy in breast cancer: The Stockholm experience. *In*: Ames FC, Blumenschein GR, Montague ED (eds.): Current Controversies in Breast Cancer. Austin: University of Texas Press, 1984.

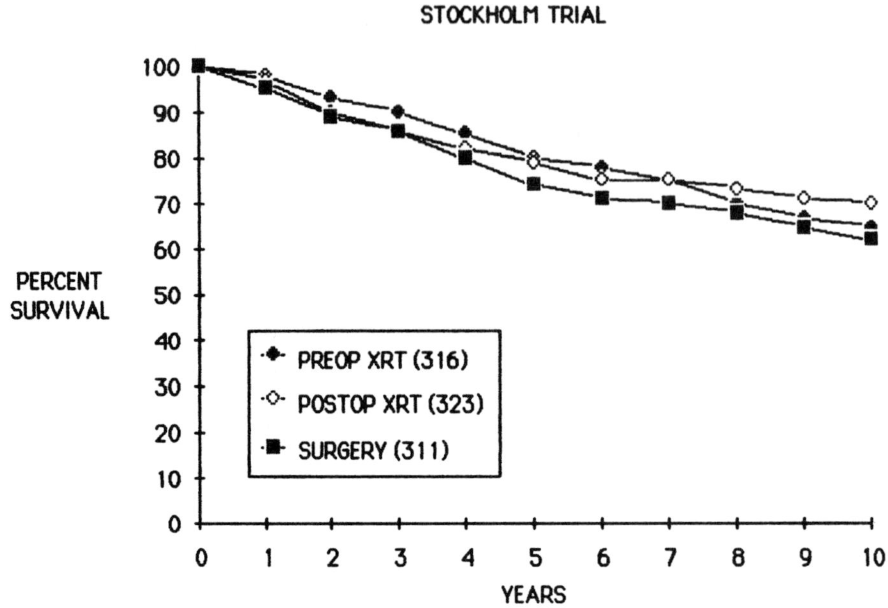

FIGURE 8–18. Results of the Stockholm trial, 1971 to 1976. No significant differences among groups were seen. (From Bedwinek J: Adjuvant irradiation for early breast cancer: An ongoing controversy. Cancer 53:729, 1984.)

this regard are the group from the M.D. Anderson Hospital in Houston. They have reported their results in literally dozens of papers, and their bias is strongly in favor of postoperative radiation therapy.[20, 46, 79, 85–88] Their irradiation technique has evolved over the years. Their current recommendations are to irradiate the apex of the axilla, the supraclavicular fossa, and the internal mammary lymph nodes in patients with positive axillary lymph nodes or in patients with central or inner quadrant primary tumors with or without positive lymph nodes. If the central or medially placed tumor is 2 cm in diameter or less, with negative axillary lymph nodes, only the internal mammary node chain is irradiated. Chest wall irradiation is added only when the tumor is greater than 5 cm in diameter, when signs of locally advanced carcinoma are present, or when there is 20 percent or more axillary node positivity (Table 8–11). The lymph nodes are irradiated with a 5000-rad applied dose over four weeks, and the chest wall is irradiated with

TABLE 8–10. Ratio of Mortality Rates of Irradiated Patients to Those of Surgical Controls—The Stockholm Trial

	No. of Patients	*No. of Deaths*	*Ratio of Mortality Rates (Range)**
PREOPERATIVE XRT			
All patients	316	90	0.85 (0.64–1.13)†
Medial tumors	74	17	0.70 (0.37–1.32)
POSTOPERATIVE RT			
All patients	323	89	0.85 (0.64–1.13)
Medial tumors	58	14	0.76 (0.39–1.47)
SURGERY ONLY			
All patients	321	102	1.00
Medial tumors	70	22	1.00

*Treatments versus surgical controls
†Ninety-five percent confidence limit
With permission from Wallgren A, Glas U, Strender LE, et al.: Adjunctive therapy in breast cancer: The Stockholm experience. *In*: Ames FC, Blumenschein GR, Montague ED (eds.): Current Controversies in Breast Cancer. Austin: University of Texas Press, 1984.

TABLE 8–11. Guidelines for Postoperative Irradiation (M.D. Anderson Hospital)

Location of Tumor and Size	Node Status	Other Signs	Region Irradiated
Inner, central, T_1	Negative	None	Internal mammary nodes
Any, T_2	Negative	None	Peripheral lymphatics*
Any	Fewer than 20% positive	None	Peripheral lymphatics
Any	More than 20% positive	None	Lymphatics and chest wall
Any, T_3–T_4	Any	None	Lymphatics and chest wall
Any	Any	Fixation to pectoral fascia; skin fixation; edema; multiple primary tumors; vascular, lymphatic, or perineural invasion	Lymphatics and chest wall

*Include axilla if (1) fewer than ten nodes are recovered, (2) extranodal disease is present, or (3) matted or fixed nodes are present.

With permission from Brady LW, Fletcher GH, Levitt SH: Cancer of the breast: The role of radiation therapy after mastectomy. Cancer 39:2868, 1977.

a 5500-rad surface dose over four weeks. The percentage of recurrences in the supraclavicular fossa and in the chest wall for the two irradiation techniques are presented in Table 8–12. When more than four positive lymph nodes were found in the axilla, the percentage of chest wall treatment failure ranged from 11 to 20 percent, despite postoperative irradiation. The results show that patients who were irradiated either preoperatively or postoperatively had an overall survival rate identical with patients treated with radical mastectomy alone. However, only 12 percent of the radical mastectomy patients had positive nodes, whereas nearly 60 percent of the postoperative irradiation patients and 30 percent of the preoperative irradiation patients had positive nodes. When analyzed by nodal status (Fig. 8–19), patients who had irradiation survived significantly longer than patients treated with surgery alone. The postoperative radiation technique can produce major complications in some patients, including multiple telangiectasia, fibrosis, radiation pneumonitis, and chest wall necrosis.[85, 86] The incidence of arm edema is doubled in the postoperatively irradiated group compared with the mastectomy alone group and is tripled in the preoperative irradiation series.[85]

Nonetheless, the disease-free survival rates in node-positive patients treated without adjuvant chemotherapy at the M.D. Anderson Hospital are among the highest reported in the literature. The entire node-positive group has a 44 percent ten-year disease-free survival rate, broken down as 56 percent in patients with one to three positive nodes and 33 percent in patients with four or more positive nodes. The radiotherapists at the M.D. Anderson Hospital claim that such a good outcome is the direct result of postoperative or preoperative adjuvant irradiation. However, there could be other factors contributing to these excellent results. There is never enough information in any of their papers to completely rule out potentially im-

TABLE 8–12. Incidence of Locoregional Recurrence Following Postoperative Irradiation (M.D. Anderson Hospital)

Region Irradiated	No. of Positive Axillary Nodes	No. of Patients	Locoregional Recurrence Rate (%)
Peripheral lymphatics	0	207	6
	1–3	221	9
	4 or more	79	20
Lymphatics and chest wall	0	53	2
	1–3	102	8
	4 or more	257	11

With permission from Tapley N, Spanos WJ, Fletcher GH, et al.: Results in patients with breast cancer treated by radical mastectomy and post-operative irradiation with no adjuvant chemotherapy. Cancer 49:1316, 1982.

Harris Methodist Health Sciences Library 1301 Pennsylvania Ave. Fort Worth, TX 76104

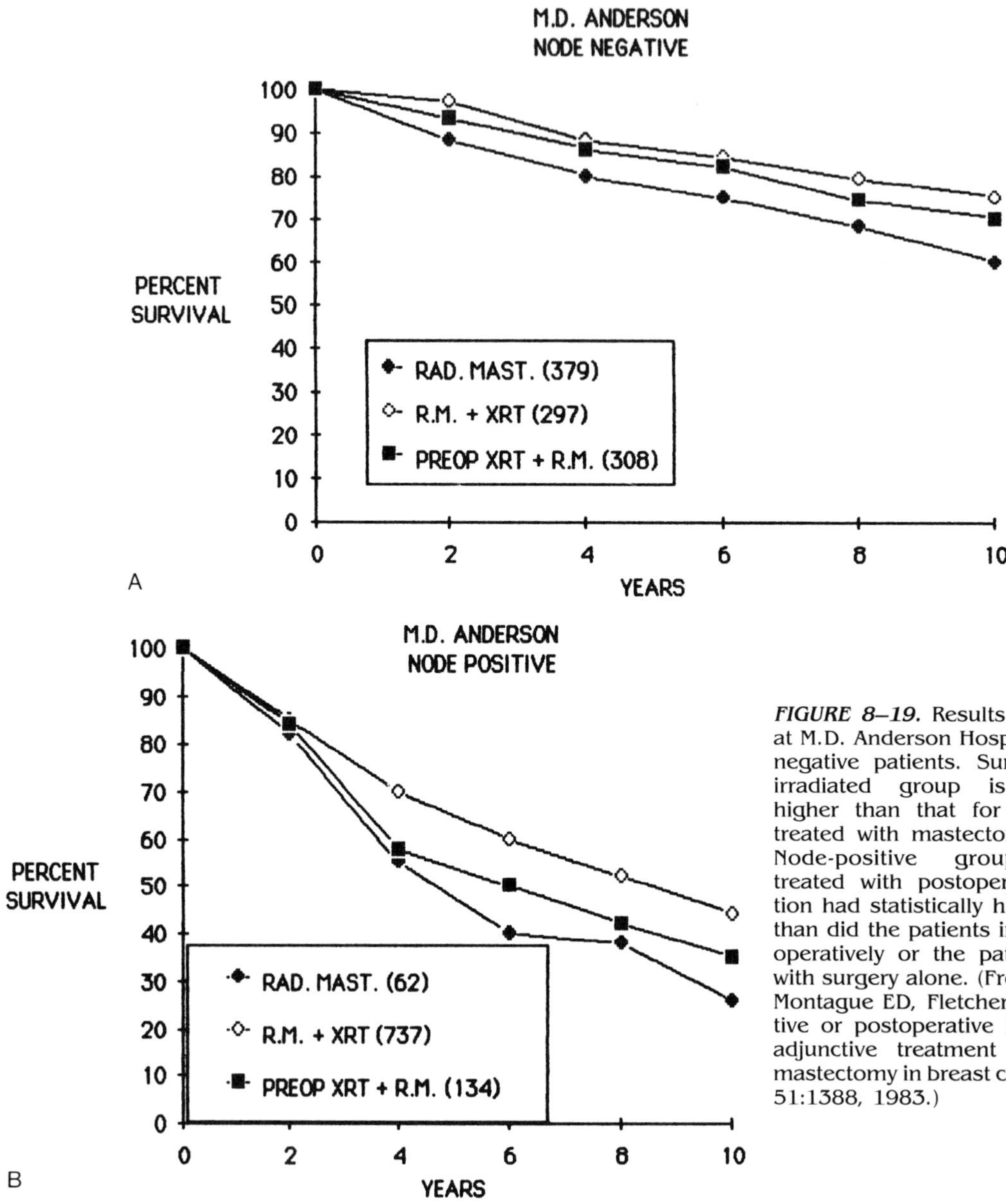

FIGURE 8–19. Results of treatment at M.D. Anderson Hospital. *A,* Node-negative patients. Survival for the irradiated group is statistically higher than that for the patients treated with mastectomy alone. *B,* Node-positive group. Patients treated with postoperative irradiation had statistically higher survival than did the patients irradiated preoperatively or the patients treated with surgery alone. (From Rodger A, Montague ED, Fletcher G: Preoperative or postoperative irradiation as adjunctive treatment with radical mastectomy in breast cancer. Cancer 51:1388, 1983.)

portant patient selection bias. For example, no discussions are presented concerning known outcome parameters such as patient age, tumor grade, menopausal status, or additional supplemental treatment such as estrogen therapy or oophorectomy. Almost two thirds of the patients who received postoperative irradiation at the M.D. Anderson Hospital had their surgery at an outside institution and were referred to Houston for treatment. It is possible that patients who have the economic wherewithal and the general medical status capable of supporting a trip to a distant referral center may be a "better" group of patients than those generally seen at most medical centers where therapy is performed on consecutive patients. Much of the follow-up of these patients is performed at outside institutions and is available to the M.D. Anderson group only through referring physician notes. While it is hard to argue that survival figures could be misleading from such follow-up at a distance, disease-free survival figures could certainly reflect the diligence and thoroughness of follow-up. One hint that the groups of patients treated with mastectomy or treated with adjuvant radiation were, in fact, different populations of patients relates to the average age of patients. While this number is never directly stated, in one publication the "expected" survival of patients extrapolated from life-table analysis is quoted.[89] In all categories, the adjuvant radiation therapy patients have a longer expected survival than their mastectomy counterparts, indicating that they were a younger group of patients. Since the reports deal with over a thousand patients, it is difficult to ascribe a difference in average patient age to chance alone. Rather, it probably reflects referral patterns for patients who are seen at the M.D. Anderson Hospital for mastectomy versus patients who have their mastectomy elsewhere and are referred for adjuvant irradiation. The M.D. Anderson group frequently compares the outcome of their irradiated patients with the outcome of the NSABP patients with similar nodal status. Because of the aforementioned considerations concerning referral patterns and patient selection, it is hazardous to make such a comparison. Until the physicians at the M.D. Anderson Hospital show in a randomized prospective trial on their own patient population that postoperative irradiation is better than mastectomy alone, their treatment results must be interpreted with caution.

ADJUVANT POSTOPERATIVE IRRADIATION IN COMBINATION WITH SYSTEMIC CHEMOTHERAPY

Most studies testing the value of postoperative adjuvant irradiation had been done in the era before chemotherapy. Such studies have generally shown, as summarized in the previous sections of this chapter, that postoperative adjuvant irradiation reduces the incidence of locoregional failure but fails to statistically improve the overall survival rate. Since the survival of patients is related to the presence or absence of systemic disease, it has been theorized that if systemic control can be achieved through the use of adjuvant chemotherapy, reduction in local chest wall failures may be critical to producing maximum long-term survival. It must be emphasized that this theory may not be valid. The NSABP trial B-04[74] has shown that leaving microscopic disease behind in axillary nodes does not necessarily influence the overall survival rate if axillary treatment is instituted at the time of failure. Similarly, a local recurrence in the breast following tumor excision with or without breast irradiation may not jeopardize survival if adequate local treatment is administered at the time of recurrence.[24] Thus, a local chest wall failure may be treatable at the time of failure with no adverse effect on outcome, provided that the patient is systemically free of disease.

The ability of chemotherapy to reduce disease recurrence in the chest wall is a controversial topic. Some investigators report that disease recurrences in the chest wall are reduced equally well by radiation therapy or chemotherapy,[90–92] while others suggest that chemotherapy has, at best, a small effect on the expected rate of local failure in the chest wall following mastectomy, with 15 to 20 percent of patients having recurrences of locoregional disease.[93–97] In order to test whether the combination of local chest wall irradiation plus systemic chemotherapy is better than systemic chemotherapy alone, a number of clinical trials have been performed.

Ahmann and colleagues from the Mayo Clinic performed a trial randomizing patients to treatment with L-PAM alone versus cyclophosphamide, 5-FU, and prednisone (CFP) versus CFP plus postoperative radiation therapy.[93, 98] When this trial was first begun in 1974, a surgery alone and a radiation therapy alone arm were included in the study, and the single-agent L-PAM arm was absent. After 33 patients were entered, early evidence supporting an effect of postoperative chemotherapy in node-positive patients caused the investigators to drop the surgery alone and postoperative radiation therapy alone arms and to substitute single-agent L-PAM treatment. A subsequent interim analysis suggested that L-PAM alone was inferior to combination chemotherapy in the premenopausal subset of patients, and the L-PAM arm was closed for that subset. All three arms in the postmenopausal group continued to accrue patients until the end of the trial, and from 1974 to 1980, 293 patients were randomized. Eligible participants included patients who were less than 70 years of age, had completed a total mastectomy with axillary dissection, and had either positive lymph nodes or the presence of unfavorable local signs such as tumor invasion of the skin, muscle, fascia, or nipple. The radiation therapy consisted of split-course treatment: 5000 rad was delivered to the supraclavicular and internal mammary lymph node chains, using an L-shaped portal; and 2500 rad was given over two weeks, followed by a four-week break and then the second two weeks of treatment. Chest wall radiation was given only to patients with cutaneous involvement or with involvement of pectoral muscle or fascia. The number of patients who received chest wall radiation appears to be less than 10 percent of the total group.

Results from this study (Fig. 8–20) showed that in postmenopausal patients there was no difference in disease-free or overall survival rates for any of the treatment arms. In premenopausal patients, the L-PAM alone arm performed significantly worse in terms of disease-free survival and overall survival rates. There was no difference between the combination chemotherapy alone arm and the chemotherapy plus irradiation arm in premenopausal disease-free or overall survival rates. It should be pointed out that in the premenopausal group of patients, slightly more than half of the patients who were randomized to CFP or CFP plus irradiation had four or more positive lymph nodes, while 75 percent of the patients randomized to L-PAM had this adverse finding. The groups were more evenly balanced in the postmenopausal subset. This imbalance in nodal status for the premenopausal patients could have strongly influenced the results of this trial concerning the poor performance of single-agent L-PAM.

As with many trials employing adjuvant postoperative irradiation, a dramatic effect was seen on the incidence of locoregional failures through the use of this treatment. Overall, 4 percent (4 of 108) patients treated with CFP plus irradiation had a locoregional recurrence, versus 19 percent (19 of 104) of patients treated with CFP alone ($p < 0.01$). Thus, in this randomized trial, radiation therapy was successful in producing fewer locoregional failures, compared with chemotherapy alone, but this did not translate into a change in the overall survival rate in the presence of combination chemotherapy.

Investigators at the University of Arizona studied the effect of adding postoperative irradiation to chemotherapy in node-positive patients.[99] From 1974 until 1980, 159 patients received eight courses of adjuvant Adriamycin-Cytoxan (AC) at three-week intervals. Sixty-three patients received AC plus postoperative radiation therapy, while 96 patients received AC alone. This was a nonrandomized study, and therefore, the two treatment arms were not exactly balanced. There was also an imbalance in the distribution of the number of positive lymph nodes between the two groups, with 57 percent of the com-

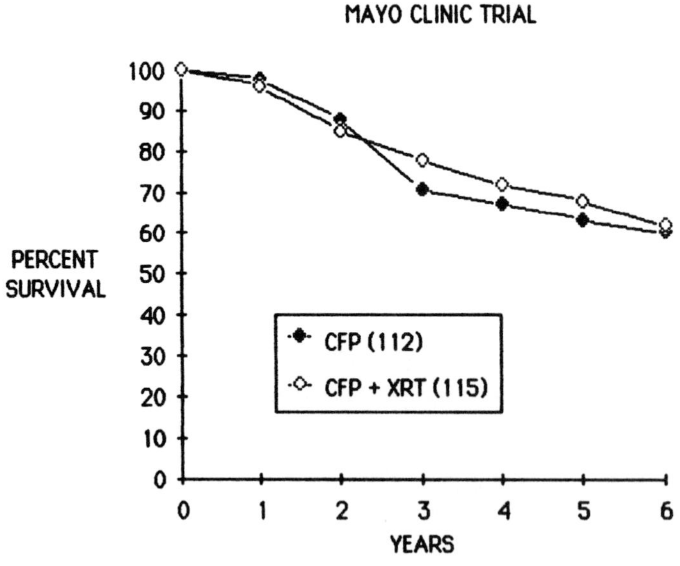

FIGURE 8–20. Results from the Mayo Clinic trial, 1974 to 1980. No statistically significant differences between groups were seen. (From Ahmann DL: Status of adjuvant chemotherapy in patients with breast cancer. Cancer 53:724, 1984.)

bined-modality group having four or more positive nodes, versus 34 percent of the chemotherapy alone group.

Radiation therapy consisted of 4400 rad delivered to the chest wall, supraclavicular and axillary regions, and internal mammary lymph nodes. Radiation therapy was started one week after the second dose of AC, and chemotherapy was resumed one week after completion of the irradiation. There are no further details on the radiation given in the publication concerning this series.[99] There is also no indication as to whether the chemotherapy alone group received the same delay between the second cycle and the third cycle of chemotherapy that the radiation patients were subjected to. The investigators state that there was no difference in the relapse-free survival rate between the pre- and the postmenopausal patients, and so they were grouped together and the population analyzed by nodal status. Results have shown no difference in the relapse-free survival rate between the entire two treatment groups. However, when broken down by nodal status, there was a statistically significant improvement in the survival rate of the patients treated with combined-modality therapy who had one to three positive lymph nodes ($p = 0.05$) (Fig. 8–21). In those patients with four or more positive nodes, there was no difference in the relapse-free survival rate between the two groups. Locoregional recurrences were also analyzed, and in both groups, they stood at 11 percent.

The results of this trial contradict the conventional wisdom concerning the use of postoperative radiation therapy. It has generally been believed that patients with a higher number of positive lymph nodes have a greater chance of a local recurrence and have a higher local tumor burden. Thus, it is in this group that radiation therapy is believed to be most beneficial. However, it appears from this trial that just the opposite is true. Patients with a high number of positive lymph nodes have systemic failure so often that it is possible that no amount of local treatment can affect that result. On the other hand, patients with a small number of positive lymph nodes have a reasonable expectation of systemic control with chemotherapy. In theory, this subset of patients may benefit from postoperative radiation therapy. It must be cautioned, however, that there were only 24 patients in the AC plus irradiation group for the subset of patients with three or fewer lymph nodes. The results from this trial should be sufficient to stimulate other groups to perform similar studies so that this interesting and provocative finding can be either confirmed or refuted.

Another clinical trial of adjuvant chemotherapy with or without postoperative irradiation was performed at the M.D. Anderson Hospital by Buzdar and colleagues.[91] Between May 1977 and May 1980, 238 node-positive patients were randomized to receive combination chemotherapy with 5-FU, Adriamycin, and Cytoxan (FAC) with or without

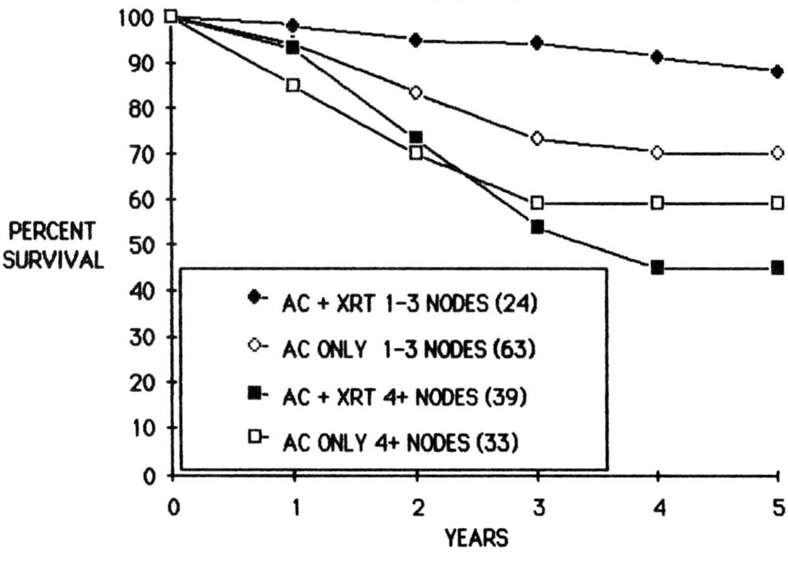

FIGURE 8–21. Results from the University of Arizona trial, 1974 to 1980. Patients with one to three positive nodes, treated with chemotherapy plus irradiation, had statistically higher survival than did patients treated with chemotherapy alone. No significant differences were observed in the group with four or more positive nodes. (From Allen H, Brooks R, Jones SE, et al.: Adjuvant treatment for stage II [node positive] breast cancer with Adriamycin-cyclophosphamide [AC] + radiotherapy [XRT]. *In* Salmon SE, Jones SE [eds.]: Adjuvant Therapy of Cancer III. New York: Grune & Stratton, 1981, pp. 453–462.)

nonspecific immunotherapy with bacillus Calmette-Guérin (BCG). For the first year of the study, all patients received routine postoperative irradiation, but after May 1978, the irradiation was also randomized. In addition, a number of patients received postoperative radiation therapy prior to arriving at the M.D. Anderson Hospital for inclusion in the chemoimmunotherapy trial. These patients have been analyzed in the radiation therapy subgroup. There are no details given concerning the type of radiation therapy employed.

Results from the study showed no difference between the groups treated with or without BCG, with a slightly higher survival rate in patients treated without immunotherapy. Thus, the chemotherapy-immunotherapy arms were folded together, and the entire trial was reanalyzed using radiation therapy as the treatment variable. Seventy-five patients received no postoperative radiation, while 163 patients did. It should be pointed out that patients treated with irradiation had a significantly prolonged delay in starting adjuvant chemotherapy, versus patients treated with chemotherapy only. Eighty-four percent of the nonirradiated patients began their chemotherapy within ten weeks after surgery, versus only 15 percent of the irradiated group. Conversely, only 5 percent of the nonirradiated group had a delay of greater than 14 weeks from surgery to the start of chemotherapy, whereas this lengthy delay occurred in 45 percent of the irradiated patients. Irradiation did not produce a change in the disease-free survival rate, compared with the nonirradiated group (Fig. 8–22). Locoregional recurrences were quite low for both irradiated (2 percent) and nonirradiated (5 percent) patients. However, the median length of follow-up in this study was only 33 months, and it is somewhat premature to draw firm conclusions from this trial. There is no indication as to how many patients received their radiation outside the M.D. Anderson Hospital, and the authors know nothing about the quality of the irradiation that was performed prior to patients being referred to Houston. Thus, while there is no suggestion that radiation therapy had an influence on locoregional recurrence or disease-free survival rates in this study, there are too many uncontrolled variables concerning the radiation therapy to make this conclusion with a great deal of certainty.

In 1976, a trial in Stockholm, Sweden, was instituted to explore adjuvant system chemotherapy or hormonal therapy with or without irradiation in pre- and postmenopausal women. A preliminary analysis of the postmenopausal subset in this trial has been submitted for publication.[95] Between November 1976 and December 1982, 331 patients 70 years of age or younger, with tumors 3 cm in diameter or greater and with or without

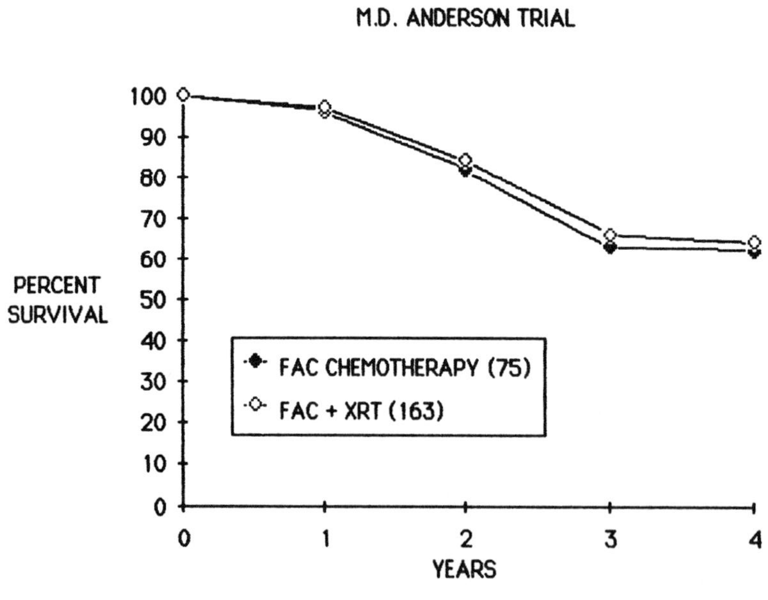

FIGURE 8–22. Results of the M.D. Anderson trial, 1977 to 1980. No statistically significant differences between groups were seen. (From Buzdar AU, Blumenschein GR, Smith TL, et al.: Adjuvant chemotherapy with fluorouracil, doxorubicin, and cyclophosphamide, with or without bacillus Calmette-Guerin and with or without irradiation in operable breast cancer. Cancer 53:384, 1984.

positive axillary nodes, were randomized. The primary randomization was to receive adjuvant chemotherapy with cyclophosphamide, methotrexate, and 5-FU (CMF) versus postoperative radiation therapy. Patients then went on to a further randomization to receive or not receive tamoxifen. Thus, there were four treatment groups in the study. Eighty-nine percent of the patients were lymph node–positive, and 72 percent were estrogen receptor–positive. Chemotherapy dosages were similar to those given by Bonadonna and colleagues[100] and were reduced for women 65 years of age or older.

With a mean follow-up period of 49 months, results have shown significantly more locoregional recurrences in the chemotherapy group versus the irradiation group. Tamoxifen did not seem to make any difference in the likelihood of local control. Overall, 24 percent (42 of 173) of the chemotherapy patients experienced a local failure, versus 9 percent (14 of 158) of the radiation therapy patients. Tamoxifen treatment also reduced the rate of systemic recurrence, especially when it was added to adjuvant chemotherapy.

Results in terms of the disease-free survival and overall survival rates are presented in Figure 8–23. The disease-free survival rate was improved with the use of radiation therapy, compared with CMF in premenopausal women ($p = 0.09$) and postmenopausal women ($p = 0.01$). However, the overall survival rate in this trial was identical when CMF was compared with radiation therapy.

The inferences from this study are rather intriguing. The trial suggests that chemotherapy is not effective in controlling local chest wall disease when compared with irradiation, and the 24 percent recurrence rate seen with CMF chemotherapy is relatively similar to that seen with surgery alone. Since numerous randomized trials have not suggested a survival advantage to the administration of postoperative radiation therapy when compared with surgery alone, the fact that postoperative radiation therapy in this study resulted in a survival rate equal to that of CMF may indicate that CMF does not have a survival advantage over surgery alone. While this lack of survival advantage from CMF has been published for postmenopausal patients,[90] such has not been the case for premenopausal patients. It should be noted, however, that while the postoperative radiation therapy was given in acceptable doses (4600 rad over four and one-half weeks comprehensively to the chest wall and lymph node regions), the chemotherapy was delivered in rather low doses. For example, only 27 percent of Wallgren's patients received 85 percent of protocol dose or greater. Since the women over 65 had a built-in dose reduction, only 18 percent of those patients received 85 percent or greater of the prescribed dose. Although the researchers state that an analysis of the outcome versus chemotherapy dose did not show any significance, full-dose chemotherapy would have been a desirable addition to this study.

The Southeastern Cancer Study Group began a clinical trial in node-positive breast cancer patients in September 1976.[92] Patients with T_1 to T_3 primary breast cancer with positive lymph nodes were randomized following radical or modified radical mastectomy. Patients with fewer than four positive lymph nodes received CMF for 6 or 12 months. Those with more than four positive nodes were randomized to one of those two treatment arms plus a third arm that involved postoperative radiation therapy, followed by six months of CMF. Radiation therapy was delivered comprehensively to the chest wall and regional nodes at a dose of 5000 rad over five weeks. There were, however, some significant differences in the way the chemotherapy was administered to patients who received postoperative radiation therapy versus those who did not receive such therapy. The radiation therapy preceded chemotherapy, and thus, the median time from mastectomy to initiation of chemotherapy in the irradiation group was 96 days, whereas it was 37 days in the nonirradiation group. In addition, the study had a built-in dose reduction for the first two cycles of CMF that were initiated after irradiation. These were given at 75 percent of standard dose levels, and then patients were eligible for escalation to full dose during their third cycle.

The most recent report of this study involved 375 patients who had been randomized and reviewed.[92] Twenty-one percent of these patients were deemed unevaluable, and thus 303 patients were analyzed. The median time of the study was relatively short, being only 33 months. Focusing on the results of patients with four or more positive nodes, the overall relapse rates for patients with six months of chemotherapy

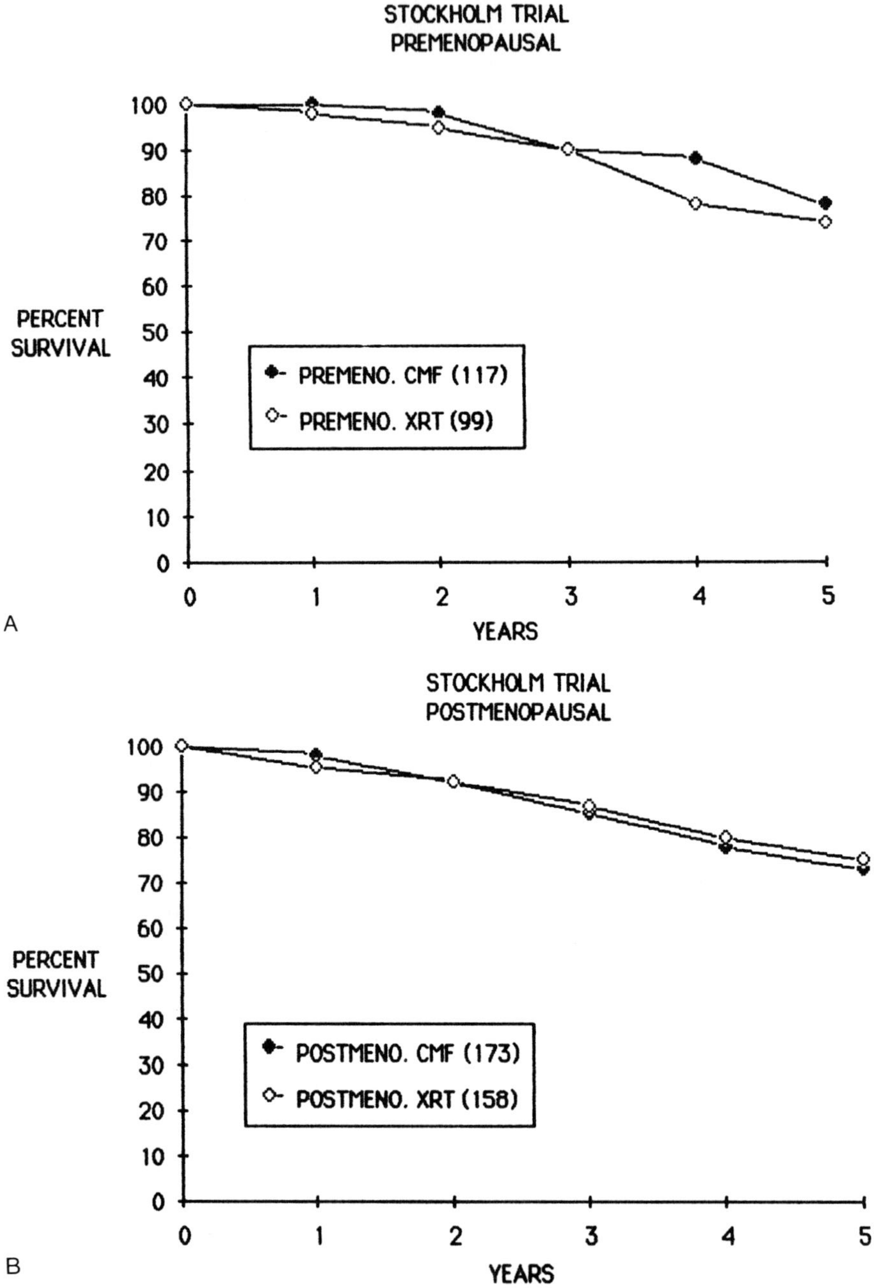

FIGURE 8–23. Results from the Stockholm chemotherapy trial, 1976 to 1982. *A*, Premenopausal patients. *B*, Postmenopausal patients. No statistically significant differences between groups were seen. (From Wallgren A, Baral E, Beling U, et al.: Tamoxifen and combination chemotherapy as adjuvant treatment in postmenopausal women with breast cancer. Recent Results Cancer Res 96:197, 1984.)

was 36 percent; with 12 months of chemotherapy, 45 percent; and with irradiation plus six months of chemotherapy, 28 percent. While this figure was not statistically significant, there were statistically significant reductions in relapse rates for the subset of patients with ten or more lymph nodes involved and for patients with T_1 and T_2 primary tumors (Table 8–13). In premenopausal patients, there was a nonsignificant trend toward improved survival in the radiation-treated patients (Fig. 8–24*A*). Such a trend was not seen in the postmenopausal patients (Fig. 8–24*B*). Analysis of locoregional recurrence figures showed no difference whether or not radiation therapy was added. The chemotherapy alone group had a locoregional failure rate of 10 percent, while the irradiation group had a locoregional relapse rate of 6 percent.

It is difficult to draw firm conclusions from this study with such a short median follow-up time. There were also relatively few patients analyzed: A total of 174 patients with four or more positive nodes were divided among the three treatment groups. Longer follow-up on larger numbers of patients will be most interesting. It is unfortunate that the study design built in a lengthy chemotherapy time delay for patients receiving adjuvant irradiation and also built in a dose reduction for such patients. Thus, one is comparing standard-dose chemotherapy against reduced-dose, delayed chemotherapy for the adjuvant irradiation patients. If such time-dose factors are important in the effectiveness of chemotherapy, the adjuvant irradiation group would be greatly disadvantaged. It is also unfortunate that patients with one to three positive lymph nodes were not irradiated in this trial. This is the subset of patients for which the University of Arizona study showed an advantage for adjuvant irradiation.

The Piedmont Oncology Association performed a clinical trial testing the effectiveness of L-PAM with and without postoperative irradiation versus CMF with and without postoperative irradiation.[101] Patients whose tumors were smaller than 5 cm with positive axillary lymph nodes were eligible. Chemotherapy was started no sooner than four weeks but no later than six weeks following surgery for the drug alone groups, whereas in the irradiated patients, chemotherapy was not instituted until after all radiation therapy was completed. The radiation treatment portals included the chest wall, internal mammary nodes, and supraclavicular fossa. A dose of 4500 to 5000 rad was delivered over six weeks.

Results of the study with a median follow-up time of 24 months (range 2 to 49 months) showed no difference in frequency of recurrence between patients treated with L-PAM versus L-PAM plus postoperative radiation therapy. There was a statistically significant lower rate of recurrence in patients treated with CMF alone versus patients treated with CMF plus postoperative irradiation (Fig. 8–25). The local recurrence rate was low in irradiated groups, three recurrences appearing in 72 patients. A slightly higher local recurrence rate was seen for CMF alone (4 of

TABLE 8–13. Relapse Rates in Patients With Four or More Positive Nodes

	6 Months CMF	*12 Months CMF*	*XRT + 6 Months CMF*
MENOPAUSAL STATUS			
Pre	12 of 30 (40%)	7 of 16 (44%)	4 of 19 (21%)
Post	15 of 46 (33%)	13 of 28 (46%)	11 of 35 (31%)
NODAL STATUS			
4–9	12 of 40 (30%)	7 of 20 (35%)	8 of 31 (26%)
10 or more	14 of 30 (47%)	12 of 19 (63%)*	6 of 20 (30%)*
SIZE OF PRIMARY			
5 cm or smaller	17 of 51 (33%)	4 of 29 (48%)†	8 of 39 (21%)†
Larger than 5 cm	8 of 16 (50%)	3 of 7 (43%)	7 of 13 (54%)
TOTAL	27 of 76 (36%)	20 of 44 (45%)	15 of 54 (28%)

*p = 0.07
†p = 0.02
With permission from Velez-Garcia E, Moore M, Vogel CL, et al.: Postmastectomy adjuvant chemotherapy with or without radiation therapy in women with operable breast cancer and positive axillary lymph nodes: The Southeastern Cancer Group experience. Breast Cancer Res Treat 3:49, 1983.

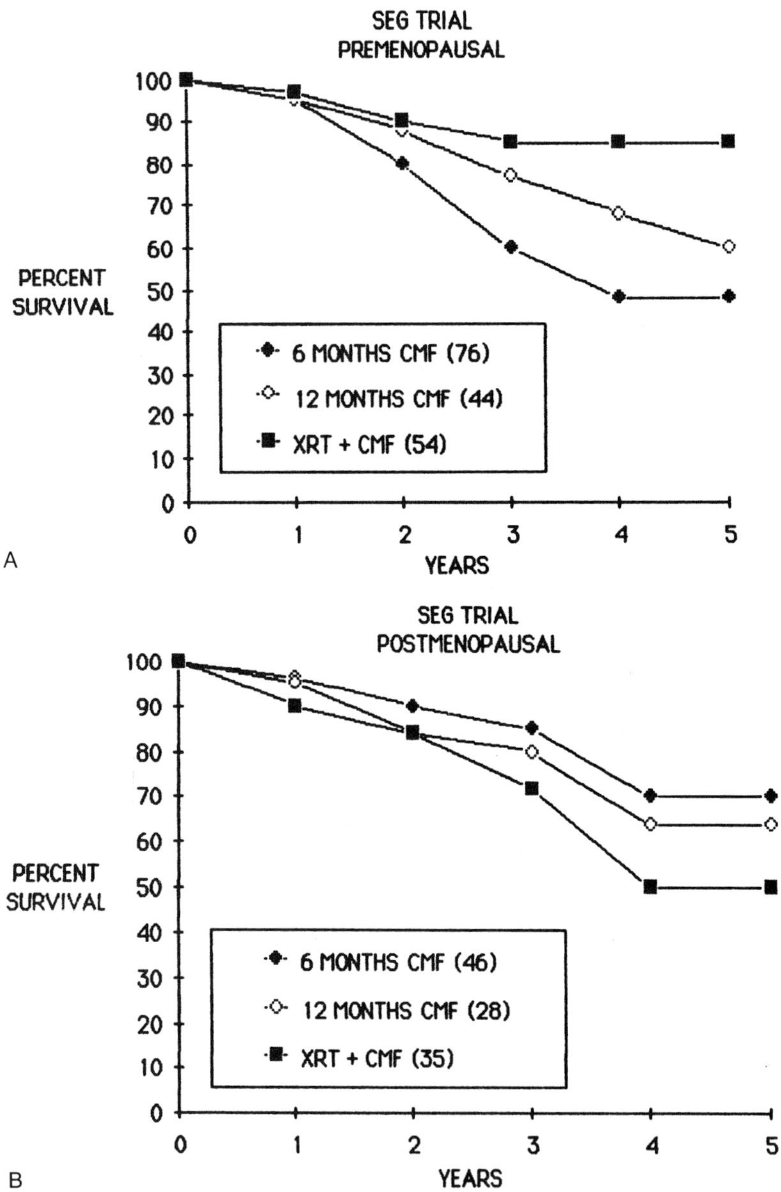

FIGURE 8–24. Results from the Southeastern Cancer Study Group trial, 1976 to 1982. No statistically significant differences between groups were seen. *A,* Premenopausal patients. *B,* Postmenopausal patients. (From Velez-Garcia E, Moore M, Vogel CL, et al.: Postmastectomy adjuvant chemotherapy with or without radiation therapy in women with operable breast cancer and positive axillary lymph nodes: The Southeastern Cancer Group experience. Breast Cancer Res Treat 3:49, 1983.)

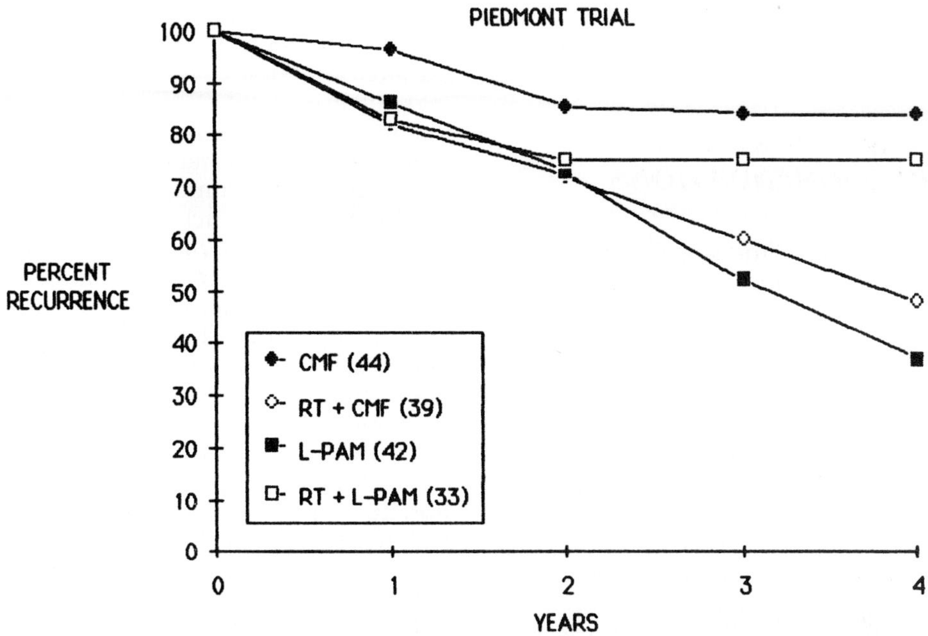

Figure 8–25. Results from the Piedmont Oncology Association trial. Chemotherapy with CMF alone yielded significantly fewer recurrences than did treatment with CMF plus irradiation. (From Cooper MR, Rhyne AL, Muss HB, et al.: A randomized comparative trial of chemotherapy and irradiation therapy for stage II breast cancer. Cancer 47:2833, 1981.)

44) and an even higher rate was seen for L-PAM alone (7 of 42). The number of local recurrences on the L-PAM alone arm was significantly greater than on the other three treatment arms. In comparing the dose of chemotherapy received, patients who were given postoperative irradiation received statistically less drug in both the L-PAM and the CMF treatment groups than did their drug alone counterparts. While this study was small (158 patients divided among four groups) and median follow-up was short (24 months), it certainly suggests no improvement in recurrence rate for patients receiving radiation therapy in addition to chemotherapy. Whether radiation therapy is detrimental to patients awaits further follow-up from this study on larger numbers of patients as well as publication of a disease-free survival curve and an overall survival curve, which were not included in the original publication.

Discussion

A definitive study addressing the question of whether postoperative irradiation is beneficial in node-positive patients who are receiving chemotherapy has yet to be performed. The study from the University of Arizona suggesting an advantage to irradiating patients who had one to three positive nodes was nonrandomized and based on small patient numbers. All other published studies have had major design flaws. They were nonrandomized as regards the radiation,[91] used very unusual dose fractionation,[98] or introduced lengthy time delays or drug dose reduction, or both, into the irradiation arm of the trial.[92, 95, 101] A proper trial would hold the chemotherapy schedule and dose constant between the two arms of the study, a task that can be performed if radiation is not given directly into the mediastinum.[102] Careful radiation treatment planning and dose delivery are essential.

Until such a trial is performed, recommendations based on available data must be made. It does not appear that irradiation offers a survival benefit to node-positive women receiving adjuvant chemotherapy. However, the local recurrence rate is reported to be unaffected by adjuvant chemotherapy in a number of trials.[93–98] Thus, the indications for postoperative irradiation in women who are at high risk for local recurrence (e.g., those with multiple positive nodes, positive surgical margins, or skin involvement) should not change, and those centers that employ irradiation for these types of patients should continue to do so.

SUMMARY AND RECOMMENDATIONS

The literature and clinical experience with postoperative irradiation in the treatment of primary breast cancer are vast and highly controversial. However, a number of firm conclusions can be supported by the available data. Foremost among these conclusions is that the use of routine postoperative irradiation for all patients with breast cancer cannot be supported,[103–105] and its use, especially in node-negative patients, is rapidly and appropriately declining.[106] The long-term survival rate in node-negative patients exceeds 75 percent,[106] and locoregional failures occur in approximately 5 percent of such cases.[107] Thus, adjuvant irradiation has little to offer such patients, even those with medial quadrant tumors.[108] However, it is true that axillary node–negative patients with medial quadrant tumors have a higher incidence of internal mammary node involvement than do those with lateral tumors.[109] If internal mammary nodes are positive, patients have a poor prognosis compared with patients in the same axillary node category without internal mammary node involvement.[110, 111] Lymphoscintigraphy may be able to identify patients with a high likelihood of having internal mammary lymph node involvement,[111] and a useful area of investigation may be postoperative irradiation in those women with abnormal parasternal nodes on lymphoscintigraphy, the sole group of node-negative patients who might benefit from such therapy.

Another firm conclusion that can be supported by the literature is that postoperative irradiation does not increase the survival rate in surgically treated breast cancer. No study has been able to document a survival advantage for the irradiated group as a whole. In some studies, a nonstatistically significant advantage has been suggested for patients with medial quadrant tumors and positive axillae.[49, 55, 84] This subset of patients represents only about 15 percent of breast cancer patients, and it is difficult even for large clinical trials to accumulate enough cases to make a firm statement. If irradiation is to be given with the idea of enhancing survival, it is only in this group that a case can be made for such therapy.

A third well-substantiated fact is that irradiation decreases the incidence of locoregional failure. Certain subsets of patients have an overwhelmingly high incidence of local recurrence. Such subsets include those patients with locally advanced signs such as skin involvement, chest wall involvement, and fixed axillary adenopathy. These groups demonstrate local failure rates of over 40 percent.[113] Similarly, any patient with positive tumor margins or dermal lymphatic involvement has a high risk of local failure. Even though most of these patients will receive chemotherapy, postoperative irradiation to the peripheral nodes and the chest wall to decrease the local recurrence rate from these locally advanced tumors is recommended.

The evidence in the literature supports the concept that clinically negative axillary lymph nodes can be dissected, irradiated, or left alone without altering survival.[60, 74] However, 15 to 20 percent of patients who have not had axillary treatment will need a therapeutic axillary procedure for local recurrrence.[60, 74] Primary therapy with simple mastectomy and irradiation is entirely justifiable if histologic data on axillary lymph node status is not desired.

Finally, many investigators report that adjuvant chemotherapy has not had a significant impact on local recurrence rates.[93–97] Many investigators are questioning whether adjuvant chemotherapy significantly benefits any group of breast cancer patients, especially postmenopausal patients.[114, 115] Thus, decisions regarding the use of postoperative irradiation should be made independent of the patient's treatment with adjuvant cytotoxic drugs or hormones.

REFERENCES

1. Halsted WS: The results of operations for the cure of cancer in the breast performed at the Johns Hopkins Hospital from June 1889 to January 1894. Johns Hopkins Hosp Rep 4:297, 1895.
2. Meyer W: An improved method of the radical operation for carcinoma of the breast. Med Rec 46:746, 1894.
3. Baum M, Edwards MH: Management of early carcinoma of the breast. Lancet 2:85, 1972.
4. DeMoulin D: A short history of breast cancer. Boston: Martinus Nijhoff, 1983, p. 98.

5. Harrington SW: Carcinoma of the breast—surgical treatment and results. JAMA 92:208, 1929.
6. Pfahler GE, Woodman BP: Statistical study of radiation therapy in 1801 cases of carcinoma of the breast. Am J Roentgenol 14:550, 1925.
7. Pfahler GE, Parry LD: Results of roentgen therapy in carcinoma of the breast. JAMA 94:101, 1930.
8. Pfahler GE, Parry LD: Roentgen therapy in carcinoma of the breast—a statistical study of 977 private cases. Ann Surg 93:412, 1931.
9. Pfahler GE: Results of radiation therapy in 1022 private cases of carcinoma of the breast from 1902–1928. Am J Roentgenol 27:497, 1932.
10. Pfahler GE: The treatment of carcinoma of the breast—Caldwell Lecture, 1937. Am J Roentgenol 39:1, 1938.
11. Gratzek FR, Stenstrom KW: Roentgen therapy of mammary carcinoma: Survival study based on 731 cases. Radiology 44:44, 1945.
12. Lee BJ: The therapeutic value of radiation and the treatment of mammary cancer—a survey of 5-year results in 335 cases treated at the Memorial Hospital of New York. Ann Surg 88:26, 1928.
13. Evans WA, Leucutia T: Deep roentgen ray therapy of mammary carcinoma—15-year results in a formally published group and a statistical analysis of 1200 cases treated between 1922 and 1937. Am J Roentgenol 42:866, 1936.
14. Portmann UV: Post-operative roentgen therapy for cancer of the breast—report of 103 consecutive cases. Am J Roentgenol 27:512, 1932.
15. Adair FE: The role of surgery and irradiation in cancer of the breast. JAMA 121:553, 1943.
16. Greenough RB: Treatment of malignant diseases with radium and x-ray—report of the Committee on the Treatment of Malignant Diseases with Radium and X-Ray of the American College of Surgeons. Surg Gynecol Obstet 49:247, 1926.
17. Pendergrass EP, Hodes PG: Some observations on carcinoma of the breast. Am J Roentgenol 39:397, 1938.
18. Lee BJ, Herendeen RE: An evaluation of pre-operative and post-operative radiation in the treatment of mammary carcinoma. Ann Surg 82:404, 1925.
19. Edland RW, Maldonado LG, Johnson RO, et al.: Post-operative radiation in breast cancer. Radiology 92:905, 1969.
20. Tapley N, Spanos WJ, Fletcher GH, et al.: Results in patients with breast cancer treated by radical mastectomy and post-operative irradiation with no adjuvant chemotherapy. Cancer 49:1316, 1982.
21. Fisher B, Slack N, Katrych D, et al.: Ten year follow-up results of patients with carcinoma of the breast in a co-operative clinical trial evaluating surgical adjuvant chemotherapy. Surg Gynecol Obstet 140:528, 1975.
22. Atkins H, Hayward JL, Klugman DJ, et al.: Treatment of early breast cancer: A report after ten years of a clinical trial. Br Med J 2:423, 1972.
23. Veronesi U, Saccozzi R, Del Vecchio M, et al.: Comparing radical mastectomy with quadrantectomy, axillary dissection, and radiotherapy in patients with small cancers of the breast. N Engl J Med 306:6, 1981.
24. Fisher B, Bauer M, Margolese R, et al.: Five-year results of a randomized clinical trial comparing total mastectomy and segmental mastectomy with or without radiation in the treatment of breast cancer. N Engl J Med 312:665, 1985.
25. Bross ISD, Blumenson LE: Predictive design of experiments using deep mathematical models. Cancer 28:1637, 1971.
26. Levitt SH, Potish RA: The role of radiation therapy in the treatment of breast cancer: The use and abuse of clinical trials, statistics, and unproven hypotheses. Int J Radiat Oncol Biol Phys 6:791, 1980.
27. Potish RA, Boen J, Levitt SH: The distinction between statistical significance and clinical importance. Int J Radiat Oncol Biol Phys 6:941, 1980.
28. Potish RA, Boen J, Levitt SH: Statistical inference in the analysis of radiation compliance and its relation to treatment outcome. Cancer Clin Trials 4:475, 1981.
29. Hughes LE, Forbes JF: Early breast cancer: Part I: Surgical pathology and preoperative assessment. Br J Surg 65:753, 1978.
30. Baum M: Scientific empiricism in clinical medicine. Experientia (Suppl) 41:35, 1982.
31. Patterson R: Clinical trials in malignant disease: Part 1: Principles of random selection. J Fac Radiologists 9:80, 1958.
32. Patterson R, Russell MH: Clinical trials in malignant disease: Part 3: Breast cancer: Evaluation of post-operative radiotherapy. J Fac Radiologists 10:175, 1959.
33. Patterson R: Breast cancer: A report of two clinical trials. J R Coll Surg Edinb 7:243, 1962.
34. Cole MP: The place of radiotherapy in the management of early breast cancer—a report of two clinical trials. Br J Surg 51:216, 1964.
35. Eason EC: Post-operative radiotherapy in breast cancer. *In* Forrest AP (ed.): Prognostic Factors in Breast Cancer. Baltimore: Williams & Wilkins, 1968, pp. 118–127.
36. Brinkley D, Haybittle JL: Treatment of stage two cancer of the female breast. Lancet 2:291, 1966.
37. Brinkley D, Haybittle JL: Treatment of stage two cancer of the female breast. Lancet 2:1086, 1971.
38. Fischer B, Slack NH, Cavanaugh PJ, et al.: Post-operative radiotherapy in the treatment of cancer—results of the NSABP trial. Ann Surg 172:711, 1970.
39. Fisher B: Cooperative clinical trials in primary breast cancer: A critical appraisal. Cancer 31:1271, 1973.
40. Harris JR, Hellman S: Local and regional management of carcinoma of the breast. *In:* Carter S, Glatstein E, Livingston R (eds.): Principles of Cancer Treatment. New York: McGraw-Hill, 1982, p. 306.
41. Kaae S, Johansen H: Breast cancer—a comparison of the results of simple mastectomy with post-operative roentgen irradiation by the McWhirter method to those of extended radical mastectomy. Acta Radiol (Suppl) 188:155, 1959.
42. Kaae S, Johansen H: Simple mastectomy plus post-operative irrradiation by the method of McWhirter for mammary carcinoma. Prog Clin Cancer 1:453, 1965.
43. Kaae S, Johansen H: Simple mastectomy followed by irradiation offers survival comparable to radical procedures. Int J Radiat Oncol Biol Phys 2:1163, 1977.
44. Anglem TJ, Leber RE: The dubious case for conservative operation in operable cancer of the breast. Ann Surg 176:625, 1972.
45. McWhirter R: Simple mastectomy and radiotherapy

in the treatment of breast cancer. Br J Radiol 28:128, 1955.

46. Fletcher GH, Montague ED: Does adequate irradiation of the internal mammary chain and supraclavicular nodes improve survival rates? Int J Radiat Oncol Biol Phys 4:481, 1978.
47. Høst H, Brennhovd IO: Combined surgery and radiation therapy versus surgery alone in primary mammary carcinoma—the effect of orthovoltage radiation. Acta Radiol Ther Phys Biol 14:25, 1975.
48. Høst H, Brennhovd IO: The effect of post-operative radiotherapy in breast cancer. Int J Radiat Oncol Biol Phys 2:1061, 1977.
49. Høst H: Post-operative radiotherapy in breast cancer. Experientia (Suppl) 41:580, 1982.
50. Carter SK: Clinical trials in primary breast cancer—the therapeutic implications. Cancer 53:740, 1984.
51. Bruce J: Operable cancer of the breast—a controlled clinical trial. Cancer 28:1443, 1971.
52. Hamilton T, Langlands AO, Prescott RJ: The treatment of operable cancer of the breast: A clinical trial in the southeast region of Scotland. Br J Surg 61:758, 1974.
53. Langlands AO, Prescott JR, Hamilton T: A clinical trial in the management of operable cancer of the breast. Br J Surg 67:170, 1980.
54. Lacour J, Bucalossi P, Caceres E, et al.: Radical mastectomy versus radical mastectomy plus internal mammary dissection. Five-year results of an international cooperative study. Cancer 37:206, 1976.
55. Tubiana M, Sarrazin D: A reappraisal of radiotherapy in the treatment of operable breast cancer. The new light on the internal mammary chain roll. Eur J Cancer (Suppl) 1:243, 1980.
56. Burn JI: Early breast cancer: The Hammersmith trial. Br J Surg 61:762, 1974.
57. Stjernsward J: Decreased survival related to irradiation postoperatively in early operable breast cancer. Lancet 2:1285, 1974.
58. Baum M, Edwards MH, Magarey CJ: Organization of a clinical trial on a national scale: Management of early cancer of the breast. Br Med J 4:476, 1972.
59. Cancer Research Campaign Working Party: Management of "early" cancer of the breast. Report of an international multi-center trial supported by the CRC. Br Med J 1:1035, 1976.
60. Cancer Research Campaign Working Party: Cancer Research Campaign (King's/Cambridge) trial for early breast cancer. A detailed update at the tenth year. Lancet 2:55, 1980.
61. Brinkley D, Haybittle JL, Houghton J: The Cancer Research Campaign (King's/Cambridge) trial for early breast cancer: An analysis of the radiotherapy data. Br J Radiol 57:309, 1984.
62. Cancer Research Campaign Working Party: Trials and tribulations: Thoughts on the organization of multi-center clinical studies. Br Med J 281:918, 1980.
63. Elston CW, Gresham GA, Rao GS, et al.: The Cancer Research Campaign (King's/Cambridge) trial for early breast cancer: Clinical pathologic aspects. Br J Cancer 45:655, 1982.
64. Forrest APM, Roberts MM, Preece P, et al.: The Cardiff–St. Mary's trial. Br J Surg 61:766, 1974.
65. Forrest APM, Roberts MM, Stewart HJ: Selection of local therapy for primary breast cancer by lower axillary node histology. Eur J Cancer (Suppl) 1:237, 1980.
66. Forrest APM, Stewart JH, Roberts MM, et al.: Simple mastectomy and axillary node sampling (pectoral node biopsy) in the management of primary breast cancer. Am J Surg 196:371, 1982.
67. Fisher B, Redmond C, Fisher ER: The contribution of recent NSABP clinical trials of primary breast cancer therapy to an understanding of tumor biology: An overview of findings. Cancer 46:1009, 1980.
68. Turnbull AR, Chant ADB, Buchanan RB, et al.: Treatment of early breast cancer. Lancet 2:7, 1978.
69. Lythgoe JP: Manchester regional breast study. Lancet 1:744, 1978.
70. Lythgoe JP, Palmer MK: Manchester regional breast study—five and ten year results. Br J Surg 69:693, 1982.
71. Brady LW, Fletcher GH, Levitt SH: Cancer of the breast: The role of radiation therapy after mastectomy. Cancer 39:2868, 1977.
72. Hughes LE: Does local treatment affect the outcome of breast cancer?—an alternative view of the Manchester Regional Breast Study. Br J Surg 70:391, 1983.
73. Fisher B, Montague ED, Redmond C, et al.: Comparison of radical mastectomy with alternative treatments for primary breast cancer: A first report of results from a prospective randomized clinical trial. Cancer 39:2827, 1977.
74. Fisher B, Redmond C, Fisher E, et al.: Ten-year results of a randomized clinical trial comparing radical mastectomy and total mastectomy with or without radiation. N Engl J Med 312:674, 1985.
75. Fisher B, Wolmark N, Bauer M, et al.: The accuracy of clinical nodal staging and of limited axillary dissection as a determinant of histologic nodal status in carcinoma of the breast. Surg Gynecol Obstet 152:765, 1981.
76. Fisher B, Montague ED, Redmond C, et al.: Findings from NSABP protocol B-O4—comparison of radical mastectomy with alternative treatments for primary breast cancer. 1. Radiation compliance and its relation to treatment outcome. Cancer 46:1, 1980.
77. Balawajder I, Antich PP, Boland J: An analysis of the role of radiotherapy alone and in combination with chemotherapy and surgery in the management of advanced breast carcinoma. Cancer 51:574, 1983.
78. Zucali R, Uslenghi C, Kena R, et al.: Natural history and survival of inoperable breast cancer treated with radiotherapy and radiotherapy followed by radical mastectomy. Cancer 37:1422, 1976.
79. Montague ED, Fletcher GH: The curative value of irradiation in the treatment of nondisseminated breast cancer. Cancer 46:995, 1980.
80. Wallgren A: A controlled study: Pre-operative versus post-operative irradiation. Int J Radiat Oncol Biol Phys 2:1167, 1977.
81. Wallgren A, Arner O, Bergstrom J, et al.: Preoperative radiotherapy in operable breast cancer: Results in the Stockholm Breast Cancer Trial. Cancer 42:1120, 1978.
82. Wallgren A, Arner O, Bergstrom J, et al.: The value of pre-operative radiotherapy in operable mammary carcinoma. Int J Radiol Oncol Biol Phys 6:287, 1980.
83. Strender LE, Wallgren A, Arndt J, et al.: Adjuvant radiotherapy in operable breast cancer: Correlation between dose in internal mammary nodes and prognosis. Int J Radiat Oncol Biol Phys 7:1319, 1981.

advancement at the time of diagnosis, thus permitting the selection of appropriate therapy before treatment is rendered and facilitating the comparison of results for definitive therapies between comparable patient groups. Numerous staging classifications, devised in this century, describe the disease from very early stages to that of widespread metastases. Included within this spectrum is locally advanced, nonmetastatic breast cancer. The precise definition of this disease entity has varied with different staging schemata and investigators. Hence, understanding these various staging systems becomes essential for comparison of different investigators' reports of prognostic variables and therapeutic results in locally advanced breast cancer.

Recognizing the need for a practical clinical classification, in 1905 Steinthal of Stuttgart described certain clinical disease situations in which surgical therapy was futile.[1] These situations, which he termed "Stage 3," included patients whose tumors involved a great part of the breast, extended to the skin as well as the underlying tissues, or involved the supraclavicular nodes. In 1940, the Manchester classification was developed at the Christie Hospital and Holt Radium Institute in Manchester, England, as a purely clinical method of staging breast cancer.[2] This system included the features of locally advanced breast cancer within Stages III and IV. Stage III was defined as tumor growth extending beyond the mammary parenchyma, as shown by skin invasion or fixation over an area large in relation to the size of the breast or by skin ulceration or tumor fixation to the underlying muscle or fascia. Axillary nodes, if present, were mobile. Stage IV included tumors that extended beyond the breast area, as shown by fixation or matting of axillary nodes, complete fixation of the tumor to the chest wall, metastases to supraclavicular nodes or the opposite breast, satellite nodules, or distant metastases. Three years later, Portmann at the Cleveland Clinic introduced a four-stage system based upon both clinical and pathologic features, in which he defined locally advanced disease in the highest two stages.[3] Stage III comprised tumors diffusely infiltrating the breast, fixation of the tumor or the breast to the chest wall, breast edema, and secondary tumors. Skin involvement was characterized by edema; brawny red induration and inflammation not obviously due to infection; extensive ulceration; and multiple secondary nodules. Metastases included many axillary lymph nodes involved or fixed but no clinical or roentgenologic evidence of distant metastases. Stage IV incorporated the aforementioned tumor and skin characteristics, with metastases defined as axillary and supraclavicular lymph nodes extensively involved and with clinical or roentgenologic evidence of distant metastases.

In 1943, Haagensen and Stout published their criteria of operability of breast cancer after reviewing the treatment results at Presbyterian Hospital from 1915 to 1935.[4] They reviewed a group of patients who presented with locally advanced disease and were treated with radical mastectomy, with no apparent benefit. Three local clinical features were identified that conferred this poor prognosis: extensive edema of the skin over the breast, satellite tumor nodules in the skin, and inflammatory carcinoma. Patients with such features were never cured with radical surgery; these features formed the basis of the classification of "categorically inoperable." From further correlations of the clinical features of breast carcinoma with the results of operation, a list of clinical criteria of operability was compiled. These criteria called for radical mastectomy in all situations, except when there was extensive edema of the skin over the breast, satellite nodules in the skin over the breast, inflammatory carcinoma, parasternal tumor, supraclavicular metastases, arm edema, distant metastases, and any two or more grave signs of locally advanced carcinoma. These grave signs included ulceration of the skin, edema of less than one third of the skin over the breast, solid fixation of the tumor to the chest wall, axillary lymph nodes measuring 2.5 cm or more in transverse diameter, and fixation of axillary lymph nodes to the skin or the deep axillary structures. In reviewing 120 patients treated with radical mastectomy (77 of whom were considered categorically inoperable, and 43, inoperable because of two or more grave signs), the investigators observed local recurrence in half of these patients, with no patient cured of her disease.[2] On the basis of this careful work by Haagensen and Stout, the Columbia Clinical Classification (see Table 4–2) was established and became the most widely used staging classification through the early 1970's.

TABLE 9–1. TNM Classification

*Primary Tumor (T)**

Definitions for the primary tumor (T) for clinical-diagnostic classification are the same as those for postsurgical classification.

T_X	Minimum requirements to assess primary tumor cannot be met.
T_0	No evidence of primary tumor.
TIS	*In situ* cancer (*in situ* lobular cancer, pure intraductal cancer, and Paget's disease of the nipple without palpable tumor).
Note:	Paget's disease with a demonstrable tumor is classified according to size of the tumor. Inflammatory carcinoma should be reported separately.
T_1	Tumor 2 cm or less in greatest dimension.
T_{1a}	No fixation to underlying pectoral fascia or muscle.
T_{1b}	Fixation to underlying pectoral fascia or muscle.
i	Tumor $\leq$ 0.5 cm.
ii	Tumor $>$ 0.5 $\leq$ 1.0 cm.
iii	Tumor $>$ 1.0 $\leq$ 2.0 cm.
T_2	Tumor more than 2 cm but not more than 5 cm in greatest dimension.
T_{2a}	No fixation to underlying pectoral fascia or muscle.
T_{2b}	Fixation to underlying pectoral fascia or muscle.
T_3	Tumor more than 5 cm in greatest dimension.
T_{3a}	No fixation to underlying pectoral fascia or muscle.
T_{3b}	Fixation to underlying pectoral fascia or muscle.
T_4	Tumor of any size, with direct extension to chest wall or skin. (Chest wall includes ribs, intercostal muscles, and serratus anterior muscle, but not pectoral muscle.)
T_{4a}	Fixation to chest wall.
T_{4b}	Edema (including peau d'orange), ulceration of the skin of the breast, or satellite skin nodules confined to the same breast.
T_{4c}	Both of the above.
T_{4d}	Inflammatory carcinoma.

Nodal Involvement (N)

N_X	Regional lymph nodes cannot be assessed clinically.
N_0	Homolateral axillary lymph nodes not considered to contain growth.
N_1	Movable homolateral axillary nodes considered to contain growth.
N_2	Homolateral axillary nodes considered to contain growth and are fixed to one another or to other structures.
N_3	Homolateral supraclavicular or infraclavicular nodes considered to contain growth, or edema of the arm. (Edema of the arm may be caused by lymphatic obstruction, and lymph nodes may not then be palpable.)

Distant Metastasis (M)

M_X	Minimum requirements to assess the presence of distant metastasis cannot be met.
M_0	No (known) distant metastasis.
M_1	Distant metastasis present. Specify____________________.

*Dimpling of the skin, nipple retraction, or any other skin changes, except those in T_{4b}, may occur in T_1, T_2, or T_3 without changing the classification.

The most widely used clinical classification of breast cancer is based upon the TNM system (Table 9–1) and has been adopted by the International Union Against Cancer (UICC) and the American Joint Committee for Cancer Staging and End Results Reporting (AJC).[5] In 1972, the AJC and UICC established staging groups such that patients with locally advanced disease, comprising TNM stages T_3–T_4 N_0–N_1 M_0 and T_1–T_4 N_2–N_3 M_0, would be included in Stage III (Table 9–2).[6] In 1978, the AJC revised its staging groups, including most patients with locally advanced disease in Stage IV (Table 9–3); however, T_3 N_0–N_1 M_0 and T_1–T_2 N_2 M_0 patients remained in Stage III.[6] Additional modifications in 1978 by the UICC[7] and in 1983 by

TABLE 9–2. AJC-UICC 1972 Stage Grouping

Stage III	Any T_3, Any N, M_0
	Any T_4, Any N, M_0
	Any T, N_2, M_0
	Any T, N_3, M_0
Stage IV	Any T, Any N, M_1

the AJC[5] divided Stage III into a and b subclassifications and moved patients with locally advanced breast cancer entirely within this stage (Table 9–4). Inflammatory carcinoma is considered a T_4 tumor and is included in Stage III_b.

FREQUENCY OF LOCALLY ADVANCED BREAST CANCER AND DISTRIBUTION OF PATIENT SUBSETS

The frequency of locally advanced breast cancer is not easy to estimate. Heterogeneity among staging systems, coupled with multiple changes within each staging classification, have contributed to much of the difficulty in interpreting the older literature and in comparing various series. In addition, many series fail to report the total number of patients presenting with all stages of breast cancer from which the study population was drawn, making estimates of the denominator uncertain. Table 9–5 shows the frequency of locally advanced breast cancer compiled from five series in which both staging criteria and total presenting patient populations were described.[2, 8–11] The frequencies range from 10 to 29 percent, with an average frequency in 8754 patients of 20.0 percent. Most of these series preceded the era of modern diagnostic technology and the public's heightened awareness of and concern regarding cancer; since then, estimates of the frequency of locally advanced nonmetastatic breast cancer have been lower.

The distribution of clinical TNM stages for patients with locally advanced breast cancer is shown in Table 9–6 for seven reported series and collectively.[10–16] Using current AJC staging criteria for Stage III patients, 62.5 percent of patients are Stage III_b and 37.5 percent of patients are Stage III_a, a ratio of approximately 2:1. The distribution of T_3 and T_4 tumors is 35.7 and 58.4 percent, respectively. Of interest is the fact that N_0 patients constitute 27.4 percent of this collective patient population, with 12.5 percent T_3 N_0 and 14.7 percent T_4 N_0. The distribution of N_1, N_2, and N_3 nodal disease is 46.6, 15.6, and 10.4 percent, respectively. An estimate of the frequency of pathologic nodal involvement can be obtained from reported series in which patients with locally advanced breast cancer were treated with radical mastectomy. Fracchia and colleagues[17] reviewed the case records of 488 patients treated with radical mastectomy at Memorial Hospital and found that 88 percent of these patients had pathologically involved axillary nodes. The clinical stage of these patients prior to surgery was Stage III, according to the 1972 AJC criteria; they would be included in Stages III_a and III_b, according to 1983 criteria. Of those patients with pathologically positive nodes, 3.5 percent had only microscopic involvement, 24.2 percent had fewer than four involved nodes, and 72.3 percent had greater than four involved nodes. Haagensen[2] reported a 76.5 percent frequency of pathologic nodal involvement in 63 Stage C patients. Similar results have been cited for Stage C patients by Butcher in St. Louis and Miller in Detroit, with an 89.5 and a 76.7 percent frequency of documented axillary metastases.[2]

TABLE 9–3. AJC 1978 Stage Grouping

Stage III	T_{1a} or T_{1b}, N_2, M_0
	T_{2a} or T_{2b}, N_2, M_0
	T_{3a} or T_{3b}, N_0 or N_1 or N_2, M_0
Stage IV	Any T_4, Any N, Any M
	Any T, N_3, Any M
	Any T, Any N, M_1

TABLE 9–4. UICC 1978–AJC 1983 Stage Grouping

Stage III_a	T_0, N_2, M_0
	T_{1a} or T_{1b}, N_2, M_0
	T_{2a} or T_{2b}, N_2, M_0
	T_{3a} or T_{3b}, N_0, M_0
	T_{3a} or T_{3b}, N_1, M_0
	T_{3a} or T_{3b}, N_2, M_0
Stage III_b	Any T, N_3, M_0
	Any T_4, Any N, M_0
Stage IV	Any T, Any N, M_1

Node Status

The prognostic significance of various staging criteria has been examined by several investigators. Axillary node involvement has been consistently found to exert a major influence on relapse and survival rates. Zucali and associates,[12] in an analysis of 454 patients treated with either irradiation alone

TABLE 9–5. Frequency of Locally Advanced Breast Cancer (LABC)

Investigator	Inclusive Period	Staging System	No. of Patients with LABC	No. of Patients with All Stages of Breast Cancer	Percentage of Patients with LABC
Haagensen[2]	1915–1942	Columbia	120	1135	11.6
McWhirter[8]	1941–1947	Manchester	546	1882	29.0
Rubens et al.[9]	1961–1973	TNM	184	1083	17.0
Arnold and Lesnick[10]	1961–1973	TNM	228	2218	10.3
Donegan and Lewis[11]	Up to 1957	TNM	673	2424	27.8
Total			1751	8754	20.0

or irradiation followed by mastectomy, found that the survival time for clinical N_0 patients was almost twice as long as that of N_1–N_3 patients, with a median survival of 4.0 versus 2.3 years. Relapse within the first 18 months was higher in patients with node involvement, with frequencies of 27 percent for T_3 N_0 versus 46 percent for T_3 N_1–N_3 and of 29 percent for T_4N_0 versus 50 percent for T_4 N_1–N_3. Patients with N_3 disease had the worst survival times, with a median of 1.4 years. Treurniet-Donker and colleagues[18] showed a similar trend in a group of 129 patients treated with irradiation alone, with five-year survival rates of 30, 12, and 0 percent for patients with N_0, N_1–N_2, and N_3 disease, respectively. Rao and associates[19] reported that in patients treated with irradiation alone, the regional failure rate increased from 9 percent for N_0–N_1 patients to 58 percent for N_2–N_3 patients, with a concomitant decrease in five-year disease-free survival rates from 30 to 4 percent, respectively. These trends were not observed in similar patients treated with surgery followed by irradiation. In a series of 228 surgically treated patients, Arnold and Lesnick[10] reported overall five- and ten-year survival rates of 33 and 22 percent, respectively. For patients with T_3N_0 disease, the five- and ten-year survival rates were 77 and 63 percent, respectively, while the respective survival rates for T_4N_0 patients were 65 and 34 percent. In Fracchia's series detailing pathologic node involvement, the respective survival rates at five and ten years were 50 and 23 percent if fewer than four nodes were involved, versus 35 and 17 percent if more than four nodes were involved.[17] Bulk node disease, as manifested clinically by matting or fixation to the skin or the chest wall, was not observed to have an effect on the survival rate. In contrast, those patients with only microscopic nodal involvement had a 41 percent ten-year survival rate. Pa-

TABLE 9–6. Distribution of TNM for All Patients Presenting with Locally Advanced Breast Cancer

Stage	Donegan and Lewis[11]	Zucali et al.[12]	Balawajder et al.[13]	Hortobagyi et al.[14]*	Bedwinek et al.[15]	Harris et al.[16]	Arnold and Lesnick[10]†	Total (%)
T_1N_2	—	—	—	—	2	—	—	2 (0.1)
T_1N_3	—	—	—	—	2	—	—	2 (0.1)
T_2N_2	15	—	11	2	3	7	25	63 (3.6)
T_2N_3	24	—	—	5	2	5	—	36 (2.1)
T_3N_0	132	37	9	—	11	16	13	218 (12.5)
T_3N_1	141	76	15	1	12	22	34	301 (17.3)
T_3N_2	—	3	14	3	2	7	38	67 (3.9)
T_3N_3	11	11	3	4	3	2	—	34 (2.0)
T_4N_0	76	80	17	—	40	26	19	258 (14.8)
T_4N_1	169	208	10	11	35	25	51	509 (29.3)
T_4N_2	14	16	18	12	14	18	48	140 (8.1)
T_4N_3	30	23	11	14	21	9	—	108 (6.2)
Total	612	454	108	52	147	137	228	1738 (100)

*Excluding node-negative patients and patients with inflammatory carcinoma.
†Surgical series excluding N_3 patients.

tients who were pathologically node-negative had five- and ten-year survival rates of 82.2 and 75.3 percent, respectively. Of note was the fact that patients with negative nodes displayed a high percentage of histologic types other than infiltrating ductal carcinoma, with 19 percent of these patients having papillary, lobular, or medullary carcinomas. In addition, of 11 node-negative patients who had estrogen receptors (ER) determined, 91 percent were ER positive, compared with 48 percent ER-positivity in 75 patients with involved nodes who underwent estrogen receptor evaluation.

Tumor Characteristics

Tumor size, according to Rao and associates,[19] influenced local failure and survival rates in patients treated with irradiation alone in the absence of an excisional biopsy only when the tumor was larger than 8 cm. Local failure rates increased from 44 percent for tumors of 0 to 8 cm to 76 percent for tumors larger than 8 cm, while the five-year disease-free survival rates decreased from 30 to 4 percent, respectively. This difference was not appreciated in patients undergoing surgery followed by irradiation. The presence of grave signs such as skin ulceration, skin fixation, chest wall fixation, and edema had no significant effect upon failure rates or five-year disease-free survival rates in this study. The presence of skin infiltration was a poor prognostic factor in the Fracchia series, with five- and ten-year survival rates of 30 and 13.2 percent, compared with 43.7 and 24.1 percent if these features were absent.[17] Skin edema also adversely affected survival rates, but only in node-positive patients, with five- and ten-year survival rates of 17 and 9.2 percent, as opposed to 44.1 and 22.3 percent in patients without skin edema. Surprisingly, invasion of the pectoral muscle did not influence the survival rate in the node-positive patients. In the Zucali series, no significant difference in relapse rate was noted between T_3 and T_4 tumors when inflammatory histology was excluded.[12] Likewise, Treurniet-Donker and associates[18] did not observe any significant difference in local relapse rates between tumors smaller than and those greater than 6 cm; however, there was a tendency for patients with the smaller tumors to do somewhat better.

Inflammatory Histology

Inflammatory carcinoma of the breast is a relatively rare disease but holds ominous prognostic implications. It began to evolve as a unique clinical entity as early as 1814, when Bell described the clinical course of a breast mass presenting with pain and overlying skin discoloration.[20] The inflammatory features of this disease were emphasized by Klotz in 1869 when he coined the term "mastitis carcinomatosa."[21] Subsequent reports by Leitch[22] and Learmonth[23] described the fulminant course of this process, which was termed acute mammary carcinoma. The first collection of cases was from Schumann and was designated carcinoma mastitoides.[24] However, it was the reports of the case series of Lee and Tannenbaum[25] and Taylor and Meltzer[26] that described the currently accepted clinical picture and established the entity of "inflammatory carcinoma" as the neoplastic process underlying these inflammatory changes. These changes, as classically described, include erythema, warmth, edema, peau d'orange, diffuse and ill-defined swelling, and sometimes pain and tenderness.

Histologic definition of this entity was advanced by Bryant,[27] who observed dermal lymphatic invasion by carcinoma and postulated that the obstruction produced by such invasion could result in the clinical inflammatory appearance. This concept was popularized by Taylor and Meltzer and was held as pathologic proof of inflammatory breast cancer.[26] Of great interest to some pathologists was the fact that while almost all patients with inflammatory carcinoma displayed a rapidly fulminant course, an occasional patient would be reported to survive five years. Ellis and Teitelbaum[28] were prompted by this to review the pathology on all available five-year survivors with inflammatory carcinoma and found that none of these patients showed dermal or subcutaneous lymphatic invasion, even though they had clinical inflammatory features. On this basis, the investigators decided that tumor emboli in dermal lymphatics must be present before a diagnosis of inflammatory carcinoma could be made and suggested using the term "dermal lymphatic carcinomatosis of the breast." Saltzstein[29] approached this same issue by examining the clinical courses of patients who had dermal lymphatic invasion in their pathology specimens but who had no clinical inflammatory features. He found that these patients exhibited a rapidly progressive deteriorating course compatible with that traditionally associated with inflammatory carcinoma. Therefore, he proposed the term "clinically occult inflammatory carcinoma" and suggested that inflammatory breast cancer be a pathologic rather than a clinical diagnosis. Lucas and Perez-Mesa[30] attempted to resolve this controversy by following the clinical courses of three groups of patients: patients with dermal lymphatic invasion with clinical inflammatory signs, patients without dermal lymphatic invasion but with clinical inflammatory signs, and patients with dermal lymphatic invasion with no inflammatory signs. In all groups, they observed similar gross and microscopic growth patterns, histologic types, degrees of axillary involvement, and patterns of metastases. Rapid deterioration characterized the course in all three groups. Hence, they suggested that either clinical or pathologic criteria could be used to define this disease entity.

With the previous controversies over the definition of inflammatory carcinoma in mind, the frequency of this form of breast cancer has been reported to be 1.5 to 4 percent.[26, 31–35] Despite the varying size and oftentimes ill-defined nature of these tumors, for TNM staging purposes they are included within the T_4 category. Clinically involved axillary nodes are the rule, with estimates in the range of 90 percent.[2, 30] In those cases available for histologic correlation, the frequency of pathologic nodal involvement was approximately 97 percent.[30] Survival in this group of patients has been very poor, with early local relapse and distant metastatic disease. A review of 12 series in the literature between 1924 and 1980 showed a range of mean survival time of 4 to 30 months for all these series, regardless of whether the patients received mastectomy alone, irradiation alone, or a combination of surgery and irradiation.[2, 25, 26, 32, 33, 35–40, 71] Less than 4 percent of the patients in these collective series survived five years.

Thus, within the heterogeneous population of patients with locally advanced breast cancer, there exist subsets of patients with relatively favorable and less favorable prognostic features. The prognosis of patients with T_3 or T_4 tumors but with clinically negative axillary nodes or only microscopic nodal involvement is better than that of a significant number of Stage II patients and may even approach that of some Stage I patients. In contrast, patients with advanced nodal metastases or inflammatory histology have the worst outcome. Hence, these subsets of patients must be carefully examined when comparing different treatment strategies reported in the literature, since subtle changes in the proportions between these groups may dramatically alter the patterns of relapse and survival among different series.

LOCAL THERAPEUTIC MODALITIES

Untreated Patients

The clinical course of untreated breast cancer provides a baseline against which to assess the value of various therapies. In modern times, almost all patients with breast cancer receive some form of treatment; hence, most available information regarding the course of untreated patients comes from the nineteenth and early twentieth centuries. The patient populations from which these data are derived are those whose cancers were too locally advanced for the surgical treatments of that time, those who refused therapy, and those who were institutionalized in the terminal phases of their illness. Bloom[41] studied the records of 250 patients at the Middlesex Hospital seen between 1805 and 1933 who died of untreated breast cancer. By the Manchester staging criteria, 97.6 percent of these patients were either Stage III or IV (23.2 percent Stage III, and 74.4 percent Stage IV). The proportion of Stage IV patients with metastatic disease at the time of presentation is not available. All patients had their diagnosis confirmed at autopsy. The survival patterns showed 44, 18, and 4 percent alive at three, five, and ten years, respectively. The median survival time was 2.7 years. These survival times compare closely with those reported for untreated patients by Greenwood,[42] Daland,[43] Nathanson and Welch,[44] and Forber.[45] In a collection of 1091 patients studied by five different authors, Bloom[41] reported a mean survival time of 3.2 years, with a range of 2.5 to 3.3 years. In his own series, no case of spontaneous regression was noted. Seventy-three percent of his patients developed marked ulceration of the breast; in 21 percent, this ulceration was so extensive that it sometimes destroyed the breast and the chest wall, exposing the pleura. Thus, until the time when patients with locally advanced breast cancer die of metastatic disease, they may endure significant local morbidity that will detract from the quality of life during their time of survival. Consequently, in evaluating the efficacy of various individual therapeutic modalities or combinations of modalities, both quality of survival and local control of the primary lesion should be considered.

Surgery

In the treatment of breast cancer, radical surgery has traditionally been the standard by which other modalities or combinations of modalities have been judged and, as such, provides the first treatment data for patients with locally advanced breast cancer. Table 9–7 summarizes the results of seven different series in which radical surgery was used as the primary and only treatment modality in patients with locally advanced breast cancer.[4, 10, 17, 46–49] All patients who received postoperative therapy of any type are excluded from this tabulation. Comparisons are complicated by the different staging classifications used in each series. Local relapse rates ranged between 6 and 50 percent, with an average of approximately 34 percent. Five-year survival rates ranged from 9 to 53 percent, with an average of approximately 47 percent. Ten-year survival rates ranged from 7 to 34 percent, with an approximate average of 26 percent. Local control and survival rates were higher in Columbia Stage C versus D. The survival rate was also higher in patients with N_0 nodal status. Of importance is the fact that when this purely local form of therapy was rendered to patients with these disease stages, the rate of development of subsequent distant metastases was in the range of 56 to 81 percent.

Radiation Therapy Alone

As investigators realized the futility of radical surgery in all but a few select patients with locally advanced breast cancer, radiation therapy assumed the primary role in the treatment of this disease. Table 9–8 summarizes the results of 16 series in which radiation therapy was the primary and only treatment modality in patients with locally advanced breast cancer.[9, 12, 13, 15, 16, 18, 49–58] All patients, reported by these investigators, who received postirradiation surgery or chemotherapy are excluded from this tabulation. Comparisons are complicated not only by different staging classifications but also by changing radiotherapeutic techniques, equipment, and doses. Local relapse rates vary from 22 to 87 percent, with an approximate average of 50 percent. Five-year survival rates range from 10 to 41 percent, with an approximate average of 25 percent. Median survivals, when reported, have been similar. Within given series, patients with advanced nodal status did worse than those with N_0 disease. The range of development of sub-

TABLE 9–7. Local Therapy with Surgery Alone

				Relapse (%)			*Survival (%)*			
Author	*Period*	*No. of Patients*	*Clinical Stage*	Local	Local & Distant	Distant	Median (Years)	3-Year	5-Year	10-Year
Haagensen and Stout[4]	1965–74	120	C and D (Columbia)	49.2	—	—	—	—	2.3*	—
Donegan[46]	—	130	C (Columbia)	35	—	58	—	—	52	30
		80	D (Columbia)	50	—	81	—	—	22	7
Schottenfeld et al.[47]	1960	62	T_3 N_0–N_2	6	—	56	—	68.5	53	33.9
		21	T_3N_0	—	—	—	—	—	—	42.9
		41	T_3 N_1–N_2	—	—	—	—	—	—	30.8
Arnold and Lesnick[10]	1937–75	50	III (AJC)	—	57	—	4.5	—	40	31
Handley[48]	—	52	III (TNM)	—	—	—	—	—	48	26.9
Fracchia et al.[17]	1965–74	207	III (UICC)	25	—	—	—	—	43	27
		58	T_3–T_4 N_0	—	—	—	—	—	82.2	75.3
Cade[49]	1932–38	—	III (Portmann)	—	—	—	—	—	9	7

*Disease-free survival.

TABLE 9–8. Local Therapy with Irradiation Alone

Author	*Period*	*No. of Patients*	*Clinical Stage*	*Relapse (%)* Local	*Relapse (%)* Distant	Median (Years)	*Survival (%)* 3-Year	*Survival (%)* 5-Year	*Survival (%)* 10-Year	*Radiation Therapy—Dose (rad), Technique*
Cade[49]	1932–38	—	III (Portmann)	—	—	—	—	15	13	3500 (breast & axilla), orthovoltage
Pearlman et al.[50]	1960–69	49	Inoperable	57	—	—	—	12*	—	Not stated
Langland et al.[51]	1969–73	165	III (UICC)	67	—	—	32	14	—	3000–4500 (breast & nodes), 2 or 6 MV
Atkins and Horrigan[52]	1950–61	56	Inoperable†	87	—	—	31.7	10.7	—	4250 (breast & nodes), orthovoltage 5000 (breast & nodes), 22.5 MV betatron
Golding[53]	1960–69	138	III (unspecified)	—	—	—	—	29	—	6000 (breast & internal mammary), ^{60}Co, 3000 (supraclavicular nodes), ^{60}CO
Yarom et al.[54]	1968–72	33	Inoperable	—	89	—	36	24‡	—	6000 (breast & nodes), ^{60}Co
Bouchard[55]	1941–57	42	III (Portmann)	—	—	—	—	36	—	6000–8000 (breast & nodes), orthovoltage
Baclesse[56]	Before 1964	95	C (Columbia)	—	—	—	—	41	—	4100–9000 (breast),§ orthovoltage 6000–7000 (axilla), orthovoltage
		200	D (Columbia)†	—	—	—	—	13	—	Same
Rubens et al.[9]	1961–72	184	III (UICC)	72	66	2.1	28	13	—	3600–4000, 4 MV 3000 boost, orthovoltage
Balawajder et al.[13]	1962–79	38	III (UICC)	62	86	—	—	38	—	4500 (breast & axilla), ^{60}Co 500–2000 boost, ^{60}Co or e^-
Bedwinek et al.[15]	1960–75	54	III and IV (AJC)	61	65	—	—	—	—	4000–5000 (breast), ^{60}Co or 4 MV 5000 (nodes), ^{60}Co or 4 MV 1500–2500 boost, ^{60}Co, 4 MV, e^-
Zucali et al.[12]	1968–72	321	T_3–T_4 N_x M_0	—	—	2.1	36*	21	—	6000–7000 (breast & axilla), ^{60}Co 4000–4500 (breast & axilla), orthovoltage 3000 (axilla), orthovoltage
Harris et al.[16]	1968–78	137‖	III (UICC)	46	72	—	—	30	—	5000–6500 (breast & nodes), megavoltage; 1500–3500 boost, ^{192}Ir
Amalric et al.[57]	1960–74	341	III (UICC)¶	41	—	—	—	45	33	4500–6500 (axilla), megavoltage 6000 (breast), megavoltage 2000 boost, megavoltage
Treurniet-Donker et al.[18]	1965–74	129	III (TNM)**	22	—	2.0	—	17	—	4500–6000 (nodes), megavoltage 2000–7000 (breast & nodes), orthovoltage 2900–6300 (breast & nodes), megavoltage
			T_3–T_4 N_0	—	—	—	—	30	—	
			T_3–T_4 N_1–N_2	—	—	—	—	12	—	
			T_3–T_4 N_3	—	—	—	—	0	—	
Spanos et al.[58]	1960–72	158	III and IV (AJC)	28	—	—	—	—	—	6000 (breast), ^{60}Co 1000–4000 boost, ^{60}Co, e^-, implant 5000 (axilla), ^{60}Co

*Determined from graph.
†Number of patients with distant metastases not stated.
‡Four-year survival.
§Protracted technique.
‖Some patients received adjuvant chemotherapy.
¶Only T_3 N_0–N_1 patients.
**T_3–T_4 N_x M_0; T_1–T_2 N_2–N_3 M_0.

sequent distant metastases was 65 to 89 percent.

Radiation dose appears to exert some effect on local control when external beam radiation alone is used. While comparison between each series is difficult, some authors have reported dose-response relationships within their treated patient groups. Langlands and colleagues[51] noted improvement in local control rates, from 19 to 41 percent when the dose was increased from 3000 rad to 4500 rad. Treurinet-Donker and associates[18] noted an improved effect on the survival rate when patients receiving greater than 1700 ret were compared with those receiving less than 1500 ret total dose (ret is a unit of radiation incorporating total dose, number of fractions, and total time). In contrast, no effect was observed by Bedwinek and colleagues[15] when they analyzed local failure rates in response to different total doses from 4000 to 7000 rad. Some authors have emphasized the importance of radiation dose delivered with a local implant. Table 9–9 shows the results in four series.[59–62] The local relapse rate was reduced to the range of 0 to 24 percent. Bruckman and associates[62] reported 100 percent local control in a select group of seven patients who had had excisional biopsies performed on their tumors before external beam and implant.

The dose of radiation that can be given to the breast is not limitless. Spanos and colleagues[58] examined the frequency of late local complications in patients receiving high doses of radiation to their breasts and found an increasing trend toward severe fibrosis and necrosis above 8100 rad. There was no difference in the frequency of these complications according to whether the radiation boost was given by reduced tangential photon fields, electron beam, or interstitial implant.

Pre- and Postoperative Radiation Therapy

Table 9–10 summarizes the results of 13 series in which preoperative radiation therapy was followed by surgery.[10, 12, 13, 15, 49, 50, 52–55, 63, 64, 69] No systemic therapy was given following local therapy. Comparisons are complicated by different staging classifications, radiation doses, radiation techniques, x-ray equipment, and types of surgery. Local relapse rates range from 11 to 45 percent, with an approximate average of 18 percent. Five-year survival rates range from 10 to 55 percent, with an approximate average of 37 percent. The range of development of subsequent distant metastases was 65 to 89 percent.

Pathologic evaluation of mastectomy specimens that were treated preoperatively with irradiation provides a measure of the ability of radiation therapy to sterilize gross disease in locally advanced breast cancer. Table 9–11 shows sterilization rates from 0 to 38 percent.[12, 53, 55, 64–67] In the Zucali series, sterilization rates of breast specimens varied with tumor size, as 75 percent of sterilized specimens were T_3 and 25 percent were T_4.[12] There appears to be a trend toward increasing degrees of sterilization with increasing radiation dose.

Table 9–12 summarizes the results of four series in which either simple or radical mastectomy was followed by radiation therapy alone.[8, 10, 17, 68] Local relapse rates vary from 14 to 30 percent, with an approximate average of 22 percent. Five-year survival rates range from 30 to 45 percent, with an approximate average of 34 percent. The subsequent development of distant metastases is not well documented in these series; however, Arnold and Lesnick[10] reported a 69 percent overall relapse rate.

Local Therapy for Inflammatory Breast Cancer

As previously mentioned, a review of the literature from 1924 to 1980 showed a range of mean survival times of 4 to 30 months for patients with inflammatory breast cancer, regardless of whether patients were treated with mastectomy alone, irradiation alone, or a combination of surgery and irradiation (Table 9–13). Barker and associates[70] treated 69 patients with 6000 rad plus a 1000 to 2000 rad boost, using ^{60}Co and conventional fractionation, and reported a 46 percent rate of local relapse. When twice-daily fractionation was used, giving 5100 to 5400 rad in 40 fractions over a four-week period plus a 2000 rad boost in 16 fractions, the local relapse rate decreased to 33 percent. However, the rates of development of subsequent distant metastases remained high, with 77 and 82 percent in each group, respectively. Chu and colleagues[71] treated 62 patients with 6000 rad

TABLE 9–9. Local Therapy with External Beam Irradiation Plus ^{192}Ir Implant

Author	Period	No. of Patients	Clinical Stage	Relapse (%) Local	Relapse (%) Distant	Survival (%) 5-Year	External Radiation Dose (Rad) Technique	^{192}Ir Implant Dose (Rad)
Pierquin et al.[59]	1961 and beyond	43	T_3 N_0–N_1	23	16	70	4500 (breast & nodes), ^{60}Co	2500–3700
Syed et al.[60]	1974–79	79*	III (UICC)	9	45	63†	5000 (breast & nodes), megavoltage	3000–4000
Alderman[61]	—	18	C & D (Columbia)	0	—	—	5000 (breast & nodes), ^{60}Co, 1000 boost, ^{60}Co	4000
Bruckman et al.[62]	1968–76	54	III (UICC)	24	—	—	5000–6500 (breast & nodes), megavoltage	1500–3500
		7‡	III (UICC)	0	—	—	Same	Same

*Some patients received adjuvant chemotherapy.
†Determinted from graph.
‡All patients had a complete excisional biopsy.

TABLE 9–10. Local Therapy with Preoperative Irradiation and Surgery

Author	Period	No. of Patients	Clinical Stage	Relapse (%) Local	Relapse (%) Distant	Median (Years)	Survival (%) 3-Year	Survival (%) 5-Year	Survival (%) 10-Year	Radiation Therapy—Dose (rad), Technique
Cade[49]	1932–38	—	III (Portmann)	—	—	—	—	10	9	3500 (breast & axilla), orthovoltage
Pearlman et al.[50]	1960–69	26	Inoperable	37	—	—	—	12	—	Not stated
Atkins and Horrigan[52]	1950–61	23	—	16.7	—	—	47.6	33.3	—	4250 (breast & nodes), orthovoltage
Golding[53]	1960–69	45	III (unspecified)	—	—	—	—	51	—	5000 (breast & nodes), 22.5 MV betatron 6000 (breast & internal mammary), ^{60}Co 3000 (supraclavicular nodes), ^{60}Co
Yarom et al.[54]	1968–72	12	Inoperable	—	75	—	58	33*	—	6000 (breast & nodes), ^{60}Co
Bouchard[55]	1941–57	18	III (Portmann)	—	—	—	—	55	—	6000–8000 (breast & nodes), orthovoltage
Balawajder et al.[13]	1962–79	17	III (UICC)	45	79	—	—	44	—	4500 (breast & axilla), ^{60}Co 500–2000 boost, ^{60}Co or e^-
Bedwinek et al.[15]	1960–75	93	III and IV (AJC)	13	68	—	—	—	—	4000–5000 (breast & nodes), ^{60}Co, 4 MV 1500–2500 boost, ^{60}Co, 4 MV, e^-
Zucali et al.[12]	1968–72	133	T_3–T_4 N_x M_0	—	—	3.9	57†	45	—	6000–7000 (breast & axilla), ^{60}Co 4000–4500 (breast) 3000 (axilla), orthovoltage
Townsend et al.[63]	—	45	III and IV (TNM)	11	89	—	—	—	—	5000 (breast & nodes), ^{60}Co
Stoker and Ellis[64]	1962–70	24	T_4N_x (UICC)	13	65	—	—	—	—	6000 (breast & nodes), 2 MV
Arnold and Lesnick[10]	1937–75	54	III (AJC)	—	69‡	2.6	—	33†	17	Not stated
Delarue et al.[69]	1937–56	28§	III (TNM)	—	—	—	—	28.6	4.3	4500 (breast & nodes), orthovoltage
		192‖	III (TNM)	—	—	—	—	33.1	16.1	4500 (breast & nodes), orthovoltage

*Four-year survival.
†Determined from graph.
‡Local plus distant relapse.
§Received simple mastectomy after irradiation.
‖Received radical mastectomy after irradiation.

TABLE 9–11. Pathologic Sterilization of Tumor After Irradiation

Investigator	*No. of Specimens*	*No. of Specimens Without Tumor (%)*	*Dose*
Terz et al.[65]	35 (breast)	4 (11)	4000 rad, ^{60}Co
	35 (axilla)	8 (22)	5000 rad, ^{60}Co
Golding[53]	45	5 (11.1)	6000 rad, ^{60}Co
Lenz[66]	38 (breast)	0 (0)	4500 rad, 200 kV
	38 (axilla)	7 (18.4)	4500 rad, 200 kV
Stoker and Ellis[64]	24	1 (4)	6000 rad, 2 MV
Bouchard[55]	36 (breast)	10 (27.7)	6000–8000 rad, orthovoltage
	36 (axilla)	8 (22.2)	6000–8000 rad, orthovoltage
Zucali et al.[12]	131 (breast)	33 (25)	6000–7000 rad, ^{60}Co or 4000–4500 rad, 222 kV
	131 (axilla)	42 (32)	6000–7000 rad, ^{60}Co or 3000 rad, 222 kV
Vaeth et al.[67]	16 (breast)	6 (38)	4500–6500 rad, ^{60}Co
	11 (axilla)	4 (36)	4500–6500 rad, ^{60}Co

TABLE 9–12. Local Therapy with Surgery and Postoperative Radiation Therapy

				Relapse (%)		*Survival (%)*				
Author	*Period*	*No. of Patients*	*Clinical Stage*	LOCAL	DISTANT	MEDIAN (YEARS)	5-YEAR	10-YEAR	MASTECTOMY TYPE	*Radiation Therapy—Dose (rad), Technique*
Brown et al.[68]	1955–69	189	III	14	—	—	45.5	21.5	Simple	4500–5000 (chest wall), orthovoltage and megavoltage 5000 (axilla), orthovoltage and megavoltage
McWhirter[8]	—	564	III and IV (Manchester)	—	—	—	30	15	Simple	3750 (chest wall & nodes), orthovoltage
Fracchia et al.[17]	1965–74	179	III (UICC)	30	—	—	34.3	13	Radical	4000–5500 (internal mammary & supraclavicular nodes)
Arnold and Lesnick[10]	1937–75	122	III (AJC)	—	69*	3.0	31†	21	Radical	Not stated

*Local plus distant.
†Determined from graph.

TABLE 9–13. Results of Treatment of Inflammatory Breast Carcinoma in the Literature

	Local Therapy (No. of Patients)			*Survival*	
Author	Radical Mastectomy	Radiation Therapy	Radical Mastectomy Radiation	Mean (Mo.)	5-Yr. (No. of Patients)
Haagensen[2]	29	—	—	19	1
	—	29	—	14.7	0
Lee and Tannenbaum[25]	4	—	—	15	0
	—	13	—	11	0
Taylor and Meltzer[26]	6	—	—	21	0
	—	19	—	9.2	0
Barber et al.[32]	—	—	50	25	5
Richards and Lewison[33]	2	—	—	14	0
	—	—	11	11	0
Wang and Griscom[35]	—	23[a]	—	14.3	0
	—	10[b]	—	30	2
Chris[36]	—	—	7	13.3	0
	—	9	—	16	0
Meyer et al.[37]	—	—	47	28	3
Rogers and Fitts[38]	—	—	20	20.7	1
	—	24	—	15.7	1
Spratt and Donegan[39]	—	—	11	15.1	0
	—	17	—	20.2	0
Dao and McCarthy[40]	—	—	6	13	0
	—	3	—	4	0
Chu et al.[71]	—	62	—	24.2	2

[a]Orthovoltage
[b]Supervoltage

plus a 2000 to 3000 rad boost, using megavoltage equipment and conventional fractionation, and observed a local recurrence rate of 69 percent. Dose-response analysis showed improved local control with increasing dose for lesions 10 cm or smaller. In a small group of patients, twice-daily fractionation reduced that local recurrence rate to 33 percent. The rate of development of distant metastases still remained high at 77 percent.

Summary of Local Therapy

An extensive amount of data is available regarding treatment of the primary disease in locally advanced breast cancer; however, the optimum modality or combination of modalities has still not been determined. Table 9–14 summarizes the results of surgery alone, radiation therapy alone, irradiation followed by mastectomy, and mastectomy followed by irradiation with respect to local recurrence, distant recurrence, and five-year survival rates for the data presented in the preceding sections. Radiation therapy alone is effective in controlling a large number of locally advanced breast cancers; however, it has the highest rate of local recurrence. Maximum local control appears to have been achieved in series coupling surgery with either pre- or postoperative irradiation. Since all of these studies are retrospective, it is quite possible that patients treated with irradiation alone were those who had the most unfavorable prognoses and that a selection bias was used in deciding which more favorable patients could undergo combined therapy. Patients reported to have undergone postoperative radiation therapy of necessity had a surgical

TABLE 9–14. Results of Local Therapy Alone in Locally Advanced Breast Cancer

	Local Relapse		*Distant Relapse*		*5-Year Survival*	
Treatment	Range (%)	Average (%)	Range (%)	Average (%)	Range (%)	Average (%)
Surgery	6–50	34	56–81	65	9–53	47
Irradiation	22–87	50	65–89	71	10–41	25
Preoperative irradiation	11–45	18	65–89	73	10–55	37
Postoperative irradiation	14–30	22	—	—	30–45	34

option at the outset of treatment, which implies certain more favorable disease characteristics for this subset of patients. Likewise, patients reported to have undergone preoperative radiation therapy may not have had an initial surgical option but were rendered operable after achieving a good response to radiation therapy. Consequently, the response to radiation therapy may have provided the selection bias for picking which patients would complete combined treatment.

An alternative explanation for the improved local control reported in combined surgery–radiation therapy series can be made. The low sterilization rate of gross disease by irradiation points out the ineffectiveness of radiation therapy alone in controlling bulk disease. Optimizing the radiation dose with a boost from a reduced tangential photon beam, electron beam, or interstitial implant may further increase local control rates; however, there are practical limits to radiation dosage after which local complications of tissue necrosis will ensue. In light of the data showing improved local control in patients undergoing excisional biopsy compared with incisional biopsy prior to definitive radiation therapy, surgical removal may provide the best "boost" for gross disease. Consequently, the increased local control rates observed in combined-modality series may reflect this cytoreductive effect.

While improved local control may have resulted in the slight increases in five-year survival rates observed in combined-modality series, the five-year survival rates in general for all series have been poor. This can be explained by the high rates of development of subsequent distant metastases, which range from 56 to 89 percent. Such rates suggest quite strongly that disseminated micrometastases are present at the time of diagnosis and that further refinements in local therapy alone will do little toward improving survival.

SYSTEMIC CHEMOTHERAPY PLUS LOCAL THERAPY

Adjuvant Chemotherapy

Although variable degrees of local recurrence have followed therapy with the previously mentioned local treatment modalities, high rates of distant relapse have consistently resulted, emphasizing the systemic nature of this problem at the time of diagnosis and suggesting the need for the integration of systemic therapy in the management of this disease. The influence of adjuvant chemotherapy in locally advanced breast cancer can be seen in several retrospective studies. In Bruckman's series[62] of patients treated with primary radiation therapy, 26 patients received some form of chemotherapy after irradiation, 10 of whom also had an endocrine ablative procedure. Chemotherapy consisted of single-agent melphalan, cyclophosphamide-doxorubicin, or cyclophosphamide, methotrexate, and 5-fluorouracil (CMF). When a matched-pair analysis was performed, with patients receiving radiation therapy without chemotherapy, a significant improvement in the local control rate was seen at four years for those patients receiving chemotherapy versus those patients who did not (85 versus 63 percent). The relapse-free survival rate was also significantly higher in the patients receiving chemotherapy, compared with the matched control subjects, with four-year relapse-free survival rates of 51 and 29 percent, respectively. For patients with inflammatory breast cancer, Chu and colleagues[71] observed that in those receiving either CMF (cyclophosphamide, 100 mg/m^2 PO on days 1 to 14; methotrexate, 40 mg/m^2 IV on days 1 and 8; and 5-fluorouracil, 600 mg/m^2 IV on days 1 and 8) or CMFVP (cyclophosphamide, 2 mg/kg PO daily for six weeks; methotrexate, 0.3 mg/kg IV once weekly for six weeks; 5-fluorouracil, 12 mg/kg IV once weekly for six weeks; vincristine, 1 mg IV once weekly for six weeks; and prednisone, 0.75 mg/kg PO daily for for six weeks) after radiation therapy, the rate of distant metastases was 56 percent, compared with 100 percent in patients not receiving postirradiation chemotherapy.

Sponzo and associates[72] prospectively gave CFP chemotherapy (cyclophosphamide, 150 mg/m^2 IV on days 1 to 5; 5-fluorouracil, 300 mg/m^2 IV on days 1 to 5; and prednisone, 10 mg PO daily) to 13 patients with T_3–T_4 N_x M_0 breast cancer, either concurrently with or immediately following radiation therapy (5000 rad to the breast and adjacent draining nodes, with a 2000- to 4000-rad boost to the breast). A complete response was achieved in 12 patients, with a median duration of 38 or more months. Seven patients underwent a mastectomy at the conclusion of the aforementioned treatment, with no microscopic evidence of tumor in six patients. In a subsequent two-arm ECOG (Eastern Cooperative Oncology Group) trial with nonresectable Stage III patients, one group received CMFP chemotherapy (cyclophosphamide, 100 mg/m^2 PO on days 1 to 14; methotrexate, 40 mg/m^2 IV on days 1 and 8; 5-fluorouracil, 600 mg/m^2 IV on days 1 and 8; and prednisone, 40 mg/m^2 PO on days 1 to 14) for 18 cycles after completing radiation therapy to the breast (7500 rad) and nodal areas (5000 rad).[73] The objective response rate with this combined therapy was 69 percent, with a median time to progression and survival time of 10.9 and 24.6 months, respectively. Serrou and associates[74] initially treated 80 patients with T_3–T_4 N_x M_0 breast cancer with radiation therapy with or without mastectomy and then randomly assigned them to no further therapy, BCG (150 mg PO weekly for one year), or CVF chemotherapy for 12 cycles (cyclophosphamide, 300 mg/m^2 IV on days 3 to 6; vincristine, 1 mg/m^2 IV on days 1 and 2; and 5-fluorouracil, 400 mg/m^2 IV on days 3 to 6). No differences were seen favoring the BCG arm. Of note, in the group receiving CVF at 30 months, only 43 percent of patients relapsed, compared with 78 percent of patients in the control group; however, the results were not statistically significant.

In a series of 120 patients with operable Stage III breast cancer (T_3N_0–N_2), Gröhn and colleagues[75] randomized patients, after treating them with modified radical mastectomy, to radiation therapy alone, six cycles of CAV chemotherapy (cyclophosphamide, 200 mg/m^2 PO on days 1 to 5; Adriamycin [doxorubicin], 45 mg/m^2 IV on day 1; and vincristine, 1.2 mg/m^2 IV on day 1), or radiation therapy followed by six cycles of CAV chemotherapy. All patients were also randomized to receive or not to receive levamisole. Patients receiving radiation alone had a five-year survival rate of 57 percent, with a 17 percent local relapse and a 50 percent distant relapse rate. The five-year survival rate was better in the group receiving chemotherapy (73 percent), with a concomitant decrease in distant metastases to 12.5 percent; however, local control was poorer, with 40 percent of patients having local relapse. Patients receiving combined therapy had the best five-year survival rate (90 percent), with the lowest local (2.6 percent) and distant relapse rates (10.2 percent). Levamisole was found to be of no benefit in any subgroup.

Induction Chemotherapy

In both retrospective and prospective studies, the addition of adjuvant chemotherapy following local therapy seems to have had a favorable impact on the management of locally advanced breast cancer, with decreased distant metastases, increased survival rates, and even enhanced local control. These results have led some investigators to question the optimum sequencing of local and systemic therapy in this disease, pointing out that waiting until local therapy has been completed may allow a considerable amount of time to elapse before the critical issue of micrometastatic disease is addressed. In fact, in one series it was documented that an appreciable number of patients had relapses in distant sites during the time of irradiation.[12] This concern has led to the proposal that chemotherapy precede local therapy in an effort to attack systemic disease as early as possible and to enhance the efficacy of subsequent local therapy by providing initial primary tumor regression. Support for this sequencing of therapy can be found in the retrospective review of Balawajder and associates.[13] Thirty-eight patients received radiation therapy alone, resulting in five-year local control, freedom from metastases, and survival rates of 38 percent, 14 percent, and 38 percent, respectively. In 23 patients who received three cycles of chemotherapy (cyclophosphamide, 100 mg PO on days 1 to 14; methotrexate, 40 mg/m^2 IV on days 1 and 8; and 5-fluorouracil, 40 mg/m^2 IV on days 1 and 8) before irradiation and 30 patients who received this chemotherapy before irradiation and surgery, the freedom from metastases rates increased to 41 and 36 percent, respectively; however, the five-year survival rates remained at 46 and 38 percent. Local control at five years was 54 and 88 percent for each group, respectively. At 7.5 years, the freedom from metastases rate for patients receiving chemotherapy before irradiation remained at 41 percent. Within this group of patients, those receiving over 4800 to 5000 rad in 24 to 25 fractions had an 80 percent local control rate. This was comparable with the local control rate in patients receiving sequential treatment with chemotherapy, irradiation and surgery, emphasizing the beneficial effect of chemotherapy plus adequate radiation therapy in improving local control.

Combination chemotherapy, given in a prospective manner prior to local therapy, was introduced by the Milan group.[76] In a series of 110 consecutive patients with T_{3b}–T_4 N_x M_0 breast cancer, four cycles of AV chemotherapy (Adriamycin [doxorubicin], 75 mg/m^2 IV on day 1, and vincristine, 1.4 mg/m^2 IV on days 1 and 8) were given prior to local radiation therapy. An objective response rate with chemotherapy of 70 percent was observed, with 15 percent complete response (CR) and 55 percent partial response (PR). Thirty-six percent of these patients had inflammatory breast cancer; however, no difference in response rate was noted between these patients and those with noninflammatory carcinoma. Patients with no response or with progressive disease (10.9 percent) were removed from the study and received alternative chemotherapy regimens. At the completion of combined therapy, 73.6 percent of all patients starting treatment were considered to have a CR, with 10.9 percent, a PR. Those patients exhibiting a CR to combined therapy were randomized to receive maintenance chemotherapy for six cycles with either AV or CMF. The median duration of complete response was 15 months overall; however, there was a statistical difference between those who received maintenance therapy and those who did not (19 versus 11 months, respectively). Interestingly, the local recurrence rate was lower in the group receiving maintenance chemotherapy; however, no difference in the rate of distant relapse was observed between these two groups. When compared with their historical control group,[12] the present combined-modality approach significantly improved the overall survival rate at three years, from 40.7 to 52.8 percent. The median survival at three years was not determined for the patients with noninflammatory cancer and was 25 months for the patients with inflammatory disease. No improvement in survival at three years was noted for the patients with inflammatory cancer (24.9 percent), compared with the historical control subjects (29 percent). Since local failure constituted 37.5 percent of patients in this series, a subsequent trial was conducted to randomly compare radiation or radical mastectomy as local therapy in a combined-modality setting.[77] A total of 132 consecutive patients with T_{3b}–T_4 N_o–N_2 M_x breast cancer (i.e., excluding patients with inflammatory breast cancer or N_3 nodes) received three cycles of AV chemotherapy (Adriamycin [doxorubicin], 60 mg/m^2 IV on day 1, and vincristine, 1.2 mg/m^2 IV on days 1 and 8) followed by randomization to radiation therapy or surgery. All patients subsequently received seven cycles of AV maintenance chemotherapy. The objective response rate with chemotherapy was 53 percent, with CR and PR rates of 4 and 49 percent, respectively. It should be noted that this AV regimen used a 20 percent reduction in the doxorubicin dose, compared with the earlier study. After combined therapy, 64.4 percent of all patients starting treatment achieved a CR, with 50.7 percent in the radiation group and 78.5 percent in the surgery group. The locoregional failure rate was 31.1 percent in the radiation group and 29.6 percent in the surgery group. Recurrence in supraclavicular nodes was greater in the surgery arm, while recurrence in the chest wall was greater in the radiation arm. Survival at four years was almost identical in both groups, with 51.7 percent in the group receiving radiation and 49.1 percent in the group receiving surgery.

Rubens and associates[78] gave four cycles of AV chemotherapy (Adriamycin [doxorubicin], 70 mg/m^2 IV on day 1, and vincristine, 1.4 mg/m^2 IV on days 1 and 8) to 12 patients with inoperable breast cancer (excluding T_3 N_0–N_1 M_0) prior to local radiation therapy, followed by eight cycles of CMF maintenance therapy after completion of local therapy.[78] They reported a 50 percent objective response to induction chemotherapy, with 17 percent CR and 33 percent PR. The rates of local and distant recurrence were each 25 percent. The duration of objective response was 33 months, which was significantly longer than the 10.5 months for their historical control group. The median survival time was 36 months, which was not significantly different from the 25 months for their historical control subjects.

Perloff and Lesnick[79] treated 17 patients with T_3 N_1–N_2 M_0 and T_4 N_0–N_2 M_0 breast cancer with two to four cycles of CMF, CMFP, CMFVP, or CAF (cyclophosphamide, Adriamycin [doxorubicin], and 5-fluorouracil) prior to modified radical mastectomy and an additional 24 months of maintenance chemotherapy. They observed a 59 percent objective response to induction chemotherapy, with the cancers of all of these patients becoming technically operable. Local recurrence was observed in only one patient (6 percent), with 59 percent of patients developing distant metastases. The median disease-free interval and survival time were 29 and 40 months or more, respectively.

At the M.D. Anderson Hospital, 52 patients with T_3–T_4 N_2–N_3 M_0 breast cancer (excluding inflammatory carcinoma) were treated with three cycles of FAC chemotherapy plus BCG (5-fluorouracil, 500 mg/m^2 IV on days 1 and 8; Adriamycin [doxorubicin], 50 mg/m^2 IV on day 1; and cyclophosphamide, 500 mg/m^2 IV on day 1; plus BCG, 6 $\times$ 10^8 units by scarification on days 9, 13, and 17) prior to local therapy.[14] An objective response to chemotherapy of 82 percent was achieved, 15 percent CR and 67 percent PR. Local therapy was then guided by chemotherapy response. Patients exhibiting a CR or no change (NC) after three cycles of induction chemotherapy would then receive local radiation therapy, while patients with a PR underwent mastectomy followed by local radiation therapy. Radiation therapy consisted of 5000 rad to the breast or the chest wall and adjacent nodal areas, with a 1500- to 2000-rad boost to areas of gross disease. This was followed by a planned 24 months of maintenance chemotherapy. Following induction chemotherapy and local therapy, 94 percent of all patients were rendered disease free. First relapse occurred locally in 21 percent of patients and distantly in 38 percent. There was no statistical difference in relapse rates as analyzed by the type of local therapy, age, menopausal status, race, or initial chemotherapy response. In the 16 patients who had estrogen receptor data, all four ER-negative patients had had relapses while 3 of 12 ER-positive patients remained disease free. Treatment compliance was poor in this series, with only 61 percent of all patients completing the entire planned course of treatment. Excluding those who died of intercurrent disease, overall three- and five-year survival rates were 65 and 55 percent respectively. The median survival time was 65 months. In 32 patients with inflammatory breast cancer treated with the same induction regimen, response rates to chemotherapy were similar to those of the patients with noninflammatory carcinoma.[80] This was followed by local radiation therapy consisting of 5100 rad in 40 fractions to the breast and adjacent nodal areas, with a 2000-rad boost to the breast in 16 fractions. The local recurrence rate was decreased to 26 percent, compared with 43 percent for historical control subjects receiving radiation therapy alone. The systemic recurrence rate was decreased to 21 percent compared with 44 percent for control subjects. The overall median disease-free survival time was 22.8 months for the group receiving combined-modality therapy and 9 months for the group receiving irradiation only; the overall median survival times were 30.1 months and 18 months, respectively. In a recent report from the M.D. Anderson Hospital in which 21 patients with inflammatory breast cancer and 69 patients with noninflammatory locally advanced breast cancer were treated with three cycles of FAC chemotherapy prior to mastectomy, 15 patients (17 percent) had no evidence of gross disease in their pathology specimens and six patients (7 percent) had no evidence of microscopic disease.[81] The disease-free rate at 36 months and the survival rate at 48 months were no different for patients exhibiting a pathologic CR versus those showing residual microscopic disease, with greater than 80 percent reported for both groups. The survival rate for the rest of the series at 48 months was 55 percent for the patients with noninflammatory cancer and 45 percent for the patients with inflammatory carcinoma.

Zylberberg and associates[82] treated 15 patients with inflammatory breast cancer with initial chemoimmunotherapy (doxorubicin, 45 mg/m^2 IV on day 1; vincristine, 1 mg/m^2 IV on day 2; cyclophosphamide, 500 mg/m^2 IV on days 3 and 4; 5-fluorouracil, 500 mg/m^2 IV on days 3 and 4; melphalan, 4 mg PO on days 3 to 9; and BCG by scarification on days 10 to 18 and on day 26) followed by radical mastectomy. In contrast with other series using induction chemotherapy, local therapy was not started after a fixed number of chemotherapy cycles but after serial thermographic measurements of the involved breast showed no further signs of thermal gradient, compared with the opposite breast. Clinical inflammatory phenomena and pain disappeared after one to three cycles of chemotherapy; however, it required four to seven cycles before thermographic measurements dictated the start of local therapy. The objective response rate with induction therapy was 93 percent, with 20 percent CR and 73 percent PR. Histologic evaluation of the surgical specimens showed no tumor in 3 of 15 breast specimens (20 percent) and 9 of 15 axillary specimens (60 percent). Local therapy was followed by ten cycles of chemoimmunotherapy. Local relapse occurred in 2 of 15 patients; however, both of these patients had only tumorectomy rather than radical mastectomy. Distant relapse occurred in 20 percent of patients. The disease-free interval ranged from 44 to 77 months, with the median survival not reached by 56 months.

Since 1977, the NCI has treated women with locally advanced breast cancer with combination chemotherapy given to the point of best objective clinical response, to maximally reduce the tumor bulk prior to definitive local therapy and to destroy occult micrometastatic disease. Concomitant endocrine therapy was employed with chemotherapy by giving tamoxifen and premarin sequentially before the administration of cell cycle–specific agents, in the hopes of synchronizing DNA synthesis in a proportion of these tumor cells and thus making them more susceptible to CAMF cytotoxic chemotherapy (cyclophosphamide, 500 mg/m^2, and Adriamycin [doxorubicin], 30 mg/m^2 IV on day 1; tamoxifen, 40 mg PO on days 2 to 6; premarin, 0.625 mg PO q 12 hr for three doses beginning on day 7; methotrexate, 300 mg/m^2 IV, followed in 1 hr by 5-fluorouracil, 500 mg/m^2 IV on day 8; and leucovorin, 10 mg/m^2 PO q 6 hr for six doses beginning 2 hr after methotrexate).[83, 84] Patients showing a pathologic complete response, as determined by multiple biopsies in the area of prior disease, received radiation therapy, while patients with residual disease and PR or NC status received debulking surgery to minimize tumor burden prior to radiation therapy. Maintenance chemotherapy was given for an additional six months. Forty-three patients with locally advanced breast cancer, 15 with Stage III$_a$ and 28 with Stage III$_b$, have been treated in this manner. Of these, 42 are currently evaluable with respect to response, time to progression, and survival. The objective response rate with chemotherapy was 90 percent, with 50 percent CR, 40 percent PR, and 10 percent NC. The median number of cycles of chemotherapy to achieve a CR, PR, or NC was five, four, and four, with a range of cycles of three to 11, three to nine and four to six, respectively. Figure 9–1 shows the time course from the start of treatment to these patients' exhibiting their best response to chemotherapy. If only three or four cycles of chemotherapy were given, as was done in prior combined-modality trials, then anywhere from 75 to 40 percent of these patients, respectively, would not have shown their best possible response to chemotherapy before the end of induction therapy. Eighteen patients with a CR to chemotherapy were assessed histologically; 14 of these patients (33 percent of the entire series) were proved to be pathologic complete responders. Thirty patients thus far have completed combined therapy, and all have been rendered disease free. Eight pa-

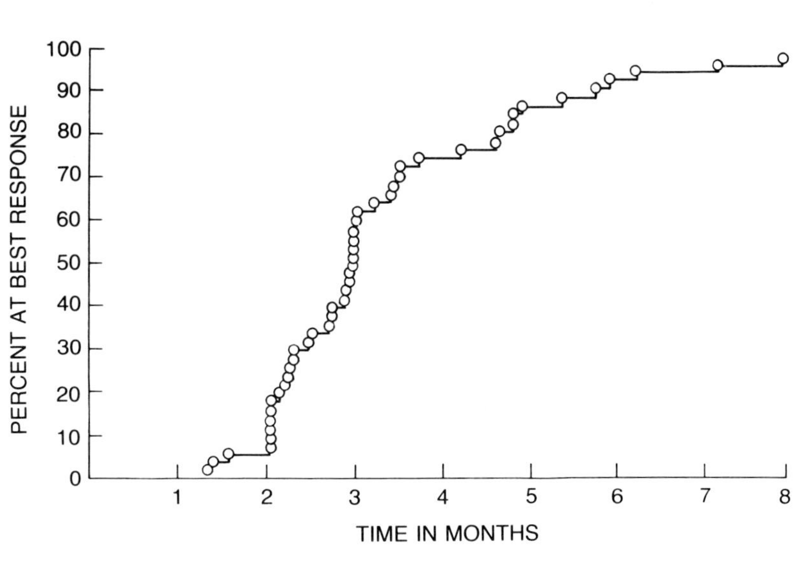

FIGURE 9–1. Time from start of therapy to best response.

tients have had relapses, seven having Stage III_b disease, with six of these patients having inflammatory histology. One Stage III_a patient has had a relapse. Median survival and time to progression have not been reached in Stage III_a patients and were 33 and 18 months, respectively, in Stage III_b patients.

The use of debulking surgery prior to induction chemotherapy and local radiation therapy has been reported by Loprinzi and colleagues.[85] Thirty-two patients received initial aggressive surgery to remove as much gross disease as was feasible, followed by two cycles of CMF chemotherapy. This was followed by radiation therapy with 5000 rad to the chest wall and adjacent draining nodes, with a 1500- to 2000-rad boost if gross disease was present. Maintenance chemotherapy was given for 16 cycles with CMF, alternating with AV. The three-year actuarial survival rate was 65 percent with the median not reached. The median disease-free interval was 29.5 months. Patients who had gross residual disease after mastectomy were at greater risk of recurrence, with a death rate about twice as high as that of patients who had all gross disease removed. Metastatic disease developed in 50 percent of patients, as the first site of relapse.

Treatment Guidelines

As stated at the outset, the optimum therapy for locally advanced breast cancer has not been reached. The data reviewed in the preceding sections is largely retrospective and, as such, does not definitively settle this issue. However, this information can provide a framework for some rational treatment guidelines and for constructing appropriate clinical trials. The following discussion outlines treatment recommendations for the various subsets of patients with locally advanced disease.

T_3N_0 Patients

Patients with T_3 N_0 disease constitute approximately 12 percent of all patients with locally advanced breast cancer and are the subset with the most favorable prognosis. The natural tumor biology of these patients may be inherently different from that of Stage II or III patients with nodal disease, as these tumors grow to such a large local size without metastasizing to regional lymph nodes. These tumors are technically operable and, as such, in skilled hands, should be treatable by surgical therapy with radical or modified radical mastectomy. Lumpectomy followed by primary radiation therapy may be a viable option in selected patients, provided that the amount of tissue that would have to be removed to perform a complete excisional biopsy did not result in a significant deformity of the remaining breast. If a major deformity resulted from such a procedure, the cosmetic outcome would be poor after primary radiation therapy and would negate the benefits of this approach, compared with primary surgical treatment followed by reconstructive surgery. Likewise, as the ratio of tumor size to breast size increases, the relative proportion of residual breast tissue in the tumor bed that would need to be boosted with a high dose of radiation therapy will increase, and this could further adversely affect the cosmetic outcome.

Adjuvant therapy following primary surgery in these patients is still controversial, in that each of the reported retrospective series on locally advanced breast cancer had small numbers of patients in this subset and, in many instances, did not analyze these patients separately with respect to survival, local control, and distant metastases rates. Using the sole criterion of tumor size, the routine use of postoperative radiation therapy in these patients who are successfully managed with primary surgical treatment has not been definitively established. Patients who undergo radical or modified radical mastectomy with adequate surgical margins may not need further local therapy. While one could not be faulted for using postoperative radiation therapy in such a situation, given the limited data, radiation therapy may be more appropriately reserved for patients with close or positive surgical margins. The details of this radiation therapy are discussed separately at the end of this chapter.

The use of adjuvant chemotherapy in these patients is also unclear. Since nodal involvement correlates with distant metastases and poor survival rates, the absence of this feature may confer a favorable prognosis by tremendously reducing the likelihood of disseminated micrometastatic disease. Therefore, with the limited data available, the routine use of adjuvant chemotherapy in this subset of patients, simply on the basis of the size of the lesion, is an unsettled issue. Sampling errors in obtaining and sectioning all the lymph nodes may compound the uncertainty in this situation. Until further information becomes available, the use of adjuvant chemotherapy in this patient subset will need to be decided on an individual basis, with appropriate counseling of the patient and family.

T_3N_1 AND SELECTED T_1–T_3 N_2 PATIENTS

This group constitutes approximately 25 percent of the patients with locally advanced breast cancer, with the majority having T_3N_1 disease. These cancers are technically operable, if there are no lymph nodes fixed to the chest wall, and should respond to primary surgical therapy with radical or modified radical mastectomy. Lumpectomy and primary radiation therapy may be a viable alternative, with the stipulations mentioned in the previous section. Postoperative radiation therapy to the chest wall and the adjacent draining nodal areas should be given to these patients, since this can optimize locoregional control. Since nodal involvement correlates with distant metastases and poor survival rates, these patients, of necessity, should be considered as having disseminated micrometastatic disease at the time of diagnosis and, therefore, as candidates for adjuvant chemotherapy. The optimum sequencing of postoperative radiation therapy and adjuvant chemotherapy has not been determined. The traditional sequence of events has been for chemotherapy to follow all local therapy. However, by analogy to the situation in earlier stage breast cancers in which the sooner adjuvant chemotherapy is instituted after surgery, the better the results, this may be the best sequence of adjuvant therapies in this patient group, especially since the likelihood of disseminated micrometastases is higher in Stage III_a disease. Therefore, chemotherapy should be started as early as possible, with postoperative radiation therapy to follow or to be sandwiched within the chemotherapy course after at least the first cycle of chemotherapy is complete. Whether the chemotherapy alone would be sufficient adjuvant therapy to prevent locoregional recurrence in the absence of radiation therapy awaits further study. By analogy to earlier stage breast cancer patients treated with adjuvant chemotherapy, the locoregional recurrence rate appears to be higher than originally estimated and may approach that of comparable patients receiving surgery without chemotherapy. Therefore, postoperative radiation therapy should continue in the management scheme of this subset of patients with locally advanced breast cancer.

An alternative form of treatment for this subset of patients consists of primary induction chemotherapy followed by definitive local therapy, as detailed in the following section. This would provide the earliest opportunity to sterilize occult micrometastatic disease, while effecting locoregional cytoreduction that could facilitate the subsequent administration of definitive local therapy.

T_3N_2, T_xN_3, AND T_4N_1–N_3 PATIENTS

This group comprises approximately 50 percent of patients with locally advanced breast cancer. With few exceptions, the tumors of these patients will be technically inoperable and, therefore, the patients will have no definitive surgical option available at the time of diagnosis. Traditionally, these patients have been treated with radical radiation therapy alone, with the shortcomings as outlined in previous sections. Those patients who were reported in retrospective series to have undergone combined therapy with either pre- or postoperative irradiation were most likely patients in the more favorable subsets and were not representative of the group as a whole.

The high rate of subsequent distant metastases in this subset of patients suggests that disseminated micrometastases were present at the time of diagnosis and emphasizes the systemic nature of this disease process from the outset. Aggressive initial measures to ensure local control in these patients will in no way circumvent the necessity of addressing this systemic issue. Therefore, the early institution of systemic chemotherapy in the treatment of these patients provides a rational management basis for approaching this problem and a framework for optimizing subsequent locoregional therapy. Primary induction chemotherapy may be given for a fixed number of cycles before definitive local therapy or can be continued to the point of best response, to make optimum use of this modality's antitumor effects in the locoregional area. This approach also has the added benefit of enabling the physician to visually monitor the clinical efficacy of the chemotherapeutic agents selected. Combination chemotherapy with AV, CMF, CMFP, CMFVP, or FAC can achieve a substantial objective response rate when given for a fixed number of cycles, usually two to four, and each would be a suitable induction regimen. As noted earlier, CAMF with hormone synchronization, when given until best response, has the highest reported objective response rate with the highest percentage of patients showing clinical and pathologic complete responses. These other regimens may achieve similar response rates if given until best response; however, there are no published reports on these regimens used in such a manner.

Subsequent local therapy can then be guided by the best response to induction chemotherapy. Patients showing a pathologic CR, as determined by repeat biopsy in sites of previous gross disease, have had their tumor burdens reduced to the magnitude of minimal microscopic levels and, therefore, are good candidates for consolidative local therapy with definitive radiation therapy alone to the intact breast and adjacent draining nodal areas. Patients with residual gross disease can subsequently have debulking surgery to further reduce their tumor burdens to minimal levels (in a attempt to achieve ideally only microscopic residual disease) and then receive consolidative radiation therapy to the chest wall and adjacent draining nodal areas. Chemotherapy should continue during this phase of therapy, with doxorubicin withheld, to prevent radiation sensitization of normal tissues in the irradiated field. Maintenance chemotherapy should also be given, after local therapy, for a period of 6 to 12 months with either the induction regimen alone or, perhaps, an alternating non–cross-resistant regimen. In appropriate study situations, tumor clonogenic assays may facilitate the selection of the optimum maintenance regimen.

A special note should be made regarding patients with T_4N_0 lesions. In selected cases such as tumors with only limited skin involvement with no chest wall fixation, these tumors may be technically operable and could be managed in the manner described for T_3N_0 lesions.

Inflammatory Carcinoma

Inflammatory breast cancer is the most aggressive and rapidly fulminant form of locally advanced breast cancer but fortunately constitutes only 1.5 to 4 percent of all cases. These tumors are frequently ill defined locally and diffusely invasive, involve axillary nodes in excess of 90 percent and develop distant metastases in a high percentage of patients. These lesions must be approached as systemic problems from the outset and, as such, there is no role for initial curative radical surgical measures. Radical radiation therapy may be successful in controlling locoregional disease but will not have an impact upon the almost certain occult micrometastatic disease. This will, of necessity, require the integration of adjuvant chemotherapy to complete a comprehensive treatment strategy. Alternatively, induction chemotherapy followed by local therapy can be utilized in the manner described for T_4 lesions in the preceding section. Such an approach should be ideally suited to the treatment of this problem, since it provides for the earlier introduction of systemic therapy into the management scheme.

Radiation Therapy Guidelines

Guidelines for the radiation therapy described in the preceding section are as follows. For patients who have undergone simple, modified radical or radical mastectomy and who require postoperative radiation therapy, the chest wall and the adjacent draining nodal sites are irradiated. The chest wall is treated using coplanar tangential fields that include the ipsilateral internal mammary node chain. The ipsilateral supraclavicular node area is treated with an anteroposterior half-beam blocked field, matched to the superior borders of the tangents using a pedestal angle to remove the divergence into the supraclavicular field. The axilla is excluded from treatment if a full node dissection was performed but is included in the supraclavicular field if no dissection or an axillary sampling was done. If the axilla is treated, it will be necessary to supplement the midplane axillary dose with a posterior axillary boost. The chest wall and nodal sites should receive 5000 rad, using 180- to 200-rad daily fractions, five times a week. Bolus should be applied to the chest wall every other day to avoid underdosing the skin surface. Computerized treatment planning with lung-density corrections should be used for all tangential fields. If close margins are an issue, an additional 1000 rad should be given with an *en face* electron field to the local areas at risk. If residual gross disease is an issue, a 1500- to 2500-rad boost, using either reduced tangential fields or electrons, or both, should be given to these sites. For patients with inflammatory breast cancer, the tangential fields should be taken to 6000 rads, with the same fractionation.

For patients who exhibited a pathologic CR to induction chemotherapy, the intact breast and the adjacent draining nodal sites are irradiated. The breast, chest wall, and ipsilateral internal mammary node chain are treated using coplanar tangential fields. The supraclavicular nodal area and the axilla are treated as outlined earlier. The intact breast and nodal sites should receive 5000 rad, using 180- to 200-rad daily fractions, five times a week. The tumor bed should receive a 1500- to 2000-rad boost, using electrons or an interstitial implant. For patients with inflammatory breast cancer, twice-a-day treatment giving 5100 rad over a four-week period may be beneficial.

FUTURE DIRECTIONS

The issues that need to be resolved in the treatment of locally advanced breast cancer are many and involve basic biologic as well as clinical questions. Among the greatest concerns that will affect practicing medical, surgical, and radiation oncologists are the following. What adjuvant therapy is needed following resection in T_3N_0 patients? What is the role of induction chemotherapy in technically operable stage III_a disease? What is the optimum regimen and format for the administration of induction chemotherapy in inoperable stage III_a and III_b disease? What is the optimum local therapy for patients undergoing induction chemotherapy? What is the optimum systemic regimen for inflammatory carcinoma? These issues are of major importance for clinical oncologists and will be settled only as a result of prospective controlled trials using uniform staging classification for reliable comparison.

REFERENCES

1. Steinthal CF: Zur Dauerheilung des Brustkrebses. Beitr Z klin Chir 47:226, 1905.
2. Haagensen CD: Diseases of the Breast, 2nd ed. Philadelphia: W.B. Saunders Co., 1971, pp. 617–668.
3. Portmann UV: Clinical and pathologic criteria as a basis for classifying cases of primary cancer of the breast. Cleve Clin Q 10:41, 1943.
4. Haagensen CD, Stout AP: Carcinoma of the breast; criteria of operability. Ann Surg 118:859–870, 1032–1051, 1943.
5. Beahrs OH, Myers MH (eds.): Manual for Staging of Cancer—American Joint Committee on Cancer. Philadelphia: J.B. Lippincott Co., 1983.
6. American Joint Committee for Cancer Staging and End Results Reporting: Manual for Staging of Cancer, Chicago, 1978.
7. Harmer MH: TNM Classification of Malignant Tumors, 3rd ed. Geneva: UICC, 1978.
8. McWhirter R: Simple mastectomy and radiotherapy in the treatment of breast cancer. Br J Radiol 28:128, 1955.
9. Rubens RD, Armitage P, Winter PJ, et al: Prognosis in inoperable stage III carcinoma of the breast. Eur J Cancer 13:805, 1977.
10. Arnold DJ, Lesnick GJ: Survival following mastectomy for Stage III breast cancer. Am J Surg 137:362, 1979.
11. Donegan WL, Lewis JD: Clinical diagnosis and staging of breast cancer. Semin Oncol 5:373, 1978.
12. Zucali R, Uslenghi C, Kenda R, et al.: Natural history and survival of inoperable breast cancer treated with radiotherapy and radiotherapy followed by radical mastectomy. Cancer 37:1422, 1976.
13. Balawajder I, Antich PP, Boland J: An analysis of the role of radiotherapy alone and in combination with chemotherapy and surgery in the management of advanced breast carcinoma. Cancer 51:574, 1983.
14. Hortobagyi GN, Blumenschein GR, Spanos W, et al.: Multimodal treatment of locoregionally advanced breast cancer. Cancer 51:763, 1983.
15. Bedwinek J, Rao DV, Perez C, et al: Stage III and localized Stage IV breast cancer: Irradiation alone versus irradiation plus surgery. Int J Radiat Oncol Biol Phys 8:31, 1982.
16. Harris JR, Sawicka J, Gelman R, et al: Management of locally advanced carcinoma of the breast by primary radiation therapy. Int J Radiat Oncol Biol Phys 9:345, 1983.
17. Fracchia AA, Evans JF, Eisenberg BL: Stage III carcinoma of the breast: A detailed analysis. Ann Surg 192:705, 1980.
18. Treurniet-Donker AD, Hop WCJ, Hoed-Sijtsema S: Radiation treatment of Stage III mammary carcinoma: A review of 129 patients. Int J Radiat Oncol Biol Phys 6:1477, 1980.
19. Rao DV, Bedwinek J, Perez C, et al.: Prognostic indicators in Stage III and localized Stage IV breast cancer. Cancer 50:2037, 1982.
20. Bell CA: A System of Operative Surgery, Vol. 11. Hartford, CT: Kale & Hosmer, 1814, p. 136.
21. Klotz ID: Ueber Mastitis Carcinomatosa Gravidarum et Lactantium. Thèse, Halle, 1869.
22. Leitch A: Peau d'orange in acute mammary carcinoma: Its cause and diagnostic value. Lancet 1:861, 1909.

23. Learmonth GE: Acute mammary carcinoma (Volkmann's mastitis carcinomatosa). Can Med Assoc J 6:499, 1916.
24. Schumann EA: A study of carcinoma mastitoides. Ann Surg 54:69, 1911.
25. Lee BJ, Tannenbaum NE: Inflammatory carcinoma of the breast: A report of twenty-eight cases from the breast clinic of the Memorial Hospital. Surg Gynecol Obstet 39:580, 1924.
26. Taylor GW, Meltzer A: "Inflammatory carcinoma" of the breast. Am J Cancer 33:33, 1938.
27. Bryant T: Diseases of the Breast. New York: Wood's Medical and Surgical Monographs, 1889, pp. 35–322.
28. Ellis DL, Teitelbaum SL: Inflammatory carcinoma of the breast: A pathologic definition. Cancer 33:1045, 1974.
29. Saltzstein SL: Clinically occult inflammatory carcinoma of the breast. Cancer 34:382, 1974.
30. Lucas FV, Perez-Mesa C: Inflammatory carcinoma of the breast. Cancer 41:1595, 1978.
31. Donnelly BA: Primary "inflammatory" carcinoma of the breast. A report of five cases and a review of the literature. Ann Surg 128:918, 1948.
32. Barber KW, Dockerty MB, Clagett OT: Inflammatory carcinoma of the breast. Surg Gynecol Obstet 112:406, 1961.
33. Richards GJ, Lewison EF: Inflammatory carcinoma of the breast. Surg Gynecol Obstet 113:729, 1961.
34. Byrd BF, Stephenson SE: Inflamed or inflammatory carcinoma of the breast. Am Surg 28:303, 1962.
35. Wang CC, Griscom NT: Inflammatory carcinoma of the breast. Results following orthovoltage and supervoltate radiation therapy. Clin Radiol 15:168, 1964.
36. Chris SM: Inflammatory carcinoma of the breast: Report of 20 cases and a review of the literature. Br J Surg 38:163, 1950.
37. Meyer AC, Dockerty MB, Harrington SW: Inflammatory carcinoma of the breast. Surg Gynecol Obstet 87:417, 1948.
38. Rogers CS, Fitts WT: Inflammatory carcinoma of the breast: A critique of therapy. Surgery 39:367, 1956.
39. Spratt JS, Donegan WL: Cancer of the Breast. Philadelphia: W.B. Saunders Co., 1967, p. 167.
40. Dao TL, McCarthy JD: Treatment of inflammatory carcinoma of the breast. Surg Gynecol Obstet 105:289, 1957.
41. Bloom HJC: The natural history of untreated breast cancer. Ann NY Acad Sci 114:747, 1964.
42. Greenwood M: The natural history of cancer. London: Ministry of Health Reports of Public Health and Medical Subjects, His Majesty's Stationery Office, 1926, No. XXVI.
43. Daland EM: Untreated cancer of the breast. Surg Gynecol Obstet 44:264, 1927.
44. Nathanson IT, Welch CE: Life expectancy and incidence of malignant disease: Carcinoma of the breast. Am J Cancer 28:40, 1936.
45. Forber JE: Incurable cancer. London: Ministry of Health Reports on Public Health and Medical Subjects, His Majesty's Stationery Office, 1931, No. LXVI.
46. Donegan WL: Cancer of the Breast, 2nd ed. Philadelphia: W.B. Saunders Co., 1979, p. 263.
47. Schottenfeld D, Nash AG, Robbins GF, et al.: Ten-year results of the treatment of primary operable breast carcinoma. Cancer 38:1001, 1976.
48. Handley RS, from Haagensen CD: Diseases of the Breast, 2nd ed. Philadelphia: W.B. Saunders Co., 1971, p. 634.
49. Cade S: Treatment and results in cancer of the breast. Am J Roentgenol 62:326, 1949.
50. Pearlman NW, Guerra O, Fracchia AA: Primary inoperable cancer of the breast. Surg Gynecol Obstet 143:909, 1976.
51. Langlands AO, Kerr GR, Shaw S: The management of locally advanced breast cancer by x-ray therapy. Clin Oncol 2:365, 1976.
52. Atkins HL, Horrigan WD: Treatment of locally advanced carcinoma of the breast with roentgen therapy and simple mastectomy. Am J Roentgenol 85:860, 1961.
53. Golding P: The treatment of inoperable carcinoma of the breast in Portsmouth, 1960–69. Proc Soc Med 69:701, 1976.
54. Yarom J, Assa J, Robinson E: The survival of inoperable breast cancer treated with radiotherapy and radiotherapy followed by mastectomy. J Surg Oncol 9:203, 1977.
55. Bouchard J: Advanced cancer of the breast treated primarily with irradiation. Radiology 84:823, 1965.
56. Baclesse F: Five-year results in 431 breast cancers treated solely by roentgen rays. Ann Surg 161:103, 1965.
57. Amalric R, Santamaria F, Robert F, et al: Radiation therapy with or without primary limited surgery for operable breast cancer. Cancer 49:30, 1982.
58. Spanos WJ, Montague ED, Fletcher GH: Late complications of radiation only for advanced breast cancer. Int J Radiat Oncol Biol Phys 6:1473, 1980.
59. Pierquin B, Owen R, Maylin C, et al: Radical radiation therapy of breast cancer. Int J Radiat Oncol Biol Phys 6:17, 1980.
60. Syed AMN, Puthawala AA, Orr LE, et al: Primary irradiation in the management of early and locally advanced carcinoma of the breast. Br J Radiol 57:317, 1984.
61. Alderman SJ: Combination teletherapy and iridium implantation in the treatment of locally advanced breast cancer. Cancer 38:1936, 1976.
62. Bruckman JE, Harris JR, Levene MB, et al.: Results of treating Stage III carcinoma of the breast by primary radiation therapy. Cancer 43:985, 1979.
63. Townsend CM, Fish JC, Olson MH, et al.: Management of locally advanced breast cancer. Proc Am Soc Clin Oncol 22:427, 1981.
64. Stoker TAM, Ellis H: Post-irradiation toilet mastectomy in the management of locally advanced carcinoma of the breast. Br J Radiol 45:851, 1972.
65. Terz JJ, Romero CA, Kay S, et al.: Preoperative radiotherapy for Stage III carcinoma of the breast. Surg Gynecol Obstet 147:497, 1978.
66. Lenz M: Tumor dosage and results in roentgen therapy of cancer of the breast. Am J Roentgenol Radium Ther 56:67, 1946.
67. Vaeth JM, Clark JC, Green JP, et al.: Radiotherapeutic management of locally advanced carcinoma of the breast. Cancer 30:107, 1972.
68. Brown GR, Horiot JC, Fletcher GH, et al.: Simple mastectomy and radiation therapy for locally advanced breast cancer technically suitable for radical mastectomy. Am J Roentgenol 120:67, 1974.
69. Delarue NC, Ash CL, Peters V, et al.: Preoperative irradiation in management of locally advanced breast cancer. Arch Surg 91:136, 1965.
70. Barker JL, Montague ED, Peters LJ: Clinical experi-

ence with irradiation of inflammatory carcinoma of the breast with and without elective chemotherapy. Cancer 45:625, 1980.

71. Chu AM, Wood WC, Doucette JA: Inflammatory breast carcinoma treated by radical radiotherapy. Cancer 45:2730, 1980.
72. Sponzo RW, Cunningham TJ, Caradonna RR: Management of nonresectable (Stage III) breast cancer. Int J Radiat Oncol Biol Phys 5:1475, 1979.
73. Sponzo RW, Gray R, Damsker JI, et al: The management of non-resectable (Stage III) breast cancer. Proc Am Soc Clin Oncol 2:110, 1983.
74. Serrou B, Sancho-Garnier H, Cappelaere P, et al.: Follow-up results from a randomized trial for T_3 and T_4 breast cancer patients: Previous BCG immunotherapy improves response to chemotherapy in the relapse patient. Recent Results Cancer Res 80:157, 1982.
75. Gröhn P, Heinonen E, Klefström P, et al.: Adjuvant postoperative radiotherapy, chemotherapy, and immunotherapy in stage III breast cancer. Cancer 54:670, 1984.
76. DeLena M, Zucali R, Viganotti G, et al. Combined chemotherapy-radiotherapy approach in locally advanced (T3b–T4) breast cancer. Cancer Chemother Pharmacol 1:53, 1978.
77. DeLena M, Varini M, Zucali R, et al.: Multimodal treatment for locally advanced breast cancer. Cancer Clin Trials 4:229, 1981.
78. Rubens RD, Sexton S, Tong D, et al.: Combined chemotherapy and radiotherapy for locally advanced breast cancer. Eur J Cancer 16:351, 1980.
79. Perloff M, Lesnick GJ: Chemotherapy before and after mastectomy in stage III breast cancer. Arch Surg 117:879, 1982.
80. Buzdar AU, Montague ED, Barker JL, et al.: Management of inflammatory carcinoma of the breast with combined modality approach—an update. Cancer 47:2537, 1981.
81. Feldman L, Hortobagyi G, Buzdar A, et al.: Pathologic complete remission in patients with inflammatory breast cancer and locally advanced breast cancer. Proc Am Soc Clin Oncol 25:197, 1984.
82. Zylberberg B, Salat-Baroux J, Ravina JH, et al.: Initial chemoimmunotherapy in inflammatory carcinoma of the breast. Cancer 49:1537, 1982.
83. Lippman ME, Cassidy J, Wesley M, et al: A randomized attempt to increase the efficacy of cytotoxic chemotherapy in metastatic breast cancer by hormonal synchronization. J Clin Oncol 2:28, 1984.
84. Sorace RA, Bagley CS, Lichter AS, et al.: The management of nonmetastatic locally advanced breast cancer using primary induction chemotherapy with hormonal synchronization followed by radiation therapy with or without debulking surgery. World J Surg 9:775, 1985.
85. Loprinzi CL, Carbone PP, Tormey DC, et al.: Aggressive combined modality therapy for advanced local-regional breast carcinoma. J Clin Oncol 2:157, 1984.

Intraepithelial Carcinoma of the Breast: Lobular Carcinoma in Situ *and Ductal Carcinoma* in Situ

SANDRA M. SWAIN, M.D.
MARC E. LIPPMAN, M.D.

10

The concept of carcinoma *in situ* was proposed by Broders in 1932.[1] He described carcinoma *in situ* as "a condition in which malignant epithelial cells and their progeny are found in or near positions occupied by their ancestors before the ancestors underwent malignant transformation. At least they have not migrated beyond the juncture of the epithelium and connective tissue or the so-called basement membrane." He also makes a statement relevant to intraepithelial breast carcinoma: "In adenocarcinoma *in situ* the malignant cells often completely replace the nonmalignant cells in what were once normal acini, ducts, or tubules."

Intraepithelial breast cancers consist of lobular carcinoma *in situ* (LCIS) and ductal carcinoma *in situ* (DCIS), which is more commonly referred to as intraductal carcinoma. The intraepithelial phase of breast cancer is felt to represent a malignancy that has not yet invaded basement membrane and therefore does not have metastasizing potential. Important questions relating to the natural history of these cancers include: Are they really malignant? Do they eventually become invasive cancers having metastatic potential? What is the clinical significance of the diagnosis of intraepithelial, or noninvasive, cancer? The goal of this chapter is to summarize published studies on the subject of LCIS and DCIS and, from the studies, attempt to answer these important questions.

Intraepithelial cancers represent 1.4 to 12.0 percent[2–5] of all breast cancer reported. However, these cancers are an important subset, since with better mammographic screening techniques, increased numbers are being diagnosed. Furthermore, with therapeutic recommendations ranging from surveillance to local excision to bilateral mastectomies, it can be seen that a clear understanding of the disease process is mandatory for patient management.

The discussion will begin with screening studies that have allowed an increased detection of noninvasive, or intraepithelial, cancers. Next, the topic of precancerous or proliferative breast disease as a precursor to intraepithelial carcinoma will be reviewed along with the concept of minimal breast cancer. Then, the general pathology of noninvasive cancer will be described (for a more detailed discussion, please refer to Chapter 3). Specifically, LCIS and DCIS will be considered, including age at diagnosis, etiology, clinical findings, presence of invasive disease at mastectomy, incidence of bilaterality, incidence of multicentricity, risk of subsequent invasive cancer, incidence of axillary node positivity, and treatment.

DETECTION

It is the hope of proponents of screening techniques such as mammography that the noninvasive and more curable forms of breast cancer will be detected. This is analogous to the routine Papanicolaou smear done for early detection of cervical carcinoma. Several large screening trials have been completed to try to determine the effect of early detection on breast cancer mortality. The most widely quoted study, performed by the Health Insurance Plan of New York (HIP), was begun in 1963 and followed women for nine years.[6, 7] This randomized study entered women 40 to 64 years of age into either a study group that was screened or a control group. Screened women were followed by yearly physical examination and two-view mammography for five years.

Both screening by physical examination and mammography contributed to earlier detection of cancers in this study. Mammography was suggestive of or positive for cancer in patients with normal results on physical examination in a significant proportion of women diagnosed as having breast cancer: 19 percent of women with cancer aged 40 to 49; 42 percent of those aged 50 to 59; and 31 percent of those 60 or older. On the other hand, many patients with normal mammograms had cancers discovered by physical examination alone: 61 percent of women with cancer aged 40 to 49; 40 percent of those aged 50 to 59; and 31 percent of women aged 60 or older. It can be seen that screening played a particularly important role in the detection of cancer in women aged 50 or older. Lymph node involvement, an important prognostic indicator, was present in 29 percent of cancers detected by screening and 55 percent of those detected in the control group. It should be noted that *in situ* cancers constituted 12 percent of all cancers diagnosed in the screened group and 8.4 percent of those in the control group. There was an overall decrease in breast cancer mortality by over 30 percent in the screened group. More specifically, there was a decrease in mortality by 40 percent in women over age 50, which was statistically significant. There was no impact on mortality in women under age 50.

While the HIP study is important, it should be remembered that with current mammographic technique, image definition has improved markedly while radiation dose has decreased. Therefore, many smaller cancers can now be detected. Also, it is difficult to evaluate the individual contribution of mammography, as compared with physical examination, in the HIP study. It was evident after the HIP study that further studies were needed, especially to determine the impact of screening mammography on younger women.

One of the largest and most comprehensive nonrandomized studies was done by the Breast Cancer Detection Demonstration Project (BCDDP) in 1973, sponsored by the National Cancer Institute and the American Cancer Society.[8, 9] Twenty-seven projects each enrolled 10,000 women aged 35 to 74. These women were volunteers and therefore self-selected, with 25 percent having a family history positive for breast cancer. Screening physical examination, mammography, and thermography were performed annually for five years with no nonscreened control group. One hundred cancers were discovered. Of these, 44 percent were referred for biopsy on mammographic grounds alone (44 percent in the 40 to 49 year age group and 48 percent in the 50 to 59 year age group), 48 percent were suspected because of physical examination and abnormal mammograms, and 7.4 percent were referred for biopsy by abnormal physical examination findings alone. In contrast with the HIP project, the 40 to 49 year age group had a higher detection rate by mammography alone. Twenty-six percent of all cancers found were noninvasive, and of those that were invasive,

40 percent were less than 1 cm in diameter. Of patients with noninvasive cancer, 65 percent had negative nodes; 3 percent, positive nodes; and 32 percent, unknown. Of patients with invasive cancers, 63 percent had negative nodes; 24 percent, positive nodes; and 13 percent, unknown. The conclusions were that detection of breast cancer was increased, in the 40 to 49 year age group as well as in the 50 to 59 year age group. Many cancers with favorable prognostic factors were discovered, and the investigators believed that mortality would consequently be decreased.

Another study emphasizing earlier detection of cancers, especially in the noninvasive form, is a nonrandomized British trial, the Guilford Breast Screening Project, begun in 1979.[10] Of the 24,069 women aged 45 to 64 who were invited, 16,586 (69 percent) attended screening. Single-view mammography and physical examination were done, with 91 percent of subjects having negative results. The 9 percent with positive results were sent on to have two-view mammography. Two percent of the total were referred to a surgeon for biopsy, and 91 cancers were diagnosed, of which 14 were noninvasive. In the control (nonrandomized) population, who were not screened, none of the cancers detected was noninvasive. Twenty-seven percent of cancers in the screened group were suspected on mammographic grounds alone. These investigators concluded that screening diagnosed cancers with a more favorable prognosis.

Sweden has a breast cancer incidence comparable with that of the United States. A different breast cancer screening approach was taken by the Swedish group. A randomized, controlled trial was begun in 1977 in two counties in Sweden, using single-view mammography alone as the screening technique.[11, 12] Women aged 40 to 74 were included and screened every two to three years. There were 78,085 women in the screened group, while 56,782 were in the control. A total of 1068 cancers were found in the screened group and 595 in the control. Fifty-eight percent, or 616, of the cancers in the screened group were Stage I, while 35 percent, or 209, in the control were Stage I. There were 98 cases (9.1 percent) of DCIS in the screened group and 15 (2.5 percent) in the control group. The breast cancer mortality was statistically decreased in the screened women aged 50 to 74. It is felt that mortality was decreased by the increased detection of noninvasive and Stage I cancers, which are more likely to be cured by local therapy.

These studies all indicate a trend toward detection by screening (including, specifically, mammography) of more prognostically favorable cancers, such as noninvasive and smaller invasive cancers. It is hoped that early detection will be translated into decreased mortality.

Several specific studies have been directed toward correlating mammographic findings with a known diagnosis of LCIS. Finely stippled calcifications in tight clusters have been seen on mammography in cases of LCIS.[13] The calcifications rarely occur in the cancer itself but usually in the adjacent lobule, which is felt to be an area of benign disease. For example, calcifications are also seen with cystic disease, duct ectasia, sclerosing adenosis, duct papillomatosis, ductal stasis, and other benign diseases.[14]

Snyder[13] retrospectively studied 35 breasts of 27 patients with a pathologic diagnosis of LCIS who had a preoperative mammogram in the 1960's at Memorial Sloan-Kettering Cancer Center. In ten cases (37 percent of patients) the diagnosis of carcinoma was made by mammography alone, and in eight cases the x-ray report was suggestive but not diagnostic of cancer. The finding most consistent with cancer was calcification consisting of three or more small punctate or linear flecks in a random pattern. An addition to this series was made in 1968 by Hutter and colleagues[15] from the same institution. The report consisted of findings from 109 breasts of 61 patients with LCIS. Seventy-seven breasts contained LCIS; seven, DCIS; and ten, infiltrating cancer. Forty-three percent of patients with LCIS had positive mammograms. Twelve percent were diagnosed on the basis of mammography alone. Fifty-seven percent had negative mammograms and were diagnosed on the basis of physical examination. The investigators' conclusion was that mammography can be helpful in diagnosing LCIS but is positive in less than 50 percent of cases.

Another series describing indications for biopsy of LCIS from mammography is by Tulusan.[16] Of 52 cases of LCIS, 27 (52 percent) were positive on mammogram for microcalcifications, and six, for microcalcifications and a breast mass. The pathology of these areas of microcalcifications is not described.

On the other hand, one small study by Morris and associates[17] refuted the utility of mammography in LCIS. Mammograms of 26 breasts from 14 patients were reviewed. The mammograms were positive in 5 to 26 breasts, three of which contained LCIS. Thirteen of the remaining 21 breasts with negative mammograms and positive clinical findings underwent biopsy and were found to contain LCIS. In this study, the incidence of positive mammograms in LCIS was 3 of 16 breasts, or 19 percent. This is considerably less than in the previous data.

In conclusion, LCIS may be detected by mammography in a screening situation, but calcifications are usually in areas of benign disease. The association of these calcifications with LCIS is frequent enough to justify biopsy. Also, mammography is extremely important in the follow-up of patients with LCIS, since they are at higher risk for the development of invasive cancers.

PRECURSOR LESIONS OF INTRAEPITHELIAL CANCER

Many pathologists now propose that there is a continuum of change from normal breast epithelium to carcinoma *in situ*.[18–20] The lesions that occur prior to an *in situ* cancer may have some of the same cytologic features but lack the complete criteria for that diagnosis.[18] Specifically, for the diagnosis of LCIS to be made, the major part of the lobule must be involved, the nuclei must have a homogeneous pattern and be hyperchromatic, no intercellular lumina should be apparent, and lobules must be distended and distorted by these cells.[18, 21] in DCIS, nuclei are hyperchromatic and round, and the cells are moderately pleomorphic and proliferate within and distend ducts[18, 21] in one of four growth patterns: solid, comedo, papillary, or cribriform.[21, 22] Lesions that do not fully meet these criteria are borderline lesions and are called atypical lobular or ductular hyperplasia.[18] The biologic and prognostic significance of these lesions has been studied systematically by several investigators.

Rush and Kramer[23] examined 40 breasts from 20 patients at random at autopsy to correlate findings with the development of cancer. Approximately 50 slides per breast were examined. Microcysts were found in 19 of 20 cases and apocrine metaplasia in 17 of 20 cases. Fourteen of 20 had some ductal hyperplasia, with 10 of 20 being severe hyperplasia. Two of 20 patients had bilateral carcinoma: three breasts contained DCIS, and one, infiltrating ductal carcinoma. Both of these patients had associated severe benign hyperplasia. The investigators updated their study in 1972 with an additional 50 cases, for a total of 70 patients, or 140 breasts.[24] All women were age 70 or older. Forty-eight patients (69 percent) had intraductal hyperplasia, 19 patients (27 percent) had severe hyperplasia, and seven (10 percent) had atypical hyperplasia. Adenosis or severe branching proliferation was seen in 40 (57 percent). There were four patients (5.7 percent) with intraductal carcinoma, one with a small area of microinvasion. All four of these patients had associated adenosis and atypical hyperplasia. Only 3 of 66 patients (4.5 percent) without carcinoma had associated atypical findings. The actual yearly incidence quoted for comparison in this study for new breast cancers is 0.3 percent. The 5.7 percent incidence of occult carcinoma in their autopsy patients was 19 times that of expected clinical breast cancer. The high incidence of epithelial hyperplasia (69 percent) in older women is associated with a relatively much lower incidence of occult carcinoma (5.7 percent). However, since (1) all women who had carcinoma had associated atypical hyperplasia, (2) most women without carcinoma did not have atypical findings, and (3) both patients with carcinoma had bilateral cancer, authors of the study felt that the same systemic factors were operative in the development of both atypical hyperplasia and carcinoma. It may be that these women were at high risk for developing neoplastic lesions and that the atypical lesions and carcinomas developed independently.

Ashikari and colleagues[25] have also studied atypical lobular hyperplasia and atypical ductal papillomatosis and their relationship to breast cancer. The study included 296 patients diagnosed from 1960 to 1972 at Memorial Sloan-Kettering Hospital as having atypical breast lesions. These patients were followed by physical examinations every four months and yearly mammograms. Twenty patients were found to have breast cancer, with three having axillary metastases and one eventually dying of her disease. The investigators calculated the risk of breast cancer in patients with atypical lesions to be 18 times that of the general population.

The most extensive study to determine the risk of cancer in women who have had a breast biopsy for benign disease was done by Dupont and Page.[26] They retrospectively reviewed 10,366 breast biopsies, for which median follow-up was 17 years. Sixty-eight percent of cases were diagnosed as nonproliferative benign disease, and 30 percent, as proliferative disease. Proliferative breast disease included atypical lobular hyperplasia, atypical ductal hyperpalsia, moderate and florid hyperplasia of the usual type (epitheliosis), papillomas, sclerosing adenosis, or ductal involvement with cells of atypical lobular hyperplasia. The overall relative risk for developing breast cancer in patients both with and without proliferative disease who had had a breast biopsy was one and one-half times greater than that in the general population in the Third National Cancer Survey in Atlanta. Patients with proliferative disease had a 1.9 risk, and those with nonproliferative disease had a risk of 0.89. Patients with proliferative disease without atypia (PDWA) had a risk of developing cancer 1.9 times that of the women with nonproliferative disease in their study. Patients with atypical hyperplasia had 5.3 times the risk of those with nonproliferative disease. This risk increased to 11 times in those patients with a family history of breast cancer. Women with cysts and a family history had 2.7 times the risk of women without either of these factors, while women with cysts alone had no increased risk. Also, patients with PDWA had a risk of 2.7 times that of patients with nonproliferative disease without a family history. In conclusion, this study shows that the majority of women who have undergone breast biopsy are not at highly increased risk for developing breast cancer, unless a lesion with atypia is present. Also, a family history elevates the cancer risk.

Fisher and associates[27] reviewed the pathologic findings of NSABP Protocol B-04 (radical versus total mastectomy) and found a 13.4 percent incidence of multicentric cancer, with 9.3 percent being noninvasive. Multicentric cancer was more frequently associated with proliferative breast disease (67.8 percent) than with nonproliferative (22.3 percent). This indicated that each of the two entities may have been initiated by the same stimulus and that one may not necessarily be the precursor to the other.

In summary, the diagnosis of atypical hyperplasia places the patient at increased risk for developing breast cancer. Increased surveillance is warranted, but the diagnosis itself at the present time is not sufficient grounds for surgical intervention. However, with the addition of other factors, such as a strong family history or dense breasts on mammography making interpretation difficult, mastectomy might be considered.

THE CONCEPT OF MINIMAL BREAST CANCER

The definition of minimal breast cancer (MBC) as originally proposed by Gallager and Martin[28] includes LCIS, DCIS, and invasive carcinoma, either lobular or ductal, which form a mass no greater than 0.5 cm in diameter.

Gallager and Martin felt at the time they put forward their concept that it was important to define the stages of breast cancer amenable to local forms of treatment. To do this they needed to determine the upper limit in size of invasive breast cancer still associated with a low occurrence of axillary node disease and a good prognosis. Mammograms from 200 patients who subsequently had radical mastectomies were reviewed.[29] The volumes of the masses were measured, and the incidence of known nodal metastasis was plotted. The size of a mass with a volume of 0.125 cm^3 or the volume of a 0.5 cm sphere correlated with an incidence of nodal involvement of less than 10 percent. Therefore, the size of 0.5 cm was chosen as the upper limit to define minimal breast cancer. Since then, some other investigators have used the term minimal breast cancer to include tumors that are less than or equal to 1 cm.[30]

There are many investigators who accept the concept of MBC and feel that it is important prognostically.[30, 31] However, the noninvasive forms of breast cancer will be discussed separately from even those minimally invasive carcinomas that by light microscopy violate basement membranes. This is because there is a substantial incidence of node positivity reported in patients with MBC. Gallager's review[31] of the literature on this subject revealed an incidence rate of 0 to 9.6 percent node positivity in a total of 415 patients with MBC. This obviously supports his hypothesis. On the other hand, Bedwani and associates[32] reviewed the American College of Physicians breast cancer survey in 1981 and found an incidence of 23 percent node positivity in 204 patients with invasive cancer measuring less than 0.5 cm and 21 percent node positivity in those with tumors 0.6 to 1.0 cm.

An important analysis has been done of 8587 cases of breast cancer diagnosed in 1975 from the Surveillance, Epidemiology, and End Results program (SEER) of the National Cancer Institute (NCI).[4] The SEER program followed 10 percent of the United States population from nine states. Of 8587 cases of breast cancer, noninvasive cancer constituted 5.3 percent, or 456 cases, and 3.8 percent of the invasive cancers were less than 1 cm. Of the patients whose nodes were sampled, those with invasive lesions less than 0.5 cm had a 17.2 percent node positivity rate, and patients with lesions measuring 0.5 cm to 0.9 cm had a 20.2 percent node involvement with cancer. Also, of the patients who were felt to have clinically negative nodes, approximately 31.4 percent had positive nodes pathologically. Therefore, even minimal invasive cancers with nonpalpable nodes include a fair percentage of patients whose tumor has already metastasized.

Even the smallest invasive cancers will not be included in the discussion of LCIS and DCIS because, as can be seen by the previous data, size is not all that determines biologic behavior and metastatic potential. Therapeutic interventions are different for invasive versus noninvasive disease. It is clear that any invasive cancer requires definitive local treatment by radiation therapy or surgery and careful evaluation for additional systemic treatment.

PATHOLOGY OF INTRAEPITHELIAL CANCER

It is important to remember the normal anatomy of the breast before discussing LCIS and DCIS. A lobule contains an entire intralobular duct, terminal ducts, alveoli, and connective tissue.[21]

Lobular carcinoma *in situ* arises from ducts within the lobule. Microscopically, the nuclei are round and uniform, the cells are two times normal size, cytoplasmic margins are indistinct, and there is a loss of cellular cohesiveness.[21] Some pathologists feel that LCIS can be diagnosed only with the presence of more than one involved lobule,[33] whereas others feel that involvement of 75 percent of one lobule is adequate for diagnosis.[34]

The origin of ductal carcinoma has been thought to be small, medium, and large ducts. However, a study done by Wellings and Jensen[35] of 60 whole-human breasts disputes this issue. They found that the earliest foci of DCIS were localized to what they call the solitary terminal ductal lobular units (TDLUs). By their definition, the terminal duct has an extralobular and an intralobular component ending in ductules or tubelike structures. They proposed that DCIS begins in the extra- and intralobular units, with progressive expansion of proliferative neoplastic cells. Eventually, the neoplastic cells involve the ductules, which distend and coalesce to form a tumor.

LCIS and DCIS by definition have intact basement membranes by light microscopy.[36] Infiltrating tumors lack basement membranes.[36] Ozzello[22, 37] studied DCIS by PAS staining and found defective basal laminae in almost all cases. This ranged from variations in thickness to areas of discontinuity of the basememt membrane. Ozzello also studied DCIS by electron microscopy.[38, 39] In many cases of DCIS, gaps were present and cells protruded through the gap into the surrounding stroma, indicating invasiveness. These abnormalities of basement membranes are not observed by light microscopy. Ozzello[40] found cases of LCIS to have well-formed basal laminae and, only infrequently, gaps and cell protrusions into the stroma.

On the other hand, Barsky and colleagues[41] have studied the basement membranes of benign breast lesions, DCIS, and invasive cancers by immunofluorescence and immunoperoxidase staining. They observed apparent interrupted areas of basement membrane in cases of DCIS with microinvasive disease. Basement membranes were found to be intact in five cases of fibroadenoma, three cases of sclerosing adenosis, and five cases of DCIS. Fifteen cases of infiltrating cancers studied lacked basement membrane immunoreactivity. The denominator of patient samples studied was not stated.

Clearly, these two studies have differing results. The interpretation by Barsky is that the cases seen by Ozzello actually represented ductal carcinoma with microinvasive disease, and not carcinoma *in situ*. This is interesting; however, further studies on benign breast disease and a systematic study of cases of *in situ* cancer need to be done before the biologic significance of these findings can be determined.

LOBULAR CARCINOMA IN SITU

Cornil[42] advocated the epithelial origin of cancer, in which he used mammary carcinoma as a model. In 1865, he described carcinoma in mammary lobules. Lobular carcinoma *in situ* was described in 1919 by Ewing as a "precancerous change."[43] In 1941, Foote and Stewart[44] described this lesion pathologically in more detail and named it "lobular carcinoma *in situ*." It is at this time that lobular carcinoma *in situ* became a distinct morphologic entity. Further definition by Stewart[45] in 1950 divided lobular carcinoma into two types, noninfiltrating and infiltrating. In 1972, Haagensen and associates[46] proposed that lobular carcinoma *in situ* was a misnomer, since many lesions, as suggested by the word carcinoma, may not progress or metastasize. They felt that the lesion should be called "lobular neoplasia" and was a benign entity.

There have been more than 1000 patients with lobular carcinoma *in situ* reported in the literature.[2, 5, 16, 47–63] Many of the cases have been discovered by retrospective reviews of biopsies of benign lesions not originally diagnosed as LCIS.[47, 54, 59, 62] Also, many reports include those patients who have a mixture of invasive and noninvasive cancer.[51, 56, 62, 64] Treatment varies widely from radical mastectomy to bilateral mastectomy to biopsy alone with surveillance. These variations make it difficult to compare different studies and to extrapolate the findings to the general population. The incidence of LCIS ranges from 0.5 to 12.3 percent of reported cases of breast carcinoma.[2, 4, 5, 48, 50, 59]

Age at Diagnosis

Haagensen and colleagues[54] believed that lobular neoplasia or LCIS was a disease of premenopausal women that regressed during menopause. This is similar to the involution of normal lobules in a woman of advancing age. In his series of 211 patients, 90 percent were premenopausal. Of the premenopausal patients, 50 percent had LCIS alone and 5 percent had associated ductal carcinoma *in situ*, with 45 percent having both. In the postmenopausal patients, LCIS alone occurred in 22 percent, DCIS alone in 22 percent, and both in 56 percent. Therefore, they concluded that the ductal phase was more prominent in older women and that both diseases, DCIS and LCIS, were closely related.

Other series support the lower age incidence of LCIS compared with that of invasive lobular cancer (Table 10–1).[47–49, 54, 55, 57–59, 62] The average age at diagnosis of LCIS ranges from 43 to 47 years. The average age of patients with infiltrating lobular cancer ranges from 48 to 68 years,[21, 65, 66] suggesting that LCIS could be a precursor to the invasive lobular cancer.

Etiology

It is postulated that LCIS is a hormone-dependent tumor.[46] It occurs largely in younger women who still have lobules in their breast that respond to the normal changes of the menstrual cycle. On the other hand, most postmenopausal women have atrophic lobules. One study looked at exogenous hormone usage in postmenopausal patients with the diagnosis of LCIS.[67] Of a total of 39 patients with LCIS, nine patients (23 percent) were postmenopausal. Seven of these nine had never taken hormone-contain-

TABLE 10–1. Age at Diagnosis of Lobular Carcinoma in Situ (LCIS)

Author	*No. of Patients*	*Mean Age*
Andersen[47]	52	46
Benfield et al.[48]	13	46
Carter and Smith[49]	49	47.2
Haagensen et al.[54]	211	90% premenopausal
Lewison and Finney[55]	40	46
Newman[57]	26	45
Ringberg et al.[58]	16	46
Rosen et al.[59]	99	45
Wheeler et al.[62]	38	43.9

ing medication. Therefore, Rosen and colleagues felt that there was no link between LCIS and estrogen use in postmenopausal women. This experience is too small to be convincing.

There has been little written in the literature documenting the estrogen receptor status of lobular carcinomas and none concerning LCIS. Rosen and associates[68] studied 13 patients with lobular carcinoma and found 12 of 13 specimens (92.3 percent) to be positive in a dextran-coated charcoal assay for estrogen receptor. They suggest that lobular carcinoma may be a more hormonally dependent tumor. Antoniades and Spector[69] also assayed 13 cases of lobular carcinoma for estrogen receptor in the dextran-coated charcoal assay and found 84 percent to be positive. Clearly, more patients with LCIS and lobular carcinoma need to be assayed for estrogen receptor before a conclusion can be reached.

Clinical Findings

LCIS is almost always a nonpalpable lesion.[54] As discussed previously, mammography is of limited value in the diagnosis of LCIS because the mammogram is positive in areas of benign disease. LCIS is usually discovered only after biopsy for other clinically palpable lesions such as fibroadenoma,[48, 54, 57, 59, 70, 71] cysts,[5, 53, 54, 59, 71] breast abscess,[48, 54] papilloma,[5, 54, 57, 59, 71] papillomatosis,[54, 55, 57, 59] fat necrosis,[53, 59, 71] and periductal mastitis.[53, 55, 57, 59, 71] For example, in Haagensen's series of 211 patients with LCIS, 73 percent of the patients had gross cysts leading to the diagnosis of LCIS.[54] In 5.7 percent of patients, a fibroadenoma was the lesion leading to the diagnosis. Andersen[71] found a 43 percent incidence of gross cysts associated with LCIS in his series of 52 patients. Rosen and colleagues[59] found an 81 percent coincidence of cysts and LCIS in their series of 99 patients. In summary, the diagnosis of LCIS is made on the basis of microscopic findings, usually as a result of the discovery of benign lesions.

Multicentricity and Bilaterality

Bilaterality and multicentricity in LCIS are related phenomena. The presence of bilateral or multicentric lesions indicates that all lobules of the breast are susceptible to the initiating stimulus. This concept is important, especially in the planning of treatment for patients so affected.

Multicentricity

Multicentricity is defined in LCIS as areas of disease in the breast separate from the site in which the original diagnosis was made. Some physicians require that the areas of disease be in entirely different quadrants,[72] and others require only a separation by normal lobules.[58] This, however, should always exclude residual disease in the mastectomy specimen alone. Unfortunately, most series in the literature do not make a distinction between residual disease and separate areas of disease (Table 10–2).

All of the following series use the term multicentricity to mean residual disease in the mastectomy specimen. Benfield and colleagues[48] quote an incidence of 8 of 13, or 62 percent, multicentricity; Carter and Smith,[49] 31 of 49, or 63 percent; and Dall'Olmo and associates,[50] 14 of 25, or 56 percent.

Other authors state that there is multicentricity of the LCIS in the mastectomy specimen, including some areas of disease distinct and distant from the original area of diagnosis. However, they do not separate these patients from patients with residual disease. The studies that fall into this category include those by Farrow,[5] with 142 of 227, or 63 percent, "multicentric"; Lewison and Finney,[55] 21 of 34, or 62 percent, "multicentric"; and Newman,[57] 28 of 30, or 93 percent, "multicentric."

Haagensen makes a statement in his treatise on LCIS: "We conclude that lobular neoplasia is a multicentric disease affecting both lobules and ducts, usually in a number of foci, and often in both breasts."[54] However, he does not discuss the number of patients in whom he has seen this and how he comes to this conclusion.

Ringberg and colleagues[58] studied 16 patients with LCIS, 11 of whom had separate foci of LCIS in the mastectomy specimen for a multicentricity incidence of 69 percent. Two other patients had invasive carcinoma in the mastectomy specimens and one, DCIS.

In Rosen's series of 50 patients with LCIS treated with mastectomy, 30 patients had

TABLE 10–2. Bilaterality and Multicentricity of Lobular Carcinoma* in Situ *(LCIS)

	No. of Patients	*Bilateral LCIS (simultaneous)—No. Positive/No. Biopsies*	*Multicentricity or Residual LCIS in Mastectomy Specimen—No. Positive/No. of Mastectomy Specimens*
Andersen[71]	52	8/25 (32%)	9/19 (47%) (R and M)
Benfield et al.[48]	13	2/5 (40%)	8/13 (62%) (R)
Carter and Smith[49]	49	17/44 (39%)	31/49 (63%) (R)
Dall'Olmo et al.[50]	24	5/?	41/25 (56%) (R)
Erdreich et al.[52]	31	12/?	NA
Farrow[5]	270	33/?	142/227 (63%) (R and M)
Lewison and Finney[55]	40	7/15 (47%)	21/34 (62%) (R and M)
Newman[57]	26	4/18 (22%)	28/30 (93%) (R and M)
Ringberg et al.[58]	16	11/16 (69%)	11/16 (69%) (M)
Rosen et al.[72]	50	NA	30/50 (60%) (R and M) 24/50 (48%) (M)
Rosen et al.[73]	108	22/63 (35%)	NA
Sunshine et al.[63]	36	14/21 (67%)	NA
Urban[74]	26	9/26 (35%)	NA

R, residual; M, multicentric; NA, not available

persistent LCIS in the breast.[72] Twenty-four of these, or 48 percent of the total, had LCIS in quadrants other than the one in which the biopsy had been done. This is interesting, but there may be a selection bias in this study. Rosen and associates[59] also have a series of 99 patients, many of whom were retrospectively discovered and were treated by biopsy alone. It may be that their conservatively treated patients had less extensive disease and less multicentricity, but this is unknown. The reasons for treating some patients with mastectomy and not others is not explained in their study.

These data all suggest that LCIS has a high incidence of multicentricity in the breast containing the initially diagnosed lesion. However, more detailed and specific reporting of pathologic findings in these cases is necessary before an absolute conclusion can be drawn.

BILATERALITY

The issue of bilaterality has been discussed extensively in the literature, with a reported incidence of 12 to 69 percent (Table 10–2). There are many problems with most series discussing this feature of LCIS. These problems include small numbers of patients; inconsistency of sampling of the opposite breast; inclusion of previously, simultaneously, or subsequently occurring invasive disease as bilateral disease; and no distinction between noninvasive and invasive disease.

Farrow's series[5] has the largest number of patients for whom the status of the contralateral breast is known. His series included 270 patients with LCIS; 207 had unilateral LCIS, 29 bilateral LCIS, 30 ipsilateral LCIS and DCIS, and 4 contralateral LCIS and DCIS. There were 33 bilateral simultaneous lesions of LCIS and 16 subsequent contralateral lesions of LCIS, for a bilaterality incidence of 18 percent (49 of 270). Also, 70 patients had prior (34 patients), simultaneous (30 patients), or subsequent (6 patients) invasive cancer. The number of patients who had a contralateral biopsy is not given. This number probably underestimates the incidence, since many patients probably had no contralateral biopsy. Also, it must be pointed out that 34 of these patients also had DCIS.

One of the most widely quoted studies dealing with bilaterality is that of Newman,[57] who reported on 26 patients. Eighteen patients had contralateral biopsies; 4 of 18 (22 per cent) were positive for simultaneous bilateral LCIS. Two other patients had delayed (15 months and 24 months) contralateral biopsies, which were positive for LCIS. He recommended routine random biopsy of the contralateral breast, preferably in the upper outer quadrant, on the basis of his findings.

Subsequently, there have been several systematic approaches to the determination of bilaterality in LCIS. In 1977, Carter and Smith[49] reported on 49 patients with LCIS. Thirty-nine patients had a contralateral biopsy, of which 14 were positive for LCIS. An additional three of five patients who had bilateral mastectomies had bilateral LCIS. A total of 17 of 44 patients, or 39 percent, for whom the status of the contralateral breast was known had bilateral disease.

Urban[74] most consistently performs contralateral biopsies on patients with breast cancer. He reported on 26 patients with LCIS who had a contralateral biopsy. Ten of 26, or 38 percent, had a positive biopsy (nine positive for noninvasive disease, and one positive for invasive disease).

In Rosen's series of 125 patients with LCIS, 108 were treated with ipsilateral mastectomy.[73] Sixty-three of the 125 patients had contralateral biopsy. Twenty-two, or 35 percent, were positive for LCIS, and six invasive cancers were also discovered.

Ringberg's study of 73 patients with unilateral breast cancer is also quoted in bilaterality statistics.[58] Patients with *in situ* disease were treated with bilateral subcutaneous mastectomy and breast reconstructive surgery. However, not all patients with *in situ* disease agreed to this treatment; therefore, these data may be biased. Sixteen patients with LCIS were studied, and 11 (69 percent) of these had LCIS in the contralateral breast at mastectomy, and three more had DCIS.

Sunshine and associates[63] recently reported on a retrospective series of 36 patients with LCIS. Thirty-five patients had some form of ipsilateral mastectomy as treatment. Twenty-one of 36 patients (58 percent) had a simple mastectomy with low axillary dissection of the contralateral breast. LCIS was present in 14 of these contralateral mastectomy specimens (67 percent). This represents a bilaterality incidence of 39 percent of total patients in this series.

Evidence indicates that there is a substantial incidence of bilaterality of LCIS; thus, both breasts are at risk to develop LCIS at the same time. This is an important point to consider when making decisions about therapeutic intervention.

Incidence of Invasive Disease at Mastectomy for LCIS

Several reports exist in the literature regarding patients with LCIS who have been treated with mastectomy alone. The incidence of invasive cancer in the mastectomy specimen ranges from 0 to 13 percent. Carter and Smith[49] found 3 of 49, or 6 percent; Benfield,[48] 0 of 13, or 0 percent; Dall'Olmo,[50] 0 of 23, or 0 percent; Ringberg,[58] 2 of 16, or 13 percent; and Rosen,[72] 2 of 50, or 4 percent. This may seem low and may be so, since most series excluded those patients who had coincident invasive cancer at mastectomy in their reports.

Risk of Subsequent Invasive Carcinoma

The question as to whether LCIS is a precursor to invasive disease has been studied in detail. Obviously, the natural history of the disease is the most important issue regarding LCIS. If LCIS remains dormant, therapeutic intervention would be unnecessary. However, if invasive disease is the end point of LCIS or, alternatively, a larger proportion of patients with LCIS also develop coincident invasive cancer, measures to reduce lifetime mortality from breast cancer are needed. This could be either close clinical surveillance or surgical treatment.

Godwin[53] is credited with the first case report of a patient with a previous history of LCIS who developed lobular carcinoma. His patient was found to have lobular carcinoma in 1947, and in retrospect, a breast biopsy done in 1935 was reviewed. The specimen had contained cysts and LCIS. He felt that this case represented the evolution of an *in situ* cancer to an infiltrative phase of cancer over a 12-year period.

There appears to be a substantial incidence of invasive cancer associated with LCIS (Table 10–3). Based on a review of all series in the literature, the number of patients with LCIS developing invasive cancer either ipsilaterally or contralaterally is 2 to 38 percent.

The best way of determining the natural history of a disease is by following untreated patients for a prolonged period of time. Several series in the literature have followed untreated patients with LCIS. Unfortunately, these are largely retrospective studies of benign breast biopsies, in which the diagnosis of LCIS was missed at the time of the original biopsy. This may mean that the lesions of LCIS were very small, borderline, or otherwise "good actors." Obviously, this biases these studies of the natural history of LCIS.

The largest series of untreated LCIS is Haagensen's, consisting of cases from Co-

TABLE 10–3. Development of Invasive Cancers in Lobular Carcinoma *in Situ* (LCIS)

Author	No. of Patients	Average Follow-up (Years)	Subsequent Ipsilateral Invasive Cancer	Subsequent Contralateral or Previous Invasive Cancer	No. of Patients Developing Invasive Cancer
Andersen[75]	52	16	9/44 (20%)	9/52 (17) (5 previous)	15/52 (29%)
Carter and Smith[49]	49	8	1/49	?	1/49 (2%)
Farrow[5]	270 (34 patients LCIS and DCIS)	NA	?	70/270 (26%) (5 previous)	70/270 (26%)
Giordano and Klopp[76]	124	5	3/124 (2)	0	3/124 (2)
Haagensen et al.[54]	211 (1 lost)	14	19/193 (10%)	20/205 (10%) (1 previous)	36/210 (17%)
Hutter and Foote[77]	53 (46) (7 exclusions)	4–27	10/40 (25%)	4/40 (10%) (3 previous)	14/46 (30%)
Rosen et al.[59]	99 (84) (15 inevaluable)	24	19/84 (23%)	19/84 (23%) 3 previous	32/84 (38%) (1 unknown side)
Sunshine et al.[63]	36	10	?	?	1/36 (3%)
Webber et al.[61]	68	9	0	3/68 (4%)	3/68 (4%)
Wheeler et al.[62]	38	17.5	1/25 (4%)	5/34 (15%) (2 previous)	6/38 (16%)

lumbia-Presbyterian Medical Center.[54] A retrospective review of 5560 benign breast biopsies was undertaken, and 211 patients were found to have "lobular neoplasia" without invasion. The series included patients with bland, lobular neoplasia, which may have been classified by others at that time as atypical hyperplasia or borderline lesions.[34] Therefore, some physicians argue that the incidence of subsequent invasive disease may actually be higher than that which Haagensen reported in the series.[34]

The patients in Haagensen's series were treated with biopsy alone, with a mean follow-up time of 14 years. Seventeen percent of patients were followed for 20 years, and only two were lost to follow-up. Thirty-six patients, or 17 percent, had 38 cases of subsequent invasive cancer. There was one case in which a carcinoma had been diagnosed prior to the lobular neoplasia. There were 19 ipsilateral cancers and 20 contralateral cancers. The invasive cancer occurred up to 40 years after diagnosis (one patient had a prior diagnosis of carcinoma). The histology of the invasive cancers was not consistent and varied from small-cell neoplasia (lobular invasive) in 12 patients, to tubular cancers in three, intraductal cancers in nine, intraductal with other cancers in five, and other unspecified cancers in seven.

Haagensen and associates carefully looked at the variations in all their cases of lobular neoplasia. The extent of involvement or quantitative analysis did not predict subsequent invasive disease. They tried to determine which histologic features would indicate the patients most likely to develop invasive carcinoma. Microscopic variations, differing from the typical bland lobular neoplasia they had noted, frequently occurred. They described four patterns of these variations: loss of cohesiveness; increase in cell size; macroacinar pattern; and hyperchromatic, closely packed cell masses. Then, the extent of qualitative variations was tabulated for three different groups of patients: patients who subsequently developed invasive carcinoma; patients who did not develop invasive carcinoma; and those who had the persistence of lobular neoplasia when invasive carcinoma developed. No indication could be found in this analysis as to which patients were likely to develop invasive cancer. The only positive correlation was that the variations, either alone or in combination, were more likely to occur in patients with persisting lobular neoplasia at the time of diagnosis of invasive cancer. Another point that Haagensen and associates make about their microscopic analysis is that in the series, patients with what they called bland lobular neoplasia were just as likely to develop invasive cancer as those with the more florid microscopic variations. Their conclusion was that the presence of bland lobular neoplasia, which others have called atypical hyperplasia,[34] indicated a predilection to develop invasive cancer and that both conditions were part of the spectrum of the same disease.

As stated previously, 39 cancers were diagnosed in 36 patients, from 0 to 42 years after the diagnosis of LCIS. Six patients died of metastatic disease and two were alive with metastatic disease. None of these 36 patients had been given the diagnosis of LCIS at the time of their original biopsy and, therefore, had not received regular follow-up. Twenty-six patients were treated with radical mastectomy and were free of disease at the time of the report. Two patients died of intercurrent disease.

Haagensen and colleagues summarized the study by saying that patients with LCIS who were followed for 15 years had a cumulative probability of developing invasive cancer in the ipsilateral breast of 10 percent and in the contralateral breast of 9 percent. In those followed for 16 to 25 years, the risk in the ipsilateral breast was 22 percent and in the contralateral breast, 15 percent. Since the predisposition to cancer was equal in both breasts, the interval to cancer was long, and the cancers developing had favorable prognoses, the investigators recommended close clinical surveillance, which included breast palpation every four months.

There are several problems apparent in this study. First, it was a retrospective study. Second, the study included lesions diagnosed by many pathologists as atypical hyperplasia.[34] However, the investigators seem to have justified this, as previously discussed, by the finding that in either case the risk of subsequent invasive cancer was the same. Patients with bland lobular hyperplasia did not have a lower risk of developing invasive cancer, as suggested by other pathologists. Third, only patients with excisional biopsy alone were included in the series, indicating that those with the more aggressive-looking disease may have been treated with mastectomy. Also, there was only a small number of patients followed for 20 years (17 percent), making the projection of risk at 20 years tenuous. In spite of these objections, the study is carefully and thoughtfully done and indicates that both breasts are equally predisposed to invasive cancer. This does occur in a substantial proportion of patients.

Another series of largely untreated patients was reported by Hutter and Foote.[77] It consisted of 46 patients with LCIS, diagnosed at Memorial Sloan-Kettering Cancer Center (MSKCC) between 1940 and 1952. There were originally a total of 53 patients, with seven exclusions: three with a history of previous mastectomy, three lost to follow-up, and one because no current records were available. Of the 46 patients, 40 were treated with biopsy alone and six with radical mastectomy. Fifteen of 46 patients (33 percent) developed 20 cancers (noninvasive and invasive). Ten of 40 evaluable patients (six with previous mastectomy not included), or 25 percent, developed ipsilateral invasive cancer, and four of 40, or 10 percent, developed contralateral invasive cancer. Interestingly, only one half of the invasive cancers occurred within the first ten years of follow-up. The others occurred after more than ten years, indicating that there was still an increased risk many years after the initial diagnosis of LCIS. Hutter and Foote concluded that LCIS was a preinvasive form of cancer with high risk of subsequent invasive disease. They felt that modified radical mastectomy was the appropriate form of treatment.

Rosen and associates[59] have also reviewed and studied noninvasive breast cancer. They reviewed 8609 breast biopsies performed between 1940 and 1950 at MSKCC. Sixty-four patients with previously unrecognized LCIS, plus the 53 patients with the known diagnosis of LCIS reported by Hutter and Foote, were included, for a total of 117 patients. Eighteen patients were excluded for the following reasons: ipsilateral mastectomy in nine; intraductal carcinoma and LCIS in seven; and contralateral invasive carcinoma in two. This left 99 patients, of whom only 84 were evaluable and were followed for an average of 24 years. Therefore, in their analyses, a total of 33 patients, or 28 percent, were excluded.

The patients in Rosen's series were followed after biopsy alone. Twelve patients (14 percent) of 84 developed subsequent ipsilateral carcinoma; 12 (14 percent), contralateral carcinoma alone; seven (8 percent), bilateral carcinoma; and one, carcinoma unknown side. Thus, a total of 32 patients (38 percent) developed a subsequent carcinoma. The average interval to detecting invasive ductal cancer was 16.3 years and to detecting invasive lobular cancer, 20.4 years. Thirty-eight percent of subsequent invasive cancers were diagnosed 20 years after the biopsy was done for LCIS.

The histologic types of the subsequent carcinomas were varied and occurred in combination. This included DCIS in five patients; invasive ductal in 20; invasive lobular in 13; LCIS in ten; colloid in one; and tubular in one. The most frequent carcinoma was invasive ductal, seen in 11 ipsilateral cancers and nine contralateral cancers.This is an interesting finding, indicating that LCIS itself may not become invasive but that its presence indicates predisposition to cancer. It is also possible, since there was such a long time to diagnosis of invasive cancer, that the LCIS and invasive cancer were entirely unrelated.

Rosen and colleagues felt that it was important to determine whether the incidence of breast cancer increased subsequent to the diagnosis of LCIS. They compared their patients with a representative population from the Connecticut Tumor Registry. To do this analysis, they excluded patients with previous or simultaneous contralateral carcinoma, unknown age at diagnosis of subsequent cancer, unknown age of diagnosis of LCIS, and unknown age at last follow-up. This left 77 patients from the original 117. Therefore, for this analysis, 40 patients with the known diagnosis of LCIS (34 percent) were excluded from the original 117 patients. Twenty-eight patients of these 77 (36 percent) developed breast cancer. In a normal population of women similar to those in the Connecticut Tumor Registry, 3.1 cases of breast cancer would be expected. Therefore, this was nine times greater. Since 1.5 deaths due to breast cancer would be expected, the 16 patients who died of breast cancer from this group of 77 represented a 10.7 times increase in breast cancer deaths. The conclusion was that a significantly increased risk of developing invasive cancer and of dying from it occurs subsequent to the diagnosis of LCIS.

While these findings are provocative, it must be emphasized that this was a retrospective analysis, and many exclusions occurred. It can be said from Rosen's study that there does seems to be a trend for increased incidence of invasive cancer in these patients, with equal distribution between breasts.

Another series of patients that addresses the development of invasive cancer in patients with LCIS was reported by Andersen in 1974.[47] He retrospectively reviewed 3299 benign breast biopsies from the Institute of Pathology, Bispebjerg Hospital, Copenhagen, with a mean follow-up of 15.9 years. There were 52 cases of LCIS without evidence of invasion that involved at least a single lobule. Forty-four patients had been treated with biopsy alone. Eleven patients (25 percent) developed 13 invasive cancers: nine ipsilateral (20 percent) and four contralateral (9 percent) (two bilateral). The histology included seven invasive lobular cancers, five invasive other, and one invasive lobular with invasive other. The incidence of development of invasive cancer was 12 times the expected frequency. The average interval to the development of invasive cancer was nine years. Five of these patients developed metastatic disease, with four deaths. It must be remembered that these patients were retrospectively found to have LCIS and did not have careful follow-up. Andersen felt that treatment of LCIS with close follow-up (four clinical examinations a year and yearly mammograms) was a viable alternative to mastectomy.

Wheeler and colleagues[62] retrospectively reviewed 4898 benign breast biopsies performed from 1948 to 1960 at the Hospital of the University of Pennsylvania. Also included were other cases diagnosed from 1960 to 1963. Thirty-eight patients were found to have had LCIS alone, and 57, associated invasive cancer. The discussion includes the 38 patients with LCIS alone. Thirteen underwent mastectomy, with no evidence of invasive cancer in any of the mastectomy specimens. The remaining 25 patients were the subject of the paper. They were followed for an average of 17.5 years after biopsy alone. Only one woman of 25 (4 percent) developed ipsilateral invasive cancer. Thirty-two patients had an evaluable contralateral breast, and three (9.7 percent) developed invasive cancer. This was a much lower incidence of ipsilateral invasive cancer than that in previous studies. However, it must be remembered that 57 patients with a combination of LCIS and invasive cancer were excluded. This may have biased the results toward patients with less aggressive disease, thus improving the eventual outcome.

The subset of Wheeler's patients with LCIS and associated invasive cancer is interesting. Thirteen of 57 patients had associated lobular carcinoma, and 8 of 57, invasive lobular and invasive ductal carcinomas. Therefore, a total of 21 of 57 (37 percent) had associated invasive lobular cancer. Thirty-five patients with LCIS had associated intraductal cancer, and eight, intraductal and invasive lobular cancers. Forty-three patients (75 percent) had invasive ductal cancer associated with LCIS. The point of looking at the histology of invasive cancers associated with LCIS is to try to determine whether LCIS is a preinvasive form of cancer leading to lobular carcinoma or whether the presence of LCIS indicates a general tendency of the breasts to develop cancer. Wheeler's study revealed a high incidence of intraductal cancer as the only form of invasive cancer associated with LCIS.[62] This would seem to indicate that these patients are in general at increased risk to develop cancer. However, Wheeler and colleagues concluded that since the association of LCIS with lobular invasive cancer was frequent in the study and also was well documented in the literature, this was an indication that LCIS was a preinvasive form of cancer. This conclusion was based on Newman's study of 73 patients with lobular carcinoma:[66] of these 73 patients with lobular carcinoma, 72 had associated LCIS.

Haagensen and associates[64] present a series of 237 patients with lobular neoplasia (LCIS) coexisting with invasive breast carcinoma. All patients were treated with mastectomy. The associated invasive cancers were: 32 percent small cell (lobular invasive) cancers alone; 31 percent DCIS alone; 18 percent small-cell and other forms; and the remainder ranging from mucoid to no particular type. It was felt that small-cell (lobular) carcinoma evolved directly from lobular neoplasia. The investigators made this statement on the basis of their own microscopic examination of these specimens. Also, it was felt that in this series, DCIS evolved directly from lobular neoplasia.

Another fact supporting the nature of the LCIS as a precursor to other cancers is that LCIS can spread in a pagetoid manner.[78] This occurs by centripetal movement toward the nipple. In this way, LCIS extends into the larger ducts and can appear as DCIS or infiltrating ductal carcinoma.

Rosen and colleagues,[59] on the other hand, present data that subsequent cancers may not be related to the original LCIS. A group of 75 of their patients with LCIS treated at diagnosis with mastectomy had an 11 percent incidence of DCIS in other areas of the mastectomy specimen. Therefore, it was concluded that two distinct types of cancer were present at diagnosis. In patients who had been followed after biopsy alone for LCIS, the foci of DCIS in the remainder of the breast may be the site that exhibits the cancer in the future.

In conclusion, the development of subsequent invasive cancer in patients with LCIS has been reported to range from 2 to 38 percent. Most series report an equal incidence in both breasts. These series, along with the high incidence of multicentricity and bilaterality suggested by other studies, support the hypothesis that both breasts should be considered as one organ in patients with LCIS and both have an equal breast cancer risk. Also, the histologies of the invasive cancers that do occur vary. If LCIS is a precursor to invasive cancer, infiltrating lobular carcinoma should be the result in all cases. Since all types of cancer are seen, it would appear that these patients are in general at increased risk to develop cancer.

Axillary Lymph Node Metastases

Cases of LCIS with axillary metastases have rarely been documented in the literature. The earliest recorded case was in 1949 by Cogswell.[79] He illustrated a case that would be classified as LCIS today. The patient was reported to have multiple axillary node metastases. A 1-cm tumor was described, and it is not clear whether this lesion was carefully examined for evidence of invasive disease. Next, the BCDDP's data document 1 of 50 cases (2 percent) of LCIS to have one to three axillary node metastases.[9] Rosen[80] describes four patients who presented with axillary node metastases, which led to the diagnosis of LCIS. Exhaustive microscopic review of the mastectomy specimen revealed no evidence of invasive disease.

One other series reports one case of axillary node metastases in LCIS. Carter and Smith[49] report an incidence of 2 percent node positivity (1 of 49 patients). However, they do have three patients in the series with invasive carcinoma in the mastectomy specimen and do not state that one of these patients had positive nodes. It appears that none of the patients with LCIS alone had node positivity.

There are no other reported cases with node positivity in LCIS. Therefore, it can be seen that the presence of positive lymph nodes in patients with LCIS alone is a rare occurrence.

Treatment

The treatment of LCIS has varied widely and, to date, there is no consensus on the optimal treatment. The reason for this is that the natural history of LCIS has not been determined conclusively, as can be seen by the previous data. Therapy has been based on the opinions of various physicians as to the natural history of the disease. On one side, there are those who feel that LCIS is a preinvasive form of cancer, leading eventually to invasive cancer.[77] On the other side are those who feel that LCIS is a benign entity, occurring in patients predisposed to cancer.[54]

Another problem confounding treatment decision making in these patients is the different thresholds used by pathologists for making the diagnosis of LCIS. There are many borderline lesions that would be called atypical hyperplasia by some pathologists and LCIS by others. If the pathologist knows that no treatment will be undertaken besides biopsy, the diagnosis of LCIS may be made more readily. However, if treatment with mastectomy is the policy, the diagnosis of LCIS in these borderline cases will be made more reluctantly. These problems can obviously bias selection of patients.

The treatment options discussed next include (1) observation after excisional biopsy, with frequent follow-up; (2) re-excision for microscopically clear margins and then surveillance, (3) hormonal treatment after excisional biopsy, (4) ipsilateral mastectomy, (5) ipsilateral mastectomy, with contralateral biopsy and mastectomy if biopsy is positive, and (6) bilateral mastectomies.

Several studies support biopsy alone as treatment for LCIS. They will be discussed first. The American College of Surgeons conducted a survey of noninvasive breast carcinoma in 1978.[2] They identified 121 cases of LCIS, which amounted to 1.4 percent of the breast carcinomas reported in that survey. Patients were treated with eight different surgical procedures, ranging from biopsy alone to superradical mastectomy. Thirty-one patients had wedge excision, and two had biopsy alone, with no recurrences in either group. There was no statistically significant difference in the five-year disease-free survival rates in patients treated with conservative versus more radical surgical treatments. As discussed previously, Haagensen also believed in conservative management by biopsy alone and physical examination every four months.[54] He felt that LCIS was a benign entity with a predisposition to subsequent carcinoma to a limited degree, frequently after a long interval. It was believed that both breasts were at equal risk and, therefore, should be treated equally in this disease. Bilateral mastectomies were not seen as justified because of the belief that there was a low likelihood of these patients' presenting with noncurable disease and dying of metastatic disease. However, this statement is not documented by Haagensen's series because of the limited follow-up of these patients. It was the *hope* that the mortality would be small after follow-up alone. Wheeler and colleagues[62] also felt that biopsy alone was the treatment of choice. Their series reported a low incidence of subsequent ipsilateral (1 of 25, or 4 percent) and contralateral (3 of 37, or 9.7 percent) invasive carcinomas. Giordano and Klopp[76] followed 19 patients with LCIS treated with excisional biopsy alone. Two of these 19 patients developed ipsilateral invasive lobular cancer. They both were treated with radical mastectomy, had negative nodes, and remained free of disease. Therefore, there was no increase in mortality in these patients followed by biopsy alone.

There are several disadvantages with this treatment approach. Studies such as Andersen's[47] support a fairly substantial incidence of subsequent invasive carcnoma. Of his 44 patients treated with biopsy alone, 11 patients developed 13 invasive cancers. Five (11 percent) of these patients developed metastases, with four deaths from invasive breast carcinoma. Another problem concerns the follow-up of these patients. It is hoped that with current mammographic techniques, subsequent carcinomas will be detected while small enough to have a low node positivity and a high cure rate. However, it is unlikely that all will be detected early. Also, even those detected early have about a 10 to 20 percent incidence of node positivity.[4, 32] Finally, to ensure close, lifelong follow-up, as is recommended, the patient and the physician must be well motivated and willing to continue close surveillance.

Most researchers do not discuss the surgical margins in their series of LCIS treated with biopsy alone. However, re-excision to obtain microscopically clear surgical margins is important. Re-excision is necessary to remove all known disease and, thus, enable pathologists to search for invasive disease and associated cancers such as DCIS or infiltrating ductal carcinoma.

No medical therapeutic trials, such as that with an antiestrogen or possibly danazol (a synthetic androgen that also suppresses LH and FSH output), are being undertaken in the study of LCIS. Theoretically, if the lesions of LCIS are hormonally dependent, this may be an effective form of treatment. Prospective trials in this area are needed.

Ipsilateral mastectomy has been the treatment of choice of many physicians.[48–50, 55, 57, 59, 73, 76, 77] Rosen and colleagues[72] feel that because of the multicentricity of the disease (48 percent in their series) and the possibility of coexistent invasive disase (0 to 6 percent), total mastectomy with low axillary dissection is the treatment of choice. It is their belief that the mortality from breast cancer in these patients will be decreased with such an approach. In Rosen's own series of 99 patients treated with excisional biopsy alone, 32 developed subsequent invasive carcinoma.[59] Sixteen of these patients died of the disease. Of these 16, six had developed invasive disease in their ipsilateral breast, five in the contralateral, and five bilaterally. Because of the increased risk in the contralateral breast, contralateral biopsy in the upper outer quadrant was recommended. According to Rosen's experience, women with negative contralateral biopsies are at a lower risk to develop carcinoma. The pitfall of this treatment is the possibility of sampling error with a random biopsy. Also, since both breasts have an equal cancer risk, only half of the disease is being treated.

Recurrences of cancer after mastectomy for LCIS are rare. Giordano and Klopp[76] reviewed all breast biopsies done at George Washington University from 1953 through 1971 and found 124 cases of LCIS among 8000 biopsies. In 105 patients, the treatment was simple mastectomy with low axillary dissection, and the other patients previously discussed were treated with excision alone. One of 105 patients developed a chest wall lesion four years after treatment. It was felt to be a recurrence in a focus of breast tissue not removed by the original surgery. This patient died of metastatic disease. This series supports the use of a surgical technique that will remove all breast tissue possible, if mastectomy is chosen as treatment. In Sunshine's series of 36 patients (97 percent treated with mastectomy), there was one recurrence four years postoperatively.[63] This patient had had an ipsilateral radical and contralateral simple mastectomy. The histology of recurrent disease is not given.

The ideal surgical procedure is total mastectomy with a low axillary dissection. The axillary dissection is done not to remove nodes but to remove any breast tissue that may be in the tail of the axilla. Hicken[81] studied 385 breasts mammographically and found mammary ducts in 95 percent of the axillas and 15 percent of the epigastric areas. Therefore, to ensure a thorough removal of all breast tissue, a low axillary dissection should be done. If this is done, the patient with LCIS has an almost 100 percent chance of cure in the ipsilateral breast.

However, again the problem with this choice of treatment is the substantial risk of contralateral LCIS and invasive cancer. The last treatment option is bilateral mastectomies, recommended by at least two groups of investigators.[58, 63] The arguments in favor of this treatment have already been given, even by those physicians who recommend excision alone, such as Haagensen,[54] that is, that LCIS is a bilateral and multicentric disease, putting both breasts at equal risk for the development of invasive cancer. Bilateral mastectomies obviate the risk of future invasive cancer. As previously mentioned, with mastectomy thoroughly performed, there is essentially a 100 percent cure of LCIS. This option should be considered, especially in a patient who cannot live comfortably with the knowledge of her increased risk for developing cancer. Also, this option may be more justified in a patient who also has a positive family history or diffusely nodular breasts that make physical examination and mammography more difficult to interpret. The obvious problem with this radical surgical approach is that the woman loses a valued part of her body, which can interfere with her self-image and sexuality. Such radical treatment is certainly unnecessary in many cases, since the natural history of LCIS clearly shows that the majority of women will not develop subsequent invasive cancer.

The patient should be made aware of the

available breast reconstruction procedures, if bilateral mastectomies are done. Breast reconstruction has been a very positive force in breast cancer surgery. It can make the loss of breasts less frightening to a patient, and after simple mastectomy, cosmetic results are excellent.

The treatment of LCIS is by no means clear-cut. Re-excision is recommended if necessary for clear surgical margins and close clinical follow-up, including physical examination at least every four to six months and yearly mammography in most patients. The patient should be made aware of the controversial nature of the treatment for this disease and should participate in the decision making. She should also be made aware of the potentially increased risk of developing invasive carcinoma. The physician and the patient must be willing to commit themselves to close lifelong follow-up. A viable alternative is that of bilateral total mastectomies with low axillary dissections, especially in the patients described earlier, such as those with a positive family history, dysplastic breasts on examination, multiple biopsies for suspicious lesions, or unremitting anxiety about the development of invasive cancer. Ipsilateral mastectomy is not recommended in any patient, because of the predisposition of both breasts to the development of invasive cancer.

DUCTAL CARCINOMA IN SITU

Intraepithelial, noninvasive carcinoma of the mammary ducts is most commonly referred to as intraductal carcinoma. This can be confusing to clinicians who frequently understand this to mean "duct" carcinoma and consider it to be invasive. We prefer to use the term ductal carcinoma *in situ*, which is more specific and indicates the noninvasive character of the lesion.

Unlike LCIS, DCIS is generally accepted to be a malignant disease that will become invasive and will metastasize if left untreated.[22] This section will discuss the development of DCIS, the presence of coexistent invasive disease in mastectomy specimens, the status of axillary nodes, the occurrence of multicentricity and bilaterality, the progression to invasive cancer, and finally, treatment.

Two physicians are responsible for the most important early literature concerning DCIS. In 1934, Bloodgood, a surgeon at Johns Hopkins University, described comedocarcinoma and "comedo with areas of fully developed cancer of the breast."[82] Among his patients with pure comedocarcinoma, none had axillary node metastases and one died of breast cancer. Bloodgood recommended radiation therapy after local excision for these patients.

Cheatle of King's College Hospital, London, studied DCIS by doing whole-organ sectioning of breasts in the early twentieth century.[34] He found that comedocarcinoma rarely occurred in a pure form but usually in coexistence with other forms that he described as cribriform, micropapillary, and papillary. Today four growth patterns of ductal carcinoma *in situ* are described: solid, comedo, papillary, and cribriform.[22] Others also include intracystic.[21] Usually, a mixture of these subtypes is seen in lesions of DCIS.

The incidence of DCIS diagnosed in women ranges from 0.8 to 5 percent of breast cancers.[2–4] DCIS has also been reported in 3 to 9 percent of cases of male breast cancer.[83] The actual frequency of DCIS in the general population is unknown. Nielsen and colleagues[84] studied 83 consecutive, unselected, female autopsy cases with a median age of 67 years to try to determine the actual frequency of preinvasive breast cancer. This study was done in Denmark, where autopsies are performed in 52 percent of all deaths. At autopsy, bilateral total mastectomies with partial axillary dissections were done on all patients. The results revealed seven cases of infiltrating ductal cancer (six diagnosed during the patient's lifetime), and 14 cases of *in situ* cancer (eight DCIS, three LCIS, and three DCIS and LCIS). The frequency of DCIS was eight times the expected incidence. It is conceivable that the actual incidence is this high in the general population but that lesions either regress or are not detected during a lifetime. Other autopsy studies do not report such a high incidence of DCIS,[23, 24, 85] but they may not have been done as carefully and in unselected autopsy cases.

Development

It has been postulated that DCIS is a preinvasive stage of cancer that is present for a prolonged period and eventually evolves to an invasive cancer. Gallager and Martin[20] proposed that breast carcinoma begins in the normal mammary epithelium. They felt that normal epithelium became hyperplastic and, after a latent period, became *in situ* carcinoma and eventually invasive cancer. This hypothesis was tested by studying 60 breasts from radical mastectomies by whole-organ sectioning.[86] Forty-seven of the 60 specimens contained invasive carcinomas, while eight contained noninvasive carcinoma. Of these 47 breasts, 22 contained multiple invasive sites. In most cases, the invasive cancer was located along the course of a duct containing atypical hyperplasia or carcinoma *in situ*, or both. It was concluded that atypical hyperplasia was a precursor to DCIS and that DCIS was a stage occurring prior to the development of invasive cancer.

Silverberg and Chitale[87] did an extensive study in 1973 attempting to quantify the spectrum of changes occurring from pure intraductal, or DCIS, to pure invasive ductal cancer. They retrospectively studied 267 mastectomy specimens containing DCIS or invasive ductal cancer and divided the carcinomas into six groups, based on relative amounts of invasive cancer present (pure DCIS to pure invasive). There were 14 cases of pure DCIS; 14 with less than 10 percent infiltration; 16 with 10 to 49 percent infiltration; 26 with 50 to 89 percent infiltration; 64 with 90 to 99 percent infiltration; and 133 with pure invasive carcinoma. Fifty percent of the patients had pure invasive cancer. The average age of the patients was essentially the same in all groups (58.1 years in the pure DCIS and 57.1 in the pure invasive). The researchers looked at the size of tumors relative to infiltration and found no tendency for tumors with greater degrees of invasiveness to be larger. The proportions of tumors greater than 5.5 cm in diameter were equal in all six groups: 21 to 25 percent. Next, lymph node involvement was examined. Patients with pure DCIS had no positive nodes, and with increasing amounts of invasive cancer, the involvement of lymph nodes increased to 67.9 percent in patients with pure invasive cancer. Survival was related to degree of invasiveness, with a 78.6 percent five-year survival rate for pure DCIS and a progressive decrease in the survival rate to 45 percent in patients with pure invasive cancer. There were no deaths from cancer in the pure DCIS group or the group with less than 10 percent infiltration. The breast cancer death rate was 20 percent in the group with 10 to 49 percent infiltration; 26.1 percent in the group with 50 to 89 percent infiltration; 37.5 percent in the group with 90 to 99 percent infiltration; and 44.1 percent in the group with pure infiltrating ductal carcinoma. In summary, survival decreased with increasing amounts of invasion.

These data could be interpreted in two ways. One is that the time period for transition from preinvasive to invasive carcinoma is very short. This is supported by the observation that there was not a progression of age as the amount of invasiveness increased. If there was a long latent period, one would expect an age difference in the group. The second possibility is that pure DCIS and infiltrating cancer arise by two different mechanisms. Arguments against this include the work of Ozzello, who describes microinvasion by electon microscopy in almost all cases of DCIS that he reviewed.[38, 39] Also, as will be discussed later in the chapter, there is a high incidence of progression to invasive cancer if DCIS is left untreated.[34, 88, 89]

Age at Diagnosis

The age at diagnosis of patients with DCIS ranges from 51 to 59 years (Table 10–4).[2, 49, 88, 90–93] This is similar to the average age at diagnosis of patients with invasive ductal cancer in the United States, which ranges from 50 to 60 years.[21, 94]

Clinical Findings

Most patients reported in the literature have presented with a palpable mass containing the DCIS (Table 10–5).[88, 90–93, 95–97] In reviewing eight series, 281 of 376 patients (75

TABLE 10–4. Age at Diagnosis of Patients with Ductal Carcinoma in Situ (DCIS)

Author	No. of Patients	Mean Age (Years)
Ashikari et al.[90]	87	53
Brown et al.[91]	40	59
Carter and Smith[49]	38	54
Page et al.[88]	28	52
Rosner et al.[2]	202	54
von Rueden and Wilson[92]	53	51
Westbrook and Gallager[93]	64	55

TABLE 10–5. Presenting Symptoms in Patients with Ductal Carcinoma in Situ (DCIS)

Authors	Mass	Nipple Discharge
Ashikari et al.[90]	98/112 (88%)	26/112 (23%)
Betsill et al.[95]	13/15 (87%)	0/15 (0%)
Brown et al.[91]	34/40 (85%)	1/40 (3%)
Gillis et al.[96]	15/36 (42%)	9/36 (25%)
Millis and Thynne[97]	24/28 (86%)	5/28 (18%)
Page et al.[88]	26/28 (79%)	0/28 (0%)
von Rueden and Wilson[92]	38/53 (72%)	11/53 (21%)
Westbrook and Gallager[93]	33/64 (52%)	16/64 (25%)
Total	281/376 (75%)	68/376 (18%)

percent) presented with a mass. Sixty-eight of 376 (18 percent) presented with a nipple discharge, which in most cases was bloody.

However, with better mammographic screening techniques, more occult *in situ* ductal cancers are being diagnosed before they become palpable. In the BCDDP study, 143 of 212 cases of DCIS (67 percent) were detected by mammography alone.[8, 9] Only four (1.8 percent) were detected by physical examination alone, whereas 60 (28 percent) were found by a combination of mammography and physical examination. Schwartz and associates[98] retrospectively reviewed 557 cases of clinically occult breast lesions, which were detected only by mammography. All patients had biopsies performed, and 31 percent were positive for carcinoma. Twenty-six percent of the cancers were DCIS. These studies emphasize the importance of screening mammography in detecting lesions with a good prognosis, such as DCIS.

Multicentricity and Bilaterality

MULTICENTRICITY

Multicentricity is defined differently among pathologists. The general definition given by McDivitt is "the presence of two or more separate foci of carcinoma within the breast which are thought to have arisen independently in response to the same carcinogenic stimulus."[99] Some pathologists require separation of areas of disease into different breast quadrants,[84, 92, 98] while others require separation only by areas of normal tissue.[58, 90] Multicentricity has been reported to occur in 19 to 76 percent of patients with the diagnosis of DCIS.[22, 49, 58, 72, 84, 90–92, 98, 100] The most carefully reported studies done in this area are by Brown,[91] von Rueden,[92] Nielsen,[84] Lagios,[100] and Schwartz.[98]

Brown and colleagues[91] retrospectively analyzed 52 patients with DCIS, excluding 12 cases from the multicentricity assessment because of inadequate samples (two cases) or change of diagnosis (eight to invasive and two to benign). Multicentricity was defined as tumor in more than one quadrant or when in the same quadrant, within one or more major lactiferous ducts. Multicentricity was found in 13 of 40 cases (33 percent).

Von Rueden and Wilson[92] also did a retrospective review of 55 patients with DCIS (two male) and were able to evaluate 47 for multicentricity after mastectomy. They found multicentricity (more than one quadrant involved, by their definition) in 18 of 47 (38 percent).

Lagios and associates[100] defined multicentricity as a lesion at a distance of 5 cm from the primary tumor. In very careful and extensive studies, they employed whole-organ sectioning on specimens from mastectomies that had been done for DCIS. Multicentricity was found in 17 of 53 (32 percent) of the mastectomy specimens. Multicentricity increased with the increasing size of the primary lesion and occurred in 4 of 29 tumors (14 percent) 25 mm or less in diameter and in 13 of 25 (54 percent) of those 26 mm or larger.

Nielsen and colleagues[84] studied multicentricity of DCIS in their autospy series of 83 women. Fourteen cases of *in situ* cancer were diagnosed, eight with DCIS alone and three with DCIS and LCIS. Multicentricity, defined as lesions in more than one quadrant of the breast, was present in 4 of 11 cases of DCIS (36 percent).

Schwartz and associates[98] have been interested in the incidence of multicentricity in nonpalpable or clinically occult breast cancers that have been detected by mammography. In a series of 52 cancers detected by mammography alone, 14 (27 percent) were DCIS. Eleven of the 14 patients were treated with mastectomy, while three refused further therapy after biopsy. Multicentricity was defined as disease in a quadrant other than that of the primary tumor. Five of these 11 patients had multicentric disease: four DCIS and one LCIS. Therefore, in the specimens studied, 45.5 percent had multicentric carcinoma, or more specifically, 36 percent had multicentric DCIS.

Ringberg and associates[58] also commented on the presence of multicentricity in their patients with DCIS, describing it as "microscopically clearly separated foci of carcinoma." Of their 23 patients with DCIS, 16 (70 percent) had multicentric carcinoma. Two patients had invasive cancer (many authors would exclude these patients), two LCIS, and 12 DCIS. Multicentric DCIS alone occurred in 12 of 23, or 52 percent of patients.

Ashikari and associates[90] at MSKCC described multifocal disease as carcinoma in more than one tissue block. This is not necessarily multicentric disease as defined by McDivitt.[99] There were 143 patients with DCIS. However, 30 patients with associated Paget's disease of the nipple and one male were excluded, leaving 112 patients in the report. Eighty-eight had pure DCIS, classified according to subtype as 41 cribriform, 28 solid, 12 papillary, 6 comedo, and 1 intracystic. The remaining 24 had associated LCIS. Multifocal carcinoma was reported in 36 of 112 patients (32 percent). It was not specified whether the disease was DCIS or LCIS.

Rosen and colleagues[72] described 53 cases of DCIS also drawn from the MSKCC experience. Thirty patients had residual DCIS alone at mastectomy, and ten of these included foci of disease in other quadrants. Therefore, the incidence of multicentricity of DCIS was 19 percent.

Wanebo reports residual foci of DCIS in 60 percent of breasts after excisional biopsy.[22] Contesso and Petit reported residual disease in 76 percent of 47 patients with DCIS in the mastectomy specimen.[22] One other study done by Carter and Smith[49] included 38 cases of DCIS. They found residual DCIS in 25 mastectomy specimens (66 percent) and occult Paget's disease in five patients (13 percent). In these three studies, residual disease is not equal to multicentricity as defined by McDivitt.

In summary, evidence both from meticulously done studies with whole-organ sectioning and from careful reporting of findings in the literature reveals about a 35 percent incidence of multicentricity in DCIS. This incidence is taken from series that define multicentricity as carcinoma in more than one quadrant.

BILATERALITY

Bilaterality of DCIS has been reported to occur in 0 to 30 percent of patients. These data are very fragmentary. The important points to consider in these studies are the number of patients who had a contralateral biopsy, the reason for the biopsy, and the type of disease present in the contralateral breast.

Von Rueden's study of 53 patients reported bilaterality in nine patients (17 percent).[92] Three of these patients had contralateral DCIS, and six invasive cancer. However, it is not stated how many patients had biopsies performed on the contralateral side and why they were performed. It is possible that the patients who had biopsies had symptoms or signs leading to a diagnostic procedure or that they were high-risk patients with a positive family history.

In Carter's series of 38 patients with DCIS, only ten of the patients (26 percent) had a contralateral biopsy.[49] In only one of these patients was the biopsy positive for DCIS (3 percent of total patients in the study).

Westbrook's study of 64 patients, which excluded patients with previous or concurrent ipsilateral invasive disease and LCIS, reported contralateral biopsy information on 14 patients (22 percent).[93] Five of these 14 had DCIS, and three invasive cancer. Again, the reasons for biopsy in these patients are not given.

Ashikari and colleagues[90] reported that 16 of 112 of their patients (14 percent) had a simultaneous contralateral biopsy that was positive (11 for invasive cancer, four for LCIS, and one for DCIS). Seventeen more patients had had previous contralateral mastectomy for cancer (15 invasive and two DCIS). Again, the reasons for contralateral biopsy as well as the number of patients with biopsies are not given. Furthermore, 24 of the 112 patients had both LCIS and DCIS.

Urban[74] reported an incidence of simultaneous bilateral cancer in DCIS of 0 percent in 16 women who had a contralateral biopsy also treated at MSKCC. Three of these women, however, had had a previous contralateral mastectomy (two for invasive cancer and one for noninvasive).

Rosen[34] studied 64 patients with DCIS also drawn from the MSKCC population. The overlap among his, Urban's and Ashikari's data is not known. The status of the opposite breast was known in 34 cases (53 percent). Five of 34 (15 percent) had previous carcinoma and 4 of 34 (12 percent) had concurrent contralateral carcinoma (described as ductal) for a total incidence of 26 percent (9 of 34).

Ringberg's study of 23 women with DCIS is different in that the recommendation for treatment of DCIS was bilateral mastectomies.[58] The study encompassed 102 unilateral cancers of all kinds, for which 73 patients (72 percent) had bilateral operations ranging from subcutaneous mastectomy to reduction mammoplasty in the contralateral breast. Five patients with DCIS refused a bilateral operation but had at least a unilateral subcutaneous mastectomy. Therefore, bilateral information was available on 18 of the patients (78 percent) with DCIS. Seven of these patients (30 percent) had bilateral carcinoma (two invasive, two LCIS, and three DCIS). It should also be noted that examination of the ipsilateral mastectomy specimens in these 23 patients revealed two patients with invasive disease (9 percent), two with coincident LCIS, and 12 with residual DCIS.

Sunshine and associates[63] recently reported on 70 patients with DCIS. The recommendation for treatment was also bilateral mastectomies. Twenty-three of 70 patients (33 percent) had a contralateral mastectomy. The mastectomy specimen was positive for DCIS in seven, or 30 percent, of those treated with bilateral mastectomies. This represents a bilaterality incidence of 10 percent of total patients.

In summary, these studies are inconclusive and too highly biased to determine the actual incidence of simultaneous bilateral DCIS. However, it can be said that patients with a diagnosis of unilateral DCIS need careful follow-up of the contralateral breast. These patients may have an increased risk of developing cancer in that breast, but the exact incidence is unknown.

Incidence of Invasive Disease Coexistent with DCIS

If carefully examined pathologically, a substantial number of patients originally diagnosed as having DCIS will be found to have areas of invasion. This is exemplified by the following two reports. Gillis and colleagues[96] reviewed a total of 50 cases diagnosed as DCIS at the Mayo Clinic. In many instances, new blocks were cut to look for any evidence of invasion. In 14 of the cases (28 percent), areas of invasion were discovered. Also, Brown and associates[91] reviewed 52 cases diagnosed as DCIS and found that 8 (15 percent) actually had areas of invasion. These studies stress the importance of a thorough and extensive review of specimens that appear to contain DCIS alone. The diagnosis of DCIS should be rendered only after multiple cuts of a biopsy specimen are made. The recommendation is that at least eight to ten slides be cut and examined.[21]

The frequency of finding invasive disease at mastectomy in patients with a biopsy diagnosis of DCIS ranges from 6 to 21 percent (Table 10–6). One of the most carefully done studies was by Lagios, using whole-organ sectioning.[100] The incidence of occult invasive disease was found to be 21 percent. Of the 24 lesions 25 mm in diameter or larger, 11 (46 percent) showed invasion, while among the 20 lesions less than 25 mm in diameter, there were no instances of occult invasion. The conclusion was that the extent of the noninvasive lesions is an important predictor of occult invasion. This conclusion is in contrast with that of Silverberg and Chitale,[87] who found no difference in the amount of invasiveness relative to the size of the tumor.

Rosen's series of 53 patients with DCIS found invasive carcinoma in 3 of 50 patients (6 percent) at mastectomy.[72] Von Rueden and Wilson[92] found invasion in 6 of 47 mastectomy specimens (11 percent). Carter and Smith[49] found invasion in 7 of 38 (18 percent). In summary, with careful scrutiny of the biopsy alone or of the mastectomy specimen, occult invasive carcinoma is found in 6 to 21 percent of patients diagnosed as having DCIS.

Development of Subsequent Invasive Cancer

The natural history of a disease is an important factor in deciding on treatment.

TABLE 10–6. Invasive Cancer in Patients with Ductal Carcinoma *in Situ* (DCIS) at Mastectomy

Author	*No. of Patients*	*Mastectomy Specimens with Invasive Cancer*
Carter and Smith[49]	38	7 (18%)
Lagios et al.[100]	53	11 (21%)
von Rueden and Wilson[92]	47	6 (11%)
Rosen et al.[72]	50	3 (6%)
Ringberg et al.[58]	23	2 (9%)
	191	27 (14%)

There are two large retrospective studies that include patients followed after original biopsy only.

Betsill and colleagues[95] retrospectively reviewed 8609 benign breast biopsies and found 25 patients with previously undiagnosed DCIS. Ten patients were available for long-term follow-up. Seven of ten patients developed subsequent ipsilateral invasive carcinoma after an average interval of 9.7 years, with five having positive axillary nodes. Four of seven patients had cancers in the same quadrant as the original biopsy, one in an adjacent quadrant, and two unknown. Two of these patients died of metastatic breast cancer, and two others were alive with metastatic cancer. The conclusion reached was that DCIS was a preinvasive disease, and it was felt that mastectomy would be an effective form of treatment.

Rosen[34] recently updated this series in his article on intraepithelial carcinoma. He states that there were 30 women with DCIS who had been treated with biopsy alone. Follow-up information was available on 15 patients. The average follow-up was 21.6 years. Ten women developed ipsilateral carcinomas, eight had infiltrating ductal, one medullary, and one DCIS. Five patients had positive axillary lymph nodes. There were no cases of contralateral cancer. Four patients died of metastatic breast carcinoma, and one was alive with disease recurrence.

Page and associates[88] retrospectively reviewed 11,760 benign breast biopsies and found 28 patients with undiagnosed DCIS treated with biopsy alone. Seven patients (25 percent) developed invasive cancer in the ipsilateral breast, presenting an average of 6.1 years after the original biopsy. Six of seven invasive cancers occurred in the same quadrant as the original lesion, and one in an adjacent quadrant. Three of these seven died of metastatic disease, and one was alive with metastatic disease.

The retrospective nature of these two studies creates a bias; that is, these lesions were originally diagnosed as benign, making it possible that they included only minute foci of DCIS. Lagios and colleagues[100] have shown that the incidence of occult invasion increases with the increasing size of the lesion. Therefore, it is possible that these retrospective studies included lesions that were less likely to have occult invasion. There have been no studies that have prospectively watched all patients after biopsy alone. It may be that if biopsy alone were done in all cases of DCIS, the subsequent occurrence of invasive carcinoma would be much greater than that reported.

Farrow's series[5] contained 25 patients with DCIS treated with excisional biopsy alone. Five (20 percent) developed recurrent cancer, one to eight years after the diagnosis, all in the area of the original biopsy. The type of cancer that developed is not stated.

Lagios and associates[100] followed 20 patients with lesions averaging 8 mm in diameter treated with excision alone (equivalent to a wedge resection), for an average of 44 months. There were three ipsilateral breast cancer recurrences. Two patients had recurrences of DCIS in the previous biopsy site and were treated with re-excision. The third disease recurrence was a 4-mm invasive lesion, which was managed by modified radical mastectomy, with negative nodes. All patients were free of disease at the time of the report.

Other reports of patients treated with biopsy alone have included very small numbers. In Millis and Thynne's report[97] of 28 patients with DCIS, eight patients were treated with wide local excision. There was no difference in survival, compared with patients treated with mastectomy. Two of the eight conservatively treated patients had breast cancer recurrences with DCIS, 6 and 84 months postoperatively, respectively. At the time of recurrence, the former patient was treated with mastectomy, and the latter with local excision. A second breast cancer recurrence appeared in the latter patient at 96 months and was then treated with mastectomy. Both patients were still alive and without disease at the time of the report. One other patient with severe congestive heart failure was treated with radiation therapy alone after biopsy. She died seven years later, after developing skeletal metastases.

Von Rueden and Wilson[92] treated three patients with excisional biopsy and three with primary radiation therapy (surgical treatment prior to radiation treatment unstated). None of these patients developed invasive cancer. Ashikari's series had two patients treated with wide local excision, neither of whom developed invasive cancer.[90] In Carter's report, two patients deferred mastectomy.[49] One had a mastectomy 20 months after biopsy alone, and DCIS was found in the mastectomy specimen. A second patient had a mastectomy 63 months later, revealing infiltrating ductal carcinoma. Neither the symptoms present nor the reasons for the mastectomy were commented upon. Also, the area in which the subsequent carcinoma developed was not described. Both patients were alive without disease at the time of the report.

The American College of Surgeons National Survey in 1978 makes the point that recurrences following conservative treatment with wedge resection are equal to those following treatment with more extended surgical procedures.[2, 32] Fifteen patients had wedge resection, with a recurrence rate of 6.7 percent. Mastectomy patients had recurrence rates from 6.4 to 15.5 per cent. Five patients treated with biopsy alone had a recurrence rate of 20 percent. This rate was statistically higher than that of patients treated with all other modalities. One could conclude that a biopsy should be done with negative surgical margins (wide local excision) to ensure the lowest recurrence rate.

In summary, when DCIS is treated with excisional biopsy alone, there appears to be at least a 25 percent incidence of subsequent invasive cancer in the ipsilateral breast. These cancers have been reported to occur mostly in the area of previous biopsy, which would indicate that residual foci of DCIS remained after excisional biopsy alone. Since many of these cases were originally diagnosed as benign, no attempt was made to obtain clear margins or an adequate sample size to rule out occult invasion.

One other rare group of DCIS, the intracystic papillary carcinomas, should be mentioned here. Carter and colleagues[101] collected a series of 41 patients with intracystic papillary carcinoma of the breast. This tumor was defined as that which involved a cystically dilated duct alone. Twenty-nine patients were treated with mastectomy, one with radiation therapy after excisional biopsy, and 11 with excisional biopsy alone. There were no recurrences in the group receiving mastectomy. There were three recurrences in the group undergoing biopsy alone: one with recurrent *in situ* disease and two (18 percent) with invasive ductal cancer. These patients were all alive without evidence of disease at the time of the report. One interesting aspect of the study is that 19 of the 41 patients (46 percent) had associated DCIS (15 treated with mastectomy and four with biopsy). All these patients who developed recurrence had associated DCIS. This led the researchers to conclude that DCIS found in cases of intracystic papillary carcinoma was a precursor to invasive carcinoma. One other point brought out by the study is that cases of intracystic papillary carcinoma without associated DCIS treated with biopsy alone showed no predilection to developing invasive cancer.

Data on subsequent contralateral cancer patients with DCIS is limited. Webber's series of 116 cases of DCIS followed for an average of nine years demonstrated four contralateral cancers (one DCIS, one LCIS, and two invasive ductal).[61] Ashikari and associates[90] also report a low incidence of contralateral invasive cancers in their series, with follow-up time ranging from one to nine years. They reported the development of contralateral invasive cancers in 4 of 112 patients (4 percent). Conclusions are difficult to make from these studies. It is possible that patients with DCIS in one breast may have an increased risk of contralateral invasive cancer, but there are no data to support this at the present time.

Axillary Lymph Node Metastases

The frequency of axillary node metastases reported in patients with DCIS alone ranges from 0 to 9 percent (Table 10–7). A cumulative figure of 2.1 percent node positivity can be derived from the available literature.

As discussed previously, Silverberg and Chitale[87] have done the careful series in this area. They studied lesions of DCIS and infiltrating carcinoma by whole-organ sectioning. By this method, 14 cases of pure DCIS were found. These 14 patients had no positive nodes. Lagios and colleagues[100] also carefully studied breasts with DCIS by whole-organ sectioning. In their study of 53 patients with DCIS, only one patient had positive nodes. This patient had a lesion that measured 160 mm in diameter and had one area of occult invasion at mastectomy. Of her twelve axillary nodes, one was positive.

A group of patients described by Rosen should be mentioned in this section.[80] His report included three patients who presented with axillary node metastases and were found to have DCIS at modified radical mastectomy. Each mastectomy specimen was ex-

TABLE 10–7. Lymph Node Status in Patients with DCIS

Authors	*No. of Patients*	*No. of Axillary Dissections*	*No. of Positive Nodes (% of Total Patients)*
Ashikari et al.[90]	112	113	1 (0.9%)
BCDDP[9]	212	?	2 (1.0%)
Brown et al.[91]	40	21	1 (2.5%)
Carter and Smith[49]	35	26	1 (2.5%)
Gillis et al.[96]	36	?	1 (2.8%)
Kouchoukos et al.[102]	24	24	1 (4.2%)
Lagios et al.[100]	53	53	1 (1.9%)
Ozzello[22]	22	?	2 (9.0%)
Rosner et al.[2]	210	210	8 (3.8%)
Silverberg and Chitale[87]	14	12	0 (0%)
Sunshine et al.[63]	70	61	0 (0%)
von Rueden and Wilson[92]	53	32	0 (0%)
Westbrook and Gallager[93]	64	60	1 (1.5%)
	875		18 (2.1%)

amined in more than 100 sections, and no evidence of invasion was seen. It may be that these lesions of DCIS had areas of microinvasion not seen by conventional light microscopy but visible by electron microscopy.

The data suggest that in cases in which positive nodes are discovered, areas of microinvasion were missed in the diagnosis of the primary tumor. In any case, the incidence of axillary lymph node positivity is low in DCIS, indicating a good prognosis with low mortality.

Treatment

DCIS is not a benign lesion that will regress but a lesion with the potential to become invasive. Therefore, DCIS requires definitive therapy. There are several factors that must be taken into consideration when making a treatment decision. First, retrospective studies have shown that patients treated with biopsy alone develop invasive cancer in the ipsilateral breast in at least 25 percent of cases.[34, 88, 95] Second, DCIS appears to be multicentric in about 35 percent of cases.[84, 91, 92, 98, 100] Third, the incidence of occult invasion at mastectomy for DCIS ranges from 6 to 21 percent.[49, 58, 72, 92, 100] Fourth, the incidence of bilaterality is unclear but does not seem to be greater than that in patients with invasive ductal cancer.[61, 68] Finally, the incidence of axillary node positivity in these patients is about 2.1 percent (Table 10–7).

These factors suggest that biopsy alone is not adequate treatment. Also, bilateral mastectomies, as treatment for DCIS alone with no other risk factors for cancer, are not justified in this disease. This leaves several options for the treatment of DCIS: (1) wide excision alone, with close follow-up, (2) wide excision and radiation therapy, or (3) ipsilateral mastectomy.

The previous data discussed under development of subsequent invasive cancer support wide local excision alone as a viable treatment option. The American College of Surgeons survey in 1978 revealed that the five-year disease-free survival rate was no different in those patients treated with radical mastectomy versus wedge excision.[2, 32] There was a recurrence in 1 of the 15 patients (16.7 percent) treated with wedge excision alone. Patients having total mastectomy had a recurrence rate of 14.2 percent; those with modified radical mastectomy 6.4 percent; and those with radical mastectomy 10.1 percent.

Millis and Thynne's study[97] of eight patients treated with wide local excision also reveals no survival rate difference in these patients compared with those treated with mastectomy. Two of the eight patients had recurrence (25 percent) but with further surgical therapy remained free of disease.

Lagios's study of 20 patients with lesions of DCIS less than 8 mm in diameter, following what it calls tylectomy (an equivalent to wedge excision), also supports wide excision alone.[100] There were three recurrences (15 percent) with no deaths from breast cancer. Lagios and associates feel that wide local excision can be done in patients with lesions measuring less than 25 mm in diameter. This group is singled out because in their study of mastectomy specimens of patients with

DCIS, the patients with smaller lesions had a 0 percent incidence of occult invasion and a lower incidence of multicentricity (14 percent compared with 54 percent in larger lesions). The researchers also required adequate margins of resection, breasts that would be easy to examine in follow-up, breasts of low radiographic density to enable adequate mammographic follow-up, and no risk factors such as prior contralateral cancer or a family history of cancer in a first-degree premenopausal relative or of bilateral cancer in a first-degree relative. All patients were informed of the potential risks of this treatment strategy.

One recent paper gives information that could argue against wide local excision alone for treatment of DCIS. Holland and colleagues[103] studied 32 cases of DCIS. The study included consecutive breast specimens; however, ten cases had been excluded because the lesions were nonpalpable and radiologically occult. At diagnosis, nine tumors (28 percent) were pathologically 2 cm or smaller, 19 tumors (59 percent) were 5 cm or smaller, and 13 tumors (41 percent) were larger than 5 cm. In 21 of 32 cases (66 percent), the diagnosis was made by discovery of microcalcifications on mammography. In 8 of the 21 (38 percent), the radiologic size of the tumor was less than the pathologic size. The researchers argue that since 41 percent of the patients had tumors larger than 5 cm, wide local excision would leave a large cosmetic defect and thus would not be the optimal treatment. This certainly is true, but it must be remembered that ten patients (24 percent) were excluded because of the occult nature of their disease. If these were included, the number of patients with tumors larger than 5 cm would probably be much smaller.

There are many physicians who feel that wide local excision alone is inadequate treatment, because of the substantial incidence of multicentricity and occult invasive disease at mastectomy. Therefore, they would choose one of the following two treatments: wide local excision with radiation therapy or ipsilateral mastectomy with or without low axillary dissection. The experience of treating DCIS with radiation therapy after local excision is limited. Is DCIS radiosensitive? Data from the National Surgical Adjuvant Breast and Bowel Project (NSABP) studies will eventually address this question.[104]

A randomized trial in patients with invasive breast carcinoma, comparing segmental mastectomy (with negative microscopic margins) with or without radiation therapy versus the standard modified radical mastectomy has recently been reported.[104] As of 1986, there was no survival rate difference between the different treatment arms. However, there was a 28 percent incidence of breast cancer recurrence in those patients treated with segmental mastectomy alone, compared with an 8 percent incidence in those receiving segmental mastectomy plus radiation therapy. This would indicate that there was a substantial incidence of multicentricity or inadequate excision. Previous work by Fisher and colleagues[27] supports this hypothesis. They define multicentricity as disease in more than one quadrant. In their evaluation of 904 mastectomy specimens from protocol B-04 (radical mastectomy versus total mastectomy), multicentricity occurred in 13.4 percent of cases. The multicentric cancers were noninvasive in 9.3 percent of cases and invasive in 4.1 percent. Therefore, the facts that multicentricity was noninvasive in 9.3 percent of cases and that there were fewer breast cancer recurrences in patients receiving radiation therapy might indicate that *in situ* lesions are radiosensitive. However, it must be kept in mind that the median follow-up time was only 39 months in this study, and more recurrences might appear in the future in a follow-up of at least 10 to 15 years.

The rationale for treatment of DCIS with more conservative surgical measures is that it is cosmetically and psychologically more appealing to most women. Several reports describe a collection of patients with DCIS treated with local excision and radiation therapy. Montague[105] treated 34 patients with DCIS with simple excision followed by radiation therapy. Irradiation consisted of 5000 rad to the breast over five weeks and a boost to the tumor bed of 1000 to 2000 rad. The follow-up time was 3 to 17 years. One patient (3 percent) had a recurrence in the axilla and was successfully treated with surgery.

Findlay and Goodman's series[106] includes 14 patients treated with total excision of the breast abnormality (either a mass detected on physical examination or microcalcifications found on mammography), limited or classic axillary dissection, and radiation therapy. Radiation therapy consisted of 4200 to

5000 rad to the breast and, for large tumors, an interstitial implant was done, delivering 1500 rad to the tumor bed. Cosmetic results were reported to be excellent. The follow-up time was short, with a median of 23.5 months. Two patients (14 percent) required subsequent mastectomy for recurrence: the first, for Paget's disease of the nipple, and the second, for DCIS and invasive ductal carcinoma in the original biopsy site.

Recht and colleagues[107] have combined the Philadelphia experience described earlier with that at Boston. They report on 40 patients with DCIS treated with radiation therapy after excisional biopsy. The total dose to the primary tumor was less than 5000 rad in one patient, between 5000 and 5999 rad in 20 patients, and greater than 6000 rad in 19 patients. The median follow-up time was 44 months. There were four recurrences (10 percent), all in the same area as the original biopsy site. Three of these patients had presented with a nipple discharge and a central primary tumor. Two recurrences were DCIS alone, and two were DCIS and invasive cancer. All four patients were treated with mastectomy and were without disease at the time of the report.

Zafrani and associates[108] describe 55 patients with DCIS treated with local excision and radiation therapy. These patients received 5000 rad to the breast, with 1000 to 1500 rad to the tumor bed. The median follow-up time was 55 months. One patient (2 percent) developed a recurrence at 14 months (histology not stated) and died of disease.

There has been one other report, which includes only one case.[109] A patient with DCIS was treated with wedge resection and external radiation therapy to the breast and nodal regions, for a total dose of 5100 rad. Three years later, she was found to have minute calcifications on a follow-up mammogram. Excision of these revealed DCIS. Her treatment at this time consisted of mastectomy, the results of which contained no evidence of cancer. She remained free of disease. This study stresses the importance and usefulness of follow-up mammograms in patients who have had procedures less extensive than mastectomy as their treatment for this disease.

These studies would indicate that the recurrence rate after local excision and radiation therapy ranges from 1 to 14 percent. This is not dissimilar to the recurrence rate with local excision alone, 6.7 to 25 percent. Patients who have recurrences after local excision or radiation therapy do not have a decreased survival rate. However, the follow-up time in those patients who have had radiation therapy is too short to make a definitive statement about the efficacy of this treatment for DCIS.

For many physicians, the procedure of choice for DCIS remains mastectomy. The recurrence rate following mastectomy ranges from 0 to 10 percent (Table 10–8). The largest number of patients for whom recurrence rate data are available are included in the series by the American College of Surgeons, as reported by Rosner.[2] The total recurrence rate in 182 patients who all received mastectomy (ranging from total to radical mastectomy) was 10 percent. Details, such as the presence of invasive disease in the mastectomy specimen and the number of patients who died of disease, are not given.

Most other studies show a low incidence of recurrences after mastectomy. Carter's[49] and Lagios's[100] sets of three recurrences each included two patients who had had invasion at mastectomy. Other studies report a very low recurrence rate, from 0 to 5 percent.

TABLE 10–8. Recurrence and Mortality after Mastectomy for Ductal Carcinoma* in Situ *(DCIS)

Authors	*No. of Patients*	*Patients with Recurrence*	*Patients Dead of Disease*
Ashikari et al.[90]	112	1 (1%)	1 (1%)
Brown et al.[91]	40	0	0
Carter and Smith[49]	38	3 (8%)	3 (8%)
Lagios et al.[100]	53	3 (6%)	1 (2%)
Millis and Thynne[97]	20	0	0
Ozzello[22]	22	1 (5%)	1 (5%)
Rosner et al.[2]	182	19 (10%)	?
Sunshine et al.[63]	70	3 (4%)	3 (4%)
von Rueden and Wilson[92]	47	1 (2%)	0
Westbrook and Gallager[93]	60	2 (3%)	?

The next question is whether axillary dissection should be done to determine which patients have a need for adjuvant chemotherapy. These patients are already known to have a good prognosis. The node positivity rate should be no more than 2 percent if careful sectioning of the primary lesion is done to rule out invasion. Therefore, axillary dissection would not seem necessary for prognostic purposes.

What type of mastectomy should be done? The reasons for selecting the mastectomy treatment are the physician's concerns about multicentric disease and occult invasion. If this is the reasoning, the physician should want all breast tissue removed. Without a low axillary dissection, about 95 percent of patients will have some remaining breast tissue in the axilla.[81] Therefore, total or simple mastectomy with low axillary dissection is the procedure of choice. The axillary dissection is important not prognostically but to ensure thorough removal of the maximum amount of breast tissue.

It is obvious that prospective randomized trials for the treatment of DCIS need to be done. Not only will treatment plans become clearer, but also questions about the natural history will be answered. The NSABP implemented a new protocol, NSABP B-17, in October 1985.[110] This protocol accepts patients with DCIS or mixed DCIS and LCIS. Treatment options include segmental mastectomy with clear histologic margins and Levels I and II axillary dissection versus segmental mastectomy with axillary dissection and postoperative radiation therapy. Radiation therapy consists of 5000 rad to the breast, without a boost. Patients will be randomized after segmental mastectomy and axillary dissection. If the nodes are positive, patients are ineligible and are not randomized. If the surgical margins are positive, one further procedure is allowed to obtain clear margins, and then patients are randomized. This study will undoubtedly answer questions about the natural history and optimal treatment of DCIS. It is the hope that a large number of patients with DCIS in the United States will be included in this study.

In summary, the recurrence rates after local excision alone obtained from retrospective studies are 6.7 to 25 percent; after wide excision and irradiation, 1 to 14 percent; and after mastectomy 0 to 10 percent. These recurrence rates are very similar, with no decrease in the survival rates for more conservative procedures.

Since no definitive study results are available for treatment of this disease, it is highly recommended that patients be placed on a protocol such as NSABP B-17, where they will be studied and followed meticulously. In the event that a patient has a lesion 25 mm or smaller and no risk factors, is reliable for follow-up, has nondysplastic breasts on mammography, and cannot be placed on a protocol, that patient could have wide local excision alone to obtain negative surgical margins. Also, frequent follow-up by physical examination and a yearly mammogram should be done. For the patients who have a mass greater than 25 mm, risk factors, difficult or unreliable follow-up, or nipple involvement, the treatment options of either simple mastectomy with low axillary dissection or wide excision and radiation therapy are acceptable. This more extensive treatment is felt to be necessary for such patients because of the higher incidence of multicentricity and occult invasion that occurs with larger lesions.

CONCLUSIONS

Intraepithelial breast carcinomas are an important subset of breast carcinoma because of the increasing frequency of their diagnosis with screening mammography and because of their good prognosis. It is essential that patients with intraepithelial breast carcinoma be studied prospectively in large series to unravel the mysteries of the disease's natural history and to establish uniform guidelines for treatment.

REFERENCES

1. Broders AC: Carcinoma *in situ* contrasted with benign penetrating epithelium. JAMA 99:1670, 1932.
2. Rosner D, Bedwani RN, Vana J, et al.: Noninvasive breast carcinoma: Results of a national survey by the American College of Surgeons. Ann Surg 192:139, 1980.
3. Rosen PP: The clinical significance of preinvasive breast carcinoma. Cancer 46:919, 1980.
4. Smart CR, Myers MH, Gloeckler LA: Implications from SEER data on breast cancer management. Cancer 41:787, 1978.

5. Farrow JH: The James Ewing lecture: Current concepts in the detection and treatment of the earliest of the early breast cancers. Cancer 25:468, 1970.
6. Shapiro S: Evidence on screening for breast cancer from a randomized trial. Cancer 39:2772, 1977.
7. Feig SA: Mammographic screening: Benefit and risk. *In*: Feig SA, McLelland R (eds.): Breast Carcinoma: Current Diagnosis and Treatment. New York: Masson Publishing USA, Inc., 1983, pp. 351–363.
8. Beahrs OH, Smart CR: The Breast Cancer Detection Demonstration Projects as viewed by the clinician. *In*: Feig SA, McLelland R (eds.): Breast Carcinoma: Current Diagnosis and Treatment. New York: Masson Publishing USA, Inc., 1983, pp. 307–314.
9. Report of the working group to review the NCI/ACS Breast Cancer Detection Demonstration Projects. J Natl Cancer Inst 62:641, 1979.
10. Thomas BA, Price JL, Boulter PS: The Guilford Breast Screening Project. Clin Oncol 9:121, 1983.
11. Tabar L, Gad A, Akerlund E, et al.: Screening for breast cancer in Sweden. *In*: Feig SA, McLelland R (eds.): Breast Carcinoma: Current Diagnosis and Treatment. New York: Masson Publishing USA, Inc., 1983, pp. 315–326.
12. Tabar L, Fagerberg CJ, Gad A, et al.: Reduction in mortality from breast cancer after mass screening with mammography. Lancet 1:829, 1985.
13. Snyder RE: Mammography and lobular carcinoma *in situ*. Surg Gynecol Obstet 122:255, 1966.
14. Gershon-Cohen J, Berger SM, Curcio BM: Breast cancer with microcalcifications: Diagnostic difficulties. Radiology 87:613, 1966.
15. Hutter RVP, Snyder RE, Lucas JC, et al.: Clinical and pathologic correlation with mammographic findings in lobular carcinoma *in situ*. Cancer 23:826, 1969.
16. Tulusan AH, Egger H, Schneider ML, et al.: A contribution to the natural history of breast cancer: Lobular carcinoma *in situ* and its relation to breast cancer. Arch Gynecol 231:219, 1982.
17. Morris DM, Walker AP, Coker DC: Lack of efficacy of xeromammography in preoperatively detecting lobular carcinoma *in situ* of the breast. Breast Cancer Res Treat 1:365, 1981.
18. Page DL, Dupont WD, Rogers LW, et al.: Atypical hyperplastic lesions of the female breast: A long term follow-up study. Cancer 55:2698, 1985.
19. Gallager HS: The developmental pathology of breast cancer. Cancer 46:905, 1980.
20. Gallager HS, Martin JE: Early phases in the development of breast cancer. Cancer 24:1170, 1969.
21. McDivitt RW, Stewart FW, Berg JW: Tumors of the breast. Atlas of Tumor Pathology, 2nd series, fascicle 2. Washington, DC: Armed Forces Institute of Pathology, 1968, pp. 22–86.
22. Ozzello L: Intraepithelial carcinomas of the breast. *In*: Hollman KH, Verley JM: New Frontiers in Mammary Pathology. New York: Plenum Press, 1983, pp. 147–164.
23. Rush BF, Kramer WM: Proliferative histologic changes and occult carcinoma in the breast of the aging female. Surg Gynecol Obstet 117:425, 1963.
24. Kramer WM, Rush BF: Mammary duct proliferation in the elderly: A histopathologic study. Cancer 31:130, 1973.
25. Ashikari R, Huvos AG, Snyder RE, et al.: A clinicopathologic study of atypical lesions of the breast. Cancer 33:310, 1974.
26. Dupont WD, Page DL: Risk factors for breast cancer in women with proliferative breast disease. N Engl J Med 312:146, 1985.
27. Fisher ER, Gregorio R, Redmond C, et al.: Pathologic findings from the National Surgical Adjuvant Breast Project (Protocol No. 4): I. Observations concerning the multicentricity of mammary cancer. Cancer 35:247, 1975.
28. Gallager HS, Martin JE: An orientation to the concept of minimal breast cancer. Cancer 28:1505, 1971.
29. Gallager HS: Minimal breast cancer: Origin of concept and definition. *In*: Feig SA, McLelland R (eds.): Breast Carcinoma: Current Diagnosis and Treatment. New York: Masson Publishing USA, Inc., 1983, pp. 251–255.
30. Hartmann WH: Minimal breast cancer: An update. Cancer 53:681, 1984.
31. Gallager HS: Minimal breast cancer: Results of treatment and long-term follow-up. *In*: Feig SA, McLelland R (eds.): Breast Carcinoma: Current Diagnosis and Treatment. New York: Masson Publishing USA, Inc., 1983, pp. 291–294.
32. Bedwani R, Vana J, Rosner D, et al.: Management and survival of female patients with "minimal" breast cancer: As observed in the long-term and short-term surveys of the American College of Surgeons. Cancer 47:2769, 1981.
33. Hutter RVP: The pathologist's role in minimal breast cancer: An update. Cancer 53:681, 1984.
34. Rosen PP: Lobular carcinoma *in situ* and intraductal carcinoma of the breast. *In*: McDivitt RW, Oberman HA, Ozzello L, et al. (eds.): The Breast. Baltimore: Williams & Wilkins, 1984, pp. 59–105.
35. Wellings SR, Jensen HM: On the origin and progression of ductal carcinoma in the human breast. J Natl Cancer Inst 50:1111, 1973.
36. Ozzello L, Speer FD: The mucopolysaccharides in the normal and diseased breast: Their distribution and significance. Am J Pathol 34:993, 1958.
37. Ozzello L: The behavior of basement membranes in intraductal carcinoma of the breast. Am J Pathol 35:887, 1959.
38. Ozzello L, Sanpitak P: Epithelial-stromal junction of intraductal carcinoma of the breast. Cancer 26:1186, 1970.
39. Ozzello L: Ultrastructure of intraepithelial carcinomas of the breast. Cancer 28:1508, 1971.
40. Ozzello L: Benign and malignant proliferations of the mammary epithelium: Ultrastructural observations. *In*: McDivitt RW, Oberman HA, Ozzello L, et al. (eds.): The Breast. Baltimore: Williams & Wilkins, 1984, pp. 106–138.
41. Barsky SH, Siegal GP, Jannotta F, et al.: Loss of basement membrane components by invasive tumors but not by their benign counterparts. Lab Invest 49:140, 1983.
42. Cornil AV: Contributions a l'histoire du developpement histologique des tumeurs epitheliales (squirrhe, encephaloide, etc.) J Anat Physiol 2:266, 1865.
43. Ewing J: Neoplastic Diseases, 2nd ed. Philadelphia: W. B. Saunders Co., 1928, p. 562.
44. Foote FW, Stewart FW: Lobular carcinoma *in situ*: A rare form of mammary cancer. Am J Pathol 17:491, 1941.

45. Stewart FW: Tumors of the Breast. Atlas of Tumor Pathology, Section IX, fascicle 34. Washington, DC: Armed Forces Institute of Pathology, 1950, p. 43.
46. Haagensen CD, Lane N, Lattes R: Neoplastic proliferation of the epithelium of the mammary lobules: Adenosis, lobular neoplasia, and small cell carcinoma. Surg Clin North Am 52:497, 1972.
47. Andersen JA: Lobular carcinoma *in situ*. A long-term follow up in 52 cases. Acta Pathol Microbiol Scand [A] 82:519, 1974.
48. Benfield JR, Jacobson M, Warner NE: *In situ* lobular carcinoma of the breast. Arch Surg 91:130, 1965.
49. Carter D, Smith RL: Carcinoma *in situ* of the breast. Cancer 40:1189, 1977.
50. Dall'Olmo CA, Ponka JL, Horn RC, et al.: Lobular carcinoma of the breast *in situ*: Are we too radical in its treatment? Arch Surg 110:537, 1975.
51. Donegan WL, Perez-Mesa CM: Lobular carcinoma—An indication for elective biopsy of the second breast. Ann Surg 176:178, 1972.
52. Erdreich LS, Asal NR, Hoge AF: Morphologic types of breast cancer: Age, bilaterality, and family history. South Med J 73:28, 1980.
53. Godwin JT: Chronology of lobular carcinoma of the breast: Report of a case. Cancer 5:259, 1952.
54. Haagensen CD, Lane N, Lattes R, et al.: Lobular neoplasia (so-called lobular carcinoma *in situ*) of the breast. Cancer 42:737, 1978.
55. Lewison EF, Finney GG: Lobular carcinoma *in situ* of the breast. Surg Gynecol Obstet 126:1280, 1968.
56. Macaulay RAA, Mitchinson MJ: Lobular carcinoma *in situ* of the breast. Br J Surg 60:527, 1973.
57. Newman W: *In situ* lobular carcinoma of the breast: Report of 26 women with 32 cancers. Ann Surg 157:591, 1963.
58. Ringberg A, Palmer B, Linell F: The contralateral breast at reconstructive surgery after breast cancer operation: A histopathological study. Breast Cancer Res Treat 2:151, 1982.
59. Rosen PP, Lieberman PH, Braun DW, et al.: Lobular carcinoma *in situ* of the breast: Detailed analysis of 99 patients with average follow-up of 24 years. Am J Surg Pathol 2:225, 1978.
60. Schwartz GF, Feig SA, Rosenberg AL, et al.: Staging and treatment of clinically occult breast cancer. Cancer 53:1379, 1984.
61. Webber BL, Heise H, Neifeld JP, et al.: Risk of subsequent contralateral breast carcinoma in a population of patients with *in situ* breast carcinoma. Cancer 47:2928, 1981.
62. Wheeler JE, Enterline HT, Roseman JM, et al.: Lobular carcinoma *in situ* of the breast: Long-term follow-up. Cancer 34:554, 1974.
63. Sunshine JA, Moseley HS, Fletcher WS, et al.: Breast carcinoma *in situ*. A retrospective review of 112 cases with a minimum 10 year follow-up. Am J Surg 150:44, 1985.
64. Haagensen CD, Lane N, Bodian C: Coexisting lobular neoplasia and carcinoma of the breast. Cancer 51:1468, 1983.
65. Haagensen CD: Small cell carcinoma. *In*: Haagensen CD (ed.): Diseases of the Breast. Philadelphia: W. B. Saunders Co., 1971, pp. 526–527.
66. Newman W: Lobular carcinoma of the female breast: Report of 73 cases. Ann Surg 164:305, 1966.
67. Rosen PP, Senie RT, Farr GH, et al.: Epidemiology of breast carcinoma: Age, menstrual status, and exogenous hormone usage in patients with lobular carcinoma *in situ*. Surgery 85:219, 1979.
68. Rosen PP, Menendez-Botet CJ, Nisselbaum JS, et al.: Pathological review of breast lesions analyzed for estrogen receptor protein. Cancer Res 35:3187, 1975.
69. Antoniades K, Spector H: Correlation of estrogen receptor levels with histology and cytomorphology in human mammary cancer. Am J Clin Pathol 71:497, 1979.
70. Pick PW, Iossifides IA: Occurrence of breast carcinoma within a fibroadenoma: A review. Arch Pathol Lab Med 108:590, 1984.
71. Andersen JA: Multicentric and bilateral appearance of lobular carcinoma *in situ* of the breast. Acta Pathol Microbiol Scand [A] 82:730, 1974.
72. Rosen PP, Senie R, Schottenfeld D, et al.: Noninvasive breast carcinoma: Frequency of unsuspected invasion and implications for treatment. Ann Surg 189:377, 1979.
73. Rosen PP, Braun DW, Lyngholm B, et al.: Lobular carcinoma *in situ* of the breast: preliminary results of treatment by ipsilateral mastectomy and contralateral breast biopsy. Cancer 47:813, 1981.
74. Urban JA: Biopsy of the "normal" breast in treating breast cancer. Surg Clin North Am 49:291, 1969.
75. Andersen JA: Lobular carcinoma *in situ* of the breast: An approach to rational treatment. Cancer 39:2597, 1977.
76. Giordano JM, Klopp CT: Lobular carcinoma *in situ*: Incidence and treatment. Cancer 31:105, 1973.
77. Hutter RVP, Foote FW: Lobular carcinoma *in situ*: Long-term follow-up. Cancer 24:1081, 1969.
78. Azzopardi JG: *In situ* and invasive lobular carcinoma of the breast. *In*: Hollman KH, Verley JM: New Frontiers in Mammary Pathology. New York: Plenum Press, 1983, pp. 127–145.
79. Cogswell HD: Hidden carcinoma of the breast. Arch Surg 58:780, 1949.
80. Rosen PP: Axillary lymph node metastases in patients with occult noninvasive breast carcinoma. Cancer 46:1298, 1980.
81. Hicken NF: Mastectomy—a clinical pathologic study demonstrating why most mastectomies result in incomplete removal of the mammary gland. Arch Surg 40:6, 1940.
82. Bloodgood JC: Comedo carcinoma (or comedo-adenoma) of the female breast. Am J Cancer 22:842, 1934.
83. Wertheimer MD, Johnson PR: Carcinoma *in situ* of the male breast: A case report and review. Breast 8:7, 19182.
84. Nielsen M, Jensen J, Andersen J: Precancerous and cancerous breast lesions during lifetime and at autopsy: A study of 83 women. Cancer 54:612, 1984.
85. Frantz VK, Pickren JW, Melcher GW, et al.: Incidence of chronic cystic disease in so-called "normal breasts." Cancer 4:762, 1951.
86. Gallager HS, Martin JE: The study of mammary carcinoma by mammography and whole organ sectioning. Cancer 23:855, 1969.
87. Silverberg SG, Chitale AR: Assessment of significance of proportions of intraductal and infiltrating tumor growth in ductal carcinoma of the breast. Cancer 32:830, 1973.
88. Page DL, Dupont WD, Rogers LW, et al.: Intra-

ductal carcinoma of the breast: Follow up after biopsy only. Cancer 49:751, 1982.

89. Shah JP, Rosen PP, Robbins GF: Pitfalls in local excision in the treatment of carcinoma of the breast. Surg Gynecol Obstet 136:721, 1973.
90. Ashikari R, Hajdu SI, Robbins GF: Intraductal carcinoma of the breast (1960–1969). Cancer 28:1182, 1971.
91. Brown PW, Silverman J, Owens E, et al.: Intraductal "noninfiltrating" carcinoma of the breast. Arch Surg 111:1063, 1976.
92. von Rueden DG, Wilson RE: Intraductal carcinoma of the breast. Surg Gynecol Obstet 158:105, 1984.
93. Westbrook KC, Gallager HS: Intraductal carcinoma of the breast: A comparative study. Am J Surg 130:667, 1975.
94. Stamler FW, Berg JW: Breast cancer in Iowa women. *In*: Correa P, Johnson WD (eds.): An International Survey of Distributions of Histologic Subtypes of Breast Cancer. Geneva: International Union Against Cancer, 1978, pp. 93–100.
95. Betsill WL, Rosen PP, Lieberman PH, et al.: Intraductal carcinoma: Long term follow up after treatment by biopsy alone. JAMA 239:1863, 1978.
96. Gillis DA, Dockerty MB, Clagett OT: Preinvasive intraductal carcinoma of the breast. Surg Gynecol Obstet 110:555, 1960.
97. Millis RR, Thynne GSJ: *In situ* intraduct carcinoma of the breast: A long term follow-up study. Br J Surg 62:957, 1975.
98. Schwartz GF, Feig SA, Rosenberg AL: Staging and treatment of clinically occult breast cancer. Cancer 53:1379, 1984.
99. McDivitt RW: Breast cancer multicentricity. *In*: McDivitt RW, Oberman HA, Ozzello L, et al. (eds.): The Breast. Baltimore: Williams & Wilkins, 1984, pp. 139–148.
100. Lagios MD, Westdahl PR, Margolin FR, et al.: Duct carcinoma *in situ*. Relationship of extent of noninvasive disease to the frequency of occult invasion, multicentricity, lymph node metastases, and short-term treatment failures. Cancer 50:1309, 1982.
101. Carter D, Orr SL, Merino MJ: Intracystic papillary carcinoma of the breast: After mastectomy, radiotherapy, or excisional biopsy alone. Cancer 52;14, 1983.
102. Kouchoukos NT, Ackerman LV, Butcher HR: Prediction of axillary nodal metastases from the morphology of primary mammary carcinomas: Guide to operative therapy. Cancer 20:948, 1967.
103. Holland R, Veling SHJ, Mravunac M, et al.: Histologic multifocality of Tis, T1–2 breast carcinomas. Implications for clinical trials in breast-conserving surgery. Cancer 56:979, 1985.
104. Fisher B, Bauer M, Margolese R: Five-year results of a randomized clinical trial comparing total mastectomy and segmental mastectomy with or without radiation in the treatment of breast cancer. N Engl J Med 312:665, 1985.
105. Montague ED: Conservative surgery and radiation therapy in the treatment of operable breast cancer. Cancer 53:700, 1984.
106. Findlay PA, Goodman R: Radiation therapy for treatment of intraductal carcinoma of the breast. Am J Clin Oncol 6:281, 1983.
107. Recht A, Danoff B, Solin LJ, et al.: Intraductal carcinoma of the breast: Results of treatment with excisional biopsy and irradiation. J Clin Oncol 4:716, 1986.
108. Zafrani B, Fourquet A, Vilcoq JR et al.: Conservative management of intraductal breast carcinoma with tumorectomy and radiation therapy. Int J Radiat Oncol Biol 10:140, 1984.
109. Wecksell A, Attkiss MJ, Shahamatpour M: Recurrent intraductal breast carcinoma following radiation therapy: A case report. Breast 8:13, 1982.
110. Fisher B: NSABP Protocol No. B-17. Twenty-eighth semiannual meeting of the National Surgical Adjuvant Project for Breast and Bowel Cancers (NSABP), February 17–19, 1986.

Steroid Hormone Receptors and Mechanisms of Growth Regulation of Human Breast Cancer

MARC E. LIPPMAN, M.D.

For nearly a century, the value of endocrine therapy for breast cancer has been appreciated. A dramatic advance in the understanding of steroid hormone action was achieved in the 1970's and has allowed improved selection of those patients who are likely to benefit from endocrine therapy, thus offering them a potentially safer, less toxic alternative to chemotherapy. The importance of such endocrine therapy cannot be emphasized enough, since patients with metastatic disease who respond to hormone manipulations not only have significant palliation of symptoms but also have longer survival when compared with nonresponders. In older women (over the age of 50), prophylactic endocrine therapy can prevent disease recurrences and increase survival. Since the first attempt by Beatson,[1] 90 years ago, to develop an endocrine treatment for breast cancer and his demonstration that ovariectomy could indeed induce regression of an advanced breast tumor, a wide variety of endocrine therapies, both ablative and additive, have been tried more or less empirically.

This chapter will consist of two parts. We will initially consider some facets of steroid hormone action and growth regulation of human breast cancer. This will be followed by a more detailed consideration of the clinical utility of steroid receptor analyses.

11

STEROID HORMONE ACTION

Major progress in the understanding of steroid hormone action at the cellular and molecular levels has been made, beginning with the demonstration in the mid 1960's of a so-called receptor protein in the rat uterus that could specifically bind estradiol.[2] This discovery had been preceded by the synthesis of tritiated estrogens with highly specific activity. These reagents made possible the detection of specific retention of hormone in target tissues and, later, the detection of the receptor protein by competitive protein-binding techniques.[3, 4] Soon thereafter, cytoplasmic estrogen receptor was detected in human breast cancer tissue,[5] in several other organs including human uterus[6] as well as brain,[7, 8] skin,[9] liver,[10, 11] thymus,[12] and prostate,[13] and in different cancerous tissues.[14–17]

The interest in the estrogen receptor protein increased further when it became clear that after binding of estrogen to its receptor, the steroid-receptor complex underwent a change termed activation or transformation, which permitted its translocation and binding to nuclei. This led to the concept that the nucleus was the primary site of action of this class of steroids.[18, 19] More recently, data have accumulated that suggest that estrogen receptor, even when unoccupied and unactivated, may reside in the nucleus.[20] However, activation still represents the acquisition by the steroid-receptor complex of increased affinity for nuclear components. Since then, many studies have demonstrated that a key role for the steroid receptors is the induction of numerous genes coding for secreted or intracellular proteins or enzymes.[21–24] These inductions appear to occur by an increase in the rate of transcription of specific genes into messenger RNAs.[25, 26] In some systems, regulation may possibly occur by a decrease in the rate of transcription.[27, 28] In addition, several sites of post-transcriptional regulation, including those controlling stabilization of these messenger RNAs, may exist.[29] The exact locus at which the steroid receptor molecule can exert control of specific genes is not clear. Considerable attention has been given to receptor binding sites in chromatin. The nature of these "acceptor" sites is not certain. Much evidence suggesting that they are localized to certain acidic fractions of nonhistone chromosomal proteins has accumulated.[30] Evidence for receptor interactions with histones also exists.[31] Recent reports indicate that direct binding to specific DNA segments can occur.[32] Recognition of specific DNA sequences by receptor proteins may alter their transcription in as yet unknown ways.[33] Since the rates of induction of steroid-controlled genes vary as a function of the steroid or combination of steroids tested and of the time of induction,[21] more complex regulatory pathways become highly probable. These possibilities may include receptor heterogeneity, acceptor site heterogeneity as well as numerous post-transcriptional sites.

Growth Regulation of Human Cancer

Multiple lines of investigation all suggest that estrogens are critically responsible for continued growth of hormone-dependent breast cancers. Removal of sources of estrogens such as the ovary and the adrenal results in worthwhile clinical responses, as does therapy with antiestrogens. Response to these endocrine therapies is highly associated with the presence of specific cellular receptors for estrogens. Administration of physiologic doses of estrogens to castrated or postmenopausal women can stimulate tumor proliferation *in vivo*. While all these data clearly demonstrate that estrogens are mitogens for human breast cancer, they do not identify the exact mechanism of estrogens' action or even prove that estrogens act directly on tumor cells to stimulate growth.

This chapter will review some recently accumulated information that supports the following three hypotheses:

1. Estrogens directly interact with human breast cancer cells and can directly alter gene expression at the level of transcription. This results in increased activity of many enzymes involved in cell growth as well as increased activities of other intracellular proteins such as progesterone receptor.
2. Part of this alteration in gene expression induced by estrogens results in alterations in specific proteins secreted by hormone-responsive breast cancer cells. Some of these secreted proteins serve as autocrine and paracrine growth stimulators capable of initiating growth of quiescent cells, further stimulating growth of cells already in proliferative cycle, and finally, inducing reversible acquisition of the malignant phenotype in nontransformed cells.
3. Conversion of hormone-responsive breast cancer to the hormone-independent phenotype is accompanied by increased and non–hormone-regulated (constitutive) secretion of a similar or identical collection of autocrine and paracrine growth factors. Thus, strategies directed against hormonally

regulated growth factors or their specific receptors could alter growth properties and clinical progression of both hormone-dependent and hormone-independent human breast cancer.

In order to test these hypotheses, it was initially necessary to develop a suitable *in vitro* model system for human breast cancer. This decision was made because of two inherent difficulties in performing and interpreting such experiments *in vivo*. First, *in vivo* it is impossible to alter the concentration of a hormone such as estradiol without altering the activities or concentrations of many other hormones or potential growth factors. Furthermore, if one hypothesizes that there is an unknown substance secreted by some other tissue in the body under estrogenic control that then alters breast cancer growth (a putative estromedin),[34, 35] it follows that an *in vitro* system will not respond to estrogen directly (although it would provide a suitable assay system for an estromedin). Second, even if a stimulatory or inhibitory response is observed in a tumor following a hormonal manipulation *in vivo*, it is not possible to conclude that this is due to a direct effect of the substance on the tumor cells. An intervening or mediating effect on the immune system or supporting stroma or vasculature is just as plausible and may be responsible for altered tumor behavior. In certain circumstances, such as androgen-induced mammary gland regression, an indirect mechanism has been shown to be the cause of hormonal effects *in vivo*.[36]

In our own studies, cloned lines of human breast cancer cells have been employed to address these questions. The human and mammary nature of these cells has been extensively discussed.[37] Approximately ten years ago, we first succeeded in showing that these cell lines would respond to direct stimulation with physiologic concentrations of estradiol by increasing their rate of proliferation.[38, 39] We subsequently showed that these results could be duplicated in defined medium devoid of unknown serum constituents.[40] Furthermore, potent antiestrogens were capable of inhibiting estrogenic stimulation. The effects of antiestrogens were shown to be specific, because only cell lines containing estrogen receptor responded; antiestrogen effects were prevented by simultaneous estrogen administration or were reversed by subsequent estradiol administration. This latter effect has led to successful clinical trials in patients with breast cancer.[41, 42] While some initial controversy arose because of occasional difficulties in obtaining direct effects of estrogens on breast cancer cell growth *in vitro*,[43, 44] subsequently numerous groups have succeeded in confirming that estradiol can serve as a proximate mitogen for human breast cancer.[45–56] Physiologic concentrations of estradiol have been shown to promote nucleoside incorporation into DNA and increase the thymidine-labeling index, net DNA synthesis, and cell number. Estradiol induces a large number of enzyme activities specifically involved in nucleic acid synthesis, including those of DNA polymerase, thymidine and uridine kinases, thymidylate synthetase, carbamyl-phosphate synthetase, aspartate transcarbamylase, dihydroorotase, and dihydrofolate reductase.[57, 58] We have demonstrated that physiologic concentrations of estradiol stimulate DNA synthesis by both scavenger and *de novo* biosynthetic pathways. It has also been shown that estrogens regulate both thymidine kinase and dihydrofolate reductase mRNA concentrations.[59–61]

In addition to controlling these essential growth-regulating enzymes, estrogens alter the activity of several other proteins whose functions remain unknown. These include progesterone receptor,[62] plasminogen activator,[63] and several secreted proteins including a 24-kilodalton protein described by Ciocca and colleagues,[64] 52- and 160-kilodalton glycoproteins described by Westley and colleagues,[65] and a 7-kilodalton protein identified initially by Jakowlew and colleagues[66] by detection of an estrogen-induced mRNA species, using differential hybridization techniques. The exact function of these latter secreted proteins is unknown, although several lines of experimental evidence have suggested that they do not act as major autostimulatory growth factors. The 52 kilodalton protein described by Westley and colleagues appears to be a protease similar to cathepsin D. We have used similar strategies of differential hybridization to identify several estrogen-induced genes. The conditions of short-term stimulation prior to nucleic acid isolation were designed to increase the likelihood of obtaining nonabundant genes induced at early points in time by estradiol. The preliminary results in this direction have been successful.[67] Thus, while estrogens undoubtedly affect many tissues of the body, which may in turn alter breast cancer progression, direct effects of estrogens on isolated breast cancer cells, including important growth-regulating effects, are well established, placing hypothesis I on firm footing.

Observations by Sporn and Todaro led them to propose that important aspects of growth control of tumors were mediated by factors, secreted by cancer cells, which could be either autostimulatory (autocrine factors) or stimulatory of surrounding tissues such as connective tissue or vasculature (paracrine factors).[68] Either of these classes of growth factors could be under endocrine control or could be released constitutively. Of course, endocrine stimulation of breast cancer growth need not necessarily involve such paracrine or autocrine mechanisms.

Three sets of observations support the possibility that such secreted growth factor activities could be important in the pathogenesis and progression of human breast cancer. First, we and others have shown growth regulation and other phenotypic responses of breast cancer cells to a long list of other trophic substances, aside from estrogens. These include glucocorticoids, androgens, progestins, iodothyronines, vitamin D, retinoids, epidermal growth factor (EGF), insulin-like growth factor 1 (IGF-1), calcitonin, and prolactin.[69] This multiplicity of effector molecules suggested that some estrogenic responses *in vivo* could be indirectly modulated by effects on these other growth factors. Alternatively, similar or identical growth factors could be elaborated by the breast cancer.

Second, the response of MCF-7 human breast cancer cells *in vitro* in cell culture versus *in vivo* in a nude mouse model system was quite different. Under the former set of conditions, estrogens can directly stimulate growth, but the cells will grow in the absence of estradiol. In the presence of optimal stimulation by serum and insulin and other growth supplements, estradiol will have little if any additional growth-promoting properties. *In vivo* in the athymic nude mouse, estradiol has, up until now, been an absolute requirement for tumor growth.[58, 70, 71] Huseby and colleagues[72] have further defined this system by showing that estradiol need not enter the systemic circulation in nude mice to promote MCF-7 cell tumor formation; elevation of local estradiol concentration near the tumor was sufficient. This suggested that although estrogens might be required to induce other mediating factors needed by the tumor (or host) for tumorigenesis, the production and action of such factors is probably restricted to the local area of the tumor. These observations argue strongly against the view that estromedins (estrogen-induced products acting as endocrine factors) are of substantial importance in estrogen-evoked tumor formation.

Third, it was noticed that the initial growth rate of breast cancer cells in culture was proportional to the number of cells plated.[73] While multiple interpretations of this observation are possible, they are consistent with the production of autostimulatory growth factors. Work with 3T3 cells has also supported such a hypothesis.[74] In a series of preliminary experiments, we found that crude conditioned medium prepared from human breast cancer cell lines was capable of stimulating proliferation of other breast cancer cell lines, as compared with replenishment with fresh unconditioned medium. At the same time, Vignon and colleagues[75] had also observed that MCF-7 cells showed enhanced stimulation by estradiol when medium was changed less frequently.[75] This led them to also hypothesize that estrogens acted, at least in part, by inducing secretion of autocrine growth factors, which were diluted out by more frequent medium changes. These investigators also supported this hypothesis by crude conditioned medium experiments.

In order to be able to identify and purify the components, secreted by breast cancer cells, required for both autostimulation and *in vivo* tumorigenesis, it was necessary to develop a serum-free culture system that supported the growth of hormone-responsive and hormone-unresponsive human breast cancer cell lines. Previous work was of great assistance in this regard.[40, 45] We found that Richter's Improved Minimal Essential Medium, supplemented with 2 mg/l transferrin and 2 mg/l fibronectin, supported cell growth for at least a week. Cells were grown in this medium with or without 10^{-9} mol/l estradiol for four days; subsequent two-day collection periods in fresh identical medium provided a source of secreted protein activity. These collected media were harvested, filtered to remove cellular debris, dialyzed extensively against 1 mol/l acetic acid, lyophilized, and reconstituted in phosphate-buffered saline. We found that extraction removes greater than 99.98 percent of the residual estradiol. This material was the starting material for biologic assays and purification procedures and was also the material used for *in vivo* infusions to stimulate tumor growth, to be described later.

We initially examined breast cancer cell line–conditioned medium for insulin-like growth factor 1 (somatomedin C) (IGF-1). IGF-1 was chosen because it was already known that some breast cancer cell lines responded to IGF-1 and had IGF-1 receptors on their surface.[76] Using a sensitive and specific radioimmunoassay, we were able to determine (in collaboration with E.M. Spencer of Children's Hospital of San Francisco) that all the human breast cancer cell lines tested (MCF-7, ZR-75-1, MDA-MB-231, and Hs578T) produced IGF-1 immunoreactive material.[77] Secreted levels were as follows: MCF-7, 11.6 ng/ml, 65 pg/μg DNA; ZR-75-1, 9.7 ng/ml, 103 pg/μg DNA; MDA-MB-231, 30.3 ng/ml, 342 pg/μg DNA; and Hs578T, 48.8 ng/ml, 534 pg/μg DNA. The first two cell lines, both estradiol-responsive, produced substantially less IGF-1 than did the latter two estrogen-independent cell lines. In initial experiments, estradiol did not stimulate IGF-1 secretion, although glucocorticoids and antiestrogens, which both inhibit the growth of MCF-7 cells, strongly inhibit IGF-1 secretion. Later, using more stringent means of removing estradiol from culture medium, we were able to show estrogenic effects of IGF-1 activity. This activity was inhibited by antiestrogen treatment of hormone-dependent breast cancer cells. All four cell lines respond to exogenous authentic IGF-1 with enhanced proliferation. Using acid-extracted medium, IGF-1 migrates on a Biogel P60 column as a high molecular weight species, but upon acid-ethanol extraction, this high molecular weight activity converted to a lower molecular weight activity, which co-migrated with authentic IGF-1 standard. In studies we have performed in collaboration with Kenneth Gabbay (Baylor College of Medicine), it has been shown that a human cDNA probe for IGF-1 identifies a single mRNA species identical in size to that seen in non-transformed human fibroblasts, thus confirming that human breast cancer cells synthesize and secrete apparently authentic IGF-1. However, both with unfractionated conditioned medium and after medium chromatography on Sephacryl S-200 columns, it was observed that conditioned medium derived from estrogen-treated cells contained three to eight times the autostimulatory activity of medium derived from non–estrogen-treated cells, and this activity was distributed in multiple peaks. Therefore, it appeared likely that other activities were contributory to tumor growth.

Because epidermal growth factor (EGF) had also been shown previously to stimulate the growth of human breast cancer cells,[78] these cell lines were next examined for the production of EGF-related materials. We used the A431 human carcinoma cells as a source of EGF receptor for these radioreceptor assays.[79] All the human breast cancer cell lines tested produced material that competed with iodinated EGF for binding to EGF receptor. None of the several peaks of activity (30 Kd to Vi) corresponded to the position of authentic EGF after fractionation on Biogel P60 columns. Depending on assay conditions, estradiol induced a four- to sixfold increase in EGF receptor reactive material. The principal peak of activity, at approximately 30 Kd, however, did not correspond to the reported molecular weight of sequenced TGF_{α}, a transforming growth factor with amino acid homology to EGF that has been shown to bind with high affinity to EGF receptor. While transforming growth factors may have other activities, they have been defined by their ability to induce anchorage-independent growth (colonies in soft agar) in nontransformed fibroblasts.[79] MCF-7 cells had been reported to secrete transforming factors in this assay.[80] Therefore, we assayed conditioned medium from human breast cancer cell lines for TGF activity, using assay of normal rat kidney (NRK) fibroblast colony formation as an end point. At least two classes of TGF activity exist. First, assay conditions were employed that measured TGF_{α}-like activity only. TGF_{α}-like peptides compete with EGF for binding to EGF receptor. TGF_{α}-like peptides contain a sequence homologous with EGF but are not recognized by anti-EGF antibodies. Anti-EGF receptor antibodies, which block EGF binding, block TGF_{α} activity.[81]

A second class of complementary TGF activity, that of TGF_{β}, has been described.[82, 83] This peptide does not bind to EGF receptor. Both TGF_{α} and TGF_{β} are acid- and heat-stable peptides that are sulfhydryl reagent sensitive. Both TGF_{α} and TGF_{β} are required for anchorage-independent growth of NRK cells; however, in the assay conditions employed, TGF_{β} activity was supplied so that we measured estrogen induction of either TGF activity or an activity that could replace it. All breast cancer cell lines except Hs578T were positive in this assay.[84] It should be noted that the Hs578T cell line is not derived from an epithelial tumor but rather a carcinosarcoma. Once again, hormone-independent (in this case, MDA-MB-231) cells produced substantially more TGF_{α} activity than did the hormone-responsive MCF-7 and ZR-75-1 cells. Using this assay, TGF_{α}-like activity was increased up to eight fold by estradiol treatment of MCF-7 cells. Whether this activity is due to authentic TGF_{α} or some alternative EGF receptor–reactive material is not as yet clear.

In order to assay TGF_{β}, A549 human carcinoma cells were used as a source of TGF_{β} receptor for a radioreceptor assay.[85] In collaboration with Sporn and colleagues at the NIH, we have found that all of the human breast cancer cell lines tested secrete TGF_{β} receptor–reactive material. Once again, the two hormone-unresponsive cell lines, Hs578T and MDA-MB-231, produced the highest concentrations of TGF_{β} activity. An important point to keep in mind is that although the TGFs are named (and defined) by their ability to induce anchorage-independent growth of nontransformed cell lines, this may not be their only important activity. For example, Hanauske and colleagues[86] have shown that authentic TGF_{α} can stimulate clonogenic growth of tumor samples of the breast as well as other neoplasms, and Ibbotson and colleagues and Sporn and associates have shown that TGF_{β} is a growth inhibitor for certain established tumor cell lines including MCF-7 and that TGF_{β} has activity in bone resorption[87] and wound healing assays.[88] Thus, it is interesting to note that TGF_{β} activity, as measured by radioreceptor assay in conditioned medium, is increased by estrogen withdrawal in MCF-7 cells and is stimulated still further by antiestrogen treatment. Furthermore, TGF_{β} inhibits growth of several human breast cancer cell lines with TGF_{β} receptor. Interestingly, a variant of MCF-7, which was selected for growth resistance to antiestrogens, secretes lower concentrations of TGF_{β}, and antiestrogens do not increase TGF_{β} secretion. Whether or not this is the mechanism by which these cells escape antiestrogen inhibition is under investigation. In collaboration with Sporn and colleagues, we have been able to show that a cDNA for human TGF_{β} identifies a single mRNA species of identical size to that found in other human tissues, establishing that these human breast cancer cells are a source of apparently authentic TGF_{β}.

Growth factors may conveniently be divided into at least two classes: competency factors and progression factors.[89] These were defined operationally by their ability to stimulate quiescent, contact-inhibited, nontransformed fibroblasts. These cells will undergo a single wave of DNA synthesis if refed with fresh serum-containing medium. If serum derived from platelet-poor plasma is used instead, no stimulation is seen. Reconstitution of platelet-poor plasma with an extract derived from platelets led to growth stimulation. Platelet-derived growth factor (PDGF) (the active moiety later purified from platelets) was required only for 30 minutes, after which it could be removed, and the continuous presence of platelet-poor plasma would be sufficient for subsequent DNA synthesis 24 hours later. Much of the growth stimulatory effect of the platelet-poor plasma could be replaced by addition of EGF. Thus in such an assay system, PDGF would be defined as a competency factor, EGF as a progression factor. IGF-1, EGF, and TGF_{α} cannot function as competency factors. We established an assay for competency factors produced by human breast cancer cells, using contact-inhibited fibroblasts and platelet-poor plasma. This assay was responsive to either exogenously added PDGF or fibroblast growth factor (FGF), another competency factor. All the human breast cancer cell lines secreted factors producing competency activities. Studies aimed at identification of these factors are under way. Immunoprecipitation studies and direct measurement of specific mRNA have suggested that much of this activity is due to authentic PDGF.

Halper and Moses[90] have recently described an adrenal carcinoma cell line (SW-13) whose growth in soft agar is stimulated by conditioned medium from various cancer cell lines and extracts from primary tumors. The SW-13 cell line's spectrum of response is such that FGF is strongly stimulatory, whereas insulin, IGF-1, EGF, TGF_{α}, and

TGF_β are inactive. We employed this assay and found that breast cancer cell lines are secreting a high-molecular-weight, acid-stable factor that is highly stimulatory of SW-13 colony formation. Whether our competency assay and SW-13 colony formation assay are scoring distinct or overlapping growth factors is currently under study. Preliminary experiments suggest that peaks of competency activity and SW-13 growth stimulatory activity are distinct. This suggests that these may represent a separable class of transforming growth factor activities that act on carcinoma.

In any event, the aforementioned studies clearly demonstrate that human breast cancer cells secrete multiple, discrete growth factors, at least some of which are clearly under estrogenic control. Obviously, a great deal of effort will be required to identify specifically each of these separable growth stimulatory activities.

But what, if any, is the physiologic significance of these observations? In order to be able to answer this question, we took advantage of the observation, previously alluded to, that hormone-responsive MCF-7 cells will not form tumors in oophorectomized nude mice unless the animals receive supplemental estrogen pellets.[58, 70, 71] Reconstituted concentrated conditioned medium and conditioned medium derived from E_2-treated cells were infused into oophorectomized nude mice, using ALZA minipumps. The equivalent of 10 ml of conditioned medium or conditioned medium from E_2-treated cells was infused daily for four weeks from a middorsal subcutaneous location. A total of 2 to 5 $\times$ 10^6 MCF-7 cells was injected into each of four different mammary fat-pad locations in each mouse. Tumors of up to 0.5 cm in diameter appeared at MCF-7 sites within two weeks. In animals infused with conditioned medium from non–estrogen-treated cells, tumors appeared with a frequency of 11 percent, while conditioned medium from E_2-treated cells supported tumors with a frequency of 25 percent. Animals infused with concentrated control medium had a tumor incidence of less than 5 percent. Conditioned medium and conditioned medium from E_2-treated animals stimulated tumor growth for two to three weeks, after which time tumors usually declined in size. Reimplantation with pumps containing fresh conditioned medium did not prevent this regression. Histologic examination prior to regression revealed adenocarcinomas that were morphologically identical to tumors found in animals treated with an estrogen pellet instead of the conditioned medium. We do not as yet know why the adenocarcinomas induced by conditioned medium are not maintained and eventually regress. Growth factors may not all be present in sufficient concentration when administered by an endocrine route. Alternatively, during the purification of conditioned medium, labile components may be eliminated. Finally, conditioned medium may possibly not replace some other action of estradiol on other tissues, for example, natural labile-cell activity.

Conditioned medium from E_2-treated animals had no effect on ovariectomized mouse uterine weight or histology. Conditioned medium from E_2-treated animals was inactivated by trypsin treatment, reducing agents, and heating at 56°C for one hour. These observations, together with direct measurements of estradiol concentration in the conditioned medium, eliminate the possibility that the enhanced effects of conditioned medium from E_2-treated animals were due to contamination with estradiol. The absence of stimulation of uterine weight suggests that the peptides produced upon estrogen stimulation do not function as generalized estromedins but retain tumor specificity even when administered by an endocrine route, as opposed to their usual diffusion-limited effects. These results also clearly suggest that a substantial fraction of estrogen-induced tumor growth is mediated at the level of alterations in secreted polypeptide growth factors. This has obvious potential therapeutic implications; for example, antibodies directed against either the secreted growth factors or their receptors would certainly be expected to alter rates of tumor progression.

An additional implication of these observations is that a plausible mechanism by which breast tumors may become hormone-independent is through loss of hormonal regulation of growth factor production. If acquisition of the ability to constitutively synthesize growth factors is an important mechanism for loss of hormone dependence, therapies directed against such growth factors or their receptors might be equally effective for hormone-dependent and hormone-independent breast cancers.

Support for this viewpoint is provided by some recent experiments in which the hormone dependency of MCF-7 human breast cancer cells was altered by activated oncogenes introduced by DNA-mediated gene transfer.[91] We transfected the cells with the ras oncogene derived from the Harvey sarcoma virus (v-ras^H) by a co-selection methodology using a bacterial gene as a selectable gene marker. Stably transfected MCF-7 cells were obtained, in which several copies of the v-ras^H gene were integrated into the host cellular DNA. These cells (MCF-7_{ras}) expressed v-ras^H mRNA and had detectably phosphorylated p21 (the protein that is the ras gene product). MCF-7_{ras} cells (as compared with MCF-7 cells transfected with only the selectable gene encoding the bacterial xanthine-phosphoribosyl-transferase enzyme activity—MCF-7_{gpt}) were essentially unresponsive to antiestrogens *in vitro*. In addition, unlike wild-type MCF-7 cells or MCF-7_{gpt}, which require estrogen supplementation for tumorigenesis in nude mice, MCF-7_{ras} formed tumors with about 85 percent efficiency in oophorectomized athymic nude mice. The ras oncogene conferred hormone-independence on the tumorigenicity of the MCF-7_{ras} cells. We have begun studies on the mechanism of the development of hormone-independence by MCF-7_{ras}. Conditioned medium prepared from MCF-7_{ras} contains three- to fourfold increases in EGF receptor–reactive material and anchorage-independent growth-promoting activity for fibroblasts (TGF_α-like) as wild-type cells. A single peak of EGF receptor–reactive material with transforming activity was eluted at an apparent molecular weight of about 30 Kd after acid gel chromatography of MCF-7_{ras}-conditioned medium. In addition, both IGF-1 radioimmunoassayable material and TGF activity (as measured by radioreceptor assay) were augmented three to four fold in MCF-7_{ras} cells. Thus, ras gene activation appears to induce phenotypic activities and tumorigenic changes, which are induced in wild-type MCF-7 cells only after estrogen stimulation.

Therefore, strong evidence exists that human breast cancer cells secrete a collection of separable growth factors (IGF-1, TGF_α-like material, TGF_β, a competency factor, and an additional epithelial anchorage-independent growth-promoting factor). Some of these activities are estrogen inducible. Taken together, they are capable of promoting *in vivo* tumorigenesis of hormone-dependent breast cancer cells in nude mice, although not to the same extent as estrogen treatment of the mice. Hormone-independent breast cancer cells, whether spontaneously arising in culture or constructed by DNA-mediated gene transfer, appear to secrete such growth factors in increased amounts. Such an externalized system of autocrine and paracrine cell regulation obviously suggests multiple interventions, which may eventually have clinical applicability in the control of neoplastic breast cancer growth.

Although our knowledge of how steroids and steroid receptor proteins affect DNA synthesis and cell growth is still incomplete, an accumulation of clinical data demonstrates a close correlation between receptor presence and tumor regression following hormonal manipulations. We will now evaluate the clinical use of steroid receptor assays as well as review the methods available for their quantification, describing the pitfalls that may be encountered in receptor measurement and in the interpretation of the results. First, there will be a brief discussion of how the presence of estrogen and progesterone receptors (ER and PR, respectively) correlates with a response to endocrine and cytotoxic chemotherapy.

ER IN BREAST CANCER: DISTRIBUTION

Since the discovery of specific cytosolic estrogen-binding proteins, a great deal of information has accumulated concerning the value of these receptor determinations in breast cancer.[92] About two thirds of primary breast cancers contain detectable concentrations of ER, while a somewhat smaller proportion (50 percent) of metastatic samples are positive for estrogen receptor in untreated patients. Males represent approximately 1 percent of all breast cancer patients. Approximately 85 percent of all male breast cancers are ER positive.[93] Premenopausal female patients have tumors that are less frequently estrogen receptor positive (ER+) and contain, on average, lower concentrations of receptor than patients whose breast cancers are evaluated after menopause (Table 11–1). These observations are partially explained by the fact that the higher concentrations of endogenous estrogens in plasma of premen-

TABLE 11–1. Incidence of Estrogen Receptor Positivity (ER+) and Menopausal Status*

Author	Stage of Disease	Total No. of Patients	Type of Assay	Cutoff Value	Premenopausal ER+ (%)	Postmenopausal ER+ (%)
Hubay et al.	II	296	DCC	3 fmol/mg	68	74
Osborne et al.	II	1366	DCC	3 fmol/mg	61	78
Brooks et al.	—	105	DCC	3 fmol/mg	48	83
Stewart et al.	Primary tumor	278	DCC	3 fmol/mg	62	73
					58	74
Allegra et al.	Primary tumor	182	DCC	10 fmol/mg	41	65
Kiang and	Primary tumor	171	SDG	+8 S	29	61
Kennedy	Metastatic tumor	79			40	60

*Modified from refs. 195 and 196.

opausal women may lead to receptor occupancy, tight nuclear binding and processing, or down regulation of binding sites. Other evidence additionally suggests that the presence or absence of ER may reflect a different biologic potential of the tumor cells.[94, 95]

The presence of ER and PR is correlated with tumors that are histologically better differentiated and less aggressive.[94–96] Attempts to correlate the presence of ER with a specific histologic type of tumor have been confounded, mainly by the vast preponderance of infiltrating ductal carcinomas. In a series of 500 patients,[13] a greater percentage of the intraductal, tubular, and lobular carcinomas contained 10 fmol/mg protein of ER and PR, as compared with other types of carcinomas. The nuclear grade related more closely to the presence of sex steroid receptor than did any other single histologic factor. A modification of the grading as it was established by the National Surgical Adjuvant Breast Project (NSABP) was developed by McCarty and associates.[94] Their histologic Grades I to III attempt to assess cellular differentiation through both nuclear grade and histomorphologic patterns. Better differentiated histologic Grades I and II were more responsive to endocrine therapy. The relative cellularity of the invasive neoplasms did not consistently correlate with the quantity of receptor observed.[94] Several studies showed an absence of correlation between the size of the tumors and the receptor content,[38, 39] but ER-positive patients show a tendency for less lymph node involvement compared with ER-negative patients.[97] The location of the tumor in the breast also was not correlated with receptor presence.[98]

Seasonal variations of ER in breast cancer (BC) of postmenopausal women have been described; this coincides with similar variations in other species.[99] Known fluctuations in adrenal steroid secretion[100] have been thought responsible for this pattern. Although obvious seasonal variations in reproductive patterns in animals would point to a link between seasons and sex hormone receptor levels, these data could not be confirmed for human BC samples in our laboratory (unpublished observations) or by McGuire and colleagues (personal communication). Whether these divergent results may be due to climatic or latitude differences, or both, remains to be established.

A diurnal rhythm of cytoplasmic estrogen receptors in the rat brain can be demonstrated in ovariectomized rats. Pentobarbital was shown to decrease the reduction of receptors that occurred in the dark; melatonin injection in the light partially mimicked the action of darkness in reducing receptor levels.[101] Menstrual variations of receptor levels were demonstrated in a study on benign breast disease (BBD).[102] Although a relation between BBD and BC is not firmly established, common etiologic factors exist.[103] It is difficult to assess physiologic variations of receptor levels in premenopausal breast cancer patients, because of the known heterogeneity of breast cancer cells as well as the variations in receptor pattern that occur throughout the course of the disease and following treatment.[104] Variations observed in receptor levels between the primary mastectomy specimen[105] and metastatic samples of the same patient are not infrequent. The variations found between metastatic lesions at the same time in the same patient[105] may reflect genetic instability of the cancer cell.

ER AND BENIGN BREAST DISEASE

A relationship between benign breast disease (BBD) and cancer has long been known, but as Mauvais-Jarvis and colleagues[106] and others point out, knowledge of an exact relationship remains extremely imprecise as a result of differing definitions of the disease by the radiologist, the pathologist, or the physician as well as the incompleteness of epidemiologic studies. Most studies are retrospective and although many women with breast cancer do not give histories of benign mastopathy, previous benign lesions may have gone unnoticed because in the past, systematic breast examination during the reproductive years was not widespread. Regardless of these difficulties, cystic disease appears to be positively correlated with mammary carcinoma, increasing the risk of such carcinoma two to seven fold.[107–109] Fibrocystic disease is found with a high frequency in the vicinity of mammary cancer.[110] In order to identify subgroups of patients with a higher risk for developing subsequent cancer, studies have been conducted to evaluate the relative risk of associated ductal papillomatosis. Although the presence of ductal papillomatosis with atypical features as well as lobular hyperplasia has been found to correlate with carcinoma,[110–113] only a negligible incidence of intraductal papillomas was found in the vicinity of cancer in a study of 1000 cases.[110] Chromosomal as well as ultrastructural studies in proliferative fibrocystic disease have shown abnormalities that clearly resemble those encountered in cancer, thus stressing a close association between those two diseases, with a possible evolution from one to the other. Of interest is the fact that a majority of cancers observed in patients with a previous history of cystic disease became clinically apparent five to ten years after the benign disease was diagnosed.[109] Common etiologic features have been found in BBD and mammary carcinoma,[114] as well as common hormonal patterns. Estradiol is the hormone initially responsible for the differentiation and development of the ductal epithelium, acting by increasing mitotic activity in the cylindrical cells of the internal layer of the ducts.[115–117] Progesterone is the hormone that antagonizes the action of estradiol on duct cells by changing the proliferative estrogen effects into a phase of cellular differentiation and mitotic rest.[118] Thus, ovarian function is of special interest in patients with various benign breast diseases. Plasma levels of progesterone and estradiol evaluated on three different days between the first and last day of the thermal plateau in 109 patients with BBD show significantly lower progesterone levels in patients ($p < 0.001$) as compared with those of 50 normal control subjects. In adenofibroma patients whose ER levels were examined as a function of cellularity of the tumor and of length of evolution, the greatest concentration of estradiol-binding sites was observed in tumors that had developed recently and had high epithelial cellularity. PR levels were determined from breast tissue obtained at midfollicular phase and showed a linear relation with ER levels in the highly cellular adenofibromas, whereas the group with the intermediate, more fibrous, less cellular tumors had almost undetectable PR levels, although the ER levels were between 10 and 50 fmol/mg protein. When the cellular components were minimal, neither of the receptors was detected.

The percentage of ER positivity in BBD in the literature is also quite variable and may in fact be underestimated in most cases. ER positivity ranged from 7 percent, as reported by Menendez-Botet and associates,[119] and 21 percent, as reported by Hawkins and colleagues,[120] to 55 percent in our series.[121] When the cytosol to be assayed was pretreated for 21 minutes at 4°C with a 0.5 percent dextran-coated charcoal solution before incubating it with various concentrations of hormone, 14 of 18 ER-negative PR-positive breast cancer samples of patients under the age of 51 were moved to the ER-positive PR-positive category.[122] Whether this procedure removes only unbound cytosolic hormones or unknown inhibitors of binding is unclear.

ER AND RESPONSE TO ENDOCRINE THERAPY

The presence of ER has a highly significant association with the likelihood of response to endocrine therapy. While only about one third of unselected breast cancer patients can be expected to respond to any endocrine therapy, a stratification by presence or absence of ER in the cytosol yields a response rate of 50 to 70 percent for ER+ patients, whereas lack of detectable ER is usually associated with a response rate between 0 and 10 percent.[92, 123, 124]

Quantification can substantially improve the predictive accuracy of the test,[125] but whereas high levels are strongly predictive of a response, low levels are not predictive of an absence of response. In a retrospective study including 109 post- and 50 premenopausal patients, ER levels have been compared with the number of patients responding to therapy.[105] In the premenopausal group, all patients with receptor levels above 250 fmol/mg tissue had a remission, whereas 83 percent of those who failed to respond had receptor levels below this value. Similarly, in postmenopausal patients, levels above 750 fmol/mg tissue were associated with a response to therapy in 86 percent, whereas 80 percent of the patients failing to respond had ER levels below this value. Although changes in ER content over time and between two metastatic sites at the same time are not uncommon,[105] there exists an approximately 85 percent correlation between the ER assay of the primary tumor and that at the time of recurrence.[105, 126] No significant relationship between the site of the metastases and the presence or absence of ER was established in a study including 500 patients, but there was a trend toward soft tissue or bone metastases being more often ER positive.[94, 127] Soft tissue and bone metastases tend to respond more often than viscera to endocrine therapy.[94]

ER, DISEASE-FREE INTERVAL, AND ADJUVANT THERAPY

The presence of ER in primary tumor has been shown not only to be predictive of a response to endocrine therapy but also to predict a better prognosis with lower recurrence rates (Table 11–2) and a longer disease-free interval.[94] Much of this effect is accounted for by correlations with nuclear and histologic-grade and proliferative indices. Progesterone receptor concentrations appear to provide an even more accurate prediction of disease-free interval. Most of the correlation between receptor content and disease-free interval is lost following systemic adjuvant therapy.

Treatment with tamoxifen (in combination with chemotherapy) has been shown to improve the prognosis for patients with ER-positive primary tumors. In a recent study including 214 patients having a median follow-up time of 36 months, Hubay and associates[128] found a decrease in recurrence rates in ER-positive patients, from 37 to 11 percent in the tamoxifen-treated group. Although in another study done by Fisher and colleagues,[129] treatment with tamoxifen did not change disease-free survival rates in ER-positive patients younger than 49 years, a significantly better disease-free survival rate is found in older women at a median follow-up time of 36 months. The same study showed higher ER levels to be significantly correlated with longer disease-free survival in tamoxifen-treated ER-positive patients. No difference in disease-free survival rates was

TABLE 11–2. Recurrence According to ER Status*

Author	No. of Patients		ER+ (%)	ER− (%)	Median Follow-up (Months)
Maynard et al.	232		32	39	36
Osborne et al.	281	Premenopausal	18	35	24
		Postmenopausal	15	38	
Furmanski et al.	422	Premenopausal	9	38	40
		Postmenopausal	12	26	
Lippman and Allegra	182	ER status of primary breast cancer	8	30	27
		ER status of all patients	35	58	27
Hubay et al.	214		13	33	36

*Modified from refs. 195 and 196.

TABLE 11–3. Relation of ER and PR Status to Response to Endocrine Therapy*

	ER− PR−	ER− PR+	ER+ PR−	ER+ PR+
McGuire	3/20	—	14/45	16/20
Degenshein et al.	0/14	1/1	3/14	26/33
Young et al.	2/9	1/2	3/14	20/29
Skinner et al.	3/30	2/3	2/6	9/12
Brooks et al.	—	—	2/7	4/6
Normura et al.	—	—	8/12	7/10
King	2/9	0/2	3/15	10/11
Manni et al.	0/2	—	3/5	15/24
Allegra et al.	0/12	0/4	8/14	11/14
Total	10/96	4/12	46/132	118/159
Percentage	10	33	34	74

*Modified from refs. 195 and 196.

seen in younger patients, despite the fact that premenopausal patients have been shown to respond to tamoxifen as well as other endocrine therapies. These results may reflect a more aggressive disease in the younger age group, as suggested by the following observations. Meyer and Hixon[130] have studied the thymidine-labeling indices (LI) of tumors and have found that high LIs appear to be associated with rapid evolution of breast carcinoma both before and after diagnosis and treatment. Women with LIs above the 2.21 median had a significantly higher rate of earlier recurrence than did patients with LIs below 2.2 ($p = 0.001$). Thirty-nine younger women (below 50) had a higher geometric mean LI (2.79) than did 89 women over the age of 50 (1.96).

As the number of sites involved with metastatic tumor increases, the objective response rate to endocrine therapy decreases.[131] In the NSABP study, increased numbers of micrometastases in premenopausal patients may account for the absence of a difference in disease-free survival rates in the younger age group following tamoxifen treatment.

OTHER MEASURES OF HORMONE DEPENDENCY, INCLUDING PR

In an attempt to better delineate the patients likely to benefit from hormonal therapy, it is reasonable to look for evidence of tumor responsivity to hormone treatment, such as nucleoside incorporation,[132] peroxidase induction,[133] or PR synthesis. In 1972, Milgrom and colleagues[134] first demonstrated that estradiol induces PR in the rat uterus. This observation was found to be true for breast cancer cell lines.[135] Thus, it appears that the presence of PR can give at least partial information on the integrity of ER-mediated pathways. In discriminating between ER-positive patients likely to respond to endocrine treatment and those who are not, the concomitant presence of PR and ER appears to be a better indicator than are ER values alone. PR is detected in approximately two thirds of ER-positive tumors; it is exceptional in ER-negative tumors. Its presence has been shown to improve the prediction of an objective response to endocrine therapy by up to 80 percent (Table 11–3).

Interestingly, about 30 percent of ER-positive but PR-negative tumors respond to endocrine therapy. Since the induction of PR is under estrogenic control, extremely low amounts of circulating estrogens, as occur in postmenopausal women, may be responsible for the failure to find PR in some elderly women with hormone-dependent tumors. On the other hand, in premenopausal women, high circulating levels of progesterone during the luteal phase of the menstrual cycle may mask the receptor sites.[136] In both cases, the absence of detectable PR does not argue against the hormone responsiveness of the tumor, and perhaps many of these responders could be reclassified as ER positive PR positive if nuclear exchange assays were employed or estrogen stimulation used.

TABLE 11–4. Response to Different Endocrine Therapies in ER+ Patients

	Oophorectomy	*Surgical Adrenalectomy*	*Ovariectomy Plus Adrenalectomy*	*Hypophysectomy*	*Estrogens*	*Antiestrogens*	*Aromatase Inhibitor*	*Corticosteroids*	*Androgens*
Maass et al.	12/14			3/7	24/36	7/12		9/12	9/12
De Sombre and Jensen	9/12	4/6		2/4	4/5	1/2		0/1	5/13
De Sombre and Jensen			14/19						
Manni et al.				20/28		43/77			
McGuire et al.						39/77			
Rubens and Hayward	5/25			3/8	8/21	21/42		5/6	4/29
Lawrence et al.							19/38		
Total	26/51	4/6	14/19	28/47	36/62	111/210	19/38	14/29	18/54
Percentage	50	67	74	59	58	52	50	48	33

*Modified from refs. 195 and 196.

ER AND RESPONSES TO SPECIFIC ENDOCRINE THERAPY

Although great progress has been made in selecting those patients likely to respond to an endocrine therapy, the mechanisms of cell kill are as yet unknown. Identical responses can be achieved by either ablative or additive therapies (Table 11–4). In general, premenopausal patients are initially treated with castration, although in one study, tamoxifen has been suggested to be as effective.[137] About 50 percent of patients having a response to oophorectomy will benefit from subsequent adrenalectomy;[138] this therapy is intended to remove the small amounts of estrone secreted by the adrenals as well as the source of androstenedione, which can be aromatized to estrone by peripheral tissues.[139] One study suggests that aminoglutethimide combined with hydrocortisone may be equivalent to surgical adrenalectomy.[140]

Additive endocrine therapy, mostly reserved for postmenopausal patients, encompasses pharmacologic doses of estrogens, antiestrogens, androgens, glucocorticoids, and progestins. The observation that some patients with breast cancer respond to pharmacologic doses of estrogens was not anticipated, but following the initial observation by Kennedy,[141] remission rates of 30 to 37 percent were reported in two larger series.[142,143] It could be argued that the effects of pharmacologic concentrations of estrogens are not mediated solely through the high-affinity, low-capacity cytosolic receptor but through a different class of lower-affinity binding sites or else by direct actions on enzymes or lysosomal membranes.[144–146] One cannot rule out an indirect action occurring via secretion of so-called estromedins by other organs under estrogen stimulation,[147] which in turn modulate growth of classic estrogen target organs. While antiestrogens induce no greater proportion of responses than do estrogens, antiestrogens' lower toxicity may make them the endocrine treatment of first choice. Specific antiestrogen-binding sites, separable from classic ER-binding ones, have been detected in rat uterus and human breast cancer[148] and do not bind estradiol. Although their biologic significance is not clear, they may be important in mediating antiestrogen effects. Antiestrogens also compete efficiently with estradiol for binding to the cytosolic ER. The precise way in which antiestrogens bring about their effects remains to be elucidated. In a study performed by Sherman and colleagues,[149] the endocrine effects of tamoxifen in healthy premenopausal women were as follows: (1) induction of maturation of multiple ovarian follicles, (2) doubling of midcycle estradiol levels, (3) lack of luteal changes in the endometrium, and (4) normal gonadotrophin levels. These observations suggest an effect on multiple endocrine target organs. Tamoxifen has been shown to decrease the synthesis and the excretion of urinary metabolites of cortisol, but these effects were not related to the outcome of the endocrine therapy.[150] How different antiestrogens compare in their endocrine effects is actually unknown, but there does not appear to be a significant difference in therapeutic efficacy.[151] Specific cytosolic receptors for androgens and glucocorticoids have also been detected in breast cancer samples.[152] Again, the presence of these receptors may be necessary for their action but do not contribute to predicting response to a hormonal treatment.

Most evidence still suggests that antiestrogens act by directly antagonizing estrogen effects in target tissues.

Some chemotherapeutic agents will actually affect endocrine target organs. Schultz and associates[153] as well as others[154] have evaluated ovarian function following chemotherapy with alkylating agents, and their data show evidence of variable degrees of ovarian failure, with induction of a permanent amenorrhea in all their premenopausal patients. Although the Case Western Reserve University study,[128] which shows ER-positive premenopausal patients treated with CMF alone doing better than their ER-negative counterparts, would be in favor of endocrine-mediated effects being responsible for a better response, several points would tend to oppose this hypothesis. First, a study by Tancini and colleagues[155] comparing relapse-free survival rates at three years in ER-positive and ER-negative premenopausal women treated with CMF did not find any meaningful difference. Second, postmenopausal patients often receive less than a full dose of chemotherapy and thus are not comparable with the premenopausal group. In fact 25 percent of postmenopausal patients received less than 55 percent of the total dose, compared with less than 10 percent of premenopausal patients.[156] Third, as Carter[157] points out, it is hard to understand why an imperfect medical castration would be superior to the absolute effectiveness of castration. Since ER positivity has been shown to be an independent prognostic factor for both recurrence and survival rates and since premenopausal patients may be able to tolerate a more aggressive treatment as compared with postmenopausal patients (which, in turn, improves the prognosis of the former), it appears that no valid comparison can be made between the two groups, and the hormone hypothesis of CMF remains to be proved.

ESTROGEN RECEPTORS AND CHEMOTHERAPY

In 1978, we reported a negative correlation between ER content and response to chemotherapy in patients with disseminated breast cancer, and subsequently, contradictory findings were presented by Kiang and associates.[158] Controversy involving the subject has remained active, with many other investigators publishing their observations. Some have reported a negative correlation between ER presence and the response to chemotherapy,[159–161] others have noted a positive correlation,[162–165] and still others have not been able to demonstrate any relationship at all.[166–168] Clearly, ER should not be used in deciding on treatment with chemotherapy.

INTERPRETATION OF ASSAY RESULTS

Many clinical reports demonstrate that the presence of a receptor is a necessary but not sufficient requirement for predicting a response to hormonal therapy. There are a substantial number of reasons why a one-to-one correlation between the presence of binding activity and a response to hormone therapy does not necessarily occur. A consideration of these permits a more accurate understanding of the usefulness of receptor measurement and the effects of ER on breast cancer, despite the limitation caused by the lack of direct comparisons.

False-Positive Assay Results

It is a common observation that a not negligible number of patients (20 to 60 percent) whose tumors have been classified as ER positive do not respond to endocrine therapy. The most frequently invoked explanation for this is tumor cell heterogeneity, that is, a small number of tumor cells with abundant receptor molecules may exist within a tumor sample in which the majority of cells are actually receptor negative. Support for this hypothesis is derived from the observation that there is a direct correlation between the total concentration of estrogen-receptor molecules and the likelihood of response to endocrine manipulations.[169] Furthermore, breast tumors have been shown to be heterogeneous, being composed of both receptor-rich and receptor-poor cells.[170] Qualitative variations may exist,[171] but they have been difficult to assess. External regulatory proteins for the early steps in receptor activation and inhibition have been described.[172–175] Limited *in vitro* proteolysis of almost all steroid receptors yields a low-molecular-weight fragment (kD 25,000) termed the meroreceptor,[176] which contains the hormone-binding moiety but has lost its receptor-related functions. High proteolytic activity in the tumor cells could potentially lead to the same inactive product. Such an explanation would be compatible with a 4 S only receptor being nonfunctional as opposed to the 8 S + 4 S patterns. The progesterone receptor appears to be a dimer of two slightly different subunits.[177] Dimerization has been proposed by Notides and colleagues[140] to be part of the activation process for ER. A defect in synthesis or turnover of one subunit would explain loss of receptor function in this model. But whereas multiple agents influencing receptor-ligand interactions and subsequent activation or inhibition of activation of the receptor have been studied *in vitro*,[178–181] little is actually known about the steps following the nuclear translocation of the steroid-receptor complex.

Although, in the past, specific binding of the receptor protein to crude DNA preparation was not demonstrable, work done on cloned DNA fragments of MMTV (mouse mammary tumor virus) known to be glucocorticoid responsive demonstrates that the receptor protein interacts directly with a specific DNA segment.[32] Absence or mutation of these nuclear acceptor sites, loss of unknown regulatory substances, or mutations in the genome coding for a single gene product under steroid control may result in a steroid-resistant cell. Hormone-independent variants of an estrogen-responsive human breast cancer cell line have been developed.[182, 183] Receptor concentration and hormone binding were normal. There were no differences in activation and translocation, but analysis of binding to DNA cellulose revealed a different pattern from that seen in the wild-type, hormone-dependent cell line. These variants may represent a model of a hormone-unresponsive ER-positive tumor. Other defects, which manifest themselves after hormone-binding, may include absence of activation or translocation and abnormal or absent nuclear receptor sites or genes to be transcribed. A legion of interacting regulatory enzymes, ions, or other small molecules also might be deranged.

Yet another reason that ER-positive patients might not respond to an endocrine therapy is the choice of an inadequate therapy. Although the total percentage of responses to endocrine therapy in ER-positive patients does not vary substantially between therapies, it is conceivable that individual patients may respond to one therapy and not another. The finding that a small number of ER-positive patients who do not respond to oophorectomy may subsequently respond to adrenalectomy has been explained by the fact that the adrenals constitute a source of androgens, which can serve as a substrate for peripheral aromatization to estrogens. Postmenopausal concentrations of estrogens in plasma have been shown to be capable of stimulating the growth of human breast cancer cells.[184] ER-positive premenopausal patients seem to respond as well to tamoxifen as to oophorectomy,[137, 185] despite an increase in plasma estradiol levels following tamoxifen treatment. Our understanding of drug-induced alterations of the hormonal milieu is incomplete, and progress in this area might also help explain why some ER-negative patients do worse when treated with a combination of chemotherapy and tamoxifen as compared with chemotherapy alone,[129] especially since tamoxifen is known to have little toxicity by itself. These apparent paradoxes reflect the complexity of endocrine interregulations and suggest that endocrine therapies need not work only through a given receptor system at the level of the cancer cells but that endocrine target organs as well as metabolically important organs such as liver or kidney may play an important role. Further understanding of the regulation of ER in benign and malignant cells as well as the mechanism of endocrine treatment will be needed to individualize therapies and optimize results.

Methodological defects that may lead to false-positive results include the choice of the ligand and the competitor previously discussed, as well as the somewhat arbitrary designation of receptor positive versus receptor negative, which is generally based on the individual laboratory's direct experience with the response to endocrine therapy. Furthermore, it seems intuitively obvious that an aneuploid malignant cell line might not be stable genetically and that spontaneous variants occur, which may or may not have measurable steroid hormone receptors and may or may not be endocrine responsive.

This hypothesis is supported by the lack of concordance regarding receptor status between two distinct sites of tumor metastases, which occurs with a frequency of approximately 10 percent, as well as by the decrease of responsiveness to endocrine treatment as the number of metastatic sites increases.

False-Negative Receptor Assays

Although occurring infrequently, false-negative results represent a potentially disastrous situation, since highly beneficial therapy may be withheld. The result is puzzling if the axiom that a receptor is a necessary element for endocrine response is correct. Several technical problems may account for these inappropriate results. Steroid receptors are unstable, thermolabile proteins, and any delay in the transport of the sample as well as incorrect storage may destroy the binding properties, resulting in a falsely negative assay. Other circumstances hazardous to the measurement of these proteins include faulty selection of ligand concentrations, ligand metabolism, and correct pH or ionic conditions. The choice of a method requiring a large amount of tissue may contribute to an incorrect negative classification of the tumor sample. In samples that are correctly quantitated, there may nonetheless be an incorrect assignment to a negative receptor category, since that designation is based on a correlation with past therapeutic results of a given laboratory. Many laboratories do not develop clinical correlations with their own data and simply presume their method to be valid and quantitatively in agreement with others.

Another error is introduced through the variable properties of malignant and benign cells in a given tumor. Since the surrounding fat and connective tissue contain little, if any, estrogen receptor, incorrect sampling may increase the uneven distribution of cancerous and benign cells. This may result in a false-negative result in the presence of a low proportion of strongly positive malignant cells when binding is normalized against total cytosol protein.

Another situation in which the tumor cells are potentially hormone responsive but in which most of the commonly employed hormone-binding assays would fail to detect any receptor protein is occupancy of this protein by endogenous hormone. Higher circulating levels of estrogen in premenopausal women may mask (occupy and process) estrogen receptor sites and account for the generally lower ER levels in premenopausal women. Saez and colleagues[136] have shown that progesterone receptor is undetectable during the luteal phase in premenopausal breast tumors, presumably because of occupancy and nuclear translocation by endogenous hormone. Similarly, tamoxifen and its active metabolites, which have been shown to have plasma half-lives of between 10 and 14 days,[186] make it difficult to re-evaluate ER levels in patients discontinuing tamoxifen therapy. Although exchange assays are available, they are technically difficult, and they will not detect processed receptor. Progesterone receptor synthesis in breast cancer was shown to be under estrogen control[187] as well as to be a predictor of response to endocrine therapy. Postmenopausal patients may have too low an estrogen concentration to induce progesterone receptor fully, and thus, PR assay may result in an inaccurate assessment of the biologic potential of the tumor.

Quality Control

In order to be able to compare the clinical outcomes of endocrine therapies in a meaningful way, it appears necessary to standardize and optimize the methods for quantitation of receptor and to adopt measures both in the assays and in specimen collection that minimize variance. Interlaboratory standardization procedures, which had been hampered by the thermolability of the receptor proteins, can be performed on lyophilized calf uterine and human breast cancer samples, which do not show any reduction in binding activity after 14 days' storage at room temperature.[188, 189]

Important factors in specimen collection have been shown to be:

1. Immediate and proper cooling of the tissue samples after removal.

2. Storage at $-79°C$ of the complete tissue sample (freezing of cytosol results in a loss of 25 to 50 percent of the binding activity.[190]

3. The use of a frozen-section specimen for receptor assays. In fact, a study of 13 cases comparing assay results of an initial frozen-section biopsy specimen with those of the final mastectomy specimen shows levels 1.6 to 6.5 times greater for the former assay.[191] These important differences are attributed to devitalization of the breast during mastec-

tomy, mechanical and possibly chemical injury, and the greater delay in obtaining the mastectomy specimens.

4. Tissue pulverization at the temperature of liquid nitrogen.

5. The presence of a sulfhydryl-protecting agent in the buffer.

6. The use of a simple, reproducible assay procedure.[192]

Accurate quantification of a discrete high-affinity receptor protein appears to be best guaranteed by a multiple-point procedure such as the charcoal adsorption method combined with a Scatchard plot. Most other techniques are set up using the DCC assay as a reference. In a recent study of inter- and intralaboratory variation including six laboratories experienced in the analysis of receptors, significant divergencies could be observed.[193] Not only were variations obtained through assaying a given sample by different methods in each laboratory, but also even greater differences were arrived at when identical samples were analyzed in separate laboratories. Furthermore, 29 to 42 percent of the total assays of standard samples containing low ER concentrations were misclassified as being negative. Similarly, when data from PR analysis were calculated in 18 different laboratories, six different methods were employed and substantial variation in affinity and number of binding sites was noted.[194]

CONCLUSIONS

ER and PR assays have proved invaluable in predicting prognosis in patients with both early and advanced breast cancers. These assays consititute a basis for selecting hormone-dependent tumors and thus help the physician to individualize and optimize therapy.

REFERENCES

1. Beatson GT: On treatment of inoperable cases of carcinoma of mamma: Suggestions for a new method of treatment with illustrative cases. Lancet 2:104, 1896.
2. Toft D, Gorski J: A receptor molecule for estrogens: Isolation from the rat uterus and preliminary characterization. Proc Natl Acad Sci USA 55:1574, 1966.
3. Glascock RF, Hoekstra WG: Accumulation of tritium-labelled hexoestradiol by the reproductive organs of immature female goats and sheep. Biochem J 72:673, 1959.
4. Jensen EV, Jacobson HI: Basic guides to the mechanism of estrogen action. Recent Prog Horm Res 18:387, 1962.
5. Jensen EV, De Sombre ER, Jongblut PW: Estrogen receptors in hormone-responsive tissues and tumors. *In* Wissler RW (ed.): Endogenous Factors Influencing Host Tumor Balance. Chicago: University of Chicago Press, 1967, p. 68.
6. Bayard F: Cytoplasmic and nuclear estradiol and progesterone receptors in human endometrium. J Clin Endocrinol 46:635, 1978.
7. Attardi B, Ohno S: Androgen and estrogen receptor in the developing mouse brain. Endocrinology 99:1279, 1976.
8. Adashi EY, Hsueh AJW, Yen SSC: Alterations induced by clomiphene in the concentrations of oestrogen receptors in the uterus, pituitary gland and hypothalamus of female rats. J Endocrinol 87:383, 1980.
9. Hasselquist MB, Goldberg N: Isolation and characterization of the estrogen receptor in human skin. J Clin Endocrinol Metab 50:76, 1980.
10. Eisenfeld AJ, Aten R, Weinberger M, et al.: Estrogen receptor in the mammalian liver. Science 191:862, 1976.
11. Dickson RB, Eisenfeld AJ: Estrogen receptor in liver of male and female rats: Endocrine regulation and molecular properties. Biol Reprod 21:1105, 1980.
12. Malcarne P, Piffanelli A, Fumero S, et al.: Estrogen receptors in rat thymus lymphocytes. *In* Wittliff JL, Dapunt O (eds.): Steroid Receptors and Hormone-Dependent Neoplasia. New York: Masson Publishing USA, 1980, p. 181.
13. Murphy JB, Emmott RC, Hicks LL, et al.: Estrogen receptors in the human prostate, seminal vesicle, epididymis, testis and genital skin: A marker for estrogen responsive tissues? J Clin Endocrinol Metab 50:938, 1980.
14. Fisher RI, Neifeld JP, Lippman ME: Oestrogen receptors in human malignant melanoma. Lancet 2:337, 1976.
15. Kasantikul V, Brown WJ: Estrogen receptor in acoustic neurilemmomas. Surg Neurol 15:105, 1981.
16. Pollow K, Lubbert H, Boquol E, et al.: Characterization and comparison of receptors for 17 beta estradiol and progesterone in human proliferative endometrium and endometrial carcinoma. Endocrinology 96:319, 1975.
17. Pizzocaro G, Valento M: Preoperative irradiation and surgery for oesophageal cancer: Causes of failure. Tumori (Milan) 66:739, 1980.
18. Jensen EV, Suzuki T, Kawashima T, et al.: A two step mechanism for the interaction of estradiol with rat uterus. Proc Natl Acad Sci USA 59:632, 1968.
19. Gorski J, Toft D, Shyamala G, et al.: Hormone receptors: Studies on the interaction of estrogen with the uterus. Recent Prog Horm Res 24:45, 1968.
20. Zava DT, McGuire WL: Estrogen receptor. Unoccupied sites in nuclei of a breast tumor cell line. J Biol Chem 252:3703, 1977.
21. Palmiter RD, Mulvihill ER, Shepherd JH, et al.: Steroid hormone regulation of ovalbumin and covalbumin gene transcription. J Biol Chem 256:7910, 1981.
22. Philipp BW, Shapiro DJ: Estrogen regulation of hepatic 3-hydroxy-3-methylglutaryl coenzyme A reductase and acetyl-CoA carboxylase in Xenopus laevis. J Biol Chem 256:2922, 1981.

23. Butler WB, Kirkland WL, Jorgensen TL: Induction of plasminogen activator by estradiol in a human breast cancer cell line (MCF-7). Biochem Biophys Res Commun 90:1328, 1979.
24. Westley B, Rochefort H: A secreted glycoprotein induced by estrogen in human breast cancer cell lines. Cell 20:353, 1980.
25. Swaneck GE, Nordstrom JL, Kreuzaler F, et al.: Effect of estrogen on gene expression in chicken oviduct: Evidence for transcriptional control of ovalbumin gene. Proc Natl Acad Sci USA 76:1049, 1979.
26. Schütz G, Nguyen-Huu MC, Giesecko K, et al.: Hormonal control of egg white protein messenger RNA synthesis in the chicken oviduct. Cold Spring Harbor Symp Quant Biol 42:617, 1977.
27. Ivarie RD, O'Farrell PH: The glucocorticoid domain: Steroid-mediated changes in the rate of synthesis of rat hepatoma proteins. Cell 13:41, 1978.
28. Commer P, Schwartz C, Tracy S, et al.: Dexamethasone inhibits alphafetoprotein gene expression in developing mouse liver. Biochem Biophys Res Commun 89:1294, 1979.
29. McKnight GS, Palmiter RD: Transcriptional regulation of the ovalbumin and covalbumin genes by steroid hormones in chick oviduct. J Biol Chem 254:9050, 1979.
30. Scott RW, Frankel FR: Enrichment of estradiol-receptor complexes in a transcriptionally active fraction of chromatin from MCF-7 cells. Proc Natl Acad Sci USA 77:1291, 1980.
31. Kallos J, Fasy TM, Hollander VP: Assessment of estrogen receptor–histone interaction. Proc Natl Acad Sci USA 78:2874, 1981.
32. Payvar F, Wrange O, Carlstedt-Duke J, et al.: Purified glucocorticoid receptors bind selectively in vitro to a cloned DNA fragment whose transcription is regulated by glucocorticoids in vivo. Proc Natl Acad Sci USA 78:6628, 1981.
33. Lee F, Mulligan R, Berg P, et al.: Glucocorticoids regulate expression of dihydrofolate reductase cDNA in mouse mammary tumor virus chimaeric plasmids. Nature 294:228, 1981.
34. Ikeda T, Sirbasku DA: Purification and properties of a mammary-uterine-pituitary tumor cell growth factor from pregnant sheep uterus. J Biol Chem 259:4049, 1984.
35. Shafie SM: Estrogen and growth of breast cancer. New evidence suggests indirect action. Science 209:701, 1980.
36. Dornberger H, Neuberger B, Schwartz P, et al.: Mesenchyme-mediated effect of testosterone on embryonic mammary epithelium. Cancer Res 38:4066, 1978.
37. Engel LW, Young NA: Human breast carcinoma lines in continuous culture: A review. Cancer Res 38:4327, 1978.
38. Lippman ME, Bolan G, Huff K: The effects of estrogens and antiestrogens on hormone responsive human breast cancer in long-term tissue culture. Cancer Res 36:4595, 1976.
39. Lippman ME, Bolan G, Huff K: Interactions of antiestrogens with human breast cancer in long term tissue culture. Cancer Treat Rep 60:1421, 1976.
40. Allegra JC, Lippman ME: Growth of a human breast cancer cell line in serum-free hormone receptors and response to cytotoxic chemotherapy in patients with metastatic breast cancer. Cancer Res 38:3823, 1978.
41. Lippman ME, Cassidy JC, Wesley M, et al.: A randomized attempt to increase the efficacy of cytotoxic chemotherapy in metastatic breast cancer by hormonal synchronization. J Clin Oncol 2:28, 1984.
42. Lippman ME, Sorace R, Bagley C, et al.: Effective systemic management of locally advanced breast cancer (LABC). *In*: Proc Am Soc Clin Oncol, 4, (Abstract 249), 1985.
43. Butler WB, Kelsey WH, Goran N: Effects of serum and insulin on the sensitivity of the human breast cancer cell line MCF-7 to estrogens and antiestrogens. Cancer Res 41:82, 1981.
44. Edwards DP, Murphy SR, McGuire WL: Effect of estrogen and antiestrogens on DNA polymerase in human breast cancer. Cancer Res 40:1722, 1980.
45. Barnes D, Sato G: Growth of a human mammary tumour cell line in a serum-free medium. Nature 281:388, 1979.
46. Chalbos D, Vignon F, Keydar I, et al.: Estrogens stimulate cell proliferation and induce secretory proteins in a human breast cancer cell line (T47D). J Clin Endocrinol Metab 55:276, 1982.
47. Darbre P, Yates J, Curtis S, et al.: Effect of estradiol on human breast cancer cell in culture. Cancer Res 43:349, 1983.
48. Noguchi S, Kitamura Y, Uchida N, et al.: Growth-stimulative effect of estrogen on androgen-dependent Shionogi carcinoma 115. Cancer Res 44:5644, 1984.
49. Katzenellenbogen B, Norman MJ, Eckert RL, et al.: Bioactivities, estrogen receptor interactions, and plasminogen activator–inducing activities of tamoxifen and hydroxy-tamoxifen isomers in MCF-7 human breast cancer cells. Cancer Res 44:112, 1983.
50. Leung BS, Qureshi S, Leung JS: Response to estrogen by the human mammary carcinoma cell line CAMA-1. Cancer Res 42:5060, 1982.
51. Natoli C, Sica G, Natoli V, et al.: Two new estrogen-supersensitive variants of the MCF-7 human breast cancer cell line. Breast Cancer Res Treat 3:23, 1983.
52. Page M, Field J, Everett N, et al.: Serum regulation of the estrogen responsiveness of the human breast cancer cell line MCF-7. Cancer Res 43:1244, 1983.
53. Weichselbaum RR, Hellman S, Piro A, et al.: Proliferation kinetics of a human breast cancer cell line in vitro following treatment with 17 beta-estradiol and 1-beta-D-arabinofuranosylcytosine. Cancer Res 38:2339, 1978.
54. Whitehead RH, Quirk SJ, Vitali AA, et al.: A new human breast carcinoma cell line (PMC42) with stem cell characteristics. III. Hormone receptor status and responsiveness. J Natl Cancer Inst 73:643, 1984.
55. Simon WE, Albrecht M, Trams G, et al.: In vitro growth promotion of human mammary carcinoma cells by steroid hormones, tamoxifen, and prolactin. J Natl Cancer Inst 73:313, 1984.
56. Calvo F, Brower M, Carney DN: Continuous culture and soft agarose cloning of multiple human breast carcinoma cell lines in serum-free medium. Cancer Res 44:4553, 1984.
57. Cowan KH, Goldsmith ME, Levine RM, et al.: Dihydrofolate reductase gene amplification and possible rearrangement in estrogen-responsive methotrexate-resistant human breast cancer cells. J Biol Chem 257:15079, 1982.

58. Aitken SC, Lippman ME: Hormonal regulation of net DNA synthesis in MCF-7 human breast cancer cells in tissue culture. Cancer Res 42:1727, 1982.
59. Kasid A, Davidson N, Gelmann E, et al.: Transcriptional control of thymidine kinase gene expression by estrogen and antiestrogens in MCF-7 human breast cancer cells. J Biol Chem 261:5562, 1986.
60. Cowan HK, Goldsmith ME, Levine RM, et al.: Dihydrofolate reductase gene amplification and possible rearrangement in estrogen-responsive methotrexate-resistant human breast cancer cells. J Biol Chem 257:15079, 1982.
61. Levine RM, Rubalcaba E, Lippman ME, et al.: Effects of estrogen and tamoxifen on the regulation of dihydrofolate gene expression in a human breast cancer cell line. Cancer Res 45:1644, 1985.
62. Horwitz KB: Is a functional estrogen receptor always required for progesterone receptor induction in breast cancer? Biochemistry 15:209, 1981.
63. Huff KK, Lippman ME: Hormonal control of plasminogen activator secretion in ZR-75-1 human breast cancer cells in culture. Endocrinology 114:1665, 1984.
64. Ciocca DR, Adams DJ, Edwards DP, et al.: Distribution of an estrogen-induced protein with a molecular weight of 24,000 in normal and malignant human tissues and cells. Cancer Res 43:1204, 1983.
65. Westley B, Rochefort H: A secreted glycoprotein induced by estrogen in human breast cancer cell lines. Cell 20:353, 1980.
66. Jakowlew SB, Breathnach R, Jeltsch JM, et al.: Sequence of the pS2 mRNA induced by estrogen in the human breast cancer cell line MCF-7. Nucleic Acids Res 12:2861, 1984.
67. Davidson N, Wilding G, Lippman ME, et al.: Isolation of estrogen regulated cDNA clones from human breast cancer cells. Proceedings of American Society of Clinical Investigation. Clin Res 33:577, 1985.
68. Sporn MB, Todaro GJ: Autocrine secretion and malignant transformation of cells. N Engl J Med 303:878, 1980.
69. Lippman ME: Hormonal regulation of human breast cancer cells in vitro. *In*: Pike MC, Siiteri P, Welsch CW (eds.): Hormones and Breast Cancer. Cold Spring Harbor, NY: Cold Spring Harbor Laboratory, 1981, pp. 171–184.
70. Soule HD, McGrath CM: Estrogen-responsive proliferation of clonal human breast carcinoma cells in athymic mice. Cancer Lett 10:177, 1980.
71. Seibert K, Shafie SM, Triche TJ, et al.: Clonal variation of MCF-7 breast cancer cells in vitro and in athymic nude mice. Cancer Res 43:2223, 1983.
72. Huseby RA, Maloney TM, McGrath CM: Evidence for direct growth-stimulating effect of estradiol on human MCF-7 cells *in vivo*. Cancer Res 44:2654, 1984.
73. Jakesz R, Smith CA, Aitken S, et al.: Influence of cell proliferation and cell cycle phase on expression of estrogen receptor in MCF-7 breast cancer cells. Cancer Res 44:619, 1984.
74. Dunn GA, Ireland GW: New evidence that growth in 3T3 cell cultures is a diffusion-limited process. Nature 312:63, 1984.
75. Vignon F, Derocq D, Chambon M, et al.: Les protéines oestrogéno-induites sécrétés par les cellules mammaires cancéreuses humaines MCF7 stimulent leur prolifération. C R Seances Acad Sci 296:151, 1983.
76. Furlanetto RW, DiCarlo JN: Somatomedin C receptors and growth effects in human breast cells maintained in long term culture. Cancer Res 44:2122, 1984.
77. Huff KK, Lippman ME, Spencer EM, et al.: Secretion of immunoreactive IGF-1 by cultured human cancer cells. Cancer Res 46:4613, 1986.
78. Osborne CK, Hamilton B, Titus G, et al.: Epidermal growth factor stimulation of human breast cancer cells in culture. Cancer Res 40:2361, 1980.
79. DeLarco JW, Todaro GJ: Growth factors from murine sarcoma virus–transformed cells. Proc Natl Acad Sci USA 75:4001, 1978.
80. Salomon DS, Zweibel JA, Mozeena S, et al.: Presence of transforming growth factors in human breast cancer cells. Cancer Res 44:4069, 1984.
81. Carpenter G, Stoscheck CM, Preston YA, et al.: Antibodies to the epidermal growth factor receptor block the biological activities of sarcoma growth factor. Proc Natl Acad Sci USA 80:5627, 1983.
82. Anzano MA, Roberts AB, Smith JM, et al.: Sarcoma growth factor from conditioned medium of virally transformed cells is composed of both type alpha and type beta transforming growth factors. Proc Natl Acad Sci USA 80:6264, 1983.
83. Tucker RF, Shipley GD, Moses HL, et al.: Growth inhibitor from BSC-1 cells closely related to platelet type B transforming growth factor. Science 226:705, 1981.
84. Dickson RB, Huff KK, Spencer FM, et al.: Induction of epidermal growth factor–related polypeptides by 17β-estradiol in MCF-7 human breast cancer cells. Endocrinology 118:138, 1986.
85. Roberts AB, Anzano MA, Wakefield CM, et al.: Type B transforming growth factor: A bifunctional regulator of cellular growth. Proc Natl Acad Sci USA 82:119, 1985.
86. Hanauske AR, Pardue R, Van Hoff DD: Rat transforming growth factor improves growth of human tumors in vitro. Clin Res 33:452A, 1985.
87. Ibbotson KJ, D'Souza SM, Smith DD, et al.: EGF receptor antiserum inhibits bone resorbing activity produced by a rat Leydig cell tumor associated with the humoral hypercalcemia of malignancy. Endocrinology 116:469, 1985.
88. Sporn MB, Roberts AB, Shull JH, et al.: Polypeptide transforming growth factos isolated from bovine sources and used for wound healing in vivo. Science 219:1329, 1983.
89. Leof EB, Wharton W, Van Wyk JJ, et al.: Epidermal growth factor (EGF) and somatomedin C regulate GI progression in competent BALb/c-3T3 cells. Exp Cell Res 141:107, 1982.
90. Halper J, Moses HL: Epithelial tissue-derived growth factor–like polypeptides. Cancer Res 43:1972, 1983.
91. Kasid A, Lippman ME, Papageorge AG, et al.: Harvey murine sarcoma virus DNA transfected into MCF-7 human breast cancer cells bypasses their dependence on estrogen for tumorigenicity. Science 228:725, 1985.
92. McGuire WL (ed.): Breast Cancer: Advances in Research and Treatment, Vols. 1–4. New York: Plenum Press, 1980.
93. Everson RB, Lippman ME: Male breast cancer. *In*: McGuire WL (ed.): Breast Cancer: Advances in Research and Treatment, Vol. 3. New York: Plenum Press, 1979, p. 239.
94. McCarty KS, Jr., Barton TK, Fetter BF, et al.:

Correlation of estrogen and progesterone receptors with histologic differentiation in mammary carcinoma. Cancer 46:285, 1980.
95. Meyer JS, Rao BR, Stevens SC, et al.: Low incidence of estrogen receptor in breast carcinomas with rapid rates of cellular replication. Cancer 40:2290, 1977.
96. Parl FF, Wagner RK: The histopathological evaluation of human breast cancers in correlation with estrogen receptor values. Cancer 46:362, 1980.
97. Allegra JC, Lippman ME, Simon R, et al.: Association between steroid hormone receptor status and disease-free interval in breast cancer. Cancer Treat Rep 63:1271, 1979.
98. Heuson JC, Le Clercq G, Longeval E, et al.: Estrogen receptors: Prognostic significance in breast cancer. *In:* McGuire WL, Carbone PP, Vollmer EP (eds.): Estrogen Receptors in Human Breast Cancer. New York: Raven Press, 1975, p. 57.
99. Wagner RK, Jongblut PW: Improved biochemical characterization of breast cancer as a guide to hormonal treatment. *In:* Henningen B, Lindner F, Steichele C (eds.): Endocrine Treatment of Breast Cancer. Heidelberg: Springer-Verlag, 1980, p. 3.
100. Curtis CG: Long-term changes in corticosteroid excretion. *In*: Ferin M, Halberg F, Richart RM, et al. (eds): Biorhythms and Human Reproduction. New York: John Wiley & Sons, Inc., 1974, p. 417.
101. Roy EJ, Wilson MA: Diurnal rhythm of cytoplasmic estrogen receptors in the rat brain in the absence of circulating estrogens. Science 213:1525, 1981.
102. Kuttenn F, Fournier JC, Mauvais-Jarvic P: Estradiol and progesterone receptors in human breast fibroadenomas. J Clin Endocrinol 52:1225, 1981.
103. Mauvais-Jarvis, P, Sitruk-Ware R, Kuttenn F, et al.: Luteal phase insufficiency: A common pathophysiological factor in development of benign and malignant breast diseases. *In*: Bulbrook RD, Taylor DJ (eds.): Commentaries on Research in Breast Disease. New York: Alan R. Liss, 1979, p. 25.
104. Allegra JC, Barlock A, Huff KK, et al.: Changes in multiple or sequential estrogen receptor determinations in breast cancer. Cancer 45:792, 1980.
105. De Sombre ER, Jensen EV: Estrophilin features and application to the mastectomy specimen. Cancer 46:2783, 1980.
106. Mauvais-Jarvis P, Sitruk-Ware R, Kuttenn F: Benign breast disease. *In* McGuire WL (ed.): Breast Cancer: Advances in Research and Treatment, Vol. 4. New York: Plenum Press, 1977, p. 51.
107. Swerdlow M, Humphrey LJ: Fibrocystic disease and carcinoma of the breast. Arch Surg 87:457, 1963.
108. Davis H, Simons M, Davis JB: Cystic disease of the breast: Relationship to carcinoma. Cancer 17:957, 1964.
109. Donnelly PK, Baker KW, Carney JA, et al.: Benign breast lesions and subsequent breast cancer in Rochester, Minnesota. Mayo Clin Proc 50:650, 1975.
110. Fisher ER: Pathology of the breast. *In*: McGuire WL (ed.): Breast Cancer: Advances in Research and Treatment, Vol. 1. New York: Plenum Press, 1977, p. 43.
111. Humphrey LJ, Swerdlow M: Relationship of benign breast disease to carcinoma of the breast. Surgery 52:841, 1962.
112. Black MM, Barclay THC, Cutler SJ, et al.: Association of atypical characteristics of benign breast lesions with subsequent risk of breast cancer. Cancer 29:338, 1972.
113. Wellings SR, Jensen HM, Marcum RG: An atlas of subgroup pathology of the human breast with special reference to possible precancerous lesions. J Natl Cancer Inst 55:231, 1975.
114. MacMahon B, Cole P, Brown J: Etiology of human breast cancer: A review. J Natl Cancer Inst 50:21, 1973.
115. De Brux J: Histoire naturelle et diagnostic de quelques lesions mammaires. Rev Fr Gynecol 68:365, 1973.
116. Bassler R: Morphology of hormone induced structural changes in the female breast. Curr Top Pathol 53:1, 1970.
117. Mauvais-Jarvis P, Kuttenn F: Les mastopathies bénignes. Nouv Presse Med 3:993, 1976.
118. Vorherr H, Messer RH: Breast cancer: Potentially predisposing and protecting factors. Role of pregnancy, lactation, and endocrine status. Am J Obstet Gynecol 130:335, 1978.
119. Menendez-Botet CJ, Nisselbaum JS, Fleischer M, et al.: Correlation between estrogen receptor protein and carcinoembryonic antigen in normal and carcinomatous human breast tissue. Clin Chem 22:1366, 1976.
120. Hawkins RA, Hill A, Freedman B: A simple method for the determination of oestrogen receptor concentrations in breast tumors and other tissues. Clin Chim Acta 64:203, 1975.
121. Allegra JC, Lippman ME, Green L, et al.: Estrogen receptor values in patients with benign breast disease. Cancer 44:228, 1979.
122. Sarrif AM, Durant JR: Evidence that ER negative, PR positive breast and ovarian carcinomas contain estrogen receptor. Cancer 48:1215, 1981.
123. Thompson EB, Lippman ME (eds.): Steroid Receptors and the Management of Cancer. Boca Raton, FL: CRC Press, 1979.
124. Wittliff JL, Dapunt O (eds.): Steroid Receptors and Hormone-dependent Neoplasia. New York: Masson Publishing, USA, 1980.
125. Lippman ME, Allegra JC: Quantitative estrogen receptor analysis: The response to endocrine and cytotoxic chemotherapy in human breast cancer and the disease-free interval. Cancer 46:2829, 1980.
126. Skinner LG, Barnes DM, Ribeiro GG: The clinical value of multiple steroid receptor assays in breast cancer management. Cancer 46:2939, 1980.
127. Singhakowinta A, Mohindra R, Brooks SC, et al.: Clinical correlation of endocrine therapy and estrogen receptor. *In*: McGuire WL, Vollmer EP, Carbone PP (eds.): Estrogen Receptors in Human Breast Cancer. New York: Raven Press, 1975, p. 131.
128. Hubay CA, Peterson OH, Marshal JS, et al.: Antiestrogen, cytotoxic chemotherapy and bacillus Calmette-Guérin vaccination in stage II breast cancer: A preliminary report. Surgery 52:841, 1980.
129. Fisher B, Redmond C, Brown A, et al.: Treatment of primary breast cancer chemotherapy and tamoxifen. N Engl J Med 305:1, 1981.
130. Meyer JS, Hixon B: Advanced stage and early relapse of breast carcinomas association with high thymidine labelling indices. Cancer Res 39:4042, 1979.
131. De Wys WD, Allegra JC, Simon R, et al.: A proposed model for the prediction of response to endocrine therapy in breast cancer from the estrogen receptor status of one site and the number of metastatic sites. Cancer Res 40:2423, 1980.

132. Nicole I, Saez S: Human breast cancer isolated cells in short-term culture: Relation between steroid receptor content and the response to hormone addition. Cancer Res 38:4314, 1978.
133. Anderson WA, Kang YH, De Sombre ER: Endogenous peroxidase: A specific marker enzyme for tissues displaying growth dependency on estrogens. J Cell Biol 64:668, 1975.
134. Milgrom E, Atger M, Perrot M, et al.: Progesterone in uterus and plasma: Uterine progesterone receptors during the estrous cycle and implantation in the guinea pig. Endocrinology 90:104, 1972.
135. Rao BR, Meyer JS: Estrogen and progestin receptors in normal and cancer tissue. *In*: McGuire WL, Raynaud JP, Baulieu EE (eds.): Progesterone Receptors in Normal and Neoplastic Tissues (Progress in Cancer Research and Therapy, Vol. 4). New York: Raven Press, 1977, p. 155.
136. Saez S, Martin PM, Chouver CD: Estradiol and progesterone receptor levels in human breast adenocarcinoma in relation to plasma estrogen and progesterone levels. Cancer Res 38:3468, 1978.
137. Pritchard KI, Thomoson DB, Myers RE, et al.: Tamoxifen therapy in premenopausal patients with metastatic breast cancer. Cancer Treat Rep 64:787, 1980.
138. Fracchia AA, Randall HT, Farrow JH: The results of adrenalectomy in advanced breast cancer in 500 consecutive patients. Surg Gynecol Obstet 125:747, 1967.
139. Grodin JM, Siiteri, PK, MacDonald PC: Source of estrogen production in postmenopausal women. J Clin Endocrinol 36:207, 1973.
140. Notides AC, Lerner N, Hamilton DC: Positive cooperativity of the estrogen receptor. Proc Natl Acad Sci USA 78:4926, 1981.
141. Kennedy BJ: Diethylstilbestrol versus testosterone propionate therapy in advanced breast cancer. Surg Gynecol Obstet 120:1246, 1965.
142. Stoll BA: Castration and oestrogen therapy. *In:* Stoll BA (ed.): Endocrine Therapy in Malignant Disease. London: W.B. Saunders Co., 1972, p. 139.
143. Kennedy BJ: Hormone therapy in inoperable breast cancer. Cancer 24:1345, 1969.
144. Tomkins GN, Maxwell ES: Some aspects of steroid hormone action. Annu Rev Biochem 12:677, 1963.
145. Williams-Ashman HG: New facets of the biochemistry of steroid hormone action. Cancer Res 25:1096, 1965.
146. Grant JK: Actions of steroid hormones at cellular and molecular levels. Essays Biochem 5:1, 1969.
147. Sirbasku DA: Estrogen-induction of growth factors specific for hormone-responsive mammary pituitary and kidney tumor cells. Proc Natl Acad Sci USA 75:3786, 1978.
148. Sutherland RL, Murphy LC, Foo MS, et al.: High-affinity anti-oestrogen binding site distinct from the oestrogen receptor. Nature 288:273, 1980.
149. Sherman BM, Chapler FK, Crickard K, et al.: Endocrine consequences of continuous antiestrogen therapy with tamoxifen in premenopausal women. J Clin Invest 64:398, 1979.
150. Levin J, Markham MJ, Greenwald ES, et al.: Effect of tamoxifen treatment on cortisol metabolism and the course of the disease in advanced breast cancer. Cancer 47:1394, 1981.
151. McGuire WL, Horwitz KB, Zava DT, et al.: Hormones in breast cancer: Update 1978. Metabolism 27:487, 1978.
152. Allegra JC, Lippman ME, Thompson EB, et al.: Relationship between the progesterone, androgen, and glucocorticoid receptor and response rate to endocrine therapy in metastatic breast cancer. Cancer Res 39:1973, 1979.
153. Schultz KD, Schmidt-Rhode P, Waymar P, et al.: The effect of combination chemotherapy on ovarian, hypothalamic and pituitary function in patients with breast cancer. Arch Gynecol 227:293, 1979.
154. Carter SK: Integration of chemotherapy into combined modality treatment of solid tumors. VII. Adenocarcinoma of the breast. Cancer Treat Rev 3:141, 1976.
155. Tancini G, Bajetta E, Marchina S, et al.: Preliminary 3-year results of 12 versus 6 cycles of surgical adjuvant CMF in premenopausal breast cancer. Cancer Clin Trials 2:85, 1979.
156. Rossi A, Valagussa P, Bonadonna G: Combined modality management of operable breast cancer. Recent Results Cancer Res 68:80, 1979.
157. Carter SK: Surgery plus adjuvant chemotherapy—a review of therapeutic implications. I. Breast cancer. Cancer Chemother Pharmacol 4:147, 1980.
158. Kiang DT, Frenning DH, Goldman AI, et al.: Estrogen receptors and responses to chemotherapy and hormonal therapy in advanced breast cancer. N Engl J Med 229:1330, 1978.
159. Janet W, Maass H: Some comments on the necessity of receptor determinations in human breast cancer. Cancer Res 38:4305, 1978.
160. Hilf R, Feldstein ML, Gibson SL, et al.: The relative importance of estrogen receptor analysis as a prognostic factor for recurrence or response to chemotherapy in women with breast cancer. Cancer 45:1993, 1980.
161. Blamey RW, Bishop HM, Blake JRS, et al.: Relationship between primary breast tumor receptor status and patient survival. Cancer 46:2765, 1980.
162. Young PCM, Ehrlich CE, Einhorn LH: Relationship between steroid receptors and response to endocrine therapy and cytotoxic chemotherapy in metastatic breast cancer. Cancer 46:2961, 1980.
163. Rosenbaum C, Marslam TA, Stolbach LL, et al.: Estrogen receptor status and response to chemotherapy in advanced breast cancer: The Tufts-Shattuck-Pandville experience. Cancer 46:2919, 1980.
164. Samal BA, Brooks SC, Cummings G, et al.: Estrogen receptors and responsiveness of advanced breast cancer to chemotherapy. Cancer 46:2925, 1980.
165. Mortimer J, Reimer R, Greenstreet R, et al.: Influence of estrogen receptor status on response to combination chemotherapy for recurrent breast cancer. Cancer Treat Rep 65:763, 1981.
166. Rubens RD, King RJB, Sextan S, et al.: Oestrogen receptors and response to cytotoxic chemotherapy in advanced breast cancer. Cancer Chemother Pharmacol 4:43, 1980.
167. Janet W, Maass H, Stolzenbach G, et al.: Estrogen receptor status and response to polychemotherapy in advanced breast cancer. Cancer 46:2809, 1980.
168. Bonadonna G, Valagussa P, Tancini G, et al.: Estrogen receptor status and response to chemotherapy in early and advanced breast cancer. Cancer Chemother Pharmacol 4:37, 1980.
169. McGuire WL: Steroid receptors in human breast cancer. Cancer Res 38:4289, 1978.
170. Poulsen HS, Jensen J, Hermansen C: Human breast

cancer: Heterogeneity of estrogen binding sites. Cancer 48:1791, 1981.

171. Wittliff JL, Savlov ED: Estrogen-binding capacity of cytoplasmic forms of the estrogen receptors in human breast cancer. *In*: McGuire WL, Vollmer EP, Carbone PP (eds.): Estrogen Receptors in Human Breast Cancer. New York: Raven Press, 1975, p. 73.
172. Thampan TW, Clark JH: An oestrogen receptor activator protein in rat uterine cytosol. Nature 290:152, 1981.
173. Nishizawa Y, Maeda Y, Noma K: A modulator which converts activated estrogen receptor to a biologically inactive aggregated form. Endocrinology 109:1403, 1981.
174. Sato B, Maeda Y, Noma K: Estrogen binding component of mouse Leydig cell tumors: An in vitro conversion from nonreceptor to receptor-like molecule. Endocrinology 108:612, 1981.
175. Okulicz WC, Macdonald RG, Leavitt WW: Progesterone-induced estrogen receptor–regulatory factor in hamster uterine nuclei: Preliminary characterization in a cell-free system. Endocrinology 81:2273, 1981.
176. Sherman M, Pickering L, Rollwagen FM, et al.: New receptors: Proteolytic fragments of receptors containing the steroid binding site. Fed Proc 37:167, 1978.
177. Clark JH, Schrader WT, O'Malley BW: Mechanisms of steroid hormone action. *In*: Wilson J, Foster D (eds.): Textbook of Endocrinology. Philadelphia: W. B. Saunders, 1985, pp. 33–75.
178. Schneider SL, Dao TL: Effect of CA2+ and salt on forms of estradiol cytoplasmic receptor in human neoplastic breast tissue. Cancer Res 37:382, 1977.
179. Tilzer LL, McFarland RT: Different ionic forms of estrogen receptor in rat uterus and human breast carcinoma. Cancer Res 41:1508, 1981.
180. Miller LK, Tuazon FB, Niu EM, et al.: Human breast tumor estrogen receptor: Effects of molybdate and electrophoretic analyses. Endocrinology 108:1369, 1981.
181. Redeuilh G, Secco C, Baulieu EE, et al.: Calf uterine estradiol receptor. Effects of molybdate on estrogen receptor. J Biol Chem 256:11496, 1981.
182. Nawata HJ, Bronzert D, Lippman ME: Isolation and characterization of tamoxifen-resistant cell line derived from MCF-7 human breast cancer cells. J Biol Chem 256:5016, 1981.
183. Nawata H, Chong MT, Bronzert D, et al.: Estradiol-independent growth of a subline of MCF-7 human breast cancer cells in culture. J Biol Chem 256:6895, 1981.
184. Lippman ME, Bolan G, Huff K: The effects of estrogens and antiestrogens on hormone-responsive human breast cancer in long-term tissue culture. Cancer Res 36:4595, 1976.
185. Manni A, Pearson O: Antiestrogen-induced remissions in premenopausal women with stage IV breast cancer: Effects of ovarian function. Cancer Treat Rep 64:779, 1980.
186. Fabian C, Sternson L: Clinical pharmacology of tamoxifen in patients with breast cancer: Comparison of traditional and loading dose schedules. Cancer Treat Rep 64:765, 1980.
187. Horwitz KB, McGuire WL: Specific progesterone receptors in human breast cancer. Steroids 25:497, 1975.
188. Bojar H, Wittliff WC, Balzer K, et al.: Properties of specific estrogen-binding components in human kidney and renal carcinoma. Acta Endocrinol (Suppl) 193:51, 1980.
189. Benraad T, Koenders A: Estradiol receptor activity in lyophilized calf uterus and human breast cancer tissue. Cancer 46:2762, 1980.
190. Thompson J, Haven MC, Langdon SM, et al.: Stability of 8 S molecular form in frozen cytosols and practical criteria for its confirmation. Am J Clin Pathol 73:340, 1979.
191. Hasson J, Luhan PA, Kohl MW: Comparison of estrogen receptor levels in breast cancer samples from mastectomy and frozen section specimens. Cancer 48:138, 1981.
192. Wagner RK, Jungblut PW: Quality control in steroid hormone receptor analyses. Cancer 46:2950, 1980.
193. Cohen JC, Gelman R, Raam S, et al.: A blinded study in the performance of estrogen receptor assay. Proc Am Soc Clin Oncol 21:325, 1980.
194. Braunsberg H, Hammond KD: Methods of steroid receptor calculation: An interlaboratory study. Acta Endocrinol (Suppl) 193:51, 1975.
195. Siebert IT, Lippman ME: Hormone receptors in breast cancer. Clin Oncol 1:735, 1982.
196. Scholl S, Lippman ME: Methods and clinical use of receptor assay. *In*: Bonadonna G (ed.): Breast Cancer: Diagnosis and Management. London: John Wiley & Sons, 1984, pp. 75–108.

Adjuvant Therapy for Breast Cancer

NANCY E. DAVIDSON, M. D.
MARC E. LIPPMAN, M. D.

12

Of the 120,000 women who were found to have breast cancer in the United States in 1985, over 90 percent presented with disease apparently localized to the breast and axillary lymph nodes. Yet nearly one half of these women will develop and eventually die of metastatic disease, despite advances in early diagnosis and primary treatment modalities. It is now commonly believed that breast cancer is often a systemic disease at diagnosis and therefore no longer curable by local therapy alone. Thus, the desire to identify those women at high risk for disease recurrence and to develop effective forms of systemic therapy to supplement their therapy has led to intense study of adjuvant forms of therapy over the last 25 years. This chapter will review the scientific principles underlying adjuvant therapy; the results of a variety of clinical trials using endocrine, chemotherapeutic, or immunotherapeutic approaches; and the impact of various prognostic factors on outcome in order to elucidate the role of adjuvant therapy in the treatment of breast cancer.

SCIENTIFIC PRINCIPLES UNDERLYING ADJUVANT THERAPY TRIALS

Treatment of breast cancer was first predicated on the Halstedian view that breast cancer spread in an orderly fashion from primary tumor to involvement of local lymphatics and finally to disseminated disease. Trials of local radiation therapy have refuted this view, because sterilization of the axilla has not prevented the development of metastatic disease. Similarly, extensive local surgical procedures such as the extended radical mastectomy have failed to prevent disease spread. It had also been believed that disease spread via tumor seeding during surgery; the finding of a strong relationship between the number of involved axillary nodes and the likelihood of subsequent disease recurrence makes this unlikely. Nonetheless, several trials of perioperative chemotherapy designed to eradicate tumor cells that were presumably disseminated during surgery have demonstrated a benefit for patients treated with short courses of chemotherapy during the immediate postoperative period. These results suggest that even brief courses of adjuvant therapy may be effective.

The design of most recent trials has been influenced by a few crucial scientific principles. Cells with the clonogenic potential to result in gross metastatic disease are shed from a tumor relatively late in its life span but early in terms of its clinical detectability. Of patients with nonpalpable breast tumors, 5 to 10 percent have pathologically positive axillary lymph nodes. Of patients with tumors 3 cm in diameters, about half will already have axillary lymph node metastases.

Systemic drugs are used in an effort to eradicate cancer cells remaining after primary local treatment. Drug-induced cell kill is best described by first-order kinetics; a drug kills a constant fraction of cells rather than a constant number. Thus, therapy would theoretically be most effective when the number of cells is the smallest—after the bulk of the tumor burden has been treated by primary surgery with or without radiation therapy.[1, 2]

Growth of malignant tumors can be described by a gompertzian equation. As tumor size increases, its growth fraction decreases and the tumor-doubling time lengthens. Since most cytotoxic agents are more effective against dividing cells than resting cells, chemotherapy should be most effective against small tumors with high growth fractions and, by extrapolation, against micrometastatic disease.[3] This concept has been tested in transplantable animal tumor models. Macroscopic disease was initially resected, and chemotherapy was administered immediately after surgery. Combined therapy was more effective in increasing survival than was surgery or chemotherapy alone. If surgery was delayed after tumor implantation, resulting in increased tumor burden, surgery and chemotherapy were less effective. Chemotherapy that was delayed after surgery was also less effective, presumably because of increased growth of micrometastatic tumor. Finally, more aggressive chemotherapy resulted in a higher disease-free survival rate.[2]

As a final point, Goldie and Coldman[4–6] have proposed that tumor cells have a finite rate of mutation that will result in the development of drug-resistant cells. The probability that a tumor will contain drug-resistant cells is thus directly related to tumor burden: large tumors will be more likely to contain drug-resistant cells. Therefore, systemic therapy should be administered as early as possible in the life span of a tumor to avoid development of drug-resistant cells and, theoretically, to increase the possibility of cure. Though none of these ideas have been thoroughly substantiated in humans, these concepts have been crucial in the development of adjuvant chemotherapy trials in the modern era.

PROBLEMS OF TRIAL DESIGN AND ASSESSMENT OF OUTCOME

In reviewing results of trials, it is important to recognize the pitfalls one may encounter in analyzing a particular trial or comparing results between trials. These may include (1) differences in patient eligibility, (2) variation in type and timing of local therapy, (3) different times for initiation of adjuvant therapy, (4) differences in patient prognostic variables, both recognized and unrecognized, (5) variations in definition of menopausal status, (6) differences in attitude regarding aggressiveness of therapy, and (7) methodological considerations such as the use of historical versus concurrent randomized control groups or the exclusion of patients from analysis because of ineligibility, loss to follow-up, or protocol violations. In addition, the difficulty in determining what constitutes a response to therapy in these patients without evidence of disease is readily apparent. Nearly all studies use relapse-free survival (RFS) as a short-term and imperfect index of efficacy of therapy. However, the ultimate goal of adjuvant therapy is obviously prolongation of overall survival (OAS), but the lengthy follow-up required for analysis of survival means that such information is available for fewer trials at present. In addition, subsequent therapy in the event of recurrent disease is frequently not standardized or reported, further complicating interpretation of any survival data.

EARLY TRIALS OF POSTOPERATIVE CHEMOTHERAPY

Several trials begun more than 20 years ago examined the usefulness of short courses of chemotherapy with cyclophosphamide (C), thiotepa, or nitrogen mustard in the immediate postoperative period. Many of these studies were designed to kill tumor cells presumed to have been dislodged during the surgical procedure. Although the theory underlying these trials has since fallen into disfavor, the results of several remain positive after long periods of follow-up. An early study examined the use of thiotepa for three days postoperatively.[7, 8] That regimen resulted in a decrease in the relapse rate of premenopausal women with involvement of more than three axillary nodes. In another trial,[9–12] cyclophosphamide, 5 mg/kg/day, was given intravenously for six days to 507 evaluable patients, while 519 randomized control subjects underwent radical mastectomy alone. At 15 years' follow-up, a significant decrease in relapse rates and an increase in OAS of about 15 percent were noted in the treated cohort. The benefit extended to both premenopausal and postmenopausal patients and was independent of axillary lymph node status. It was absent only in a subgroup of patients treated in a single institution where chemotherapy was delayed about one month to permit completion of postoperative radiation therapy. After 20 years of follow-up, the increase in survival rate persisted but was no longer statistically significant because of an increase in deaths not due to breast cancer in this now elderly population. Results of six early trials, which included a surgical control group, are summarized in Table 12–1.[8, 12–18] Although predicated on apparently outmoded notions of tumor biology, the success of some of these trials provided some of the impetus for the next generation of trials examining the effect of prolonged courses of chemotherapy.

TRIALS OF CHEMOTHERAPY WITH CONCURRENT SURGICALLY TREATED CONTROL SUBJECTS

The modern era of adjuvant chemotherapy for breast cancer was ushered in by a series of trials designed to evaluate the effects of lengthy courses of chemotherapy in high-risk axillary lymph node–positive patients through comparison of treated patients with randomized surgical control subjects. The two most influential trials were those of the National Surgical Adjuvant Breast Project (NSABP) using melphalan (P) for two years[8, 19] and the National Cancer Institute of Milan using cyclophosphamide, methotrexate, and 5-fluorouracil (CMF) for one year.[20, 21] Both trials have consistently shown an increase in RFS and OAS that is limited to premenopausal women receiving treatment. Indeed, a lack of benefit in postmenopausal women was noted in many of the surgically controlled trials. Of great concern, too, was the observation that while RFS was frequently increased in treated women, in only a few studies was a significant improvement in OAS reported. This suggested that administration of chemotherapy served only to delay disease recurrence rather than to prevent it. Nonetheless, these studies strongly supported the idea that at least a subset of women could clearly benefit from prolonged courses of adjuvant chemotherapy (Table 12–2).[8, 21–29]

In fact, a recent summation of results from all available trials has shown that all women may profit from adjuvant chemotherapy. Peto[30] has reviewed the results from virtually all randomized trials of adjuvant cytotoxic chemotherapy that included an untreated

TABLE 12–1. Controlled Studies of Perioperative Chemotherapy

Therapy	*Duration*	*No. of Patients*	*Relapse Rate*	*Survival*	*Reference*
Thiotepa	2 d	826	↓ premenopausal > 3 nodes	↑ premenopausal > 3 nodes	8
C	10 d	83	↑	↓ stage II only	13
C	4–6 mo	113*	—	↑ stage I only	14
Thiotepa	q wk for 1 yr	166	—	↑ stage I only	15, 16
C	1 mo	287	↓ node + only	↓ node + only	17
C	6 d	1026	↓ all groups	↑ all groups	12
Nitrogen mustard	q 3 mo for 1 yr	156	↓ all groups	↑ all groups	18

*Historical control subjects.

TABLE 12–2. Adjuvant Chemotherapy Studies in Axillary Node–Positive Patients with Surgical Control Arm

			Significant Benefit in				
			Relapse-Free Survival		Overall Survival		
Treatment	No. of Patients	Follow-up (Yr)	PRE	POST	PRE	POST	Reference
P	370	10	yes	no	yes	no	8
CMF	386	10	yes	no	yes	no	21
LMF + BCG	118	8	no	yes	no	no	24, 26
CMF ± XRT	322	3.5	yes	yes	no	no	27
CMF	327	4	yes	no	no	no	28
P	370	4	no	no	no	no	23
VACMF	462	4.5	yes	no	no	no	25
CMFV	252	3	no	yes	—	—	29
P	215	3	no	yes	—	—	22
CMF			yes	yes	—	—	

surgical control group. A total of nearly 15,000 women participated in these studies. In this review, patients from a particular trial were compared with their peers in that trial only; no comparison between trials was made. In each trial, patients were grouped into subsets based on age and axillary node status. For the general review, results of individual trials were then combined to give an overall result. A 14 percent reduction in early mortality was observed with all types of cytotoxic therapy (CMF, other combinations, and single agent) compared with no adjuvant treatment. An equal reduction in mortality was observed for patients with negative and positive axillary nodes. Analysis by age showed that in women younger than 50, there was a 24 percent reduction in short-term mortality with any type of cytotoxic therapy as compared with untreated patients; those older than 50 demonstrated an 8 percent reduction, which was statistically significant in this large patient population. The reduction in mortality rate was 24 percent with CMF chemotherapy, 13 percent with non-CMF polychemotherapy, and 8 percent with single-agent chemotherapy. It is clear, then, from this review that women belonging to all age and nodal groups may benefit from administration of adjuvant cytotoxic therapy. Possible explanations for the discrepancy in results between premenopausal and postmenopausal women, including adequacy of drug dosage and role of drug-induced suppression of ovarian function, will be discussed later.

Further support for the benefit of adjuvant chemotherapy may be obtained from the studies of Jones and colleagues,[31] who compared the results of trials from the National Cancer Institute in Milan, the Southwest Oncology Group (SWOG), the University of Arizona, and the M.D. Anderson Memorial Hospital with a Natural History Data Base (NHDB). Because many second-generation trials did not include an untreated control group, these investigators compiled data on nearly 2000 patients who had undergone surgery with or without irradiation only at the NCI-Milan, M.D. Anderson, and Royal Marsden institutions. These patients could then be used as a historical control group for comparison of results of various adjuvant programs. This data collection is known as the NHDB, and comparison of the results from the trials of the groups previously listed has confirmed that combination chemotherapy resulted in a significant survival advantage. Analysis by patient subset is not yet available.

STUDIES COMPARING ADJUVANT CHEMOTHERAPY REGIMENS

The recognition that at least some patients benefited from adjuvant chemotherapy in early trials, coupled with the observation that multidrug therapy resulted in higher response rates than single-agent therapy in advanced disease, resulted in a series of studies comparing single-drug treatment with multiple-drug approaches. Two of the most influential trials were undertaken by the NSABP, which examined P versus PF,[8, 32] and by the SWOG, which evaluated P against CMFVPr.[33, 34] The NSABP trial compared two years of P (6 mg/m^2 for five days every six weeks) with P (4 mg/m^2) and F (300 mg/m^2) IV for five days every six weeks. The SWOG trial is of particular interest, as it continues to show one of the best outcomes with adjuvant chemotherapy. In that trial, 366 evaluable women with involved axillary nodes were randomized to receive either two years of P (5 mg/m^2 PO for five days every six weeks) or one year of CMFVPr (C, 60 mg/m^2 PO daily; M, 15 mg/m^2 IV weekly; F, 300 mg/m^2 IV weekly; vincristine, 0.625 mg/m^2 IV weekly for ten weeks; and prednisone, 30 mg/m^2 PO daily for two weeks, with a taper over the next four weeks). At a median follow-up of eight years, 65 percent of patients who received CMFVPr were alive, while 54 percent of those who received melphalan survived. Both of these studies strongly supported the use of combination chemotherapy over single agents. Several other studies have failed to confirm this, but they have generally included smaller numbers of patients, different drug combinations, or less intensive drug dosing in the multidrug arm (Table 12–3).[8, 33, 35–42]

A few studies have addressed the question of what constitutes the ideal number of drugs in a combination. In two studies[43, 44] comparing CMF and CMFVPr or AVCF, the RFS with CMF was found to be inferior after three or five years' follow-up, respectively, However, no significant prolongation of OAS has been observed. The NSABP study of PF versus PMF[8] showed no advantage for the three-drug regimen. Available information, then, suggests that combination regimens tend to be superior to single agents, but the ideal number of drugs is not known. As mentioned previously, Peto's review also shows a superior reduction in mortality with multiagent therapy compared with single-agent therapy.[30]

The choice of drugs for adjuvant therapy has been largely dictated by rates of response to individual agents in metastatic disease. Cyclophosphamide, methotrexate, 5-fluorouracil, and doxorubicin (A) are included most commonly in adjuvant regimens, while other useful agents have included melphalan, chlorambucil (L), thiotepa, and mitomycin C. Most drug combinations have been derived from results of treatment of advanced disease. However, adjuvant therapy may represent the ideal setting for therapy tailored to the individual patient through testing in the human tumor clonogenic assay or in other *in vitro* drug activity systems. *In vitro* drug sensitivity information for a primary tumor could be obtained within a relatively short period of time and perhaps result in more appropriate drug choices for a particular patient.

Doxorubicin is the most active single agent for treatment of advanced breast cancer, and use of doxorubicin-containing regimens has led to about a 10 percent increase in response rates over those obtained with non–doxorubicin-containing combinations. Thus, several investigators have sought to take advantage of the drug's increased activity by using it in adjuvant therapy. Two groups have pioneered in this use of doxorubicin: the Uni-

TABLE 12–3. Single Agent Versus Multiple Agents in Adjuvant Chemotherapy

Treatment	*No. of Patients*	*Follow-up (Yr)*	*Benefit of Combination Over Single Agent*	*Reference*
P PF	741	9	yes	8
P CMFVPr	366	8	yes	33
P CFPr	185	2	yes	35, 36
P CFPr ± BCG	194	2	no	37, 38
P CMF	171	3	no—P better	39
P CMF	87	5	no	40, 41
C CMF	843	3	no	42

versity of Arizona, with the AC regimen,[45] and the M.D. Anderson Memorial Hospital, with FAC.[46] In two studies using FAC with or without BCG immunotherapy or local irradiation, Buzdar and associates[46] demonstrated a significant increase in RFS and OAS in nearly all patient subsets afer six to eight years' median follow-up, using a historical control group from their own institution. In fact, comparison with other regimens included in the evaluation of the NHDB showed FAC to be the most active regimen studied, a finding that may be related to its aggressive drug dosing and scheduling.[47] Myocardial dysfunction associated with the doxorubicin dose of 300 mg/m^2 used in these studies was about 1 percent.[48] Trials[45] using AC chemotherapy have also uniformly shown an increase in RFS for all groups of treated patients; again, a historical control group of surgical patients was used. Clinical cardiac toxicity has been slight for the regimen, which gives a total dose of doxorubicin of 240 mg/m^2. Results of these trials are very encouraging, but their impact is lessened somewhat by the use of historical control groups, with all of their inherent difficulties.

Three randomized trials of a regimen without doxorubicin compared with one containing doxorubicin are in progress. Misset and associates[43] have found a significant improvement in RFS but not OAS after five years of therapy with AVCF compared with CMF. How much of the improvement can be attributed to doxorubicin is not clear, but it should be noted that vincristine has been found to contribute little to multidrug combinations in the treatment of metastatic disease. The NSABP[8] is currently conducting two trials comparing the efficacy of PF with PAF or PFT (P, F, and tamoxifen) with PAFT. About 1800 patients have been enrolled in the two studies. Early results of both studies suggest a significant improvement in RFS and OAS in both studies after three years of follow-up. Of particular importance is the observation that women older than 49 sustain a significant prolongation of RFS ($p = 0.005$) and OAS ($p = 0.01$) with the addition of doxorubicin.

Two anthracycline derivatives, dihydroxyanthracenedione and bisantrene, appear to have an efficacy similar to that of doxorubicin, with possibly fewer side effects, in early trials in advanced disease. It remains to be established whether they will be useful in adjuvant therapy.

TIMING AND DURATION OF CHEMOTHERAPY

In most trials, adjuvant therapy begins within four weeks of surgery. No randomized trials examining the optimal time to initiate therapy are available, but several studies provide potentially useful information concerning the effects of treatment delay. In a randomized trial of cyclophosphamide given over six days postoperatively, Nissen-Meyer[9] noted a significant improvement in OAS at 15 years in treated patients, except in those patients treated in a single collaborating institution where chemotherapy was delayed about one month to permit completion of postoperative radiation therapy. The University of Arizona has retrospectively analyzed the effect of delay in instituting AC chemotherapy.[49] Patients with one to three positive axillary nodes were found to have a significantly higher RFS at four years when therapy was begun within four weeks (85 percent versus 59 percent), while those with more than three positive nodes showed, if anything, a trend in the opposite direction. RFS was 46 percent for patients treated early, compared with 61 percent for those whose treatment began more than four weeks postoperatively. Finally, in the M.D. Anderson Memorial Hospital trial of FAC with or without BCG and radiation therapy,[50] delays of 10 weeks or less, 10 to 13 weeks, 14 to 17 weeks, and more than 17 weeks were found to lead to similar results; the early postoperative period, where one might plausibly expect to see the most difference, given other results cited, was not examined in more detail. Unfortunately, in this trial, patients who had disease recurrence before institution of adjuvant chemotherapy were excluded from analysis, introducing into the study a major bias toward patients with a better prognosis. There is some suggestion, then, that chemotherapy is best initiated in the early postoperative period and that delays of even a few weeks may be detrimental.

Yet to be determined is the role of neoadjuvant or preoperative chemotherapy. The use of such therapy in breast cancer has been limited to patients with locally advanced or inflammatory breast cancer, in which cases its success is becoming apparent. For example, in an ongoing study at the National Cancer Institute,[51] 76 consecutive evaluable patients (31 Stage III_a, 41 Stage III_b, 4 Stage IV) were treated with a CAMF regimen with conjugated estrogen (Premarin) and tamoxifen synchronization before receiving definitive local therapy. The overall response rate to induction chemotherapy was 93 percent, with 49 percent of patients attaining a complete response. Although follow-up is short, only 24 patients, mostly Stage III_b, have relapsed. That such an approach is safe as adjuvant therapy has been demonstrated in a pilot study by Ragaz,[52] in which the first course of CMF was given within a median of two days after diagnostic biopsy and ten days before mastectomy, without untoward surgical complications. A randomized study of neoadjuvant versus standard postoperative CMF is under way.

The very early studies of adjuvant chemotherapy examined the effect of short courses of single-agent therapy in the immediate postoperative period, which were designed to eradicate putative surgery-related systemic seeding of tumor. The results were variable as noted earlier but suggested that administration of therapy for even a brief time may be profitable. Most adjuvant studies since then have used an empirically chosen duration of therapy of between one and two years. Difficulty with short-term side effects and fear of long-term toxicity have led to several trials of shorter courses of therapy. All trials, save one, have shown that the shorter duration of therapy was as effective as therapy for a year or more. The single negative trial[11] compared one cycle of CMF with 12 cycles of CMF, while the positive trials all used a minimum of five or six cycles in the short-duration arm. In sum, these trials suggest that no additional benefit is accrued by prolongation of therapy beyond four to six months (Table 12–4).[11, 12, 21, 24, 33, 53, 54]

INTENSITY OF THERAPY

The impact of intensity of therapy on efficacy remains a controversial area in treatment of both primary and metastatic breast cancer. Intuitively, it would seem that administration of more drug would result in improved outcome. In fact, it is equally possible to argue that the ability to tolerate more drug is associated with improved outcome. Randomized trials of aggressive therapy in advanced breast cancer with "super CMF" or high-dose FAC, for example, have failed to result in increased survival rates. However, Hryniuk and Bush[55] have published a review of results with various CMF, CMFPr, CMFVPr, and CAF regimens in advanced disease that suggest that dose intensity is a crucial determinant in efficacy of therapy. For each study, an average relative dose intensity, derived from the dose administered over time, was calculated. For example, the Bonadonna regimen of CMF includes cyclophosphamide, 100 mg/m^2/day for days 1 to 14 or 350 mg/m^2/week, while the Cooper regimen of CMFVPr gives cyclophosphamide 80 mg/m^2/day, for a dose intensity of 560 mg/m^2/week. Thus the dose intensity of cyclophosphamide in Bonadonna's CMF therapy is 62 percent that of the dose intensity in Cooper's CMFVPr regimen. Dose intensities for each agent may be calculated similarly, and an average dose intensity for a particular regimen may thus be obtained. This value was found to be highly correlated with the published response rate of the trial, while the response rate was correlated, although not as well, with OAS. This analysis suggests that dose intensity is a crucial predictor of outcome in metastatic disease.

A similar analysis of adjuvant trials was performed.[56] This evaluation was limited to prospectively randomized trials of regimens derived from CMF, which included pre- and postmenopausal patients with one to three or more than three positive axillary nodes. Trials of therapy including doxorubicin, immunotherapy, or endocrine therapy were not considered because of small patient numbers. Over 6000 patients were enrolled in these trials and, overall, a clear linear relationship between projected dose intensity and three-year RFS was observed. A lack of information on dose reduction precluded analysis of actual dose intensity, and the impact that increased three-year RFS may have on OAS is not known. Nonetheless, the data are very suggestive that dose intensity is a critical factor in predicting outcome with adjuvant therapy as well.

Indeed, several individual studies have attempted to correlate drug dose with outcome since Bonadonna's[57] initial retrospective analysis of CMF suggested that patients who received the highest amount of drug had the

TABLE 12–4. Duration of Adjuvant Chemotherapy

Treatment	*No. of Patients*	*Follow-up (Yr)*	*Result*	*Reference*
CMF, 6 vs. 12 mo	459	8	6 = 12	21
CMF, 6 vs. 12 mo	369	3.5	6 = 12*	53
AC, 15 vs. 30 wk	286	10	15 = 30	54
CMF, 1 vs. 12 mo	369+	8	12 > 1	11, 12
LMF, 6 vs. 18 mo	386	5	6 = 18	24
CMFVP, 1 vs. 2 yr	312+	—	—	33

*Twelve better than six in premenopausal women with fewer than four nodes.

greatest benefit from treatment. In that study, the subset of postmenopausal women receiving greater then 85 percent of predicted drug dose was found to have a significant improvement in RFS and OAS compared with untreated control subjects, even though no benefit was seen in the total group of postmenopausal women. Other investigators, including Redmond and colleagues of the NSABP, have been unable to confirm this relationship and have pointed out the pitfalls one may encounter in such retrospective analyses.[58] In fact, at least one trial has shown that patients receiving the highest doses or attaining the greatest degree of myelosuppression had higher recurrence rates.[39] Further prospective trials will be necessary to evaluate this important question. For example, a current National Cancer Institute trial of adjuvant AC therapy in Stage II patients uses a design in which each patient's prescribed dose is escalated to maximally tolerated doses. In a very early appraisal, there is a trend for patients who received less drug to have recurrences more often, suggesting that drug dose intensity is indeed critical.[59]

RADIATION THERAPY AND ADJUVANT CHEMOTHERAPY

Although routine postoperative radiation therapy in the patient who has had any form of mastectomy has not been shown to have a significant impact on OAS, there has been a resurgence in the use of irradiation as an adjunct to breast-sparing surgical procedures, such as local excision for the treatment of primary breast cancer. A crucial question, then, is what effect, if any, does irradiation have on the ability to deliver adjuvant chemotherapy to the appropriate patient? For example, it is possible, although unlikely, that addition of local irradiation, because of its efficacy in preventing local recurrence, may help to prevent distant seeding and therefore improve survival. However, a number of potential disadvantages may be identified as well: (1) delay of adjuvant chemotherapy administration with resulting decrease in its effectiveness, as supported by the data of Nissen-Meyer[9] and Brooks[49] discussed earlier; (2) impairment of host immunity in some unknown fashion; and (3) decrease in the ability to deliver intense chemotherapy, because of radiation-induced marrow toxicity. A few randomized trials have examined the role of irradiation in mastectomized patients receiving adjuvant chemotherapy.[35, 36, 40, 41, 45, 50] In no case was radiation therapy found to yield substantial benefit in RFS or OAS, and in at least one case, recipients of irradiation in fact did slightly worse, a finding that was attributed to delay in initiation of chemotherapy or inability to tolerate full-dose chemotherapy, or both (Table 12–5).

In a trial comparing the efficacy of modified radical mastectomy with local excision and radiation therapy, Lippman and associates[59] analyzed the effect of radiation on the ability to deliver AC adjuvant chemotherapy. In this study, all patients received chemotherapy dose escalation or reduction until a maximally tolerated drug dose was attained. Patients undergoing radiation therapy had slightly greater myelosuppression, which was due almost entirely to lymphopenia rather than neutropenia. They required drug dose reduction twice as frequently as their surgical counterparts and received slightly less drug overall. From this, it would appear that the use of radiation therapy in the conservative management of primary breast can-

TABLE 12–5. Randomized Trials of Adjuvant Chemotherapy With or Without Postoperative Radiation Therapy in Mastectomized Patients

Treatment	No. of Patients	Dose of Chemotherapy Reduced with Radiation Therapy	Benefit with Radiation Therapy	Reference
L ± XRT	75	no	no	40, 41
CMF ± XRT	83	yes	no*	40, 41
FAC ± BCG ± XRT	238	no	no	50
AC ± XRT	159	yes	no	45
CFP ± XRT	212	yes	no	35, 36

XRT, radiation therapy.
*The relapse-free survival (RFS) rate of the CMF-alone patients was significantly better than that of patients treated with CMF plus XRT.

cer has a negligible impact on the ability to deliver adjuvant chemotherapy, although a longer period of evaluation will be necessary. The potential for an increased incidence of second malignancies, especially leukemia, in patients receiving combined-modality therapy remains a concern, however.

TOXICITY OF ADJUVANT CHEMOTHERAPY

Concerns about acute and chronic toxicity of therapy are especially pertinent in the adjuvant treatment setting, as the efficacy of therapy has not been absolutely established for all women and as treatment is administered to largely asymptomatic patients, some fraction of whom were cured by primary therapy alone. Acute treatment deaths are rare but do occur.[60] The overall incidence in published reports is less than 0.5 percent. It is conceivable that this incidence may be higher in general medical practice, as literature data refer mostly to patients treated in university settings with access to highly specialized supportive care.

Other potential side effects include those seen commonly with chemotherapy administration, such as cyclophosphamide-induced cystitis or vincristine-induced neuropathy. Nausea and vomiting are quite common and are anticipatory in nature in about 30 percent of patients.[61] Despite this, a large number of patients gain weight during the course of chemotherapy for unknown reasons.[62] The incidence of drug-induced alopecia requiring use of a wig ranges from about 15 percent with CMF regimens to nearly 100 percent with doxorubicin-containing combinations.[63]

The psychologic effects of adjuvant therapy in breast cancer have only recently come under scrutiny and are discussed in detail in Chapter 15. The negative effects of mastectomy, hair loss, and weight gain on self-image and esteem may be profound. Even so, one study suggested that while nearly 50 percent of patients reported residual effects several years after mastectomy, virtually all would advise a friend to undergo therapy if needed.[64]

Several potential chronic side effects are worthy of discussion. As nearly all regimens include alkylating agents, drug-induced amenorrhea and sterility are major concerns for premenopausal patients. The likelihood of resumption of menses diminishes with increasing age at time of therapy, such that nearly all women over age 40 are rendered permanently infertile, while most women under 35 regain normal menstrual function.[63] For those women who do retain or resume menses, there is no evidence that subsequent pregnancy in any way affects the course of the disease, nor do infants born of mothers previously treated with adjuvant chemotherapy have a higher incidence of congenital anomalies.[65]

The use of doxorubicin-containing regimens has led to concern about potential cardiotoxicity. The M.D. Anderson Memorial Hospital and University of Arizona experiences suggest that the incidence of long-term cardiotoxicity is less than 1 percent with combinations using less than 300 mg/m^2 of doxorubicin, but longer follow-up of larger patient populations will be necessary to gauge the potential negative impact of this treatment.[48] The use of new agents with less cardiotoxicity, such as mitoxantrone, may alleviate this problem.

Finally, with the description of second malignancies in patients treated with chemotherapy or radiation therapy, or both, the issue of second tumors in women receiving adjuvant therapy for breast cancer has been of major concern. Rockette[66] reported on the incidence of leukemia and myeloproliferative disorders in the NSABP trials of melphalan-containing regimens. Information was derived from 8483 patients who were treated with surgery alone, surgery and radiation therapy, or surgery and chemotherapy. At ten years, the cumulative risk of leukemia and myeloproliferative disease was 0.1 percent (1 of 2068) in surgical patients, 1.4 percent (4 of 646) in patients receiving regional radiation therapy postoperatively, and 1.5 percent (19 cases of leukemia and 5 cases of myeloproliferative disorders in 5299 patients) in patients receiving adjuvant chemotherapy postoperatively. Thus, the risk of development of hematologic disorders was 1 to 2 percent at ten years in patients receiving postoperative irradiation or chemotherapy, at least tenfold greater than after surgery alone. In another extensive review[67] of over 2500 women treated on five different studies with a surgical control arm, the incidence of extramammary tumors, including leukemias, was 3.1 percent for surgical control subjects and 2.7 percent for patients receiving adjuvant chemotherapy. Contralateral breast cancers were also equally common in the two groups, occurring in about 2.5 percent of patients. Although prolonged follow-up will continue to be necessary, as these patients have been followed for no more than 15 years, the occurrence of leukemia and myeloproliferative disorders appears to be increased only in patients receiving radiation therapy or melphalan-containing regimens; no increase in the incidence of solid tumors has been noted. In view of the proven efficacy of several regimens lacking melphalan, it seems prudent to abandon its use as an adjuvant agent.

PROGNOSTIC FACTORS FOR OUTCOME WITH ADJUVANT CHEMOTHERAPY

Although the studies outlined earlier unequivocally show that many women have profited from adjuvant therapy, it is clear that basic questions about what kind of therapy to give, to whom, and for how long remain unanswered. Whereas investigators have described relatively well the risk factors for breast cancer development,[68] prognostic factors for survival at disease presentation,[69] and factors predicting the response to endocrine therapy[69] and, to a lesser extent, chemotherapy[70] in advanced disease, the prognostic factors governing response to adjuvant therapy remain less well explored.[71, 72] This section reviews a variety of potential prognostic parameters, including patient and disease characteristics, laboratory findings, and factors of treatment itself. Such an analysis may help in the selection of therapy for the individual patient, in the design and interpretation of clinical trials, and in the identification of patient subsets for whom aggressive therapy may be indicated. This is of particular importance, as adjuvant therapy is administered to apparently healthy women, a portion of whom are already cured, and places them at risk for development of a variety of potential acute and chronic side effects.

Patient Characteristics

Age and Menopausal Status

Both age and menopausal status have been employed as stratification parameters in the design and analysis of adjuvant studies. With few exceptions, the age of 50 years has been designated as the major point of demarcation when age is used, while definitions of pre-, peri-, and postmenopausal status vary widely. Age and menstrual status cannot be considered to be entirely synonymous, as concordance between age 50 and menopause is obviously far from perfect. Although most trials are stratified by age, results have been reported on outcome relative to menstrual status, with few exceptions.

As noted earlier, the results of the trials of the NSABP[8] and the National Cancer Institute in Milan[21] comparing patients treated with melphalan or CMF versus a surgically treated control group suggested that the beneficial effects of adjuvant chemotherapy were limited to premenopausal women. Other trials, including those with untreated control groups[22, 23, 25–29] and those comparing two or more drug regimens,[8, 33, 35, 43, 44] have since examined this issue, and several have suggested that all women may derive benefit regardless of menopausal status (Table 12–6).

The failure of postmenopausal women to profit from chemotherapy in some of these trials remains somewhat puzzling. Whether it resulted from inadequacy of drug dose is

TABLE 12–6. *Menopausal Status and RFS with Adjuvant Chemotherapy*

Treatment	Follow-Up (Yr)	No. of Patients	Significant Benefit PRE	POST	Reference
O vs. P	10	380	yes	no	8
O vs. CMF	10	386	yes	no	21
O vs. LMF + BCG	9	118	no	yes	26
O vs. VCMF	3	252	no	yes	29
O vs. P	4	370	no	no	23
O vs. AVCMF	4.5	462	yes	no	25
O vs. CMF	3	327	yes	no	28
O vs. P vs. CMF	2.5	215	yes	yes	22
O vs. CMF ± XRT	3.5	322	yes	yes	27
P vs. CMFVPr	8	366	yes	no*	33
P vs. PF	9	741	no	yes	8
CMF vs. CMFVPr	3	316	no	yes	44
CMF vs. AVCF	5	325	yes	no	43
P vs. CFPr	2	185	yes	no	35

*Yes if noncancer deaths censored.
O, observation.

not known. Supporting evidence for this hypothesis is derived from an analysis of the Milan data, in which postmenopausal women receiving greater than 85 percent of projected CMF dose demonstrated a benefit, while those receiving less did not.[57] The sequential studies of melphalan-containing regimens from the NSABP[58] as well as the Ludwig Breast Cancer Study (LBCS) group trial of CMFPr[74] fail to substantiate this viewpoint, however, as they document similar results regardless of dose administered.

A second explanation for the difference in results between younger and older women is that premenopausal women show a prolongation of RFS because of drug-induced suppression of ovarian function. This is probably invalid as a sole explanation, although it may be contributory. Evaluation by both the NSABP[75] and the Milan[63] groups has shown no significant association between drug-induced amenorrhea in patients and length of RFS. In the NSABP trial, patients under 50 years of age receiving melphalan demonstrated a greater RFS than did untreated controls, but the greatest benefit was seen in those under 39. Yet, cessation of menses occurred much more frequently in the 40 to 49 age group, as did an increase in luteinizing and follicle-stimulating hormones and a decrease in estradiol, all indicators of ovarian suppression. Thus, the youngest women had the greatest improvement in RFS with the smallest effect on menstrual function. Bonadonna and Valagussa[63] also examined the relationship between age-related susceptibility to drug-induced amenorrhea and incidence of relapse. At nine years, the RFS was 35 percent in women 40 and younger who became amenorrheic and 31 percent in those whose menses continued, a difference lacking statistical significance.

On the other hand, LBCS I trial[76] of CMF and CMFP in premenopausal women with one to three positive axillary nodes demonstrated a clear difference in patients receiving CMF. At four years, 81 percent of amenorrheic patients survived disease-free, while only 58 percent of patients who continued to menstruate were free of disease. Interestingly, this difference was much less in CMFP patients—72 versus 66 percent. The Danish study[42] of no therapy versus cyclophosphamide versus CMF in premenopausal women showed that drug-induced menopause was associated with improved RFS in patients receiving cyclophosphamide but not in those receiving CMF. In summary, these studies suggest that some part of the effect of adjuvant therapy in premenopausal women is mediated by the loss of ovarian function, but it is unlikely that such loss accounts for the entire effect.

Another likely explanation for the difference in pre- and postmenopausal responses lies in an observation from Peto's analysis of trials,[30] which suggests that the improvement in RFS and OAS achieved thus far is small in postmenopausal women, at most 20 percent. Thus, trials with less than 600 women will not invariably show a statistically significant difference in outcome.

A final potential explanation lies in recent reports,[8, 21] which suggest that the benefit of adjuvant chemotherapy is seen predominantly in patients whose tumors demonstrate poor prognostic features, such as poor histologic differentiation, high nuclear grade, or hormone receptor negativity. As these findings are more characteristic of tumors in younger women than in older women, this finding may also account for part of the difference in response.

Axillary Node Status

It has long been observed that axillary node status represents the single most important prognostic factor in primary breast cancer. Substantial differences in RFS exist between patients with no, one to three, and more than three positive nodes. Most studies of adjuvant therapy have been limited to those patients with positive nodes who have a higher risk of disease recurrence. Though the risk is very great with only four nodes involved, it continues to rise with even greater degrees of nodal involvement, as demonstrated by the NSABP,[77] M.D. Anderson,[78] and Milan[72] evaluations of patients with more than four involved nodes.

An analysis of the benefit of adjuvant chemotherapy in relation to the number of positive nodes in individual randomized trials with untreated control subjects shows a trend toward greatest benefit in patients with fewer than four positive nodes, although some studies demonstrate an advantage in patients with larger tumor burden as well (Table 12–7).[32, 42, 79–81] In fact, Peto's overview analysis[30] shows an equal reduction in mortality rate for treated patients with zero, one to three, or more than three axillary node metastases. However, the effects of therapy are very small in patients with more than ten involved nodes, as demonstrated by Bonadonna and colleagues in the Milan trials.[82]

A logical extension of these findings is that node-negative patients might profit from adjuvant therapy as well. As the relapse rate for such patients is about 25 percent at ten years, significant impact may be difficult to detect. In order to observe any discernible effects, it may be important to further subdivide this group of patients to analyze particularly those women with other bad prognostic signs, such as lack of estrogen receptor or poorly differentiated histology. Nonetheless, a few trials have addressed this subset of patients, with positive results in some cases (Table 12–8)[12, 21, 26, 42, 80, 83] Both the Nissen-Meyer trial[12] of perioperative cyclophosphamide and the Senn trial[26] of chlorambucil, methotrexate, 5-fluorouracil, and BCG (LMF plus BCG) have shown an increased RFS and OAS for treated women, although the differences fail to reach statistical significance in all cases. In a third trial, Bonadonna and colleagues[21] have examined the use of an intensive intravenous CMF regimen in axillary lymph node–negative women who have ER-negative tumors, a group with a clearly worse prognosis. Although the follow-up time is very short, a striking improvement in both RFS and OAS has been noted for CMF-treated women. Further analysis showed that this benefit was limited to women whose tumors demonstrated a high score on the

TABLE 12–7. Axillary Node Involvement and Outcome with Adjuvant Chemotherapy in Node-Positive Patients

Treatment	Menopausal Status	Follow-Up (Yr)	% RFS with Positive Nodes 1–3	> 3	Reference
Control	Pre	3	64	44	42
C			78*	49	
CMF			80*	55*	
Control	Pre	2	74	38	32
P			88*	57*	
Control	Post	2	82	55	32
P			83	63	
Control	Both	4	49	35	81
LMF + BCG			54	41	
Control	Both	6	46	32	79
CMF			65*	36	
Control	Both	5	58	53	80
C + mitomycin			85*	53	

*Statistically significant difference from control subjects.

TABLE 12–8. Outcome with Adjuvant Chemotherapy in Node-Negative Patients

Treatment	Menopausal Status	No. of Patients	Follow-Up (Yr)	RFS (%)	Reference
Control	Both	229	5	90	80
C + mitomycin				94	
Control	Both	610	20	55	12
C				64	
Control	Both	122	9	62	26
LMF + BCG				68	
Control	Pre	142	3	66	42
C				89	
CMF				87	
Control	Both	467	4.5	86	83
LMF				86	
Control	Both	89	2	50	21
CMF	(ER−)			96*	

*Statistically significant difference from control subjects.

thymidine-labeling index. This suggests that this simple laboratory parameter may be a useful prognostic indicator to define further a group of patients with uninvolved axillary lymph nodes who may still have a relatively poor prognosis and who may profit from adjuvant chemotherapy. Finally, a noncontrolled study[84] of three cycles of doxorubicin-cyclophosphamide (AC) chemotherapy is in progress at the University of Arizona. With nearly five years' median follow-up, only 1 of 58 patients with T_1 lesions and 15 of 98 patients with T_2 lesions have relapsed. Thus, although adjuvant chemotherapy has not been routinely administered to patients with uninvolved axillary lymph nodes, these studies suggest that certain high-risk women (e.g., those of young age or with large tumors, ER-negative tumors, or high thymidine-labeling indices) may in fact derive considerable benefit from treatment. It is therefore appropriate to consider the use of adjuvant chemotherapy for these individuals, although every effort should be made to include them in controlled clinical trials.

Attempts have also been made to ascertain the impact of micro- versus macrometastases on prognosis in patients with a small axillary node tumor burden. Micrometastases are defined as tumor cell infiltrations less than 2 mm in diameter and account for less than 10 percent of cases with positive nodes. Information can be best obtained from three series looking at women with a single axillary node metastasis.[72, 85] In the Memorial Hospital series[85] of 147 women followed for at least ten years, those women with a single micrometastasis had a recurrence rate of 24 percent, compared with 39 percent for those with a macrometastasis. Evaluation in conjunction with tumor size showed that no difference was seen for patients with T_1 primary lesions whose prognosis was identical, regardless of size of metastasis, and inferior to that of node-negative patients. Rather it was limited to patients with T_2 lesions, among whom node-negative and micrometastatic patients had similar outcomes. The Milan group[72] failed to demonstrate any difference between micro- and macrometastatic involvement in a single node in a group of 68 women with predominantly T_2 lesions but observed a less favorable prognosis in a comparable group of node-negative women. None of those patients received adjuvant chemotherapy. Some suggestion that adjuvant chemotherapy may be most effective in micrometastatic disease may be extrapolated from a second Milan study[72] of women with T_1 lesions, in which node-positive patients received adjuvant chemotherapy. Here, patients with a single micrometastatic focus exhibited the best ten-year RFS and OAS, superior even to that of node-negative patients, while those with macrometastatic involvement did least well.

Psychologic Aspects

For years, clinicians have postulated the existence of a relationship between the psychologic characteristics of patients and their course of illness and response to therapy. Early studies in cancer patients suggested that patients' behavior was of predictive value in determining length of survival. Specifically, patients who were openly negative and angry about their disease survived significantly longer than those who were not. Studies of psychologic coping mechanisms and survival in both early and metastatic breast cancer have appeared.[86, 87] In general, patients with high measures of anxiety, anger, and denial on psychologic testing were found to survive significantly longer than their apparently more accepting and better adjusted peers. For example, in patients with primary breast cancer receiving local irradiation as their only adjuvant therapy, Greer and associates[87] found that RFS was significantly longer in those patients exhibiting denial or "fighting spirit" when compared with those who were characterized as showing stoic acceptance or helplessness/hopelessness. Based on animal studies, it has been suggested that the effect of behavioral factors on the course of breast cancer is mediated via the immune or neuroendocrine systems, or both.

However, a prospective study[88] of potential psychosocial correlates of survival in patients with cancer has questioned the validity of previous findings. In this study, seven variables found to predict longevity in other studies, including extent of adjustment to disease and degree of helplessness/hopelessness, were evaluated in a group of 60 patients with Stage II breast cancer (most receiving unspecified adjuvant chemotherapy) and 40 patients with intermediate or high-risk malignant melanoma. No relation between the psychosocial factors and time to recurrence of disease was noted for the entire group; patients with breast cancer were not analyzed separately, nor was overall survival examined.

The impact of patient attitude on outcome with adjuvant chemotherapy has yet to be examined. In an ongoing study of treatment of primary breast patients, including adjuvant AC chemotherapy in axillary node–positive patients, we have found that apathy and depression are highly associated with lower natural killer cell activity and with the occurrence of lymph node involvement in women not yet aware of their node status.[89] Further follow-up of this patient population will allow us to assess the relationship between psychologic make-up and the outcome with adjuvant therapy.

Tumor and Disease Characteristics

HISTOPATHOLOGY

Histologic grade has been shown to be of prognostic significance in newly diagnosed breast cancer. Patients with Grade I tumors have a better prognosis than do those patients whose tumors are of higher grade.[90, 91] Poorly differentiated high-grade tumors are also associated with higher thymidine-labeling index[92] and with estrogen receptor negativity,[90, 93] both prognostic factors in their own right.

Data from the sequential NSABP studies of adjuvant therapy with P, PF, and PMF suggest that women with histologically undifferentiated cancers associated with more than three positive axillary nodes have a statistically more favorable response to adjuvant therapy than do their peers with well-differentiated tumors. Patients with one to three nodal metastases were not found to exhibit particular responsiveness to any adjuvant regimen, regardless of tumor grade.[94, 95] These findings were confirmed in a study[96] of CMFVb chemotherapy in women with Stages I and II breast cancer, in which only patients with undifferentiated tumors benefited from treatment. The overall survival rate was 79 percent in those patients with undifferentiated tumors who were treated compared with 41 percent in those who were untreated; it was identical in both groups with well or moderately differentiated tumors.

TUMOR SIZE

The size of the primary tumor is an independent prognostic factor for the risk of recurrence in breast cancer, although it is highly correlated with axillary node involvement. Whether tumor size is also an independent factor in the efficacy of adjuvant therapy has been examined in a few controlled studies. Nissen-Meyer's study[9] of postoperative cyclophosphamide showed a 12-year RFS of 83 percent in treated node-negative patients with tumors smaller than 2 cm (control subject RFS was 65 percent), compared with 70 percent in their peers with tumors larger than 2 cm (control subject RFS was 65 percent), suggesting a better result with smaller tumors. At three years' follow-up, Bonadonna and Valagussa[57] demonstrated a significant reduction in failure rate with CMF in T_2 lesions but not in T_1 or T_3 lesions. The latter patient groups were quite small, however, and the extent of nodal involvement was not considered. The University of Arizona data with AC in node-negative patients suggest a higher failure rate with T_2 lesions compared with T_1 lesions: 15 percent versus 2 percent at five years.[84] This information supports the notion that tumor size is a prognostic factor for efficacy of adjuvant chemotherapy independent of its association with axillary node status. However, Fisher and associates[94] were able to attach no significance to tumor size in patients receiving P, PF, or PMF adjuvant therapy in the NSABP trials, casting some doubt on the issue.

Estrogen and Progesterone Receptor Status

With the advent of methods for measurement of estrogen and progesterone receptors, the ability to select patients with advanced disease who were likely to benefit from endocrine manipulation was markedly improved. Furthermore, absence of ER helps to identify a group of primary breast cancer patients with a higher rate of disease recurrence and a shorter survival whose tumors tend to be faster growing, as measured by parameters such as thymidine-labeling index.[97, 98] These ER-negative tumors are more likely to metastasize to sites associated with poor prognosis, such as brain and liver, than to bone and skin.[99] The idea that rapidly growing tumors would theoretically be more responsive to chemotherapy led to a series of retrospective reviews of the relationship between receptor status and response to chemotherapy in advanced disease.[100] The consensus of these reviews was that there was no significant correlation between estrogen receptor status and response to combination chemotherapy in metastatic disease.

McGuire's review[101] has provided further information on the role of steroid hormone receptors as prognostic factors in primary breast cancer. Lack of ER was found to be the most important factor in predicting earlier recurrence and poorer survival in patients with Stage I breast cancer. However, in Stage II breast cancer, lack of PR was the most important determinant of RFS and was as useful as ER in predicting OAS. The likelihood of benefit from adjuvant endocrine therapy was better predicted by PR status than ER status.

Definitive data for the relationship between receptor status and response to adjuvant chemotherapy are few, as receptor assays became routine only after many of the crucial randomized studies including an untreated control arm were initiated. However, two such studies are in progress. The ECOG study[102] of observation versus CMFP versus CMFPT in postmenopausal women showed an improvement in five-year RFS in patients with ER-negative tumors receiving CMFP or CMFPT (22 percent in control subjects versus 39 percent with CMFP versus 52 percent with CMFPT). Patients with ER-positive tumors had similar RFS with or without therapy. Similarly, in a study of CMFVb chemotherapy given to patients with Stages I and II breast cancer, Jakesz and associates[96] also demonstrated an effect of chemotherapy only in patients with ER-negative tumors. At four years, OAS in ER-positive patients was 84 percent in treated patients and 80 percent in untreated patients. Patients with tumors lacking ER, on the other hand, had an OAS of 84 percent if treated and 37 percent if untreated. These two studies suggest that ER negativity is associated with enhanced response to adjuvant chemotherapy.

Two other studies lacking an untreated control arm may provide indirect support for this finding. The Milan trial[103] of 6 versus 12 months of CMF and the NSABP trial[104] of PF versus PFT both include receptor information for most patients. Neither trial demonstrated a relationship between receptor status and RFS, and from these, it has been suggested that because ER-negative patients are at greater risk for relapse, a lack of association between estrogen receptor level and response to chemotherapy could be explained by a greater effect of therapy in ER-negative patients.

Finally, one trial[25] including an untreated control group has reported on both ER and PR status for the two thirds of patients who did have receptor assays performed. At four and one-half years, the recurrence rate in axillary node–positive patients treated with combination chemotherapy was 36 percent in ER-positive patients, compared with 42 percent in untreated control subjects. A total of 63 percent of both treated and untreated ER-negative patients had disease recurrences. Similar analysis using progesterone receptor showed recurrence rates of 29 percent in treated ER-positive patients, 37 percent in untreated PR-positive patients, 43 percent in treated PR-negative patients, and 51 percent in untreated PR-negative patients. Further follow-up will be required before any definitive conclusions can be drawn from this series, but no striking relationship between ER or PR status and response to therapy has emerged in this study.

KINETIC PARAMETERS

Cell kinetic measurements, including mitotic index, flow cytometric measurement of S-phase fraction (SPF), and tritiated thymidine-labeling index (TLI), have been applied to the study of breast cancer. The work of Meyer,[92, 97, 98, 105] Kute,[106] Silvestrini,[107] and Tubiana[108] suggests that SPF and TLI correlate well with each other. Both are higher in aneuploid cell lines, which proliferate more rapidly and are more undifferentiated histologically. They show an inverse correlation with estrogen and progesterone receptor status; a positive correlation with tumor size, degree of nuclear anaplasia, and histologic dedifferentiation; and no relation to axillary node involvement.[97, 101, 105, 106] High TLI is associated with a high risk of early recurrence after primary therapy, regardless of node status.[92] In particular, the TLI can select a subgroup of node-negative patients with an expected relapse rate of nearly 50 percent at four years, potentially a group who would benefit from adjuvant therapy.[21, 97] Meyer and colleagues[97] found that primary breast cancer patients with TLI below the median carried a probability of relapse of 20 percent at four years, compared with 52 percent for those patients with TLI above the median. Some of the patients included in Meyer's study received adjuvant chemotherapy or radiation therapy, or both; however, no analysis of the relationship between TLI and RFS in these treated patients is presented. Early results of the Milan trial[21] of CMF in patients with uninvolved axillary lymph nodes have shown that benefit is limited almost exclusively to those patients whose tumors demonstrate a high thymidine-labeling index. It appears then that high TLI, like undifferentiated tumor histology and high nuclear grade, may identify a group of patients who obtain increased benefit from adjuvant chemotherapy. Once again, this may explain in part the enhanced response of younger patients to adjuvant chemotherapy. In any case, like receptor status, it is a potent predictor of the natural history of primary breast cancer.

Laboratory Findings

The development of *in vitro* tests that correlate with *in vivo* tumor behavior has been the subject of intense study in breast cancer. Here we consider the role of conventional laboratory tests, tests of immunologic function, and biomarkers in predicting outcome with adjuvant chemotherapy.

ROUTINE LABORATORY TESTS

Information on the relationship between common laboratory tests and prognosis in primary breast cancer is almost nonexistent. This reflects the overwhelmingly normal laboratory values in this generally healthy group of patients, including those who receive adjuvant therapy, and the nearly universal requirement for normal hematologic, hepatic, and renal function for inclusion in drug trials. In a single study, Buzdar and associates[50] examined the association of pretreatment LDH and alkaline phosphatase levels with outcome in patients receiving FAC chemotherapy and found that neither correlated with RFS.

TESTS OF IMMUNOLOGIC FUNCTION

There is a paucity of literature on the relationship between prognosis in primary breast cancer and immune reactivity as measured by a variety of *in vitro* and *in vivo* test systems; no information on subsequent outcome with adjuvant therapy is available. Krown and colleagues[109] found no correlation between reactivity to a battery of common skin tests and axillary node involvement, nor did she note any relationship between DNCB reactivity and RFS. In a different approach, Cannon and associates[110] demonstrated that patients with lymphocytes capable of proliferating in response to autologous tumor extracts had a significantly longer RFS than did those with a low response to autologous extracts. More work is clearly needed in this field, with attention both to the natural history of patients with particular immunologic parameters and to their outcome with adjuvant chemotherapy.

BIOMARKERS

Identification of biomarkers useful in detecting residual disease or early metastases and in predicting response to therapy has constituted a third avenue of approach. Numerous such markers exist, with CEA,[70, 111–122] ferritin,[112, 114, 121, 122] hCG,[112, 115, 118, 121–123] ceruloplasmin,[121, 124, 125] urinary hydroxyproline,[111, 121, 126–128] calcitonin,[112, 114, 115, 121, 122] polyamines,[111, 112, 118, 121] lactalbumin, and casein[115] among the most studied in both early and late breast cancer. In general, it may be said that their usefulness is limited, because only a fraction of patients have elevated marker substances at any stage and because none of the aforementioned markers is tumor specific. When they are produced, an increased value may correlate with an increased risk of recurrence in early disease, presumably because of residual occult disease after primary therapy. For example, Myers and associates[117] found that 16 percent of patients with elevated CEA values developed recurrent disease, compared with 5 percent of patients with normal values, thus delineating a group with high risk of recurrence. If elevated in instances of advanced disease, the level frequently parallels the overall response to therapy, decreasing with response and increasing with lack thereof.

For the most part, information on biomarkers in early breast cancer patients is fragmentary. Results on only small groups of patients who underwent a variety of often poorly defined surgical, radiotherapeutic, and chemotherapeutic treatments have been reported. In one study,[125] however, Schapira and Schapira monitored ceruloplasmin levels in 52 patients with Stage II breast cancer treated with mastectomy followed by adjuvant chemotherapy. In this group, 16 patients (30 percent) had elevated ceruloplasmin levels before chemotherapy, and the levels fell within the first three months of therapy in all save one patient. Subsequently, the levels rose in seven of these patients (40 percent), and all later relapsed. Thirty-six patients (70 percent) had a normal ceruloplasmin level before therapy, and only two of those patients (6 percent) have relapsed. Seven of 56 Stages I and II patients not receiving adjuvant therapy also developed metastatic disease, each with a preceding rise in the ceruloplasmin level. This suggests, then, that an elevated biomarker may delineate a group of patients with high risk of recurrence, despite the use of adjuvant chemotherapy. Further studies of this nature will be required to identify individual biomarkers with greater discriminatory power or perhaps panels of biomarkers that may be useful in predicting risk of recurrent disease and likelihood of positive outcome with adjuvant chemotherapy.

Finally, although still in the early stages of development for clinical use, polyclonal antisera and monoclonal antibodies may play a role in evaluation of breast cancer in the future. For example, Coombes and associates[129] have developed both a polyclonal antiserum and a monoclonal antibody to milk fat globule membrane. The polyclonal antiserum was used to screen bone marrow from 269 patients with early stage breast cancer. Twenty-three percent of patients were found to have malignant cells in the marrow, despite normal Giemsa marrow smears and bone scans. The presence of malignant cells was highly correlated with primary tumor size and extent of vascular invasion. Early results have shown that 32 percent of the group with micrometastases and 17 percent of the group with normal bone marrow have had relapses. This approach clearly holds promise in the future as a means of selecting patients for adjuvant therapy.

ADJUVANT ENDOCRINE THERAPY

The earliest studies of adjuvant therapy of breast cancer focused on the role of ovarian ablation by surgery or irradiation as a means of enhancing survival. Several trials are noteworthy. In a study[130] characterized by exclusion from evaluation of over half of the patients randomized, the NSABP was unable to document any beneficial effect from oophorectomy or ovarian irradiation in premenopausal women. Contradictory results were obtained from a prospective randomized trial of oophorectomy performed on 359 patients by Bryant and Weir.[131] Here, axillary node–positive patients under the age of 50 years had a significant increase in RFS at five years and both RFS and OAS at ten years.

Women over 50 years of age showed no advantage. Nissen-Meyer,[132, 133] studying the usefulness of ovarian irradiation, failed to find any benefit for premenopausal axillary node–negative women and did not randomize axillary node–positive patients because of ethical considerations. Curiously, a concurrent small study of postmenopausal women showed a significant increase in RFS and OAS over the first two years in Stage II patients, especially those over the age of 60. Between 1948 and 1955, a crucial trial of prophylactic ovarian irradiation in premenopausal women was performed by the Manchester group.[134, 135] Results of that trial involving 293 irradiated patients and 303 concurrently untreated control subjects showed an increase in crude survival of borderline significance at 10 ($p = 0.07$) and 15 ($p = 0.06$) years of follow-up for patients with irradiation-induced menopause. This trend was noted in all patients, regardless of axillary node status. Careful analysis of the data suggested that the greatest benefit was accrued in the first year after irradiation and that, thereafter, relapse rates were similar in the two groups. It appeared then that irradiation-induced menopause did not significantly increase survival but served merely to lengthen the disease-free interval. Finally, the Princess Margaret Hospital group[136] evaluated ovarian irradiation in women under the age of 45 and ovarian irradiation with or without daily prednisone in those over 44. Prednisone was administered to decrease adrenal steroid synthesis, a secondary source of estrogen. A total of 705 evaluable axillary node–negative and node-positive patients were followed for up to 15 years. No benefit was noted with any treatment of postmenopausal women, and a nonsignificant prolongation of RFS and OAS was found for irradiated women under 45 years of age. However, the subset of premenopausal patients more than 44 years old who received both irradiation and prednisone had a significant increase in both RFS and OAS, which has persisted throughout the study. In fact, survival in the group parallels that of age-matched normal control subjects, suggesting that a subset of these patients may in fact be cured of their disease. Clearly, these findings require confirmation by other investigators. In summary, then, the results of these individual trials would suggest that prophylactic castration of premenopausal women induces, at best, a prolongation of RFS without a substantial concomitant increase in OAS. However, in Peto's trial summation,[30] ovarian ablation was found to decrease short-term mortality by 29 percent. Still, neither oophorectomy nor ovarian irradiation is routinely used as adjuvant therapy for primary breast cancer today. It is possible that the use of ER and PR status may help define a population of premenopausal women who do benefit from such therapy, and trials combining oophorectomy and chemotherapy for appropriate candidates are under way.

With the successful use of tamoxifen as treatment for advanced disease, several trials evaluating the efficacy of tamoxifen as adjuvant therapy were undertaken (Table 12–9).[136–142] Interpretation of the results is hampered by differences in patient characteristics, including axillary node, estrogen receptor, and menopausal status; variations in drug dose and duration; and the generally short follow-up time. Most of the studies have limited participation to postmenopausal

TABLE 12–9. Single-Agent Tamoxifen in Studies with Untreated Control Subjects

Daily Dose and Duration	*No. of Patients*	*Menopausal Status*	*Follow-Up (Yr)*	*Benefit of Tamoxifen*	*Reference*
20 mg for 2 yr	1129	Both	6	↑ RFS + OAS	137
30 mg for 2 yr	366	Post	3.6	↑ RFS in ER+	136
30 mg for 1 yr	1650	Post	5	↑ RFS in age 50–54 or >3 axillary nodes or ER >100	138
20 mg for 1 yr	552	Post	5	↑ OAS in >3 axillary nodes	139
40 mg for 2 yr	199	Post	4	↑ RFS for first 3 yr only	140
20 mg for 1 yr*	629	Post	4	↑ RFS with PT	141
20 mg for 2 yr	177	Post >65 yr	3	↑ RFS	142

*With prednisone, 7.5 mg daily.

women and tend to show an improvement in RFS in those receiving tamoxifen. More important, however, a trial of 1129 women conducted by the Nolvadex Adjuvant Trial Organization[137] that was limited to premenopausal women with axillary node involvement and postmenopausal women with or without node metastases has demonstrated a 34 percent reduction in deaths for all three patient groups after four years' median follow-up. This effect extended to patients with ER-positive or ER-negative tumors. In another study,[139] postmenopausal patients with more than three positive axillary nodes showed a modest survival benefit as well. Although information on estrogen and progesterone receptor status is not uniformly available, there is a suggestion that receptor-positive patients exhibit the greatest likelihood of improvement.

Peto[30] also examined the effect of tamoxifen on short-term mortality in his overview of adjuvant trials. These trials examined the outcome of about 16,000 women who were randomized to receive either local therapy alone or local therapy supplemented with one to two years of tamoxifen. At five years, RFS was 65 percent in tamoxifen-treated patients and 55 percent in control subjects, while OAS was 75 percent and 70 percent, respectively. The improvement in both RFS and OAS was highly statistically significant. As with chemotherapy, the effect was similar in women with or without axillary node involvement. However, benefit was limited to women over the age of 50; no advantage was seen in younger women.

Other endocrine interventions that have been investigated include the use of diethylstilbestrol (DES) and aminoglutethimide. The use of DES was evaluated by a Danish trial[143] comparing tamoxifen, DES, and no therapy in postmenopausal women. Although DES was found to be as effective as tamoxifen in the improvement of RFS, nearly half of all patients treated with DES stopped therapy because of side effects, including 17 percent because of thromboembolic events. In addition, 80 percent of patients suffered from vaginal bleeding. The high incidence of side effects greatly reduces the usefulness of DES, and it is rarely used. A double-blind placebo-controlled study of aminoglutethimide and hydrocortisone for two years, with a projected enrollment of 400 patients, is under way at the Royal Marsden Hospital.[144] The short duration of the study thus far precludes any interpretation.

Chemohormonal Therapy

Given the limitations of systemic adjuvant chemotherapy already outlined, many investigators have attempted to improve results by combining endocrine therapy and chemotherapy. Theoretically, the appeal of such an approach is great—improved results because of the use of agents with independent modes of antineoplastic action, with little if any additional toxicity.

Two trials have been designed to examine the role of combination chemotherapy in conjunction with oophorectomy in pre- and perimenopausal women. In the LBCS II trial,[141] those women with more than three involved axillary nodes were randomized to either adjuvant surgical oophorectomy followed by CMFP chemotherapy or to CMFP alone. At four years' median follow-up, there was no difference between RFS (54 and 51 percent, respectively) or OAS (71 and 70 percent, respectively) for the whole group nor was any difference noted in those women who had ER-positive tumors. Nearly 90 percent of women receiving chemotherapy alone became amenorrheic, suggesting that oophorectomy may have added little to the effect of chemotherapy. Another trial,[33] conducted by the SWOG, includes premenopausal patients who are randomized between CMFVPr alone and CMFVPr following oophorectomy. This trial is still accruing patients.

Several studies of adjuvant chemohormonal therapy have combined tamoxifen with conventional multidrug regimens (Table 12–10).[101, 102, 141, 145–147] The period of follow-up remains short in most of these studies, but in general, they show an increase in RFS for postmenopausal women receiving tamoxifen in addition to combination chemotherapy; in those studies for which receptor information is available, the benefit is more striking in the ER- and PR-positive subsets as a rule. Results are less promising in premenopausal women. Hubay and colleagues,[148] for example, found an increase in RFS at three years in premenopausal women receiving CMFT, while Tormey and associates[102] were unable to confirm this in a group of women receiving CMFPrT. Even more disheartening are the data from Fisher's trial of PF versus PFT,[101,

TABLE 12–10. Randomized Trials of Chemoendocrine Adjuvant Therapy

Treatment	No. of Patients	Patient Characteristics	Follow-Up (Yr)	Benefit	Reference
AC ACT	244	>3 positive nodes or 1–3 positive nodes and ER or PR negative	3	↑ RFS with ACT	145
CMF CMFPr CMFPrT	556	Premenopausal	4.5	No difference	102
Observation CMFPr CMFPrT	224	Postmenopausal, <66 yr	5	↑ RFS with CMFPr or CMFPrT if ER−	102
PF PFT	1861	<50 yr ≥50	5	↓ OAS with PFT ↑ RFS with PFT	101
CMF CMFT	124	Postmenopausal, <70 yr	2.3	↑ RFS with CMFT	146
CMF CMFT	312	All	6	No difference	147
Observation PrT CMFPrT	463	Postmenopausal, <65 yr	4	↑ RFS with CMFPrT	141

[104, 149] which showed a poorer OAS at five years for women younger than 50 years with ER-negative, PR-negative tumors (56 percent in the PF group, compared with 44 percent in the PFT group) or ER-positive, PR-negative tumors (70 percent with PF versus 56 percent with PFT). Taken as a whole, these results are discouraging with respect to the addition of tamoxifen to chemotherapy for younger women.

Few studies have addressed the crucial issue of the relative contributions of the endocrine and chemotherapeutic components to outcome with combined therapy. An ongoing randomized study[145] of tamoxifen versus CMF in low-risk women with one to three positive axillary nodes and ER- or PR-positive tumors has shown no difference in RFS after three years of follow-up. The LBCS[141] is at present comparing CMFPrT with PrT or no therapy in postmenopausal women under 66 years of age. Relapse-free survival is significantly longer in patients receiving combined therapy after four years, but no difference in OAS has been observed. However, RFS in ER-positive patients was not different between chemoendocrine and endocrine treatment groups; the advantage of combined therapy was limited to ER-negative patients. Finally, the SWOG has recently begun a trial of tamoxifen versus CMFVPr versus CMFVPr and tamoxifen in postmenopausal women with ER-positive tumors and involved axillary nodes.[33]

Of great concern are findings from several studies suggesting that the beneficial effects of tamoxifen are limited to the period of administration only, an observation consistent with the animal studies of Jordan and associates,[150] in which dimethylbenzanthracene-induced hormone-dependent breast cancer in rats is prevented by tamoxifen only so long as the drug is continued. Trials that support this notion include that of Hubay and colleagues,[147] in which the RFS of patients receiving CMFT chemohormonal therapy was superior at three and four years but equal at six years to that of CMF-treated control subjects, and that of Tormey and associates,[151] in which the relapse rates for postmenopausal women receiving CMFPr or CMFPrT were lower during the period of therapy but comparable thereafter, with those of the observation only group. These results suggest that tamoxifen acts as a cytostatic rather than a cytocidal agent and therefore should probably be continued indefinitely in the absence of definitive data.

The results just cited also suggest that negative interactions between antiestrogen therapy and chemotherapy may occur. If tamoxifen is cytostatic, it may protect breast cancer cells from the effects of drugs that are more active against dividing cells. Support

TABLE 12–11. Randomized Trials of Adjuvant Chemoimmunotherapy

Treatment	No. of Patients	Follow-Up (Yr)	Benefit	Reference
CMF ± BCG	290	4	no	152
CMFT* ± BCG	211	6	no	147
CFPr ± BCG	156	2	no	38
FAC ± BCG	238	4	no	50
AC ± LEV*	52	6	no	153
P ± LEV	135	4.5	no	154

*T, tamoxifen; LEV, levamisole.

for this concept may be derived from the overview analysis of Peto.[30] His evaluation of the effect of tamoxifen with or without cytotoxic agents showed that the combined therapy resulted in a reduction in the mortality rate of only 8 percent ± 7 percent, while tamoxifen alone resulted in a mortality rate reduction of 17 percent ± 5 percent. On subset analysis, women under the age of 50 had a −5 percent ±12 percent reduction with combined therapy and a 15 percent ± 15 percent reduction with tamoxifen alone, while women over 49 responded identically to either therapy. These data support the notion that negative interactions between the two therapeutic modalities may occur, particularly in women under 50 years of age. They also suggest that a strategy of administering tamoxifen following completion of chemotherapy cycles is worthy of consideration.

Chemoimmunotherapy

Studies of immunotherapy in primary breast cancer have focused on the use of nonspecific immunostimulants such as BCG or levamisole. Several randomized trials of chemoimmunotherapy as adjuvant therapy have clearly demonstrated a lack of benefit with the addition of these agents to conventional multidrug combinations (Table 12–11).[38, 50, 147, 152–154] In fact, in a trial examining the role of levamisole alone,[155] the recurrence rate was actually higher in treated patients than in untreated control subjects, and a high incidence of side effects led to premature discontinuation of therapy in over half of the patients.

There has been one promising study of immunotherapy alone.[156] Lacour and colleagues randomized 300 axillary node-positive and node-negative patients to placebo or six weekly injections of polyadenylic-polyuridylic acid (poly A–poly U), a modulator of both humoral and cellular immune responses. Both RFS and OAS were increased in the poly A–poly U group at seven years, the latter significantly so. Benefit was limited to axillary node–positive patients. Further study of this potentially useful and apparently nontoxic agent is in progress, with a trial comparing CMF and poly A–poly U. In the interim, there is no role for the routine use of immunotherapy in any form, outside of well-designed clinical trials.

RECOMMENDATIONS OF THE CONSENSUS DEVELOPMENT COMMITTEE ON ADJUVANT CHEMOTHERAPY FOR BREAST CANCER

In September 1985, the National Cancer Institute convened a Consensus Development Committee to review available information on the role of adjuvant therapy for breast cancer.[157] After consideration of the research data presented, the Committee made the following recommendations regarding administration of adjuvant therapy for breast cancer:

I. Optimal therapy has not been defined for any subset of breast cancer patients. Therefore, all patients and physicians are strongly urged to participate in controlled clinical trials.

II. Outside the context of a clinical trial, the Committee recommended that

   A. Premenopausal women with positive axillary nodes should receive combination chemotherapy.

   B. Premenopausal women with negative axillary nodes may be considered for adjuvant chemotherapy on an individual basis if they are felt to be at high risk for disease recurrence.

C. Postmenopausal women with positive axillary nodes and positive tumor hormone receptor levels should receive tamoxifen.

D. Postmenopausal women with positive axillary nodes and negative tumor hormone receptor levels may be considered for adjuvant chemotherapy on an individual basis.

E. Postmenopausal women with negative axillary nodes require no further treatment.

CONCLUSIONS

It is clear that the optimal systemic treatment of early breast cancer has not been established. The need for continuing clinical trials cannot be overemphasized; every effort should be made to enroll recipients of adjuvant therapy in a clinical trial. Thus far, results of trials comparing adjuvant therapy plus local therapy with local therapy alone show that adjuvant chemotherapy results in increased RFS and, in some cases, increased OAS for at least a portion of patients. Important prognostic factors for the natural history of breast cancer, including menopausal status, histopathology, estrogen and progesterone receptor status, thymidine-labeling index, and axillary node involvement, do not consistently identify groups with a good or a bad response to adjuvant chemotherapy. However, these factors do point out subsets of patients with particularly good or bad prognoses, which might then influence decisions about the type of adjuvant therapy to administer.

Administration of adjuvant chemotherapy should be considered as standard care for premenopausal patients with involved axillary nodes; its administration should be strongly considered for some premenopausal patients without axillary metastasis, especially if they have other poor prognostic characteristics such as large tumors, high growth fraction, negative receptor status, or age less than 35. Postmenopausal women with receptor-negative tumors should also be carefully considered as candidates for adjuvant chemotherapy, particularly if they demonstrate other risk factors for recurrence, such as involved axillary nodes.

It appears that combination chemotherapy is superior to single-agent treatment, but no particular combination of drugs stands out. Doxorubicin-containing regimens are probably better than non–doxorubicin-containing combinations, and special concerns about major toxicity seem unfounded. The optimal duration of therapy remains unknown, but it seems clear that several months of treatment confer essentially the same advantage as regimens lasting a year or more, with a concomitant decrease in toxicity. There is evidence that chemotherapy should be initiated as soon as possible to obtain maximal benefit, perhaps in the perioperative period, and that it may be safely interdigitated with radiation therapy. Additional information supports the idea that maximally tolerated drug doses, as measured by dose intensity over time, are most efficacious.

Tamoxifen is unequivocally indicated for therapy of postmenopausal women with hormone receptor–positive tumors and axillary node metastases. Its use should also be carefully considered in patients without axillary node involvement, given its virtual lack of toxicity. There is information to support chronic rather than short-term tamoxifen administration. The routine use of endocrine or chemoendocrine therapy remains unproven for premenopausal women. While there is some suggestion that combined chemoendocrine therapy may be beneficial for postmenopausal women, it is not clear if the benefit from such regimens is derived from the combined therapy or from the endocrine therapy alone. Appropriate trials to answer this question are under way. No role for immunotherapy outside of the research setting can be identified at present.

While much progress has been made, it is clear that much remains to be done in defining the optimal adjuvant therapy for breast cancer. The information on prognostic factors for outcome of therapy may serve to guide decision making for an individual woman, but adjuvant therapy is still best regarded as an experimental therapeutic approach, to be administered, when possible, in the setting of randomized trials. In this fashion, maximal benefit for both the individual patient and the field of study may be obtained.

REFERENCES

1. Skipper HE: Kinetics of mammary tumor cell growth and implications for therapy. Cancer 28:1479, 1971.
2. Schabel FM: Surgical adjuvant chemotherapy of metastatic murine tumors. Cancer 40:558, 1977.
3. Shackney SE, McCormack GW, Cuchural GJ: Growth rate patterns of solid tumors and their relation to responsiveness to therapy. Ann Intern Med 89:107, 1978.
4. Goldie JH, Coldman AJ: A mathematic model for relating the drug sensitivity of tumors to their spontaneous mutation rate. Cancer Treat Rep 63:1727, 1983.
5. Goldie JH, Coldman AJ: Rationale for the use of alternating non–cross-resistant chemotherapy. Cancer Treat Rep 66:439, 1982.
6. Goldie JH, Coldman AJ: Quantitative model for multiple levels of DNA resistance in clinical tumors. Cancer Treat Rep 67:923, 1983.
7. Fisher B, Slack N, Katrych D: Ten year follow-up results of patients with carcinoma of the breast in a co-operative clinical trial evaluating surgical adjuvant chemotherapy. Surg Gynecol Obstet 140:528, 1975.
8. Fisher B, Redmond C, Fisher ER, et al.: Systemic adjuvant therapy in treatment of primary operable breast cancer: National Surgical Adjuvant Breast and Bowel Project experience. NCI Monographs No. 1, p. 35, 1986.
9. Nissen-Meyer R, Kjellgren K, Mansson B: Adjuvant chemotherapy in breast cancer. Recent Results Cancer Res 80:142, 1982.
10. Nissen-Meyer R: One short chemotherapy course in primary breast cancer: 12-year follow-up in series 1 of the Scandinavian adjuvant chemotherapy study group. *In*: Jones SE, Salmon SE (eds.): Adjuvant Therapy of Cancer II. New York: Grune & Stratton, 1979, pp. 207–213.
11. Nissen-Meyer R, Kjellgren K, Malmio K, et al.: Surgical adjuvant chemotherapy: Results with one short course with cyclophosphamide after mastectomy for breast cancer. Cancer 41:2088, 1978.
12. Nissen-Meyer R, Host H, Kjellgren K, et al.: Treatment of node-negative breast cancer patients with short course of chemotherapy immediately after surgery. NCI Mongraphs No. 1, p. 125, 1986.
13. Finney R: Adjuvant chemotherapy in the radical treatment of carcinoma of the breast—a clinical trial. Am J Roentgenol Radium Ther Nucl Med 111:137, 1971.
14. Donovan IA, Powell J, Waterhouse JAH, et al.: A prolonged course of cyclophosphamide as an adjunct to mastectomy in the primary treatment of breast carcinoma. Br J Surg 63:817, 1976.
15. Donegan WL: Extended surgical adjuvant thiotepa for mammary carcinoma. Arch Surg 109:187, 1974.
16. Donegan WL, Kardinal CG: Long term results of extended adjuvant thiotepa for operable breast cancer. Proc Am Soc Clin Oncol 4:75, 1985.
17. Rieche K, Berndt H, Prahl B: Continuous postoperative treatment with cyclophosphamide in breast carcinoma—a randomized clinical study. Arch Geschwulstforsch 40S:349, 1972.
18. Mrazek RG, McDonald GO: Surgery and adjuvant chemotherapy in treatment for breast carcinoma. Abstract of the Tenth International Cancer Congress, Houston, Texas, 1970, p. 501.
19. Fisher, B, Carbone P, Economou SG, et al.: L-Phenylalanine mustard (L-PAM) in the management of primary breast cancer. A report of early findings. N Engl J Med 292:117, 1975.
20. Bonadonna G, Brusamolino E, Valagussa P, et al.: Combination chemotherapy as an adjuvant treatment in operable breast cancer. N Engl J Med 294:405, 1976.
21. Bonadonna G, Valagussa P, Tancini G, et al.: Current status of Milan adjuvant chemotherapy trials for node positive and node negative breast cancer. NCI Monographs No. 1, p. 45, 1986.
22. Howat JMT, Hughes R, Durning P, et al.: A controlled clinical trial of adjuvant chemotherapy in operable cancer of the breast. *In* Salmon SE, Jones SE (eds.): Adjuvant Therapy of Cancer III. New York: Grune & Stratton, 1983, pp. 371–376.
23. Rubens RD, Knight RK, Fentiman IS, et al.: Controlled trial of adjuvant chemotherapy with melphalan for breast cancer. Lancet 1:839, 1983.
24. Senn H-J, Jungi WF: Swiss adjuvant trials with LMF (+ BCG) in N− and N+ breast cancer. *In*: Jones SE, Salmon SE (eds.): Adjuvant Therapy in Cancer IV. Orlando, FL: Grune & Stratton, 1984, pp. 261–270.
25. Morrison JM, Howell A, Grieve RJ, et al.: The West Midlands Oncology Association trials of adjuvant chemotherapy for operable breast cancer. *In*: Jones SE, Salmon SE (eds.): Adjuvant Therapy of Cancer IV. Orlando, FL: Grune & Stratton, 1984, pp. 253–260.
26. Senn HJ, Jungi WF, Amgwerd R, et al.: Swiss adjuvant trial (OSAKO 06/74) with LMF + BCG in node-negative breast cancer patients: 9-year results. NCI Monographs No. 1, p. 129, 1986.
27. Smith DC, Crawford D, Dykes EH, et al.: Adjuvant radiotherapy and chemotherapy in breast cancer. *In*: Jones SE, Salmon SE (eds.): Adjuvant Therapy of Cancer IV. Orlando, FL: Grune & Stratton, 1984, pp. 283–289.
28. Howell A, Bush H, George WD, et al.: Controlled trial of adjuvant chemotherapy with cyclophosphamide, methotrexate, and fluorouracil for breast cancer. Lancet 2:307, 1984.
29. Wheeler TK: Four drug combination chemotherapy following surgery for breast cancer. *In*: Jones SE, Salmon SE (eds.): Adjuvant Therapy of Cancer II. New York: Grune & Stratton, 1979, pp. 269–276.
30. Peto R: Presentation to the Consensus Development Conference on Adjuvant Chemotherapy for Breast Cancer, September 9–11, 1985, Bethesda, NCI Monographs No. 1, p. 71, 1986.
31. Jones S, Moon T, Davis S, et al.: Comparative analysis of selected breast cancer adjuvant trials in relation to the Natural History Data Base (NHDB). *In*: Salmon SE, Jones SE (eds.): Adjuvant Therapy of Cancer III. New York: Grune & Stratton, 1981, pp. 483–491.
32. Fisher B, Redmond C, Wolmark N, et al.: Disease-free survival at intervals during and following completion of adjuvant chemotherapy: The NSABP experience from three breast cancer protocols. Cancer 48:1273, 1981.
33. Osborne CK, Rivkin SE, McDivitt RW, et al.: Adjuvant therapy of breast cancer: Southwest Oncology Group studies. NCI Monographs No. 1, p. 71, 1986.
34. Glucksberg H, Rivkin SE, Rasmussen S, et al.: Combination chemotherapy (CMFVP) versus L-

phenylalanine mustard (L-PAM) for operable breast cancer with positive axillary nodes. A Southwest Oncology Group study. Cancer 50:423, 1982.
35. Ahmann DL, Scanlon PW, Bisel HF, et al.: Repeated adjuvant chemotherapy with phenylalanine mustard or 5-fluorouracil, cyclophosphamide, and prednisone with or without radiation, after mastectomy for breast cancer. Lancet 1:893, 1978.
36. Ahmann DL, O'Fallon JR, Scanlon PW, et al.: A preliminary assessment of factors associated with recurrent disease in a surgical adjuvant clinical trial for patients with breast cancer with special emphasis on the aggressiveness of therapy. Am J Clin Oncol 5:371, 1982.
37. Caprini JA, Oviedo MA, Cunningham MP, et al.: Adjuvant chemotherapy for stage II and III breast carcinoma. JAMA 244:243, 1980.
38. Cohen E, Scanlon EF, Caprini JA, et al.: Follow-up adjuvant chemotherapy and chemoimmunotherapy for stage II and III carcinoma of the breast. Cancer 49:1754, 1982.
39. Carpenter JT, Jr., Maddox WA, Laws HL, et al.: Favorable factors in the adjuvant therapy of breast cancer. Cancer 50:18, 1982.
40. Muss H, Cooper R, Ferree C, et al.: Long-term follow-up of L-PAM and CMF with and without radiation therapy (RT) as adjuvant treatment for stage II breast carcinoma. Proc Am Soc Clin Oncol 3:117, 1984.
41. Cooper MR, Rhyne AL, Muss HB, et al.: A randomized comparative trial of chemotherapy and irradiation therapy for stage II breast cancer. Cancer 47:2833, 1981.
42. Brincker H, Mouridsen HT, Andersen KW: Adjuvant chemotherapy with cyclophosphamide or CMF in premenopausal women with stage II breast cancer. Breast Cancer Res Treat 3:91, 1983.
43. Misset JL, Delgado M, De Vassal F, et al.: Five-year results of the French adjuvant trial for breast cancer comparing CMF to a combination of Adriamycin (ADM), vincristine (VCR), cyclophosphamide (CPM), and 5-fluorouracil (5FU). *In*: Jones SE, Salmon SE (eds.): Adjuvant Therapy of Cancer IV. Orlando, FL: Grune & Stratton, 1984, pp. 243–252.
44. Tormey DC, Weinberg V, Holland JF, et al.: A randomized trial of five and three drug chemotherapy and chemoimmunotherapy in women with operable node-positive breast cancer. J Clin Oncol 1:138, 1983.
45. Jones SE, Salmon SE, Allen H, et al.: Adjuvant treatment of node-positive breast cancer with Adriamycin-cyclophosphamide with or without radiation therapy: Interim results of an ongoing clinical trial. Recent Results Cancer Res. 80:162, 1982.
46. Buzdar AU, Hortobagyi GN, Marcus CE, et al.: Results of adjuvant chemotherapy trials in breast cancer at M.D. Anderson Hospital and Tumor Institute. NCI Monographs No. 1, p. 81, 1986.
47. Jones SE, Moon TE, Bonadonna G, et al.: Trials for women with operable stage II (node-positive) breast cancer. Jones, SE, Salmon SE (eds.): *In* Adjuvant Therapy of Cancer IV. Orlando, FL: Grune & Stratton, 1984, pp. 235–242.
48. Hortobagyi GN, Buzdar AU, Marcus CE, et al.: Immediate and long-term toxicity of doxorubicin containing adjuvant chemotherapy regimens in the M.D. Anderson adjuvant chemotherapy trials. Cancer Treat Rep (In Press).
49. Brooks RJ, Jones SE, Salmon SE, et al.: Improved outcome with early treatment in an adjuvant breast cancer program. Proc Am Soc Clin Oncol 2:110, 1983.
50. Buzdar AU, Blumenschein GR, Smith TL, et al.: Adjuvant chemotherapy with fluorouracil, doxorubicin, and cyclophosphamide, with or without bacillus Calmette-Guérin and with or without irradiation in operable breast cancer. A prospective randomized trial. Cancer 53:384, 1984.
51. Swain S, Sorace RA, Bagley CS, et al.: Neoadjuvant chemotherapy in the combined-modality approach of locally advanced nonmetastatic breast cancer. Cancer Res (In press).
52. Ragaz J: Emerging modalities for adjuvant therapy of breast cancer—neoadjuvant chemotherapy. NCI Monographs No. 1, p. 145, 1986.
53. Velez-Garcia EO, Moore M, Vogel CCL, et al.: Postsurgical adjuvant chemotherapy with or without radiation therapy in women with breast cancer and positive axillary nodes: The Southeastern Cancer Study Group (SECSG) experience. *In*: Jones SE, Salmon SE (eds.): Adjuvant Therapy in Cancer IV. Orlando FL: Grune & Stratton. 1984, pp. 273–282.
54. Henderson IC, Gelman RS, Harris JR, et al.: Duration of therapy in adjuvant chemotherapy trials. NCI Monographs No. 1, p. 95, 1986.
55. Hryniuk W, Bush H: The importance of dose intensity in chemotherapy of metastatic breast cancer. J Clin Oncol 2:1281, 1984.
56. Hryniuk WM, Levine MN, Levin L: Analysis of dose intensity for chemotherapy in early (stage II) and advanced breast cancer. NCI Monographs No. 1, p. 87, 1986.
57. Bonadonna G, Valagussa P: Dose-response effect of adjuvant chemotherapy in breast cancer. N Engl J Med 304:10, 1981.
58. Redmond C, Fisher B, Weiand HS: The methodologic dilemma in retrospectively correlating the amount of chemotherapy received in adjuvant therapy protocols with disease-free survival. Cancer Treat Rep 67:519, 1983.
59. Lippman ME, Lichter AS, Edwards BK, et al.: The impact of primary irradiation treatment of localized breast cancer on the ability to administer systemic adjuvant chemotherapy. J Clin Oncol 2:21, 1984.
60. Carbone PP: The present dilemma of adjuvant chemotherapy: Acceptance and risk versus benefits. Recent Results Cancer Res 96:218, 1984.
61. Wilcox PM, Fetting JN, Nettesheim KM, et al.: Anticipatory nausea and vomiting in women receiving cyclophosphamide, methotrexate, and 5-FU (CMF) adjuvant chemotherapy for breast carcinoma. Cancer Treat Rep 66:1601, 1982.
62. Knobf MK, Mullen JC, Xistris D, et al.: Weight gain in women receiving adjuvant chemotherapy. Oncol Nurs Forum 10:28, 1983.
63. Bonadonna G, Valagussa P: Adjuvant systemic therapy for resectable breast cancer. J Clin Oncol 3:259, 1985.
64. Meyerowitz BE, Watkins IK, Sparks FC: Psychosocial implications of adjuvant chemotherapy. A two-year follow-up. Cancer 52:1541, 1983.
65. Wallack MK, Wolf JA, Jr., Bedwinek J, et al.: Gestational carcinoma of the female breast. Curr Probl Cancer: 7:1, 1983.
66. Rockette H, Fisher B, Fisher E, et al.: Leukemia following adjuvant chemotherapy for breast cancer. Proc Am Soc Clin Oncol 4:66, 1985.
67. Holdener EE, Nissen-Meyer R, Bonadonna G, et

al.: Second malignant neoplasms in operable carcinoma of the breast. Recent Results Cancer Res 96:188, 1984.
68. Kelsy JL: A review of the epidemiology of human breast cancer. Epidemiol Rev 1:74, 1979.
69. Henderson IC, Canellos GP: Cancer of the breast. The past decade (parts I & II). N Engl J Med 302:17–30, 78–90, 1980.
70. Swenerton KD, Legha SS, Smith T, et al.: Prognostic factors in metastatic breast cancer treated with combination chemotherapy. Cancer Res 39:1552, 1979.
71. Mouridsen HT, Palshof T: Adjuvant systemic therapy in breast cancer; A review. Eur J Cancer Clin Oncol 19:1753, 1983.
72. Bonadonna G, Valagussa P: Contribution of prognostic factors to adjuvant chemotherapy in breast cancer. Recent Results Cancer Res 96:34, 1984.
73. Smith DC, Crawford D, Dykes EH, et al.: Adjuvant radiotherapy and chemotherapy in breast cancer. *In*: Jones SE, Salmon SE (eds.): Adjuvant Therapy in Cancer IV. Orlando, FL: Grune & Stratton, 1984, pp. 283–289.
74. Goldhirsch A: Adjuvant therapy for postmenopausal women with operable breast cancer: Part I—a randomized trial of chemo-endocrine versus endocrine therapy versus mastectomy alone. *In*: Jones SE, Salmon SE (eds.): Adjuvant Therapy in Cancer IV. Orlando FL: Grune & Stratton, 1984, pp. 379–392.
75. Fisher B, Sherman B, Rockette H, et al: L-Phenylalanine mustard (L-PAM) in the management of premenopausal patients with primary breast cancer: Lack of association of disease-free survival with depression of ovarian function. Cancer 44:847, 1979.
76. Ludwig Breast Cancer Study Group: Adjuvant combination chemotherapy with or without prednisone in premenopausal breast cancer patients with metastases in 1 to 3 axillary lymph nodes: A randomized trial. Cancer Res 45:4454, 1985.
77. Fisher B, Bauer M, Wickerham DL, et al.: Relation of number of positive axillary nodes to the prognosis of patients with primary breast cancer. An NSABP update. Cancer 52:1551, 1983.
78. Buzdar A, Smith T, Blumenschein G, et al.: Adjuvant chemotherapy with fluorouracil, doxorubicin, and cyclophosphamide (FAC) for stage II or III breast cancer: 5-year results. *In*: Salmon SE, Jones SE (eds.): Adjuvant Therapy of Cancer III. New York: Grune & Stratton, 1981, pp. 419–434.
79. Bonadonna G, Valagussa P, Rossi A, et al.: Multimodal therapy with CMF in resectable breast cancer with positive axillary nodes: The Milan Institute experience. Recent Results Cancer Res 80:149, 1982.
80. Koyama H, Wada T, Takahashi Y, et al: Surgical adjuvant chemotherapy with mitomycin C and cyclophosphamide in Japanese patients with breast cancer. Cancer 46:2373, 1980.
81. Senn HJ, Amgwerd R, Jungi WF, et al.: Adjuvant chemoimmunotherapy with LMF plus BCG in node-negative and node-positive breast cancer—intermediate report at 4 years. Recent Results Cancer Res 80:177, 1982.
82. Bonadonna G, Rossi A, Tancini G, et al.: Adjuvant chemotherapy trials in resectable breast cancer with positive axillary nodes. The experience of the Milan Cancer Institute. *In*: Jones SE, Salmon SE (eds.): Adjuvant Therapy of Cancer IV. Orlando, FL: Grune & Stratton, 1984, pp. 195–208.
83. Morrison JM, Howell A, Grieve RJ, et al.: The West Midlands Oncology Association trials of adjuvant chemotherapy for operable breast cancer. *In*: Salmon SE, Jones SE (eds.): Adjuvant Therapy of Cancer III. New York: Grune & Stratton. 1981, pp. 403–410.
84. Brooks RJ, Jones SE, Salmon SE, et al.: Adjuvant chemotherapy of axillary node negative carcinoma of the breast using doxorubicin and cyclophosphamide. NCI Monographs No. 1, p. 135, 1986.
85. Rosen PP, Saigo PE, Braun DW, et al.: Axillary micro- and macrometastases in breast cancer. Prognostic significance of tumor size. Ann Surg 194:585, 1981.
86. Derogatis LR, Abeloff MD, Melisaratos N: Psychological coping mechanisms and survival time in metastatic breast cancer. JAMA 242:1504, 1979.
87. Greer S, Morris T, Pettingale KW: Psychological response to breast cancer: Effect on outcome. Lancet 2:785, 1979.
88. Cassileth BR, Lusk EJ, Miller DS, et al.: Psychosocial correlates of survival in advanced malignant disease? N Engl J Med 312:1551, 1985.
89. Levy S, Lippman M, Herberman R, et al.: Natural killer cells as mediators between stress and tumor response in primary breast cancer patients. Proc Am Soc Clin Oncol 3:70, 1984.
90. Elston CW, Blamey RW, Johnson J, et al.: The relationship of oestradiol receptor (ER) and histological tumor differentiation with prognosis in human primary breast carcinoma. Eur J Cancer (Suppl) 1:59, 1980.
91. Fisher E, Redmond C, Fisher B: Pathologic findings from the National Surgical Adjuvant Breast Project (protocol No. 4). VI. Discriminants for five-year treatment failure. Cancer 46:908, 1980.
92. Meyer JS, McDivitt RW, Stone KR, et al.: Practical breast carcinoma cell kinetics: Review and update. Breast Cancer Res Treat 4:79, 1984.
93. Rich MA, Furmanski P, Brooks SC, et al.: Prognostic value of estrogen receptor determinations in patients with breast cancer. Cancer Res 38:4296, 1978.
94. Fisher E, Redmond C, Fisher B: Pathologic findings from the National Surgical Adjuvant Breast Project. VIII. Relationship of chemotherapeutic responsiveness to tumor differentiation. Cancer 51:181, 1983.
95. Fisher ER: Prognostic and therapeutic significance of pathologic features of breast cancer. NCI Monographs No. 1, p. 29, 1986.
96. Jakesz R, Kolb R, Reiner G, et al.: Effect of adjuvant chemotherapy in Stage I and Stage II breast cancer is dependent on tumor differentiation and estrogen status. Proc Am Soc Clin Oncol 4:69, 1985.
97. Meyer JS, Friedman E, McCrate MM, et al.: Prediction of early course of breast carcinoma by thymidine labeling. Cancer 51:1879, 1983.
98. Meyer JS, Lee JY: Relationships of S-phase fraction of breast carcinoma in relapse to duration of remission, estrogen receptor content, therapeutic responsiveness, and duration of survival. Cancer Res 40:1890, 1980.
99. Stewart JF, King RJB, Sexton SA, et al.: Oestrogen receptors, sites of metastatic disease and survival in recurrent breast cancer. Eur J Cancer 17:449, 1980.

100. Corle DK, Sears ME, Olson KB: The relationship of quantitative estrogen receptor level and clinical response to cytotoxic chemotherapy in advanced breast cancer: An extramural analysis. Cancer 54:1554, 1984.
101. McGuire WL, Clark GM, Dressler LG, et al.: Role of steroid hormone receptors as prognostic factors in primary breast cancer. NCI Monographs No. 1, p. 19, 1986.
102. Tormey DC, Gray R, Taylor SG, et al.: Postoperative chemotherapy and chemohormonal therapy in women with node-positive breast cancer. NCI Monographs No. 1, p. 75, 1986.
103. Bonadonna G, Valagussa P, Tancini G, et al.: Estrogen-receptor status and response to chemotherapy in early and advanced breast cancer. Cancer Chemother Pharmacol 4:37, 1980.
104. Fisher B, Redmond C, Brown A, et al.: Treatment of primary breast cancer with chemotherapy and tamoxifen. N Engl J Med 305:1, 1981.
105. Meyer JS: Cell kinetics in selection and stratification of patients for adjuvant therapy of breast carcinoma. NCI Monographs No. 1, p. 25, 1986.
106. Kute TE, Muss HB, Anderson D, et al.: Relationship of steroid receptor, cell kinetics, and clinical status in patients with breast cancer. Cancer Res 41:3524, 1981.
107. Silvestrini R, Daidone MG, DiFronzo G: Relationship between proliferative activity and estrogen receptors in breast cancer. Cancer 44:665, 1979.
108. Tubiana M, Pejovic MJ, Renaud A, et al.: Kinetic parameters and the course of the disease in breast cancer. Cancer 47:937, 1981.
109. Krown SE, Pinsky CM, Wanebo HJ, et al.: Immunologic reactivity and prognosis in breast cancer. Cancer 46:1746, 1980.
110. Cannon G, Dean J, Herberman R, et al.: Lymphoproliferative responses to autologous tumor extracts as prognostic indicators in patients with resected breast cancer. Intl J Cancer 27:131, 1981.
111. Waalkes TP, Abeloff MD, Ettinger DA, et al.: Multiple biological markers and breast carcinoma: A preliminary study in the detection of recurrent disease after primary therapy. J Surg Oncol 18:9, 1981.
112. Waalkes TP, Tormey DC: Biological markers and breast cancer. Semin Oncol 5:434, 1978.
113. DeJong-Bakker M, Hart AAM, Persijn JP, et al.: Prognostic significance of CEA in breast cancer: A statistical study. Eur J Cancer Clin Oncol 17:1307, 1981.
114. Bezwoda W, Derman D, Bothwell T, et al.: Significance of serum concentrations of carcinoembryonic antigen, ferritin, and calcitonin in breast cancer. Cancer 48:1623, 1981.
115. Franchimont P, Zangerle PF, Colin C, et al.: Tumor associated markers in breast cancer. Eur J Cancer (Suppl) 1:17, 1980.
116. Haagensen DE, Kister SJ, Vandevoorde JP, et al.: Evaluation of carcinoembryonic antigen as a plasma monitor for human breast carcinoma. Cancer 42:1512, 1978.
117. Myers RE, Sutherland DJ, Meakin JW, et al.: Carcinoembryonic antigen in breast cancer. Cancer 42:1520, 1978.
118. Tormey DC, Waalkes TP: Biological markers and prognostic and clinical evaluation tools. Eur J Cancer (Suppl) 1:21, 1980.
119. Tormey DC, Waalkes TP: Clinical correlation between CEA and breast cancer. Cancer 42:1507, 1978.
120. Tormey DC, Waalkes TP, Snyder JJ, et al.: Biological markers in breast carcinoma III. Clinical correlations with carcinoembryonic antigen. Cancer 39:2391, 1977.
121. Coombes R, Gazet J, Sloane J, et al.: Biochemical markers in human breast cancer. Lancet 2:132, 1977.
122. Coombes R, Powles T, Gazet J, et al.: A biochemical approach to the staging of human breast cancer. Cancer 40:937, 1977.
123. Tormey DC, Waalkes TP, Simon RM: Biological markers in breast carcinoma. III. Clinical correlations with human chorionic gonadotrophin. Cancer 39:2391, 1977.
124. Lamourex G, Mandeville R, Poisson R, et al.: Biological markers and breast cancer: A multiparametric study. 1. Increased serum protein levels. Cancer 49:502, 1982.
125. Schapira DV, Schapira M: Use of ceruloplasmin levels to monitor response to therapy and predict recurrence of breast cancer. Breast Cancer Res Treat 3:221, 1983.
126. Neill HB, Palmieri GM, Neely CL, Jr., et al.: Postabsorptive urinary hydroxyproline test in patients with metastatic bone disease from breast cancer. Arch Intern Med 141:1471, 1981.
127. Gielen F, Dequeker J, Drochmans A, et al.: Relevance of hydroxyproline excretion to bone metastasis in breast cancer. Br J Cancer 34:279, 1976.
128. Powles TJ, Leese CL, Bondy PK: Hydroxyproline excretion in patients with breast cancer and response to treatment. Br Med J 2:164, 1975.
129. Coombes RC, Berger U, Mansi J, et al.: Prognostic significance of micrometastases in bone marrow in patients with primary breast cancer. NCI Monographs No. 1, p. 51, 1986.
130. Ravdin RG, Lewison EF, Slack NH, et al.: Results of a clinical trial concerning the worth of prophylactic oophorectomy for breast cancer. Surg Gynecol Obstet 131:1055, 1970.
131. Bryant AJS, Weir JA: Prophylactic oophorectomy in operable instances of carcinoma of the breast. Surg Gynecol Obstet 153:660, 1981.
132. Nissen-Meyer R: Suppression of ovarian function in primary breast cancer. *In*: Forrest APM, Kunkler PB (eds.): Prognostic Factors in Breast Cancer. Edinburgh: E. S. Livingston, Ltd., 1968, pp. 139–145.
133. Nissen-Meyer R: The role of prophylactic castration in the therapy of human mammary cancer. Eur J Cancer 3:395, 1967.
134. Cole MP: Prophylactic compared with therapeutic X-ray artificial menopause. *In*: Joslin CAF, Gleave EN (eds.): The Clinical Management of Advanced Breast Cancer. Cardiff: Alpha Omega Alpha Publishing Co., 1970, pp. 2–11.
135. Cole MP: Suppression of ovarian function in primary breast cancer. *In*: Forrest APM, Kunkler PB (eds.): Prognostic Factors in Breast Cancer. Edinburgh: E. S. Livingston, Ltd., 1968, pp. 146–156.
136. Meakin JW: Review of Canadian trials of adjuvant endocrine therapy for breast cancer. NCI Monographs No. 1, p. 111, 1986.
137. Nolvadex Adjuvant Trial Organization: Controlled trial of tamoxifen as single adjuvant agent in man-

agement of early breast cancer. Lancet 1:836, 1985.
138. Mouridsen HT, Andersen AP, Brincker H, et al.: Adjuvant tamoxifen in postmenopausal high-risk breast cancer patients. Present status of the Danish Breast Cancer Cooperative Group Trials. NCI Monographs No. 1, p. 115, 1986.
139. Ribeiro G, Palmer MK: Adjuvant tamoxifen for operable carcinoma of the breast: Report of clinical trial by the Christie Hospital and Holt Radium Institute. Br Med J 286:827, 1983.
140. Wallgren A, Baral E, Carstensen J, et al.: Should adjuvant tamoxifen be given for several years in breast cancer? *In*: Jones SE, Salmon SE (eds.): Adjuvant Therapy in Cancer IV. Orlando, FL: Grune & Stratton, 1984, pp. 331–338.
141. Goldhirsch A, Gelber R: Adjuvant treatment for early breast cancer: The Ludwig Breast Cancer Studies. NCI Monographs No. 1, p. 55, 1986.
142. Cummings FJ, Gray R, Davis TE, et al.: Tamoxifen vs. placebo: Double blind adjuvant trial in elderly women with stage II breast cancer. NCI Monographs No. 1, p. 119, 1986.
143. Palshof T, Mourisden HT, Daehnfeldt JL: Adjuvant endocrine therapy of primary operable breast cancer. Report on the Copenhagen breast cancer trials. *In*: Mouridsen HT, Palshof T (eds.): Breast Cancer: Experimental and Clinical Aspects. Oxford: Pergamon Press, 1979, pp. 183–187.
144. Coombes RC, Chilvers C, Powles TJ: Adjuvant aminoglutethimide therapy for postmenopausal patients with primary breast cancer. *In*: Jones SE, Salmon SE (eds.): Adjuvant Therapy in Cancer IV. Orlando, FL: Grune & Stratton, 1984, pp. 349–358.
145. Kaufmann M, Maass H, Kubli F, et al.: Risk adapted adjuvant chemohormonotherapy in operable nodal positive breast cancer. *In*: Jones SE, Salmon SE (eds.): Adjuvant Therapy in Cancer IV. Orlando, FL: Grune & Stratton, 1984, pp. 369–378.
146. Wallgren A, Baral E, Glas U, et al.: Adjuvant breast cancer treatment with tamoxifen and combination chemotherapy in postmenopausal women. *In* Salmon SE, Jones SE (eds.): Adjuvant Therapy of Cancer III. New York: Grune & Stratton, 1981, pp. 345–350.
147. Hubay CA, Gordon NH, Crowe JP, et al.: Antiestrogen-cytotoxic chemotherapy and bacillus Calmette-Guérin vaccination in stage II breast cancer: 72-month follow-up. Surgery 96:61, 1985.
148. Hubay CA, Pearson OH, Marshall JS, et al.: Adjuvant chemotherapy, antiestrogen therapy and immunotherapy for stage II breast cancer. *In*: Mouridsen HT, Palshof T (eds.): Breast Cancer: Experimental and Clinical Aspects. Oxford: Pergamon Press, 1979, pp. 189–195.
149. Fisher B, Redmond C, Brown A, et al.: Influence of tumor estrogen and progesterone receptor levels on the response to tamoxifen and chemotherapy in primary breast cancer. J Clin Oncol 1:227, 1983.
150. Jordan VC, Dix CJ, Allen KE: The effectiveness of long-term tamoxifen for treatment in a laboratory model for adjuvant hormone therapy of breast cancer. *In*: Salmon SE, Jones SE (eds.): Adjuvant Therapy of Cancer III. New York: Grune & Stratton, 1981, pp. 19–26.
151. Tormey DC, Taylor SG, IV, Kalish LA, et al.: Adjuvant systemic therapy in premenopausal (CMF, CMFP, CMFPT) and postmenopausal (observation, CMFP, CMFPT) women with node positive breast cancer. *In*: Jones SE, Salmon SE (eds.): Adjuvant Therapy in Cancer IV. Orlando, FL: Grune & Stratton, 1984, pp. 359–368.
152. Tormey DC: Adjuvant systemic therapy in postoperative node positive patients with breast carcinoma: The CALGB trial and the ECOG premenopausal trial. Recent Results Cancer Res 96:155, 1984.
153. Schreml W, Lang M, Betzler M, et al.: Adjuvant chemo(immuno)-therapy of primary breast cancer with Adriamycin-cyclophosphamide (and levamisole)—six-year evaluation. Eur J Cancer Clin Oncol 19:607, 1983.
154. Kay RG, Mason BH, Stephens EJ, et al.: Levamisole in primary breast cancer. Cancer 51:1992, 1983.
155. Brincker H, et al.: Increased breast cancer recurrence rate after adjuvant therapy with levamisole. A preliminary report. Lancet 2:824, 1980.
156. Lacour J, Lacour F, Spira A, et al.: Adjuvant treatment with polyadenylic-polyuridylic acid in operable breast cancer: updated results of a randomised trial. Br Med J 288:589, 1984.
157. Consensus Development Conference Committee: Adjuvant chemotherapy for breast cancer. NCI Monographs No. 1, p. 1, 1986.

Treatment of Metastatic Breast Cancer

NANCY E. DAVIDSON, M.D.
MARC E. LIPPMAN, M.D.

Breast cancer is an extremely common disease in the United States. About 120,000 cases are diagnosed annually. Fewer than 10 percent of patients will present with advanced disease initially; yet, about 40 percent of patients will develop metastatic disease despite advances in early diagnosis, local treatment, and adjuvant therapy. Thus, the treatment of metastatic disease has been the subject of intense investigation, and substantial progress has been made in both hormonal and chemotherapeutic approaches. However, recent results of treatment with combination chemotherapy have reached a plateau, such that some 40 to 70 percent of patients may be expected to respond to current first-line combination chemotherapy, with a median response duration of 7 to 13 months and a median survival time of 12 to 24 months. A similar lack of progress has been seen with endocrine therapy. About one third of unselected patients have a median response duration not in excess of one year. Unfortunately, these therapies are palliative, and virtually all patients with metastatic breast cancer ultimately die of their disease. This chapter will review the concepts underlying current approaches to therapy of advanced breast cancer and will explore new approaches that may lead to improved results.

ENDOCRINE THERAPY

The responsiveness of a subset of patients with metastatic breast cancer to endocrine manipulation has been recognized for nearly 100 years. Since Beatson's original description[1] of the efficacy of bilateral oophorectomy as treatment for premenopausal women with breast cancer, a variety of therapeutic approaches have been examined. These may be divided into ablative therapies, additive therapies, inhibitors of hormone synthesis, and antagonists of hormone action. As previously noted, about one third of unselected patients will respond to endocrine therapies. An enhanced response rate of 50 to 60 percent may be observed in women with estrogen recep-

13

tor–positive tumors, whose clinical features often include long disease-free intervals; nonvisceral sites of disease, including soft tissue, bone, and lymph nodes; good performance status; and postmenopausal status. It is also clear that patients who respond to one hormone therapy have a higher likelihood of responding to subsequent endocrine maneuvers than do nonresponders. However, both response rate and duration tend to decrease with each successive trial.

Ablative Therapies

About 25 to 30 percent of premenopausal women will have an objective response to castration, either surgical or irradiation-induced, and the median duration of response is 9 to 12 months.[2, 3] In perimenopausal and postmenopausal women, the regression rate from castration is well below that seen in women with ovarian function.[2, 3] Bilateral oophorectomy is generally preferred, as ovarian irradiation may require several months to be effective, and residual ovarian function due to incomplete follicular destruction may be observed.[4] Until recently oophorectomy was the treatment of choice for premenopausal patients receiving endocrine therapy; the role of tamoxifen as an alternative is discussed later.

The rationale for the use of adrenalectomy is the finding that estrogens persist in the blood after ovariectomy or menopause, in concentrations sufficient to stimulate growth of human breast cancer cells in culture.[5] Estrone is both secreted directly by the adrenal cortex[6] and produced via the transformation of androstenedione, a product of the adrenal cortex, to estrone in peripheral tissues.[7] Like oophorectomy, adrenalectomy has an overall response rate of 30 to 40 percent, which may be improved by patient selection.[8–10] Patients with estrogen receptor–positive tumors respond in up to 60 percent of cases, while those who have previously responded to castration demonstrate a 50 percent response rate. Lifelong glucocorticoid and mineralocorticoid replacement is required after adrenalectomy, a distinct disadvantage. The use of adrenalectomy has been virtually abandoned with the development of aminoglutethimide, as discussed later.

The mechanism of response to hypophysectomy is not known.[11–13] The removal of ACTH may account, in part, for tumor response, as suggested by the observation that response to hypophysectomy after adrenalectomy is low. A decrease in prolactin is not felt to play a role, since administration of bromocriptine or L-dopa, which lowers the prolactin level, is of no benefit as treatment for breast cancer. Also, pituitary stalk section, which increases the prolactin level, is as effective as hypophysectomy. Other as yet undefined hypothalamic or pituitary peptides may be important in tumor growth.[14] The response rate after hypophysectomy is felt to be equivalent to or perhaps slightly better than that after adrenalectomy, and the response duration after hypophysectomy was demonstrated to be superior by one study—15 months versus 8 months.[15] The use of hypophysectomy has been largely supplanted by medical therapies, discussed later, because of its disadvantages, including the need for specialized surgical skills and the requirement for chronic thyroid hormone and corticosteroid replacement.

Additive Therapies

Estrogens

Paradoxically, high doses of estrogen may induce tumor regression in about one third of patients.[16, 17] Clinical features associated with response include a long period of time after menopause and a lengthy disease-free interval. Remission rates are less than 10 percent in patients who have undergone adrenalectomy or hypophysectomy or who have failed other endocrine therapies.

Commonly used estrogen preparations include conjugated estrogen (Premarin) and diethylstilbestrol. Numerous toxicities have been reported. Vaginal bleeding secondary to endometrial hyperplasia may be controlled by administration of a progestin, followed by a short break in therapy to allow endometrial sloughing. Hypercalcemia may be observed in patients with widespread bony disease but is rare in patients who are at least ten years postmenopausal. Estrogen withdrawal and saline diuresis are usually sufficient to control the calcium level, and mithramycin is infrequently needed. Gradual resumption of administration of the drug may result in disease regression without recurrent hypercalcemia, and patients who develop hypercalcemia have been found to have a higher response rate than do those who do not become hypercalcemic.[18] Other lesser side effects include salt and water retention, nausea, vomiting, anorexia, and changes in pigmentation and libido.

The phenomenon of disease regression following cessation of estrogen or androgen therapy has been noted.[19, 20] Withdrawal responses can be seen, even in patients who failed to respond to either therapy initially; however, they are more common after a primary response. The mechanism of the withdrawal response is not known. Its existence suggests that patients should be observed without any therapy for at least six weeks after estrogen or androgen withdrawal, unless clinical considerations dictate an immediate change in treatment.

ANDROGENS

Androgens have been used in the treatment of metastatic breast cancer for over 30 years. Their mechanism of action is unknown[21]; in particular, the role of androgen receptors present in some tumors has yet to be clarified.[22] The response rate to androgens is lower than that seen with most other endocrine therapies: 21 percent in one study of testosterone propionate administered to 521 women. It was less than 10 percent in perimenopausal patients and highest in those at least five years postmenopausal. The median duration of remission was about eight months.[23]

All androgen preparations are equally effective when given in high doses. Because of the severe virilization associated with standard agents such as testosterone or fluoxymesterone, efforts have been made to identify new androgens that cause minimal masculinization but retain their antineoplastic properties. Two such drugs are testolactone[24] and danazol.[25, 26]

PROGESTINS

Interest in progestins for treatment of metastatic breast cancer has been rekindled by their relative lack of toxicity and improved efficacy in high doses. The mechanism of action of progestational agents is also not known.[21] Binding to progesterone receptor, interference with estrogen receptor synthesis, and other effects (for example, on the immune system) have all been postulated to play roles. Response rates of 20 to 30 percent have been observed and may be seen in patients previously treated with any other endocrine measure, even in the absence of a primary response. Improvement is most marked in patients with soft-tissue disease; osseous metastases rarely regress. The two commonly used preparations are medroxyprogesterone acetate and megestrol acetate; both are without significant side effects, except for edema and weight gain. Recent studies have focused on the use of high-dose regimens, which may result in higher response rates.[27, 28]

GLUCOCORTICOIDS

High doses of glucocorticoids equivalent to 200 to 300 mg of cortisol daily result in a 10 to 15 percent response rate in metastatic breast cancer.[29] Remission is generally of short duration but may be of rapid onset, making glucocorticoids useful in treatment of rapidly advancing disease. In contrast with other endocrine therapies, response to glucocorticoids is not associated with an increased likelihood of response to other endocrine modalities. Because of the low response rate and numerous side effects of chronic therapy, glucocorticoids should be used only (1) as supportive treatment for disease-related complications such as central nervous system metastases, (2) in conjunction with combination chemotherapy, or (3) for a short time in the treatment of fast-growing tumors, as mentioned earlier.

Inhibitors of Steroid Synthesis

The morbidity and mortality associated with adrenalectomy resulted in efforts to develop a medical adrenalectomy. The use of aminoglutethimide to suppress adrenal function was first reported in 1973.[30] Aminoglutethimide, an inhibitor of adrenal steroid synthesis, blocks the first step in *de novo* steroid synthesis, the conversion of cholesterol to pregnenolone.[31] Its second critical effect is to inhibit the conversion of androstenedione to estrone in peripheral tissues, a pathway that is the principal source of estrogen in the postmenopausal woman.[32] Because aminoglutethimide results in adrenal suppression and a concomitant fall in cortisol level leading to a rise in ACTH level and subsequent override of adrenal blockade, the drug was initially administered with dexamethasone to suppress the pituitary response. This therapy was effective in some women, but later studies[33] showed that aminoglutethimide shortened the plasma half-life of dexamethasone, leading to failure of the blockade of steroid synthesis. Substitution of hydrocortisone, whose metabolism is not altered by aminoglutethimide, led to the development of a regimen that effectively suppresses adrenal function in most patients. Aminoglutethimide combined with hydrocortisone is capable of inducing falls in plasma estrone and estradiol levels similar to those seen after adrenalectomy, and a randomized trial of aminoglutethimide versus surgical adrenalectomy showed that response rates and durations were equivalent.[34]

As with most other endocrine therapies, the response rate in unselected patients is about 30 percent, with an increase to 40 to 50 percent in patients with estrogen receptor–positive tumors and a response duration time of about one year. The drug is administered at 250 mg four times daily with 40 mg of hydrocortisone given in divided doses. Early side effects may include lethargy, fever, blurred vision, dizziness, and rash, all of which generally resolve over the first few weeks of treatment. The ready reversibility of its metabolic effects is an obvious advantage of aminoglutethimide, as adrenal function returns to normal within a day or two after discontinuation of therapy.[35] Another inhibitor of peripheral aromatization, 4-hydroxyandrostenedione, has gone into clinical trials.[36] Preliminary results suggest that it is less toxic than aminoglutethimide but effective nonetheless.

Antagonists of Hormone Action

Although any substance that will antagonize the action of estrogen may be termed an antiestrogen, only a few such compounds are clinically relevant. These include nafoxidine, clomiphene, and tamoxifen, all derivatives of triphenylethylene. Of these, only tamoxifen is used in the treatment of breast cancer, and discussion will be limited to that agent.

Despite intense study, tamoxifen's mechanism(s) of action is unclear.[37, 38] The drug is known to compete with estradiol for binding to the estrogen receptor, possibly activating the estrogen receptor and facilitating its binding to an as yet unidentified nuclear acceptor site(s), which may be involved in mediating estrogenic effects. In fact, antiestrogens have many estrogenic effects. Some premenopausal patients continue to have normal menstrual cycles throughout therapy, even concurrent with objective tumor regression.[39] The vaginal epithelium of postmenopausal women often shows an estrogenic effect. Finally, some women exhibit a "flare" of tumor growth after administration of antiestrogen therapy.[40] Thus, a competition with estradiol for receptor binding fails to account for all of tamoxifen's actions.

Distinct antiestrogen binding sites have been described.[41–43] These sites have limited affinity for estrogens and do not translocate from cytoplasm to nucleus. In addition, the binding affinity for various antiestrogens does not correlate well with antiestrogenic activity. Thus, any role of these sites in mediating the effects of antiestrogens remains to be defined.

Tamoxifen has been extremely valuable in the management of postmenopausal breast cancer where the overall response is about 34 percent.[44–47] Some 60 percent of patients with estrogen receptor–positive tumors respond, whereas those with receptor-negative tumors respond in less than 10 percent of cases. A few trials have addressed the use of tamoxifen in premenopausal women. Three trials[48–51] have shown a response rate of about 30 percent, comparable with that seen with oophorectomy in this patient population. Two of those studies[48, 49, 51] also showed that those women who progressed after a response to tamoxifen had a relatively high likelihood of response to subsequent oophorectomy compared with nonresponders. These results suggested that a tamoxifen trial could identify those patients who were good surgical candidates. Two randomized trials[52, 52a] of tamoxifen and oophorectomy in premenopausal women yielded similar response and overall survival rates with the two modes of therapy.

A comprehensive review of results of tamoxifen treatment was published by Patterson and colleagues.[53] In 2889 patients treated with tamoxifen in 45 studies, the overall response rate was 34 percent, with less than 7 percent achieving a complete response.

Response rates ranged from 14 to 57 percent, pointing out again the importance of patient selection and prognostic variables in determining treatment outcome. Response was virtually independent of age, with response rates of 31, 30, and 36 percent in women under 50, aged 51 to 60, and aged 61 to 70, respectively. The sole exception was in women over 70, who responded in 46 percent of cases. Previously untreated patients had a response rate of 43 percent. Those who had responded to prior endocrine therapy responded in nearly 60 percent of cases, while endocrine nonresponders demonstrated a 21 percent response rate. The response rate was not affected by previous chemotherapy; 41 percent of patients so treated responded.

The usual dose of tamoxifen ranges from 20 to 40 mg daily. No dose-response relationship has been identified,[54] a finding consistent with the drug's pharmacology and metabolism.[55, 56] Tamoxifen has a terminal elimination half-life of seven to ten days. Thus, plasma levels of 300 ng/ml, or 10 μM, are reported after a month of tamoxifen at 20 mg b.i.d., at least a 1000-fold excess over premenopausal plasma concentrations of estradiol. Also, a major metabolite of tamoxifen, 4-hydroxytamoxifen, is at least ten times as potent as tamoxifen and has a relative binding affinity equal to that of estradiol. Thus, sufficient tamoxifen and 4-hydroxytamoxifen are probably present to antagonize the effect of plasma estrogens, even in premenopausal women.

Tamoxifen is a remarkably nontoxic agent. Minor side effects may include nausea and vomiting. Leukopenia and thrombocytopenia occur in 10 to 15 percent of patients but rarely require dose modification.[54] A dose-related retinitis has been observed in patients receiving high drug doses but has not been seen with standard doses of 20 to 40 mg daily for up to five years.[57] Finally, an early treatment-related hypercalcemia may occur, particularly in patients with extensive bony disease, necessitating careful monitoring of these women for the first few weeks of therapy.[54]

Because of its efficacy and lack of toxicity, we consider tamoxifen the agent of choice for first-line endocrine therapy in postmenopausal women. Trials comparing tamoxifen with estrogens and aminoglutethimide have shown equivalent response rates but less toxicity with tamoxifen. A randomized trial[58] of DES and tamoxifen showed response rates of 41 and 33 percent ($p = 0.37$), respectively; but 12 percent of patients receiving DES stopped therapy because of adverse reactions, whereas no patients on tamoxifen stopped therapy because of toxicity. Two trials[59, 60] comparing aminoglutethimide with tamoxifen showed response rates of 36 and 30 percent for aminoglutethimide versus 38 and 30 percent for tamoxifen, again with greater toxicity in the aminoglutethimide arms. Studies[61, 62] comparing tamoxifen with high-dose progestational agents, particularly megestrol acetate, also document equivalent response rates of about 30 percent, but toxicity associated with both drugs is similar, suggesting that progestins may be acceptable first-line agents as well. However, the need for administration four times daily makes them less convenient than tamoxifen, which can be administered once daily. Patient compliance is likely to be better with the latter schedule of drug administration.

Combination Endocrine Therapy

Because of the limitations of single agents in endocrine therapy, several attempts have been made to combine hormonal therapies in order to increase therapeutic efficacy. A randomized trial[63] of tamoxifen alone or combined with aminoglutethimide and hydrocortisone has been performed. The response rate to tamoxifen was 43 percent, compared with 49 percent with the combination. However, toxicity was more severe in the combined therapy arm. Twenty percent of patients receiving two drugs stopped therapy because of side effects, while only 2 percent of tamoxifen-treated patients stopped because of toxicity. Twenty-four patients received aminoglutethimide after tamoxifen failure, with a 12 percent response rate. In another trial,[54] single-agent tamoxifen was compared with tamoxifen and fluoxymesterone. The response rate was better with the combination—15 percent for tamoxifen and 38 percent for combined therapy—but median survival time was only modestly longer, 380 versus 330 days. Patients receiving tamoxifen were not switched to fluoxymesterone therapy upon tamoxifen failure. The unusually low response rate with tamoxifen was attributed to low tamoxifen dose and to patient selection, as a number of patients had visceral disease and had been heavily pretreated. Toxicity was similar in the two treatment groups, except for a 39 percent incidence of masculinization in the group receiving androgen. In a third trial,[64] the efficacy of tamoxifen was compared with that of a combination of tamoxifen, aminoglutethimide, and danazol in 107 women. A superior response rate of 50 percent over 33 percent was observed with the three-drug regimen, without significantly increased toxicity. However, neither response duration nor survival time was improved with the combination. From these studies, it appears that routine administration of combined endocrine therapy is not warranted, as toxicity is generally increased, without any clear advantage over sequential administration of single agents.[65]

Recommendations for Endocrine Therapy

Endocrine therapy is a rational initial treatment for many women with advanced breast cancer. Good candidates include those patients whose pattern of disease is not life threatening and who have estrogen receptor–positive tumors or clinical characteristics suggestive of a hormonally responsive tumor. These clinical correlates include a long disease-free interval, nonvisceral metastases, increased age (over 35), nonperimenopausal status, good performance status, and prior response to endocrine therapy.

Oophorectomy or tamoxifen is recommended as the first intervention for premenopausal and probably perimenopausal women. Tamoxifen is the drug of choice for postmenopausal women because of its efficacy and low toxicity. Studies with high-dose progestins suggest that they are reasonable alternatives. Second-line therapies including aminoglutethimide and progestational agents are recommended for those who progress after an initial tumor regression, but lower response rates and shorter response duration times are usually observed. Estrogens, androgens, or surgical procedures may be indicated as tertiary therapies in selected patients. Combination endocrine therapy is under investigation, but initial studies suggest that it provides little advantage over sequential single agents.

CHEMOTHERAPY

While experience with single agents in metastatic breast cancer dates back to the 1940's, the advent of multiple-drug approaches was heralded by the reports of Greenspan[66] and Cooper[67] in the late 1960's. Initial enthusiasm over the 88 percent response rate noted by Cooper with his five-drug regimen was tempered by the results of several studies of closely related regimens, which produced response rates of 40 to 60 percent, with median response duration times of about ten months. Multiple studies have since addressed the issues of drug type, dosage, scheduling, and number; the role of concomitant hormonal or immunotherapy; and the usefulness of so-called non–cross-resistant approaches in an effort to improve on these results. The impact of these treatment variables on outcome is discussed next.

Choice of Drugs

Doxorubicin (A), cyclophosphamide (C), 5-fluorouracil (F), and methotrexate (M) are the most active single agents in breast cancer and are the mainstays of most drug combinations. Other frequently used agents include L-phenylalanine mustard (L-PAM), vincristine (V), mitomycin C, prednisone (P), and vinblastine (Vb). Individual response rates to these drugs vary between 20 and nearly 50 percent, but median response duration times are brief, perhaps four months (Table 13–1). Further information may be obtained from several excellent reviews of drug activity in breast cancer.[68–72]

At least ten drugs have been found to be active as single agents for treatment of metastatic breast cancer. One major question to be answered is which drugs contribute most in combination regimens? Early studies concentrated on identification of the critical drugs in the Cooper regimen of cyclophosphamide, methotrexate, 5-fluorouracil, vincristine, and prednisone. No study has clearly shown vincristine to be of additional benefit in combinations derived from the parent CMFVP combination.[73–77] In fact, a series of studies by Ahmann and associates[75] has demonstrated a decrease in response and survival rates when vincristine is added to

TABLE 13–1. Single-Agent Therapy for Metastatic Breast Cancer

Drug	Response Rate (%)
Cyclophosphamide	34
L-Phenylalanine mustard	23
Chlorambucil	20
5-Fluorouracil	26
Methotrexate	34
Vincristine	21
Vinblastine	20
Adriamycin	37
Mitomycin C	38
Hexamethylmelamine	28
Dibromodulcitol	27
Thiotepa	30
cis-Platinum	54

Modified from Broder LE, Tormey DC: Combination chemotherapy of carcinoma of the breast. Cancer Treat Rev 1:183, 1974, and from Kolaric K, Roth A: Phase II clinical trial of *cis*-dichlorodiamine platinum (*cis*-DDP) for antitumorigenic activity in previously untreated patients with metastatic breast cancer. Cancer Chemother Pharmacol 11:108, 1983.

CFP. At best, then, the drug appears to confer little advantage, at the expense of sometimes considerable neurotoxicity. The addition of prednisone, on the other hand, may be of more benefit. Ramirez and colleagues[78] demonstrated improved response rates with unchanged survival rates with the use of CMFVP versus CMFV, while Tormey and associates[79] noted better survival rates and response duration times with similar response rates upon comparison of CMFP with CMF. The actual role of cyclophosphamide is difficult to ascertain, as it has been included in virtually all combinations derived from the parent CMFVP regimen. Finally, studies on combinations without 5-fluorouracil by Brunner and colleagues[74] show results equivalent to those of Ahmann's regimen[75] lacking methotrexate, suggesting that either agent is equally effective when combined with cyclophosphamide and prednisone.

The role of doxorubicin deserves special consideration. Clearly the most effective single agent, with response rates as high as 50 percent in previously untreated patients,[80] its median response duration time is still only about four months. There has been great interest in defining its role in combination therapy. Several randomized studies have examined multiple-drug regimens in which doxorubicin is substituted for another agent in otherwise identical combinations (Table 13–2).[81–83] Contradictory information has emerged. Muss and associates[83] noted similar response rates, with improvement of response duration and median survival, for CAFVP responders compared with CMFVP responders, while Bull and colleagues[82] noted increased response rates with a trend toward longer survival in patients receiving CAF versus CMF. Finally Bezwoda and associates[81] noted no advantage with inclusion of doxorubicin in place of vinblastine. Review of a number of other studies comparing doxorubicin and non–doxorubicin-containing combinations substantiates these observations that addition of doxorubicin is of marginal value, adding at best 10 percent to overall response rates.[79, 84–93]

Drug Number

Cooper's use of a five-drug regimen immediately raised questions about whether combination chemotherapy was indeed superior to single-agent therapy and, if so, what constituted the ideal number of drugs

TABLE 13–2. Role of Doxorubicin (Adriamycin) in Combination Chemotherapy

Drug Regimen	No. of Patients	Response Rate (%)	Response Duration (Months)	Median Survival (Months)	Reference
CAMF	51	55	—	13	81
CVbMF	57	44	—	12	
CAF	38	82	10	27	82
CMF	40	62	8	17	
CAFVP	44	58	16	33*	83
CMFVP	41	57	14	20	

*Responders only.

TABLE 13–3. Single-Drug versus Combination Chemotherapy in Metastatic Breast Cancer

Drug Regimen	No. of Patients	Response Rate (%)	Median Response Duration	Median Survival (Months)	Reference
L-PAM	91	20	13 wk	9	94
CMF	93	53	25 wk	12	
5-FU	67	18	6 mo	5	97
CMFVP	68	69	12.5 mo	16	
C	27	25	210 d	—	95
CMFVP	28	63	400 d	—	
C	49	55	2 mo	6	96
CMFVb	50	62	3 mo	6	

in a combination. Several studies addressed the first question with randomized trials of L-PAM versus CMF,[94] C versus CMFVP,[95] C versus CMFVb,[96] and F versus CMFVP (Table 13–3).[97] In general, they demonstrate, although by no means conclusively, improved response rates, response duration times, and, in one case, survival without markedly increased toxicity in the combination chemotherapy arms. A more pertinent question, however, was whether multiple-drug therapy offered any advantage over sequential administration of the same drugs, particularly with regard to the ultimate goal of increased survival. Three studies[98–100] have shown that combination chemotherapy tended to improve response frequency and duration, but in none was overall survival significantly different between the two arms (Table 13–4). Thus, it is questionable whether all patients with metastatic breast cancer benefit from aggressive combination therapy, although it seems clear that a large group of patients will have an improved response rate and, in some cases, prolonged survival.

If combination therapy is indeed seen as preferable to single-agent therapy for the majority of patients, the optimal drug number remains to be determined. In an elegant analysis, Carbone and Tormey[69] evaluated response rate and duration as a function of drug number in more than 70 published trials. They noted that a plateau for both parameters is reached with three drugs. Several randomized trials comparing combinations with different numbers of drugs have confirmed their findings that four- or five-drug combinations offer no advantage over two- or three-drug regimens (Table 13–5).[73, 74, 84, 86]

Frequency of Therapy

Cooper's original five-drug regimen was administered on a continuous basis. With time, continuous scheduling has given way to drug administration in an intermittent fashion, frequently day 1–day 8, as popularized by Bonadonna[101] and Cannellos.[102, 103] The efficacy of this simplified approach has been the subject of several investigations.

TABLE 13–4. Sequential Single-Agent versus Combination Chemotherapy in Metastatic Breast Cancer

Drug Regimen	No. of Patients	Response Rate (%)	Median Survival	Reference
CFV	46	44	7 mo	98
F—C—V*	30	53	13 mo	
CMFPT3†	61	56	15 mo	99
F—C—P+T3—M*	60	32	11 mo	
CMFVP (continuous)	35	46	50 wk	100
CMFVP (intermittent)	33	27	50 wk	
F—M—C—V—P*	34	18	25 wk	

*Sequential administration.
†T3 = tri

TABLE 13–5. Number of Drugs and Response Rate

Drug Combination	No. of Patients	Response Rate (%)	Response Duration	Median Survival	Reference
AF	105	42	22 wk	64 wk	86
AFC	103	43	33 wk	64 wk	
AFCM	105	49	35 wk	64 wk	
CMF	38	34	23 wk	—	73
CMFVP	34	50	26 wk	—	
AC	26	50	10 mo	—	84
ACMF	22	55	10 mo	—	
CMP	78	64	7 mo	15 mo*	74
CMFVP	91	75	8 mo	16 mo*	

*Responders only.

Data to support the use of longer intervals between drug doses are available for doxorubicin as a single agent; five-week and three-week schedules gave similar results in all respects.[104] However, Hoogstraten and colleagues[80] showed response rates of 59 and 40 percent, respectively, for CMFVP schedules of every week and every four weeks, with similar median response duration times and an increase in neutropenic deaths with the intermittent schedule of every four weeks. Another study[100] showed response rates of 46 percent for continuously treated patients, compared with 27 percent for patients treated monthly, with median survival equal for the two groups. Thus, while clearly more convenient for patient and physician, intermittent drug administration is, if anything, inferior to the original continuous approach when examined in a randomized prospective fashion. It is worth noting that among the best results with adjuvant chemotherapy have been those obtained by the Southwest Oncology Group, whose continuous schedule of CMFVP has resulted in a 65 percent relapse-free survival rate at more than 60 months' median follow-up.[105] As will be discussed next, these observations may actually stem from the finding that many intermittent schedules, while administering higher drug dosages per treatment, in fact have lower dose intensities, that is, less drug administered per unit of time.

Drug Dosage and Dose Intensity

In addition to studies of optimal frequency of drug administration, attention has been focused on aspects of drug dose. Both high- and low-dose approaches have been examined; unfortunately, few randomized comparisons of either with standard dose therapy exist. Low-dose therapy (therapy using customary drugs at about 50 percent of the generally prescribed doses) has been promulgated most by Creech,[106, 107] who has obtained response rates of 46 and 49 percent with low-dose CMF regimens in two published studies, results within the realm of those obtained with standard CMF. Other investigators providing support for these observations have included Irwin and colleagues,[90] who noted equal response rates, response duration times, and survival rates in a randomized evaluation of a standard-dose CAMF combination versus a low-dose combination with half as much cyclophosphamide and doxorubicin. Still others[108] have noted a diminished response rate with such low-dose regimens but without a concomitant change in the survival rate. Thus, the evidence supporting the use of standard-dose therapy over low-dose regimens is not compelling, especially in view of the risk of increased toxicity with the more intensive regimens. Several low-dose regimens have been published in recent years and could be considered as alternative treatment strategies in selected patients.[109, 110]

The use of extremely aggressive induction therapy has received some, albeit less, attention as well. Such an approach is founded on the hope that a higher drug dose will increase the likelihood of complete remission and thereby increase the chance of prolonged survival, as has been observed in other malignancies such as lymphoma. "Super-CMF," a combination of cyclophosphamide, doxorubicin, 5-fluorouracil, and high-dose methotrexate with leucovorin rescue, resulted in a response rate of 78 percent (27 percent complete responses) with a median duration of two years, both somewhat higher than those reported in representative studies of CMF, CAF, or CA but probably not justifying the additional patient and physician inconvenience, expense, and potential toxicity.[111] An uncontrolled evaluation of high-dose cyclophosphamide and 5-fluorouracil gave a response rate of 93 percent, with 40 percent complete responders.[112] However, a randomized study of conventional-dose FAC compared with high-dose therapy including 5-fluorouracil, 500 mg/m^2 for five days, doxorubicin, 85 mg/m^2, and cyclophosphamide, 1500 mg/m^2 on day one, showed similar response rates of 82 percent for the former and 84 percent for the latter. The median survival time was 22 months for the intensively treated patients and 19 months for those treated with conventional therapy.[113] On the basis of these studies, then, high-dose therapy is not recommended over standard-dose therapy.

However, a new evaluation of the importance of dose intensity in chemotherapy of metastatic breast cancer addresses the crucial question of whether administration of intensive chemotherapy in fact results in a better outcome. An equally plausible alternative would be that the ability of a patient to tolerate higher doses of chemotherapy is a good prognostic factor resulting in a better response to therapy.

Spurred by the apparent discordance between the 88 percent response rate to Cooper's CMFVP regimen and the consistently lower response rates to subsequent CMFVP, CMF, and CFP combinations, Hryniuk and Bush[114] devised a method for calculating the dose intensity of a combination that considered dose to be administered over unit of time. They then compared the projected dose intensity with the response rate in over 30 studies using CMFVP- or CAF-like regimens and showed a highly statistically significant positive correlation between dose intensity and response rate. The correlation was even more striking in those studies in which the actual dose administered was reported, permitting a comparison of actual dose intensity with response rate. A third analysis of the relationship between median survival time and response rate for all studies demonstrated a positive correlation as well, suggesting indirectly that increased dose intensity was associated with increased survival. This study points to the possibility that dose intensity may be an important determinant of outcome; further properly designed randomized trials will be necessary to establish this hypothesis. In the interim, it seems reasonable to suggest that individual patients be treated to maximal tolerance.

Non–Cross-Resistant Therapy

The rationale for the use of non–cross-resistant drug combinations is twofold. First, it has been suggested that fixed alternation of treatment regimens might improve response rate and duration by preventing the emergence of a second population of tumor cells that are resistant to the first drug combination. Second, alternating regimens might decrease the frequency of administration of drugs such as doxorubicin (Adriamycin) and vincristine, thereby decreasing cumulative toxicity and extending the period of time over which they may be safely used. In brief, with the exception of one study of fewer than 20 patients in which an improved response rate was noted,[91] fixed non–cross-resistant therapy has failed to show any advantage in terms of response rate, response duration, or survival over the use of a selected regimen until failure, followed by the alternate non–cross-resistant regimen (Table 13–6).[115–119]

Chemoimmunotherapy

Studies of immunotherapy in metastatic breast cancer have focused on the use of nonspecific immunostimulants such as BCG or levamisole in conjunction with standard drug combinations. Investigators at the M. D. Anderson Memorial Hospital have conducted a series of historically controlled studies of FAC with immunotherapy including BCG by scarification, methanol-extracted residue of BCG (MER-BCG), or levamisole.[117, 120–122] They concluded that immunotherapy, while not affecting response rate, improves response duration and survival in responding patients. All three agents were equally effective in their hands, making levamisole the favored agent because of its lesser toxicity. These observations have not held up in two randomized trials of chemotherapy with

TABLE 13–6. Alternating Non–Cross-Resistant Therapy in Metastatic Breast Cancer

Drug Regimen	No. of Patients	Response Rate (%)	Median Response Duration (Months)	Median Survival	Reference
AC×4→MF×3/AC×1	34	56	7	16 mo*	116
VAC+IT×3/FM+IT×3†	156	67	13	21	117
AV×2/CMF×2	55	53	11	—	118
CMF×2/AV×2	55	60	12	—	
CAVFP	52	56	16	25	119
CA/MF	53	43	12	26	
CAF	46	63	10	—	115
DAV×3/CMF×3‡	48	71	10	—	

*Responders only.
†IT, immunotherapy.
‡D = dibromodulcitol

and without MER-BCG. Neither Muss[119] nor Britell[123] noted enhanced response rate, response duration, or survival or diminished myelosuppression in patients subjected to immunotherapy in conjunction with combination chemotherapy. Thus, a role for immunotherapy remains to be established (Table 13–7).

Chemohormonal Therapy

Given the limitations of systemic chemotherapy already outlined, many investigators have attempted to improve results by combining endocrine therapy and chemotherapy. Superficially, the appeal of such an approach is great—theoretically improved results because of use of agents with independent modes of antineoplastic action, with little, if any, additional toxicity. In fact, it has been estimated that addition of endocrine therapy to existing chemotherapy regimens would improve response rates by 10 per cent at best. This estimate is derived from the observation that about one third of patients receiving cytotoxic chemotherapy will fail to respond, while two thirds of unselected patients treated with endocrine therapy will not benefit from that approach. Assuming no interaction between these populations, the chance of a patient being resistant to both is the product of one third and two thirds or two ninths. This represents a decrease in the fraction of patients resistant to chemotherapy from one third or three ninths to two ninths,

TABLE 13–7. Chemoimmunotherapy in Metastatic Breast Cancer

Drug Regimen	No. of Patients	Response Rate (%)	Median Response Duration	Median Survival (Months)	Reference
CFP	31	52	261 d	20	123
CFP + MER†	34	39	385 d	20	
CAFVP	52	56	16 mo	25	119
CAFVP + MER	50	54	14 mo	23	
CA/MF	53	43	12 mo	26	119
CA/MF + MER	42	43	16 mo	26	
FAC*	44	73	9 mo	15	122
FAC*/BCG	105	76	14 mo	21	122
FAC*/LEV‡	114	72	13 mo	24	122

*Sequential studies; not randomized.
†Methanol-extracted residue of BCG.
‡Levamisole.

TABLE 13–8. Chemohormonal Therapy for Metastatic Breast Cancer

Drug Regimen	Menopausal Status	No. of Patients	Response Rate (%)	Median Response Duration	Median Survival	Reference
Ox + VPCMF	Pre	54	72	17 mo	26 mo	127
Ox + C		56	65	16 mo	23 mo	
Ox→VPCMF		38	18, 50	5, 8 mo	30 mo	
Ox + CFP	Pre	36	39	13 mo	33 mo	125, 129
Ox→CFP		36	25, 21	4 mo	22 mo	
CMF	Post	105	49	12 mo	19 mo	133, 134
CMF + T		115	75	18 mo	24 mo	
CMF→CMF + T	Post	71	51, 31	47 wk	118 wk	130
CMF + T		62	74	51 wk	84 wk	
Ox→Chemo	Pre	54	43	—	21 mo	126
Ox + Chemo		55	46	—	25 mo	
T→Chemo	Post	145	33	—	28 mo	126
T + Chemo		152	40	—	24 mo	
CMFVP	Pre	23	43	8 mo	13 mo	133
Ox + CMFVP		19	74	10 mo	20 mo	
CMFVP	Post	48	54	11 mo	19 mo	131
DES + CMFVP		48	63	8 mo	27 mo	
AV	Post*	33	61	10 mo	15 mo	132
AV + MPA†		36	53	10 mo	8 mo	
AC	Any	36	53	12 mo	14 mo	128
AC + Calusterone		20	65	22 mo	24 mo	

*Prior endocrine therapy.
†Medroxyprogesterone acetate.

or a one ninth increase in response rate.[124] In addition, there is no reason to believe that combined therapy would be more effective in the long run than sequential therapy, a question frequently overlooked in trial designs. These objections notwithstanding, a large body of literature exists on this topic. In general, a variety of studies[125–134] examining chemotherapy combined with oophorectomy or continuous use of antiestrogens, androgens, diethylstilbestrol, or progestins have demonstrated moderately improved response rates without a significant positive effect on survival (Table 13–8).

A second approach has been to take advantage of the proven ability of certain endocrine therapies to perturb cell cycle kinetics *in vitro*, so as to synchronously stimulate cell proliferation. Cytotoxic chemotherapy administered thereafter might induce a greater proportion of cell kill. Three such studies in progress use varying regimens of tamoxifen followed by conjugated estrogen (Premarin) to synchronize cells, followed by the cell-cycle–specific agents methotrexate and 5-fluorouracil.[135–137] Preliminary results of the controlled trial examining CAMF with or without tamoxifen and conjugated estrogen priming showed that a single subset, partial responders to the combined regimen, had longer time to progression and improved survival.[135] Of note in this trial, inoperable Stage III and nonmetastatic Stage IV patients had a 94 percent response rate, with 40 percent complete responses.

Effect of Prior Therapy on Response to Chemotherapy

The vast majority of patients with metastatic breast cancer have undergone one or more prior therapies, including treatment for the primary cancer, adjuvant chemotherapy for potential micrometastatic disease, and medical or surgical endocrine therapy for advanced disease, before receiving combination chemotherapy. The impact of previous treatment on the response to chemotherapy is examined here.

SURGERY

Surgery remains an integral part of the treatment of primary breast cancer, with procedures for local control ranging from excisional biopsy to some form of mastectomy. There is no evidence that the type of surgical procedure for primary disease affects the response rate or length of survival once the disease has spread.[138, 139]

RADIATION THERAPY

Patients who have received extensive radiation therapy have lower response rates and shorter survival times in general. In one study, nonirradiated patients had a 69 percent response rate with a median survival of two years versus patients receiving irradiation to more than three sites, who responded only 50 percent of the time with a 76-week median survival time.[138] Part of this effect may reflect the fact that those patients with a history of extensive radiation therapy for metastatic disease are likely to have a larger tumor burden, in itself an important negative prognostic factor. It is unlikely that primary breast irradiation as part of a breast-conserving therapy will have any discernible effect on patient response to chemotherapy in the event of development of metastatic disease.

ENDOCRINE THERAPY

For many years oophorectomy, adrenalectomy, and hypophysectomy were therapeutic mainstays in the treatment of metastatic disease. Published response rates to chemotherapy for patients having previously undergone ovariectomy for treatment of metastatic disease range from 20 to 65 percent, suggesting little decrement in efficacy of the chemotherapy.[125–127, 140] Similar data are available for patients receiving second-line chemotherapy after adrenalectomy or adrenalectomy-oophorectomy. Nemoto and associates[141] showed a response rate of 35 percent with CFP chemotherapy in patients who previously underwent adrenalectomy, compared with 43 percent in patients without prior adrenalectomy. In a small series, Oberfield and colleagues[142] demonstrated a CMF-induced response rate of 75 percent in patients relapsing after adrenalectomy-oophorectomy as initial treatment for metastatic disease.

Surgical ablative endocrine therapy has largely given way to medical therapies including all classes of sex steroids, aminoglutethimide, and tamoxifen. Appropriate information from crossover studies is limited for many of these agents, but for tamoxifen and diethylstilbestrol, at least, there is some evidence to suggest that prior therapy with either agent does not substantially affect subsequent response to combination chemotherapy.[143–145] The one group noting an association between history of prior endocrine therapy of any type and poor response to combination chemotherapy attributed the effect, in part, to larger tumor burden in the pretreated patients.[146] It has also been suggested that patients who responded previously to endocrine therapy have a chemotherapy-induced response duration time nearly twice that of their unresponsive peers, despite equivalent response rates.[144, 145] Confirmation of these findings is needed.

ADJUVANT CHEMOTHERAPY

With the increased use of adjuvant chemotherapy in patients felt to be at high risk for recurrence after primary therapy, the problem of metastatic disease in patients previously exposed to chemotherapy will undoubtedly become more prevalent. Several studies have evaluated response to subsequent chemotherapy in this group. The largest reported experience is derived from the Milan Tumor Institute studies of CMF. Valagussa and associates[147] reviewed results of salvage therapy in 442 patients who failed primary therapy in the first two CMF trials, CMF-treated patients versus untreated control subjects and 6 versus 12 months of CMF. A total of 38 percent of control patients who were treated with chemotherapy at relapse responded to that therapy with a median survival time of 16 months. Eighty-four patients who had previously received CMF adjuvant therapy had a response rate of 39 percent, with a median survival of 17 months after salvage therapy. Of note, in women with a disease-free interval longer than one year after CMF adjuvant therapy, the response rate to retreatment with CMF was 52 percent. Lippman and colleagues[135] found that a small group of patients relapsing after adjuvant L-PAM had a combination chemotherapy–induced response rate of 52 percent and a median survival time of 20 months, not significantly different from those of their untreated counterparts (68 percent and 17 months). The Western Cancer Study Group[148] evaluated patients failing a randomized trial of single-agent 5-fluorouracil versus combined cyclophosphamide, methotrexate, and 5-fluorouracil. Although the relapse rate of 64 percent at 70 months for the 5-FU group was higher than the 53 percent relapse rate observed in the CMF arm, the survival for the 5-FU cohort was paradoxically increased at 60 percent, in contrast with 47 percent for the group receiving CMF, the result of longer survival after relapse in the former group. Response rates with chemotherapy are not available in this study.

Bitran and associates[149] reported that response rate and median survival time in failures of adjuvant chemotherapy with L-PAM plus F or CMF were similar to those of patients without previous exposure to either. In another group of patients who had initially received adjuvant doxorubicin and cyclophosphamide chemotherapy, response rate and median survival time were less in those receiving CMF at the time of disease spread when compared with those receiving hormone treatment with or without doxorubicin and cyclophosphamide.[150] A follow-up[151] from the same institution noted a 61-week median survival among metastatic breast cancer patients who had received prior adjuvant chemotherapy, compared with a 124-week median survival in previously untreated women with metastatic disease. Finally, in a second group of patients with prior doxorubicin-containing adjuvant therapy, response rates of about 40 percent were obtained with both doxorubicin and non–doxorubicin-containing regimens at the time of relapse.[152] Although some variation is noted, these data suggest, on the whole, that prior adjuvant therapy does not markedly influence the rate of response to subsequent combination therapy for metastatic disease.

Salvage Chemotherapy

Because of our inability to cure patients with metastatic breast cancer with any first-line therapy, the search for effective salvage chemotherapy regimens to palliate patients' conditions remains an active one. A number of such regimens have been published, usually as relatively small trials encompassing a heterogeneous population of women who have failed a variety of initial therapies. Women treated initially with CMF, CMFP, or CMFVP are probably best treated with doxorubicin, either as a single agent or in combination. Thereafter, no single treatment can be recommended for general usage, as all demonstrate virtually the same limited efficacy in terms of response rate and duration and survival. A representative list of some recent trials is shown in Tables 13–9 and 13–10.[153–164]

Prognostic Factors in the Response to Chemotherapy

Patient Characteristics

Age. The influence of age alone on the response to chemotherapy is infrequently examined in individual chemotherapy studies. Often, in fact, subsets of very young or elderly patients are excluded from participa-

TABLE 13–9. Salvage Chemotherapy with Non–Doxorubicin-Containing Regimens

Treatment	*Prior Therapy*	*No. of Patients*	*Response Rate (%)*	*Median Response Duration*	*Median Survival*	*Reference*
MMC/VLB	AC, CMF	22	32	164 d	—	153
MMC/VDS	AC, CMF	15	40	247 d	—	153
VP16/CTX	Various	27	41	31 wk	61 wk	154
HMM/V/M	CFP + A	11	45	6.5 mo	12 mo*	155
HMM/V/MMC	FAC + CMF	27	19	5 mo	—	156
MMC/VLB	Various	30	40	127 d	—	157

*Responders only.
MMC = mitomycin C
VDS = vindesine
HMM = hexamethylmelamine

TABLE 13–10. Salvage Chemotherapy with Doxorubicin-Containing Regimens

Treatment	*Prior Therapy*	*No. of Patients*	*Response Rate (%)*	*Median Response Duration (Months)*	*Median Survival (Months)*	*References*
VLB/A/T/H	CMF + VP + A	29	45	11	13	158
A/MMC	Unknown	27	26	7	8	159
F/V/A/MMC	CMF	25	56	6	>8	160
A/V/L-PAM	CMF	15	13	3.8	—	161
A/D/MMC	CMFVP	26	54	11	>18*	162
V/A/M	CMF	36	31	5	5.9	163
A/CCNU	CM + F + P	17	46	—	9.1	164
A/CCNU/V	CM + F + P	18	39	—	7.0	164

*Responders only.

tion, making analysis of response at either age extreme rather difficult. However, several investigators have reported pertinent findings, as part of extensive analyses of prognostic factors in composite patient groups. Swenerton and colleagues[138] found no significant difference in response or survival rates in 619 patients at the M. D. Anderson Memorial Hospital; about 20 percent of their patients were under 40 or over 65 years of age. A similar lack of correlation between age and complete response was noted by Decker and associates[165] at the Mayo Clinic. One group[166] has demonstrated that young age predicts a poorer response to chemotherapy and a poorer survival rate; however, the small number of patients under 40 makes these data suspect. Finally, Corle and colleagues[167] found a response rate of nearly 70 percent in patients aged 50 to 59, compared with 55 percent in younger or older women, in their review of 324 patients. No general trend merges then, and patient age appears not to predict response to combination chemotherapy (Table 13–11).[138, 139, 166, 167]

Race. Although the incidence of breast cancer is lower in nonwhite populations in the United States, mortality rates for white and nonwhite patients are comparable because of a poorer survival rate for nonwhites compared with that of whites.[168] Black[168] and Mexican-American[169] patients tend to present at an earlier age with tumors that are larger, more advanced, less differentiated histologically, and more frequently lacking estrogen receptors, all factors contributing to shorter survival. In addition, two major studies[138, 139] have shown that the response rate with chemotherapy is lower in nonwhite patients: 31 and 59 percent for nonwhites versus 62 and 66 percent for whites. Contradictory data are found only in a single study[81] of South African patients, in which response rates with chemotherapy were equal in blacks and whites, even though black patients generally presented with the same negative factors listed earlier. Available evidence suggests then that black or Hispanic race is a negative prognosticator for response to chemotherapy and survival. Asian patients, on the other hand, appear to have a generally better prognosis than do white patients.[170, 171] Comparison of white American and Japanese patients with any nodal status showed five-year disease-free survival rates of 75 percent for Japanese patients and 55 percent for white American patients. However, the difference

TABLE 13–11. Age and Response to Chemotherapy

Patient Age (Years)	*No. of Patients*	*Response Rate (%)*	*Reference*
< 49	109	54	167
50–59	106	70	
> 60	109	56	
< 45	34	59	139
45–54	94	59	
55–64	74	66	
> 64	40	68	
< 40	6	33	166
40–49	31	84	
> 49	101	64	
< 40	75	63	138
40–49	104	66	
50–55	119	68	
56–65	198	64	
> 65	63	56	

in the overall survival rate at five years is not nearly as great, 77 percent in Japanese patients versus 68 percent in white American patients, suggesting that survival with metastatic disease is significantly better in white American women.[170] Few data exist on chemotherapy responsiveness in the Japanese group.

Menopausal Status. The usefulness of menopausal status as a predictor of response to chemotherapy is not clear-cut. Variations in definitions of pre-, peri-, and postmenopausal states make comparison of existing data particularly difficult. Nonetheless, most randomized studies of drug combinations and several retrospective reviews of large patient populations[138, 139, 166, 167, 172] find no significant difference, regardless of definition of menopausal status. Contradictory data are found in the experience of the Milan Tumor Institute,[146] in which early postmenopausal patients (i.e., those for whom less than two years had elapsed since their last menstrual period) carried a very poor prognosis, with a 46 percent response rate, compared with about 60 percent for all other groups, and a median survival time for responders of 18 months, 10 months less than in other groups. Contrasting with these findings are studies from the Mayo Clinic, in which complete responses were most likely in those patients within five years of menopause, and the poorest response rates overall were in patients ten or more years postmenopausal.[165] This latter group is frequently not included in chemotherapy trials because of age exclusions. No obvious explanation is apparent for these divergent observations, and available data suggest that menopausal status plays little or no role in determining response to chemotherapy for patients with metastatic disease (Table 13–12).[82, 138, 146, 167, 172]

TABLE 13–12. Menopausal Status and Response to Chemotherapy

Menopausal Status at Treatment	*No. of Patients*	*Response Rate (%)*	*Reference*
Pre	34	50	167
Post	288	61	
< 1 yr post*	25	32	172
1–5 yr	22	41	
>5 yr	76	28	
< 1 yr post*	211	68	138
1–5 yr	99	59	
> 5 yr	161	61	
Pre	62	65	146
0–2 yr post	93	46	
2–10 yr	87	60	
> 10 yr	76	58	
Pre	6	83	82
Naturally post	33	61	
Oophorectomy	39	79	

*Includes premenopausal.

Performance Status and Weight Loss. The influence of general physical condition, as measured by performance status, on overall patient survival was recognized early. In fact, information on response to chemotherapy in patients with poor performance status is limited, as these patients are frequently excluded from study. Various scoring systems have been employed, with the Karnofsky[173] and ECOG[174] systems used most commonly. When the results of either individual studies of drug combinations or retrospective institutional reviews are considered, available data strongly support higher response rates and improved survival in patients with a favorable performance status. Representative figures from Swenerton and colleagues[138] show response rates of 71, 65, and 39 percent, with median survival times of 123, 90, and 42 weeks for patients with performance status of ECOG 1, 2, and 3–4, respectively (Table 13–13).[79, 82, 84, 115, 138, 175]

Although weight loss is not commonly regarded as a symptom of metastatic breast cancer, about one third of patients note some weight loss, with 6 percent losing more than 10 percent of their normal weight.[175] The negative association between weight loss and response to chemotherapy, particularly attainment of a complete response, or survival is profound and is independent of performance status or extent of disease.[175] DeWys and colleagues[175] found a 61 percent response rate in patients without weight loss, compared with only 43 percent in those noting any degree of weight loss. Similar findings were reported by Swenerton and associates (Table 13–14).[138]

Psychologic Aspects. As discussed in Chapter 15, many clinicians have postulated the existence of a relationship between behavioral patterns and the course of illness in cancer patients. In their study of patients with metastatic breast cancer, Derogatis and associates[176] found that patients who displayed anxiety, anger, and hostility on formal psychologic testing had a significantly longer

TABLE 13–13. Performance Status and Response to Chemotherapy

Performance Status	No. of Patients	Response Rate (%)	Reference
< 80*	22	59	82
80–90	28	61	
> 90	28	93	
0–1†	236	61	175
2–4	94	38	
0–1†	28	54	84
2–4	17	47	
1†	196	71	138
2	359	65	
3–4	64	39	
< 70*	19	58	115
71–85	20	65	
> 85	47	70	
0†	99	73	79
1	132	59	
2, 3	100	42	

*Karnofsky scoring system. See Karnofsky DA, Abelman WH, Craver LF, et al.: The use of nitrogen mustards in the palliative treatment of carcinoma. Cancer 1:634, 1948.

†ECOG scoring system. See Zubrod G, Schneiderman M, Frei E, et al.: Appraisal of methods for the study of chemotherapy of cancer in man: Comparative therapeutic trial of nitrogen mustard and triethylene thiophosphoramide. J Chronic Dis 11:7, 1960.

survival than did those who appeared more accepting of their illness. These long-surviving patients were overt in their expression of negative feelings, in marked contrast with the short-term survivors, whose coping style led them to internalize or deny altogether their adverse feelings. These differences were independent of standard medical parameters including response to chemotherapy; both groups responded equally well to their antineoplastic therapy. However, a recent study[177] of psychologic correlates of disease in early breast cancer patients has failed to document any correlation between psychologic make-up and the time to disease recurrence. More work will be required in this field to verify any relationship and perhaps to evaluate behavior modification as a new therapeutic approach.

TABLE 13–14. Weight Loss and Chemotherapy Response

Weight Loss (% of Baseline Wt Lost)	No. of Patients	Response Rate (%)	Median Survival (Weeks)	Reference
None	210	61	69	175
0–5	75		46	
5–10	27	43	41	
> 10	18		43	
< 5	291	71	104	138
5–10	57	56	79	
> 10	28	42	59	

TUMOR CHARACTERISTICS

Receptor Status. The capability to measure estrogen and progesterone receptors greatly enhanced our ability to select those patients likely to benefit from endocrine therapy. In addition, a lack of estrogen receptor in a tumor was found to be associated with a higher proliferative rate, as measured by thymidine-labeling index. That such rapidly growing tumors would theoretically be more responsive to combination chemotherapy led to a number of retrospective reviews of the relationship between estrogen receptor status and response to combination chemotherapy in advanced disease.[167, 178–192] Interpretation of these studies is complicated by differences in patient selection and definition of receptor positivity, but overall there appears to be no significant correlation between estrogen receptor status and response to combination chemotherapy (Table 13–15). More limited studies on the value of the progesterone receptor have suggested that it may be a more accurate predictor of response to en-

TABLE 13–15. ER Status and Response to Chemotherapy

Cut-off (fmole/mg protein)	Responders/Total (%) ER+	ER−	Reference
5	3/12 (25)	8/19 (42)	178
3	14/16 (88)	7/20 (35)	179
3	14/33 (42)	9/17 (53)	180
10	16/36 (44)	22/37 (59)	181, 182
20	13/31 (42)	17/41 (41)	183
3 or 4	24/28 (86)	13/36 (36)	184, 185
10	3/25 (12)	34/45 (76)	186
3	17/30 (57)	4/19 (21)	187
10	13/24 (54)	8/25 (32)	188
10	6/23 (26)	7/29 (24)	189
10	12/16 (75)	6/14 (43)	190
5	20/33 (62)	8/14 (57)	191
7	23/44 (52)	20/35 (57)	192
3 or 4	28/36 (78)	28/45 (62)	193
6	6/9 (67)	10/23 (44)	194

docrine therapy but equally unhelpful in determining chemoresponsiveness.[193, 194]

Histopathology and Kinetic Studies. Although a poorly differentiated histology predicts a poorer outcome in primary breast cancer and may be inversely associated with outcome after adjuvant chemotherapy, tumor grade and cell type are of no prognostic value in advanced disease. In the only study to specifically examine this question, Decker and colleagues[165] found no difference in those characteristics when comparing complete responders to chemotherapy with those not achieving a complete response. Clearly, more data on this relationship are needed.

Several investigators[195–200] have reported on kinetic studies in breast cancer, using mitotic index, flow cytometric measurement of S-phase fraction (SPF), and tritiated thymidine-labeling index (TLI) as measurements of cellular proliferation. Their work suggests that SPF and TLI are higher in tumors not histologically differentiated and correlate inversely with estrogen and progesterone receptor status. SPF and TLI appear to have prognostic value in primary breast cancer, but TLI has not been found to be a predictor of response to chemotherapy in metastatic disease. Indeed Meyer and Lee[197] found equivalent response rates with combination chemotherapy for 22 patients with high or low TLI. No such information exists for SPF, but results may be anticipated to be similar. Thus, cell kinetic parameters are useful in evaluating patients with primary disease but have no general value in predicting response to chemotherapy in advanced disease.

Disease Characteristics

Initial Tumor Size, Location, and Node Involvement. Of the several primary disease factors determining prognosis, including tumor size and location and axillary node status, none are useful in predicting response to therapy once the disease has spread.[138] In particular, the number of axillary nodes involved, the single most important predictor in early breast cancer, is of no consequence in advanced disease. The effects of tumor location have not been evaluated in advanced disease but would not be anticipated to have any bearing.

Disease-Free Interval. The disease-free interval (DFI), defined as the period of time from treatment of primary cancer to disease recurrence, has traditionally been felt to be of prognostic value and therefore is generally included as a stratification parameter in chemotherapy trials. The presumed impact of DFI on outcome is derived from its known association with overall survival rate and rate of response to endocrine therapy (i.e., long DFI correlates with long overall survival time and increased estrogen receptor positivity and, therefore, increased response to endocrine maneuvers).[201] No such relationship exists between DFI and response to chemotherapy. There is evidence to suggest that a DFI of zero years (presenting with metastatic disease) or between one and five years confers a slightly better response rate[139, 146] and that the length of DFI is positively correlated with response duration.[82] Longer DFI also correlates with improved survival rate in chemotherapy-treated patients.[138] This undoubtedly reflects, in part, its general ability to identify a subset of patients with inherently less aggressive tumors (those that are estrogen receptor positive and have favorable histologies and lower proliferative indices) rather than an impact of chemotherapy itself. Thus DFI, while a useful parameter in gauging overall survival, is of little use in predicting response to chemotherapy (Table 13–16).[82, 138, 139, 146, 172]

Sites of Metastatic Disease and Tumor Burden. Trials of breast cancer therapy commonly classify patients according to dominant site of metastatic lesion, with visceral, osseous, and soft tissue or locoregional constituting the three subsets most often used. These categories have been viewed as of prognostic import, with visceral lesions carrying the worst prognosis, bony disease an intermediate one, and soft-tissue disease the best. The influence of dominant disease on response to combination chemotherapy has been intensively studied, and many studies suggest that soft-tissue lesions are highly responsive, with visceral disease moderately so and bony lesions only poorly responsive. These interpretations are complicated by a lack of uniformity in definitions of criteria for organ involvement or response between studies. In addition, certain disease sites such as bone are notoriously difficult to evaluate for objective evidence of progression or regression. When criteria for response and involvement of a particular anatomic site are precisely defined in a large cohort of patients, as has been done in several retrospective

TABLE 13–16. Disease-Free Interval (DFI) and Chemotherapy Response

DFI	*No. of Patients*	*Response Rate (%)*	*Median Survival (Weeks)*	*Reference*
< 1 yr	39	69	—	82
1–3 yr	25	68	—	
> 3 yr	14	86	—	
0	47	60	—	139
1–11 mo	40	50	—	
12–23 mo	57	60	—	
24–59 mo	58	67	—	
> 60 mo	35	74	—	
0–12 mo	39	26	—	172
13–24 mo	29	45	—	
25–60 mo	37	34	—	
> 60 mo	18	33	—	
0	118	63	102	138
< 2 yr	252	64	83	
> 2 yr	219	66	105	
0	59	70	—	146
< 2 yr	104	54	—	
> 2 yr	82	49	—	

reviews of a single institution's experience, there appears to be surprisingly little variation in response or survival rates among the dominant site categories (Table 13–17).[82, 138, 146, 202, 203]

Attempts to correlate overall tumor burden with response to chemotherapy and survival have been more fruitful. One comprehensive system for estimation of disease extent by number of sites and amount of disease at those sites showed a clear relation between tumor burden and both response and survival rates (Table 13–18).[138, 172] The relationship was most marked in the case of complete

TABLE 13–17. Dominant Site of Disease and Response to Chemotherapy

Disease Site	*No. of Patients*	*Response Rate (%)*	*Median Survival*	*Reference*
Visceral	46	63	—	82
Osseous	21	81	—	
Soft tissue	11	91	—	
Visceral	98	50	23 mo*	146
Osseous	76	61	23 mo	
Soft tissue	126	61	25 mo	
Liver	24	58	81 wk†	138
Pleura	26	69	90 wk	
Lung	33	76	92 wk	
Osseous	59	63	96 wk	
Nodes	14	93	96 wk	
Skin–chest wall	20	65	85 wk	
Visceral	168	60	—	203
Osseous	63	64	—	
Soft tissue	102	64	—	
Visceral	85	62	—	202
Osseous	116	35	—	
Soft tissue‡	94	67	—	

*Responders only.
†All patients.
‡Includes pleura.

TABLE 13–18. Extent of Disease and Response to Chemotherapy

Site Extent Code*	No. of Patients	Response Rate (%)	Median Survival (Weeks)	Reference
< 5	112	71	146+	138
6–12	206	70	96	
13–20	182	62	80	
> 20	119	52	62	
< 5	13	69	—	172
6–12	60	35	—	
13–20	30	27	—	
> 20	20	5	—	

*Higher code correlates with greater tumor burden. For definition, see Swenerton KD, Legha SS, Smith T, et al.: Prognostic factors in metastatic breast cancer treated with combination chemotherapy. Cancer Res 39:1552, 1979.

responders, who tended to have a smaller tumor mass. Other investigators have confirmed these findings with observations that simultaneous involvement of visceral, osseous, and soft-tissue sites portends a poorer response to therapy and shorter survival time compared with involvement of a small number of sites.[139, 146, 202]

Two disease patterns are worthy of special attention, as they are frequently excluded from chemotherapy trials. The development of brain metastasis is a very poor prognostic sign, with a median survival time of three to seven months despite treatment. Chemotherapeutic agents in use cross the blood-brain barrier poorly and do not influence the course of central nervous system disease. Radiation therapy and surgical resection in suitable patients remain the only therapeutic options. Most of these patients present with systemic disease as well, and just over half die as a consequence of that disease,[204] demonstrating the need for and importance of concurrent systemic therapy. The failure of adjuvant therapy to treat micrometastatic disease in the brain and the observation that brain metastasis may develop concurrent with improving or stable systemic disease treated with combination chemotherapy suggest that this pattern of spread may become a more common entity with increasing use of drug therapy.[204, 205]

About 25 percent of patients have disease confined to bone at the time of presentation with advanced disease.[206] Such patients are often excluded from chemotherapy studies because of difficulty in objectively determining response. Nonetheless, small studies of this group suggest that they have an excellent prognosis and benefit from aggressive chemotherapy, with appropriate hematologic support in the event of bone marrow involvement. In one study, 11 of 21 patients with disease confined to bone completed a 36-week course of combination chemotherapy and remained disease-free for a mean of six months while not receiving any therapy, with a median survival time of three and one-half years.[206] A second study documented a 93 percent response rate and a ten-month median response duration time with chemotherapy in a group of 46 patients with disease confined to bone.[207] Cooperative study data suggest that patients with disease confined to bone are likely to have a longer period of disease control when compared with patients with other patterns of metastases treated in an equivalent fashion.[208] This may reflect a smaller total tumor burden or a biologically more favorable subset of disease rather than a particular responsiveness to chemotherapy. This hypothesis is supported by evidence that estrogen receptor–positive tumors, which have more favorable prognoses, metastasize more frequently to bone.[209]

Laboratory Characteristics

The identification and development of *in vitro* tests whose results correlate with *in vivo* tumor behavior have been the subject of intense study in breast cancer research, as with other cancers. Three broad categories of laboratory parameters are considered here: conventional laboratory tests, tests of immunologic function, and identification of so-called biomarkers.

Information on the relationship between common laboratory test values and prognosis in metastatic breast cancer is surprisingly limited. This reflects in part the widespread requirement for relatively normal hematologic, hepatic, and renal function in most drug trials. However, in one exhaustive review,[138] low hemoglobin, white blood cell count, absolute lymphocyte count, platelet count, and albumin level as well as elevated levels of LDH, SGOT, bilirubin, alkaline phosphatase, and calcium were associated with poor response or survival, or both. In a smaller study examining the role of hemoglobin, calcium, SGOT, LDH, and alkaline phosphatase, George and Hoogstraten[139] were able to confirm these findings only for SGOT. That such a relationship exists would seem obvious, as these laboratory abnormalities simply reflect indirectly extent and sites of tumor involvement, toxicity of previous therapy, and general nutritional state, all possible prognostic factors in their own right.

There is a growing body of literature on the relationship between prognosis in breast cancer and immune reactivity, as measured by a variety of *in vitro* and *in vivo* test systems. In 106 patients with metastatic disease, Krown and associates[210] found that several tests of immune function, including intradermal skin testing with microbial antigens, absolute lymphocyte count, lymphocyte response to mitogens *in vitro*, and dinitrochlorobenzene (DNCB) reactivity, were not useful in distinguishing groups with good prognosis or treatment response. Cunningham and colleagues,[211] on the other hand, found that patients with a strong response to DNCB has a greater probability of response to chemotherapy and a longer median survival time. Those with strong reactions had a 52 percent response rate, with a median survival time of 78 weeks, in comparison with values of 23 percent and 35 weeks for patients who did not react to DNCB. The prognostic value of six common skin tests was also examined in 200 women with metastatic disease at the M. D. Anderson Memorial Hospital.[212] The response rate to chemotherapy did not vary with the response to individual recall antigens, except in the case of keyhole-limpet hemocyanin responders, who had a better chemotherapy response rate. However, responders to any skin test except the purified protein derivative (PPD) tended to survive longer. Patients who responded to two or more skin tests had a median survival time of 118 weeks, compared with 86 weeks for those with fewer than two positive reactions. For the most part, then, skin test responsiveness to common recall antigens does not correlate with response to chemotherapy, although a correlation between ability to mount a response and survival may exist.

Identification of biomarkers useful in detecting residual disease or early metastases and in predicting and monitoring results with therapy has constituted a third avenue of investigation. Numerous such markers exist, with CEA,[138, 213–225] ferritin,[214, 218, 223, 224] β-hCG,[214, 217, 220, 223, 224, 226] ceruloplasmin,[223, 227, 228] hydroxyproline,[214, 223, 229–231] calcitonin,[214, 216, 217, 223, 224] polyamines,[213, 214, 220, 223] and casein[217] among the most studied in breast cancer, both early and advanced. In general, it may be said that their usefulness is limited as only a fraction of tumors secrete marker proteins

TABLE 13–19. Frequency of Biomarker Abnormality in Metastatic Breast Cancer

Biomarker	*Cutoff*	*Patients with Abnormal Level/Total Patients (%)*	*Reference*
Casein	>25 ng/ml	11/25 (44)	217
Calcitonin	>0.1 μg/ml	2/17 (12)	223, 224
CEA	>5 ng/ml	88/117 (75)	222
		86/132 (65)	217
Ceruloplasmin	>50 mg/ml	47/145 (32)	227
	>40 ng/ml	91/103 (88)	228
Ferritin	>150 μg/ml	15/17 (88)	223, 224
hCG	>5 mIU/ml	65/134 (48)	226
Hydroxyproline-creatinine ratio	>25	39/53 (74)	214
		11/15 (73)	223, 224
			214
Polyamines			
Putrescine		8/142 (6)	
Spermidine		35/142 (25)	
Spermine		31/141 (22)	

TABLE 13–20. Biomarkers and Response to Therapy

Biomarker	Value	CR + PR (%) Total	Reference
CEA	<10 μg/l	62/91 (68)	138
	10–49 μg/l	37/63 (59)	
	>49 μg/l	19/27 (70)	
	<5 ng/ml	12/12 (100)	222
	>5 ng/ml	14/23 (61)	
hCG	<5 mIU/ml	18/19 (95)	226
	>5 mIU/ml	15/21 (71)	

(Table 13–19) and no marker is tumor specific. When they are produced, an increased value often correlates with an increased risk of recurrence in early disease or a higher likelihood of occult metastases later in the disease course. If elevated in instances of advanced disease, the level frequently correlates with the overall response to therapy, decreasing with response and increasing with lack thereof. In only a few studies has the prognostic value of biomarker level for response to therapy for metastatic disease been addressed. Tormey and co-workers[222] found that levels of CEA above 5 correlated with poorer response rate and duration; a similar but weaker correlation existed for β-hCG as well.[226] The results with CEA were not confirmed in larger populations studied by Swenerton and colleagues[138] and Mughal and associates[225] (Table 13–20). Thus, although the appeal of biomarkers remains great, their usefulness is limited because of their lack of specificity and their lack of broad applicability. Biomarkers may perhaps be best used as an adjunctive study in predicting risk of residual or recurrent disease and in monitoring patient response to therapy when levels are abnormal.

Multivariate Analyses

Most of the information already discussed is derived from univariate analyses of prognostic factors in metastatic breast cancer. However, three groups have attempted simultaneous assessment of multiple factors to determine outcome. George and Hoogstraten[139] found that three covariates, performance status, liver involvement, and disease-free interval, constituted a model useful for prediction of response. A multivariate analysis of patients receiving doxorubicin and cyclophosphamide resulted in development of regression equations predictive for two criteria of outcome in metastatic disease.[166] Response rate was a function of age, ability to tolerate full-dose chemotherapy, and liver involvement, while survival was best determined by age, number of involved sites, and the same ability to receive full doses of drug. Most recently, Hortobagyi and colleagues[232] published a multifactorial analysis yielding two models predictive of response to therapy and a third useful in predicting survival. Factors important in response in the first model included platelet count, nodal metastases, weight loss, number of disease sites, and race and in the second model, weight loss, alkaline phosphatase level, nodal involvement, hemoglobin value, and prior radiation therapy. Survival was a function of LDH, performance status, pulmonary involvement, and disease extent. Each model demonstrated predictive ability when used prospectively in a population of 200 patients treated subsequently in the same fashion as the population from whom the equations were derived. Studies of multiple variables similar to these will be increasingly important in the analysis of patient prognosis.

TREATMENT OF SOLITARY RECURRENCES

The treatment of breast cancer patients who have a relapse at a single site at some point after primary therapy is worthy of special consideration. Traditionally, these patients, termed Stage IV NED, have been treated with local surgery or radiation therapy, or both, followed by surveillance until disease progression, a strategy that results in a five-year disease-free survival rate of not more than 20 percent and a cure rate that is vanishingly small. Because of the recognition that such a recurrence is almost always the initial manifestation of systemic disease, the role and timing of systemic therapy as an adjunct to local therapy is under active investigation. Blumenschein and associates[233] have amassed the largest experience, with a group of 136 patients who received FAC chemotherapy, in addition to local therapy, for treatment of an isolated metastasis, 77 percent of which were soft tissue. Using a retrospective control group of 62 patients treated with surgery or irradiation, or both, for a single site of recurrence (79 percent soft tissue), the investigators have reported a median disease-free survival time of 9 months for the control group, compared with 38 months for the FAC-treated patients. The median survival time was 40 months for control subjects, who received a variety of systemic therapies following the appearance of metastatic disease, while the median survival time for FAC-treated patients exceeded 60 months. A similar retrospective review by Beck and colleagues[234] examined the impact of radiation therapy and systemic therapy (hormonal or chemotherapeutic) in 42 Stage IV NED patients with locoregional recurrence compared with 43 concurrently irradiated control subjects. Those who received systemic therapy at the time of recurrence demonstrated a significantly longer disease-free interval and overall survival at five years compared with the irradiated control subjects. Although flawed by the use of historical control subjects, both studies suggest that early systemic therapy for Stage IV NED patients may lead to substantial improvement in relapse-free and total survival. A randomized trial designed to address this question is in progress at the National Cancer Institute. Patients are randomly assigned to an early treatment group that receives local therapy and systemic therapy with CMF and tamoxifen or to a surveillance group that receives local therapy initially, with identical systemic therapy only at the time of the next recurrence.

PREGNANCY AND BREAST CANCER

The effect of concurrent or subsequent pregnancy on the disease course in breast cancer remains unclear. Controversy stems from the fact that the few reports on the subject deal with heterogeneous patient populations collected over long periods of time. The coexistence of breast cancer with pregnancy or lactation is relatively rare, with 1 to 4 percent of tumors presenting in this fashion; the incidence in women of childbearing age is considerably higher, ranging from 7 to 14 percent.[235] It has been a clinical axiom that these patients constitute a group with significantly worse prognosis. Although they rarely present with Stage IV disease (1 of 330 in Clark's series[236]), there is evidence that patients in this group have an unexpectedly high incidence of axillary node involvement compared with nonpregnant, age-matched control subjects.[237] Thus, when one controls for stage and age, pregnancy alone appears to influence prognosis little, if at all.

The stage of pregnancy may exert some effect on prognosis. Women treated in the first two trimesters or post partum seem to fare better than those treated late in pregnancy. Representative results show five-year survival rates of 48 percent during the first half of pregnancy, 11 percent during the second half, and 52 percent during the early post-partum period.[237]

Mastectomy remains the treatment of choice for the pregnant patient with early breast cancer and may be safely performed.[235] Primary or postoperative irradiation should be avoided when possible, given the potential risks to the fetus.[235] There is no evidence that therapeutic abortion or prophylactic castration performed in an adjuvant setting enhances the likelihood of cure. Regarding the former, Donegan[237] cites four studies in which the combined five-year survival rate was 62 percent in patients completing their pregnancies versus 54 percent in patients undergoing therapeutic abortion, although patients who underwent therapeutic abortion may have appeared to have more aggressive disease at the time of treatment.

Axillary node involvement or the rare presentation with advanced disease may necessitate consideration of early use of combination chemotherapy; information on its use in these settings is sparse. Experience with pregnant women with a variety of cancers treated with chemotherapy (especially acute myelogenous leukemia) shows that the risk of fetal malformation is greatest during the first trimester and in those receiving antimetabolites.[238] The likelihood of hematogenous spread of disease to the fetus appears to be extremely small.[239] Nonetheless, current recommendations for women requiring immediate chemotherapy include therapeutic abortion or expeditious delivery of the fetus when possible before beginning therapy. Combination chemotherapy with its attendant risk of fetal anomaly may be considered when termination of pregnancy is not possible and immediate treatment is deemed critical. There is no reason to anticipate a poorer response in such patients compared with their nonpregnant counterparts.[235]

Finally, there is no evidence that subsequent pregnancy adversely affects outcome in patients with early stage breast cancer. In fact, women who become pregnant after mastectomy do surprisingly well. Representative five-year survival rates from three studies are 67, 77, and 50 percent.[240–242] Patient selection may play a crucial role in these results. Two case-control studies[243, 244] of mastectomy patients with and without subsequent pregnancy demonstrated a better survival rate for the patients who later became pregnant. Thus, it appears that pregnancy does not promote disease recurrence in breast cancer patients, although an uneventful pregnancy in no way reduces the possibility of recurrent disease in the future.

NEW APPROACHES

Given the general lack of progress in treatment of advanced breast cancer, attention has been turned to new approaches to disease treatment. A number of drugs have been evaluated in Phase I and Phase II trials, and potentially useful agents in breast cancer include mitoxantrone, bisantrene, 4′-epiadriamycin, vindesine, ftorafur, dibromodulcitol, platinum derivatives such as CBDCA, and prednimustine. The first three were developed as alternatives to doxorubicin. Mitoxantrone[245–247] and bisantrene[248, 249] have shown response rates of 20 to 40 per cent in studies and appear to have substantially less cardiotoxicity than does doxorubicin. Vindesine[250, 251] and ftorafur,[252] derivatives of vinblastine and 5-fluorouracil, respectively, also have single-agent response rates of 20 to 30 percent. Dibromodulcitol and prednimustine have yielded 27 to 40 percent response rates in women previously treated with alkylating agents, while the platinum derivative CBDCA is under study.[253] Further evaluation of these agents alone and in combinations will be forthcoming.

Other investigators have focused on new ways of administering old drugs so as to decrease toxicity and possibly increase therapeutic efficacy. Particularly attention has been paid to doxorubicin, which has been successfully administered in both weekly low-dose and continuous infusion regimens. A recent Phase II trial of doxorubicin[254] given weekly at 6 to 12 mg/m^2 documented a 59 percent response rate overall, with a 56 percent response rate in patients who have previously failed standard doxorubicin regimens. The median response duration was greater than one year, and no cardiomyopathy was observed, despite administration of cumulative doses of 700 to 1030 mg/m^2 in 14 patients. Studies of continuous infusion of doxorubicin and vinblastine[255] have also been promising in early trials in heavily pretreated patients.

The use of intensive chemotherapy with autologous bone marrow transplantation is under preliminary investigation. One group has reported complete tumor regression in three of four patients receiving high-dose L-PAM as a preparative regimen.[256]

Because of its relatively indolent course and its sensitivity to a variety of chemotherapeutic agents, breast cancer may represent an excellent disease for application of *in vitro* drug-selection techniques. Tissue obtained at diagnosis and, when possible, at time of relapse may be tested for drug sensitivity *in vitro* in the hope of tailoring therapy to the individual patient.

Finally, the use of hypothalamic hormone analogues is also under investigation.[257, 258] The luteinizing hormone–releasing hormone analogue, buserelin, can be shown to inhibit ovarian estrogen synthesis to postmenopausal levels in the plasma of premenopausal women and has been associated with clinical responses.[257] A second agent, leuprolide, resulted in a 44 percent response rate in a group of 25 premenopausal patients with metastatic disease.[258]

CONCLUSION

Several conclusions may be drawn from the nearly 25 years of experience with treatment of metastatic breast cancer with combination chemotherapy. It has been possible to define a relatively few factors that bode poorly for outcome by any criteria in metastatic breast cancer. Poor performance status, weight loss, black or Hispanic race, large tumor burden as judged directly by number of sites and extent of disease at each site and indirectly by abnormal laboratory parameters, and inability to tolerate full-dose therapy all define patients with lower rates of response to chemotherapy. An obvious but critical determinant of survival remains response to chemotherapy, as a large fraction of overall survival time is accounted for by response duration. Despite intensive efforts, however, the response rates for multidrug therapy remain in the 55 to 65 percent range, with a relatively small number of patients attaining a complete response, almost none of whom may be considered cured. While most researchers believe that drug combinations are of proven benefit, there remains some doubt concerning whether the use of multiple drugs results in improved survival.[259] Combination chemotherapy is probably superior to sequential single-agent drug therapy overall, but any of a number of two- to three-drug regimens are equally efficacious. The addition of doxorubicin to a regimen or the concurrent use of endocrine manipulation appears to improve response rates by at most 10 percent, without a readily discernible effect on survival.

Nonetheless, the majority of patients, especially those with one or more of the negative factors mentioned earlier, are probably best served by the early use of aggressive combination chemotherapy as a means of improving response rate and duration and, hence, survival. However, a group of "good prognosis" patients may be defined by the absence of these factors. They would be better served by initial low-dose chemotherapy or endocrine manipulation when receptor status or clinical presentation, or both, suggest that it would be appropriate. Clearly, much more remains to be done in the development and use of prognostic information in the hope that such progress may improve our ability to rationally develop therapy for individual patients or subsets of patients in the future.

REFERENCES

1. Beatson GT: On the treatment of inoperable cases of carcinoma of the mamma: Suggestions for a new method of treatment. Lancet 2:162, 1896.
2. Hall TC, Dederick MM, Nevinney HB, et al.: Prognostic value of response of patients with breast cancer to therapeutic castration. Cancer Chemother Rep 31:47, 1963.
3. Lewison EF: Castration in the treatment of advanced breast cancer. Cancer 18:1558, 1965.
4. Cole MP: Prophylactic compared with therapeutic X-ray artificial menopause. *In*: Joslin CAF, Gleave EN (eds.): The Clinical Management of Advanced Breast Cancer. Cardiff, Wales: Alpha Omega Alpha Publishing Co., 1970, pp. 2–11.
5. Cowan K, Lippman ME: Steroid receptors in breast cancer. Arch Intern Med 142:363, 1982.
6. Longcope C: Metabolic clearance and blood production rates of estrogens in post-menopausal women. Am J Obstet Gynecol 111:778, 1971.
7. Grodin JM, Siiteri PK, MacDonald PC: Source of estrogen production in postmenopausal women. J Clin Endocrinol 36:207, 1973.
8. Moore FD, VanDevanter SB, Boyden CM, et al.: Adrenalectomy with chemotherapy in the treatment of advanced breast cancer. Objective and subjective response rates: Duration and quality of life. Surgery 76:376, 1974.
9. Silverstein MJ, Byron RL, Yonemoto RH, et al.: Bilateral adrenalectomy for advanced breast cancer: A 21 year experience. Surgery 77:825, 1975.
10. Schmidt M, Nemoto T, Dao T, et al.: Prognostic factors affecting adrenalectomy in patients with metastatic cancer of the breast. Cancer 27:1106, 1971.
11. Manni A, Pearson OH, Brodkey J, et al.: Transsphenoidal hypophysectomy in breast cancer. Evidence for an individual role of pituitary and gonadal hormones in supporting tumor growth. Cancer 44:2330, 1979.
12. Bates T, Rubens RD, Bulbrook RD, et al.: Comparison of pituitary function and clinical response after transsphenoidal and transfrontal hypophysectomy for advanced breast cancer. Eur J Cancer 12:775, 1976.
13. LaRossa JT, Strong MS, Melby JC: Endocrinologically incomplete transethmoidal trans-sphenoidal hypophysectomy with relief of bone pain in breast cancer. N Engl J Med 299:1332, 1978.
14. Schally AV, Reddin TW: Inhibition of cell growth by a hypothalamic peptide. Proc Natl Acad Sci USA 79:7014, 1982.
15. Hayward JL, Atkins HJB, Falconer MA, et al.: Clinical trials comparing transfrontal hypophysectomy with adrenalectomy and with transsphenoidal hypophysectomy. *In*: Joslin CAF, Gleave EN (eds.): The Clinical Management of Advanced Breast Cancer. Cardiff, Wales: Alpha Omega Alpha Publishing Co., 1970, pp. 50–53.
16. Kennedy BJ: Diethylstilbestrol versus testosterone propionate therapy in advanced breast cancer. Surg Gynecol Obstet 120:1246, 1965.
17. Kennedy BJ: Hormone therapy in inoperable breast cancer. Cancer 24:1345, 1969.
18. Baker WH, Kelty RM, Sohier WD: Hormonal treatment of metastatic carcinoma of the breast. Am J Surg 99:538, 1960.
19. Kaufman RJ, Escher GC: Rebound regression in advanced mammary carcinoma. Surg Gynecol Obstet 113:635, 1961.
20. Baker LH, Vaitkevicius VK: Re-evaluation of rebound regression in disseminated carcinoma of the breast. Cancer 29:1268, 1972.
21. Davies P, Nicholson RI: How do androgens and progestins cause regression of breast cancer? Rev Endocrine-Related Cancer 10:19, 1981.

22. Allegra JC, Lippman ME, Thompson EB, et al.: Relationship between the progesterone, androgen, and glucocorticoid receptor and response rate to endocrine therapy in metastatic breast cancer. Cancer Res 39:1973, 1979.
23. Cooperative Breast Cancer Group: Testosterone propionate therapy in breast cancer. JAMA 188: 1069, 1964.
24. Goldenberg JS: Clinical trial of testololactone (NSC 23759), medroxyprogesterone acetate (NSC 26386), and oxylone acetate (NSC 47438) in advanced female mammary cancer. Cancer 23:109, 1969.
25. Madanos AE, Farber M: Danazol. Ann Intern Med 96:625, 1982.
26. Coombes RC, Dearnaley D, Humphreys J, et al.: Danazol treatment of advanced breast cancer. Cancer Treat Rep 64:1073, 1980.
27. Pannuti F, Martoni A, DiMarco AR, et al.: Prospective, randomized clinical trial of two different high dosages of medroxyprogesterone acetate (MAP) in the treatment of metastatic breast cancer. Eur J Cancer 15:593, 1979.
28. Beretta G, Tabiadon D, Tedeschi L, et al.: Hormonotherapy of advanced breast carcinoma: Comparative evaluation of tamoxifen citrate versus medroxyprogesterone acetate. *In*: Iacobelli S, Lippman ME, Della Cona GR (eds.): The Role of Tamoxifen in Breast Cancer. New York: Raven Press, 1983, pp. 113–120.
29. Geimer NF, Donegan WL: Role and mechanism of corticosteroid therapy in breast cancer. Rev Endocrine-Related Cancer 6:5, 1980.
30. Griffiths CT, Hall TC, Saba Z, et al.: Preliminary trial of aminoglutethimide in breast cancer. Cancer 32:31, 1973.
31. Fishman LM, Liddle GW, Island DP, et al.: Effects of aminoglutethimide on adrenal function in man. J Clin Endocrinol Metab 27:481, 1967.
32. Santen RJ, Santner S, Davis B, et al.: Aminoglutethimide inhibits extraglandular estrogen production in postmenopausal women with breast carcinoma. J Clin Endocrinol Metab 47:1257, 1978.
33. Santen RJ, Lipton A, Kendall J: Successful medical adrenalectomy with aminoglutethimide. Role of altered drug metabolism. JAMA 230:1661, 1974.
34. Santen RJ, Worgul TJ, Samojlik E, et al.: Randomized trial comparing surgical adrenalectomy with aminoglutethimide plus hydrocortisone in women with advanced breast cancer. N Engl J Med 305:545, 1981.
35. Santen RJ: Suppression of estrogens with aminoglutethimide and hydrocortisone (medical adrenalectomy) as treatment of advanced breast carcinoma. A review. Breast Cancer Res Treat 1:183, 1981.
36. Coombes RC, Goss P, Dowsett M, et al.: 4-Hydroxyandrostenedione in treatment of postmenopausal patients with advanced breast cancer. Lancet 1:1237, 1984.
37. Jordan VC: Biochemical pharmacology of antiestrogen action. Pharmacol Rev 36:245, 1984.
38. Furr BJA, Jordan VC: The pharmacology and clinical uses of tamoxifen. Pharmacol Ther 25:127, 1984.
39. Manni A, Trujillo J, Marshall J, et al.: Antiestrogen-induced remissions in stage IV breast cancer. Cancer Treat Rep 60:1445, 1976.
40. McIntosh IH, Thynne GS: Tumour stimulation by anti-oestrogens. Br J Surg 64:900, 1977.
41. Sutherland RL, Murphy LC, Foo MS, et al.: High affinity anti-estrogen binding site distinct from the oestrogen receptor. Nature 288:273, 1980.
42. Murphy LC, Sutherland RL: Modifications in the aminoether side chain of clomiphene influence affinity for a specific antiestrogen binding site in MCF-7 cell cytosol. Biochem Biophys Res Commun 100:1353, 1981.
43. Eckert RL, Katzenellenbogen BS: Physical properties of estrogen receptor complexes in MCF-7 human breast cancer cells. J Biol Chem 257:8840, 1982.
44. Legha S, Muggia FM: Antiestrogens in the treatment of cancer. Ann Intern Med 84:751, 1976.
45. Mouridsen H, Palshof T, Patterson J: Tamoxifen in advanced breast cancer. Cancer Treat Rep 62:131, 1978.
46. Heel RC, Brogden RN, Speight TM, et al: Tamoxifen: A review of its pharmacological properties and therapeutic use in the treatment of breast cancer. Drugs 16:1, 1978.
47. Pearson OH, Manni A, Arafah BM: Antiestrogen treatment of breast cancer: An overview. Cancer Res 42:3424s, 1982.
48. Pritchard KI, Thomson DB, Myers RE, et al.: Tamoxifen therapy in premenopausal patients with metastatic breast cancer. Cancer Treat Rep 64:787, 1980.
49. Pritchard K, Meakin JW, Sawka C, et al.: The role and mechanism of action of tamoxifen in premenopausal women with metastatic carcinoma of the breast. Proc Am Soc Clin Oncol 4:54, 1985.
50. Hoogstraten B, Fletcher WS, Gad-el-Mawla N, et al.: Tamoxifen and oophorectomy in the treatment of recurrent breast cancer. Cancer Res 42:4788, 1982.
51. Planting A, Wijst JM, Alexieva-Figuseh J: Tamoxifen therapy in premenopausal women with metastatic breast cancer. Proc Third EORTC Breast Cancer Conference (Abstract) 9:17, 1983.
52. Buchanan RB, Blamey RW, Durrant KR, et al.: A randomized comparison of tamoxifen with surgical oophorectomy in premenopausal patients with advanced breast cancer. J Clin Oncol 4:1326, 1986.
52a. Ingle JN, Krook JE, Green SJ, et al.: Randomized trial of bilateral oophorectomy versus tamoxifen in premenopausal women with metastatic breast cancer. J Clin Oncol 4:178, 1986.
53. Patterson JS, Battersby LA, Edwards DG: Review of the clinical pharmacology and international experience with tamoxifen in advanced breast cancer. Rev Endocrine-Related Cancer [Suppl] 9:563, 1982.
54. Tormey DC, Lippman ME, Edwards BK, et al.: Evaluation of tamoxifen doses with and without fluoxymesterone in advanced breast cancer. Ann Intern Med 98:139, 1983.
55. Adam HK, Patterson JS, Kemp JU: Studies on the metabolism and pharmacokinetics of tamoxifen in normal volunteers. Cancer Treat Rep 64:761, 1980.
56. Fabian C, Sternson L, Barnett M: Clinical pharmacology of tamoxifen in patients with breast cancer: Comparison of traditional and loading dose schedules. Cancer Treat Rep 64:775, 1978.
57. Kaiser-Kupfer MI, Lippman ME: Tamoxifen retinopathy. Cancer Treat Rep 62:315, 1978.
58. Ingle JN, Ahmann DL, Green SJ, et al.: Randomized clinical trial of diethylstilbestrol versus tamoxifen in postmenopausal women with advanced breast cancer. N Engl J Med 304:16, 1981.
59. Smith IE, Harris AL, Morgan M, et al.: Tamoxifen

versus aminoglutethimide versus combined tamoxifen and aminoglutethimide in the treatment of advanced breast cancer. Cancer Res 42:3430s, 1982.
60. Lipton A, Harvey HA, Santen RJ, et al.: Randomized trial of aminoglutethimide versus tamoxifen in metastatic breast cancer. Cancer Res 42:3434s, 1982.
61. Morgan LR, Donley PJ: Tamoxifen versus megestrol acetate in breast cancer. Cancer Treat Rep 63:1218, 1979.
62. Ingle JN, Ahmann DL, Green SJ, et al.: Randomized clinical trial of megestrol acetate versus tamoxifen in paramenopausal or castrated women with advanced breast cancer. Am J Clin Oncol 5:155, 1982.
63. Ingle JN, Ahmann DL, Long HJ, et al.: Randomized trial of tamoxifen alone or combined with aminoglutethimide and hydrocortisone in postmenopausal women with metastatic breast cancer. Proc Am Soc Clin Oncol 4:53, 1985.
64. Powles TJ, Gordon C, Coombes RC: Clinical trial of multiple endocrine therapy for metastatic and locally advanced breast cancer with tamoxifen-aminoglutethimide-danazol compared to tamoxifen used alone. Cancer Res 42:3458s, 1982.
65. Stoll BA: Combination endocrine therapy in breast cancer. Eur J Cancer Clin Oncol 21:413, 1985.
66. Greenspan EM: Combination cytotoxic chemotherapy in advanced disseminated breast carcinoma. J Mt Sinai Hosp 33:1, 1965.
67. Cooper R: Combination cytotoxic chemotherapy in hormone resistant breast cancer. Proc Am Assoc Cancer Res 10:15, 1969.
68. Broder LE, Tormey DC: Combination chemotherapy of carcinoma of the breast. Cancer Treat Rev 1:183, 1974.
69. Carbone PP, Tormey DL: Combination chemotherapy for advanced disease. *In*: McGuire WL (ed.): Breast Cancer. Advances in Research and Treatment. Vol. 1. New York: Plenum Press, 1977, pp. 165–215.
70. Carbone PP, Davis TE: Medical treatment for advanced breast cancer. Semin Oncol 4:417, 1978.
71. Carter SK: The chemical therapy of breast cancer. Semin Oncol 1:131, 1974.
72. Tormey DC, Neifeld JP: Chemotherapeutic approaches to disseminated disease. *In:* Stoll BA (ed.): Breast Cancer Management—Early and Late. Chicago: Year Book Medical Pubs., 1977, pp. 117–131.
73. Muss HB, White DR, Cooper MR, et al.: Combination chemotherapy in advanced breast cancer: A randomized trial comparing a three- vs a five-drug program. Arch Intern Med 137:1711, 1977.
74. Brunner KW, Sonntag RW, Martz G, et al.: A controlled study in the use of combined drug therapy for metastatic breast cancer. Cancer 36:1208, 1975.
75. Ahmann DL, Bisel HF, Hahn RC, et al.: An analysis of a multiple-drug program in the treatment of patients with advanced breast cancer utilizing 5-fluorouracil, cyclophosphamide, and prednisone with or without vincristine. Cancer 36:1925, 1975.
76. Rosner D, Nemoto T, Dao TL: Combination chemotherapy in the treatment of advanced breast cancer. J Surg Oncol 8:465, 1976.
77. Rosner D, Nemoto T: Sequence for developing optimal combination chemotherapy of metastatic breast cancer. Eur J Cancer 15:1197, 1979.
78. Ramirez G, Klotz J, Strawitz JG, et al.: Combination chemotherapy in breast cancer. A randomized study of 4 versus 5 drugs. Oncology 32:101, 1975.
79. Tormey DC, Gelman R, Band PR, et al.: Comparison of induction chemotherapies for metastatic breast cancer. Cancer 50:1235, 1982.
80. Hoogstraten B, George SL, Samal B, et al.: Combination chemotherapy and Adriamycin in patients with advanced breast cancer. Cancer 38:13, 1976.
81. Bezwoda WR, DeMoor NG, Derman D, et al.: Combination chemotherapy of metastatic breast cancer. A randomized trial comparing the use of Adriamycin to that of vinblastine. Cancer 44:392, 1979.
82. Bull JM, Tormey DC, Li SH, et al.: A randomized comparative trial of Adriamycin versus methotrexate in combination drug therapy. Cancer 41:1649, 1978.
83. Muss HB, White DR, Richards F, II, et al.: Adriamycin versus methotrexate in five-drug combination chemotherapy for advanced breast cancer. A randomized trial. Cancer 42:2141, 1978.
84. Kennealey GT, Boston B, Mitchell MS, et al.: Combination chemotherapy for advanced breast cancer. Two regimens containing Adriamycin. Cancer 42:27, 1978.
85. Smalley RV, Carpenter J, Bartolucci A, et al.: A comparison of cyclophosphamide, Adriamycin, 5-fluorouracil (CAF) and cyclophosphamide, methotrexate, 5-fluorouracil, vincristine, prednisone (CMFVP) in patients with metastatic breast cancer. Cancer 40:625, 1977.
86. Tranum BL, McDonald B, Thigpen T, et al.: Adriamycin combinations in advanced breast cancer. Cancer 49:835, 1982.
87. Ahmann DL, O'Fallon J, O'Connell MJ, et al.: Evaluation of a fixed alternating treatment in patients with advanced breast cancer. Cancer Clin Trials 219:1978.
88. Brambilla C, DeLena M, Rossi A, et al.: Response and survival in advanced breast cancer after two non–cross-resistant combinations. Br Med J 1:801, 1976.
89. Eagan RT, Ahmann DL, Edmonson JH, et al.: Controlled evaluation of the combination of Adriamycin (NSC-123127), vincristine (NSC-67574), and methotrexate (NSC-740) in patients with disseminated breast cancer. Cancer Chemother Rep 6:339, 1975.
90. Irwin LE, Chlebowski RT, Weiner JM, et al.: Randomized comparison of two combination chemotherapy regimens containing doxorubicin in patients with metastatic breast cancer: A Western Cancer Study Group trial. Cancer Treat Rep 64:981, 1980.
91. Nemoto T, Horton J, Simon R, et al.: Comparison of four combination chemotherapy programs in metastatic breast cancer: Comparison of multiple drug therapy with cytoxan, 5-FU, and prednisone versus cytoxan and Adriamycin, versus cytoxan, 5-FU and Adriamycin, versus cytoxan, 5-FU and prednisone alternating with cytoxan and Adriamycin. Cancer 49:1988, 1982.
92. Rainey JM, Jones SE, Salmon SE: Combination chemotherapy for advanced breast cancer utilizing vincristine, Adriamycin, and cyclophosphamide (VAC). Cancer 43:66, 1979.

93. Tranum B, Hoogstraten B, Kennedy A, et al.: Adriamycin in combination for metastatic breast cancer. Cancer 41:2078, 1978.
94. Canellos GP, Pocock SJ, Taylor SG, III, et al.: Combination chemotherapy for metastatic breast carcinoma. Prospective comparison of multiple drug therapy with L-phenylalanine mustard. Cancer 38:1882, 1976.
95. Mouridsen HT, Palshof T, Brahm M, et al.: Evaluation of single drug versus multiple drug chemotherapy in the treatment of advanced breast cancer. Cancer Treat Rep 61:47, 1977.
96. Rubens RD, Knight RK, Hayward JL: Chemotherapy of advanced breast cancer: A controlled randomized trial of cyclophosphamide versus a four-drug combination. Br J Cancer 32:730, 1975.
97. Carmo-Pereira J, Costa FO, Henriques E: Single-drug vs combination cytotoxic chemotherapy in advanced breast cancer: A randomized study. Eur J Cancer 16:1621, 1980.
98. Baker LH, Vaughn CB, Al-Sarraf M, et al.: Evaluation of combination vs sequential cytotoxic chemotherapy in the treatment of advanced breast cancer. Cancer 33:513, 1974.
99. Chlebowski RT, Irwin LE, Pugh RP, et al.: Survival of patients with metastatic breast cancer treated with either combination or sequential chemotherapy. Cancer Res 39:4503, 1979.
100. Smalley RV, Murphy S, Huguley CM, Jr., et al.: Combination versus sequential five-drug chemotherapy in metastatic carcinoma of the breast. Cancer Res 36:3911, 1976.
101. Bonadonna G, Brusamolino M, Valagussa P, et al.: Combination chemotherapy as an adjuvant treatment in operable breast cancer. N Engl J Med 294:405, 1976.
102. Canellos GP, DeVita VT, Gold GL, et al.: Cyclical combination chemotherapy for advanced breast carcinoma. Br Med J 1:218, 1974.
103. Canellos GP, DeVita VT, Gold GL, et al.: Combination chemotherapy for advanced breast cancer: Response and effect on survival. Ann Intern Med 84:389, 1976.
104. Knight EW, Horton J, Cunningham T, et al.: Adriamycin: Comparison of a 5-week schedule with a 3-week schedule in the treatment of breast cancer. Cancer Treat Rep 63:121, 1979.
105. Rivkin SE, Glucksberg H, Foulkes M: Adjuvant chemotherapy for operable breast cancer with positive axillary nodes. Proc Am Soc Clin Oncol 3:125, 1984.
106. Creech RH, Catalano RB, Mastrangelo MJ, et al.: An effective low dose intermittent cyclophosphamide, methotrexate, and 5-fluorouracil treatment regimen for metastatic breast cancer. Cancer 35:1101, 1975.
107. Creech RH, Catalano RB, Harris DT, et al.: Low dose chemotherapy of metastatic breast cancer with cyclophosphamide, Adriamycin, methotrexate, 5-fluorouracil (CAMF) versus sequential cyclophosphamide, methotrexate, 5-fluorouracil (CMF) and Adriamycin. Cancer 43:51, 1979.
108. Muss HB, Richards R, II, Jackson DV, et al.: Vincristine, doxorubicin, and cyclophosphamide versus low-dose intravenous cyclophosphamide, methotrexate, and 5-fluorouracil in advanced breast cancer. Cancer 50:2269, 1982.
109. Berken A, Greenblatt MN, Rosenthal DS, et al.: High-frequency low dose multiple-drug chemotherapy in advanced metastatic breast cancer. Cancer 49:2231, 1982.
110. Hirshaut Y, Kesselheim H: Prolonged remissions of metastatic breast cancer achieved with a six-drug regimen of relatively low toxicity. Cancer 51:1998, 1983.
111. Henderson IC, Gelman R, Canellos GP, et al.: Prolonged disease-free survival in advanced breast cancer treated with "super-CMF" Adriamycin: An alternating regimen employing high-dose methotrexate with citrovorum factor rescue. Cancer Treat Rep 65:67, 1981.
112. Israel L, Breau J, Aguilera J: High-dose cyclophosphamide and high-dose 5-fluorouracil. A new first-line regimen for advanced breast cancer. Cancer 53:1655, 1984.
113. Malik R, Blumenschein G, Legha S, et al.: A randomized trial of high-dose 5-fluorouracil (F), doxorubicin (A), and cyclophosphamide (C) vs conventional FAC regimen in metastatic breast cancer. Proc Am Soc Clin Oncol 1:79, 1982.
114. Hryniuk W, Bush H: The importance of dose intensity in chemotherapy of metastatic breast cancer. J Clin Oncol 2:1281, 1984.
115. Tormey DC, Falkson G, Simon RM, et al.: A randomized comparison of two sequentially administered combination regimens to a single regimen in metastatic breast cancer. Cancer Clin Trials 2:247, 1979.
116. Abeloff MD, Ettinger DS: Treatment of metastatic breast cancer with Adriamycin-cyclophosphamide induction followed by alternating combination therapy. Cancer Treat Rep 61:1685, 1977.
117. Blumenschein GR, Hortobagyi GN, Richman SP, et al.: Alternating non–cross-resistant combination chemotherapy and active non-specific immunotherapy with BCG or MER-BCG for advanced breast carcinoma. Cancer 45:742, 1980.
118. Brambilla C, Valagussa P, Bonadonna G: Sequential combination chemotherapy in advanced breast cancer. Cancer Chemother Pharmacol 1:35, 1978.
119. Muss HB, Richards F, II, Cooper MR, et al.: Chemotherapy vs. chemoimmunotherapy with methanol extraction residue of bacillus Calmette-Guérin (MER) in advanced breast cancer: A randomized trial by the Piedmont Oncology Association. Cancer 47:2295, 1981.
120. Gutterman JU, Cardenas JO, Blumenschein GR, et al.: Chemoimmunotherapy of advanced breast cancer: Prolongation of remission and survival with BCG. Br Med J 1:1222, 1976.
121. Hortobagyi GN, Yap HY, Blumenschein GR, et al.: Response of disseminated breast cancer to combined modality treatment with chemotherapy and levamisole with or without bacillus Calmette-Guérin. Cancer Treat Rep 62:1685, 1978.
122. Hortobagyi GN, Gutterman JU, Blumenschein GR, et al.: Combination chemoimmunotherapy of metastatic breast cancer with 5-fluorouracil, Adriamycin, cyclophosphamide, and BCG. Cancer 44:1955, 1979.
123. Britell JC, Ahmann DL, Bisel HF, et al.: Treatment of advanced breast cancer with cyclophosphamide, 5-fluorouracil, and prednisone with and without methanol-extracted residue of BCG. Cancer Clin Trials 2:345, 1979.
124. Lippman ME: Efforts to combine endocrine and

chemotherapy in the management of breast cancer: Do two and two equal three? Breast Cancer Res Treat 3:117, 1983.

125. Ahmann DL, O'Connell MJ, Hahn RG, et al.: An evaluation of early or delayed adjuvant chemotherapy in premenopausal patients with advanced breast cancer undergoing oophorectomy. N Engl J Med 297:356, 1977.
126. Cavalli F, Beer M, Martz G, et al.: Concurrent or sequential use of cytotoxic chemotherapy and hormone treatment in advanced breast cancer: Report of the Swiss Group for Clinical Cancer Research. Br Med J 2:865, 1983.
127. Falkson G, Falkson HC, Glidewell O, et al.: Improved remission rates and remission duration in young women with metastatic breast cancer following combined oophorectomy and chemotherapy. Cancer 43:2215, 1979.
128. Lloyd RE, Jones SE, Salmon SE: Comparative trial of low-dose Adriamycin plus cyclophosphamide with or without additive hormonal therapy in advanced breast cancer. Cancer 43:60, 1979.
129. Ahmann DL, Green SJ, Bisel HF, et al.: An evaluation of early or delayed adjuvant chemotherapy in premenopausal patients with advanced breast cancer undergoing oophorectomy: A later analysis. Am J Clin Oncol 5:355, 1982.
130. Cocconi G, DeLisi V, Boni C, et al.: Chemotherapy versus combination of chemotherapy and endocrine therapy in advanced breast cancer. Cancer 51:581, 1983.
131. Brunner KW, Sonntag RW, Alberto P, et al.: Combined chemo- and hormonal therapy in advanced breast cancer. Cancer 39:2923, 1977.
132. Rubens RD, Begent RHJ, Knight RK, et al.: Combined cytotoxic and progestogen therapy for advanced breast cancer. Cancer 42:1680, 1978.
133. Mouridsen HT, Palshof T, Englesman E, et al.: CMF versus CMF plus tamoxifen in advanced breast cancer in postmenopausal women. An EORTC trial. Eur J Cancer [Suppl.] 1:119, 1980.
134. Mouridsen HT, Rose C, Engelsman E, et al.: Combined cytotoxic and endocrine therapy in postmenopausal patients with advanced breast cancer. A randomized EORTC Breast Cancer Cooperative Group study of CMF versus CMF plus tamoxifen. Eur J Cancer Clin Oncol 21:291, 1985.
135. Lippman ME, Cassidy J, Wesley M, et al.: A randomized attempt to increase the efficacy of cytotoxic chemotherapy in metastatic breast cancer by hormonal synchronization. J Clin Oncol 2:28, 1984.
136. Allegra JC, Woodcock TM, Richman SP: A phase II trial of tamoxifen, Premarin, methotrexate and 5-fluorouracil in metastatic breast cancer. Breast Cancer Res Treat 2:93, 1982.
137. Bowman D: A phase II evaluation of sequential tamoxifen, Premarin, methotrexate, and 5-fluorouracil in refractory stage IV breast cancer. Proc Am Soc Clin Oncol 2:106, 1983.
138. Swenerton KD, Legha SS, Smith T, et al.: Prognostic factors in metastatic breast cancer treated with combination chemotherapy. Cancer Res 39:1552, 1979.
139. George SL, Hoogstraten B: Prognostic factors in the initial response to therapy by patients with advanced breast cancer. J Natl Cancer Inst 60:731, 1978.
140. Preda F, Oriana S, Perozziello F, et al.: Clinical response to chemotherapy and hormone therapy as first treatment after therapeutic ovariectomy in advanced breast cancer patients. Tumori (Milan) 68:161, 1982.
141. Nemoto T, Rosner D, Diaz R, et al.: Combination chemotherapy for metastatic breast cancer. Comparison of multiple drug therapy with 5-fluorouracil, Cytoxan and prednisone with Adriamycin or adrenalectomy. Cancer 41:2073, 1978.
142. Oberfield RA, Cady B, Pazianos AG, et al.: Adrenalectomy-oophorectomy and combined chemotherapy for carcinoma of the breast with metastases. Surg Gynecol Obstet 148:881, 1979.
143. Kiang DT, Kennedy BJ: Chemoendocrine therapy in advanced breast cancer. Breast Cancer Res Treat 1:105, 1981.
144. Manni A, Trujillo JE, Pearson OH: Sequential use of endocrine therapy and chemotherapy for metastatic breast cancer: Effects on survival. Cancer Treat Rep 64:111, 1980.
145. Legha SS, Buzdar AU, Smith TL, et al.: Response to hormonal therapy as a prognostic factor for metastatic breast cancer treated with combination chemotherapy. Cancer 46:438, 1980.
146. Valagussa P, Brambilla C, Bonadonna G: Advanced breast cancer: Are the traditional stratification parameters still of value when patients are treated with combination chemotherapy? Eur J Cancer 15:565, 1979.
147. Valagussa P, Rossi A, Tancini G, et al.: Is there any effective salvage treatment for relapsing operable breast cancer with N+?. Proc Am Soc Clin Oncol 4:56, 1985.
148. Chlebowski RT, Weiner JM, Luce J, et al.: Significance of relapse after adjuvant treatment with combination chemotherapy or 5-fluorouracil alone in high-risk breast cancer. Cancer Res 41:4399, 1981.
149. Bitran JD, Desser RK, Shapiro CM, et al.: Response to secondary therapy in patients with adrenocarcinoma of the breast previously treated with adjuvant chemotherapy. Cancer 51:381, 1983.
150. Wendt AG, Jones SE, Salmon SE: Salvage treatment of patients relapsing after breast cancer adjuvant chemotherapy. Cancer Treat Rep 64:269, 1980.
151. Coburn J, Ahmann FR, Moon T, et al.: The effect of prior adjuvant chemotherapy on survival in metastatic breast cancer. Breast Cancer Res Treat 3:303, 1983.
152. Buzdar AU, Legha SS, Hortobagyi GN, et al.: Management of breast cancer patients failing adjuvant chemotherapy with Adriamycin-containing regimens. Cancer 47:2798, 1981.
153. Garewal HS, Brooks RJ, Jones SE, et al.: Treatment of advanced breast cancer with mitomycin C combined with vinblastine or vindesine. J Clin Oncol 1:772, 1983.
154. Estape J, Cirera L, Milla A, et al.: VP-16-213 and cyclophosphamide in advanced breast cancer. A phase II study. Cancer Chemother Pharmacol 10:154, 1983.
155. Longacre D, Donovan M, Paladine W, et al.: Hexamethylmelamine, vincristine, and methotrexate in advanced neoplasms. Cancer Treat Rep 61:919, 1977.
156. Legha SS, Buzdar AU, Hortobagyi GN, et al.: Phase II study of hexamethylmelamine alone and in combination with mitomycin C and vincristine in advanced breast cancer. Cancer Treat Rep 63:2053, 1979.
157. Konits P, Aisner J, VanEcho D, et al.: Mitomycin

C and vinblastine chemotherapy for advanced breast cancer. Cancer 48:1295, 1981.
158. Hart RD, Perloff M, Holland JF: One day VATH (vinblastine, Adriamycin, thiotepa, Halotestin) therapy for advanced breast cancer refractory to chemotherapy. Cancer 48:1522, 1981.
159. Harris M, Byrne P, Smith F, et al.: Treatment of advanced breast cancer with two Adriamycin-containing regimens. Proc Am Soc Clin Oncol 1:81, 1982.
160. Marcus FS, Friedman MA, Resser KJ, et al.: 5-FU plus oncovin plus Adriamycin plus mitomycin C (FOAM): An effective therapy for metastatic breast cancer in patients who have failed prior chemotherapy. Proc Am Soc Clin Oncol 21:412, 1980.
161. Tormey DC, Bull JM: L-Phenylalanine mustard, doxorubicin, and vincristine in advanced breast cancer: A pilot study. Cancer Treat Rep 64:1015, 1980.
162. DiStefano A, Yap HY, Blumenschein GR: Doxorubicin, mitolactol (dibromodulcitol) and mitomycin C treatment for patients with metastatic breast cancer previously treated with cyclophosphamide, methotrexate, 5-FU, vindesine, and prednisone (CMFVP). Cancer Treat Rep 65:33, 1981.
163. Shipp SK, Muss HB, Westrick MA, et al.: Vincristine, doxorubicin, and mitomycin (VAM) in patients with advanced breast cancer previously treated with cyclophosphamide, methotrexate, and fluorouracil (CMF). Cancer Chemother Pharmacol 11:130, 1983.
164. Chlebowski RT, Pugh R, Weiner JM, et al.: Doxorubicin and CCNU with or without vincristine in patients with advanced refractory breast cancer. A randomized trial. Cancer 52:606, 1983.
165. Decker DA, Ahmann DL, Bisel HF, et al.: Complete responders to chemotherapy in metastatic breast cancer. Characterization and analysis. JAMA 242:2075, 1979.
166. Nash CH, Jones SE, Moon TE, et al.: Prediction of outcome in metastatic breast cancer treated with Adriamycin combination chemotherapy. Cancer 46:2380, 1980.
167. Corle DK, Sears ME, Olson KB: The relationship of quantitative estrogen receptor level and clinical response to cytotoxic chemotherapy in advanced breast cancer: An extramural analysis. Cancer 54:1554, 1984.
168. Mohla S, Sampson CC, Khan T, et al.: Estrogen and progesterone receptors in breast cancer in black Americans. Cancer 50:552, 1982.
169. Daly M, Osborne C, Clark G, et al.: Mexican-American breast cancer patients have a worse prognosis. Proc Am Soc Clin Oncol 2:5, 1983.
170. Nemoto T, Tuminoga T, Chamberlain A, et al.: Differences in breast cancer between Japan and the United States. J Natl Cancer Inst 58:193, 1977.
171. Morrison A, Lowe C, MacMahon B, et al.: Some international differences in treatment and survival in breast cancer. Int J Cancer 18:269, 1976.
172. Morz R, Francesconi M, Schemper M, et al.: The value of prognostic parameters for the stratification of advanced breast cancer patients. J Cancer Res Clin Oncol 102:289, 1982.
173. Karnofsky DA, Abelmann WH, Craver LF, et al.: The use of nitrogen mustards in the palliative treatment of carcinoma. Cancer 1:634, 1948.
174. Zubrod G, Schneiderman M, Frei E, et al.: Appraisal of methods for the study of chemotherapy of cancer in man: Comparative therapeutic trial of nitrogen mustard and triethylene thiophosphoramide. J Chronic Dis 11:7, 1960.
175. DeWys WD, Begg C, Band P, et al.: The impact of malnutrition on treatment results in breast cancer. Cancer Treat Rep 65:87, 1981.
176. Derogatis LR, Abeloff MD, Melisaratos N: Psychological coping mechanisms and survival time in metastatic breast cancer. JAMA 242:1504, 1979.
177. Cassileth BR, Lusk EJ, Miller DS, et al.: Psychosocial correlates of survival in advanced malignant disease? N Engl J Med 312:1551, 1985.
178. Blamey R, Bishop H, Blake J, et al.: Relationship between primary breast tumor receptor status and patient survival. Cancer 46:2765, 1980.
179. Chang JC, Wegowske G: Correlation of estrogen receptors and response to chemotherapy of cyclophosphamide, methotrexate, and 5-fluorouracil (CMF) in advanced breast cancer. Cancer 48:2503, 1981.
180. Cocconi G, DeLisi V, Mori P, et al.: Estrogen receptors and response to chemotherapy in advanced breast cancer. Tumori (Milan) 68:67, 1982.
181. Hilf R, Feldstein ML, Savlov ED, et al.: The lack of relationship between estrogen receptor status and response to chemotherapy. Cancer 46:2797, 1980.
182. Hilf R, Feldstein ML, Gibson SL, et al.: The relative importance of estrogen receptor analysis as a prognostic factor for recurrence or response to chemotherapy in women with breast cancer. Cancer 45:1993, 1980.
183. Jonat W, Maas H, Stolzenbach G, et al.: Estrogen receptor status and response to polychemotherapy in advanced breast cancer. Cancer 46:2809, 1980.
184. Kiang DT, Frenning DH, Gay J, et al.: Estrogen receptor status and response to chemotherapy in advanced breast cancer. Cancer 46:2814, 1980.
185. Kiang DT, Frenning DH, Goldman AI, et al.: Estrogen receptors and responses to chemotherapy and hormonal therapy in advanced breast cancer. N Engl J Med 299:1330, 1978.
186. Lippman ME, Allegra JC, Thompson EB, et al.: The relation between estrogen receptors and response rate to cytotoxic chemotherapy in metastatic breast cancer. N Engl J Med 298:1223, 1978.
187. Mortimer J, Reimer R, Greenstreet R, et al.: Influence of estrogen receptor status on response to combination chemotherapy for recurrent breast cancer. Cancer Treat Rep 65:763, 1981.
188. Rosenbaum C, Marsland TA, Stolbach LL, et al.: Estrogen receptor status and response to chemotherapy in advanced breast cancer: The Tufts-Shattuck-Pondville experience. Cancer 46:2919, 1980.
189. Rubens RD, Hayward JL: Estrogen receptors and response to endocrine therapy and cytotoxic chemotherapy in advanced breast cancer. Cancer 46:2922, 1980.
190. Samaan NA, Buzdar AU, Aldinger KA, et al.: Estrogen receptor: A prognostic factor in breast cancer. Cancer 47:554, 1981.
191. Samal BA, Brooks SC, Cummings G, et al.: Estrogen receptors and responsiveness of advanced breast cancer to chemotherapy. Cancer 46:2925, 1980.
192. Young PCM, Ehrlich CE, Einhorn LH: Relationship between steroid receptors and response to endocrine therapy and cytotoxic chemotherapy in metastatic breast cancer. Cancer 46:2961, 1980.
193. Bloom ND, Tobin EH, Schreibman B, et al.: The

role of progesterone receptors in the management of advanced breast cancer. Cancer 45:2992, 1980.
194. Osborne C, Yochmowitz M, Knight W, et al.: The value of estrogen and progesterone receptors in the treatment of breast cancer. Cancer 46:2884, 1980.
195. Meyer JS, McDivitt RW, Stone KR, et al.: Practical breast carcinoma cell kinetics: Review and update. Breast Cancer Res Treat 4:79, 1984.
196. Meyer JS, Friedman E, McCrate MM, et al.: Prediction of early course of breast carcinoma by thymidine labeling. Cancer 51:1879, 1983.
197. Meyer JS, Lee JY: Relationships of S-phase fraction of breast carcinoma in relapse to duration of remission, estrogen receptor content, therapeutic responsiveness, and duration of survival. Cancer Res 40:1890, 1980.
198. Kute TE, Muss HB, Anderson D, et al.: Relationship of steroid receptor, cell kinetics, and clinical status in patients with breast cancer. Cancer Res 41:3524, 1981.
199. Silvestrini R, Daidone MG, DiFronzo G: Relationship between proliferative activity and estrogen receptors in breast cancer. Cancer 44:665, 1979.
200. Tubiana M, Pejovic MJ, Renaud A, et al.: Kinetic parameters and the course of the disease in breast cancer. Cancer 47:937, 1981.
201. Allegra JC, Lippman ME, Simon R, et al.: Association between steroid hormone receptor status and disease-free interval in breast cancer. Cancer Treat Rep 63:1271, 1979.
202. Fey MF, Brunner KW, Sonntag RW: Prognostic factors in metastatic breast cancer. Cancer Clin Trials 4:237, 1981.
203. Rozencwieg M, Staquet MJ, VonHoff DD, et al.: Prognostic factors for the response to chemotherapy in advanced breast cancer. Cancer Clin Trials 2:165, 1979.
204. DiStefano A, Yap HY, Hortobagyi GN, et al.: The natural history of breast cancer patients with brain metastases. Cancer 44:1913, 1979.
205. Sparrow GEA, Rubens RD: Brain metastases from breast cancer: Clinical course, prognosis and influence of treatment. Clin Oncol 7:291, 1981.
206. Smalley RV, Scogna DM, Malmud LS: Advanced breast cancer with bone-only metastases. A chemotherapeutically responsive pattern of metastases. Am J Clin Oncol 5:161, 1982.
207. Sherry MM, Johnson DH, Greco FA, et al.: Metastatic breast cancer confined to bone: An indolent disease. Proc Am Soc Clin Oncol 4:63, 1985.
208. Smalley RV, Carpenter J, Bartolucci A, et al.: A comparison of cyclophosphamide, Adriamycin, 5-fluorouracil (CAF) and cyclophosphamide, methotrexate, 5-fluorouracil, vincristine, prednisone (CMFVP) in patients with metastatic breast cancer. Cancer 40:625, 1977.
209. Stewart JF, King RJB, Sexton SA, et al.: Oestrogen receptors, sites of metastatic disease and survival in recurrent breast cancer. Eur J Cancer 17:449, 1980.
210. Krown SE, Pinsky CM, Wanebo HJ, et al.: Immunologic reactivity and prognosis in breast cancer. Cancer 46:1746, 1980.
211. Cunningham TJ, Daut D, Wolfgang PE, et al.: A correlation of DNCB-induced delayed cutaneous hypersensitivity reactions and the course of disease in patients with recurrent breast cancer. Cancer 37:1696, 1976.
212. Hortobagyi GN, Smith TL, Swenerton KD, et al.: Prognostic value of prechemotherapy skin tests in patients with metastatic breast carcinoma. Cancer 47:1369, 1981.
213. Waalkes TP, Abeloff MD, Ettinger DA, et al.: Multiple biological markers and breast carcinoma: A preliminary study in the detection of recurrent disease after primary therapy. J Surg Oncol 18:9, 1981.
214. Waalkes TP, Tormey DC: Biological markers and breast cancer. Semin Oncol 5:434, 1978.
215. DeJong-Bakker M, Hart AAM, Persijn JP, et al.: Prognostic significance of CEA in breast cancer: A statistical study. Eur J Cancer Clin Oncol 17:1307, 1981.
216. Bezwoda W, Derman D, Bothwell T, et al: Significance of serum concentrations of carcinoembryonic antigen, ferritin, and calcitonin in breast cancer. Cancer 48:1623, 1981.
217. Franchimont P, Zangerle PF, Colin C, et al.: Tumor associated markers in breast cancer. Eur J Cancer [Suppl] 1:17, 1980.
218. Haagensen DE, Kister SJ, Vandevoorde JP, et al.: Evaluation of carcinoembryonic antigen as a plasma monitor for human breast carcinoma. Cancer 42:1512, 1978.
219. Myers RE, Sutherland, DJ, Meakin JW, et al.: Carcinoembryonic antigen in breast cancer. Cancer 42:1520, 1978.
220. Tormey DC, Waalkes TP: Biological markers as prognostic and clinical evaluation tools. Eur J Cancer [Suppl] 1:21, 1980.
221. Tormey DC, Waalkes TP: Clinical correlation between CEA and breast cancer. Cancer 42:1507, 1978.
222. Tormey DC, Waalkes TP, Snyder JJ, et al.: Biological markers in breast carcinoma III. Clinical correlations with carcinoembryonic antigen. Cancer 39:2397, 1977.
223. Coombes R, Gazet J, Sloane J, et al.: Biochemical markers in human breast cancer. Lancet 2:132, 1977.
224. Coombes R, Powles T, Gazet J, et al.: A biochemical approach to the staging of human breast cancer. Cancer 40:937, 1977.
225. Mughal AW, Hortobagyi GN, Fritsche HA, et al.: Serial plasma carcinoembryonic antigen measurements during treatment of metastatic breast cancers. JAMA 249:1881, 1983.
226. Tormey DC, Waalkes TP, Simon RM: Biological markers in breast carcinoma. II. Clinical correlations with human chorionic gonadotrophin. Cancer 39:2391, 1977.
227. Lamoreux G, Mandeville R, Poisson R, et al.: Biological markers and breast cancer: A multiparametric study. 1. Increased serum protein levels. Cancer 49:502, 1982.
228. Schapira DV, Schapira M: Use of ceruloplasmin levels to monitor response therapy and predict recurrence of breast cancer. Breast Cancer Res Treat 3:221, 1983.
229. Neill HB, Palmieri GM, Neely CL, Jr., et al.: Postabsorptive urinary hydroxyproline test in patients with metastatic bone disease from breast cancer. Arch Intern Med 141:1471, 1981.
230. Gielen F, Dequeker J, Drochmans A, et al.: Relevance of hydroxyproline excretion to bone metastasis in breast cancer. Br J Cancer 34:279, 1976.
231. Powles TJ, Leese CL, Bondy PK: Hydroxyproline

excretion in patients with breast cancer and response to treatment. Br Med J 2:164, 1975.

232. Hortobagyi GN, Smith TL, Legha SS, et al.: Multivariate analysis of prognostic factors in metastatic breast cancer. J Clin Oncol 1:776, 1983.
233. Blumenschein GR, Pinnamaneni K, Buzdar AU, et al.: Combined regional and systemic therapy in breast cancer patients with an isolated metastasis with or without prior chemotherapy. *In*: Jones SE, Salmon SE (eds.): Adjuvant Therapy of Cancer IV. Orlando, FL: Grune & Stratton, 1984, pp. 311–318.
234. Beck TM, Hart NE, Woodard DA, et al.: Local or regionally recurrent carcinoma of the breast: Results of therapy in 121 patients. J Clin Oncol 1:400, 1983.
235. Wallack MK, Wolf JA, Jr., Bedwinek J, et al.: Gestational carcinoma of the female breast. Curr Probl Cancer 7:1, 1983.
236. Clark RM, Reid J: Carcinoma of the breast in pregnancy and lactation. Int J Radiat Oncol Biol Phys 4:693, 1978.
237. Donegan WL: Breast cancer and pregnancy. Obstet Gynecol 50:244, 1977.
238. Nicholson HO: Cytotoxic drugs in pregnancy. J Obstet Gynaecol Br Commonw 75:307, 1968.
239. Potter JF, Schoeneman M: Metastasis of maternal cancer to the placenta and fetus. Cancer 25:380, 1970.
240. White T, White W: Breast cancer and pregnancy: Report of 49 cases followed five years. Ann Surg 144:384, 1956.
241. Rissaner P: Carcinoma of the breast during pregnancy and lactation. Br J Cancer 22:663, 1968.
242. Cheek JH: Cancer of the breast in pregnancy and lactation. Am J Surg 126:729, 1973.
243. Peters MV: The effect of pregnancy in breast cancer. *In*: Forrest APM, Kunkler PB (eds.): Prognostic Factors in Breast Cancer. Baltimore: Williams & Wilkins, 1968, pp. 65–80.
244. Cooper DR, Butterfield J: Pregnancy subsequent to mastectomy for cancer of the breast. Ann Surg 171:429, 1970.
245. Stuart-Harris RC, Smith IE: Mitoxantrone: A phase II study in the treatment of patients with advanced breast carcinoma and other solid tumors. Cancer Chemother Pharmacol 8:179, 1982.
246. Yap HY, Blumenschein GR, Schell FC, et al.: Dihydroxyanthracenedione: A promising new drug in the treatment of advanced breast cancer. Ann Intern Med 95:694, 1981.
247. Henderson IC, Wolff S, Allegra J, et al.: Mitoxantrone vs doxorubicin in advanced breast cancer: A randomized trial in 220 patients. Proc Am Soc Clin Oncol 4:62, 1985.
248. Yap HY, Yap BS, Blumenschein GR, et al.: Bisantrene: A promising new drug in the treatment of metastatic breast cancer. Proc Am Assoc Cancer Res 23:580, 1982.
249. Osborne CK, Von Hoff DD, Sandback JJ: Activity of bisantrene in a phase II study in advanced breast cancer. Proc Am Soc Clin Oncol 1:87, 1982.
250. Cobleigh MA, Williams SD, Einhorn LH: Phase II study of vindesine in patients with metastatic breast cancer. Cancer Treat Rep 65:659, 1981.
251. Robins HJ, Tormey DC, Shelley MJ, et al.: Vindesine: A phase II trial in advanced breast cancer patients. Cancer Clin Trials 4:371, 1981.
252. Ansfield FJ, Kallos G, Singson J: Further phase I–II studies with oral Tegafur (Ftorafur). Proc Am Soc Clin Oncol 21:347, 1980.
253. Curt GA, Grygiel JJ, Weiss R, et al.: A phase I and pharmacokinetic study of CBDCA (NSC 241240). Proc Am Soc Clin Oncol 2:21, 1983.
254. Mattsson W, Borgstorm S, Landberg T: A weekly schedule of low-dose doxorubicin in treatment of advanced breast cancer. Clin Ther 5:193, 1982.
255. Hortobagyi GN, Yap HY, Blumenschein GR, et al.: Phase II evaluation of vinblastine, methotrexate and calcium leukovorin rescue in patients with refractory metastatic breast cancer. Cancer 51:769, 1983.
256. Corringham R, Gilmore M, Prentice HG, et al.: High-dose melphalan with autologous bone marrow transplant. Treatment of poor prognosis tumors. Cancer 52:1783, 1983.
257. Klijn JGM, DeJong FH: Treatment with a luteinising-hormone–releasing hormone analogue (Buserelin) in premenopausal patients with metastatic breast cancer. Lancet 1:1213, 1982.
258. Harvey HA, Lipton A, Diaz-Perches R, et al.: Effective medical castration producd by the GnRH analog leuprolide in metastatic breast cancer. Proc Am Soc Clin Oncol 3:111, 1984.
259. Powles TJ, Smith IE, Ford HT, et al.: Failure of chemotherapy to prolong survival in a group of patients with metastatic breast cancer. Lancet 1:580, 1980.
260. Kolaric K, Roth A: Phase II clinical trial of *cis*-dichlorodiamine platinum (*cis*-DDP) for antitumorigenic activity in previously untreated patients with metastatic breast cancer. Cancer Chemother Pharmacol 11:108, 1983.

Special Situations in The Treatment of Breast Cancer

ALLEN S. LICHTER, M.D.
MARC E. LIPPMAN, M.D.

14

Any clinician who treats patients with breast malignancies will be called upon to manage patients whose conditions are outside the boundaries of routine infiltrating ductal carcinoma. This chapter will summarize the literature and make treatment recommendations for patients presenting with these special situations. The five areas that will be presented are (1) nonepithelial tumors of the breast, (2) breast cancer associated with pregnancy, (3) breast cancer presenting as axillary adenopathy, (4) Paget's disease of the breast, and (5) male breast cancer. These conditions all are relatively rare, and even the busiest clinical center is unlikely to see more than one or two cases per year in each of these categories.

NONEPITHELIAL TUMORS OF THE BREAST

A wide variety of nonepithelial tumors can occur in the breast. Of these, two of the most important are cystosarcoma phyllodes and angiosarcoma, the former because it is the most common nonepithelial breast tumor, and the latter because of its virulence. Within the stromal component of a cystosarcoma phyllodes, one can see a variety of other sarcomas including fibrosarcoma, liposarcoma,[1] rhabdomyosarcoma,[2] osteosarcoma,[3] and hemangiopericytoma.[4] The occurrence of "pure" sarcoma of the breast without an associated cystosarcoma is extremely rare but well recognized. Thus, a handful of cases of each tumor type have been reported, including rhabdomyosarcoma,[5] osteosarcoma,[6, 7] chondrosarcoma,[8] liposarcoma,[9, 10] and leiomyosarcoma.[11] Some investigators have discussed a separate entity called stromal sarcoma of the breast.[12–15] Histologically, these tumors have a spectrum of patterns duplicating the composition of mammary stroma. Thus, these tumors may contain fibrosarcoma, liposarcoma, giant-cell and spindle-cell sarcoma, and, occasionally, heterologous elements such as osteosarcoma. Barnes and Pietruszka[16] have criticized the term stromal sarcoma. They believe that these tumors can be analyzed as to the primary sarcomatous element and should be classified accordingly rather than grouped together under the rather nonspecific term stromal sarcoma.

Another sarcomatous tumor that deserves mention is carcinosarcoma. This is a true "collision" tumor, with both a clear carcinomatous and a sarcomatous component.[17, 18] However, as pointed out by Azzopardi,[19] most diagnoses of these tumors are incorrect. Many lesions that reportedly contain bony or cartilaginous tumor actually represent metaplasia within a routine carcinoma and are not true *de novo* sarcomas. Other tumors that appear to be "fibrosarcoma" often are, in reality, spindle-cell cancers with a marked desmoplastic reaction. In any event, while carcinosarcoma does occur, it is extremely rare. Another nonepithelial but nonsarcomatous lesion that can occur as a primary tumor of the breast is malignant lymphoma.[20, 21]

Cystosarcoma Phyllodes

DEFINITION

This tumor is the most common of the nonepithelial lesions of the breast, with hundreds of cases reported in the literature and probably many thousands of additional cases unreported. The term cystosarcoma phyllodes was coined by Muller in the 1830's,[22] and the gross appearance of this tumor accounts for its name. The tumor, by definition, consists of abundant *fibrous stroma surrounding epithelium-lined spaces*. An intracanalicular growth pattern can produce a tumor that, on cut section, has a cabbage-like or leafy appearance. The term phyllodes comes from the Greek word *phyllon*, meaning leaf, and thus refers descriptively to the phyllodes tumor's grossly leafy character. The epithelial spaces can have the appearance of cysts—thus the "cysto-" component of the name. The name is, nevertheless, an unfortunate one. "Cysto" may imply that the tumor always contains cysts, and this is not the case with many of these lesions. Clearly, the term sarcoma justifiably implies an aggressive malignant tumor, but most of these lesions are, in fact, benign and quite innocent in their behavior. Over the years, there has been steady pressure to change the name of this tumor. However, no one seems to be able to agree on an appropriate alternative name, and over 66 suggestions have been recorded in the literature.[22] Most authorities agree that a term that has been in the medical literature for over 150 years is unlikely to be altered.

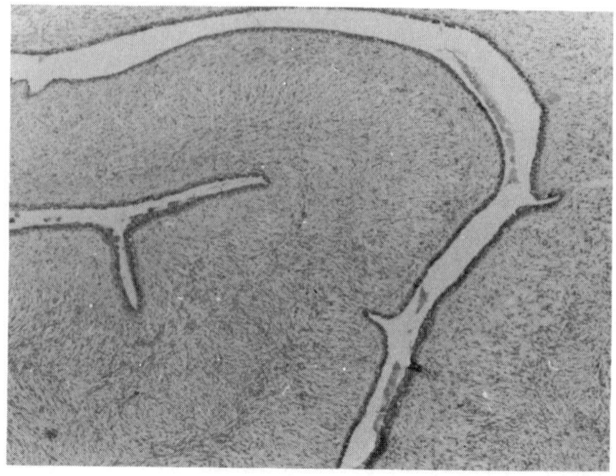

FIGURE 14–1. Typical microscopic appearance of cystosarcoma phyllodes. A dense, fibrous stroma surrounds epithelium-lined spaces.

Cystosarcoma phyllodes is a unique tumor exclusively of the female breast and has no counterpart in any other organ of the body. The tumor has two components, epithelium-lined cysts surrounded by abundant hypercellular stroma as illustrated in Figure 14–1. The two components must be admixed in order to satisfy the criteria for diagnosis. These tumors probably arise from perilobular fibrous connective tissue and can also involve periductal tissue.[23] Since the male breast does not have a well-defined lobular structure, the male breast should be immune to cystosarcoma phyllodes (as well as to lobular carcinoma), although rare case reports in men with gynecomastia have been noted (see the discussion on male breast cancer).

Grossly, the majority of these cases are sharply circumscribed, freely mobile tumors with a smooth, bosselated contour.[25] As such, there is a great temptation to remove cystosarcoma by enucleation. However, at the edge of these tumors, there can be invasion of fibrous stroma into breast fat, the so-called infiltrating border described by Oberman,[23] Pietruszka and Barnes,[4] Norris and Taylor,[26] and others. Not surprisingly, enu-

TABLE 14–1. Cystosarcoma Phyllodes—Age and Tumor Size

Author	No. of Patients	Age Range	Median Age	Size Range (cm)	Median Size (cm)
Haagensen[1]	84	14–85	44.7	—	—
Pietruszka and Barnes[4]	42	14–67	44.3	1–41	5
Treves[24]	93	16–70	45	1–20	4
McDivitt et al.[25]	73	16–68	46	1–19	5
Norris and Taylor[26]	94	15–86	45	1–45	4.5

cleation of such tumors leads to a high rate of local recurrence.[1, 26] One novel method to test the adequacy of a local excision for a cystosarcoma phyllodes is to "orange peel" the surface of the excision and look for any evidence of tumor in this thin surface section.[27]

Natural History

Patients with cystosarcoma phyllodes range from preteenagers through women in their 80's. The median age is 45, which is about 10 to 15 years older than the median age for the appearance of a fibroadenoma and about 10 years younger than the median age for the appearance of invasive carcinoma (Table 14–1). The average size of tumors is between 4 and 5 cm, ranging as low as 1 cm and as high as 30 to 40 cm in diameter, the latter filling and grossly distorting the breast and weighing more than 10 lb (Table 14–1). Many tumors that grow to a large size have been reported to do so over a few weeks. This period of rapid growth is not characteristic of the majority of cases of cystosarcoma phyllodes and has little bearing on outcome. In general, however, tumors of larger size tend to behave more aggressively than smaller tumors.[25, 26, 28]

Even tumors that grow to a large size rarely involve the skin. If there is abnormality of the skin, it represents necrosis or ulceration secondary to a stretching of the skin over a huge tumor rather than an invasion of the tumor into the skin.[1] Similarly, even large cystosarcomas rarely involve axillary nodes. The frequency of axillary lymph node positivity on histologic section is less than 1 percent (Table 14–2). On mammography and ultrasound, cystosarcomas can have a unique appearance. Mammographically, a solid well-demarcated mass with sharp borders suggestive of a benign mass is seen. On ultrasound examination, one also sees a solid mass but frequently notes small cystic spaces within the tumor.[32] The combination of these two findings is not apparent in standard infiltrating carcinoma of the breast. Putting all these clinical and radiologic factors together, it should be possible to make a clinical diagnosis of cystosarcoma phyllodes with great reliability. The clinical features that distinguish cystosarcoma from epithelial carcinoma of the breast are summarized in Table 14–3.

The clinical behavior of this tumor is variable and somewhat unpredictable. Some small and relatively innocent-appearing tumors will go on to produce metastases and will have a fatal outcome, while other very large and aggressive-looking tumors may pursue an innocent course following local excision. In an effort to make sense of this capricious clinical behavior, many researchers have attempted to histologically grade cystosarcoma into benign and malignant subtypes based on the appearance of the stromal component of the tumor; the epithelial component is malignant in very few cases.[33] The criteria that have been used are fourfold (Table 14–4). First, the tumor edge or border is considered. A well-demarcated, or pushing, border tends to be associated with benign tumors, while an infiltrative border is

TABLE 14–2. Axillary Node Involvement in Cystosarcoma Phyllodes

Author	Axillary Node Involvement*
Pietruszka and Barnes[4]	0/42
Oberman[23]	0/18
Treves[24]	0/93
Norris and Taylor[26]	2/94
Contarini et al.[28]	0/40
West[30]	0/29
Halverson et al.[31]	1/16
Total	3/332 (.9%)

*Involvement on axillary dissection or subsequent clinical involvement if axilla was not dissected.

TABLE 14–3. Clinical and Radiographic Distinction Between Cystosarcoma Phyllodes and Infiltrating Ductal Carcinoma

Criteria	*Cystosarcoma*	*Ductal Cancer*
Size	Often massive	Rarely massive
Rate of growth	Sometimes rapid	Rarely rapid
Lymph nodes	Rarely found	Frequent
Skin	Stretched, not invaded	Invaded often by large tumors
Pectoral fascia	Not fixed	Frequently fixed if tumor is large
Age	Younger	Older
Mammogram	Smooth border	Spiculated border
Ultrasound	Cystic spaces	Solid mass

more commonly associated with malignant tumors. Second, the amount of mitotic activity within the tumor should be considered. Tumors with four or fewer mitoses per high-power field have been considered benign. Third, the degree of cellular atypia in the stroma is considered. Fourth, the rapidity of growth of the cellular stroma can be considered.[23] If the stromal growth has been so rapid as to outpace that of the epithelial component, producing large areas of tumor devoid of epithelium-lined spaces, the lesion should be regarded with suspicion. Despite use of these criteria, some lesions defy inclusion into one category or another. Thus, a group of so-called borderline tumors have been defined as lying in between the obviously benign and the obviously malignant tumors. The incidence of benign, borderline, and malignant cystosarcomas is presented in Table 14–5, and the correlation of histologic grade with recurrence and survival is summarized in Table 14–6.

Estrogen receptors have been studied in two small series, with conflicting results. Kesterson and colleagues[34] studied six cases of cystosarcoma phyllodes, and none were positive for estrogen or progesterone receptors. In contrast, Porton and Poortman[35] studied eight cases, and four were positive for estrogen receptor. However, no reported responses to hormonal therapy have been published in the literature. An interesting observation concerning the degree of malignancy of cystosarcoma and its relation to fertility was made by McDivitt and associates,[25] who noted lower fertility in patients with malignant cystosarcoma. This finding was echoed by Lindquist and colleagues,[36] who studied ten patients with recurrent or metastatic cystosarcoma from the Mayo Clinic. Five of the ten had histologically malignant tumors, and all five were nulliparous. This observation may indicate some interaction between cystosarcoma and the hormonal environment, but as yet this interaction is undefined.

As difficult as it is to predict the behavior of cystosarcoma phyllodes on the basis of permanent sections of tumor, it is even more difficult to plan therapy from the results of aspiration cytology or frozen section. McDivitt and colleagues[25] looked at 35 patients with cystosarcoma who had aspiration cytology. In 18 patients (51 percent), a correct interpretation of benign or malignant tumor was made. In 12 patients (34 percent), the aspiration was labeled insufficient for diagnosis, and in five patients (14 percent), an incorrect diagnosis was made. Two benign tumors were interpreted as malignant on cytologic criteria, and three malignant tumors were interpreted as benign. These investigators then evaluated the accuracy of frozen

TABLE 14–4. Criteria for Histologic Classification

	Benign	*Borderline*	*Malignant*
Borders	Pushing	Mostly pushing	Infiltrating
Cellular atypia	Sight	Moderate	Marked
Mitoses/10 HPF	0–4	5–9	10 or more
Stromal growth	Slow	—	Rapid

From Pietruszka M, Barnes L: Cystosarcoma phyllodes: A clinicopathologic analysis of 42 cases. Cancer 41:1974, 1978, and Norris HJ, Taylor HB: Relationship of histologic features to behavior of cystosarcoma phyllodes. Cancer 20:2090, 1967.

TABLE 14–5. Distribution of Histologic Subtypes in Cystosarcoma Phyllodes

Author	No. of Patients	Benign	Borderline	Malignant
Haagensen[1]	64	58	—	6
Pietruszka and Barnes[4]	42	18	5	19
Treves[24]				
1951	77	41	18	18
1963	93	73	5	15
McDivitt et al.[25]	73	59	—	14
Contarini et al.[28]	40	23	—	17
Schmidtet al.[29]	24	21	—	3
West et al.[30]	29	23	—	6
Halverson and Hori-Rubaina[31]	16	2	6	8
Total	458	318 (69%)	34 (7%)	106 (23%)

section diagnosis in 56 patients. In 46 patients (82 percent), a correct diagnosis of benign versus malignant was made. However, 32 of these 46 patients were simply diagnosed as having benign tumor, and the fact that the tumor was a cystosarcoma phyllodes was unrecognized. Since the extent of surgical excision would be different based on whether the tumor was a benign fibroadenoma (enucleation) or a benign cystosarcoma phyllodes (wide excision), the frozen section diagnosis in these cases might have meant that the patient would have to be returned to the operating room at a later date for additional surgery. Seven patients in this series had the diagnosis of cystosarcoma phyllodes made on frozen section, but whether the tumor was benign or malignant could not be determined. Two patients had a completely erroneous frozen section diagnosis; 1 of 49 benign cystosarcomas was interpreted as malignant, and one of seven malignant tumors was interpreted as benign.

TABLE 14–6. Correlation of Histologic Factors With Recurrence and Survival in Cystosarcoma Phyllodes

Histologic Criteria	% Recurrence	% Dead of Tumor
Margin		
Pushing	15	3
Infiltrating	38	35
Atypism		
+1	27	7
+2	36	24
+3	40	25
Mitotic Activity		
0–4	18	6
5–9	31	15
Over 9	45	28

From Norris HJ, Taylor HB: Relationships of histologic features to behavior of cystosarcoma phyllodes. Cancer 20:2090, 1967.

TREATMENT

The treatment of cystosarcoma phyllodes is not completely defined, and even within the same institution, some researchers recommend radical surgery,[24] while others recommend conservative surgery.[25] The general consensus in the literature is that patients with benign cystosarcoma phyllodes should be treated with wide local excision, taking at least 1- to 2-cm margin of normal breast tissue in all directions. The margins of resection should be carefully examined for any histologic evidence of tumor. As mentioned previously, to enucleate a cystosarcoma or to excise it with very narrow margins invites local recurrence. In the literature, local recurrence following local excision is reported to occur in 10 to 20 percent of cases (Table 14–7). However, there are virtually no comments as to how wide these local excisions actually were or how carefully surgical margins were examined. In the vast majority of cases, cystosarcoma is not a multifocal disease, and a careful wide local excision should suffice for therapy, especially in a benign tumor. It must be appreciated that if a patient presents with a large tumor, a wide local excision may in fact be equivalent to a total mastectomy. In patients in whom a wide local excision would involve a grossly disfiguring operation of the breast, a total mastectomy may best serve the patient cosmetically, as she would then be a candidate for immediate or delayed surgical reconstruction of the breast. For patients with malignant cystosarcoma, the recommended therapy is either careful wide excision or total mastec-

TABLE 14–7. Local Recurrence in Cystosarcoma Phyllodes

Treatment	Histology		
	BENIGN	BORDERLINE	MALIGNANT
Local excision	24/129 (19%)	3/5 (60%)	6/21 (29%)
Total mastectomy	0/20	0/5	6/17 (35%)
Radical mastectomy	0/17	1/1	2/31 (6%)

Compiled from references 1, 4, 23, 25, 28, 29, 30, and 31.

tomy, with the latter having the greater number of recommendations in the literature. There is little need to perform a modified radical mastectomy, as the incidence of lymph node involvement in this tumor is vanishingly small. The local recurrence rate following mastectomy in malignant cystosarcoma is approximately 10 percent (Table 14–7).

The ability of radiation therapy to lower the rate of local recurrence is undefined. There is little question that for sarcomas in most other sites in the body, postoperative irradiation following wide tumor removal reduces the incidence of recurrence.[37, 38] Several series in the literature report an occasional patient with cystosarcoma treated in such a fashion. However, too few patients have been so treated to draw conclusions. Nonetheless, standard treatment for sarcomas at other sites in the body does entail the use of postoperative irradiation, and this treatment should be kept in mind for patients with malignant cystosarcomas, especially if surgical margins are close or positive. The overall survival rate in cystosarcoma phyllodes is more than 80 to 90 percent at five years, depending on the mix of benign and malignant tumors seen.

A difficult disease to treat is metastatic cystosarcoma, which is seen in approximately 25 percent of malignant cases and rarely in a histologically benign case (one fourth of the 25 percent of cases showing malignancy gives an overall metastatic rate of 5 to 10 percent). Virtually all metastases of cystosarcoma involve exclusively the sarcomatous component of the tumor, although occasional reports of both the sarcomatous and the epithelial component being present in a metastasis have been published.[24, 30] Hoover and associates[39] report a case with a transient response to cyclophosphamide and radiation therapy. Contarini and colleagues[28] describe a single patient being treated with a multidrug regimen including doxorubicin. No response data are given. Most metastatic sarcomas of other sites are treated with doxorubicin-containing regimens, with response rates of approximately 20 percent. Such therapy should be tried in metastatic cystosarcoma when systemic therapy is considered desirable. In addition, it is now clear that sarcoma metastatic to the lung is amenable to thoracotomy even if there are multiple tumor nodules. Such therapy for malignant cystosarcoma phyllodes has not been reported in the literature, most probably because of the rarity of the disease and the relatively recent onset of aggressive surgical approaches to pulmonary metastases. However, such therapy should be kept in mind for the patient with malignant cystosarcoma who is free from metastatic disease at other sites and who has a small number of pulmonary nodules that could be excised.

Angiosarcoma

DEFINITION

Angiosarcoma is the most virulent and lethal of all breast sarcomas. First described by Schmidt in 1887,[41] the tumor has since taken on a number of synonyms. Hemangioblastoma,[42] hemangiosarcoma,[43] and malignant hemangioendothelioma[44] are some of the other names used to descibe this lesion. The clinical symptoms and signs associated with this tumor are presented in Table 14–8. Noteworthy is the fact that the median age at presentation for this tumor is between 35 and 40 years, 15 to 20 years younger than for

TABLE 14–8. Symptoms and Signs of Angiosarcoma

Painless mass
Often rapid enlargement
Young age—median 35 to 40 years
Bluish discoloration if mass near skin

invasive ductal carcinoma. Patients present with a painless mass and often give a history of rapid enlargement. Although the tumor rarely invades the skin, as it approaches the skin a characteristic bluish discoloration can be seen through the skin. All of the tumors reported in the literature have presented as a gross mass, and no case of an incidental microscopic angiosarcoma has yet been published. On gross examination, the tumor is an ill-defined spongy hemorrhagic mass that is unencapsulated. Typically, these tumors are between 2 and 10 cm in diameter, with a median size of 4 to 5 cm.[45, 46]

Spread patterns from angiosarcomas of the breast are typical of other sarcomatous lesions elsewhere in the body. Nodal spread is extraordinarily rare, and there has only been one reported case in the literature.[47] The most common route of spread is systemic metastases, with the lung being the most common site. Occasionally, the tumor is bilateral,[46, 48] but it is difficult to distinguish true bilaterality from metastases to the contralateral breast.

Pathologic Diagnosis

Two of the most difficult and controversial aspects of the management of patients with angiosarcoma of the breast concern the histopathologic characteristics of the tumor. First, it is important to differentiate low-grade angiosarcoma from benign angiomas of the breast. The diagnosis of malignancy rests on three factors: the presence of interanastomosing vascular channels, the presence of hyperchromatic endothelial cells, and the presence of these vessels within the parenchyma of the breast. Benign tumors lack these interanastomosing patterns, lack hyperchromatic endothelial cells, and do not spread their vessels into the breast parenchyma. While the ability to differentiate benign from malignant lesions may sound straightforward on paper, in practice such a differentiation presents problems. In two recent reviews, over one third of the patients with angiosarcoma originally had their lesion classified as benign, and its malignant nature was brought to light only by local recurrence.[48, 49] Thus, great care must be taken when examining a gross lesion that appears to be a benign angioma to make sure that it is not, in reality, a low-grade angiosarcoma. Merino and colleagues[45] point out that most benign hemangiomas are incidental findings and are less likely to produce a gross clinically detectable mass.

The second important issue concerning the pathology of angiosarcoma is the ability to grade the tumor and the prognostic significance of such grades. Merino[45] studied 15 cases from the State of Connecticut Tumor Registry and noted that the six deaths that occurred in this series were all in patients with grades 2 and 3 tumors. The five patients who had Grade 1 tumors were all alive, although one was living with tumor. The mean survival of their Grade 1 cases was artificially prolonged by a single patient who was alive and well 24 years beyond treatment. A more convincing case for the role of tumor grade in the survival of patients with angiosarcoma is presented by Donnell and colleagues.[46] They studied 40 patients from Memorial Hospital and established a set of pathologic criteria that could be used to differentiate between low-grade and high-grade tumors (Table 14–9). The first three entries in this table form the pathologic basis for the diagnosis of angiosarcoma and are present in both low-grade and high-grade lesions, while the other criteria help to distinguish one grade from the other. The researchers emphasize that there is great variability between one area of an angiosarcoma and another, and thus, there is a need to examine multiple sections to appreciate the true grade. They report that patients with low-grade tumors had a 77 percent disease-free survival rate at five years, whereas patients with high-grade tumors had only an 11 percent survival rate.

TABLE 14–9. Pathologic Characteristics of Angiosarcoma

Characteristic	*Low Grade*	*High Grade*
Interanastomosing channels	Yes	Yes
Hyperchromatic endothelial cells	Yes	Yes
Involves parenchyma	Yes	Yes
Endothelial tufting	Minimal	Prominent
Papillary formations	No	Yes
Foci of solid and spindle cells	No	Yes
Mitoses	Rare	Yes
Blood lakes	No	Yes
Necrosis	No	Yes

From Donnell RM, Rosen PP, Lieberman PH, et al.: Angiosarcoma and other vascular tumors of the breast—pathologic analysis as a guide to prognosis. Am J Surg Pathol 5:629, 1981.

Treatment

Treatment of angiosarcoma is usually by total mastectomy. Since the lymph nodes are so rarely involved, no deliberate effort to perform axillary dissection need be made. Whether local radiation therapy to the chest wall should follow tumor excision in angiosarcoma of the breast is unclear. In the large series from Memorial Hospital,[46] approximately 25 percent of the patients had local recurrence following mastectomy, and these were mostly in patients with Grade 3 tumors. Since radiation therapy has been shown to decrease local recurrence in sarcomas of the extremities following wide tumor removal,[37, 38] some investigators are routinely adding chest wall irradiation to the treatment of angiosarcoma.[49] At the National Cancer Institute, all patients with malignant breast sarcomas receive chest wall irradiation. However, because of the rarity of this lesion, it cannot be stated with certainty that such irradiation is helpful in decreasing local recurrence or in prolonging survival.

Chemotherapy for angiosarcoma of the breast has been reported by two groups. The group at Memorial Hospital[46] tried actinomycin D as a single agent, and while there was a suggestion of activity of this agent, the number of patients was far too small to be convincing.[50] A report from Boston[49] discussed five patients who received doxorubicin as a single agent or as part of a combination of drugs. Again, with such a small number of patients it is extremely difficult to form any conclusions as to the usefulness of chemotherapy. Two of the five patients treated with doxorubicin were alive without evidence of disease at 20 and 38 months following treatment. It should be recognized, however, that metastatic spread in this tumor is so frequent and survival is so poor, especially in patients with high-grade lesions, that some form of systemic therapy will be essential to alter the natural history of this tumor. Therefore, efforts to employ adjuvant chemotherapy in treating angiosarcoma of the breast should be encouraged.

Survival

The overall survival rate in angiosarcoma of the breast is difficult to ascertain, since most published papers contain only two or three cases. A literature review by Chen and colleagues[48] stated that the three-year survival rate was 38 percent and the three-year disease-free survival rate was only 14 percent. Modern series report somewhat better results. Merino and associates[45] report a 53 percent survival rate at three years and a 40 percent disease-free survival rate. The group from Memorial Hospital[46] reports a three-year disease-free survival rate of 41 percent and a five-year disease-free survival rate of 33 percent. However, most of the long-term survivors have low-grade tumors, and the survival rate of patients with Grade 3 tumors is only 11 percent. The improvement in survival in modern series may simply be due to better recognition of low-grade tumors that were previously called benign hemangiomas. Since these patients do relatively well, addition of more Grade 1 tumors to any series would improve the overall outcome of the series without truly reflecting an improvement in treatment. Patients with low-grade tumors should be treated with total mastectomy and can probably be followed with no additional irradiation or chemotherapy. Patients with high-grade tumors should be treated with total mastectomy followed by irradiation to the chest wall to prevent local recurrence. Efforts at treating high-grade tumors with adjuvant chemotherapy should be encouraged and will require the resources of cooperative groups to accrue enough patients for meaningful analysis.

BREAST CANCER OCCURRING DURING PREGNANCY

The simultaneous occurrence of pregnancy and breast cancer represents one of the more challenging clinical problems in the treatment of breast cancer. Not only must the clinician be concerned about treating the malignancy with appropriate aggressiveness, but the effects of these therapies on the fetus must also be considered. Whether to terminate the pregnancy, treat the malignancy during the pregnancy, or delay therapy until fetal viability is likely is one of the most difficult decisions confronting oncologists. Furthermore, the relative rarity of the condition means that most reports in the literature are based on relatively few cases accrued over many years and treated in a variety of ways.

Incidence and Epidemiology

In a large retrospective literature review, Wallack and associates[51] have documented that breast cancer associated with pregnancy or lactation accounts for 1 to 2 percent of all breast cancers. Torres and Mickal[52] reviewed the literature on 416,000 pregnancies and noted 91 breast cancer cases, roughly one case in every 5000 pregnancies. The average age of patients is 34 years.

There is little question that delay in diagnosis plays a prominent role in this disease. Breast enlargement tends to obscure small masses, and many detectable and enlarging masses are attributed to benign or physiologic changes. At times, a mass detected in early pregnancy may become less prominent as the breast enlarges, giving the false impression that the mass has resolved and delaying a needed biopsy. Many clinicians are hesitant to obtain a mammogram on a pregnant patient for fear of radiation exposure to the fetus. With modern low-dose mammography, in the case of a *suspicious* finding on breast examination, such fear is unjustified. However, the density of breast tissue changes during pregnancy, making mammography less sensitive than in the nonpregnant patient.[51] Overall, delays in obtaining a biopsy average two to four months longer than in the nonpregnant population. Patient delay in seeking biopsy of a mass that is self-detected adds an additional three to six months to the diagnostic delay in pregnant and lactating females.[53–55]

Such delay probably contributes, in part, to the relatively advanced stage at presentation of pregnancy-associated breast cancer. Whereas the nonpregnant population presents with positive nodes roughly 45 to 50 percent of the time, pregnant and lactating females are discovered to have positive nodes in 65 to 85 percent of cases (Table 14–10). However, it is unlikely that simply delaying diagnosis for a few months completely accounts for the preponderance of advanced-stage gestational breast cancer.

A great deal of speculation has taken place concerning the hormonal and immunologic changes of pregnancy and their possible role in promoting breast cancer growth. Obviously, the marked elevation of estrogens and progesterone[62] may serve to stimulate a hormonally responsive tumor. However, clinical data from centers where abortion, with or without castration, has been practiced as part of the treatment of gestational breast cancer fail to show an improvement in outcome.[61] These data have suggested to some investigators that hormonally dependent breast cancers are infrequent during pregnancy.[63] Of course, it is possible that the high hormonal levels have acted as a promoter of a cancer that has become hormonally independent by the time of clinical detection.

Prolactin is another hormone whose elevation during pregnancy may influence the development of breast cancer. In rats, prolactin is protective against drug-induced breast cancer if present prior to the administration of the carcinogen.[64] However, if prolactin is introduced after the carcinogen, it may promote tumor growth. Hobbs and associates[65] have reported on a patient with gestational breast cancer whose tumor was responsive *in vitro* to prolactin and to human placental lactogen. Abortion produced a dramatic response in this instance, suggesting that hormone dependency exists in some gestational breast cancers.

Profound immunologic changes occurring during pregnancy may facilitate cancer growth. Pregnancy itself requires a state of

TABLE 14–10. Axillary Node Involvement In Pregnancy-Associated Breast Cancer

Author	*No. of Patients*	*Axilla-Positive Patients (%)*	*Axilla-Negative Patients (%)*
Haagensen[55]	48	33 (69)	15 (31)
Ribeiro and Palmer[56]	88	78 (89)	10 (11)
Clark and Reid[57]	121*	(83)	(17)
Holleb and Farrow[58]	117	86 (74)	31 (26)
White[59]	30	22 (73)	8 (27)
Rosemond[60]	37	23 (62)	14 (38)
Donegan[61]	24	17 (71)	7 (29)

*Not all patients were staged.

"immune tolerance" to avoid "rejection" of the fetus, which contains foreign (nonhost) tissue. If an occult breast cancer expressed a surface antigen that was similar to some fetal antigens, it might enjoy a measure of immunologic protection during pregnancy that would, in theory, permit rapid growth.[66] The elevation of corticosteroids and progestins that occurs in pregnant women may further compromise the immune status of the pregnant patient with breast cancer.

Diagnosis and Staging

The indications for biopsy of a breast mass during pregnancy are identical to the indications for breast biopsy in the nonpregnant patient. Needle aspiration of a benign cyst can be both diagnostic and therapeutic. Any solid mass must be biopsied, often starting with aspiration cytology but proceeding to excisional biopsy if the results of the cytologic examination are negative. Such excisions can be performed under local anesthesia, with minimal risk to mother or fetus. The chances of finding a carcinoma are similar to statistics quoted for the general nonpregnant population,[67] and the histologic types of cancers seen are no different from those in nonpregnant patients.[51]

Mammography is applicable to pregnant patients in whom clinical findings are suspicious. With appropriate abdominal shielding and modern film-screen techniques, the radiation dose to the fetus should be almost too small to measure. In one series, 368 pregnant women undergoing mammography had no apparent damage to the fetus.[68] Pregnant women have contact with physicians every one to two months. With appropriate breast examinations and a healthy index of suspicion, the unacceptable delay in diagnosis reported in most series of pregnancy-associated breast cancer could be greatly reduced or eliminated.

Once the diagnosis of breast cancer is established, the disease must be staged and a therapeutic plan developed. The tumor (T-stage) and lymph node (N-stage) examinations are no different from those for the nonpregnant patient. The amount of systemic work-up necessary and the risk of that work-up to the fetus are more controversial areas, especially in light of the fact that all staging studies, aside from blood work, involve radiation exposure. An understanding of radiation risks to the fetus is necessary to properly evaluate the role of staging x-rays and scans.

Developmental time *in utero* can be divided into three phases[69]:

1. Days 0 to 10, a preimplantation phase from fertilization to embryonic implantation in the uterine wall.
2. Days 11 to 56, the organogenesis phase, during which time the major organ systems develop.
3. Day 57 and beyond, the fetal stage when additional growth occurs.

Irradiation delivered during the preimplantation phase can result in the death of the embryo. As little as 10 rad can be lethal in the mouse.[69] However, those embryos that survive irradiation during this period appear to develop normally. Irradiation during organogenesis can lead to major developmental malformations. In humans, the most frequently noted defect is microcephaly, although other problems have been reported. Radiation doses of 10 rad or less may be sufficient to produce a measurable increase in birth defects, and doses exceeding 100 rad produced congenital abnormalities 100 percent of the time in the atomic bomb experience.[70] While exposure before week nine is most likely to produce damage, large doses of radiation at 16 to 20 weeks may lead to mental retardation and growth stunting. Irradiation after weeks 25 to 30 is far less likely to produce abnormalities.[71]

With these time frames and dose ranges in mind, it is reasonable to conclude that any radiologic staging procedure that is deemed necessary and significant for the pregnant patient with breast cancer is probably safe for the fetus, with respect to congenital malformation, especially during the second half of the gestational period. The uterine dose from a chest x-ray is less than one tenth of a rad. A liver scan will give only 20 millirad to the fetus, while a bone scan will deliver only 100 millirad.[51]

The other major risk to the fetus from radiation exposure is carcinogenesis. Several studies have shown that doses of 1 to 4 rad *in utero* can increase the risk of cancer by 40 to 50 percent.[72, 73] However, it is not clear whether these women who had abnormalities or injuries requiring x-rays are a select group of women whose children were destined to have a higher risk of malignancy secondary to the mother's illness. The association between fetal radiation exposure and cancer has not been clearly shown in data from the atomic bomb experience.[74] Conversely, in a recent study of twins, those twins who developed cancer or leukemia were twice as likely to have been exposed to x-rays *in utero* as were control sets of twins.[75] Thus, the data on the carcinogenic effect of radiation *in utero* remain controversial, and it is best to be conservative in ordering x-ray studies on pregnant patients.

Therapy

In general, mastectomy is the preferred treatment for the patient with operable gestational breast cancer. Such a procedure carries minimal risk to the mother or the fetus, and the pregnancy can be allowed to continue. There is little evidence to suggest that abortion is therapeutic in gestational breast cancer[61] (Table 14–11); thus, the decision to terminate the pregnancy must be based on considerations other than abortion's influence on the outcome of the disease, such as the overall prognosis, the need for radiation therapy, or the need for chemotherapy. Similarly, the temptation to assume that a rapidly growing gestational breast cancer is hormonally responsive and thus to recommend oophorectomy is not generally supported by clinical or laboratory data, except in isolated case reports. In a compilation of estrogen receptor data from 11 patients with pregnancy-associated breast cancer, 7 of 11 were ER-negative, 3 of 11 were borderline, and only 1 was ER-positive.[51] However, high circulating hormonal levels may have obscured receptor sites by occupation with endogenous ligand. Castration need not be performed in cases of gestational breast cancer, unless receptor data are strongly suggestive of estrogen dependency.

Some pregnant women with operable breast cancer will ask about the possibility of treatment with excision plus irradiation, preserving the intact breast. Using the standard irradiation technique of whole-breast irradiation followed by a boost dose to the tumor bed, the dose scattered to the fetus would be unacceptably high. Dose outside the radiation beam (peripheral dose) comes from two sources[76]: (1) internal scatter within the body, and (2) leakage radiation from the head of the machine. Leakage radiation must legally be below 0.1 percent of the primary dose at 1 m from the target. It is independent of field size or beam energy but can be modified by external blocking. Thus, irradiating a woman whose pelvis is protected by a block of lead can easily reduce the leakage dose by a factor of four or more. If 5000 rad is prescribed, the leakage dose can be reduced from 5 rad to less than 2 rad.

Internal scatter is dependent on field size, photon energy, and proximity to the field edge. No shielding can modify this scatter. Early in fetal life, when the distance from the breast to the top of the uterus is great, the internal scatter dose may be 10 to 20 rad for a total course of treatment. Later in the pregnancy, when the top of the uterus approaches the xyphoid, doses of 100 rad or more may be given. Obviously, the internal scatter dose carries an element of risk, and whole breast x-ray treatment is not advisable during pregnancy.

There are possible breast-conserving alternatives for women who are extremely desirous of this option and have a mass small enough to permit local excision. First, one could widely excise the tumor, perform an axillary dissection, and not give irradiation. The literature suggests that in the nonpregnant population, approximately 30 percent of patients treated in this manner will experience a local recurrence.[77] If women so treated have a recurrence in the breast, they

TABLE 14–11. Pregnancy-Associated Breast Cancer—Results of Abortion

Author	5-Year Survival	
	ABORTION*	NO ABORTION
Clark and Reid[57]	2/13 (15%)	27/93 (29%)
Holeb and Farrow[58]	2/12 (17%)	4/12 (33%)
Rissanen[88]	3/8 (38%)	10/23 (43%)

*Authors report "no bias" in selecting patients for this procedure.

are then treated with mastectomy. However, such recurrences do not appear to jeopardize survival and there is a two-thirds chance that no recurrence will develop and breast preservation will be achieved.[77] It must be emphasized that a series on partial mastectomies in the pregnant population has *not* been reported, and such treatment could be considerably more hazardous in this setting than in the nonpregnant patient.

Alternatively, one could conceivably excise the breast mass and irradiate the tumor bed with an electron beam, using a small boost field to a dose of 2000 to 2500 rad, shielding the pelvis from leakage radiation. After delivery of the fetus, whole breast irradiation with x-rays could be performed. Such a strategy would deliver less than 2 rad to the fetus, since the internal scatter dose would be very small. This scatter dose still may be too high, but it is far better than the 10 to 100 rad that would be given with standard techniques.

Finally, in women with very large primary tumors, unresectable tumors, or positive axillary nodes, one could begin treatment with systemic chemotherapy. In a nonpregnant population treated at the National Cancer Institute, such a strategy has resulted in an objective response rate of over 90 percent.[78] Women who have achieved a complete response have been treated with irradiation to the breast and regional nodes without mastectomy. The local control rate in that group has been 100 percent.[78]

The literature on the use of chemotherapy during pregnancy is rather sparse when it comes to combination chemotherapy. Single agents, when given during the second or third trimester, appear to be relatively safe, except for methotrexate.[79] However, 10 to 20 percent of infants who were exposed to chemotherapeutic agents *in utero* during the first trimester will have congenital malformations.[79, 80] Combinations of drugs given for acute leukemia, usually including cytosine arabinoside and an anthracycline, have proved safe in small numbers of patients.[81–83] Whether combinations of drugs commonly used to treat breast cancer can be employed with safety during pregnancy is as yet unknown. A recent report by Murray and colleagues[84] details a woman who received doxorubicin plus cyclophosphamide, along with radiation to the axilla and the supraclavicular and internal mammary areas, during her first trimester of pregnancy. The resulting full-term fetus had an imperforate anus, a rectovaginal fistula, and a head circumference under the fifth percentile but is "doing well" at four years of age.

As a general guide, the following treatment recommendations can be offered:

1. *Operable Breast Cancer:* Mastectomy with or without breast reconstruction. Pregnancy may continue to term if desired. A second choice would be excision alone with or without electron-beam boost, waiting until term to deliver whole-breast irradiation in a breast-conserving manner.

2. *Locally Advanced Disease:* If pregnancy is early, termination of pregnancy is desirable; breast cancer is then treated in a standard fashion. If pregnancy is late, cesarean-section delivery should be performed as soon as possible, followed by standard treatment. For the inoperable patient who refuses to terminate the pregnancy and is still many weeks from fetal viability, chemotherapy without methotrexate should be considered in an effort to shrink the tumor and possibly to permit definitive surgery. Irradiation could also be considered if the pregnancy is beyond 20 weeks. The risks of such therapy on fetal development must be weighed against the risks encountered by observing an advanced untreated breast cancer for several weeks.

3. *Node-Positive Breast Cancer:* Chemotherapy is recommended after mastectomy for node-positive patients. Since a delay between the performance of mastectomy and the institution of chemotherapy may reduce the effectiveness of adjuvant chemotherapy,[85, 86] such treatment should be employed as soon after mastectomy as possible. In pregnant patients, cesarean section followed by chemotherapy is recommended. If fetal viability is several weeks away, chemotherapy should be considered prior to delivery.

Results of Therapy

Tables 14–12 and 14–13 show the results of treatment for a number of series all performed prior to the era of adjuvant chemotherapy. The overall results of treatment are poor, with 30 to 35 percent surviving five years in most series. However, the overall total is weighted with the preponderance of node-positive patients. In node-negative patients, the five-year survival rate is 65 to 85 percent, which approaches that of the non-

TABLE 14–12. Results of Treatment of Pregnancy-Associated Breast Cancer

Author	No. of Patients	5-Year Survival Positive Nodes (%)	Negative Nodes (%)	Overall (%)
Haagensen[54]	48	3	53	19
Ribeiro and Palmer[56]	88	28	90	34
Clark and Reid[57]	121	—	—	31
Holleb and Farrow[58]	117	17	65	30
White[59]	30	5	50	16
Donegan[61]	34	31	86	48
Drosby and Barclay[87]	29	29	63	38
Rissanen[88]	88	27	80	42

pregnant population. These data present the strongest argument of all for carefully screening pregnant patients for breast masses and for proceeding with diagnostic biopsy or aspiration early rather than late. Increasing the percentage of patients who present with node-negative disease would have a marked impact on overall outcome.

BREAST CANCER PRESENTING AS AXILLARY ADENOPATHY

Carcinoma presenting in lymph nodes without an identifiable primary tumor is a well-recognized clinical situation. Most commonly, the lymph nodes contain squamous cell carcinoma and are located in the neck. The primary sites are the oral cavity, nasopharynx, oropharynx, hypopharynx, and larynx.[89] Rarely, a patient will present with axillary adenopathy that contains adenocarcinoma. Primary tumors to be considered in such cases are melanoma, thyroid carcinoma, lung carcinoma, renal cell carcinoma, gastrointestinal cancers, and ovarian carcinoma.[90] In a female patient, however, breast cancer is the most likely diagnosis for a primary site that produces axillary adenocarcinoma. Such cases were recognized as long ago as the turn of the century, when Halsted reported on three patients with axillary adenocarcinoma, all of whom subsequently developed breast cancer.[91] Since that time, a number of series have reported on this clinical situation. The relative rarity of its occurrence is summarized in Table 14–14, in which the incidences of axillary presentation of breast cancer from three large series are reported. Overall, slightly less than 0.5 percent of all breast cancer presents in this fashion. Put another way, 1 of every 227 patients with breast cancer will present with axillary metastasis and no readily identifiable primary tumor.

When confronted with a patient who has axillary adenocarcinoma, an important question is what type of work-up to order and how far to search for the primary tumor. After a careful physical examination to search for other sites of lymph node involvement and especially to look for small pigmented lesions that may represent melanoma, mammography should be the first screening test. The results of mammography in this situation are quite variable; for example, Patel and colleagues[95] report that over 50 percent of patients have their occult breast primary tumors identified by mammography. Similarly, Westbrook and Gallager[96] report a relatively high yield from mammography. However, Ashikari[90] noted that in 25 patients who had mammography following a biopsy of axillary adenocarcinoma, 22 were reported as negative, three as suspicious, and none were

TABLE 14–13. Results by Stage in Pregnancy-Associated Breast Cancer

Author	5-Year Survival Stage I	II	III	IV
Ribeiro and Palmer[56]	90%	37%	15%	0%
Crosby and Barclay[87]	63%	38%	—	0%
Rissanen[88]	90%	80%	15%	0%

TABLE 14–14. Incidence of Axillary Presentation of Breast Cancer

Author	Incidence (%)
Haagensen[92]	18/6000 (0.3)
Owen et al.[93]	25/5451 (0.46)
Fitts et al.[94]	13/1300 (1.0)
Total	56/12751 (0.44)

TABLE 14–15. Success in Finding the Primary Tumor and Results in Axillary Presentation of Breast Cancer

Author	No. of Patients	Average Age	No. of Breast Cancers/No. of Mastectomies	5-Year Survival (%)
Ashikari et al.[90]	42	51	22/34 (65%)	79
Haagensen[92]	18	52	13/14 (93%)	57
Owen et al.[93]	25	49.9	15/25 (60%)	50
Fitts et al.[94]	13	54	11/13 (85%)	71
Patel et al.[95]	29	52	16/29 (55%)	28
Westbrook and Gallager[96]	18	57	9/12 (75%)	61
Total	145		86/127 (68%)	

reported as positive. Since most of the series reporting patients with axillary adenocarcinoma have extended over many years and the technical quality of mammography has improved since the 1970's, it is difficult to make a strong statement as to how many patients with axillary adenocarcinoma would have their breast primary tumor identified today with mammography. However, it is a relatively inexpensive test, with virtually no morbidity, and since the most likely site of primary cancer is the breast, it is inconceivable to think of managing a female with axillary adenocarcinoma without obtaining bilateral mammography. Additional work-up should include chest x-ray, bone scan, routine blood studies including liver function tests, a careful pelvic and rectal examination, head and neck examinations, and a thyroid examination. If the results of these studies are negative and if the patient has no symptoms referable to other organs, further work-up will probably not yield a positive result, and the patient should be considered to have an occult undetectable breast cancer. As pointed out by Feuerman and colleagues,[97] axillary nodal metastases may originate from a variety of primary sites, but aside from breast cancer, virtually all of these primary tumors are easily identified. Thus, studying the entire gastrointestinal tract via contrast studies or performing total body CT scans is almost certainly a waste of effort and resources and serves little diagnostic purpose.

Most women presenting with axillary adenocarcinoma have been treated with mastectomy. Table 14–15 summarizes the outcome from six large series. The median age of patients is similar to that of patients presenting with frankly invasive carcinoma. Following mastectomy, only two thirds of the breast specimens are found to actually contain identifiable breast cancer. At least three reasons can be cited to explain this observation. First, some breast carcinomas can be so small that they would be missed on routine sectioning of the breast. Serial step sectioning of the breast may identify additional cancers, but this is an extremely time-consuming and costly process. Second, the primary tumor may have regressed completely and may no longer be detectable. Third, the patient might not have had breast cancer but rather another type of carcinoma. The latter is highly unlikely, as there is not a single case report in the literature of a different type of primary tumor being discovered at a later date to be the cause of the adenopathy in a woman with axillary adenocarcinoma.

Survival results are rather mixed. Overall, one would expect that a population of women with node-positive breast cancer would have a five-year survival rate in the range of 35 to 45 percent. Several series report survival rates ranging from 60 to nearly 80 percent at five years, suggesting that patients who present with an occult primary tumor and clinically detectable axillary adenopathy have a much better outlook compared with women who have the same axillary disease but a clinically detectable breast tumor. The report from Patel and colleagues[95] stands in contrast with this, with a 28 percent disease-free survival rate at five years and a 17 percent rate at ten years. However, this report stands alone. In general, one is led to the conclusion that because of biologic principles yet to be explained, patients who present only with axillary adenopathy do indeed have a significantly brighter outlook than do patients treated for routine node-positive breast cancer.

In the literature, there are two reported experiences with radiation therapy for occult

TABLE 14–16. Treatment of Axillary Adenocarcinoma With Irradiation

No. of patients	11
NED*	7
Local recurrence—mastectomy—NED*	2 (11 and 14 years after treatment)
Died of metastases—local control	1
Died of metastases—local recurrence	1

*NED, no evidence of disease.

From Vilcoq JR, Calle R, Ferme F, et al.: Conservative treatment of axillary adenopathy due to probable subclinical breast cancer. Arch Surg 117:1136, 1982.

breast cancer without mastectomy. Westbrook and Gallager[96] reported five patients so treated, four of whom subsequently died of metastatic breast cancer. This result indicates either that this treatment is not effective or that selection of patients to be treated with radiation therapy assembled an extremely poor-risk group. Vilcoq and associates[98] report an interesting series from the Institute Curie in Paris, in which 11 patients with axillary adenocarcinoma were treated with radiation therapy alone, without mastectomy or axillary dissection. Their results are summarized in Table 14–16. Of the 11 patients treated with a minimum follow-up of five years, seven are alive without disease. An eighth patient died of widely disseminated breast cancer but had locoregional control of tumor. There were three patients with local recurrences. In two patients, local recurrences appeared at 11 and 14 years following irradiation, perhaps suggesting that the tumors were new cancers. Both of these women underwent mastectomy at that point and are alive without evidence of disease. A third local recurrence at six years was reirradiated, but the patient died of widespread distant metastases. The overall survival rate in this group is 82 percent (9 of 11), and overall local control without mastectomy or axillary dissection was achieved in 8 of the 11 patients, suggesting that radiation therapy is a reasonable alternative to mastectomy in patients with occult breast cancer.

Recommendations for work-up and treatment of axillary adenocarcinoma in female patients are summarized in Table 14–17. Routine clinical investigation should complement careful history and physical examination, in ruling out likely sites of occult primary cancer. Other more sophisticated tests should be performed only on patients who are having identifiable symptoms referable to a particular organ system. Estrogen and progesterone receptor assays on the nodal tissue may further help establish the breast as the primary site. In our opinion, the axilla should be treated with complete axillary dissection. Not only will this operation treat the axilla and prevent local axillary recurrence, but also it will provide valuable prognostic information. As is basically the case in women with routine clinically evident breast cancer, women with occult breast cancer who have fewer lymph nodes have a better survival rate than that of women who have multiple positive nodes.[95] Breast treatment can be by one of two methods. Mastectomy has been used most often and has the advantage of allowing careful histologic inspection of the breast to identify the primary tumor. On the other hand, considerable experience has been gained in the treatment of breast cancer with primary irradiation (see Chapter 6). As it is almost certain that women who present with axillary adenocarcinoma have a breast cancer, it is reasonable to offer such patients breast irradiation, paralleling the philosophy of offering breast irradiation to patients who have had a clinically evident primary breast cancer excised. Although there has been reported only one small series of patients treated in that fashion, it is logical to assume that patients irradiated for occult breast cancer will have the same satisfactory outcome as patients irradiated for a clinically evident breast tumor.

TABLE 14–17. Work-up and Treatment Recommendations for Axillary Adenocarcinoma in the Female

Work-up:
- Mandatory:
  - History and physical examination
  - Careful examination of skin, thyroid, breasts, pelvis
  - Chest x-ray, blood work
  - Bilateral mammography
  - Bone scan
  - Hormone receptors on node tissue
- Optional based on symptoms:
  - CT of chest, abdomen, pelvis
  - GI tract contrast studies
  - Thyroid scan

Treatment:
- Axillary dissection with either mastectomy *or* breast irradiation

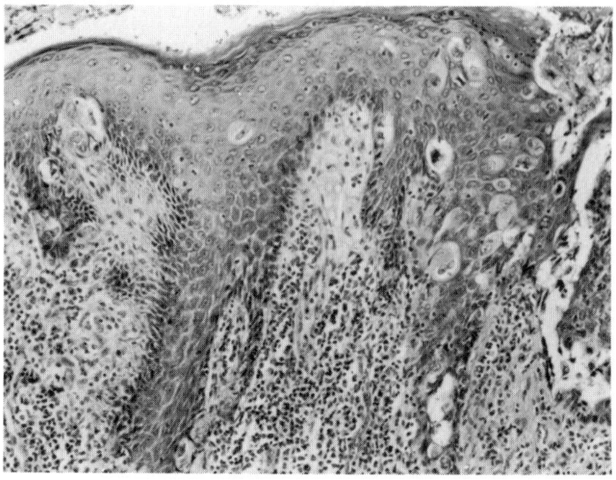

FIGURE 14–2. Paget's cells with large nuclei and abundant cytoplasm infiltrate dermis in this photomicrograph of Paget's disease.

PAGET'S DISEASE OF THE BREAST

DEFINITION

In 1874, Sir James Paget described 16 cases of a lesion of the nipple that proceeded to breast carcinoma.[99] He wrote:

> I believe it has not yet been published that certain chronic infections of the skin of the nipple and the areola are very often succeeded by the formation of scirrhous cancer in the mammary gland.... The patients were all women, various in age from 40 to 60 or more years, having in common nothing remarkable but their disease. In all of them the disease began as an eruption on the nipple and areola.... The sensations were commonly tingling, itching, and burning, but the malady was never attended by disturbance of the general health.... But it has happened that in every case which I have been able to watch, cancer of the mammary gland has followed within at the most 2 years and usually within 1 year.... In the cancers themselves I have seen in these cases nothing peculiar. They have been various in forms; some acute, some chronic, the majority following an average course, and all tending to the same end; recurring if removed, affecting lymph glands and distant parts, showing nothing which might not be written in the ordinary history of cancer of the breast. The single noteworthy fact found in all these cases is that which I have stated in the first sentence.

In essence, no more accurate description of the disease process has ever been written. The hallmark of this disease is the presence of intraepidermal Paget's cells in the nipple. Histologically, these are large cells with an abundant amount of pale cytoplasm and with large irregular hyperchromatic nuclei.[100] While these cells can appear singly, they often form clumps and are quite characteristic in their appearance (Fig. 14–2). In the overwhelming majority of cases, Paget's disease of the nipple is associated with an underlying breast cancer, of either intraductal or infiltrating type. Largely as a consequence of this association, it has been theorized that Paget's cells are special types of cells that originate from a ductal carcinoma and then, for reasons that are unknown, migrate up the large ducts toward the epidermis of the nipple. That Paget's cells stain for carcinoembryonic antigen confirms the fact that these are adenocarcinoma cells of glandular origin and eliminates some older theories that Paget's cells are altered melanocytes or that they represent an unusual form of squamous cell carcinoma.[101] However, some evidence would suggest that Paget's disease of the nipple can arise *de novo* in the epidermis of the nipple, without a direct connection to an underlying breast carcinoma. In most reported series of Paget's disease, there are one or two patients in whom a careful histologic search cannot disclose an underlying breast cancer.[102] While Haagensen states that these cases are explainable by the fact that an inadequate number of sections have been studied and the cancer simply went unnoticed,[100] in one of Haagensen's cases over 1000 sections of the breast were studied without detecting a cancer. Thus, there appear to be some cases in which an underlying carcinoma is not seen. In the series reported by Paone and Baker[103] from Johns Hopkins Hospital, six patients with Paget's disease had a tumor that was farther than 2 cm from the nipple, and no direct anatomic connection between these two lesions was seen, suggesting that the two tumors might have risen independently. In addition, cases of extramammary Paget's disease are well known and are, of course, unassociated with an underlying breast cancer, or with an underlying cancer of any type for that matter. Thus, Paget's disease can, on rare occasions, develop *in situ*.[102] As summarized by Azzopardi,[101] the two theories of the histogenesis of Paget's disease, migratory cells versus *de novo* appearance, are valid and not mutually exclusive. This type of discussion on the origin of Paget's cells is of more than aca-

TABLE 14–18. Clinical Presentations of Paget's Disease of the Breast

Author	No. of Patients	Nipple Changes Only	Nipple Changes Plus Mass	Mass Only
Haagensen[100]	133	56 (42%)	38 (29%)	39 (29%)
Maier et al.[104]	137	56 (42%)	67 (49%)	14 (10%)
Total	270	112 (41%)	105 (39%)	53 (20%)

demic interest. If all Paget's disease represents a migration of cells from deeper underlying cancer, local excision of the cancerous process would be a poor treatment choice. On the other hand, if some Paget's disease is truly a local process involving the nipple and, at most, the adjacent large ducts, local excision of the tumor may be a worthwhile treatment alternative. These considerations will be discussed later.

Diagnosis

Paget's disease should, in theory, be the easiest type of breast cancer to diagnose because it presents with early visible symptoms and signs. Patients will usually complain of pain, itching, discharge from the nipple, bleeding of the nipple, or some other significant change in sensation in the nipple. On examination, the nipple may simply be red, may show some roughness or thickening of its skin, or may show frank erosion. If the process becomes further advanced, the erosion can spread onto the areola. However, a skin lesion of the areola that does not involve the nipple cannot be Paget's disease. No doubt, an underlying tumor can involve the areola by direct extension, but Paget's disease always involves the nipple and begins with changes in the nipple.

One of the more treacherous aspects in the diagnosis of Paget's disease is the fact that the disease will often respond temporarily to symptomatic topical treatment.[100] Thus, it is not unusual for a patient to go from gynecologist to dermatologist and have a number of topical medications applied to what is thought to be a benign lesion. As stated, the lesion may actually improve but will invariably recur, only to be treated, to heal, and to recur again in continuing cycles. Haagensen noted an average duration of symptoms of 13 months, and the literature confirms that patients with Paget's disease have symptoms an average of 10 to 21 months before the disease is diagnosed.[103–106]

Clinically, patients tend to present in three broad categories: (1) the disease involves the nipple with no underlying palpable tumor; (2) the disease involves the nipple and there is a palpable mass, usually directly below the nipple; and (3) there is a mass in the breast that later shows Paget's involvement of the nipple on histologic section. The relative frequency of these presentations is summarized in Table 14–18, from two published reports. There is a slight preponderance of patients who present with nipple disease and a mass, compared with patients who present with nipple changes only. Most series do not specifically make mention of patients who have a mass only and are later found to have Paget's cells in the nipple, and in the series from Maier and colleagues[104] and Paone and Baker,[103] this occurred in only 10 percent of the patients. In contrast, in the series from Haagensen,[100] 30 percent of the patients presented with a mass only.

The importance of distinguishing patients who present with Paget's disease with or without a palpable mass is seen in Table 14–19. Clearly, the prognostic importance of this clinical finding cannot be overemphasized. If no mass is palpable in the breast, the chance of finding axillary lymph node involvement is less than 10 percent and the survival at five years is in the 80 to 90 percent range, with very few patients dying of cancer. On the other hand, if a mass is palpable in the breast, one half to two thirds of patients will have positive axillary lymph nodes and the five-year survival rate will be less than 50 percent. An explanation of these findings is presented in Table 14–20. Patients who have no palpable mass have, for the most part, a high percentage of noninvasive intraductal cancer at mastectomy. On the other hand, patients who have Paget's disease with an underlying palpable tumor almost invariably have invasive breast cancer, with the attendant risks of axillary metastasis and widespread dissemination.

The preceding information on the impor-

TABLE 14–19. Influence of Clinical Presentation on Axillary Node Positivity and on Survival in Paget's Disease

		No Mass			Mass		
Author	No. of Patients	No.	Axilla-Pos. (%)	5-Year Survival (%)	No.	Axilla-Pos. (%)	5-Year Survival (%)
Haagensen[100]	133	56	5.4	80*	77	60.0	55
Paone[103]	50	19	0	100	31	65.0	45
Maier[104]	88	40	14.0	70	48	—	38
Nance[105]	53	21	0	94	32	50.0	41
Ridenhour[106]	20	8	0	100	12	67.0	25
Ashikari[107]	209	96	14.0	92	113	65.0	45
Kay[109]	23	7	0	100	16	69.0	19
Rissanen[110]	26	13	0	83	13	77	0

*Ten-year survival rate.

tance of a palpable tumor mass to the prognosis in Paget's disease could lead one to speculate about the significance of delay in diagnosis on the outcome of this condition. Clearly, if Paget's disease is detected "early" without a palpable underlying mass, the results from therapy should improve. However, there is no clear-cut evidence supporting this concept. First, Paget's disease presenting with a mass may be a different pathophysiologic process from Paget's disease that presents without a mass. In the former, the underlying breast cancer could be the initial event, and the pagetoid changes in the nipple only a very late occurrence. Thus, discovering the disease soon after the pagetoid changes in the nipple occur would actually mean discovering the disease late in its natural history. On the other hand, some cases of Paget's disease may have nipple manifestations as the first tumor symptom, with the underlying cancer developing much later. In these cases, even with a delay of several months in diagnosing the Paget's disease, a good outcome may still be achieved. In two series that have looked at the influence of delay in diagnosis on outcome, it could not be shown that patients who had a longer delay did worse compared with patients who had a shorter delay.[104, 107]

While one can argue that lengthy delay in diagnosis of Paget's disease might not change the outcome of the illness, in general, concepts of early detection of breast cancer tend to support the fact that the earlier the breast tumor is diagnosed, the greater the frequency of noninvasive breast cancer.[108] Therefore, until proved otherwise, the prudent clinician strives to diagnose breast cancer as quickly as possible. In patients who present with redness, erosion, burning, and itching of the nipple, biopsy should be done within a few weeks of presentation rather than treating conservatively for many months. A small wedge of the nipple can be taken out under local anesthesia in the surgeon's office. This procedure is quick, virtually free of complications, relatively inexpensive, and reliably diagnostic of Paget's disease. There is little excuse for not performing this procedure in a patient who presents with suspicious nipple changes.

Treatment

Treatment for Paget's disease has most frequently involved radical mastectomy or modified radical mastectomy. However, several investigators would argue that if a patient presents without a palpable mass, it is probable that the patient has a noninvasive carcinoma and, that being the case, a lesser

TABLE 14–20. Relationship of Clinical Presentation to Invasive Histology in Paget's Disease

		No Mass		Mass	
Author	No. of Patients	No.	No. Invasive	No.	No. Invasive
Nance et al.[105]	53	21	2 (10%)	32	30 (94%)
Ashikari et al.[107]	209	96	33 (34%)	113	103 (91%)

surgical procedure could be performed. For example, Kay[109] recommends performing a simple mastectomy on those patients who have no clinically detectable tumor. If invasive carcinoma is seen on permanent sections, axillary dissection can then be performed. Lagios and associates[102] have gone even further. They have taken five patients who presented with Paget's disease and who were free of masses and had benign mammography and treated them with either partial or complete excision of the nipple-areola complex. The single patient who had a partial excision had a recurrence in 12 months, which was also conservatively resected, and the patient is without evidence of disease. The other four patients who had complete excision of the nipple-areola complex were all free of disease on follow-up that ranged from 30 to 69 months. Three of these patients had intraductal carcinoma, and two had involvement of the epidermis only, without any detectable involvement beneath the nipple. This interesting series of cases suggests that mastectomy is not necessary in all cases of Paget's disease without palpable mass.

The experience in treating Paget's disease with excision plus irradiation is scant. Rissanen and Holsti[110] treated two patients with biopsy followed by irradiation and six patients with complete excision followed by irradiation. The therapy was relatively low dose by our current standards, ranging from 1400 to 3100 rad delivered with an orthovoltage machine. Both patients who had biopsy followed by irradiation had a recurrence, but five of six patients who had excision plus irradiation were free of disease. Based on the paucity of nonmastectomy approaches to Paget's disease, mastectomy still must be considered the treatment of choice for this neoplasm. Modified radical mastectomy should be recommended for patients who present with an underlying palpable tumor, whereas total mastectomy can be performed in women who are free of palpable tumor. However, for those women who desire a nonmastectomy approach to the treatment of their breast cancer, the authors do offer patients treatment with wide local excision followed by axillary dissection and radiation therapy. In two patients so treated at the National Cancer Institute, local control has been achieved at 12 and 36 months, respectively.

MALE BREAST CANCER

About 1 of every 100 cases of human breast cancer occurs in a male, resulting in a disease both similar and dissimilar to breast cancer in females. The disorder accounts for about 0.2 percent of malignant neoplasia in men.[111] Although the basic clinical characteristics of male breast cancer (MBC) had been well characterized even before Wainwright's classic description in 1927,[112] the relative rarity of the disorder and the consequent reporting of numerous small series have led to frequent disagreement in the literature and insufficient firm data concerning its less prominent features.

Several especially notable reviews of MBC deserve citation: a review of the large (198-patient) series at Memorial Hospital by Holleb and associates,[113–115] a thorough compilation of the twentieth-century literature by Crichlow,[116] a series of articles exhaustively describing 265 Danish cases by Scheike and colleagues,[117–124] a review by Meyskens and colleagues,[125] and the review of Erlichman and associates.[126]

Incidence and Geographic Distribution

The average annual age-adjusted breast cancer incidence rates for cases reported by the United States Third National Cancer Survey were 0.7 per 100,000 males and 73.8 per 100,000 females of all races, roughly a 100-fold difference.[111] The average age at diagnosis was higher for men (64.6 years) than for women (59.8 years). Cases of MBC have been reported at ages as young as five and as old as 93 years[116] but rarely before age 35.[111] The ratio of male-to-female cases seems to be age dependent, with the percentage of cases among males increasing with age.

Worldwide, the reported annual incidence of MBC ranges more than tenfold, from a high of 1 case per 100,000 in West Germany and Connecticut to 0.1 case per 100,000 in Yugoslavia, Uganda, and Singapore. Finland and Japan, countries with relatively low rates of female breast cancer, also tend to have low MBC rates.[127] Several researchers reported a high incidence of MBC in areas of Africa and related this to chronic liver disease from malnutrition.[128, 129] Two areas in which MBC has been reported to account for a high proportion of total breast cancer cases are Egypt[130] (6 percent of all cases) and Zambia[131] (15 percent). In both these series, the age of onset was unusually young, with a mean of 41 years for the Egyptian series and between 40 and 55 years for 77 percent of the Zambian patients.

Etiology

Possible risk factors for MBC are presented in Table 14–21. Schottenfeld and associates[132] reviewed hospital charts of 120 MBC patients and interviewed 53 of these patients, comparing them with age-matched patients with gynecomastia or colon cancer. No differences in religious distribution or marital status were observed. Although numbers were small and differences not statistically significant, MBC patients had more frequent histories of infectious orchitis, x-ray exposure, gynecomastia, and breast cancer among male family members. Keller, in a case-control study based on clinical records of 181 MBC patients at United States Veterans' Administration hospitals, found no differences between MBC patients and those with urinary cancer or random control subjects in marital status, religion, race, or geographic origin; liver, endocrine, or other organ disease; and tobacco use. Two MBC patients, but no control subjects, had Klinefelter's syndrome.[133]

Lacassagne[134] produced mammary carcinoma in male mice by administering an estrogen. Several mouse strains were shown to be susceptible, although large doses were generally required.[135, 136] One study reported that castration and ovarian grafts increased the incidence of 3-methylcholanthrene–induced MBC in rats.[137] In 1942, Scarff and Smith reported a proliferative mastitis in two male stilbestrol workers, which exhibited a "dangerous" degree of epithelial proliferation.[138] Several case reports of patients' developing MBC while on estrogen therapy for prostatic carcinoma appeared subsequently, implicating estrogens in the etiology of this tumor[139]; however, only 2 of 17,000 patients with prostatic cancer treated with estrogen were reported to have developed MBC,[113] and, in another report, only 1 of more than 3000 similarly treated patients developed MBC.[140]

TABLE 14–21. Proposed Risk Factors for Male Breast Cancer

Exogenous estrogen exposure
Atypical endogenous steroid metabolism and excretion
Klinefelter's syndrome
Familial clustering
Irradiation
Gynecomastia
Other (e.g., orchitis, trauma)

Reviews by Campbell and Cummins[141] and Benson[142] suggested that many cases of carcinoma of the breast following treatment for prostatic cancer represented metastases from the prostatic primary tumors rather than induced MBC. In any case, the number of reported primary and metastatic breast neoplasms in patients with prostatic carcinoma was small. In 1976, Wilson and Hutchinson[139] could find 19 cases in the English literature, six of which they accepted as primary breast cancer and ten as metastatic prostatic lesions; in three the origin was unclear. Two autopsy studies, however, suggested that occult metastases from prostatic carcinoma are common: Malignant deposits were interpreted as being of prostatic carcinoma.[143, 144] Also, an autopsy study of breasts from 500 men found one primary MBC but ten metastases to the breast from extramammary tumors.[145] Crichlow,[116] on reviewing the literature, found only two reports of previous estrogen therapy among 457 MBC patients.

More convincing evidence for a role of estrogen in the etiology of MBC was presented by Symmers[146] in a case report describing two 30-year-old British transsexuals, both of whom died of metastatic breast carcinoma five years after surgical castration, mammoplasty, and continuous apparently massive estrogen use. The dosage used, young age, and lack of gonads are consistent with typical requirements for estrogen induction of breast cancer in male experimental animals.[137] Orentreich and Durr[147] noted two additional cases of MBC in men treated with estrogen, one in a 59-year-old man treated for ulcer disease and another in a 45-year-old man treated for myocardial infarction; their ages make association by chance more probable than in the transsexual cases.

Most studies suggest some alteration in the endocrine physiology of MBC patients. In 1966, Zumoff and associates[148] reported that six men with breast cancer produced less estrone, 2-hydroxyestrone, and 2-methoxyestrone, but more estriol, than did control subjects, following a tracer dose of estradiol. The researchers suggested that MBC patients have increased 16α-hydroxylase, leading to greater production of estriol. Five of these men had recurrent disease, and the presence of tumor may have affected the results, as some human mammary tumors can synthesize estrogens from androgens.[149]

Using chromatographic techniques, Lazarev and associates[150] and Komurdzhiev and Rogoznaia[151] reported by 1964 that MBC patients excreted more estrone, estradiol, and estriol than did control subjects. Using gas chromatography, Dao and colleagues[152] reported in 1973 that seven MBC patients excreted significantly more estrone, estradiol, and estriol than did control subjects. Three of their patients were clinically free of disease. In 1974, DeGiuli and DeGiuli[153] reported that 24 of 29 MBC patients excreted more total estrogens than did control subjects, and Calabresi and colleagues[154] subsequently showed by radioimmunoassay that 17 MBC patients (ten free of disease) had plasma levels of estrone, estradiol, and estriol higher than those of control subjects but similar concentrations of androstenedione and testosterone. Given the high rate of response of metastatic MBC to tamoxifen,[155] it is reasonable to include this as evidence for the estrogen-dependent nature of MBC. Thus, most endocrine-metabolic studies of MBC patients suggest that the disorder is linked to abnormal estrogen metabolism and excretion.

Klinefelter's syndrome is typically characterized by a 47,XXY (or mosaic) karyotype, sex-chromatin positivity, a male phenotype with poor development of male secondary sex characteristics including a female escutcheon and gynecomastia, small testes with hyalinized testicular tubules, oligo- or azospermia, Leydig-cell proliferation, and high levels of gonadotrophins.[119, 156] Breast development can include formation of acini and true lobules, typically seen in females.[145] Association of this syndrome with MBC was reported in a case report by Bauer and Erickson[157] in 1955 and in 3 of 21 patients observed by Jackson and colleagues.[156] Further case reports and the screening of MBC cases for sex chromatin have confirmed these findings. This association was reviewed by Scheike and associates.[119] By combining case series, they calculated the risk of breast cancer for patients with Klinefelter's syndrome to be roughly one fifth of the normal female and 20 times the normal male risk.

Multiple instances of familial MBC have been reported, among brothers in at least six instances,[123, 132, 158–161] and also among other relations.[153, 162, 163] The rarity of MBC makes these associations seem unlikely on a chance basis, but the extent of familial MBC risk is dificult to assess. In one study, MBC occurred in three brothers in one family, and in a man, his father, and his paternal uncle in another.[158] Male offspring of the latter family were treated with prophylactic subcutaneous mastectomies, with pathologic specimens suggesting mild dysplasia to some consultant pathologists.

Gynecomastia, or hyperplasia of epithelial or fibrous elements of male breast tissue, has been noted in case series of MBC and an association between the disorders proposed. Evidence cited to support a relationship between gynecomastia and the pathogenesis of MBC includes: (1) the frequent observation of gynecomastia among MBC patients reported by some researchers, including 7 of 40 cases in one series,[140] (2) the association of gynecomastia with epithelial atypia in some cases, (3) the association of gynecomastia with Klinefelter's syndrome, and (4) the high frequency of gynecomastia in regions (notably Egypt) where MBC accounts for a relatively high proportion of all breast cancer.[120, 164] Crichlow[116] could find only 17 reports of gynecomastia among 625 MBC cases in literature series of MBC in which gynecomastia was recorded. In summary, it appears that variable diagnostic criteria and the high frequency of gynecomastia in the general population make both its association with MBC and its role in the etiology of MBC unclear.[120]

MacKenzie[165] implicated radiation exposure from fluoroscopy required for procedures used to treat tuberculosis in the etiology of female breast cancer. The association between radiation exposure and development of breast cancer was confirmed in studies of survivors of atomic bomb explosions.[166, 167] Crichlow[116] located five instances in which MBC followed radiation exposure, including cases in which radiation was used for mediastinal lymphoma, eczema, gynecomastia, and other benign breast disease. One of these cases and a review of MBC etiology were presented by Lowell and colleagues.[168] In addition, Deutsch and associates[169] reported MBC in an 18 year old who had been exposed to an estimated 449 rads of radiation during neonatal treatments for an enlarged thymus.

Trauma has been cited, especially in the older literature, as potentially predisposing to MBC.[170, 171] Crichlow could find only 30 of 532 more recent literature cases reporting trauma preceding MBC,[116] and most evidence suggests that it is coincidental or calls attention to a preexistent malignant lesion.

In addition to a history of orchitis in 4 of 53 patients in the epidemiologic survey noted previously,[132] Nicolis and associates[172] reported MBC developing 30 years after severe mumps orchitis in one individual. A role for testicular disorders in the etiology of MBC is suggested but not proved by these findings plus the association of MBC with Klinefelter's syndrome and the note by Treves[173] that testicular "atrophy" was present in orchiectomy specimens from 24 of 40 men with MBC.

Diagnosis

A painless breast lump first noted by the patient is by far the most common presenting sign of MBC, accounting for 71 percent of cases in a Danish series of 257 patients[121] and 87 percent of another series derived from literature reports of 205 patients.[116] The other presenting signs and symptoms in the Danish series included pain and breast tenderness (8 percent) and skin ulceration, nipple retraction, and bloody or other discharges (4 percent with each). Distant metastases accounted for less than 1 percent of cases, and only 2 percent were initially discovered by physicians during routine physical examinations.[121] Presentation because of nipple discharge without an underlying mass has led to MBC diagnosis at an apparently early stage in rare cases.[174, 175] In one series of patients with breast masses and nipple discharge, a bloody discharge was present in 75 percent of MBC patients, compared with 45 percent of patients with benign disease.[174]

The duration of symptoms before presentation averaged six months in one series.[121] In a review of the literature, an 18-month duration of symptoms was noted for 1228 cases reported since 1900, with a somewhat improved ten-month delay observed for cases diagnosed since 1951.[116] This delay in seeking medical attention is reported to be longer than that for women,[176] despite the paucity of other tissue that might obscure the diagnosis in the male breast. This is possibly due to poor awareness of the possibility of MBC in the population[115] or to concerns over sexuality.

A subareolar mass is almost invariably present. Crichlow[116] could identify only two cases of occult MBC in literature reports, both presenting with regional nodes, and Cain[175] described a single case presenting with a completely normal examination but a history of bloody nipple discharge. A mass, however, is infrequently the only clinical finding. In several series, nipple ulceration was present in about 25 percent of cases and nipple retraction in 33 percent.[115, 116, 121] Nipple discharge was noted at hospital admission in only 2 percent of Scheike's patients with MBC,[121] but 14 percent of malignant and 2 percent of benign lesions reported by Treves and associates[174] had nipple discharge. At least 52 percent of MBC cases with known laterality were left-sided and about 1.5 percent bilateral.[116, 121]

Palpable homolateral nodes were present in about 50 percent of cases in a literature review. Scheike reported that tumor size in his series ranged from 1 cm to 28 × 16 cm, with 51 percent of MBC primary tumors smaller than 3 cm. He noted a significant positive correlation between tumor size and both symptom duration and frequency of ulceration.[121]

Differential Diagnosis

MBC must be differentiated from metastatic cancer, gynecomastia, and, in some cases, inflammatory lesions. Holleb[115] estimated that 65 percent of breast lesions in older males are gynecomastias, 25 percent MBC, and 10 percent other benign breast lesions. In one series of male breast lesions, 15 cases of MBC, compared with 114 of gynecomastia, were diagnosed during a 16-year period.[177] Youth and bilaterality favor gynecomastia; a firm discoid, subareolar, probably tender mass in an adolescent can be considered a normal accompaniment of puberty and is likely to disappear within one or two years.[178] A hard, poorly defined, irregular mass in an elderly man should be investigated before skin thickening, nipple

TABLE 14–22. Features Helpful in Differentiating Typical Gynecomastia from Male Breast Cancer

Male Breast Cancer	*Gynecomastia*
Increased incidence with age	Broad age distribution over most of adult life, especially puberty and senescence
Painless (unless ulcerated)	Tender
Unilateral	Bilateral in a significant minority
Eccentric	Central
Hard	Firm
Poorly defined mass	Well-defined mass
Adheres to pectoral muscles	Can adhere to areola
Associated with	Associated with
Nipple discharge, especially sanguineous	Drug use, including estrogens, androgens, corticosteroids, spironolactone, cimetidine, ergotamine, thyroid extract, reserpine, diethylpropion, phenothiazines, marijuana, thiazides, digitalis, and isoniazid
Enlarged axillary nodes	Medical conditions, including chronic liver disease, central nervous system disease, renal dialysis, thoracic disease, cardiovascular disease, and refeeding after starvation
Ulceration	Endocrine disorders, including testicular atrophy secondary to infection, trauma, or hydrocele; eunuchism; and male pseudohermaphroditism
	Neoplasms, including testicular, adrenal, pituitary, malignant lymphoma, and carcinoma of the lung, colon, or prostate
	Infections, including malaria, tuberculosis, leprosy, and bilharziasis
	Idiopathic

retraction and ulceration, adherence to the pectoral muscles, and axillary node involvement make the diagnosis obvious and the prognosis grave. Nipple discharge, especially sanguineous, should be viewed with similar suspicion. Diagnosis of benign disease frequently does not require biopsy.[162] Nevertheless, especially considering the frequency of gynecomastia associated with senescence or drugs, differentiating MBC from gynecomastia can be difficult. Table 14–22 describes features that may be of some use in making the distinction.[179–188] The frequency of conditions associated with gynecomastia varies in different reports. In a series of 126 cases of gynecomastia, it was associated with cardiovascular disorders in 23 cases (17 taking digitalis), Klinefelter's syndrome in 8, chronic liver disease in 6, central nervous system disease in 5, chronic lung disease in 15, use of various other drugs in 9, testicular and adrenocortical tumors in 1 each, miscellaneous disorders in 10, adolescent gynecomastia in 26, and no other disease in 22.[189]

Mammography

Mammography has been employed principally to distinguish gynecomastia from MBC. Radiographically, gynecomastia is characteristically smooth, fans backward from the nipple, and tends to form a symmetric cone. MBC is more likely to be eccentric, is typically dense with irregular margins with or without calcifications, and may have associated skin thickening and nipple retraction. The differential is not absolute, however, and both disorders may coexist.[185, 188, 190] Mammography should supplement, not replace, physical examination and biopsy.

Extent of Disease at Diagnosis

In the series, compiled by Scheike,[121] of 396 male patients staged according to the UICC TNM classification scheme as employed for women, 34 percent presented as Stage I; 14 percent as Stage II; 40 percent as Stage III; and 12 percent as Stage IV. The high frequency of Stage III cases is due largely to patients with skin fixation. The End Results Group of the National Cancer Institute, a large group including two state cancer registries and other hospitals (having among them 393 white MBC patients), reported that between the periods 1950 to 1954 and 1970 to 1973, the proportion of cases with localized disease at diagnosis increased from 38 to 58 percent.[191] In this report, the stage at diagnosis was similar for men and women with breast cancer.

TABLE 14–23. Comparative Histology of Male and Female Breast Cancer

Carcinoma	Male (%)	Female (%)
Infiltrating ductal, not otherwise specified	73	78.1
Nonspecified adenocarcinoma	7	
Intraductal	5	
Papillary	5	1.2
Medullary	4	4.3
Mucinous	2	2.6
Squamous	<1	
Lobular invasive	<1	8.7
Paget's disease	<1	
Sarcoma	<1	
Adenocystic	<1	
Basal-cell	<1	
Lymphoma	<1	
Tubular	<1	
Other (including comedo)	<1	4.6

In a manner analogous to staging of female breast cancer, staging of MBC should be accomplished before definitive surgery so as to aid in the planning of that surgery. A bone scan and liver function tests are the most useful tests to perform preoperatively. The finding of metastatic disease could spare a portion of the often elderly MBC patients the rigors of radical surgery.

Pathology

Except for the absence of *in situ* cases in men, reports of male and female breast pathology are similar. Table 14–23 presents a comparison of histologic subtypes for the sexes. It was adapted from Giffler and Kay's summary table including 684 MBC cases, compared with a series for females reported by the Armed Forces Institute of Pathology.[192] Major differences include the relative absence of lobular invasive carcinomas and fewer comedocarcinomas in men. Lobules are normally absent from the male breast, and whether true male lobular carcinoma exists remains subject to interpretation. Giffler and Kay[192] reported two cases and cited literature cases that they felt represented male lobular invasive carcinoma, but they stated that the *in situ* form (which in women is more common than lobular invasive carcinoma and tends to present bilaterally) has still not been described in men. Yogore and Sahgal[193] reported an additional case of lobular invasive carcinoma.

In a careful review of mastectomy specimens from 187 Danish MBC cases, Visfeldt and Scheike,[117] using the WHO classification and grading scheme, reported a direct and striking relationship between five-year survival rates and grading: 13 percent of Grade I, 54 percent of Grade II, and 94 percent of Grade III patients not dying of other causes died within five years of developing breast cancer. Haagensen[162] reported MBC to be well differentiated more often than breast cancer in women.

Paget's disease of the male breast has been the subject of several reviews.[194–196] Patients typically present because of nipple bleeding, discharge, or ulceration rather than detection of a mass: In some series, only 2 of 13 patients with detected lesions noted a lump, although a mass could usually be detected on physical examination.[194] A poorer prognosis than that for typical MBC has been suggested, with only 4 of 16 five-year survivors and only 1 known ten-year survivor.[196] Otherwise, too few cases have been reported to reliably differentiate clinical or other features of Paget's disease from those of typical MBC or to suggest treatment differing from that for typical MBC.

Inflammatory carcinoma of the male breast has been reported in as many as 2 percent of cases in some series.[197] Papillary carcinomas have been associated with a good prognosis.[115] Reports of unusual cell types have included cystosarcoma phyllodes,[198] adenoid cystic carcinoma,[199] tubular carcinoma,[200] and granular-cell tumor.[201] Most of these had a more benign course than that of typical MBC, and the latter two lesions are of special import, because their low malignant potential may indicate less radical surgical treatment.

Local excision only was employed for the two cases of granular-cell tumor in men aged 35 and 36 reported by Hart and Sisely.[201] An ultrastructural study of MBC has been made by Sirsat and colleagues.[202]

Steroid Receptors

These have been reviewed by Everson and associates,[203] who reported estrogen receptor status in tumor specimens from 34 patients with MBC and literature reports of 30 patients. Estrogen receptor was present in 84 percent of samples from MBC patients and progesterone receptor in 73 percent. A large proportion (about two thirds) of MBC patients will respond to endocrine maneuvers; thus, the proportion of receptor-positive tumors may be not unexpectedly high.

Primary Therapy

Literature reports completed by Crichlow[116] concerning 495 men with MBC revealed that 19 percent were considered inoperable, 13 percent were treated with simple mastectomy, and 68 percent were treated with radical mastectomy. Both simple[124, 204] and radical[115, 205–208] mastectomies have been advocated; no comparative trials have been attempted, and selection factors employed in electing different treatments are such that the dispute cannot be resolved by analysis of available data.[116, 122, 209] Skin grafting is frequently required and permits wider margins.[115] Postoperative radiation therapy has frequently been employed, but its efficacy has not been subjected to critical review or randomized trial, and patient-selection factors make extrapolation from literature reports of limited value. In at least one series, results were not improved by postoperative radiation therapy.[122] In nonrandomized trials it is possible, but it cannot be assumed, that radiation therapy–treated patients are selected for this therapy because of more advanced disease.

Adjuvant Therapy

Because of encouraging early reports of adjuvant chemotherapy in women with Stage II breast cancer, we began to use a similar approach in men. Since 1974, we have treated 22 men with node-positive breast cancer with adjuvant chemotherapy. All patients were staged according to the American Joint Committee Staging System (1983). All patients had pathologically positive lymph node adenopathy and were classified as having Stage II disease at presentation. The range of positive axillary nodes is from 2 to 13, with a median of two.

The treatment approach included cyclophosphamide (CTX), methotrexate (MTX), and 5-fluorouracil (5-FU). Initially, patients were treated with CTX, 100 mg/m^2 orally for 14 days, MTX, 40 mg/m^2, and 5-FU, 600 mg/m^2 intravenously on days one and eight of each cycle; beginning in 1980, the dose of CTX was changed to 500 mg/m^2 intravenously on days one and eight of each cycle, and the MTX was increased to 60 mg/m^2 intravenously. Of the 22 patients, two remain on adjuvant therapy. The median number of cycles administered for those who have completed therapy is 12. Of the 22 patients, five (23 percent) have had recurrences. The disease-free survival time is greater than 60 months, and the median survival time for this population is 108 months.

These data are highly encouraging, and if these results continue, adjuvant therapy in the male with breast cancer should be considered an efficacious approach to management. Only with longer follow-up and the accrual of more patients will one be able to make significant statements about the efficacy of treating Stage II MBC with adjuvant chemotherapy. As more data accumulate, additional subsets of patients may be identified in whom more or less aggressive forms of therapy may be indicated.

Treatment of Metastatic Disease

Available evidence suggests a similar pattern of metastases of male and female breast cancers.[171, 204, 210] Indications for systemic treatment are also similar in advanced disease. Local or isolated recurrence can be managed by excision or radiation therapy, although systemic therapy has been advocated for female patients.[211]

Reported response rates to endocrine ablation are higher for MBC than for female breast cancer. A response was reported in two thirds of patients treated with orchiectomy and in three quarters treated with adrenalectomy.[125] Other reviewers cited a duration of orchiectomy responses (45-month) that was three times longer than the ovariectomy response in breast cancer.[212]

Adrenalectomy was used after a response to orchiectomy (11 patients, 91 percent adrenalectomy responders with a 32-month median duration), after no response to orchiectomy (eight patients, 50 percent responders with a 16-month median duration), combined with orchiectomy (three patients, all responders), or as primary treatment (three patients, two responders). Hypophysectomy was also successful: A total of 10 of 17 patients responded. Responses were observed when hypophysectomy was primary treatment (two of three patients) or was used after response to orchiectomy (three of four patients). No responses to hypophysectomy were noted among three orchiectomy failures. Responders to any of these therapies tended to live longer than nonresponders. Data were too sparse to determine whether response rates differed according to metastatic site of involvement, although responses in osseous, visceral, and soft tissue were noted.[125] As in any study based on case series, it is possible that response rates were inflated by selection of favorable outcomes for publication.[213]

In his review, Crichlow[116] could find reference to only a few reports of documented responses to estrogens, and Holleb[115] reported no long-term remissions following estrogen use, despite its application to all cases with "uncontrolled breast cancer" in his series. Further details were not given, but Treves,[173] in an earlier review of the series from this same center, reported that only 2 of 14 patients responded to estrogens, although the duration of some trials was short and the response criteria were poorly defined. Kennedy and Kiang observed a patient who initially seemed to respond to diethylstilbestrol (DES) but later experienced rapid tumor growth during two trials with this same agent, with regression when the drug was discontinued. They felt that the role of estrogen therapy in the treatment of advanced MBC was not yet defined.[214]

Estrogen therapy, however, was favored in reports from European centers.[215] Scheike reported a "palliative effect" for more than six months in 20 of 63 patients treated with lower doses (generally DES, 1 mg three times a day), but response criteria and disease sites were unrecorded. Orchiectomy was not used in his large series.[122] Walach and Hochman[216] reported that 9 of 14 (60 percent) of their patients were "improved" by DES, but details were not provided.

In 1980, Patterson and colleagues[155] reviewed 31 MBC patients treated with tamoxifen. The objective response rate of this collected series was 48 percent. Four of five responders were ER positive; none of three nonresponders was ER positive. Response was not associated with dose. Toxicity was minimal. Two patients who failed to respond to prior orchiectomy failed to respond to subsequent tamoxifen; one of three responders to orchiectomy responded to subsequent tamoxifen. Though substantial series have not appeared, it is our impression that many clinicians have routinely employed tamoxifen as the endocrine therapy of choice for MBC. Given the small likelihood of a randomized trial, this is probably a reasonable decision.

Few observations of the effects of chemotherapy on MBC have been reported. Favorable response to 5-fluorouracil, cyclophosphamide, and combinations of methotrexate and thiotepa and of cyclophosphamide, doxorubicin, and 5-fluorouracil have been noted.[115, 214, 217] The high response rates of MBC to endocrine ablations, however, make them the initial treatment of choice. Whether steroid receptor status will enable selection of appropriate treatment, as appears to be the case in female breast cancer,[218] is as yet undetermined.

Many researchers state that breast cancer prognosis is poorer in males than in females.[116, 164, 219] Norris and Taylor[164] suggested that this might be attributed to the central location of most breast lesions in males, leading to a high incidence of internal mammary node metastases. Several investigators, however, developed a strong case for attributing much of the reported difference to higher mortality in males from unrelated causes.[113, 122, 220]

Other studies of breast cancer that included the experience of comparable groups from both sexes also reported similar male and female relative survival rates.[176, 221, 222] In addition, when Langlands and colleagues[223] matched male and female breast cancer cases for stage, they found equivalent age-corrected survival rates for both sexes, although the overall survival rate was higher for women.[223] Ribeiro,[224] however, reported better survival rates for women with advanced disease, in a study matching age and stage. Thus, sex differences in survival rate may favor women, but only slightly and probably without statistical certainty.

In Scheike's series, the relative survival of 246 patients was 46 percent at five years and 29 percent at ten years.[122] He reported that worsening prognosis was correlated with clinically positive axillary nodes, tumor ulceration, fixation to underlying tissues, increasing tumor stage, increasing tumor size, and worsening histologic grade. Prognosis improved from the period 1943 to 1957 compared with the period 1958 to 1971 in his series; no effect on relative survival was attributable to age at onset, duration of symptoms, or treatment employed. Norris and Taylor[164] stated that microscopic axillary involvement, tumor size greater than 1.9 cm, and skin ulceration unfavorably affect prognosis, but several histologic types including intraductal, papillary, and well-differentiated tumors had a more favorable prognosis. Corwin and associates,[177] in a series of only 15 patients, felt that patient delay in seeking treatment was the most important factor influencing prognosis.

Crichlow[116] and Satiani and Powell[225] observed a striking relationship between axillary node status and crude survival. In addition, Ribeiro[224] noted recurrences in 19 of 76 (25 percent) of Stage I and 27 of 38 (71 percent) of Stage II patients in a British series of 200 cases. Most recurrences were seen by two years after mastectomy. As noted previously, papillary MBC appeared to have a better and Paget's disease a worse prognosis than that of typical MBC. These data should be compared with the results of our uncontrolled series of node-positive MBC patients treated with adjuvant chemotherapy.

In view of the relatively long delay in seeking therapy, described previously (ten months, according to Crichlow[116]), it may be anticipated that an increasing awareness of physicians and the public as to the need for early detection and treatment of MBC may improve results.

REFERENCES

1. Haagensen CD: Diseases of the Breast, second ed. Philadelphia: W.B. Saunders Co., 1971, pp. 227–249.
2. Barnes L, Pietruszka M: Rhabdomyosarcoma arising within a cystosarcoma phyllodes. Am J Surg Pathol 2:423, 1978.
3. Sonn RL, Alpenn JB: Osteogenic sarcoma of the breast arising in a cystosarcoma phyllodes. J Am Osteopath Assoc 83:321, 1983.
4. Pietruszka M, Barnes L: Cystosarcoma phyllodes: A clinicopathologic analysis of 42 cases. Cancer 41:1974, 1978.
5. Bird CC: A breast sarcoma containing rhabdomyosarcomatous and other metaplastic elements. J Pathol 101:286, 1970.
6. Mertens HH, Langnickel D, Staedtler F: Primary osteogenic sarcoma of the breast. Acta Cytol (Baltimore) 26:512, 1982.
7. Watt AC, Haggar AM, Krasicky GA: Extraosseous osteogenic sarcoma of the breast: Mammographic and pathologic findings. Radiology 150:34, 1984.
8. Beltaos E, Banerjee TK: Chondrosarcoma of the breast. Am J Clin Pathol 71:345, 1979.
9. Kristensen PB, Kryer H: Liposarcoma of the breast. Acta Chir Scand 144:193, 1978.
10. Rasmussen J, Jensen H: Liposarcoma of the breast. Virchows Arch Pathol Anat Histol 385:117, 1979.
11. Pardo-Mindan J, Garcia-Julian G, Altuna ME: Leiomyosarcoma of the breast—report of a case. Am J Clin Pathol 62:477, 1974.
12. Berg JW, Decosse JJ, Fracchia AA, et al.: Stromal sarcoma of the breast. Cancer 15:418, 1962.
13. McDivitt RW, Stewart FW, Berg JW: Tumors of the breast. Atlas of Tumor Pathology, second series. Washington, D.C.: Armed Forces Institute of Pathology, 1968, pp. 123–124.
14. Tang PH, Petrelli M, Robechek PJ: Stromal sarcoma of breast. A light and electron microscope study. Cancer 43:209, 1979.
15. Salvadori B, Greco M, Galluzzo D, et al.: Surgery for malignant mesenchymal tumors of the breast: A series of 31 cases. Tumori (Milan) 68:325, 1982.
16. Barnes L, Pietruszka M: Sarcomas of the breast. A clinicopathologic analysis of ten cases. Cancer 40:1577, 1977.
17. Harris M, Persaud V: Carcinosarcoma of the breast. J Pathol 112:99, 1974.
18. Wayte DM, Stewart JB, McKenzie CG: A composite malignant tumor of the elderly female breast. J Clin Pathol 23:414, 1970.
19. Azzopardi JG: Problems in Breast Pathology. Philadelphia: W.B. Saunders Co., 1979, pp. 373–376.
20. Mambo NC, Burke JS, Butler JJ: Primary malignant lymphomas of the breast. Cancer 39:2033, 1977.
21. Schoaten JT, Weese JL, Carbone PP: Lymphoma of the breast. Ann Surg 194:759, 1981.
22. Fiks A: Cystosarcoma phyllodes of the mammary gland—Müller's tumor. Virchows Arch Pathol Anat 392:1, 1981.
23. Oberman HA: Cystosarcoma phyllodes; a clinicopathologic study of hypercellular periductal stromal neoplasms of breast. Cancer 18:697, 1965.
24. Treves N: A study of cystosarcoma phyllodes. Ann NY Acad Sci 114:922, 1964.
25. McDivitt RW, Urban JA, Farrow JH: Cystosarcoma phyllodes. Johns Hopkins Med J 120:33, 1967.
26. Norris HJ, Taylor HB: Relationship of histologic features to behavior of cystosarcoma phyllodes. Cancer 20:2090, 1967.
27. Grigioni WF, Santini D, Grassigli A, et al.: A clinicopathologic study of cystosarcoma phyllodes. Arch Anat Cytol Pathol 30:303, 1982.

28. Contarini O, Urdaneta LF, Hagan W, et al.: Cystosarcoma phyllodes of the breast: A new therapeutic proposal. Ann Surg 48:157, 1982.
29. Schmidt B, Lantsberg L, Goldstein J, et al.: Cystosarcoma phyllodes. Isr J Med Sci 17:895, 1981.
30. West TL, Weiland LH, Clagett OT: Cystosarcoma phyllodes. Ann Surg 173:520, 1971.
31. Halverson JD, Hori-Rubaina JM: Cystosarcoma phyllodes of the breast. Ann Surg 40:295, 1974.
32. Cole-Beuglet C, Soriano R, Kurtz AB, et al.: Ultrasound, x-ray mammography, and histopathology of cystosarcoma phyllodes. Radiology 146:481, 1983.
33. Ishida T, Izuo M, Kawai T: Breast carcinoma arising in cystosarcoma phyllodes: Report of a case with a review of the literature. Jpn J Clin Oncol 14:99, 1984.
34. Kesterson GHD, Georgiade N, Seigler HF, et al.: Cystosarcoma phyllodes: A steroid receptor and ultrastructural analysis. Ann Surg 190:640, 1979.
35. Porton WM, Poortman J: Estrogen receptors in cystosarcoma phyllodes. Eur J Cancer Clin Oncol 17:1147, 1981.
36. Lindquist KD, vanHeerden JA, Weiland LH, et al.: Recurrent and metastatic cystosarcoma phyllodes. Am J Surg 144:341, 1982.
37. Lindberg RD, Martin RG, Romsdahl MM, et al.: Conservative surgery and postoperative radiotherapy in 300 adults with soft tissue sarcomas. Cancer 47:2391, 1981.
38. Rosenberg SA, Tepper J, Glatstein E, et al.: The treatment of soft tissue sarcomas of the extremities: Prospective evaluation of limb-sparing surgery plus radiation compared with amputation. Ann Surg 196:305, 1982.
39. Hoover HC, Trestioreanu A, Ketcham AS: Metastatic cystosarcoma phylloides in an adolescent girl: An unusually malignant tumor. Ann Surg 181:279, 1975.
40. Azzopardi JG: Problems in Breast Pathology. Philadelphia: W.B. Saunders Co., 1979, p. 368.
41. Schmidt GB: Ueber das angiosarkom der mamma. Arch Klin Chir 36:121, 1887.
42. Patrick RS, Jarvis J, Miln DC: Haemangioblastoma of breast; a report of three cases. Br J Surg 45:188, 1957.
43. Steingaszner LC, Enzinger FM, Taylor HB: Hemangiosarcoma of the breast. Cancer 18:352, 1965.
44. Haagensen CD: Diseases of the Breast, second edition. Philadelphia: W.B. Saunders Co., 1971, pp. 301–303.
45. Merino MJ, Carter D, Berman M: Angiosarcoma of the breast. Am J Surg Pathol 7:53, 1983.
46. Donnell RM, Rosen PP, Lieberman PH, et al.: Angiosarcoma and other vascular tumors of the breast—pathologic analysis as a guide to prognosis. Am J Surg Pathol 5:629, 1981.
47. Gulesserian HP, Lawton RL: Angiosarcoma of the breast. Cancer 24:1021, 1969.
48. Chen KTK, Kirkegaard DD, Bocian JJ: Angiosarcoma of the breast. Cancer 46:368, 1980.
49. Antman KH, Corson J, Greenberger J, et al.: Multimodality therapy in the management of angiosarcoma of the breast. Cancer 50:2000, 1982.
50. Brennan MF: Angiosarcoma of the breast. Am J Surg Pathol 7:679, 1981.
51. Wallack MK, Wolf JA, Bedwinek J, et al.: Gestational carcinoma of the female breast. Curr Probl Cancer 7:5, 1983.
52. Torres JE, Mickal A: Carcinoma of the breast in pregnancy. Clin Obstet Gynecol 18:219, 1975.
53. Westberg SV: Prognosis of breast cancer for pregnant and nursing women. Acta Obstet Gynecol Scand (Suppl) 25:1, 1946.
54. Applewhite RR, Smith LR, DiVincenti F: Carcinoma of the breast associated with pregnancy and lactation. Am Surg 39:101, 1973.
55. Haagensen CD: Diseases of the Breast, second ed. Philadelphia: W.B. Saunders Co., 1971, pp. 660–664.
56. Ribeiro GG, Palmer MK: Breast carcinoma associated with pregnancy: A clinician's dilemma. Br Med J 2:1524, 1977.
57. Clark RM, Reid J: Carcinoma of the breast in pregnancy and lactation. Intl J Radiat Oncol Biol Phys 4:693, 1978.
58. Holleb AI, Farrow JH: The relation of carcinoma of the breast and pregnancy in 238 patients. Surg Gynecol Obstet 115:65, 1962.
59. White TT: Carcinoma of the breast associated with pregnancy. Northwest Med 57:477, 1958.
60. Rosemond GP: Carcinoma of the breast during pregnancy. Clin Obstet Gynecol 6:994, 1963.
61. Donegan WL: Mammary carcinoma and pregnancy. Major Probl Clin Surg 5:448, 1979.
62. Simpson ER, MacDonald PC: Endocrinology of pregnancy. *In:* Williams RH (ed.): Textbook of Endocrinology, sixth ed. Philadelphia: W.B. Saunders Co., 1981, pp. 412–442.
63. Diekamp U, Bitran J, Ferguson DJ: Breast cancer in young women. J Reprod Med 17:255, 1976.
64. Gala RR, Loginsky SJ: Correlation between serum prolactin levels and incidence of mammary tumors induced by 7,12-dimethylbenz (alpha)-anthracene in the rat. J Natl Cancer Inst 51:593, 1973.
65. Hobbs JR, DeSouza I, Salih H, et al.: Selection of hormone-dependent breast cancers. Br J Surg 61:785, 1974.
66. Janerich DT: The influence of pregnancy on breast cancer risk: Is it endocrinological or immunological? Med Hypotheses 6:1149, 1980.
67. Byrd BF, Bayer DS, Robertson JC, et al.: Treatment of breast tumors associated with pregnancy and lactation. Ann Surg 155:940, 1962.
68. Rickert R, Rajan S: Localized breast infarcts associated with pregnancy. Arch Pathol 97:159, 1974.
69. Hall EJ: Radiobiology for the Radiologist. New York: Harper & Row, 1978, pp. 397–410.
70. Miller R, Mulvihill S: Small head size after atomic irradiation. Teratology 14:355, 1976.
71. Dekaban AS: Abnormalities in children exposed to x-radiation during various stages of gestation: Tentative timetable of radiation injury to the human fetus, part 1. J Nucl Med 9:471, 1968.
72. MacMahon B, Hutchinson G: Prenatal x-ray and childhood cancer: A review. Acta Unio Contra Cancrum 20:1172, 1964.
73. Monson RR, MacMahon B: Prenatal x-ray exposure and cancer in children. *In:* Borce JD, Jr., Fraumeri JF, Jr. (eds.): Radiation Carcinogenesis: Epidemiology and Biologic Significances. New York: Raven Press, 1984, pp. 97–105.
74. Jablon S, Kato H: Childhood cancer in relation to prenatal exposure to atomic-bomb radiation. Lancet 2:1000, 1970.
75. Harvey EB, Borce JD, Jr., Honeyman M, et al.: Prenatal x-ray exposure and childhood cancer in twins. N Engl J Med 312:541, 1985.

76. Fraass BA, van de Geign J: Peripheral dose from megavolt beams. Med Phys 10:809, 1983.
77. Fisher B, Bauer M, Margolese R, et al.: Five-year results of a randomized clinical trial comparing total mastectomy and segmental mastectomy with or without radiation in the treatment of breast cancer. N Engl J Med 312:665, 1985.
78. Lippman M, Sorace R, Bagley C, et al.: Effective systemic management of locally advanced breast cancer (Abstract). Proc Am Soc Clin Oncol 4:65, 1985.
79. Sweet DL, Kinzie J: Consequences of radiotherapy and antineoplastic therapy for the fetus. J Reprod Med 17:241, 1976.
80. Schapira DV, Chudley AE: Successful pregnancy following continuous treatment with combination chemotherapy before conception and throughout pregnancy. Cancer 54:800, 1984.
81. Doney KC, Kraemer KG, Shepard TH: Combination chemotherapy for acute myelocytic leukemia during pregnancy: Three case reports. Cancer Treat Rep 63:369, 1979.
82. Okun DB, Groncy PK, Sieger L, et al.: Acute leukemia in pregnancy: Transient neonatal myelosuppression after combination chemotherapy in the mother. Med Pediatr Oncol 7:315, 1979.
83. Lowenthal RM, Marsden KA, Newman NM, et al.: Normal infant after treatment of acute myeloid leukaemia in pregnancy with daunorubicin. Aust NZ J Med 8:431, 1978.
84. Murray CL, Reichert JA, Anderson J, et al.: Multimodal cancer therapy for breast cancer in the first trimester of pregnancy. JAMA 252:2607, 1984.
85. Nissen-Meyer R, Kjellgren K, Malmio K, et al.: Surgical adjuvant chemotherapy results with one short course with cyclophosphamide after mastectomy for breast cancer. Cancer 41:2088, 1978.
86. Cooper RG, Holland JF, Glidewell O: Adjuvant chemotherapy of breast cancer. Cancer 44:793, 1979.
87. Crosby CH, Barclay THC: Carcinoma of the breast: Surgical management of special conditions. Cancer 28:1628, 1971.
88. Rissanen P: Carcinoma of the breast during pregnancy and lactation. Br J Cancer 22:663, 1968.
89. Krementz ET, Cerise EJ, Foster DS, et al.: Metastases of undetermined source. Curr Probl Cancer 4:4, 1979.
90. Ashikari R, Rosen PP, Urban JA, et al.: Breast cancer presenting as an axillary mass. Ann Surg 183:415, 1976.
91. Halsted WS: The results of radical operations for cure of carcinoma of the breast. Ann Surg 46:1, 1907.
92. Haagensen CD: Diseases of the Breast, second ed. Philadelphia: W.B. Saunders Co., 1971, pp. 486–491.
93. Owen HW, Dockerty MB, Gray HK: Occult carcinoma of the breast. Surg Gynecol Obstet 98:302, 1954.
94. Fitts WT, Steiner GC, Enterline HT: Prognosis of occult carcinoma of the breast. Am J Surg 106:460, 1963.
95. Patel J, Nemoto T, Rosner D, et al.: Axillary lymph node metastasis from an occult breast cancer. Cancer 47:2923, 1981.
96. Westbrook KC, Gallager HS: Breast carcinoma presenting as an axillary mass. Am J Surg 122:607, 1971.
97. Feuerman L, Attie JN, Rosenberg B: Carcinoma in axillary lymph nodes as an indicator of breast cancer. Surg Gynecol Obstet 114:5, 1962.
98. Vilcoq JR, Calle R, Ferme F, et al.: Conservative treatment of axillary adenopathy due to probable subclinical breast cancer. Arch Surg 117:1136, 1982.
99. Paget J: On disease of the mammary areola preceding cancer of the mammary gland. *In:* Corman ML (ed.): Classic articles in colonic and rectal surgery. Dis Colon Rectum 23:280, 1980.
100. Haagensen CD: Diseases of the Breast, second ed. Philadelphia: W.B. Saunders, 1971, pp. 545–569.
101. Azzopardi JG: Problems in Breast Pathology. Philadelphia: W.B. Saunders Co., 1979, pp. 258–260.
102. Lagios MD, Westdahl PR, Rose MR, et al.: Paget's disease of the nipple—alternative management in cases without or with minimal extent of underlying breast carcinoma. Cancer 54:545, 1984.
103. Paone JF, Baker RR: Pathogenesis and treatment of Paget's disease of the breast. Cancer 48:825, 1981.
104. Maier WP, Rosemond GP, Harasym EL, et al.: Paget's disease of the female breast. Surg Gynecol Obstet 128:1253, 1969.
105. Nance FC, DeLoach DH, Welsh RA, et al.: Paget's disease of the breast. Ann Surg 171:864, 1970.
106. Ridenhour CE, Perez-Mesa C, Hori JM: Paget's disease of the nipple. Cancer Bull 21:15, 1969.
107. Ashikari R, Park K, Huvos AG, et al.: Paget's disease of the breast. Cancer 26:680, 1970.
108. Baker LH: Breast Cancer Detection Demonstration Project: 5-year summary report. CA 32:194, 1982.
109. Kay S: Paget's disease of the nipple. Surg Gynecol Obstet 123:1010, 1966.
110. Rissanen PM, Holsti P: Paget's disease of the breast. Oncology 23:209, 1969.
111. Cutler SJ, Young JL, Jr. (eds.): Third National Cancer Survey: Incidence Data. National Cancer Inst Monogr 41, DHEW Publication No. (NIH) 75–787. Washington, DC: U.S. Department of Health Education and Welfare, 1975, Tables 5, 7, and 19.
112. Wainwright JM: Carcinoma of the male breast: Clinical and pathologic study. Arch Surg 14:836, 1927.
113. Holleb AI, Freeman HP, Farrow JH: Cancer of male breast. I. NY State J Med 68:544, 1968.
114. Holleb AI, Freeman HP, Farrow JH: Cancer of male breast. II. NY State J Med 68:656, 1968.
115. Holleb AI: Cancer of the male breast. *In:* Anderson Hospital (ed.): Breast Cancer: Early and Late. Chicago: Year Book Medical Publishers, 1970, pp. 245–262.
116. Crichlow RW: Carcinoma of the male breast. Surg Gynecol Obstet 134:1011, 1972.
117. Visfeldt J, Scheike O: Male breast cancer. I. Histologic typing and grading of 187 Danish cases. Cancer 32:985, 1973.
118. Scheike O, Svenstrup B, Frandsen A: Male breast cancer. II. Metabolism of oestradiol-17beta in men with breast cancer. J Steroid Biochem 4:489, 1973.
119. Scheike O, Visfeldt J, Petersen B: Male breast cancer. 3. Breast carcinoma in association with the Klinefelter syndrome. Acta Pathol Microbiol Scand (A)81:352, 1973.
120. Scheike O, Visfeldt J: Male breast cancer. 4. Gynecomastia in patients with breast cancer. Acta Pathol Microbiol Scand (A)81:359, 1973.
121. Scheike O: Male breast cancer. 5. Clinical manifes-

tations in 257 cases in Denmark. Br J Cancer 28:552, 1973.
122. Scheike O: Male breast cancer. 6. Factors influencing prognosis. Br J Cancer 30:261, 1974.
123. Scheike O: Male breast cancer. Acta Pathol Microbiol Scand (A)(Suppl) 251:13, 1975.
124. Scheike O: Factors provoking male breast cancer. *In:* Stoll BA (ed.): Risk Factors in Breast Cancer. Chicago: Year Book Medical Publishers, 1976, pp. 173–192.
125. Meyskens FL, Jr., Tormey DC, Neifeld PJ: Male breast cancer: A review. Cancer Treat Rev 3:83, 1976.
126. Erlichman C, Murphy L, Elharkin T: Male breast cancer: A 13-year review of 89 patients. J Clin Oncol 2:903, 1984.
127. Modan B, Mintz U, Finkelman J: Male breast cancer in Israel. Selected epidemiological and clinical aspects. J Chronic Dis 23:55, 1970.
128. Davies JNP: Sex hormone upset in Africans. Br Med J 2:676, 1949.
129. Sinner W: Karzinome der mannlichen Brustdruse. Beobachtungen an 27 fallen. Zurcher erfahrungen 1919 bis 1960. Strahlentherapie 115:522, 1961.
130. El-Gazayerli MM, Abdel-Aziz AS: On bilharziasis and male breast cancer in Egypt: A preliminary report and review of the literature. Br J Cancer 17:566, 1963.
131. Bhagwandeen SB: Carcinoma of the male breast in Zambia. East Afr Med J 49:89, 1972.
132. Schottenfeld D, Lilienfeld AM, Diamond H: Some observations on the epidemiology of breast cancer among males. Am J Public Health 53:890, 1963.
133. Keller AZ: Demographic, clinical and survivorship characteristics of males with primary cancer of the breast. Am J Epidemiol 85:183, 1967.
134. Lacassagne A: Hormonal pathogenesis of adenocarcinoma of the breast. Am J Cancer 27:217, 1936.
135. Gardner WU: Estrogens of carcinogenesis. Arch Pathol 27:138, 1939.
136. Pribe WA, Ockuly EA: Prostatic metastasis to the breast and the role of estrogens: Case report and review. J Am Geriatr Soc 11:891, 1963.
137. Dao TL, Greiner MJ: Mammary carcinogenesis by 3-methylcholanthrene. III. Induction of mammary carcinoma and milk secretion in male rats bearing ovarian grafts. J Natl Cancer Inst 27:333, 1961.
138. Scharff RW, Smith CP: Proliferative and other lesions of the male breast with notes on 2 cases of proliferative mastitis in stilboestrol workers. Br J Surg 29:393, 1942.
139. Wilson SE, Hutchinson WB: Breast masses in males with carcinoma of the prostate. J Surg Oncol 8:105, 1976.
140. Liechty RD, Davis J, Gleysteen J: Cancer of the male breast. Cancer 20:1617, 1967.
141. Campbell JH, Cummins SD: Metastases, simulating mammary cancer, in prostatic carcinoma under estrogenic therapy. Cancer 4:303, 1951.
142. Benson WR: Carcinoma of the prostate with metastases to breasts and testis. Cancer 10:1235, 1957.
143. Berge T: Metastases to the male breast. Acta Pathol Microbiol Scand (A)79:491, 1971.
144. Salyer WR, Salyer DC: Metastases of prostatic carcinoma to the breast. J Urol 109:671, 1973.
145. Sandison AT: An autopsy study of the adult human breast. Natl Cancer Inst Monogr 8:75, 1962.
146. Symmers WS: Carcinoma of the breast in transsexual individuals after surgical and hormonal interference with the primary and secondary sex characteristics. Br Med J 2:82, 1968.
147. Orentreich N, Durr NP: Mammogenesis in transsexuals. J Invest Dermatol 63:142, 1974.
148. Zumoff B, Fishman J, Cassouto J, et al.: Estradiol transformation in men with breast cancer. J Clin Endocrinol Metab 26:960, 1966.
149. Miller WR, Forrest APM: Oestradiol synthesis by a human breast carcinoma. Lancet 2:866, 1974.
150. Lazarev NI, Shasoukhova KS, Muravieva NI, et al.: Peculiarities specific to hormonal metabolism in males with gynecomastia and mammary carcinoma. Vestn Akad Med Nauk SSSR 24:28, 1969.
151. Komurdzhiaev KA, Rogoznaia AV: Mammary gland cancer in males. Vopr Onkol 10:87, 1964.
152. Dao TL, Morreal C, Nemoto T: Urinary estrogen excretion in men with breast cancer. N Engl J Med 289:138, 1973.
153. De Giuli G, De Giuli S: Urinary excretion of 17-KS, 17-OHCS and phenol-steroids in males with breast cancer. *In:* Davis W, Maltoni C (eds.): Characterization of Human Tumours, Vol. 1. New York: American Elsevier Publishing Co., 1974, pp. 213–217.
154. Calabresi E, De Giuli G, Becciolini A, et al.: Plasma estrogens and androgens in male breast cancer. J Steroid Biochem 7:605, 1976.
155. Patterson JS, Battersby LA, Bach BK: Use of tamoxifen in advanced male breast cancer. Cancer Treat Rep 64:801, 1980.
156. Jackson AW, Muldal S, Ockey CH, et al.: Carcinoma of male breast in association with the Klinefelter syndrome. Br Med J 1:223, 1965.
157. Bauer D de F, Erickson RL: Male breast cancer; Klinefelter syndrome with prostatic, adrenal and mammary tumors. Northwest Med 54:472, 1955.
158. Everson RB, Li FP, Fraumeni JF, Jr., et al.: Familial male breast cancer. Lancet 1:9, 1976.
159. Schmitt G, Scheffler J: Das Karzinom der männlichen Brustdrüse. Dtsch Med Wochenschr 96:931, 1971.
160. Marger D, Urdaneta N, Fischer JJ: Breast cancer in brothers. Cancer 36:458, 1975.
161. Teasdale C, Forbes JF, Baum M: Familial male breast cancer. Lancet 1:360, 1976.
162. Haagensen CD: Diseases of the Breast, second ed. Philadelphia: W.B. Saunders Co., 1971, pp. 354–379, 779–792.
163. Williams WR: Cancer of the male breast, based on the records of one hundred cases; with remarks. Lancet 2:261–263, 310–313, 1889.
164. Norris HJ, Taylor HB: Carcinoma of the male breast. Cancer 23:1428, 1969.
165. MacKenzie I: Breast cancer following multiple fluoroscopies. Br J Cancer 19:1, 1965.
166. Wanebo CK, Johnson KG, Sato K, et al.: Breast cancer after exposure to the atomic bombings of Hiroshima and Nagasaki. N Engl J Med 279:667, 1968.
167. MacMahon B, Cole P, Brown J: Etiology of human breast cancer: A review. J Natl Cancer Inst 50:21, 1973.
168. Lowell DM, Martineau RG, Luria SB: Carcinoma of the male breast following radiation. Cancer 22:581, 1968.

169. Deutsch M, Altomare FJ, Jr., Mastrian AS, et al.: Carcinoma of the male breast following thymic irradiation. Radiology 116:413, 1975.
170. Gilbert JB: Carcinoma of the male breast. Surg Gynecol Obstet 57:451, 1933.
171. Sachs MD: Carcinoma of the male breast. Radiology 37:458, 1941.
172. Nicholis GL, Sabetghadam R, Hsu CCS, et al.: Breast cancer after mumps orchitis. JAMA 223:1032, 1973.
173. Treves N: The treatment of cancer, especially inoperable cancer of the male breast by ablative surgery (orchiectomy, adrenalectomy, and hypophysectomy) and hormone therapy (estrogens and corticosteroids). Cancer 12:820, 1959.
174. Treves N, Robbins GF, Amoroso WL: Serous and serosanguineous discharge from the male nipple. A.M.A. Arch Surg 73:319, 1956.
175. Cain AS: Cancer of the male breast: Case report. Milit Med 142:892, 1977.
176. Mausner JS, Shimkin MB, Moss HN, et al.: Cancer of the breast in Philadelphia hospitals 1951–1964. Cancer 23:260, 1969.
177. Corwin JH, Ferguson EF, Jr., Moseley T, et al.: Carcinoma of the male breast. South Med J 60:777, 1967.
178. Nydick M, Bustos J, Dale JH, Jr., et al.: Gynecomastia in adolescent boys. JAMA 178:449, 1961.
179. Karsner HT: Gynecomastia. Am J Pathol 22:235, 1946.
180. Sirtoni C, Veronesi U: Gynecomastia: A review of 218 cases. Cancer 10:645, 1957.
181. Cutler M: Tumors of the Breast. Philadelphia: J.B. Lippincott Co., 1962, pp. 426–453.
182. Nicolis GL, Modlinger RS, Gabrilove JL: A study of the histopathology of human gynecomastia. J Clin Endocrinol 32:173, 1971.
183. Bannayan GA, Hajdu SI: Gynecomastia: Clinicopathologic study of 351 cases. Am J Clin Pathol 57:431, 1972.
184. Bridgman JF, Buckler JMH: Drug-induced gynaecomastia. Br Med J 3:520, 1974.
185. Kalisher L, Peyster RG: Xerographic manifestations of male breast disease. Am J Roentgenol 125:656, 1975.
186. Hall WH: Breast changes in males on cimetidine. N Engl J Med 295:841, 1976.
187. Marcus R, Korenman SG: Estrogens and the human male. Annu Rev Med 27:357, 1976.
188. Michels LG, Gold RH, Arndt RD: Radiography of gynecomastia and other disorders of the male breast. Radiol 122:117, 1977.
189. Keddie N, Morris PJ: Male breast tumors. Surg Gynecol Obstet 124:332, 1967.
190. Forman M: Roentgenography of the male breast. Am J Roentgenol 88:1126, 1962.
191. Axtell LM, Asire AJ, Myers MH (eds.): Cancer Patient Survival: Report Number 5. DHEW Publication No. (NIH) 77–992. Washington, DC: U.S. Department of Health, Education and Welfare, 1976, pp. 157–163.
192. Giffler RF, Kay S: Small cell carcinoma of the male mammary gland. Am J Clin Pathol 66:715, 1976.
193. Yogore MG, III, Sahgal S: Small cell carcinoma of the male breast. Cancer 39:1748, 1977.
194. Crichlow RW, Czernobilsky B: Paget's disease of the male breast. Cancer 24:1033, 1969.
195. Nehme AE: Paget's disease of the male breast. A collective review and case report. Am Surg 42:289, 1976.
196. Satiani B, Powell RW, Mathews WH: Paget disease of the male breast. Arch Surg 112:587, 1977.
197. Treves N: Inflammatory carcinoma of the breast in the male patient. Surgery 34:810, 1953.
198. Reingold IM, Ascher GS: Cystosarcoma phyllodes in a man with gynecomastia. Am J Clin Pathol 53:852, 1970.
199. Ferlito A, Dibonito L: Adenoid cystic carcinoma of the male breast: Report of a case. Am Surg 40:72, 1974.
200. Taxy JB: Tubular carcinoma of the male breast: Report of a case. Cancer 36:462, 1975.
201. Hart S, Sisely L: Granular cell tumour in a male breast. Med J Aust 2:1010, 1973.
202. Sirsat SM, Choksey AF, Jussawalla DJ: Ultrastructural study of mammary cancer in the human male. Indian J Cancer 13:201, 1976.
203. Everson RB, Lippman ME, Thompson EB, et al.: Clinical correlations of steroid receptors and male breast cancer. Cancer Res 40:991, 1980.
204. Greening WP, Aichroth PM: Cancer of the male breast. Br J Cancer 19:92, 1965.
205. Penettiere FJ: Cancer in the male breast. Cancer 34:1324, 1974.
206. Moss NH: Cancer of the male breast. Ann NY Acad Sci 114:937, 1964.
207. Peltokallio P, Kalima TV: Malignant tumours of the male breast in Finland. A report of 51 cases. Br J Cancer 23:480, 1969.
208. Crichlow RW, Kaplan EL, Kearney WH: Male mammary cancer: An analysis of 32 cases. Ann Surg 175:489, 1972.
209. Crichlow RW: Management of male breast cancer. *In:* Stoll BA (ed.): Breast Cancer Management—Early and Late. Chicago: Year Book Medical Publishers, 1977, pp. 167–173.
210. Huggins C, Jr., Taylor GW: Carcinoma of male breast. A.M.A. Arch Surg 70:303, 1955.
211. Tashima CK, Buzdar AU, Blumenschein GR, et al.: Adjuvant chemoimmunotherapy of stage IV (NED) breast cancer—an update. Proc Am Soc Clin Oncol (Abstract No. C–103) 19:332, 1968.
212. Neifeld JP, Meyskens F, Tormey DC, et al.: The role of orchiectomy in the management of advanced male breast cancer. Cancer 37:992, 1976.
213. Stephens RL, Muggia FM: Breast cancer in men. Am J Med 57:679, 1974.
214. Kennedy BJ, Kiang DT: Hypophysectomy in the treatment of advanced cancer of the male breast. Cancer 29:1606, 1972.
215. Juret P: Endocrine surgery in male breast cancer (translated by R. Chakravorty and E. Greenberg). *In:* Juret P (ed.): Endocrine Surgery in Human Cancers. Springfield, IL: Charles C Thomas, 1966, pp. 253–256.
216. Walach N, Hochman A: Male breast cancer. Oncology 29:181, 1974.
217. Li MC, Janelli DE, Kelly EJ, et al: Metastatic carcinoma of the male breast treated with bilateral adrenalectomy and chemotherapy. Cancer 25:678, 1970.
218. Lippman ME, Allegra JC, Thompson EB, et al.: The relation between estrogen receptors and response rate to cytotoxic chemotherapy in metastatic breast cancer. N Engl J Med 298:1223, 1978.

219. Treves N, Holleb AI: Cancer of the male breast. A report of 146 cases. Cancer 8:1239, 1955.
220. Donegan WL, Perez-Mesa CM: Carcinoma of the male breast. A 30-year review of 28 cases. Arch Surg 106:273, 1973.
221. MacKay EN, Sellers AH: Breast cancer at the Ontario cancer clinics. 1938–1956: A statistical review. Can Med Assoc J 92:647, 1965.
222. Brunet M, Janin ML, Berlie J: Carcinoma of the breast in man. Nouv Presse Med 6:721, 1977.
223. Langlands AO, Maclearn N, Kerr GR: Carcinoma of the male breast: Report of a series of 88 cases. Clin Radiol 27:21, 1976.
224. Ribeiro GG: Carcinoma of the male breast: A review of 200 cases. Br J Surg 64:381, 1977.
225. Satiani B, Powell RW: Cancer of the male breast: A thirty-year experience. Am Surg 44:86, 1978.

Psychologic Response to Breast Cancer: Direct and Indirect Contributors to Treatment Outcome

SANDRA M. LEVY, Ph.D.
WENDY S. SCHAIN, Ed.D

15

The relationship of psychosocial factors to cancer can be viewed as both cause (or at least contributor) and effect of the disease; that is, one can view behavioral and psychologic factors, or symptoms, as dependent variables or as functions of cancer and its treatments. Such factors become targets of intervention to ameliorate distressing symptoms or side effects (such as pain, anxiety, nausea, and shame), thereby restoring the patient's psychosocial quality of life. On the other hand, one can consider behavioral and psychologic factors as independent variables, or contributors to the disease process in some way. For example, life-style factors such as fatty diet potentially contribute to the risk for certain cancers, and patterns of behavioral distress responses may contribute to progression and affect the outcome of disease. An important aim in this latter area of investigation is the identification of mediating mechanisms (for example, immunologic effector mechanisms) linking higher cortical function and central nervous system input with host vulnerability and tumor response.

The first portion of the chapter will consider the psychosocial variables in a woman's life that impinge on her adaptation to breast cancer and the ensuing quality of life. The second segment of the chapter will bring to light findings regarding the correlation between a personality type, or adaptive maneuvers, immunologic response, and the progression or regression of cancer.

PSYCHOSOCIAL ADAPTATION TO BREAST CANCER

Cultural Factors

It is inappropriate to focus on the breast cancer patient in terms only of her somatic problems and the technologic aspects of her treatments. Rather, it is important to consider a much broader perspective and examine each patient as only one factor within a context of cultural, biologic, social, and psychologic forces. This is the frame of reference presented here: to discuss the woman as an individual who affects and is affected by a host of psychosocial variables, including her culture, social support network (namely, family, friends, and doctor-patient interaction), psychologic coping strategies, and attitudes about herself, her disease, and the specific types of treatment she must undergo.

Someday, anthropologists may label the current historical period as the mammocentric era, during which enormous amounts of psychic energy and capital resources went into glamorizing, idealizing, and sensationalizing the female breast. However, for centuries, artists and poets have exalted the female form and have highlighted its esthetic and symbolic meaning. While human breasts may be identified as end-organs and described as mammary glands, this part of the anatomy elicits a variety of dependent, nurturing, and sexual reactions.[1] A women's breasts are often equated with her ability to reproduce, nurture her young, attract a member of the opposite sex, and seduce and capture a mate. In many instances, they are also a major source of feminine identification and are critical to one's self-esteem. How does this critical connection get established and what are the factors that undermine or reinforce its development, and what happens to the woman (and her significant other) when she develops a breast cancer and is faced with either radical or conservative surgery on such a value-laden organ?

Susan Brownmiller[2] cogently described this phenomenon. She asked, "Where does this whole issue of femininity and sexuality start? At what age does a girl begin to view her assets and count her deficient parts? When does she close the bedroom door and begin to gaze privately into the mirror—pull in her stomach, throw out her chest, and pose again in search for the most flattering angle? At what age does the process begin? This obsessive concentration on the minutiae of her physical being...will occupy some portion of her waking hours, quite possibly, for the rest of her life." It is understandable, therefore, that a woman facing alteration or amputation of such a socially prized organ might be anguished, fearful, depressed, or enraged.

Not only does the culture in which one lives influence the weight and value placed on anatomic organs and the ability to reproduce, but also it is the tapestry into which is woven the traditions and mores of the time. Specifically, the American culture places great weight on establishment of the family and puts a premium on having a mate and children. Our society also offers the identified woman a medical system that ranges from patriarchal to egalitarian. Both these factors (the social network and the health care system) influence the breast cancer patient's choices of treatments, adaptation to her disease, and overall level of psychologic functioning.

Care Providers and Communication Patterns

The patient–care provider relationship may be one of the most crucial variables affecting patient coping,[3] and the particular nature of this relationship is shaped by the educational training of the physician or other care giver, that person's socialization experiences, and his or her own philosophic inclination. In conventional medicine, the major responsibility for treatment is given to the physician, and the therapeutic benefit is assumed to occur by the physician's doing something to or for the patient, who generally accepts what is done. Furthermore, in this approach, the focus is almost exclusively on the body and its internal organs; the mind is viewed as a separate entity that requires a separate subspecialist for treatment. For health care providers who ascribe to a holistic philosophy, a person's mind, body, and spirit are integrated into an indivisible unit and are conceived as one entity. Therefore, feelings, imagination, creativity, values, and ethics are all implicated in illness and healing and also are invoked in treatment efforts, along with more traditional kinds of medicine and interventions.

Another important aspect of the relationship between patient and physician is the degree of dominance attributed to the health care specialist. The balance of power between these two individuals has considerable impact on feelings of support, amount and type of information provided, and especially on the degree of control and sense of mastery experienced by the patient. While there are various descriptions of patient–care provider models, the distinction in this text will concentrate on exchange of information between doctor and patient and whether this process is experienced as congruent or incongruent from the patient's vantage point. To understand the issue of doctor-patient interaction more clearly, it is necessary to examine the reciprocal flow of factors that shape the doctor-patient transaction and the degree of mutuality experienced.

One line of psychosocial research in the area of doctor-patient communication has suggested that patients can be divided into MONITORS (patients who seek out and need threatening, but relevant information) and BLUNTERS (patients who need to avoid or lessen the impact of the information related to their disease).[4] Intuitively, a physician knows who is a Monitor. She is the woman who walks into the office with a pad, pencil, tape recorder, and a copy of some treatise on breast cancer. She is the type of woman who asks a hundred questions, wants a great deal of detail, is able to quote the latest statistics from medical journals, and is, in summary, determined to receive as much information as can be made available. Acquiring threat-relevant information for this type of patient may be necessary to help reduce her anxiety and increase her sense of mastery in what is beginning to be experienced as a very threatening situation, in which she is starting to feel helpless and out of control.

Blunters, on the other hand, may be distinguished by their passivity and their compliance with physician recommendations, and they seem reluctant to question or challenge what an authority figure has said. This patient's typical response (and, unfortunately, the one that is generally assumed as universal for all women) is to become noticeably anxious and distressed by too much information. Such a response pattern may prompt physicians to conclude that women do not want or cannot handle medical information in any detail. However, reports and clinical observations suggest (1) the importance of identifying the individual patient's need to know what the risks and benefits of a given therapy are and (2) the importance of providing her with the level and sophistication of information that she needs to feel gratified, in control, and psychologically safe.

Specifically, the Monitor type seems to need very detailed communication and evidence from her physician that she is welcomed as an active participant in making decisions about her treatment. The Blunter type needs to feel that her physician is taking care of her and that the physician is able to, and desires to, plan the treatment regimen with little or no input about personal needs or wishes. If too much information is disseminated to the Blunter patient, she may not be able to assimilate it effectively and may feel emotionally overloaded and have a tendency to become panicky and agitated. On the other hand, if the Monitor patient does not receive an adequate amount of information or does not experience regard for her need to be an active participant in the treatment decisions, she may feel undermined and threatened by loss of control and will search for answers elsewhere or become agitated or aggressive.

In summary, it is in both parties' best interest to optimize congruence regarding the imparting of information. Enhanced patient-physician partnership and more agreement in communication style can result in improved patient satisfaction, increased adherence to treatment regimens, reduced burdens for the doctor, and greater feelings of individuality, autonomy, and self-respect for the patient.

Coping Strategies and Types of Treatment

MASTECTOMY

The psychosocial literature reports a range in types and magnitude of emotional disturbance following mastectomy. Maguire and colleagues[5] and Morris and associates[6] report a significant degree of depression and anxiety in their study group. In addition, they respectively conclude that approximately 27 and 32 percent of the mastectomy patients acknowledged sexual problems following their surgery. Jamison and colleagues,[7] in their first study of the mastectomy patient, found that almost one fourth of their study group (23 percent) were emotionally upset and described sexual dysfunctions. A moderate number also reported depression, sleep disturbances, and occasional suicidal ideation. Upon interviewing the partners of these women in a follow-up study, Wellisch and associates[8] noted that 36 percent rated the impact of the mastectomy as negative and that approximately 17 percent of these men stated that they had not looked at their partner's unclothed body during the first year following their surgery.

Specifically in regard to male-female interaction after mastectomy, Silberfarb and colleagues[9] found that 22 to 31 percent of their study group reported sexual disturbances and reduced frequency of intercourse.[9] Frank and associates[10] reported that about one third of the mastectomy patients they investigated had not resumed intercourse for six months and that nudity and self-display became an issue for a significant proportion of women. Kolodny and colleagues[11] stated that the male superior position became preferable for these couples so that the amputated organ and the obvious physical defect was not a constant visual reminder to the male partners.

Worden and Weisman,[12] on the other hand, challenged the premise that psychosocial distress is a necessary sequel of mastectomy. In their investigation, they noted that significant depression following mastectomy was not a universal finding. In fact, they discovered that certain women fared quite well during this ordeal, some women adapted only moderately effectively, and a lesser number coped very poorly with the crisis of cancer. In a separate study conducted by this research team to investigate the "existential plight in cancer,"[13] these two researchers identified a set of psychosocial variables to predict who would and who would not cope well with this disease. In summary, patients who had higher emotional distress and were viewed as being more psychologically vulnerable were those who had many regrets about the past, were pessimistic, came from multiproblem families, and had marital problems. This same group who exhibited difficulty in coping more commonly were either widowed or divorced and anticipated little or no support from their significant others. Interestingly, the impact of social support on adaptation and coping appears over and over in the literature.[14–16]

After interviewing 300 women treated for early stages of gynecologic and breast cancer, Cobliner[17] detailed a profile of characteristics observed in women who were described as having adjusted successfully to their condition. The psychosocial characteristics include the following:

1. A high general self-image and an absence of irrational ideas about cancer.
2. A positive image of femininity, which suffers little alteration, if any, as a result of the disease or its treatments.
3. Strong faith in their doctors.
4. A high degree of trust in the clinic or hospital where they are treated.
5. A belief in the efficacy of the particular treatments they receive.
6. A desire and opportunity to confide their worries and intimate concerns to another person, usually of the same sex.
7. Involvement in an activity or occupation that provides them satisfaction.
8. Good relationships with husbands, sexual partners, or close friends, which change slightly or not at all following the onset of illness or treatment.
9. Concordance between life expectations and their degree of attainment.
10. The nature and success of any attempted resolutions of a life crisis in the past.

A list such as this can help to focus on factors facilitating adaptation and can underscore areas of potential distress in which appropriate interventions should be introduced. Clearly, successful adaptation seems to reflect past and present coping strategies that permit integration of the mastectomy experience with a gratifying life style.

Until about three years ago, the conclusions regarding psychosocial aspects of breast cancer were gleaned exclusively from mastectomy patients. Less than radical surgery for this disease was not popular or readily available in the United States and had only slowly come into prominence.[18] However, there is a paucity of information regarding adaptive reactions of conservative surgery patients and whether they face an ordeal similar to or very different from that of their mastectomy counterparts. The important issues to be explored might be described in the following ways: (1) Does elimination of amputation of the breast categorically erase negative psychologic trauma? (2) If given a choice, will all women opt to preserve this prized organ? If not, who will choose the more radical surgery, and why? and (3) What is the relationship between personality profile, environmental factors, type of treatment, and coping effectiveness?

Breast Conservation Therapy

Breast preservation in the management of this disease is fast becoming an acceptable alternative to mastectomy and a sought-after option, for obvious reasons. One might assume that breast-sparing surgery is "easy treatment" because the body is left primarily intact and the physical reminder of breast cancer is minimally in evidence to the woman and to her significant other. However, this may not be the case. The first report in the literature that investigated psychosocial sequelae of breast-sparing procedures concluded that the group receiving conservative surgery plus irradiation had a better body image following treatment than did their mastectomy counterparts.[19] On the other hand, this study showed that the two different patient populations did not exhibit major or significant differences in any of the other areas of psychosocial functioning that were assessed, including overall psychologic distress and marital discord. Contrary to popular expectation, women who were treated for this disease without removal of the breast did not escape the emotional upset formerly attributed to mastectomy in the treatment of breast cancer.

In a comprehensive study[20] comparing mastectomy and lumpectomy patients, the investigators disclosed a host of findings that more clearly reflect psychologically positive associations with breast-sparing techniques, which had been revealed only in anecdotal material. The experiences that were documented in this study revealed that, in contrast with the comparison group of mastectomy patients, the conservative surgery patients showed less disruption in feelings of femininity and attractiveness, reported no alteration in types of clothes worn either in public or in private, described less psychologic and sexual distress, and acknowledged more satisfaction with the emotional support they received. This last item, the emotional support experienced by patients, is a very critical component in quality of life and perhaps even survivorship.[21]

The reasons that lumpectomy patients might be the recipients of this beneficial social exchange are not clear and require more intensive examination. At present, one might conjecture that the woman who has a breast-sparing procedure and whose life is less obviously disrupted (at least after primary treatment is concluded) is less likely to need the constant attention, sympathy, and nurturance so often required when a woman has her life threatened by cancer and concomitantly has her body radically changed by the required treatment. It is also possible, as Peters-Golden indicated,[16] that actual support supplied by the patient's family and friends may be related to what is expected and how comfortable or "non-needy" the patient appears. Healthy well-wishers seem more able to offer support when it is not solicited from a pained, obviously ill, and emotionally needy patient. Many of the women who do not have to give up their breast may fall within the boundaries of this description.

While lumpectomy patients do not face the dual threat of a potentially lethal disease and a markedly different body, they continue to struggle with a unique set of psychosocial and sexual concerns. They may worry about whether the radiation will create long-term negative consequences, in addition to whether it really will be effective in producing control of the local disease. Some women find the axillary dissection scar very ugly and focus on it, perhaps to displace their more generalized anxiety about cancer. As a result of the changes in the texture of the breast following radiation therapy, a number of women worry about whether they should examine the treated breast and what they can tell if they do: Is the lumpiness or hardness a direct result of therapy? Is anything that feels unusual there to be considered a warning signal of recurrent disease?

A recent research investigation conducted in the Netherlands[22] reported findings directly related to the value of breast-sparing treatment and its impact on the fear of recurrence. The researchers found that in their study group of 114 BCT (breast conservation therapy) patients, there was a significant degree of positive psychologic benefit compared with the 58 RM (radical mastectomy) patients. In addition, it was found that the BCT group expressed significantly less fear of recurrence of their cancer than did their mastectomy counterparts. Whether this is related to the timeless adage "What you do not see does not bother you" is not certain. Having one's breast *intact* may reinforce the denial of an underlying malignancy or may allow a level of distance from threatening associations so that thoughts of cancer are much less frequent.

Continued investigation of underlying dynamics is essential to determining *if breast conservation therapy permits (1) a healthy level of minimization of the hazards of breast cancer or (2) an unhealthy level of denial, which could interfere with surveillance and necessary follow-up care.* One might assert that research studies are beginning to document what has been apparent in clinical case studies and anecdotal reports: Breast conservation minimizes the depression associated with the harsh visual and daily reminder of breast cancer that radical surgery elicits. This would seem to be especially true for the woman with early breast cancer who requires no adjuvant therapy and can leave behind part of her breast cancer experience after primary treatment is concluded. Whether the lessening of psychic distress and the reduction in fear of recurrence is true for all breast conservation patients or only for a certain subset with specific coping strategies (namely, avoidance or blocking) is yet to be determined.

While most psychosocial studies comparing radical mastectomy and breast conservation therapy have been retrospective assessments and have not been well controlled, similar findings were gleaned from the randomized clinical trial at the National Cancer Institute.[20] In that study, lumpectomy plus radiation therapy patients showed a distinct advantage psychologically over mastectomy patients and no increase in worry about the recurrence of their disease. Specifically, the breast conservation patients reported significantly fewer problems in the areas of sexual interest, their own body perception, anxiety, sadness, frustration, or feelings that life was not worthwhile. In summary, this group of patients was less emotionally distressed in most areas of psychologic functioning. However, it cannot be concluded that lumpectomy plus irradiation is emotionally a panacea or an "easy treatment" for all women with early breast cancer. These women reported more physical discomfort in terms of chest wall tenderness, soreness in the treated area, and concern about the size of the arm on the treated side. These complaints were subjective appraisals and are being compared with objective measures of physical parameters by the rehabilitation department.

As a result of findings from the studies previously discussed, one needs seriously to consider the potential psychologic value and medical efficacy of breast conservation therapy. The humanistic goals concerning breast cancer treatment have included extending survivorship, preserving or restoring body integrity, and safeguarding emotional well-being. While the findings are impressive, one cannot assume that BCT (with or without radiation therapy) is the only treatment of choice or that it assures psychologic equanimity. It does seem to reduce depression, anxiety about body image, and sexual dysfunction associated with breast cancer treatment. More important, it seems to be unassociated with any increased fear that keeping the treated breast will lead to additional cancer. Continued psychologic assessment of these women is necessary to evaluate their quality of life, resumption of and satisfaction with sexual activities (especially stimulation of the breast), and maintenance of health care vigilance. There seems to be little doubt that preserving the treated breast does not increase the threat of dying. However, psychologic security about survivorship and the feeling that one's disease is cured or controlled is multifaceted. The presence of one's breast may be a necessary but not sufficient condition to eliminate psychologic morbidity in the treatment of this dread disease.

Reconstruction

The physical defect created by mastectomy is no longer an irreversible state, but one that is correctable by surgical intervention and that has been demonstrated to have a beneficial effect on women's psychologic and sexual responses. A number of investigators[23–25] have documented that postmastectomy reconstruction has a positive impact on the woman's spirit, her physical appearance, her optimism about life, and often her indirect value. First, it frees the woman from anxiety about her condition being obvious, and it releases her from a preoccupation with her bodily defect, which seems to put distance between her physical condition and the underlying cancer that necessitated the radical surgery. Not to have to be worried about an external prosthesis and not having to see the ugly mastectomy scar (although the scars are, in rare instances, well repaired), which is a constant reminder of possible recurrence of disease, are welcome and revitalizing factors that facilitate the woman's return to former activities with less distraction and with fewer negative memories.

The therapeutic benefit of reconstruction is rarely challenged, but the controversy that has replaced such an issue—When, in the treatment experience, should a patient have reconstruction?—is unresolved. Reports suggest added benefits that might be associated with immediate breast reconstruction,[26] including the possibility that shortening the delay between breast amputation and repair significantly reduces hostility, anxiety, and depression.[27] In addition to the emotional relief often accompanying reconstruction, positive changes in sexual activity associated with this reparative surgery have been documented. Teimourian and Adham[28] noted that sexual activity was increased in women following their breast reconstruction, but it is not clear whether this change is due to (1) improved erotic responses in the breast region or (2) an enhanced feeling of body symmetry and restored attractiveness (especially in clothes and nighttime apparel). An interesting laboratory investigation by Gerard,[29] using a photoplethysmograph to document vaginal blood flow as an index of arousal, revealed that patients with reconstructed breasts were more sexually responsive than their mastectomy-only counterparts. While this study had a very small sample, the findings suggest that such women may be less negative about their bodies, less anxious sexually, less focused on their missing organ, and more open to responding to the sexual stimuli occurring at the moment.

The motives that prompt women to elect to have or not to have breast reconstruction vary according to the stage of disease, the information the woman gets, the support she receives from her physicians and loved ones, the availability of a reconstructive surgeon, and the internal psychologic facilitators or inhibitors that she acknowledges. We have previously presented a detailed discussion of these issues.[30] That review highlighted how little is known about this area, because most of the investigations have been conducted on women who have already chosen to have their missing breast reconstructed. Again, the controlled clinical trial at the NIH allows for serious scrutiny of psychosocial aspects of breast reconstruction. Because this population of breast cancer patients is told about the procedure at the time of initial presentation for treatment (and before any definitive surgery), plus the fact that there is no out-of-pocket expense for the patient undergoing this operation, a number of contaminating variables have been eliminated. In addition, the entire treatment team unconditionally (but without pressure) supports the fact that breast reconstruction is a freely available component in the rehabilitation of the mastectomy patient. In spite of the unconditional support for this procedure, only a limited number of the first 50 mastectomy patients opted for delayed reconstruction. However, in the last six months, intraoperative reconstruction with a tissue expander has been offered to study patients, and no mastectomy patient has chosen to decline this offer. What factors are influencing this difference in choice of reconstruction are not yet clear, but analysis of the dynamics is under way. Repeated assessment, by both standardized psychologic tests and personal interview material, is being carried out to identify the critical factors in women's choices to have or not to have their amputated breast reconstructed in a treatment protocol in which therapy is standardized and endorsement for such a choice is unchallenged. It is hoped that such an understanding will clarify a number of variables that affect breast cancer patients' adaptation and will have generalizability to patients in both clinical trials and the private sector. There is undoubtedly an interaction among a multiplicity of factors, but which are predominant for all women and which are high priorities for some women is as yet undetermined. It may be that the more assertive, energized, and effectively coping woman refuses to live with a defect that is indeed alterable. Additionally, it may be that the woman who candidly wishes to deny that she has had a breast cancer and subsequently had to have a mastectomy is the woman who opts for reconstruction. When and for whom the choice is most beneficial and in what ways restoring one's body to an intact form perhaps signifies health and physical integrity are still unknown.

We have been considering such factors as the patient's response style, motives and needs for cognitive control, social support in the treatment environment, and psychologic response to surgical intervention and reconstruction as clinical sequelae of breast cancer treatment. As was discussed in the introduction to this chapter, such behavioral and social factors can also be viewed as potential contributors to disease progression, directly or indirectly affecting the microenvironment of the tumor by way of central nervous system–endocrine–immune pathways. Behavior as a biologic response modifier relevant to at least some tumor systems will be considered in the balance of this chapter.

BEHAVIOR AS A BIOLOGIC RESPONSE MODIFIER IN BREAST CANCER PROGRESSION

The fundamental question of concern here is, Why is there variance in cancer progression? Why do two patients with apparently identical tumor types, identical stages at diagnosis, identical cellular histologies, and identical treatment histories have different disease outcomes? What proportion of this outcome variance can be attributed to behavioral and emotional factors?

We are all familiar with stories of spectacular spontaneous regressions of advanced disease and sudden eruptions of tumors after years—sometimes decades—of remission. The following case reported by Cole[31] is an example.

> Another patient—a nun—had (spontaneous) regression of cancer of the pancreas. The patient had been jaundiced for months. At exploratory celiotomy, the head of the pancreas was enlarged three times normal. A biopsy was obtained and a diagnosis of carcinoma was confirmed by three pathologists. The Sisters of the Order interceded on her behalf with prayer and so on (*sic*). She recovered rapidly from the operation and from her very weakened condition. She returned to work for 7.5 years and died suddenly. Autopsy revealed a massive pulmonary embolism but positively no evidence of tumor.

Of course, there are other stories that have appeared but have a less felicitous outcome, for example, the report of good tumor control and no evidence of disease for years, and then following a sudden trauma such as a car accident or surgical insult, a sudden eruption of the same malignancy (proved to be the same tumor by biopsy and the histologic identity).

However, in addition to such rare events as those just described, the ordinary course of tumor progression is not identical from patient to patient. Even taking into account all known biologic sources of variance, including such factors as weight and pharmacologic interventions, there may still exist unexplained disease variance. Some of this variance could be accounted for by behavioral factors, discussed in the remaining pages of this chapter.

Behavior and Cancer Progression: Human Studies

> The enormous complexity of human society and man's capacity through his symbol system to identify with more powerful beings—(gods or chosen leaders, or institutions)—give him certain invulnerability to limbic system arousal as long as he perceives himself to be socially supported here or in the hereafter. But, if as the result of early or later experience or a combination of both, he comes to perceive himself as helpless and lacking power to control his state, he may well become more vulnerable than an animal whose associational cortex is more limited.[32]

This quote from Henry captures the essence of what is emerging as important in studies of behavior and tumor progression. There seems to be a parallel behavioral pattern in studies of cancer progression in humans and animals, which we will consider in detail here. But it must be kept in mind that man and mouse differ in fundamental ways, not the least of which is man's capacity to symbolize, project future situations in fantasy, and resensitize himself continually as reaction to real or imagined stress conditions—so that the notion of acute versus chronic stress, so important a distinction in animal studies, does not so neatly hold for the human condition.

It is also important to keep in mind that the major determinant of cancer outcome is the biology of the tumor and its cellular histopathology, genetic factors, constitutional host vulnerability, and so on. However, at least for some tumors, the emotional, cognitive, and behavioral responses of the organism very probably play a role in the disease course. It is this exciting area of investigation that we will consider here.

If one is going to consider potential effects of behavior, broadly conceived, on tumor progression, there are some tumor requirements for study. First, only tumors that often (but not invariably) have a relatively *indolent course* can be considered. This would rule out the virulent types of cancer such as pancreatic or primary liver cancer, for which it is unlikely that behavioral factors would play much of a contributing role in the outcome. A second tumor requirement is that there be a rather wide interindividual variation in tumor course, despite similar cell histology, stage of diagnosis, and treatment history. This would allow for some still unexplained disease outcome variance to be potentially accounted for by behavioral and social factors. Third, there should be some evidence of hormonal or immunologic reactivity, or both, associated with the tumor in question. Both the endocrine and the immune systems have direct links with the central nervous system, and, therefore, the probability of finding contributing influences of the host's molar behavior to the tumor course is enhanced.

Several different cancers fit the foregoing requirements. These include breast cancer, melanoma and other skin cancers, prostatic and endometrial cancers, lymphomas, and colorectal malignancies. It is important for the reader to keep these tumor requirements and tumor types in mind as we consider the clinical and animal studies in this area. Nearly all the clinical studies, few as they are, have been conducted with melanoma and breast cancer patients. The animal studies have used induced and transplanted tumors of various kinds, including transplanted lymphoma and mammary cell lines, and chemical induction of mammary and colon tumors.

If the intact animal host is to be considered as a better system for understanding tumor response than an *in vitro* model, one would lean more heavily on findings from *in vivo* animal studies. And if, as Henry[32] so eloquently points out, the human host is essentially distinct from other species, one is going to weigh most heavily findings from human studies of host response and tumor progression or containment.

So, we will begin with a review of relevant clinical studies in this area and then will review recent animal studies linking behavioral patterns with increased survival in cancer patients. However, one must keep in mind all these important qualifiers (i.e., relevance to only *some* tumors, distinction between animal and human tumor systems, the necessity to understand tumor progression within the intact host, and the essential distinction between human and animal hosts).

Helplessness and Social Support in Human Studies Relevant to Cancer Progression

Since the 1950's, the clinical lore that passive patients fare worse has been part of the cancer literature. For example, Greer and colleagues[33] showed on eight-year follow-up that women who were rated as helpless or stoic had worse breast cancer outcomes than those of women who were rated as showing a fighting spirit or who denied the significance of their illness. Only tumor grade also predicted breast cancer mortality. A major problem with this study is that lymph node status was not part of the survival analysis equation, because all patients did not undergo axillary node dissection. It is therefore possible that psychologic outcome was confounded with this major biologic risk factor. Nevertheless, there is a consistency between Greer's findings and those of other investigators.

For example, Rogentine and associates[34] reported significantly greater incidence of relapse in melanoma patients who expressed little difficulty adjusting to their disease compared with those who reported more difficulty in adjustment. This reporting of few problems was interpreted as a passive or stoic response style—an insistence that life would be normal and they would get on with it. An unpublished prospective study of melanoma patients[35] demonstrated a similar association between such passivity and disease course. They showed that melanoma patients who reported higher distress, along with a "problem-solving" orientation at baseline, had reduced psychiatric disturbance, higher activity levels of a naturally occurring lymphocyte (the natural killer, or NK, cell, discussed in detail later), and reduced incidence of disease relapse nine months later. Patients who reported no distress—and no problem-solving orientation at baseline—were more disturbed, had lower levels of NK activity, and a higher rate of cancer recurrence at nine months' follow-up. These findings suggest an adaptational process over time and the need to study coping and vulnerability (biologic and psychologic) as aspects of that process.

Similarly, Derogatis and colleagues[36] reported longer survival times in breast cancer patients who were rated as distressed and who reported more psychiatric symptoms of various kinds than in women who appeared to have little psychologic difficulty. All these studies, although not fatally flawed, have some methodological weaknesses, but as an aggregate, they show consistent findings: Patients who are characterized as passive have worse cancer outcomes.

Breast Cancer Studies

As indicated earlier, the two tumors that have been the focus of human studies in this area are breast cancer and melanoma. This author's area of investigation has been breast cancer and, therefore, a discussion of this disease within the psychosocial context might be pertinent here.

Potential Endogenous Control Mechanisms

Wheelock[37, 38] and others link animal models of tumor dormancy with dramatic human clinical phenomena, such as spontaneous regression of tumors and disease recurrence latencies of 20 to 30 years. Theoretically, we could consider the notion of growth restraint and dormancy when considering the normal clinical course of time to recurrence of disease, although in humans the measures are not so precise—factors such as individual cell doubling time cannot be so readily measured or controlled. Still, given the same stage and grade of tumor, we can ask the question: What are the endogenous control mechanisms potentially functioning as restraining agents in the course of breast cancer?

For breast cancer, both *immunologic* and *hormonal* mechanisms have been implicated in such tumor growth restraint. Primary breast tumors have been reported to induce an immune response capable of modifying tumor growth by various mechanisms.[39, 40] A number of studies have shown that hormone levels play an important part in contributing to breast cancer risk as well as in modulating the course of primary breast cancer, the growth of metastatic foci, and the maintenance of the disease-free interval through endocrine therapy. This latter area concerned with endocrinologic factors and tumor response, discussed extensively in Chapter 11, will not be considered here.

Breast Cancer and Immune Containment

Many reports have been published on the prognostic significance of lymphocytic infiltration of cancer tissue.[41–43] The study of tumor immunology has been marked by both successes and failures, and the history of this area will not be discussed here. The aggregate of experimental and clinical evidence strongly suggests that cellular immune reactions are involved in the host-tumor relationship and play a modifying role related to tumor growth within the organism.

We are not concerned here with tumor immunology in general but with immunologic control of breast cancer. There have been histologic studies of *in situ* and invasive breast cancers revealing lymphoid cell infiltrations of the primary tumor.[44, 45] A study[46] showed that T-cell infiltration in breast tumors was scanty in scirrhous carcinoma but was ample in the infiltrating papillotubular carcinoma, known to have a better prognosis. There was also a significant inverse correlation between the intensity of the T-cell infiltration and the clinical stage of disease (Stage IV having practically no T-cell–relevant activity). The intensity of the T-cell infiltration was significantly higher in patients without lymph node metastasis. Although the researchers noted that these correlational data do not prove causal effects, they cited animal experiments[47] that have demonstrated that some T-cell populations have a suppressive effect on cancer cell growth.

With more advanced stage of disease, such lymphocytic infiltrate has been reported to decrease. Such decreasing responsiveness may be due to lack of competent sensitized cells, lack of tissue antigenicity, or both. In fact, one explanation for lack of containment of tumor cells is that those that slip through are antigenically modified and thus escape being targeted by sensitized effector cells. It has also been suggested that migrating tumor cells actually lose their antigenic quality and are therefore no longer detected as nonself. There are other explanations for escape from local control, including the generation of suppressor factors—T-cells or macrophages—suppressing immunologic containment of tumor cells. There is another body of literature concerned with "blocking factors" in the serum (e.g., antigen fractions that circulate as antigen-antibody complexes, combining with receptor sites on sensitized lymphocytes and blocking tumor cell lysis). These various theories and their supporting evidence will not be considered here. (The interested reader is referred to Wheelock and Robinson[37] for a more extensive discussion of this topic.)

Naturally Occurring Cytotoxicity and Tumor Control

As indicated earlier, tumor cells are very adaptive within an immunologic environment (shedding antigenic determinants, for example), and some populations within a heterogeneous tumor mass have been reported to escape specific T-cell cytolytic attack. In contrast, host cells that kill tumor cells by nonimmune (nonsensitized) mechanisms have been shown in many cases to be effective in killing such heterogeneous masses, including circulating tumor emboli.[48] Such nonspecific cells include natural killer (NK) cells and a phagocytic cell, the macrophage. Only NK cells will be discussed here, as this lymphocyte subset has direct bearing on our own work.

NK cells were discovered in the 1970's, following the observation that lymphoid cells from healthy volunteers were highly cytotoxic *in vitro* for cultured tumor cells. Since these healthy individuals could not have been exposed to tumor-associated antigen, there was clearly present a naturally occurring mechanism that was cytotoxic for tumor cells. Since that time, the nature, morphology, and function of NK cells related to cancer surveillance have been active areas of intensive investigation.[49]

One major prediction of an immune surveillance theory is that tumor growth should be preceded by depressed immunity. According to Herberman and Santoni,[50] several laboratory and clinical observations are consistent with this theory. In a colony of beige mice having a selective defect in NK activity, a high incidence of lymphomas was found, and patients with Chédiak-Higashi syndrome, with a marked and selective defect in NK activity, also have a high incidence of lymphoproliferative diseases. Further, kidney allograft recipients having received immunosuppressant drugs, who have a high risk of developing lymphomas and other tumors, have significantly lower levels of NK activity.[49]

Much of the evidence for the role of NK cells *in vivo* has come from studies of transplanted tumor growths correlated with levels of NK cells within the recipient. Most of these studies have shown a strong inverse correlation between levels of NK activity and transplanted tumor cell clearance, but such evidence does not indicate whether NK cells play a similar role in defense against spontaneous tumors. It has been found, however, that most of the spontaneous mammary tumors in C_3H mice as well as the spontaneous lymphomas in AKR mice have detectable susceptibility to NK lysis. In addition, some human leukemias, carcinomas, sarcomas, and melanomas have been lysed with NK cells.[49]

Therefore, NK cells have been shown to have spontaneous cytolytic activity against a wide range of tumors, including breast cancer tumors, as well as some normal cells. These lymphocytes have characteristics distinct from other types of lymphocytic cells but are closely associated with large granular lymphocytes, the latter composing approximately 5 percent of blood or splenic leukocytes.

Direct evidence has been supplied demonstrating that NK cells inhibit tumor metastases *in vivo*. Studies have characterized the role of NK cells in the destruction of circulating sarcoma and melanoma cells.[48] Systemic, adoptive transfer of normal spleen cells to cyclophosphamide-treated recipients 24 hours before tumor inoculation reduced the cyclophosphamide-mediated enhancement of pulmonary tumor metastases by transplanted melanoma or sarcoma tumor cells.[51] Reconstituted cells provided to the cyclophosphamide-treated animals were demonstrated to be NK cells, as the addition of anti-NK-1.2 antibodies prevented control of metastatic spread. In the *in vivo* model described in this latter work, the NK cells were most effective during a limited time period (up to 24 hours) after tumor inoculation, and the investigators concluded that their target, most probably, was the circulating tumor cell.

While most of the evidence for NK activity against cancer cell spread has been supplied by experimental investigation—with limited correlational evidence for an NK role in rare, clinical subpopulations such as patients with Chédiak-Higashi (NK-deficient) disorder—other clinical evidence for their role is emerging. It has been reported that patients with a variety of advanced cancers (including advanced breast cancer) exhibited lower NK activity against standard target cells (K562) than did patients with localized malignancy or normal control subjects. NK cells from these patients with advanced disease were normal in number but had reduced functional capacity to kill cancer cell targets.[40] Findings from our study of breast cancer patient prognosis[52] revealed a significant association between NK activity at baseline testing and disease prognosis for these patients. We will consider these findings in further detail later.

Therefore, based on the extensive animal literature as well as emerging clinical evidence, it is becoming increasingly apparent that naturally occurring lymphocyte cytotoxicity may play an important role in controlling the spread of micrometastases within the organism. In addition, since lymphocytes including NK cells are modulated by various neuropeptides such as the endogenous opioids,[53–55] central nervous system links are likely to be relevant to tumor restraint or progression.

Studies of Coping and Breast Cancer Prognosis

Unpublished research carried out at Yale[56] showed more rapid progression of breast cancer in patients to be associated with a defensive coping style characterized by lower levels of self-reported distress and higher self-report of helplessness, accompanied by symptoms of chronic stress (e.g., symptoms of constant tension and inability to relax). Jensen[56] speculated that inattention to biologic signals of distress among individuals identified as having a repressive coping style might be associated with poorer outcome at follow-up.

Ongoing work[52] has revealed similar patterns of association between passive, "helpless" response style and worse breast cancer prognosis and outcome. An early, pilot study conducted with advanced breast cancer patients (first-recurrence patients, with a disease-free interval of at least two months) replicated Derogatis's findings.[36] Findings from this study are displayed in Table 15–1. In general, patients reporting little in the way of psychiatric stress at baseline testing (at the beginning of their treatment for recurrent disease) and who were rated by others as "well adjusted" tended to be dead at one-year follow-up. On the other hand, patients who reported higher levels of psychiatric symptoms and were rated as being "disturbed" by observers tended to still be alive at one year. The only biologic factor differentiating outcome groups was the disease-free interval, with a positive correlation between the length of the disease-free interval and the survival time. Importantly, psycho-

TABLE 15–1. Self-Report Symptom and Disability Measures for Stable Versus Progressing Versus Dead at One Year

Variable	*Stable*	*Progressing*	*Dead*	*Statistic*	*p*
SCL-90-R					
Somatic	0.80	0.48	0.56	1.29	NS
O-C	0.84	0.47	0.40	1.56	NS
Interpersonal	0.89	0.26	0.08	5.9	0.01
Depression	1.18	0.55	0.29	3.55	0.05
Anxiety	1.10	0.32	0.40	4.78	0.02
Hostility	0.46	0.18	0.20	1.5	NS
Phobia	0.62	0.09	0.02	2.45	0.11
Paranoid	0.60	0.09	0.03	7.7	0.004
Psychotic	0.50	0.25	0.16	1.7	0.20
PST	0.75	0.29	0.26	3.60	0.05
Karnofsky	88	91	90	0.16	NS
GAIS	55.2	72.2	72.4	2.7	0.09

logic response factors were statistically independent of any biologic factor differentiating outcome groups. This finding suggests that the psychologic factors might be independently contributing to outcome rather than merely being confounded with biologic status and hence adding little to outcome variance.

In late 1981, we began gathering data on early-stage breast cancer patients. In that study, we added the measurement of an immunologic mediator—the natural killer cell—and found NK functional activity to have prognostic significance in our sample. When the median NK activity level of the sample was found (NK activity ranged from 8 percent cytolytic activity to 61 percent, median equal to 26 percent target cell lysis), patients who had higher levels of NK activity at the time of primary treatment had significantly fewer positive nodes (a mean of 0.26 positive nodes versus a mean of 2.7 positive nodes, respectively; $F[1,50] = 6.3$, $p < 0.01$).

Of course, a causal association can be considered only if NK activity is fairly stable over time, and lower functional levels of NK activity presumably precede the spread of tumor cells to the region. Test-retest correlation for NK activity in a subset of these patients ($N = 36$ over a three-month period) was approximately $r = +0.5$ ($p < 0.003$). Therefore, it is certainly possible that lower levels of NK activity preceded diagnosis and were present at the time of regional spread. These data suggest that NK cells are a relevant immunologic effector cell in our patient sample.

We then investigated the relative contribution of both clinically and theoretically derived behavioral, psychologic, and demographic variables to NK activity at the time of primary treatment by a stepwise multiple regression analysis.[58] As displayed in Table 15–2, it was found that patients who were rated as "adjusted" by independent observers (that is, patients who made no complaints and had no apparent psychologic difficulties), who complained about a lack of social support from their families, and who responded with a listless apathetic response style tended to have significantly lower levels of NK activity than patients who appeared more disturbed. These latter patients, while perceiving themselves to be emotionally supported by family and friends, tended to be more negatively reactive at the time of interview. In fact, on the basis of these three factors—observer rating of adjustment, perceived social support, and level of reported listlessness—we could account for 51 percent of the NK variance in these patients.

Results from this prospective study are consistent with other clinical investigators' findings[33, 35, 36, 56] as well as being consistent with laboratory *in vitro* and *in vivo* data.[59, 60] Suppression of affect and a passive, stoic response style seem to be associated with worse biologic outcome. Animal research that will be considered later in more detail has shown that a passive, apathetic behavioral response pattern is a potent elicitor of endogenous opioids, and opioids have been shown to have immunoregulatory effects. Clearly, this is one possible mediating pathway to explain our and other investigators' findings related to tumor containment by endogenous host mechanisms.

The effects of *social support* have also been studied in other cancer patient samples, but very few investigators have looked at biologic advantage as the end point. And even fewer have looked at possible mediating mecha-

TABLE 15–2. Step-Wise Multiple Regression Analysis Predicting NK Activity*

	Summary Table					
Variable	MULTIPLE R	R SQUARE	RSQ CHANGE	SIMPLE R	B	BETA
GAIS	0.56	0.31	0.32	−0.56	−0.67	−0.70
Interpersonal perception	0.68	0.46	0.15	−0.13	−1.73	−0.38
Fatigue-POMS	0.71	0.51	0.05	−0.24	−0.30	−0.14
Onset of symptoms to diagnosis in days	0.71	0.51	0.00	0.08	0.62	0.07
Total POMS	0.71	0.52	0.00	−0.19	−0.36	−0.07
Age	0.71	0.52	0.00	0.32	−0.37	−0.03
PST-SCL-90	0.72	0.52	0.00	−0.12	−2.84	−0.03
					83.88	

*From Levy S, Herberman R, Maluish A, et al.: Prognostic risk assessment in primary breast cancer by behavioral and immunological parameters. Health Psychol 4:99, 1985.

nisms linking social support and host vulnerability. Berkman and Syme[21] and, more recently, Kaplan (personal communication) showed that intact social support systems were associated with reduction of mortality in prospectively followed, large community samples. The Kaplan study specifically looked at cancer mortality figures. Studies have also looked at the effects of various environmental support systems on recovery from breast cancer surgery[61] and on survival from breast cancer.[62] The latter study showed that social involvement was independently related to survival time. In fact, when only younger and older patients were considered, both stress and social involvement independently accounted for twice as much variance in survival as stage of disease at diagnosis.

In our study of early-stage breast cancer, the perceived quality of intrafamilial social support turned out to be quite significant in the analyses. Women who complained about a lack of social support in their environment (i.e., decreased communication with spouse, poor quality of spousal relationship, and general inadequacy of family social support system) tended also to be in the worst prognostic category. This variable accounted for nearly 15 percent of the NK variance in our sample.

The whole area of social support research has been fraught with methodological difficulties. However, the sense of the research that has been done, particularly considering the studies that have examined biologic sequelae and host vulnerability as end points, suggests that the quality of perceived social support plays a role in host vulnerability to stress and, hence, disease risk.

Summary of Clinical Findings

The aggregate of clinical findings based on decades of clinical lore—that the passive patients fare worse—and based on early empirical studies and on more recent, rigorous clinical investigations suggests that a passive, stoic response style in human patient populations (at least breast cancer and melanoma populations) is associated with worse cancer outcome. Of course, these findings are correlational. We cannot make any statement regarding direction of causation. However, animal studies using an analogue or behavioral model of human helplessness have demonstrated a causal effect between behavior within a stress context and tumor course.

Animal Studies

For years, there have been studies on various forms of stress, primarily physical in nature, and tumor growth.[31, 63] Many of these studies have suggested the important role of glucocorticoids in mediating such responses. Evidence has emerged demonstrating that such effects are observed as a function of behavioral *response* to the stress, rather than exposure to the stressors per se. Predictability of aversive stimuli or control over such stressors can markedly reduce the stressful effects (e.g., elevated corticosterone or immune suppression) of such conditions. For example, rats able to terminate shock by lever pressing demonstrated less severe physiologic sequelae (gastric lesions or weight loss) than did yoked partners who could not terminate the stressors. Both groups of animals, nevertheless, received identical shock stress.

Numerous investigators have used this yoked, "helpless" model to examine the physiologic effects of lack of behavioral control over stressors. In general, it has been found that animals exposed to such uncontrollable (and acute) stress conditions have depleted brain norepinephrine levels and depletion of dopamine and serotonin levels in some brain areas. The extent and duration of such effects have been shown to vary as a function of age, strain of animal, and social housing conditions.[64] Short-term behavioral effects of such uncontrollable experience include the inability to learn and perform complex tasks; long-term effects include sensitization and perhaps conditioning of amine changes; that is, re-exposure to the originally uncontrolled stressor (or the cues associated with the stressor) may result in the re-induction of the neurochemical events associated with the original trauma. Such conditioned biologic sequelae may profoundly influence subsequent behavior, as a function of the neurochemical disruption, and may make the organism chronically vulnerable to disease processes through, for example, suppression of immune response by hormone activation.

As indicated earlier, a series of studies have been reported since 1982 from three separate laboratories[53, 59, 60] suggesting a causal relationship between behavioral helplessness in murine systems, suppression of lymphocyte function, and faster tumor growth. This relationship seems to be modulated by endogenous opioids, as the investigators reported reversal of the experimental effects with the injection of an opioid antagonist. These investigators also examined NK activity in the modulation of NK-specific tumors (YAC-1.3 and SL2-5 NK–sensitive lymphoma cell lines). One group[53] also tested *in vivo* development and elimination of implanted mammary tumors in female rats (Fisher 344) and found enhanced tumor growth positively correlated with higher levels of opioid release.

There are currently at least two controversies in this area of investigation: first, which endogenous opioids might play a role in lymphocyte modulation? While Greenberg and colleagues[59] spoke of beta-endorphin as the peptide of action in their study, when one considers the peripheral surveillance of NK cells, it is much more likely that the enkephalins, being more widely distributed than the endorphins, are playing a significant, biologically relevant role here. Many peripheral nerves have been shown to contain enkephalins, and, specifically, the high concentration in the adrenal medulla makes them a likely candidate for study in the area of coping, helplessness, and tumor response.[65]

Second, as indicated earlier, it is not clear whether opioids play an enhancing or inhibiting role related to NK activity. Shavit and associates[53] suggested that suppression of NK activity was a function of elevated opioids, and two studies have reported a suppression of tumor growth with the injection of opioid antagonists.[66, 67] Others have reported opposite effects of opioid activity, that is, lymphocyte enhancement.[54, 55] If more weight is going to be put on *in vivo* evidence, then one might lean toward the possibility of opioids playing a suppressive role in natural immunity; that is, most of the evidence suggesting that possibility has been derived from looking at tumor clearance in intact systems. In considering the host as representing a dynamic interplay of systems that function together as a homeostatic network, this may be the more appropriate model to consider. Relevant in this regard is work reported by Miczek and Thompson,[68] which showed a direct link between *victim* behavior and opioid-like analgesia. Victimized, "helpless" behavior in animals exposed to predator bites was more effective in eliciting an analgesic response than objective number of bites received. Begging and victim behavior was a potent elicitor of analgesia in a situation in which the animal *perceived* itself as biologically vulnerable.

Therefore, the weight of the evidence in animals strongly suggests that helpless behavior—at least in the acute condition (for humans, it is hard to make a distinction between acute and chronic)—causes faster tumor growth and is probably mediated by lymphocyte suppression, including NK suppression. These effects are probably modulated by endogenous opioids and other stress-related hormones (e.g., steroids). Lack of perceived control as a biologically significant form of stress may trigger this vulnerability.

Social Support as Stress Reducers in Animals

Several investigators have shown physiologic "stress effects" when animals, primarily primates, are robbed of their accustomed social support systems. For example, Coe and Levine[69] showed that when separating an infant monkey from its mother by placing it alone in a new environment, permitting it to remain in the home cage with familiar conspecifics, or placing it in a similar cage with unfamiliar mothers and infants, the typical pituitary-adrenal stress response to separation was reduced only in the presence of the familiar social environment. Others[70] also demonstrated such findings.

A study by Coe and associates[71] showed a dissociation between behavior response and physiologic indices of distress. The primates who failed to develop major behavioral "despair" responses to peer separations still showed a "distressed" physiologic pattern of response. Such a dissociation between observable distress behavior and physiologic distress markers may provide a clue to host vulnerability seen in human subjects who appear "adjusted" but have the worst biologic outcome.[35, 52]

Therefore, in addition to helpless behavior in the face of stress, intact social support systems may play a buffering role against such stress. In fact, Laudenslager and Reite[70] link the two phenomena by suggesting that the intact social group may provide, through information and group-supported expectation, a sense of control over life stressors.

CONCLUDING NOTES

It is important to keep in mind that all the work discussed in this chapter—clinical as well as animal laboratory investigations—is investigatory. The limits are obvious: In clinical studies, only associations have been reported. In animal studies, many tumor models are more or less remote from the human condition. There is a general sense—an aggregate of findings—that gives us confidence as to the nature and character of behavioral risk factors associated with poor tumor response, one characterized as passive, repressive, and stoic. Nevertheless, these studies are under way, and certainly no clinical advice or patient prescription should be made yet. Now that this cautionary note has been raised, some speculations will be hazarded. The first part of this chapter concerned with psychosocial sequelae of breast cancer and its treatment and the latter part concerned with behavior as biologic response modifier potentially contributing to tumor progression have convergent themes that bear pointing out.

First, there is enough animal evidence, as well as human research and clinical findings, to suggest that intact social support systems may have survival value. Of course, the patient has to be able to reach out for and use such support systems, and social support clearly cannot be disengaged from the patient's coping resources, skills, and strategies. Still, social support is conceivably an important piece of the puzzle explaining host vulnerability or stamina and has been demonstrated to be associated with reduced mortality in at least one large population study.[21] Therefore, its presence or absence and quality are important clinical factors to be determined.

Second, emotional passivity may not be a very adaptive response in the face of clinically negative events. While it is certainly easier for families, nurses, and physicians to deal with a smiling face, this may not be the most adaptive response on the part of the patient in an objectively difficult and dangerous situation. The expression of complaint—the articulation of distress—may not only be psychologically adaptive but *may* have survival value. Do our medical care environments foster passivity?

A final note: Humans exist as living systems within systems, with connecting links from cell to society. We began the chapter with a discussion of cultural factors influencing self-perception and beliefs about one's body and one's worth. Such self-perceptions potentially affect self-esteem in the quality of social interactions, the give and take of social support systems. In turn, evidence exists that perceived social support and the individual's belief in causes of and control over life's vicissitudes modulate important biological sequelae such as catecholamine utilization and steroid release, among other effects. These hormones can have direct and indirect effects at the cellular level, including effects on tumor cell behavior, by way of or independent of immune containment. There is even evidence[71] that stressors affect DNA repair at the intracellular level. Uncovering and understanding these pathways of influence in the intact organism remain major research challenges.

REFERENCES

1. Schain WS: Breast cancer surgeries and psychosexual sequelae: Implications for remediation. Semin Oncol Nurs 1:200, 1985.
2. Brownmiller S: Femininity. New York: Simon and Schuster, 1984, p. 25.
3. Bloom J: Cancer-care procedures and the medical care system: Facilitators or inhibitors of patient coping responses. *In* Ahmed P (ed.): Living and Dying with Cancer. New York: Elsevier, 1981.
4. Miller SM: Coping with impending stress: Psychophysiological and cognitive correlates of choice. Psychophysiology 16:572, 1979.
5. Maguire GP, Lee EG, Bevington EJ, et al.: Psychiatric problems in the first year after mastectomy. J Psychiatry Med 1:963, 1978.
6. Morris T, Greer S, White P: Psychological and social adjustment to mastectomy: A two-year follow-up study. Cancer 40:2381, 1977.
7. Jamison KR, Wellisch DK, Pasnau RO: Psychosocial aspects of mastectomy. I. The women's perspective. Am J Psychiatry 135:432, 1978.
8. Wellisch DK, Jamison KR, Pasnau RO: Psychosocial aspects of mastectomy. II. The man's perspective. Am J Psychiatry 135:543, 1978.
9. Silberfarb P, Maurer L, Crouthamel C: Psychosocial aspects of neoplastic disease. I. Functional status of breast cancer patients during different treatment regimens. Am J Psychiatry 137:450, 1980
10. Frank D, Dornbrush R, Webster S, et al.: Mastec-

tomy and sexual behavior: A pilot study. Sexuality and Disability 1:16, 1978.
11. Kolodny R, Masters W, Johnson V: Textbook of Sexual Medicine. Boston: Little Brown & Company, 1979.
12. Worden W, Weisman A: The fallacy of post-mastectomy depression. Am J Med Sci 273:169, 1977.
13. Weisman A, Worden W: The existential plight in cancer: Significance of the first 100 days. Int J Psychiatry Med 7:1, 1977.
14. Bloom J: Social support, accommodation to stress and adjustment to breast cancer. Soc Sci Med 16:1329, 1982.
15. Northouse L: Mastectomy patients and the fear of cancer recurrence. Cancer Nurs 4:213, 1981.
16. Peters-Golden H: Breast Cancer: Varied perceptions of social support in the illness experience. Soc Sci Med 16:483, 1982.
17. Cobliner W: Psychosocial factors in gynecological or breast malignancies. Hosp Physician 10:38, 1977.
18. Fisher B, Bauer M, Margolese A, et al.: Five-year results of a randomized clinical trial comparing total mastectomy and sequential mastectomy with or without radiation in the treatment of breast cancer. N Engl J Med 312:665, 1985.
19. Sanger C, Reznelsoff M: Comparison of the psychological effects of breast-saving procedures with the modified radical mastectomy. Cancer 48:2341, 1981.
20. Schain W, Edwards B, Gorrell R, et al.: Psychosocial and physical outcomes of primary breast cancer therapy: Mastectomy vs. excisional biopsy and irradiation. Breast Cancer Res Treat 3:377, 1983.
21. Berkman L, Syme L: Social networks, host resistance, and mortality: A nine-year follow-up study of Alameda County residents. Am J Epidemiol 2:186, 1979.
22. Bartelink H, Van Dam F, Van Denegan P: Psychological effects of breast-conserving therapy in comparison with radical mastectomy. Int J Radiat Oncol Biol Phys 11:381, 1985.
23. Clifford E: The reconstructive experience. The search for restitution. *In:* Georgiade NG (ed.): Breast Reconstruction Following Mastectomy. St. Louis: C.V. Mosby Co., 1979.
24. Noone RB, Frazier TG, Hayward CZ, et al.: Patient acceptance of immediate reconstruction following mastectomy. Plast Reconstr Surg 69:632, 1982.
25. Goin J, Goin M: Changing the Body: Psychological Effects of Plastic Surgery. Baltimore: Williams & Wilkins, 1981.
26. Dowden RV, Blanchard JM, Greenstreet RL: Breast reconstruction—selection, timing, and local recurrence. Ann Plast Surg 10:265, 1983.
27. Schain WS, Wellisch DK, Pasnau RO, et al.: The sooner, the better: A study of psychological factors in women undergoing immediate vs. delayed breast reconstruction. Am J Psychiatry 142:40, 1985.
28. Teimourian B, Adham MN: Survey of patients' responses to breast reconstruction. Ann Plast Surg 9:321, 1982.
29. Gerard O: Sexual functioning after mastectomy: Life vs. lab. J Sex Mar Ther 8:305, 1982.
30. Schain WS, Jacobs E, Wellisch DK: Psychosocial issues in breast reconstruction. Intrapsychic, interpersonal, and practical concerns. Clin Plast Surg 11:237, 1984.
31. Stoll B: Mind and Cancer Prognosis. New York: John Wiley & Sons, 1979, pp. 24–25.
32. Henry J: The relation of social to biological processes in disease. Soc Sci Med 6:369, 1982.
33. Greer S, Morris T, Pettingale K: Psychological Response to Breast Cancer and 8 Year Outcome. Paper presented at American Psychological Association Meetings, San Francisco, 1981.
34. Rogentine N, Van Kammer D, Fox B, et al.: Psychological factors in the prognosis of malignant melanoma: A prospective study. Psychosom Med 41:647, 1979.
35. Visintainer M, Casey R: Adjustment and Outcome in Melanoma Patients. Paper presented at the American Psychological Association Meeting, Toronto, 1984.
36. Derogatis LR, Abeloff MD, Melisaratos N: Psychological coping mechanisms and survival time in metastatic breast cancer. JAMA 242:1504, 1979.
37. Wheelock E, Robinson M: Endogenous control of the neoplastic process. Lab Invest 48:120, 1983.
38. Yunas J, Tarleton A: Dormancy and spontaneous recurrence of human breast cancer *in vitro*. Cancer Res 38:3584, 1978.
39. Lewison E: Spontaneous regression of breast cancer. Natl Cancer Inst Monogr 44:23, 1976.
40. Steinhauer E, Doyle A, Reed J, et al.: Defective natural cytotoxicity in patients with cancer: Normal number of effecter cells but decreased recycling capacity in patients with advanced disease. J Immunol 129:2255, 1982.
41. Pross H, Baines M: Spontaneous human lymphocyte-mediated cytotoxicity against tumour target cells. I. The effect of malignant disease. Int J Cancer 18:593, 1976.
42. Cochran A: Man, Cancer, and Immunity. New York: Academic Press, 1978.
43. Frost P, Kerbel R: Immunology of metastasis: Can the immune response cope with disseminated tumor? Cancer Metastasis Rev 2:239, 1983.
44. Moore O, Foote F: The relatively favorable prognosis of medullary carcinoma. Cancer 2:635, 1949.
45. Nathanson L: Immunology and immunotherapy of human breast cancer. Cancer Immunol Immunother 2:209, 1977.
46. Shimakowara I, Imamura M, Yamanaka N, et al.: Identification of lymphocyte subpopulations in human breast cancer tissue and its significance. Cancer 49:1456, 1982.
47. Kikuchi K, Ishii Y, Veno H, et al.: Cell-mediated immunity involved in autochthonous tumor rejection in rats. Ann NY Acad Sci 276:188, 1976.
48. Hanna N, Fidler I: Role of natural killer cells in the destruction of circulating tumor emboli. J Natl Cancer Inst 65:801, 1980.
49. Herberman A, Ortaldo J: Natural killer cells: Their role in defenses against disease. Science 214:24, 1981.
50. Herberman R, Santoni A: Regulation of natural killer cell activity. *In:* Mihich E (ed.): Biological Responses in Cancer. Vol. 2. New York: Plenum Publishing Company, 1984.
51. Hanna N, Burton R: Definitive evidence that natural killer (NK) cells inhibit experimental tumor metastasis *in vivo*. J Immunol 127:1754, 1981.
52. Levy S, Herberman R, Maluish A, et al.: Prognostic risk assessment in primary breast cancer by behavioral and immunological parameters. Health Psychol 4:99, 1985.
53. Shavit J, Lewis J, Terman G, et al.: Opioid peptides

mediate the suppressive effect of stress on natural killer cell cytotoxicity. Science 223:188, 1984.
54. Miller, G, Murgo A, Plotnikoff N: Enkephalins—Enhancement of active T-cell rosettes from normal volunteers. Clin Immunol Immunopathol 31:132, 1984.
55. Mathews P, Froelich D, Sibbitt W, et al.: Enhancement of natural cytotoxicity by beta-endorphin. J Immunol 130:1658, 1983.
56. Jensen M: Psychobiological Factors in the Prognosis and Treatment of Neoplastic Disorders. Ph.D. dissertation, Department of Psychology, Yale University, 1984.
57. Schwartz G: Disregulation theory and disease: Applications to the repression/cerebral disconnection/cardiovascular disorder hypothesis. Int Rev Appl Psychol 32:95, 1983.
58. Cohen J, Cohen P: Applied Multiple Regression/Correlation Analysis for the Behavioral Sciences. New York: John Wiley & Sons, 1975.
59. Greenberg A, Dyck D, Sandler L: Opponent processes, neurohormones and natural resistance. *In:* Fox B, Newberry B (eds.): Psychoneuroendocrine Systems in Cancer and Immunity. Toronto: Hogrefe, 1984.
60. Laudenslager ML, Ryan SM, Drugan SM, et al.: Coping and immunosuppression: Inescapable but not escapable shock suppresses lymphocyte proliferation. Science 221:568, 1983.
61. Funch D, Mettlin C: The role of support in relation to recovery from breast surgery. Soc Sci Med 16:91, 1982.
62. Funch D, Marshall J: The role of stress, social support and age in survival from breast cancer. J Psychosom Res 27:177, 1983.
63. Levy SM: Biological mediators of behavior and neoplasia: Animal models. *In:* Levy S (ed.): Biological Mediators of Behavior and Disease: Neoplasia. New York: Elsevier Science Publishing Co., Inc., 1982.
64. Sklar L, Anisman H: Stress and cancer. Psychol Bull 89:369, 1981.
65. Cox B: Endogenous opioid peptides: A guide to structure and terminology. Life Sci 31:1645, 1982.
66. Aylsworth C, Hodson C, Meites J: Opiate antagonists can inhibit mammary tumor growth in rats. Proc Soc Exp Biol Med 161:18, 1979.
67. Zagan I, McLaughlin P: Naloxone prolongs the survival time of mice treated with neuroblastoma. Life Sci 28:1095, 1981.
68. Miczek K, Thompson M: Analgesia resulting from defeat in a social confrontation: The role of endogenous opioids in brain. *In:* Bandler R (ed.): Modulation of Sensorimotor Activity During Altered Behavioral States. New York: Alan R. Liss, 1984.
69. Coe C, Levine S: Normal responses to mother-infant separation in nonhuman primates. *In:* Klein D, Rabkin J (eds.): Anxiety: New Research and Changing Concepts. New York: Raven Press, 1981.
70. Laudenslager M, Reite M: Coping and separations: Immunological consequences and health implications. *In:* Sharer P (ed.): Review of Personality and Social Psychology, Vol. 5 (Special Issue on Emotions, Relationships, and Health). Beverly Hills: Sage Publications, 1984.
71. Coe C, Wiener S, Levine S: Psychoendocrine responses of mother and infant monkeys to disturbance and separation. *In:* Moltz H, Rosenblum L (eds.): Symbiosis in Parent-Young Interactions. New York: Plenum Press, (In press).
72. Kiecolt-Glaser J, Speicher CE, Holliday JE, et al.: Distress and DNA repair in human lymphocytes. J Behav Med 7:1, 1984.

Rehabilitation of the Patient With Breast Cancer

CAROL WOOD, R.P.T.
LYNN H. GERBER, M.D.

16

INTRODUCTION

Historically, rehabilitation of the patient with breast cancer has meant ameliorating pain, reducing or controlling arm edema, and restoring shoulder motion. Members of the rehabilitation specialties of physiatry, physical therapy, and occupational therapy have had the opportunity only to react to problems that develop as a result of irradiation and/or surgery, rarely being able to provide comprehensive or preventive measures to help women with breast cancer to reach their maximal potential for function.

A multidisciplinary approach, the model by which rehabilitation departments function, is well suited to addressing the very complex issues that are associated with the diagnosis and treatment of breast cancer. Efficacy can be further enhanced by routine early intervention. This approach offers a mechanism for identifying and treating the multitude of physical problems following breast cancer surgery and irradiation as well as some of the emotional and other treatment-related problems that may arise.

As part of a group of investigators studying the treatment of primary breast cancer, we have had the unique opportunity of following nearly 200 women in a prospective fashion over the past six years. During this time, they have been evaluated preoperatively, during their postoperative hospitalization, and yearly thereafter. Using this approach, the natural history of the disease and its postoperative rehabilitative complications have been documented. Based on these observations and the work of many others, a program to meet the needs of our patient population has been devised.

While the great majority of our patients receive either modified radical mastectomy or lumpectomy and irradiation, additional treatment options are available. In addition, we see patients with advanced or inflammatory breast cancer. Since many diverse treatment options exist for this group of patients, we have had to be cognizant of the differences among various treatment groups in order to provide the most appropriate rehabilitation. Treatment choices include modified radical mastectomy, simple mastectomy, lumpectomy with axillary dissection followed by radiation therapy, simple or modified radical mastectomy followed by irradiation, or irradiation alone. Three different kinds of reconstructive procedures are also offered to patients. Each treatment presents slightly different clinical problems and complications, and each requires slightly different rehabilitation interventions.

Review of Literature

A review of the published information on rehabilitation of the breast cancer patient has identified three general areas for intervention: (1) programs to restore shoulder motion, (2) programs to treat or prevent lymphedema, and (3) programs to educate, to relieve anxiety, and to restore functional activity in mastectomy patients. It is interesting to note that the greatest bulk of available information is on the evaluation and treatment of lymphedema.

One study established a direct relationship between a physical therapy (PT) program designed to mobilize the shoulder immediately postoperatively and good shoulder motion. The incidence of stiff, painful, or immobile shoulders in patients who have not received any physical therapy is not precisely known, but if PT was delayed as long as seven to ten days postoperatively, abduction was moderately to severely limited in 33 percent of patients.[1] Two studies suggest that immediate shoulder motion following surgery may result in increased drainage and delayed wound healing.[2, 3]

A prospective study demonstrated that arm motion was more restricted at three months in patients who underwent radical mastectomy when compared with patients receiving lumpectomy.[4] All patients received radiation therapy, but no information is presented as to what constituted the radiation ports. Axillary dissection was not performed in patients from either group. There were no differences between groups at 15 months. Physical activity was good in 49 percent of the mastectomy patients and 77 percent of the lumpectomy group at three months. These differences were not present at 15 months. There was no edema in 19 percent of the radical mastectomy and 44 percent of the lumpectomy patients at three months and no edema in 26 and 43 percent of patients in these groups, respectively, at seven months and 15 months after surgery. The researchers suggest that mastectomy patients have more disability than do lumpectomy patients when more disability is defined as more lymphedema and less arm motion.[4]

A large questionnaire survey was performed by the Connecticut Health Department.[5] In this survey, lymphedema, arm function, and activity status were determined by an initial postoperative interview and a follow-up interview at 18 months. There were 252 women interviewed, of whom 229 had radical mastectomy and 23 had modified radical mastectomy with irradiation. Those with radical mastectomy had the following degrees of lymphedema at 18 months: Twenty-five percent had no edema, 49 percent had slight edema, 11 percent had moderate edema, and 11 percent had severe edema. In those with modified radical mastectomy, 35 percent had no edema, and 50 percent had slight edema; for 15 percent there were no follow-up data. When evaluating arm function, patients were asked if they had "wide and free arm motion and were able to perform normally." If they did, they had "good function." If there was moderate restriction and the patient was unable to perform many tasks, she had "fair" function. Severe restriction of motion was considered "poor" function. At the time of the 18-month follow-up, 75 percent of the patients who underwent radical mastectomy had good arm function, 23 percent had fair, and 1 percent had poor arm function. Ninety percent of the patients with modified radical mastectomy had good arm function, and 10 percent had fair. Clearly, at 18 months, patients with modified radical mastectomy have less arm edema and better arm function than those patients receiving radical mastectomy. This study also identified a direct relationship between arm function and degree of lymphedema, a finding in disagreement with the work of others.[6]

Lymphedema. A considerable body of literature exists on postmastectomy edema of the arm, with the majority of works having been written by surgeons in an attempt to address questions about the relationship of surgical technique to the incidence of edema. The incidence of edema following radical mastectomy ranges from 6.7 percent to 62.5 percent.[7] The wide range in reported incidence is a function of the inconsistent definition of significant lymphedema. Some define it as a 3 cm or larger increase in the maximum forearm circumference, as compared with the unoperated side.[8] Others report it as a volume increase greater than the normal extremity.[9] Zero to 150 ml is insignificant, 150 to 400 ml is slight, 400 to 750 is moderate, and more than 750 ml greater than normal is considered severe edema. Still others suggest that it should be a percentage of the volume greater than normal.[10]

Relatively little comparative information exists on the incidence of lymphedema in patients receiving a variety of treatments for breast cancer. The greatest amount of literature pertains to radical mastectomy. There is one study in which both radical and modified radical mastectomies are evaluated,[11] but not comparatively. Another compared irradiated with nonirradiated patients and showed that the latter had less postoperative edema.[12]

TYPES OF LYMPHEDEMA. A number of types of mastectomy lymphedema have been described, based on their clinical course and morphologic characteristics.[13] The first is acute, transient, and mild, occurring immediately postoperatively as a result of the acute ablation of lymphatics. This edema usually responds to elevation and hand pumping and resolves in seven to ten days. The second type is acute, painful, transient edema, occurring two to six weeks postoperatively. Thought to be due to thrombophlebitis or perivascular lymphangitis, it usually responds to elevation and anti-inflammatory medication within two weeks of onset. The third type of edema is an acute, erysipeloid, painful edema usually occurring in a chronically edematous arm. Occasionally, this follows minor trauma or an insect bite. This cellulitis requires elevation and antibiotic therapy. Compression is contraindicated in the presence of active infection. The fourth type of edema is the one most frequently seen. It is painless and usually develops insidiously without erythema. The cause of this edema is generally considered to be lymphatic ablation and subsequent insufficiency. As interstitial pressure increases, flow of lymph is impeded and the edematous limb can enlarge considerably without getting tense.[14] There is some evidence that transected lymphatics grow back within a month of surgery.[15] The contribution of venous obstruction to postoperative lymphedema has been measured in several studies. Preservation of the axillary vein has been associated with decreased lymphedema,[16] and decompression of the vein results in much improvement in edema.[17] In general, venous obstruction is not a common cause of lymphedema and is present only in cases of severe edema.[18] Other causes of lymphedema have been described, including radiation, by its direct damage to small blood vessels[19]; infection, which augments the severity of edema; and obesity.[20, 21]

In addition to physical measurements of the upper extremity, rehabilitation specialists are concerned with overall resumption of functional activity and are dedicated to maximizing the patient's potential for physical, psychologic, and social function. Information about resumption of previous activities, be they vocational or avocational, has been reported.[22] Factors influencing functional outcome are many, including the extent of surgery, age, and a relative closeness to age of retirement. One study suggests that patients who worked outside the home returned to work more quickly than homemakers returned to homemaking activities. Patients who had more extensive surgery took longer to return to work than did those with more limited surgery.[22]

CLINICAL EXPERIENCE. Our clinical observations at the National Institutes of Health (NIH) have been made mainly upon patients who have participated in a prospective trial designed to evaluate the comparative efficacy of modified radical mastectomy versus lumpectomy plus irradiation. Both groups receive complete axillary dissections. These patients are seen preoperatively by a physical therapist for orientation to the rehabilitation program and evaluation of the affected side. This evaluation includes range of motion measurements of the shoulder, manual muscle testing of the shoulder complex, and bilateral circumferential arm measurements. Approximately 200 patients from this study have been observed over a six-year period. All patients received the same postoperative rehabilitation regimen, designed to maximize motion, prevent edema, and educate them about what they should expect during the intraoperative, postoperative, and recovery periods. (A full discussion of the treatment appears later in the chapter.)

The diverse postoperative sequelae seen in these patients are summarized in Table 16–1. The natural history of upper extremity lymphedema in our patients is similar to that reported by others.[12] There is often transient, painful swelling in the arm, usually along the medial border, associated with a fullness along the medial humeral epicondyle. The swelling usually resolves within eight weeks of surgery. Persistent painless swelling requiring a compression garment of the arm has occurred as early as two months postoperatively. The longest time from surgery to prescription of a compression garment was 48 months, and this occurred in a patient who had metastatic disease. The average time between surgery and prescription of a compression garment for persistent swelling greater than 2 cm is 11.6 months.

Erysipeloid edema is very infrequently seen in our population. Much more common is lymphedema described as being painful, transient, and associated with soreness along the brachial vein. This may be a variant of a syndrome in which cordlike structures develop along the inner aspect of the upper arm and over the anterior elbow two to three weeks postoperatively. These structures feel like fibrous bands and are quite superficial and not discolored (Figs. 16–1 and 16–2). Often the patient complains that it feels like a sore muscle. Pains from these cords limit shoulder flexion when it is performed with the elbow fully extended. The cords either break or spontaneously resorb by three months. We believe that these cords are a result of sclerosing lymphangitis, although this has not been confirmed with biopsy.

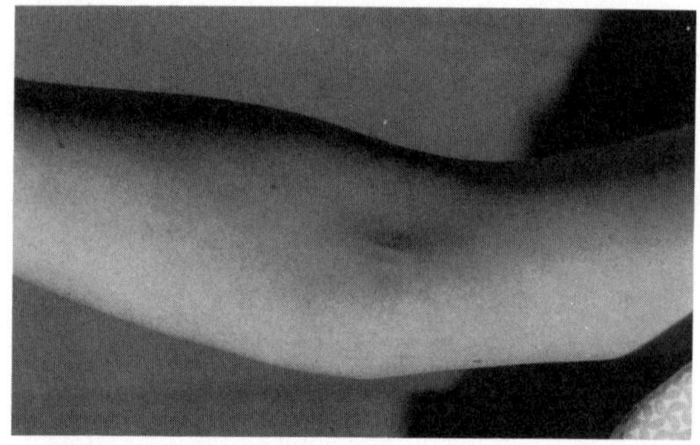

FIGURE 16–1. Cordlike structures over anterior elbow, following axillary dissection.

Approximately 85 percent of our patients requiring compression sleeves have minimal edema, a 2-cm to 4-cm increase in circumferential measurement of the arm at 30 cm above the ulnar styloid. Of the remaining 15 percent, two thirds have moderate edema (greater than 4 cm but less than or equal to 6 cm). All patients with severe edema

TABLE 16–1. Common Sequelae of Mastectomy or Axillary Dissection, or Both

Sequelae	*Patients Affected (%)*	*Weeks After Operation* 1	2	3	4	5	6	7	8	*Months After Operation* 3	6	9	12	*Years After Operation* 1	2	3	4
PAIN/DISCOMFORT																	
Incisional	90–100	†	†	†													
Paresthesia—arm	90–100	†	†	†	†	†	†	†	†								
Hypesthesia—arm	90–100	†	†	†	†	†	†	†	†	†	†	†	†	†	†	†	†
Cords	40–50			†	†	†	†	†	†								
Pectoralis spasm	20–30	†	†	†													
Chest wall	25–35									†	†	†	†	†	†		
Trigger point	<10	†	†	†													
EDEMA																	
One arm, transient	up to 50		†	†	†	†	†										
Arm requiring Jobst (increase > 2 cm)	18							†	†	†	†	†	†	†	†	†	†
Breast	90–100	†	†	†	†	†	†	†	†	†	†	†	†	†			
NEURAPRAXIA																	
Serratus anterior	15	†	†	†	†	†	†	†	†	†							
Others	15	†	†	†	†	†	†	†	†	†							
ROM LIMITATION	initial 100 > 9 mo 2	†	†	†	†	†	†	†	†								

Key: †, sequelae present.

Note: Percentage of patients with the sequelae noted above are based on actual data collection: chest wall pain, arm edema requiring Jobst, neurapraxias, and ROM limitations. Other percentages are estimates of occurrence based on clinical observation by the rehabilitation staff.

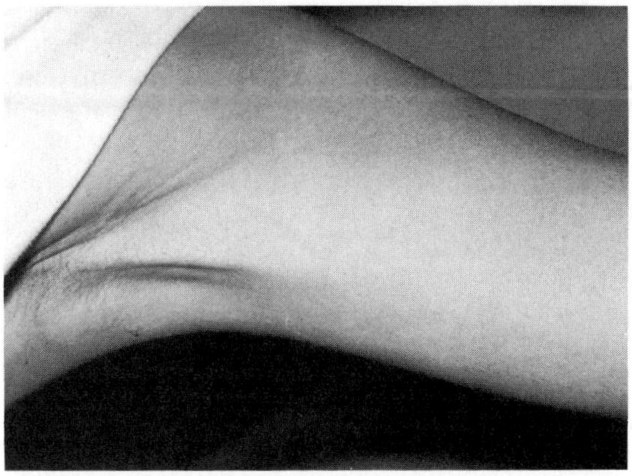

FIGURE 16–2. Cordlike structures from axilla into upper arm, following axillary dissection.

(greater than 6 cm), of whom there were three, had recurrence of their breast cancer. Forty-four percent of those receiving Jobst garments had wrist or hand edema in addition to arm edema.

The rehabilitation team often follows the patients intensively over the first several months, and then less frequently. Over a long period of follow-up, we have observed a significant number of problems that follow mastectomy or lumpectomy and irradiation for breast cancer. Many of these complications have been reported as surgical complications by others.[23] These complications include division of the long thoracic nerve, seroma, and lymphedema, all of which occurred more frequently in radical than in modified radical mastectomy. Arm edema was noted more often in patients with mastectomy and irradiation than in those with mastectomy alone.[22]

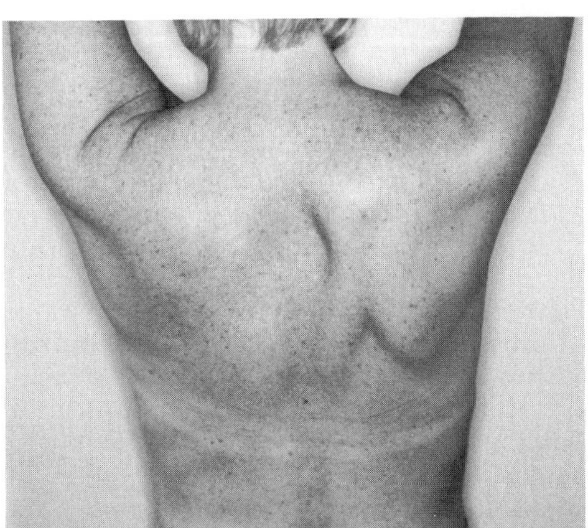

FIGURE 16–3. Serratus anterior weakness following axillary dissection. Note "winging" of right scapula.

Historically, in patients undergoing axillary dissection as part of their treatment for malignant melanoma or breast cancer, we have observed a high incidence of serratus anterior palsy (Fig. 16–3).[24] This form of neurapraxia, by which we mean a temporary neurologic deficit of the sensory or motor type, or both, is usually due to stretch of the long thoracic nerve. It is seen in 25 percent of these patients, and spontaneously resolves in all patients within three months. The incidence of neurapraxias in the current series of patients referred for treatment of primary breast cancer is lower. In addition to serratus anterior palsy, we have seen deltoid and latissimus dorsi weakness. Return to near-normal muscle strength occurs in all patients by six months.

Paresthesias are experienced by virtually all patients undergoing axillary dissection. These begin with postoperative anesthesia in the axilla and along the medial and posterior arm. Often, this anesthesia resolves and is replaced by hypesthesia or dysesthesia. Rarely will normal sensation return. Two patients in our series have had carpal tunnel syndrome requiring release of the median nerve. Both patients had received lumpectomy and irradiation. In one patient, the carpal tunnel syndrome was bilateral. This finding has been reported by others.[25]

Chest wall tenderness is experienced by 17 percent of patients in our population. The majority of those affected have received irradiation. The location of the pain is within the radiation field, is experienced upon palpation of the anterior rib cage, and is occasionally associated with rib fracture. This is not due to metastatic disease but probably radiation-induced infarction and repair of bone. Chest wall tenderness resolves slowly over time and is often symptomatically controlled using nonsteroidal anti-inflammatory medications.[19]

A variety of pain syndromes are reported by breast cancer patients following surgery. Pectoralis major spasm occurs acutely postoperatively in many patients but may be a long-term complication of radiation to the anterior chest wall. Radiation may also cause a significant amount of fibrosis and tightness in the pectoralis muscle, limiting arm abduction. Another common complaint is trapezius spasm and trigger points, which may result from postural changes or shoulder tightness.

MANAGEMENT OF METASTATIC DISEASE

Metastatic breast cancer presents in a variety of ways and the rehabilitation team must often provide long-term management. When recurrent tumor involves the chest wall and axilla, significant arm edema and chest wall pain are often seen. As mentioned earlier, arm edema that occurs in this setting is usually significant and somewhat refractory to therapy. The chest wall syndrome associated with recurrence differs from that induced by radiation in that the former is painful all the time. Recurrent disease of the chest wall will occasionally involve the pectoralis major and its underlying structures, such that shoulder motion is painful and limited. The development of arm swelling and the loss of shoulder range of motion (ROM) two years or more after surgery suggests recurrent disease. Pain is often significant in this setting.

If bone metastasis is present, the rehabilitation team is often asked to evaluate the patient's risk with respect to possible fracture and is also asked if the patient should be kept immobilized or should be provided with gait aids such as crutches, canes, or a walker. Braces may be prescribed for protected weight bearing. Little is known about the correlation between x-ray appearance and the likelihood of fracture, but most orthopedists agree that if there is cortical interruption in a weight-bearing bone, it is likely to fracture. Such patients are managed with protected weight bearing.

Rib fractures are also associated with metastatic breast cancer. Pain and its effect on movement require rehabilitation intervention. Rarely is there significant compromise of upright activity or respiratory function. When the pain is significant enough to compromise function, transcutaneous electrical nerve stimulation (TENS) may be very effective in controlling it.

REHABILITATION TREATMENT

Motion

Standard rehabilitation for postoperative breast cancer patients has generally included range of motion exercises for the shoulders and an edema prevention and treatment program. Initiation of motion depends, in part, on the clinical experience and preference of the operating surgeons. One study compared early (one day postoperative), intermediate (three to four days postoperative), and delayed (seven to ten days postoperative) motion. The authors of this study demonstrated better ROM in those patients receiving early motion.[1]

A comprehensive program offered at Memorial Hospital[26] begins on POD (postoperative day) 1 with hand squeezing. On POD 2, patients receive exercise to the shoulder for 30 to 40 minutes. The nurse provides general discussion of the surgery, the "do's" and "don't's" twice each week, and three times per week the social worker and Reach-to-Recovery volunteer discuss the psychologic and emotional problems the patients may be having. Follow-up data from this study obtained from 1700 questionnaires indicated that arm flexion returned to normal in more than 90 percent of the patients with radical or modified radical mastectomy[22] and that 75 and 78 percent undergoing radical and modified radical mastectomy, respectively, returned to work. It took the radical mastectomy group 8.6 weeks and the modified radical group 7.1 weeks to return to work. Those who received simple mastectomy returned to work in three weeks, and 100 percent did so.[22]

At the National Institutes of Health (NIH), the patients on the primary breast study start their rehabilitation on POD 1. Patients, all of whom have received an axillary dissection, are provided with a standardized program using routine physical therapy techniques. There is a definite treatment plan for the first week (Table 16–2). After the first week the therapist individualizes the program so that motion is advanced to the patient's tolerance and takes into account her particular needs.

Our regimen has a more rapid progression than is recommended by several other groups. Lotze and colleagues[2] demonstrated in a prospective randomized study that with early motion following axillary dissection, there are increases in the incidence of wound breakdown, infection, seromas, and increased duration and amount of drainage. The findings of Flew[3] were similar, in a prospective randomized study of 64 patients undergoing modified radical mastectomy.

TABLE 16–2. Range of Motion Program, Postoperative Progression

POD	Flexion	Abduction	Internal and External Rotation
1–2*	40°	40°	to tolerance
3*	45°	45°	to tolerance
4–6*	45–90°	45°	to tolerance
7	to tolerance	to tolerance	to tolerance
Drains out†	to tolerance	to tolerance	to tolerance

*Gentle accessory mobilization of glenohumeral joint may also be included.

†Active assistive range of motion exercises are added, and/or overhead pulley is used at this time when needed.

Our treatment schedule is very similar to the "early motion" of Lotze's study. The reason we use this more aggressive approach is that the target date for radiation simulation is nine to ten days postoperatively. By that time, patients in the radiation group need approximately 120° flexion, 80 to 90° abduction, and 70 to 80° external rotation. The delayed-motion program does not assure this motion in the time allowed. Rather than differentiating the exercise program according to procedure, we have found it a more practical approach to proceed with all patients in a unified manner.

As an adjunct to our range of motion program, we frequently recommend the use of a simple overhead pulley system, both in the clinic and at home. Pulley exercises are not started until the patient is allowed range of motion to tolerance, and these are continued as long as the therapist and patient feel they are beneficial. Our recommendations for follow-up exercise programs emphasize the need for a long-term commitment by the patient and probably a lifelong commitment by those patients who have received radiation, as this group is at risk of developing a slowly progressive tightening of the shoulder. Before a patient is discharged on a home program, the Department of Rehabilitation Medicine requires that the patient have a minimal ROM of 110° of flexion, 90° of abduction, and 55° of external rotation. If it is felt that the patient will have difficulty in reaching functional ROM after discharge, arrangements are made for follow-up physical therapy. If the serratus anterior, latissimus, or deltoid is weak, we assure the patient of the likelihood of return of strength based upon prior observations[24] and recommend that exercises be done while supine, without the use of weights.

In order to maintain a reasonable progression of range of motion, the rehabilitation specialist must be able to recognize and treat motion-limiting complications that may arise. Muscle spasm, usually restricted to the pectoralis major, interferes with pain-free ROM. Resolution of this is required before adequate increase in ROM can be achieved. Effective treatment includes moist heat or ice and, frequently, electrotherapeutic approaches. These approaches include transcutaneous nerve stimulation (TNS) to acupressure points for muscle relaxation and/or the application of high-voltage electrical stimulation using a high pulse rate (at least 80 per second) to fatigue the muscle, thus reducing spasm. This latter method is well tolerated and is the method of choice in our clinic. Heat or cold is not used on any tissue that is being actively irradiated, but these modalities are used before and after irradiation. Occasionally, reactive muscle spasm is successfully treated with the patient using active movement against manual resistance. In addition to muscle spasm and neurapraxias, paresthesias and trigger points will occasionally interfere with return of ROM. Since the most significant gains in ROM are made in the first six weeks, a very careful assessment should be done during that time, in order to prevent the development of a tight, painful, dysfunctional shoulder.

Other investigators have taken a different approach to this problem and have recommended arm immobilization using a sling to hold the arm in 90 degrees of flexion[27] or beginning functional arm activities to gain range, such as suggested in the pamphlet *Help Yourself to Recovery* published by the American Cancer Society. Variations on these programs have also been reported.[8]

Edema

Management of upper extremity lymphedema depends in part upon the cause. The acute transient type occurring immediately postoperatively resolves spontaneously and requires no treatment. Increasing ROM and a progression to preoperative activity should proceed uninterrupted. However, for the acute, painful, cellulitic type, treatment with antibiotics and analgesics is recommended, and ROM should be maintained to tolerance. Neither of these types of lymphedema should be treated with a compression device or sleeve.

Prevention of lymphedema is an attainable and a worthwhile goal. Suggested programs for prevention of lymphedema that have been described include: (1) elevation of the extremity in conjunction with exercise and massage,[28] (2) use of antiseptic soap baths preoperatively to prevent infection, (3) early arm mobilization, (4) postoperative compression of the arm with an elastic bandage and good wound care,[12] and (5) the prophylactic early prescription of a compression garment.[5] There is some evidence that preventive measures are effective.[28] In addition, protection of the hand and the arm is beneficial.

Close follow-up of patients undergoing mastectomy or lumpectomy with irradiation is necessary to identify the development of lymphedema. Most investigators suggest that if the arm circumference increases by more than 3 cm, steps should be taken to control the swelling. The patient is educated about arm elevation to obtain gravity assistance in decreasing arm swelling and about using isometric, antigravity arm exercises. Patients are encouraged to be aware of arm position during routine daily activity and to minimize dependency. They are taught to perform local massage and, when edema is maximally reduced, to fit themselves with a compression bandage.[4, 5, 28–31]

Refractory edema often requires a pneumatic pump. One group reports a reduction from moderate or marked edema to minimal edema in three months.[32] Another group demonstrated a twofold reduction in edema, using the pneumatic pump, compared with bandage wrapping,[33] and another demonstrated reduction in arm swelling to one half the prepump volume.[34]

Our treatment for prevention of arm edema includes many of the measures common to other programs. Arm care is discussed with each patient by the rehabilitation staff and the nursing staff. Patients also receive written material. Because we do circumferential measurements preoperatively (bilaterally) and routinely repeat them postoperatively, we are able to intervene in a more timely fashion, before significant edema develops. Although early, transient edema usually resolves, it is impossible to predict which patients may go on to have more significant edema. At a minimum, these patients are put on a hand-pumping program, along with elevation of the involved extremity. The Jobst stockinette, which does provide a limited amount of compression, is worn by some patients. If hand edema is present, the patient is fitted with an off-the-shelf compression glove. If it appears that this problem is going to persist, an appropriate custom-made compression sleeve is ordered. We have had to use the compression pump on relatively few of our primary breast cancer patients, but when we do, we want to get a maximum reduction within a reasonable time frame and then fit them with a compression sleeve. A small number of patients are not compliant in the use of their sleeves, while others have been able to discontinue wearing them because their edema has been controlled. Antibiotics have also played a role in our treatment program.

The protocols used for treating edema vary widely. Some use the compression device for five to ten days and then fit with a sleeve[36]; others suggest antibiotics, pumping for six hours, fitting with a sleeve, and in several months repumping. These patients did well in terms of edema control.[38] The common adjustment settings for the Jobst intermittent compression apparatus are 45 seconds pressure on and 15 seconds pressure off. The pressure setting should be slightly lower than the patient's diastolic blood pressure. A linear pump has been designed that uses pressures higher than diastolic pressure, but for a very short time. This linear pump has been used for several patients with severe edema, according to a protocol established by Dr. M. A. Alexander at D. T. Watson Rehabilitation Hospital.[37] It was reported that significant volumes of fluid can be removed from the limb using this technique.[39] Hence, fluid balance should be maintained. After the volume of the arm is stabilized, a garment is provided, which should be worn daily to maintain the reduction in swelling. Occasionally, salt restriction and diuretic therapy may be useful.[30, 36]

An outline summarizing the evaluations that are a standard part of the rehabilitation management and some brief recommendations for what should be done at key postoperative milestones is presented in Table

TABLE 16–3. Schema for Clinical Management of Rehabilitation Needs of Breast Cancer Patients

Problem	*Preoperative Evaluation*	*Postoperative Evaluation—0–2 Weeks*	*Postoperative Evaluation—2–12 Weeks*	*Postoperative Evaluation—3–6 Months*	*Postoperative Evaluation—6–12 Months*	*Postoperative Evaluation—More Than 1 Year*
Edema	Obtain baseline measurements If edema present, determine cause	Instruct in preventive arm care If edema present: <2 cm without erythema. Rx: elastic stockinette, elevation, hand pumping → >2 cm <4 without erythema. Rx: Jobst sleeve → >4 cm without erythema. Rx: compression pump → Any, with erythema. Rx: antibiotic →	→	>2 cm—compression sleeve, overhead hand pumping, arm elevation >4 cm—compression sleeve, compression pump >6 cm—compression pump; with erythema, Rx: antibiotics	Same as 3–6 months	→ → →
			Also maintain antigravity position as much as possible		With pain R/O metastasis	With pain R/O metastasis
Shoulder motion	Obtain baseline measurements If <145° flexion or abduction <60° ER/IR Rx: Heat and ROM exercise N.B.: Precautions for proper arm position intraoperatively	See Table 16–2	Begin use of pulley If <145° flexion/abduction <60° ER/IR Use of heat, ice (except when patient is being actively irradiated). Active and passive stretch. If no progress by eighth week, add NSAIDS to regimen and check monthly	Determine ROM If <160° flexion, 145° abduction, 60° ER/IR, Rx: ROM exercises with assistance from physical therapist	Determine ROM If <160° flexion, 145° abduction, or 60° ER/IR and if ROM exercises not effective, Rx: Scan, NSAIDS, intra-articular steroids	Same as 6–12 mos
Muscle strength	Obtain baseline measurement of shoulder complex strength, particularly stabilizers of scapula	Evaluate strength If weakness, especially serratus anterior, support scapula during ROM exercises	Evaluate strength of shoulder girdle muscle. Strength should be returning by end of this period. Maintain ROM If weakness—continue to support scapula during exercises	Evaluate strength of shoulder girdle muscles If abnormal strength, determine cause. Postoperative weakness should be resolved by 6 mos	Same as 3–6 mos	Same as 3–6 mos
Prosthesis	N/A	Fluff, or when wound heals, permanent prosthesis →	→	Consider reconstruction	Same as 3–6 mos	Same as 3–6 mos
Psyche support	Orientation to surgery/radiation and common postoperative problems	Support group/relaxation techniques, if appropriate →	→	→	Same as 3–6 mos	Same as 3–6 mos

16–3. While this outline should be a useful guide for the practitioner, it would be most beneficial to refer patients with problems pertaining to shoulder motion and strength as well as with arm edema and disability to rehabilitation specialists.

Prostheses

The Department of Rehabilitation Medicine at the National Institutes of Health is responsible for providing each mastectomy patient with a temporary prosthesis—usually a Dacron-filled "fluff." Nearly all of our patients are interested in having a fluff before they leave the hospital. Even if they are unable to wear a bra, the fluff can be pinned onto an undershirt, slip, or camisole. We have had patients pin them onto their hospital gowns. If the incision is well healed, with little or no swelling in the chest, most patients are ready to be fitted for their permanent prosthesis by three to six weeks postoperatively. Our fitters will not provide a prosthesis for any patient who has significant postoperative chest edema, because as the edema resolves, the prosthesis may no longer be appropriate. The permanent prostheses that we provide are silicone filled, but there are many different types available.[42]

Stress Management

The diagnosis of breast cancer as well as its associated treatment introduces a significant life status change for all women. Deciding between the choices that are often available at each step of the diagnosis and treatment chain either may be experienced by the patient as a positive active role in health care or may confuse the patient. Determining a proper treatment course may be very stressful; this, added to the stress of having cancer, may result in maladaptive or dysfunctional behavior.

Many programs offer comprehensive rehabilitation,[22, 28, 36] and part of these programs include therapy in stress management and vocational guidance as well as psychiatric and psychologic support. Evidence supports the improved outcome with a multidisciplinary approach to the management of breast cancer.[22, 39] There are significant data indicating that return to normal function after mastectomy is often slow, and occasionally, patients do not resume normal premorbid activities because of depression, physical incapacity, self-image distortion, and other psychosocial difficulties.[40]

Data have been presented indicating that women with physical complaints at four years after mastectomy had a high number of depressive symptoms.[41] Those who had more physical complications were more likely to be depressed, and support was influential in relieving depression.[41]

Frequent follow-up visits for evaluation of shoulder ROM, pain, and lymphedema are made to the Department of Rehabilitation Medicine (DRM) at the NIH. During these visits and therapeutic sessions, patients often describe their daily activities and the difficulties they may be experiencing in carrying out these activities. This offers our staff an opportunity to determine if patients are adjusting to their perceived role or status change.

If a patient is having a problem coping, a referral to our Occupational Therapy Service is made. The service performs an evaluation of function for the patient. If sleep patterns have been disrupted or if there has been an inability to return to work or other previous roles, therapy may be recommended. Relaxation techniques are helpful in lowering anxiety and in giving the patient a sense of mastery and control. This can be a very useful adjunct to physical therapy intervention, because it may reduce tension and muscle tightness to a degree that will permit greater physical gains to be made.

Careful evaluation and treatment monitoring of arm motion, limb edema, and physical and psychologic function should be done by the rehabilitation specialists. This approach will assure a rapid return of function and will help prevent or minimize disability. The identification and treatment of maladaptive behaviors indicative of stress or other dysfunction may help maximize the patient's level of performance and may reduce anxiety. The rehabilitation team is in an excellent position to monitor the patient carefully and to address problems promptly.

REFERENCES

1. Pollard K, Callum KG, Altman DG, et al.: Shoulder movement following mastectomy. Clin Oncol 2:343, 1976.

2. Lotze MT, Duncan MA, Gerber LH, et al.: Early vs delayed shoulder motion following axillary dissection. Ann Surg 193:288, 1981.
3. Flew TJ: Wound drainage following radical mastectomy: The effect of restriction of shoulder movement. Br J Surg 66:302, 1966.
4. Atkins H, Hayward JL, Klugman DJ, et al.: Treatment of early breast cancer: A report after 10 years of a clinical trial. Br Med J, 2:423, 1972.
5. Eisenberg HS, Goldenberg IS: Measurement of quality of survival of breast cancer patients. *In*: Hayward JL, Bulbrook RD (eds.): Clinical Evaluation in Breast Cancer. New York: Academic Press, 1966, pp. 93–106.
6. Lewison FF: Surgical treatment of breast cancer: Historical and collective review. Surgery 34:904, 1953.
7. Britton RC, Nelson PA: Causes and treatment of postmastectomy lymphedema of the arm. JAMA 180:95, 1962.
8. Sonneland J: Postmastectomy edema of arm: Causes and treatment. West J Surg 70:230, 1962.
9. Tracy GD, Reeve TS, Fitzsimmons E, et al.: Observations on the swollen arm after radical mastectomy. NZ J Surg 30:204, 1961.
10. Stillwell GK: Treatment of postmastectomy lymphedema. Modern Treatm 6:396, 1969.
11. Markowski J, Wilcox JP, Helm PA: Lymphedema incidence after specific postmastectomy therapy. Arch Phys Med Rehabil 62:449, 1981.
12. Swedborg I, Wallgren A: The effect of pre- and postmastectomy radiotherapy on the degree of edema, shoulder-joint mobility, and gripping force. Cancer 47:877, 1981.
13. Leis HP, Bowers WF, Dursi J: Postmastectomy edema of the arm. NY State J Med 66:618, 1966.
14. Guyton AC, Granger HJ, Taylor AE: Interstitial fluid pressure. Physiol Rev 51:527, 1971.
15. Danese C, Howard JM, Bowr R: Regeneration of lymphatic vessels: A radiographic study. Ann Surg 156:61, 1962.
16. Haagensen CD: Diseases of the Breast, 2nd ed. Philadelphia: W.B. Saunders Co., 1971, p. 718.
17. Larson NE, Crampton AR: A surgical procedure for postmastectomy edema. Arch Surg, 106:475, 1973.
18. Timossi G: L'edema del braccio consequenti ad intervento di mastectomia radicale. Minerva Chir 24:277, 1969.
19. Hirshowitz B, Mahler D, Goldan S: Surgical treatment of chronic radiation injuries of the axilla and shoulder. Plast Reconstr Surg 44:261, 1969.
20. Treves N: An evaluation of the etiological factors of lymphedema following radical mastectomy: An analysis of 1007 cases. Cancer 10:444, 1957.
21. Hughes JG, Patel AR: Swelling of the arm following radical mastectomy. Br J Surg 53:4, 1966.
22. Winick L, Robbins GF: Physical and psychological readjustment after mastectomy. Cancer 39:478, 1977.
23. Say CC, Donegan W: A biostatistical evaluation of complications from mastectomy. Surg Gynecol Obstet 138:370, 1974.
24. Duncan MA, Lotze M, Gerber LH, et al.: Incidence, recovery, and management of serratus anterior muscle palsy after axillary node dissection. Phys Ther 63:1243, 1983.
25. Ganel A, Engel J, Sela M, et al.: Nerve entrapments associated with postmastectomy lymphedema. Cancer 44:2254, 1979.
26. Winick L, Robbins GF: The postmastectomy rehabilitation group program. Structure, procedure and population demography. Am J Surg 132:599, 1976.
27. Parbash S, Anathakrishnan N, Mohan CR: Postoperative positioning after mastectomy and other procedures in the pectoral region. Aust NZ J Surg 52:293, 1982.
28. Stillwell GK: Management of arm edema. *In*: Stoll BA: Breast Cancer Management—Early and Late. Chicago: Year Book Medical Publishers, 1977.
29. MacCaughey AM: A comprehensive physical therapy program for the postmastectomy lymphedema patient. Scientific Exhibit, American Physical Therapy Association Conference, Chicago, June 1968.
30. Nelson PA: Recent advances in treatment of lymphedema of the extremities. Geriatrics 21:162, 1966.
31. Brush WE, Wylie JH, Beninson J, et al.: Treatment of postmastectomy lymphedema. Arch Surg 77:561, 1958.
32. Wilhelm MC, Saul PB, Morgan JA: Postmastectomy lymphedema. Va Med Mon 101:465, 1974.
33. LeClaire R, Dupuis M: Traitement physiatrique du lymphoedeme postmastectomie. Union Med Can 101:2702, 1972.
34. Brush BE, Wylie JH, Beninson J: Some devices for the management of lymphedema of the extremities. Surg Clin North Am 39:1493, 1959.
35. Brush BE, Wylie JH: The management of the swollen arm following mastectomy. West J Surg 72:64, 1964.
36. Zeissler RH, Rose GB, Nelson PA: Postmastectomy lymphedema: Late results of treatment in 385 patients. Arch Phys Med Rehabil 53:159, 1972.
37. Alexander MA: personal communication, 1984.
38. Alexander MA, Wright ES, Wright JB, et al.: Lymphedema treated with a linear pump: Pediatric case report. Arch Phys Med Rehabil 64:132, 1983.
39. Sachs S, Davis JM, Reynolds SA, et al.: Comparative results of postmastectomy rehabilitation in a specialized and a community hospital. Cancer 48:1251, 1981.
40. Talbott EE, Marino LB, Mueller DP: The evaluation of postmastectomy morbidity: A review of the literature. Prev Med 8:429, 1979.
41. Woods NF, Earp JAL: Women with cured breast cancer. Nurs Res 27:85, 1978.
42. After Mastectomy: Finding the right prosthesis. Consumer Report, November, 1975, pp. 652–654.

Reconstruction of the Breast

17

HAROLD D. McDONALD, M.D., F.A.C.S.

HISTORY

The history of breast reconstruction stretches back to the late 1800's, with many milestones in the development of reconstructive techniques. The earlier methods of breast reconstruction often had results that were not esthetically pleasing and that were limited by the fact that a number of operative procedures were required. However, the development of new techniques for breast reconstruction since the mid-1970's has been rapid and has enabled us to reconstruct symmetric, esthetically pleasing breasts. In 1895, Czerny[1] described a breast reconstruction using the free transplant of a lipoma from the lumbar region. The transplant only partially survived, but this is generally considered to be the earliest attempted breast reconstruction. In 1906, Tansini[2] described the use of the latissimus muscle in breast surgery. This procedure was, however, forgotten until it was rediscovered in the mid-1970's.[3] In 1932, Reinhardt[4] reconstructed a breast by using a shared part of the opposite normal breast. He moved the shared tissue across to the mastectomy site as a pedicle flap. This type of reconstruction has since been used by others,[5–7] but there is some question concerning its medical safety, based on the possibility that a breast cancer patient might develop carcinoma in the contralateral breast.

In 1937, Webster[8] used thoracoepigastric tubed pedicle flaps for breast reconstruction. Tubed pedicle flaps involve raising tissue from its normal site and fashioning it into a tube by sewing the underside edges together, leaving the two ends attached to the body to preserve the blood supply. The raising of the tissue in this fashion deprives the tissue of some of its blood supply and is called a delay. Reconstructive surgeons can move tubed pedicle tissue from one area in the body to another by "waltzing" it. Waltzing the tissue is carried out by sequentially detaching one end of the tubed pedicle flap and moving it forward, one end over at a time. Each sequential move requires a time delay for new blood vessels to grow into the freshly attached end. In 1945, Gillies[9] described reconstruction of a breast using a tubed pedicle of abdominal tissue including the umbilicus. He described eversion of the umbilicus to simulate the nipple in conjunction with this procedure. In 1953,

Longacre[10] used local pedicle flaps from the lower thoracic area to reconstruct the breast, thereby eliminating the lengthy time needed to move tissue by delay and waltzing from a distance. In 1963, Kiricuta[11] described the use of the transposed greater omentum in breast reconstruction. Transposing the omentum allowed him to move well-vascularized tissue to the chest area for breast reconstruction in a single procedure. In 1963, Cronin and Gerow[12] reported the use of a silicone rubber prosthesis in breast surgery. This type of prosthesis was first used in breast reconstruction by Snyderman and Guthrie.[13] It is widely used today to simulate the breast mound. In 1973, Orticochea[14] used a buttock flap carried on a wrist carrier to the chest to reconstruct a breast. This represented an attempt to reconstruct a breast by using tissue from a relatively inconspicuous donor site and utilizing a wrist attachment for temporary blood supply. In 1974, Tai and Hasegawa[15] described the transverse thoracoepigastric flap for reconstruction of the breast. This was a further refinement of the use of adjacent tissue for breast reconstruction. It is occasionally employed today for deficiencies in the lower chest wall area. However, its use is limited, because the blood supply will not support a flap long enough to reach into the infraclavicular area or to the axilla.

In 1976, Arnold and colleagues[16] reported the use of a transposed greater omental flap to cover a prosthesis in reconstruction of the breast. This was a further refinement of the use of distant well-vascularized tissue to cover an implant in order to reconstruct the breast contour. In 1976, Fugino and associates[17] described the use of free microvascular flaps in breast reconstruction. Free microvascular flaps allow the transfer of large amounts of tissue during a single operation. One of the more significant developments in reconstructive surgery came about in the mid-1970's, when the myocutaneous flap was discovered and multiple myocutaneous sites were described by McGraw and colleagues.[3] This included a rediscovery of Tansini's latissimus dorsi flap originally described in 1906.[2] A myocutaneous flap is a muscle flap with its attached overlying skin, with blood supplied by the artery or arteries to that muscle. The use of these flaps allows the reliable transfer of large amounts of tissue in one operative procedure. The latissimus dorsi myocutaneous flap was first used in breast reconstruction by Schneider and associates[18] and in a separate instance by Muhlbauer and Olbrisch in 1977.[19] In 1977, Drever[20] reported the use of a rectus abdominis myocutaneous flap with a vertical skin island in breast reconstruction. Robbins[21] used a similar flap in 1979. In 1979, Lewis[22] described a sliding flap of the abdomen and lower thoracic tissues, which was a further refinement of the use of adjacent tissue.

In 1980, Lapin and colleagues[23] reported the use of a tissue expander as a method of reconstructing the breast. The tissue expander was placed beneath the tissue on the anterior chest wall and gradually was expanded so that the tissue would cover a prosthesis symmetric with the opposite breast. This increased the usefulness of the remaining tissue in reconstruction. In 1982, Ryan[24] modified the sliding thoracic abdominal flap, first described by Lewis, by adding a definite inframammary crease and thereby enhancing its use in breast reconstruction. In 1982, Hartrampf and associates[25] described the use of a transverse paddle of skin and subcutaneous tissue carried on the rectus abdominis muscle for reconstruction of the breast. This procedure had a secondary benefit, as the tissue used for reconstruction of the breast is from an area of the lower abdomen in which removal of tissue creates an esthetically pleasing abdominoplasty. This chapter will describe in further detail the techniques generally used today in breast reconstruction. The discovery and evolution of these techniques have made it increasingly possible to reconstruct an esthetically pleasing breast for nearly any woman who has had breast surgery or irradiation, ranging from lumpectomy with irradiation through the mastectomies, from simple type to extended radical mastectomy, in which there may be an extensive deficit of tissue on the anterior chest.

PSYCHOLOGIC BENEFITS OF BREAST RECONSTRUCTION

Clifford[26] was one of the earliest investigators to note a psychologic benefit from breast reconstruction following mastectomy. He reported that patients experienced an improved sense of well-being and psychologic comfort associated with this procedure.

In his study, 70 percent of the women reported feeling restored to "normal" or "feeling whole again." Fifty percent said that they were grateful to be relieved of the problems associated with wearing an external prosthesis. Forty-two percent acknowledged feeling less self-conscious and more like a woman. Teimourian and Adham[27] further noted that breast reconstruction had both psychologic and sexual benefits for their patient population. Reconstructing the breast contour appeared to encourage evaluation of the remaining breast because the fear of treatment was lessened. Reconstruction was clearly associated with reducing the trauma generally attributed to amputation of the breast. In addition, reconstruction improved the woman's sense of femininity, liberated her choice of clothes, elevated her self-esteem, and encouraged sexual expressiveness. The question of psychologic value derived from breast reconstruction poses less conflict professionally today than does the issue of when in the treatment planning the procedure should be performed. It has been documented that additional benefits may be derived from immediate breast reconstruction.[28–31] Reasons for this seem to include the following: (1) The patient can anticipate a restored physical state from the outset of treatment, (2) she does not have to grieve the loss of a breast, and (3) she experiences less disruption psychologically and in the general activities of daily life. Three studies[27, 28, 31] have documented that irrespective of the time at which reconstruction is carried out, 92 percent of those women having breast reconstruction described satisfaction with the results.

TIMING OF BREAST RECONSTRUCTION

Immediate reconstruction can be carried out, with beneficial results, if one has a well-informed patient with a small tumor and clinically negative nodes.[28, 32] The patient needs to be well informed, in advance of the mastectomy, about the limitations of immediate reconstruction in terms of the possible complications and possible compromise of the outcome. If the patient and her physicians agree that she is a candidate for immediate reconstruction, she can go through the mastectomy and have the reconstruction and, thus, avoid mourning the loss of the breast with its accompanying psychologic trauma. If there is a small nonptotic breast on the opposite side, one can place a small implant at the time of mastectomy and thereby effect an immediate reconstruction. In the case of a moderate-sized nonptotic breast on the opposite side and a relative shortage of tissue to cover an appropriate-sized prosthesis, another technique may be more suitable. When a relative lack of tissue is noted, an esthetic match to the opposite side can be achieved by placing a tissue expander at the time of mastectomy and, after the surgical wound has healed, gradually expanding the prosthesis so that the tissue will cover an implant of the required size. Alternatively, a latissimus dorsi flap or rectus abdominis flap may be immediately made.

Delayed reconstruction (1) allows the wounds to heal and mature; (2) permits an in-depth study of permanent pathology specimens to determine the exact nature of the tumor and the margins of the resection and to ascertain the status of the axillary nodes; (3) allows evaluation of the deficit of tissue at the mastectomy site; and (4) provides the patient with time to express her wishes and individual needs in relation to which reconstructive technique is best for her. Most local recurrences arise in the scar or the skin in the subcutaneous tissue at the site of the mastectomy; thus, placement of the prosthesis under the muscles will not obscure detection of a recurrence in this area. In fact, submuscular placement of the prosthesis will push the remaining tissues forward and make them easier to examine. In the case of a flap that brings tissue into the area, there is some possibility of masking a local recurrence. However, in most patients, a local recurrence indicates systemic disease, and earlier treatment of the local recurrence may not influence the survival rate in breast cancer.

Timing Related to Adjuvant Treatment. Breast reconstruction is usually delayed until one month following the cessation of chemotherapy. This allows blood counts to return to normal and obviates the deleterious effects of chemotherapeutic agents on wound healing.[33] Breast reconstruction is also usually delayed until four to six weeks after radiation therapy has ceased, to permit resolution of some of the local effects of radiation on the tissues and to allow better wound healing.

The Defect. The tissue deficit on the treated side of the patient's chest varies with the type of therapeutic modality or modalities that have been carried out. When a lumpectomy has been performed, there may be only a slight to moderate deficit in the breast contour. There is a greater loss in size in the breast mound with a quadrantectomy. Irradiation, used in conjunction with these procedures, will cause some tissue fibrosis, with the possibility of further distortion in size and shape and of changes in the color and softness of the overlying skin. In a patient who has had a simple mastectomy or a modified radical mastectomy with preservation of both pectoral muscles, there is no breast mound or nipple-areola complex, but there may be good-quality skin remaining on the chest wall. In some modified radical mastectomies, the pectoralis minor muscle is removed and, with it, the medial pectoral nerve to the pectoralis major muscle. This results in denervation atrophy of the lateral edge of the pectoralis major muscle. In this situation, there is a relative lack of bulk in the infraclavicular area and some deficiency in the anterior axillary fold. The breast mound and the nipple-areola complex are missing, and the remaining skin may be tight. In the case of radical mastectomy, the pectoralis minor and pectoralis major muscles are removed. This results in an infraclavicular hollow and the absence of an anterior axillary fold, in addition to the lack of a breast mound and a nipple-areola complex. The remaining skin may be very tight, or, in fact, there may even be a skin graft left on the chest wall, which exposes the washboard appearance of the underlying ribs. The type and extent of tissue deficit dictate the method of reconstruction that is both necessary and desirable in each individual case.

SILICONE PROSTHESIS

Cronin and Gerow[12] developed the first silicone rubber implantable breast prosthesis in 1963. This development has made it possible to re-establish a breast contour, using a generally well-tolerated foreign body. Silicone prostheses are made of polymers of dimethylsiloxane.[34] The formula for dimethylsiloxane is:

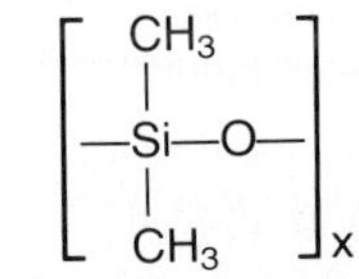

Silicone rubber is made by vulcanizing polymers of dimethylsiloxane and adding silica to increase the strength of the rubber. In a silicone gel, the more units of dimethylsiloxane that are strung together in a polymer, the more viscous the liquid becomes, varying from the viscosity of water to that of very thick honey. Silicone prostheses are of two basic types or a combination of these two types. A silicone rubber envelope filled with silicone gel is called a gel-filled prosthesis (Fig. 17–1). A silicone rubber envelope that can be filled through a valve with physiologic saline is referred to as an inflatable prosthesis. One commonly used combination of these two types has a gel-filled center and a surrounding inflatable lumen, which allows the surgeon some latitude in increasing or decreasing the size of the implant at the time of surgery (Figs. 17–2 and 17–3). Another variation of the prosthesis is to cover the silicone envelope with polyurethane foam. Some surgeons feel that this has the advantage of decreasing the incidence of capsular contracture and thereby improving the softness of the reconstructed breast. Silicone products are especially well tolerated by the body, and, in general, the patient's body has a mild fibroblastic reaction, resulting in a thin

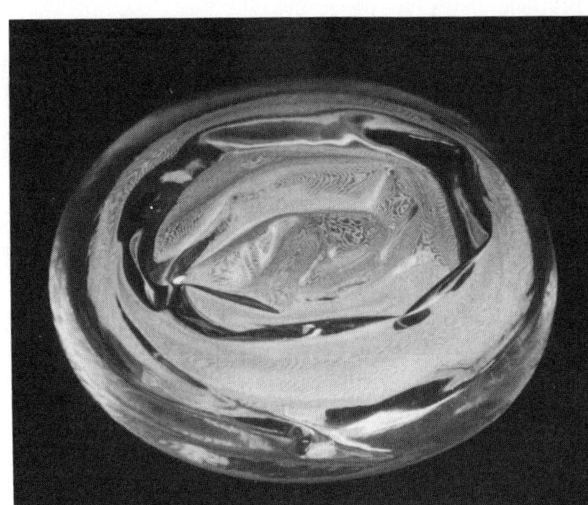

FIGURE 17–1. A gel-filled prosthesis. The lumen of this silicone rubber envelope is filled with silicone gel.

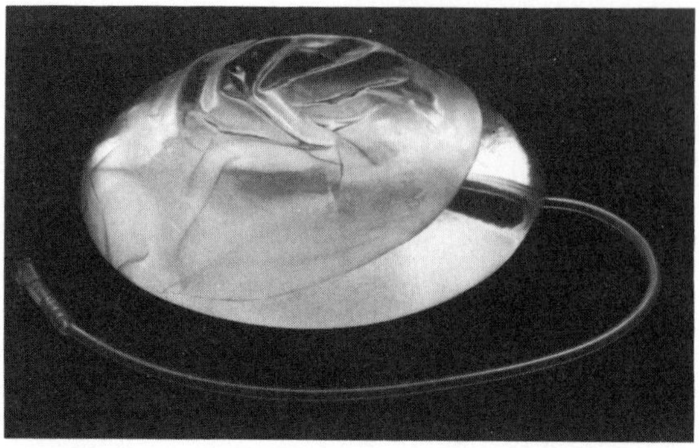

FIGURE 17–2. A two-lumen breast prosthesis. The outer lumen is filled with saline via a fill-tube inserted through a self-sealing valve on the back of the prosthesis. One can vary the volume of saline and the outer lumen. The inner lumen is filled with a soft silicone gel.

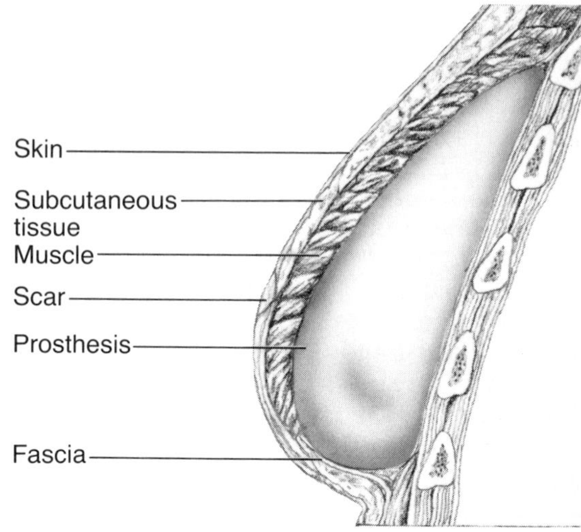

FIGURE 17–4. Position of the breast prosthesis in cross section. Note that the prosthesis is placed beneath the skin, subcutaneous tissue, and muscle. The muscle layer is composed of the pectoralis major above, the serratus anterior laterally, and the fascia of the rectus abdominis below.

encapsulation. There is almost no adherence of live tissue to the silicone rubber envelope, and there have been no substantiated reports of cancer caused by implantation of silicone in humans in over 20 years of experience using silicone prostheses in augmentation mammoplasty. One major difficulty with the use of these implantable devices is contracture of a thickened capsule, which causes the reconstructed breast to become very firm to palpation. Sometimes, these encapsulated reconstructions are not only hard but also spherical and, therefore, appear distorted. Many attempts have been made to delineate the cause of this capsule contracture, but no absolute reason for it has been determined. This particular problem is noted in approximately 25 percent of patients having one of these implants. One technique to reduce the frequency of contracture is to place the prosthesis beneath a muscle cover at the time of surgery.[35] Submuscular placement has become the method of choice in breast reconstruction whenever possible, in order to protect the prosthesis from extrusion and to decrease the incidence of capsule contracture (Fig. 17–4). Inclusion of methylprednisolone in the saline solution of an inflatable prosthesis or of triamcinolone in the prosthesis pocket may also decrease the rate of capsule contracture.

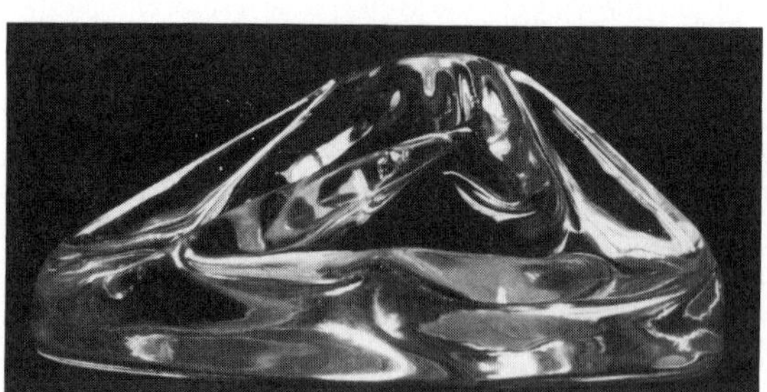

FIGURE 17–3. A three-lumen breast prosthesis. The innermost lumen is filled with a very viscous silicone gel, which gives the prosthesis a high profile. This can be used to match the contour of a projecting opposite normal breast. The next, or second, lumen is filled with a softer silicone gel, and the outermost lumen can be filled with different amounts of saline to vary its volume.

RECONSTRUCTION WITH AVAILABLE TISSUE

Indications. The indication for reconstruction using available tissue, with placement of a prosthetic device under the available tissue, is the presence of an adequate quality and quantity of skin, subcutaneous tissue, and muscle to cover an implant of a size to match the opposite breast and to establish a symmetric reconstruction. This method is most often used after a modified radical mastectomy in which the pectoralis major muscle is left intact, resulting in preservation of the infraclavicular tissue and the anterior axillary fold in the patient with a small nonptotic opposite breast.

Advantages. The advantages of reconstruction with available tissue are that it can be carried out through existing scars, so that no new scars are created. It is a relatively short and uncomplicated operative procedure compared with other reconstructive techniques. Another benefit of this type of operation is that it does not mask local recurrence of disease, because the prosthesis is placed under the muscle on the anterior chest wall, below the plane of the mastectomy.

Procedure. A small segment of the mastectomy scar is reopened, and a pocket is dissected beneath the pectoralis major, the serratus anterior, and the external oblique muscles and the fascia of the rectus abdominis muscles. A silicone prosthesis is then placed in the pocket. This allows the prosthesis to be covered with muscle, subcutaneous tissues, and skin, thereby reducing the possibility of extrusion of the prosthesis and decreasing the incidence of capsular contracture (Fig. 17–4).

Disadvantages. The disadvantages of this technique are that it is generally not usable (1) when there has been a skin graft, (2) when the skin is tight or irradiated, (3) when the pectoralis major muscle has been denervated because the medial pectoral nerve was removed at mastectomy, and (4) in radical mastectomy patients who have had both pectoral muscles removed. The use of this procedure is limited also to patients who have a small nonptotic opposite breast or who are willing to have surgery on the remaining breast to adjust the size or position for symmetry.

Complications. There are several possible types of complications with this type of reconstruction, including infection, hematoma, prosthesis deflation, necrosis of tissue with extrusion of the prosthesis, and capsule contracture. If an infection should occur around the silicone prosthesis, the prosthesis must be removed and must not be reinserted for approximately three to six months, to allow for complete resolution of the infection. The prosthesis can usually then be safely replaced, thereby providing reconstruction of the breast contour. Hematoma formation may necessitate reopening the incision to control bleeding. Prosthesis deflation can occur spontaneously or secondary to direct trauma to the device. This would require removal and replacement of the deflated prosthesis. Necrosis of skin usually does not result in extrusion of the prosthesis, unless there is no muscle covering the prosthesis. Capsule contracture occurs in approximately 25 percent of patients who have a silicone prosthesis. This complication can sometimes be treated with closed capsulotomy (squeezing the implant and splitting the capsule) or it may require open surgical lysis of the capsule.

BREAST RECONSTRUCTION WITH THE USE OF TISSUE EXPANDERS

Indications. The use of tissue expanders in breast reconstruction was introduced by Lapin and colleagues in 1980.[23] This method has been further defined by Radovan[36] and Agenta and associates.[37] The use of the tissue expander for breast reconstruction is indicated in those patients who have tissue of adequate quality but inadequate quantity on the chest wall following mastectomy. These conditions are usually found in the patient who has had modified radical mastectomy in which the pectoralis muscle was left intact and in whom there has been no radiation therapy to the chest wall or to the skin graft placed there. The tissue expander is a silicone rubber envelope that has a self-sealing valve connected either directly to it (Fig. 17–5) or remotely by a silicone fill-tube (Fig. 17–6). These devices can gradually be expanded by inflating them with saline through the self-sealing valve. An experimental self-filling model is under investigation.[38] The envelope of this type of device fills itself by way of an osmotic gradient, which draws extracellular fluid into the envelope, eliminating the need to fill it externally.

Advantages. This method of breast reconstruction requires less extensive surgery than do flap procedures. It can be carried out through existing scars, so there are no new scars on the chest wall and no donor-site scars or deformity with which to contend.

Procedure. This method can be used immediately at the time of mastectomy in the patient with a small tumor and clinically negative nodes, or it can be employed in a delayed procedure. The tissue expander generally is placed in a submuscular pocket be-

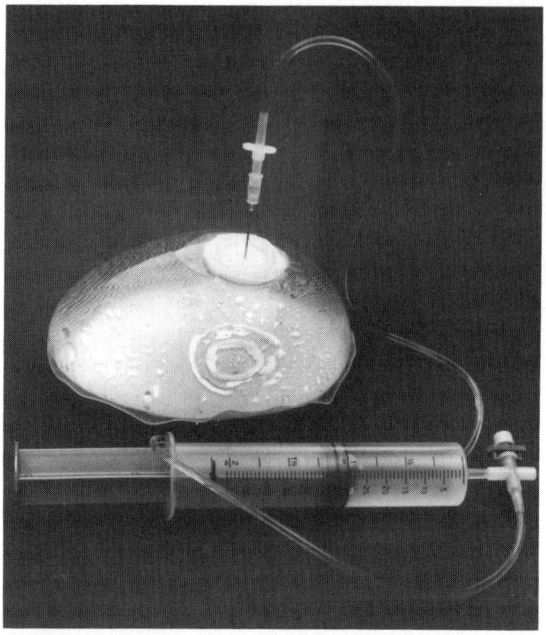

FIGURE 17–5. A tissue expander demonstrating the self-sealing valve on the front of the device, with a needle protruding through the metal-backed valve. Note the syringe connected via the extension tubing to the needle.

neath the pectoralis major, serratus anterior, and external oblique muscles and the fascia of the rectus abdominis (Fig. 17–7). The incision is allowed to heal for about two weeks; then weekly or biweekly inflation is carried out through the self-sealing valve (Figs. 17–5 and 17–6). The surgeon ultimately fills the inserted expander to a volume greater than that of the anticipated size of the permanent prosthesis. This is done to simulate ptosis of a mature breast and also to try to limit the incidence of capsular contracture around the permanent prosthesis. After the tissue expander has been inflated to the desired size, a second operation is carried out, usually with the patient receiving local anesthesia, to replace the expander with a permanent prosthesis. The nipple-areola complex can be reconstructed during this second operative procedure if so desired.

Disadvantages. One disadvantage of this type of reconstruction is that it requires two operative procedures. The first is to insert the tissue expander, and the second to implant the permanent prosthesis. Another limitation is that multiple visits to the doctor's office are required for inflation. Often, patients find this annoying. This latter problem may be obviated if experimental self-filling devices become clinically available.

Complications. Possible complications of this procedure include the following. Deflation can occur in different ways: (1) Spontaneously, (2) the envelope can be punctured with a needle at the time of filling, or (3) if a significant amount of direct trauma is applied to the prosthesis, it may rupture. If it ruptures or becomes deflated, it must be removed and replaced with either another expander or the permanent prosthesis. There is generally a two-week period during which this replacement can be done without loss of the distending action already achieved by the use of the expander. Infection can be introduced at the time of insertion or with one of the inflations or can be related to a remote infection elsewhere in the body. If the expander becomes infected, it must be removed and left out until the infection is controlled. This delay period is generally three to six months. Another complication associated with this procedure, as with all other breast reconstructions using a permanent prosthetic device, is the possibility of capsular contracture. If this problem arises, the capsule may be manually split by squeezing and twisting the prosthesis, or a surgical procedure may be required to lyse it.

LOCAL FLAPS IN BREAST RECONSTRUCTION

The use of local flaps in breast reconstruction is limited to those patients for whom only a small amount of tissue augmentation

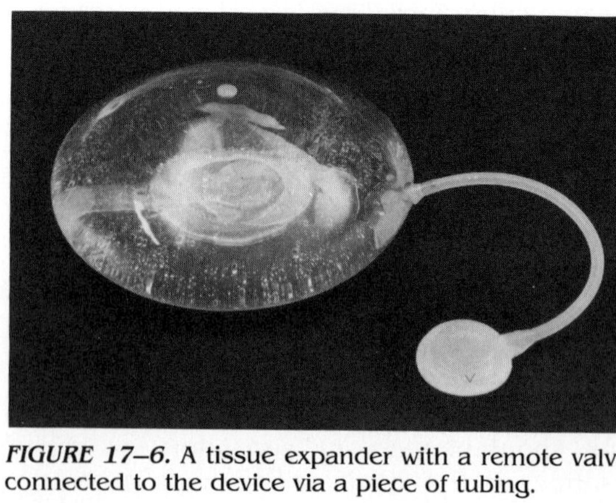

FIGURE 17–6. A tissue expander with a remote valve connected to the device via a piece of tubing.

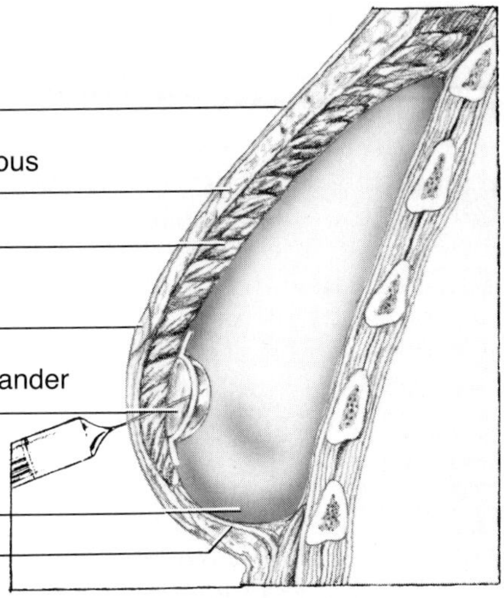

FIGURE 17–7. The position of a tissue expander with a self-sealing valve, and a syringe with the needle placed through the self-sealing valve.

is necessary and for whom this need exists only in the lower aspect of the mastectomy site. Transposition flaps from the upper abdomen and direct advancement flaps from the lower chest wall and upper abdominal tissues are included in this type of reconstruction.

The Thoracoepigastric Flap

Tai and Hasegawa[15] first described the thoracoepigastric transposition flap, and it was modified subsequently by Cronin and colleagues by delaying it to increase the usable flap length.[39]

Indications. This procedure has been used to augment a shortage of tissue in the lower portion of the chest wall in breast reconstruction, and while it continues to be used by some surgeons, it is not frequently the operation selected when a flap procedure is required.

Advantages. The advantage of a local flap is that it uses adjacent ventral body tissue, which is more likely to match the color of breast skin than are distant flaps.

Procedure. A transposition flap is raised, while based on perforators, from the upper aspect of the rectus abdominis muscle. The flap can be delayed by first incising the flap and undermining it; this extends the length of the flap that will survive the transfer. The flap is then raised after ten days to two weeks and is transposed onto the lower chest wall to release tightness and augment a tissue shortage in that area. The donor site is closed directly by undermining the surrounding tissue.

Disadvantages. A disadvantage of this flap is that it is usually too short to significantly augment tissue in the axillary or infraclavicular area. It also leaves a sizable scar in the upper abdomen and lower chest area.

Complications. The most frequent complication of this procedure is necrosis of the distal end of the flap, especially if it is taken beyond the anterior axillary fold without delay.

Direct Advancement Flaps

Direct advancement flaps of the abdomen for breast reconstruction were first described by Lewis.[22] Ryan refined this technique by adding a distinct inframammary crease.[24]

Indications. Direct advancement flaps of the abdomen are indicated when there is a shortage of tissue limited to the lower aspect of the mastectomy site.

Advantages. The use of abdominal tissue usually allows a close match of the color of the breast skin and is an operation of less magnitude than a distant flap.

Procedure. An incision is made in the skin and subcutaneous tissue on the lower chest, in a position that will permit the advancement of tissue to augment a shortage and serve as an inframammary crease. The skin and subcutaneous tissue over the lower chest and upper abdomen are then undermined and advanced onto the anterior chest wall. A pocket is developed on the chest wall, using the advanced tissue for partial cover, and a prosthesis is placed. A crescent of skin just above and just below the incision are deepithelialized, and these are sutured together and anchored to the underlying chest wall to reconstruct an inframammary crease.

Disadvantages. The disadvantage of this procedure is that it is useful only when there is a small deficit of tissue on the lower aspect of the mastectomy site.

Complications. The major complications

are those associated with the use of a silicone prosthesis, infection, hematoma, deflation, extrusion, and capsule contracture.

BREAST RECONSTRUCTION WITH THE LATISSIMUS DORSI FLAP

The latissimus dorsi flap is a muscle flap, and the latissimus dorsi flap with a skin island is a musculocutaneous flap. The concepts of muscle and musculocutaneous flaps are important in understanding the use of these flaps. The blood supply to a muscle flap is by way of a dominant direct vessel, and the entire muscle can be moved as long as the dominant vessels to it remain intact. This makes it possible to move the tissue safely in one stage. The skin over the muscle is nourished by vessels that come from the muscle and go directly to the skin and subcutaneous tissue. This makes it possible to move the skin over the muscle when one moves the muscle, without relying on the random inclusion of indirect vessels in the skin and subcutaneous tissue. Therefore, one can transfer the overlying tissue in one stage, without a delay step for enhancing the tissue's blood supply. The concepts of muscle and musculocutaneous flaps were developed by investigators in the mid-1970's.[3]

In 1906, Tansini[2] suggested the use of the latissimus dorsi muscle in breast surgery, but the concept was lost until the 1970's, when it was rediscovered in conjunction with the development of the muscle and musculocutaneous flaps. The latissimus dorsi muscle was first used in breast reconstruction in this century by Schneider and colleagues[18] and Muhlbauer and Olbrisch.[19]

Indications. The latissimus dorsi flap is indicated in a patient who has a deficiency in the quantity or quality, or both, of soft tissue on the chest wall, such as a patient who has had a radical mastectomy in which the pectoralis muscles have been excised and in which the skin is of inadequate quantity or poor quality. It may be indicated in a patient who has had a modified radical mastectomy, and whose pectoralis major muscle has been denervated secondary to the cancer surgery, or in those women who have received radiation to, or have thin skin over, the mastectomy site.

Advantages. The advantages of the latissimus dorsi flap are as follows: (1) It is a large flat muscle and, when transferred to the front of the chest, can simulate the shape of the pectoralis muscle. (2) It can be used to replace the deficiency in the axillary fold by moving the insertion from the back of the humerus to the front. (3) It may also carry skin with it to release tightness. (4) It is a hearty flap, which can usually be transferred without tissue loss.

Procedure. The latissimus dorsi muscle is a flat, fan-shaped muscle, which originates from the spinous processes of the lower sixth thoracic and the lumbar vertebrae and from the spine of the ilium through the thoracolumbar fascia. It also originates from slips from the lower four ribs and inserts into the intertubercular groove of the humerus. The latissimus dorsi muscle receives its blood supply via the thoracodorsal artery, which is a branch of the subscapular artery that comes off the third part of the axillary artery, and is innervated by the thoracodorsal nerve, a branch of the posterior cord of the brachial plexus. An incision is made over the muscle on the back, and if a skin island is to be brought with the muscle, it should be outlined at the time of this incision. The muscle is then freed from its origins on the spinous processes of the vertebrae, the spine of the ilium, and the lower four ribs. During the elevation, it is important to protect the thoracodorsal artery (or if this has been severed, the collateral vessel from the serratus anterior muscle). A tunnel is then developed under the skin of the axilla, and the muscle and skin flap are passed onto the anterior chest wall. The donor site can usually be closed directly, without any skin grafts. The patient is then turned into the supine position, so that the opposite breast can be used as a guideline for the placement of the transferred tissue. The old mastectomy site is reopened. The muscle is sutured into a position that simulates the missing pectoralis tissue and the skin island. If the skin island is brought along with the muscle, it is placed in the optimum orientation to release the tightness resulting from the mastectomy. This is most often accomplished by placing the skin island in the lower outer quadrant to simulate the ptosis contour of the opposite breast (Fig. 17–8).

Disadvantages. The use of this flap does result in additional scars on the back. It may

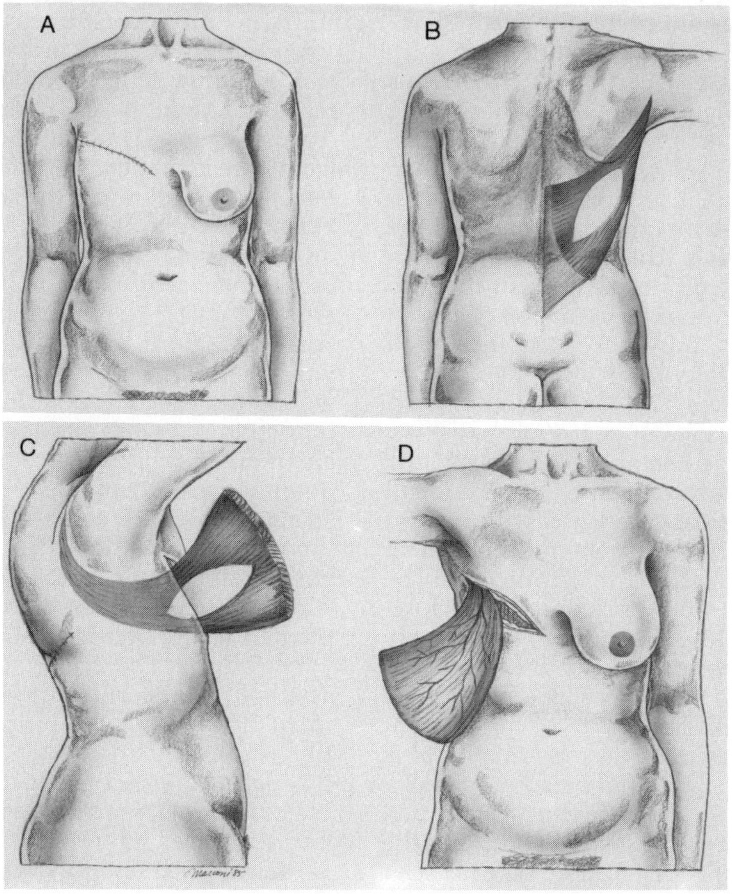

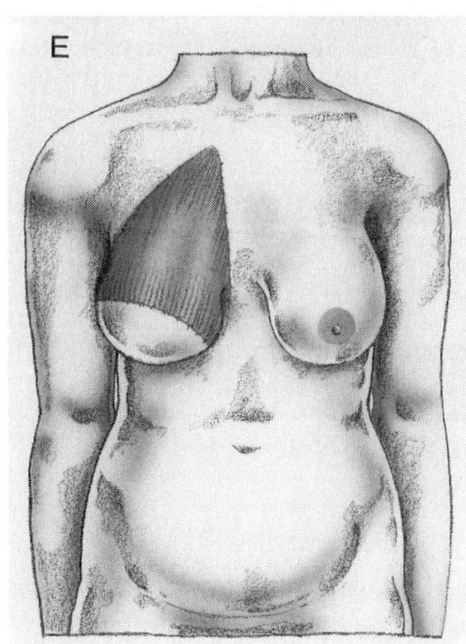

FIGURE 17–8. *A*, The postmastectomy defect with the scar. *B*, The broad, flat latissimus dorsi muscle with the proposed skin island outlined. *C*, Latissimus dorsi flap with overlying skin island passed through a tunnel in the axilla. *D*, Latissimus dorsi muscle, with arborizing thoracodorsal vessels on the underside, as it is passed through the reopened mastectomy scar. *E*, Latissimus dorsi muscle sutured into place to simulate the pectoralis major muscle where necessary, and the skin island is used to release the tightness that may result from removal of tissue during the mastectomy (see text).

weaken the shoulder girdle in a patient who already has some deficit secondary to mastectomy. This type of weakness may be noted by patients when they attempt to push themselves up out of a chair. While this procedure has been successfully carried out in tennis players and golfers without a noticeable change in their performance, it is not recommended for professional athletes. Another drawback to this operation is that it can result in a patchwork appearance on the reconstructed breast. This is because the sun exposure and, therefore, the color of the skin on the back is different from that on the front of the chest. This drawback, combined with the fact that the latissimus dorsi flap results in additional scars on the reconstructed breast, may reduce its appeal.

Limitations. The use of this flap is limited when the thoracodorsal pedicle has been cut during the cancer surgery. If the nerve and artery have been severed, the muscle can be transferred on collateral circulation from the serratus anterior and teres muscles. However, it will be atrophic and will not supply much bulk for the reconstruction. Nevertheless, it will support a piece of skin, which can be used to release tightness on the anterior chest wall. The use of this flap is limited in patients who have had a posterior lateral thoracotomy, because the incision cuts across the latissimus muscle, interrupting the blood supply to the lower part of the muscle.

Complications. This procedure provides a reliable flap with a good tissue to blood supply ratio and only occasionally results in complications, the most common of which are loss of a small portion of the flap and seroma formation in the donor site on the back.

BREAST RECONSTRUCTION USING THE RECTUS ABDOMINIS FLAP

The transverse rectus abdominis muscle flap procedure in breast reconstruction was described by Hartrampf and colleagues in 1982.[25] This was a major contribution to breast reconstructive surgery. It allows for the most natural-appearing, normal-feeling, reconstructed breast.

Indications. The rectus abdominis flap is indicated in patients with a moderate excess of tissue on the abdomen and in those women who desire breast reconstruction without the use of a silicone prosthesis. In addition, this procedure can be used to reconstruct the breast in patients who have had multiple failures of other methods of reconstruction.

Advantages. The major advantage of this technique is that the transferred tissue closely matches the color and texture of the opposite breast. In addition, the transferred tissue brought from the abdomen can simulate breast ptosis and has movement and flow approximating a natural breast. Donor-site scars are more easily hidden beneath the panty line. One of the most acclaimed benefits of this procedure is that associated with reduction of excess abdominal tissue and the creation of a slimmer look. Another frequently cited advantage of this type of reconstruction is that it can be performed without the use of a prosthetic device under the flap, eliminating the possible complications accompanying having a foreign device implanted in the breast area.

Procedure. The rectus abdominis muscle, a straplike muscle on the front of the abdomen, has two blood supplies: one through the superior epigastric artery and one through the inferior epigastric artery. Either one of these blood supplies will carry the entire muscle and overlying tissue. The transverse rectus abdominis flap procedure relies on the superior epigastric artery (Fig. 17–9). With the patient in a supine position, the desired ellipse of skin and subcutaneous fat is outlined from the suprapubic area to just above the umbilicus. The flap is usually based on the rectus muscle opposite the side of the breast to be reconstructed. The use of the contralateral muscle makes the anatomic angles that are encountered during the folding of the pedicle less likely to restrict the blood supply. If only one half of the abdomen is available, such as in the case of a midline incision, the ipsilateral muscle is used. Incisions are made around the ellipse, and the dissection is started on the side opposite the carrier muscle. The skin and subcutaneous tissue are reflected off the underlying fascia to the midline of the abdomen on the noncarrier side. The position of the perforators is noted, so they can be better protected on the carrier side. The dissection is then carried out from the lateral side to the edge of the rectus sheath. This leaves the ellipse of skin

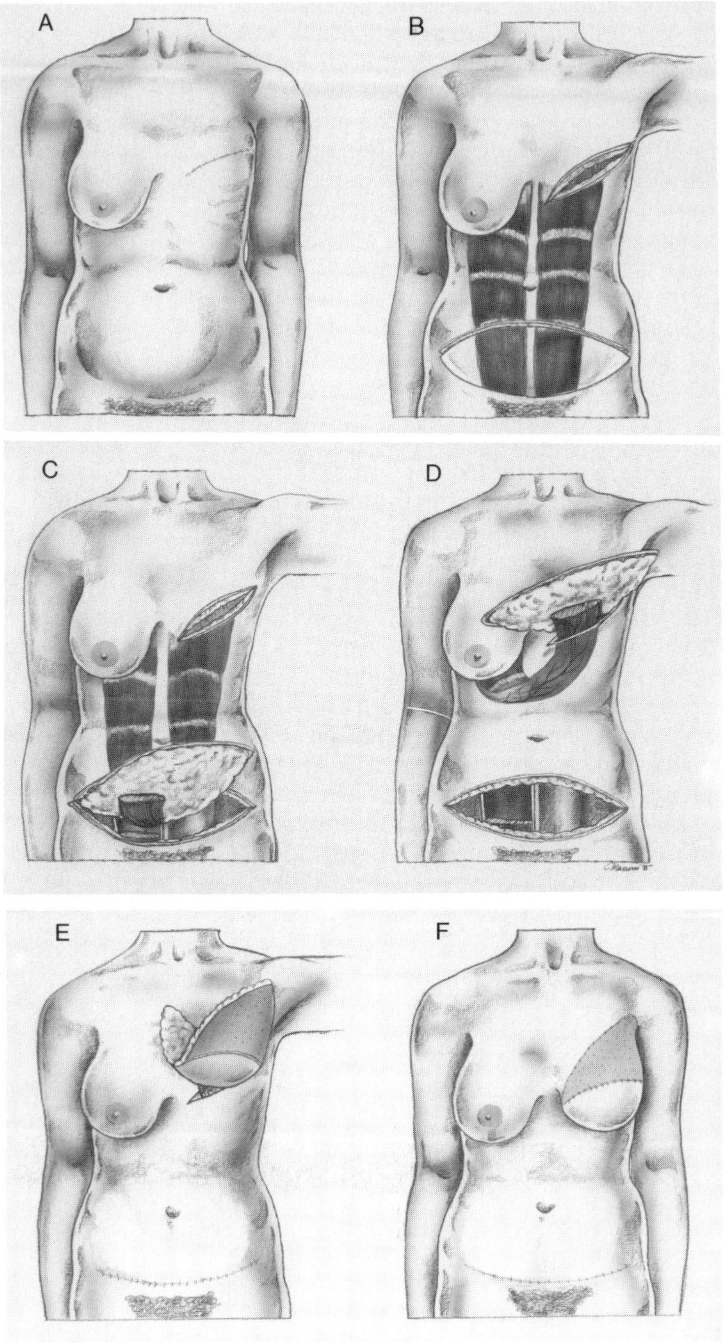

FIGURE 17–9. Breast reconstruction with the rectus abdominis flap. *A,* Defect following mastectomy, with tissue deficit on the anterior chest wall. *B,* Straplike rectus abdominis muscles. Mastectomy scar is reopened, and the skin island on the lower abdomen outlined. *C,* Skin and subcutaneous tissue left attached to the contralateral rectus abdominis muscle. *D,* Skin and subcutaneous tissue island passed through tunnel on the upper abdomen and lower chest. *E,* Donor site sutured together and the neoumbilicus brought through the upper abdominal flap. Part of the island is used to release tightness. *F,* Flap inset on chest wall effecting reconstruction of breast. (Please see text.)

and subcutaneous tissue attached to the rectus sheath, thereby protecting the perforating vessels that constitute the blood supply to the flap. The rectus sheath is then opened, and the rectus muscle reflected out of the sheath. At this time the inferior epigastric vessels are ligated, as are the segmental intercostal vessels. The posterior sheath is left intact. A portion of anterior rectus sheath is taken with the muscle to protect the integrity of the blood supply. Then, the skin and subcutaneous tissue on the upper abdomen are reflected off the underlying fascia, and a tunnel is dissected into the area on the chest wall. The old mastectomy site is then reopened, and the tissue is shaped and deepithelialized as necessary to simulate the breast contour. The rectus sheath is repaired, and the abdominal flap is brought down. The umbilicus is brought through the flap, in the same relative position on the abdomen. The final step is to suture the flap to the tissue along the lower edge of the abdomen, where the tissue for the reconstruction was harvested.

Disadvantages. The disadvantages are related to the magnitude and length of the procedure and the fact that it requires a general anesthetic. It may also involve loss of blood, with a possible need for transfusions.

Complications. The complications of this procedure include loss of some of the transferred tissue, weakness, and possible herniation of the abdominal wall and loss of some of the skin and subcutaneous tissue raised and brought down to close the donor site. The ratio of tissue to blood supply is large in this flap, and partial loss of transferred tissue is more probable, especially in smokers, obese patients, and those with arteriosclerosis. Weakness in the area of the donor site of the rectus muscle is also possible, predisposing to hernia formation. This can be lessened by preconditioning of the remaining muscles by doing sit-ups, by using only part of the muscle in the transfer, and by reinforcing the donor area with a prolene or Marlex mesh.

BREAST RECONSTRUCTION USING MICROSURGICAL FREE FLAPS

Fugino and colleagues[17] first reported using free microsurgical gluteal flaps for reconstruction of a breast in 1976. Since that time, other free flaps have been described, including the free groin flap, the free contralateral latissimus dorsi flap,[40] and the free flap of lower abdominal skin and rectus muscle.[41] Shaw has refined the technique with the use of a free gluteus myocutaneous flap. He has demonstrated good results using this method in ten patients.[42]

Indications. The indication for this type of reconstruction is failure of other methods of breast reconstruction or the patient's desire to have reconstruction without the use of a prosthesis.

Advantages. The advantages are that it allows one to reconstruct the breast with autogenous tissue, thereby obviating the difficulties found in using a silicone prosthesis. It also allows one to reconstruct a breast in a patient in whom other methods have failed one or more times.

Procedure. In the superior gluteal musculocutaneous flap, a free flap of skin, subcutaneous tissue, and muscles is designed using the superior gluteal artery and vein as donor vessels. The tissue is separated from the body at the donor site over the upper buttock area. The donor area is then closed directly, and the patient is turned to the supine position. The free flap is then transferred to the anterior chest wall, where the superior gluteal artery and vein are reanastomosed to the internal mammary vessels or to other vessels in the area. The vascular anastomosis is done with microsurgical instruments and with an operating microscope.

Disadvantages. The disadvantage of this method is that it requires special equipment and special skills for successful completion.

Complications. The main complication with free-tissue transfer is the failure of the vascular anastomosis, resulting in loss of the tissue. In experienced hands, however, this should not exceed 5 to 10 percent.

RECONSTRUCTION AFTER LUMPECTOMY AND RADIATION THERAPY

Breast reconstruction may be necessary after lumpectomy and radiation therapy. The complexity of the reconstruction is related to the post-treatment defect.[43] With a mild defect, one might find a slight distortion in the contour or a decrease in volume of the breast following a lumpectomy. Radiation therapy may result in mild fibrosis and a decrease in the size or a change in the breast contour. With a mild defect, reconstruction may be carried out by placing a small breast prosthesis beneath the treated breast, to attempt to restore the size and contour of the breast. With a moderate defect, surgery may result in a moderate distortion of the contour or the size of the breast. Radiation may also cause a moderate amount of fibrosis and disruption of the normal size and contour of the breast. With a moderate defect, reconstruction may require bringing in skin and tissue to restore the contour and size of the treated breast. In such a case, a latissimus dorsi flap with a skin pedicle may be required to restore a skin shortage after a lumpectomy and to restore volume loss resulting from the treatment. This may be done with or without the addition of a prosthetic implant. Lumpectomy and radiation therapy can cause a marked change in the treated breast. This marked change can result from a lumpectomy that has required removal of a large amount of tissue, with a considerable reduction in the size of the breast. A very large amount of radiation can cause extensive radiation change in the tissue, with fibrosis, pigmentation, and telangiectasia. When there is a dramatic change in the breast, one may need to consider replacing a large volume of tissue, with possible excision of radiation-damaged tissue. In this case, reconstruction may require the use of flap tissue, such as the transverse rectus abdominis flap, to restore a breast contour.

Techniques are available to achieve a satisfactory breast reconstruction in nearly any woman desiring one, irrespective of the type of treatment she has had for breast cancer. These techniques permit the reconstruction of defects ranging from a slight distortion of contour with a small volume deficit after lumpectomy all the way to defects left by modified radical and extended radical surgery and extensive radiation damage. Immediate breast reconstruction is available to and useful in some patients whose breast cancer is treated with surgery, and it has been helpful in reducing the psychologic trauma of mastectomy. Prophylactic mastectomy with immediate reconstruction may be beneficial in some patients who have a preponderance of risk factors for developing breast cancer.

THE CONTRALATERAL BREAST

Management of the opposite breast is of crucial concern, because symmetry is a high priority issue in breast reconstruction. The first option is to do nothing and leave the existing breast alone. It is relatively easy to reconstruct a breast to match a small or moderate-sized, nonptotic opposite breast. However, many patients do not have this type of breast structure, and surgery on the contralateral breast is often necessary. Augmentation can be done in patients with hypoplastic, atrophic, or involuted breasts. Some patients will request this in order to enhance the esthetic outcome in a reconstruction. If the other breast is large, heavy, and pendulous, it may be necessary to decrease it in size in order to match a reconstructed breast on the opposite side. If the breast is of a desirable size but is ptotic, one can carry out a mastopexy, moving the breast tissue back up to a more youthful position on the chest wall.

Prophylactic mastectomy of the remaining breast with immediate reconstruction can be considered in some patients, especially in those women who possess a large number of risk factors for developing carcinoma in the remaining breast. The decision to have or not to have this operation should be seriously discussed among the patient, her oncologist, surgeon, and plastic surgeon, and significant family members, in order to determine her specific risk-benefit ratio for the surgery.

PROPHYLACTIC MASTECTOMY

Indications. Prophylactic mastectomy is a controversial subject. There are strong proponents[44–46] of the procedure, and there are those who feel that no indications for this procedure exist.[47] We think that there are patients who can benefit from prophylactic mastectomy if they are carefully selected and are fully informed about the pros and cons of the procedure, so they and their family can participate in the decision for or against it.

The major factors that influence the choice of this procedure are a strong family history of carcinoma of the breast, histologic evidence of precancerous mastopathy, and a history of carcinoma in the contralateral breast. Anderson[48] has demonstrated that a positive family history of carcinoma of the breast is an important risk determinant. The histologic findings associated with an increased incidence of breast cancer are epithelial hyperplasia with atypia, atypical lobular hyperplasia, and diffuse papillomatosis with atypia.[49–51] A history of carcinoma in one breast has been associated with an increased risk of developing cancer in the contralateral breast.[52, 53]

Minor factors that should be considered include cancerphobia, breasts that are difficult to examine, a history of multiple biopsies, and mastodynia. Cancerphobia is a subjective phenomenon that is difficult to quantitate, but in some individuals, it can be very intense and, when coupled with a realistic risk of breast cancer, may weigh heavily in the decision for prophylactic mastectomy. Some patients have very dense breast tissue, which is difficult to examine by either physical examination or mammographic techniques. This can lead to multiple biopsies. The multiplicity of biopsies then results in scarring, which can further complicate examination of the breast tissue. Mastodynia is a subjective complaint that may or may not be relieved by prophylactic surgery and should be given only a small amount of weight in the decision for the procedure. If mastodynia is a major problem in an individual patient, consideration should be given to pharmacologic management before surgery. The pharmacologic management may include limiting intake of xanthine-containing compounds such as coffee, tea, cola, and chocolate and the use of vitamin E. It can also include the use of medications, such as a norethynodrel-mestranol combination for estrogen-progesterone balance, or the use of antiestrogens such as danazol and tamoxifen.[54]

Method. The methods recommended for prophylactic mastectomy have ranged from nearly total removal of the mammary gland and lower axillary contents, including a free graft of the areola (without the nipple),[55] to dissecting the glandular tissue out, leaving thick skin flaps and the nipple and areola undisturbed.[56] With the former technique, the complication rate is higher, with tissue necrosis and extrusion of the prosthesis and a much less desirable cosmetic outcome. The problem with the latter technique is that one is more likely to leave breast tissue behind, and in a prophylactic operation, this would be undesirable. A middle ground with respect to the extent of operation seems acceptable, with excision of as much gland as possible, but leaving flaps thick enough to obviate necrosis. With respect to the nipple-areola complex, Georgiade[45] has made the reasonable recommendation that the nipple site on the specimen be tagged and examined histologically; if atypia is found, the nipple is removed. Immediate reconstruction, with placement of the prosthesis beneath the pectoralis major and serratus anterior muscles, is usually carried out after the removal of the gland. Covering the prosthesis with muscle decreases the incidence of capsule contracture and also the possibility of prosthesis extrusion.

Early data indicate that the incidence of breast cancer after prophylactic mastectomy is less than 1 percent.[57]

NIPPLE-AREOLA RECONSTRUCTION

As more improved methods of reconstructing the breast contour have become available, the feasibility of reconstructing a breast that is more realistic in appearance and texture increases. With this objective realized, there has come a heightened interest in reconstruction of the nipple-areola complex. The goals of nipple-areola reconstruction include symmetry in size, color, and position of the areola and symmetry in color, texture, and projection of the reconstructed nipple. Reconstruction of the nipple-areola complex either can be done immediately, with reconstruction of the breast contour, or can be delayed for a period to allow the reconstructed breast to settle into its new position. The advantage of doing an immediate nipple-areola reconstruction is that it may eliminate one surgery for the patient. However, this is done usually at a cost in terms of the final outcome, as it is difficult to establish the most symmetric position for the nipple-areola complex on the reconstructed breast until it has settled.

Delayed reconstruction of the nipple-areola complex allows the new breast to settle into its ultimate position. This permits the patient and the surgeon to determine the best location for the nipple-areola complex and to attempt the best match possible. Theoretically, the best source for reconstruction of the nipple would be the original nipple-areola complex itself. Millard and associates[58] have proposed banking of the nipple-areola complex at the time of mastectomy for later reconstruction. They suggested frozen-section control to eliminate the possibility of transplanting the tumor to any other location. The incidence of involvement of the nipple-areola complex in carcinoma of the breast has been documented to range from 8 to 38 percent.[59–62] There are reports in the literature of transplantation of tumor with banking of the nipple,[63] both in procedures done with frozen-section control[64, 65] and without frozen-section control.[66] The other major objection to banking of the nipple-areola complex is an esthetic one. If the nipple-areola complex is first transplanted to the groin and then is retransplanted to the chest wall, there is a revascularization process required in both instances. This usually results in scarring and pigment loss, so that the banked nipple-areola complex does not match the opposite side in color, texture, or size. Some patients also object to the scar left at the site of the banking procedure and to the experience of having a nipple placed elsewhere on the body. For these reasons, many surgeons have abandoned banking the nipple-areola complex as a method of reconstruction. As a result, there have been several methods suggested for reconstruction of the areola. Adams[67] suggested the use of the labia minora. Conway and associates[68] used tattoo pigments. Kiskadden[69] noted that a nipple-areola complex could be transferred using a split-thickness graft. Gillies[9] used an everted umbilicus, transferred via a pedicle flap to reconstruct a nipple. Rapin[70] suggested the use of pigmented axillary skin, transferred to the breast by a tubed pedicle. Some of the procedures just described are of historical interest and are infrequently used today in nipple-areola reconstruction.

The remaining nipple-areola complex on the opposite breast is one possible donor site.[71, 72] It does require that the opposite areola be large enough to allow for reconstruction of a reasonable-sized areola of about 30 to 40 mm on each side. Other sources of reconstructive material are related to the color of the normal areola. In the case of a pink or light-colored opposite areola, postauricular skin with its pink blush can be used for a reasonable color match.[73] For a tan opposite areola, upper inner thigh skin has been found to be the most satisfactory match.[74] In a dark brown or black patient, labial tissue seems to be the best color match. Tattoo pigments are also used today to simulate the areola.

METHODS OF RECONSTRUCTING THE NIPPLE

The primary aim in nipple reconstruction is to simulate the opposite nipple in color, texture, and projection. One of the useful areas for donor material to reconstruct the nipple is the opposite nipple. If the remaining nipple is very salient, one can take a horizontal full-thickness or vertical V-shaped graft, close the donor site primarily, and graft that onto the new breast. If it is only moderately salient, a vertical halving procedure or V-shaped wedge can be done with direct closure, and this can be used to reconstruct the nipple. These methods will decrease the projection of the donor nipple, thereby achieving more symmetric projection. Composite grafts of the ear lobe[75] or toe pad[76] have been used. These sources do give some projection, but their color is often too light to match the opposite side. Local traction flaps, similar to those used to correct the deformity of inverted nipples, have been used.[77] These techniques are designed to pull the tissue into a projecting position and hold them there by surgical manipulation of the surrounding tissue.[78] Local pedicle flaps with split-thickness skin-graft coverage have been found to give good nipple projection and also a satisfactory color match.[79] In situations in which the reconstructed nipple does not match the color of the opposite side, various techniques have been employed to attempt to bring about a better color match. These include using a sun lamp to darken the grafted side[80] and dermabrasion to darken the nipple-areola complex. Dermabrasion has been especially useful in black patients.[81] In situations in which the pigment is splotchy, overgrafting has been used.[80]

REFERENCES

1. Czerny V: Plastischer ersatz der brustdruse durch ein lipom. Zentralbl F Chir 27:72, 1895.
2. Tansini I: Sopra il mio nuovo processo di amputazione della mamella. Gazetta Medica Italiana 57:141, 1906.
3. McGraw JB, Dibbell DG, Carraway JH: Clinical definition of independent myocutaneous vascular territories. Plast Reconstr Surg 60:341, 1977.
4. Reinhardt W: Reconstruction with sharing of opposite breast. Zeikchr F Chir, 1932.
5. Alexander JE, Block LI: Breast reconstruction follow-

ing radical mastectomy. Plast Reconstr Surg 40:175, 1967.
6. Holdsworth WG: A method of reconstructing the breast. Br J Plast Surg 9:161, 1956.
7. Pontes R: Single stage reconstruction of the missing breast. Br J Plast Surg 26:377, 1973.
8. Webster JP: Thoraco-epigastric tubed pedicles. Surg Clin North Am 17:145, 1937.
9. Gillies HD: Practical use of tubed pedicle flap. Br J Surg 30:477, 1945.
10. Longacre JJ: The use of local pedicle flaps for reconstruction of breast after subtotal or total extirpation of the mammary gland and for correction of distortion and atrophy of the breast due to excessive scar. Plast Reconstr Surg 11:380, 1953.
11. Kiricuta I: L'emploi du grand epiploon dans la chirurgie du sein cancereux. Presse Med 71:15, 1963.
12. Cronin TD, Gerow FJ: Augmentation mammoplasty: A new "natural feel" prosthesis. *In*: Transactions of the Third International Congress of Plastic Surgery. Amsterdam: Excerpta Medica Foundation, 1963, pp. 41–49.
13. Snyderman RK, Guthrie R: Reconstruction of the female breast following radical mastectomy. Plast Reconstr Surg 47:565, 1971.
14. Orticochea M: Use of the buttock to reconstruct the breast. Br J Plast Surg 26:304, 1973.
15. Tai Y, Hasegawa HA: A transverse abdominal flap for reconstruction after radical operations for recurrent breast cancer. Plast Reconstr Surg 53:52, 1974.
16. Arnold PG, Hartrampf CR, Jurkiewicz MJ: One-stage reconstruction of the breast, using the transposed greater omentum. Plast Reconstr Surg 57:520, 1976.
17. Fugino T, Harashina T, Enomoto K: Primary breast reconstruction after a standard radical mastectomy by a free flap transfer. Plast Reconstr Surg 58:371, 1976.
18. Schneider WJ, Hill HL, Brown RG: Latissimus dorsi myocutaneous flap for breast reconstruction. Br J Plast Surg 30:277, 1977.
19. Muhlbauer W, Olbrisch R: The lattisimus dorsi myocutaneous flap for breast reconstruction. Chir Plast (Berlin) 4:27, 1977.
20. Drever JM: The epigastric island flap. Plast Reconstr Surg 59:343, 1977.
21. Robbins TH: Rectus abdominis myocutaneous flap for breast reconstruction. Aust NZ J Surg 49:527, 1979.
22. Lewis JR, Jr.: Use of a sliding flap from the abdomen to provide cover in breast reconstruction. Plast Reconstr Surg 64:491, 1979.
23. Lapin R, Daniel D, Hutchins H, et al.: Primary breast reconstruction following mastectomy using a skin-expander prosthesis. Breast 6:20, 1980.
24. Ryan JJ: A lower thoracic advancement flap in breast reconstruction after mastectomy. Plast Reconstr Surg 70:153, 1982.
25. Hartrampf CR, Scheflan M, Black PW: Breast reconstruction with a transverse abdominal island flap. Plast Reconstr Surg 69:216, 1982.
26. Clifford E: The reconstructive experience, the search for restitution. *In*: Georgiade NG (ed.): Breast Reconstruction Following Mastectomy. St. Louis: C.V. Mosby, 1979.
27. Teimourian B, Adham MN: Survey of patients' responses to breast reconstruction. Ann Plast Surg 9:321, 1982.
28. Noone RB, Frazier TG, Hayward CZ, et al.: Patient acceptance of immediate reconstruction following mastectomy. Plast Reconstr Surg 69:632, 1982.
29. Stevens LA, McGrath MH, Druss RG, et al.: The psychological impact of immediate breast reconstruction for women with early breast cancer. Plast Reconstr Surg 73:619, 1984.
30. Noone RB, Murphy JB, Spear SL, et al.: A 6-year experience with immediate reconstruction after mastectomy for cancer. Plast Reconstr Surg 76:258, 1985.
31. Schain WS, Wellisch DK, Pasnau RO, et al.: The sooner the better: A study of psychological factors in women undergoing immediate versus delayed breast reconstruction. Am J Psychiatry 142:1, 1985.
32. Georgiade GS, Georgiade NG, McCarty KS, Jr., et al.: Rationale for immediate reconstruction of the breast following modified radical mastectomy. Ann Plast Surg 8:20, 1982.
33. Schamberger RC, Devereux DF, Brennan MF: The effect of chemotherapeutic agents on wound healing. Int Adv Surg Oncol 4:15, 1981.
34. Blocksma R, Braley S: The silicone in plastic surgery. Plast Reconstr Surg 35:366, 1965.
35. Gruber RP, Kahn RA, Lash H, et al.: Breast reconstruction following mastectomy: A comparison of submuscular and subcutaneous techniques. Plast Reconstr Surg 67:312, 1981.
36. Radovan C: Breast reconstruction after mastectomy using the temporary expander. Plast Reconstr Surg 59:69, 1982.
37. Agenta LC, Marks MW, Grabb WL: Selective use of serial expansion in breast reconstruction. Ann Plast Surg 11:188, 1983.
38. Austad ED, Rose GI: A self-inflating tissue expander. Plast Reconstr Surg 70:588, 1982.
39. Cronin TD, Upton J, McDonough JM: Reconstruction of the breast after mastectomy. Plast Reconstr Surg 59:1, 1977.
40. Serafin D, Voci VE, Georgiade NG: Microsurgical composite tissue transplantation: Indications and technical considerations in breast reconstruction following mastectomy. Plast Reconstr Surg 70:24, 1982.
41. Pennington DG, Lai MF, Pelly AD: The rectus abdominis myocutaneous free flap. Br J Plast Surg 33:277, 1980.
42. Shaw WW: Breast reconstruction by superior gluteal microvascular free flaps without silicone implants. Plast Reconstr Surg 72:490, 1983.
43. Pearl RM, Wisinicki J: Breast reconstruction following lumpectomy and irradiation. Plast Reconstr Surg 76:83, 1985.
44. Pennisi VR: The prevention of breast cancer by subcutaneous mastectomy. Surg Clin North Am 57:1023, 1977.
45. Georgiade NG, Serafin D, Georgiade G, et al.: Subcutaneous mastectomy: An evolution of concept and technique. Ann Plast Surg 8:8, 1982.
46. Buehler PK: Patient selection for prophylactic mastectomy: Who is a high risk? Plast Reconstr Surg 72:324, 1983.
47. Love SM, Gelman RS, Silen W: Fibrocystic "disease" of the breast—a nondisease? N Engl J Med 307:1010, 1982.
48. Anderson DE: Genetics and the etiology of breast cancer. Breast 3:37, 1977.
49. Hutchinson WB, Thomas DB, Hamlin WB, et al.: Risk of breast cancer in women with benign breast disease. J Natl Cancer Inst 65:13, 1980.
50. Black MM, Kwon S: Precancerous mastopathie:

Structural and biological considerations. Pathol Res Pract 166:491, 1980.
51. Page DL, Vander Zwaag R, Rogers W, et al.: Relation between component parts of fibrocystic disease complex and breast cancer. J Natl Cancer Inst 61:1055, 1978.
52. Robbins GF, Berg JW: Bilateral primary breast cancer: A prospective clinicopathological study. Cancer 17:1501, 1964.
53. Leis HP, Jr.: Selective, elective prophylactic contralateral mastectomy. Cancer 28:956, 1971.
54. London RS, Sundaram GS, Goldstein PJ: Medical management of mammary dysplasia. Obstet Gynecol 59:519, 1982.
55. Maliniac JW: Use of pedicle dermo-fat flap in mammaplasty. Plast Reconstr Surg 12:110, 1953.
56. Freeman BS: Subcutaneous mastectomy for benign breast lesions with immediate or delayed prosthetic replacement. Plast Reconstr Surg 30:676, 1962.
57. Pennisi VR, Capozzi A: Subcutaneous mastectomy—an interim report on 1,244 patients. Ann Plast Surg 12:340, 1984.
58. Millard DR, Devine J, Jr., Warren WD: Breast reconstruction: A plea for saving the uninvolved nipple. Am J Surg 122:763, 1971.
59. Andersen JA, Pallesen RM: Spread to the nipple and areola in carcinoma of the breast. Ann Surg 189:367, 1979.
60. Lagios MD, Gates EA, Westdahl PR, et al.: A guide to the frequency of nipple involvement in breast cancer. A study of 149 consecutive mastectomies using a serial subgross and correlated radiographic technique. Am J Surg 138:135, 1979.
61. Parry RG, Cochra TC, Jr., Wolfort FG: When is the nipple involved in carcinoma of the breast? Plast Reconstr Surg 59:535, 1977.
62. Smith J, Payne WS, Carney JA: Involvement of the nipple and areola in carcinoma of the breast. Surg Gynecol Obstet 143:546, 1976.
63. Allison AB, Howorth MB: Carcinoma in a nipple preserved by heterotopic auto-implantation. N Engl J Med 298:1132, 1978.
64. Bouvier B: Problems in breast reconstruction. Med J Aust 1:937, 1977.
65. Rose JH: Carcinoma in a transplanted nipple. Arch Surg 115:1131, 1980.
66. Khandekar JD: Carcinoma in a heterotopically autoimplanted nipple. Cancer 43:2502, 1979.
67. Adams WM: Labial transplant for correction of loss of nipple. Plast Reconstr Surg 4:295, 1949.
68. Conway H, Hugo NE, Tulenko JR (eds.): Surgery of Tumors of the Skin, 2nd ed. Springfield, IL: Charles C Thomas, 1966.
69. Kiskadden WS: Case report on split grafting of the nipple. Plast Reconstr Surg 5:184, 1950.
70. Rapin M: Reconstruction of the nipple. Br J Plast Surg 7:372, 1955.
71. Wexler MR, O'Neal RM: Areola sharing to reconstruct the breast nipple. Plast Reconstr Surg 51:176, 1973.
72. Georgiade GS, Riefkohl R, Georgiade NG: To share or not to share. Ann Plast Surg 14:180, 1985.
73. Brent B, Bostwick J: Nipple-areola reconstruction with auricular tissues. Plast Reconstr Surg 60:353, 1977.
74. Broadbent TR, Woolf RM, Metz PS: Restoring the mammary areola by a skin graft from the upper inner thigh. Br J Plast Surg 30:220, 1977.
75. Brent B: Nipple-areola reconstruction following mastectomy: An alternative to the use of labial and contralateral nipple-areola tissues. Clin Plast Surg 6:85, 1979.
76. Klatsky SA, Manson PN: Toe pulp free grafts in nipple reconstruction. Plast Reconstr Surg 68:245, 1981.
77. Skoog T: Inverted nipples. *In*: Skoog T (ed.): Plastic Surgery. Philadelphia: W.B. Saunders Co., 1974, pp. 384–389.
78. Little JW, Munasifi T, McCulloch DF: One-stage reconstruction of a projecting nipple: The quadrapod flap. Plast Reconstr Surg 71:126, 1983.
79. Hartrampf CP, Culbertson JH: A dermal-fat flap for nipple reconstruction. Plast Reconstr Surg 73:982, 1984.
80. Gruber RP: Nipple-areola reconstruction: A review of techniques. Clin Plast Surg 6:71, 1979.
81. Cohen IK: Reconstruction of the nipple-areola by dermabrasion in a black patient. Plast Reconstr Surg 67:238, 1981.

Nursing Care of the Patient with Breast Cancer

CATHERINE RICE GORRELL, R.N., M.S.N.
TERESA M. d'ANGELO, R.N., B.S.N.
CAROLINE STOKES BAGLEY, R.N., M.S.N.

18

INTRODUCTION

Cancer nursing, an essential subspecialty within nursing, has developed as a result of the recognition of cancer as a major health problem. The scope of practice in cancer nursing includes aspects of prevention, detection, and education of people with pathologic processes and covers all areas of nursing practice. The application of the roles of cancer nursing can be found in this chapter.[1]

The goals of cancer nursing are to help the patient and family to function optimally, both physically and psychologically, anywhere in the continuum of the disease process. Nursing intervention takes place in all health care settings, and the focus is on the patient, family, and community. In 1976, Donovan and Pierce[2] described the four qualities they believe the nurse who cares for people with cancer should have: "The oncologic nurse needs to be more than an experienced technician. She needs to be a human being reaching out to her fellow man and offering herself with her knowledge, her skills, and her humanity. To be able to do this the oncologic nurse needs four things: (1) knowledge, (2) a philosophy of life compatible with cancer nursing, (3) satisfaction (positive reinforcement), and (4) supportive guidance (peer support)."

Beginning with prevention, early detection, and diagnosis, nurses are actively involved in ensuring that patients and their families possess adequate information about breast cancer detection and diagnosis. Although there are no proven methods for preventing breast cancer, it is important for nurses to have knowledge of the risk factors as well as the signs and symptoms and significance of breast abnormalities. Also important is information about methods of appropriate screening and diagnostic tools and procedures.

Once the diagnosis of breast cancer is made, an important role for the nurse is to provide information so that the patient and family "possess knowledge about the disease and therapy in order to attain self-management, participation in therapy, optimal living and peaceful death."[1] During definitive breast cancer treatment such as surgery, radiation therapy, and chemotherapy, nurses are instrumental in assisting the patient in the identification and management of the side effects of treatment as well as making decisions related to their disease. In the person undergoing a mastectomy, this includes the pre- and postoperative teaching and review of nursing care required for the rehabilitation, such as preventing or managing lymphedema, selecting a prosthesis, or deciding to have breast reconstruction. In caring for the patient having radiation therapy, the role of the nurse is to provide general skin care guidelines, to assist in the management of altered skin integrity, and to identify other side effects and supply strategies for management. When a patient's treatment includes a radioactive implant, the role of the nurse is to provide information to the patient, family, and other nurses regarding the special safety precautions required. Frequently patients with breast cancer undergo chemotherapy during the course of their illness. Special challenges face nurses in the areas of obtaining venous access and in preventing, identifying, and managing the side effects often associated with chemotherapy or the disease itself.

Assisting the patient and the family to live with the diagnosis of breast cancer and its treatment is an area in which nurses provide immeasurable information and support to their clients. Insight into family dynamics and the relationships of family members is important in developing patient support systems. Knowledge of available resources, such as patient education materials and community oncology resources, is an essential part of the cancer nurse's practice.

DETECTION AND DIAGNOSIS

People are more concerned with their health today than ever before. They are better informed as a result of mass media efforts. The combined effect of these factors has enabled women to recognize the need for assuming an active role in their health care. People recognize more frequently their right to seek information, to learn about treatment options, and to participate in making treatment-related decisions. The nurse plays an important role in providing this information to patients, directing them to appropriate resources and offering support to them and their family members throughout the diagnostic, treatment, and follow-up phases of the disease. Nurses caring for people with breast cancer must, therefore, have a broad knowledge about breast diseases and their management. Specifically, a nurse needs to be knowledgeable about the assessment of an individual with a newly detected breast mass, benign and malignant breast diseases, counseling of people with a strong family history of breast cancer, the risk factors associated with breast cancer, and the treatment options for early-stage breast cancer.

Breast Self-Examination (BSE)

To be knowledgeable about all aspects of breast diseases, the nurse must be aware of the current literature in each of these areas. Studies have evaluated what women know about breast self-examination (BSE) and what factors influence the actual practice of BSE.[3,4] These studies revealed the following about the actual practice behaviors and beliefs of women concerning BSE. First, contrary to previous beliefs, fear of finding a lump was reported to be a barrier to the practice of BSE by less than 30 percent of women. Second, the more confidence that a woman had in her skill in detecting a lump, the greater the frequency of BSE practice. Third, the more confidence she had that the actual practice of BSE was an effective method of detection, the greater the likelihood that she would practice BSE. Having a knowledge of some of the barriers to the practice of BSE enables the nurse to target her assessment, eliciting specific information concerning the reasons that an individual does not practice BSE, and then to plan nursing interventions accordingly. Included in information required for an accurate assessment is the patient's knowledge of the techniques and recommended frequency of BSE practice. This assessment is followed by education and counseling as needed.

One of the nurse's roles in all health care settings is to assess the patient's knowledge of, and skill in performing, BSE. Verbal instruction, supplemented by written BSE ed-

TABLE 18–1. Guidelines for Breast Self-Examination

Breast self-examination should be part of a woman's monthly routine.
All natural breast tissue (including reconstructed breast tissue, irradiated tissue, and surgical incisions) should be examined once a month, noting changes in appearance and feeling.
Surgical procedures (including breast reconstruction) and radiation therapy cause changes in breast tissue, so women will have to relearn what is a "normal" finding during BSE.
In menstruating women, BSE should be performed two to three days after their period ends, when their breasts are less likely to be tender or swollen. For women who do not menstruate, BSE should be performed regularly on one day, such as the first day of each month.

Six Steps in Performing Breast Self-Examination

1. Stand before a mirror. Inspect the breasts for anything unusual, such as any discharge from the nipple (reconstructed nipple need not be checked) or puckering, dimpling, or scaling of the skin. In front of the mirror, inspect all surgical incisions for swelling, lumps, redness, or color change. The irradiated skin may be slightly darker in color. Incisions often are reddened for several months after surgery.

The next two steps are designed to emphasize any change in the shape or contour of the breasts. As these two steps are performed, a woman should be able to feel her chest muscles tighten.

2. Watching closely in the mirror, clasp hands behind the head and press hands forward.
3. Next, press hands firmly on the hips and bow slightly toward the mirror, pulling shoulders and elbows forward.

The next part of the examination is done while standing. Some women do it in the shower because fingers glide over soapy skin, making it easy to concentrate on the texture underneath.

4. Raise the arm of the untreated side. Using three or four fingers of the other hand, explore the breast firmly, carefully, and thoroughly. Beginning at the outer edge, press the flat part of your fingers in small circles, moving the circles slowly around the breast. Gradually work toward the nipple. Be sure to cover the entire breast. Pay special attention to the area between the breast and the armpit, including the armpit itself. Feel for any unusual lump or mass under the skin.
5. Gently squeeze the nipple and look for a discharge. Repeat the examination on the treated breast. Raise the arm on the treated side. Using three or four fingers of your other hand, examine your scar from the lymph node surgery. Examine any additional surgical incisions. Begin at the top of the incision. Press gently, using small circular motions, and feel the entire length of the incision. Look for thickenings, lumps, or hard places. As with the breasts, familiarity with your incision makes it easier to notice any changes.
6. Steps 4 and 5 should be repeated while lying down. Lying on your back, raise the arm on the treated side over your head and place a pillow or folded towel under your shoulder. This position flattens the breast and makes it easier to examine. Use the same circular motion described earlier.

ucation material, should be routinely provided to patients. Patients unfamiliar with practicing BSE should give a return demonstration, using a breast model or, preferably, using their own breast tissue. The patient should contact her physician for any signs and symptoms of breast cancer. They include a lump or thickness in the breast, swelling, skin irritation, dimpling, distortion, retraction or scaliness of the nipples, and nipple discharge or tenderness.

There is strong evidence that regular breast self-examination in the general population has assisted in identifying lumps and breast abnormalities and may facilitate the early identification of breast cancer. However, the importance of BSE following breast cancer has not been well documented in the literature.

Guidelines and techniques for practicing breast self-examination are the same for the general population, those at high risk for developing breast cancer, and those women with a history of breast cancer. Table 18–1 summarizes the steps in performing BSE.

Many women report that their reluctance to perform BSE is due to their fear of discovering a possible abnormality, or worse yet, a lump that is breast cancer. Although having a history of breast cancer is reported to be a risk factor for the development of breast cancer, there is little support for regular BSE practices within the breast cancer population. Generally, people with breast cancer are followed closely by physicians in the early years following diagnosis and treatment. As the disease-free interval increases, the frequency of follow-up decreases, even though breast cancer recurrences are diagnosed many years following treatment. As the number of follow-up visits decreases, one would think that the potential for early discovery of recurrent or metastatic disease would increase when BSE is regularly performed after breast cancer treatment. Therefore, it seems essential to target this group of women as well as the women without breast cancer.

As physically important as BSE is following breast cancer treatment, it can also be psychologically distressing. The guidelines for BSE advocate visual and manual examination of the breast tissue, axillae, and supraclavicular areas, comparing the two breasts for similar or dissimilar characteristics. When a woman discovers a possible abnormality in one breast, she is encouraged to look for the same characteristic in the contralateral breast. Breast cancer treatment, as we know it today, results in physical changes in the treated or cancerous breast. Women treated for unilateral breast cancer are subject to increased anxiety when they identify characteristics in their treated, or untreated, breast or chest wall that are dissimilar to their contralateral side. Both surgery and radiation therapy, therefore, have a series of effects on the breast and chest wall that range from subtle to dramatic and that may change in the months and years after local treatment. It is important for nurses, when instructing patients in BSE after breast treatment, to emphasize the changes that patients should expect to see after breast surgery or radiation therapy. The actual methods used in performing BSE are the same for women with a diagnosis of breast cancer and the general population. Table 18–1 includes the guidelines and steps recommended by the National Cancer Institute in performing breast self-examination.

Assessment

Assessment is an integral part of nursing practice. The data generated from a comprehensive assessment provide members of the health care team with information critical to adequate care planning. In order to adequately assess patients faced with a breast problem, whether it be benign breast disease, a strong family history, or breast changes suggestive of cancer, the nurse should address many similar areas. The assessment guidelines presented in Table 18–2 provide a suggested format for approaching this population. In general, these guidelines include demographic variables, a risk-factor profile, an assessment of knowledge, past medical history, and a general section that identifies reasons for seeking health care, expected outcomes, and other factors that might be significant for comprehensive care planning.

The emphasis placed on any one of the general areas will vary, depending on the purpose of the assessment, the patient's expected goals of the contact with the health care professional, and the diagnosis. It is important to emphasize that having this baseline data will allow planning of future health care to flow smoothly. For the woman who needs counseling on risk factors or recommended follow-up for benign breast disease or the woman with a diagnosis of breast cancer, the nurse must be aware of the extent of the patient's knowledge about breast disease, her attitudes toward therapy and follow-up, and where health care intervention is appropriate. Table 18–2 can be used for, and adapted to, any stage of the diagnostic treatment phase, providing the nurse with data sufficient to design nursing interventions appropriate to each individual.

Breast Cancer in Men

Although breast cancer is far more prevalent in women, nurses may encounter men with this disease. Male breast cancer accounts for only 1.0 percent of all cases of the disease and only 0.2 percent of all malignant neoplasia in men. However, for the nurse who does care for a man with breast cancer, there are additional assessment factors that should be addressed.

There have been no reports or studies that address the nursing care requirements of male breast cancer patients. For men with breast cancer, nurses must draw on their general knowledge of assessment and on their specific knowledge of assessment of persons with cancer. Probably, a man's reactions to a diagnosis of breast cancer will be similar to those experienced by men and women with various types of cancer. The potential for complications from therapy and for side effects from chemotherapy are also similar. Additional assessment factors may include:

1. Reactions to a diagnosis of breast cancer: Does a man perceive this diagnosis differently because it is a predominantly female disease?
2. Sexual and body image changes. Even though the male breast does not have the

TABLE 18–2. Nursing Assessment

Demography—Chronologic and developmental
- Age
- Race
- Religion
- Marital status

Socioeconomic Aspects
- Educational and experiential backgrounds
- Career responsibilities
- Family responsibilities
- Community involvement and resources

Support Systems
- Spouse or significant other(s)
- Children
- Parents
- Extended family
- Friends
- Colleagues

Risk-Factor Profile
- Previous history of breast cancer or other cancer
- Family history of breast cancer (especially first-degree relative)
- History of benign breast disease, exposure to radiation, or hormone therapy
- Age at menarche
- Age at first full-term pregnancy
- Age at menopause
- Obesity (high fat diets, high sugar intake)

Knowledge about Breast Disease
- What is benign breast disease?
- Does benign breast disease increase one's risk for breast cancer?
- What is the most common symptom of breast cancer?
- What screening tests for breast cancer are most frequently performed?
- What is the only definitive way of diagnosing breast cancer?
- What are the most common risk factors?
- What is breast self-examination (BSE)?
- Who should practice breast self-examination?
- What is known about treatment options for breast cancer?
- What is the patient's own risk profile for breast cancer?

Past Health History
- Major illnesses and surgeries
- Previous hospitalizations
- Problems with breasts
  - History of benign breast disease
  - Previous biopsies
  - Previous diagnostic studies for breast disease
- Previous/current hormonal ingestion
- Other health problems
- Practice breast self-examination
- Physical examination

General
- Purpose for seeking health care
  - Evaluation of breast disease
  - Learn BSE
  - Counseling
  - Treatment options
- What sources of information are used
  - Health care personnel
  - Friends, relatives
  - Written—books, pamphlets, audio-visual
  - Organizations, e.g., American Cancer Society and National Cancer Institutes' Office of Cancer Communications
- Psychosocial
  - Support systems
  - Psychologic variables
  - Coping strategies
- Goals
  - What she wants to achieve

same sexual importance as does the female, it is an organ that may have significance to the male in sexual foreplay.

3. Men's feeling conscious of changes in their physical appearance. Will they go without a shirt; if so, what, if any, reactions do they display?

4. Differences that may exist in the family for a male with breast cancer. Does the wife view him differently because he has "breast cancer"?

5. The family members' perceptions of his disease. Do they understand that male and female breast cancers are similar diseases, with similar treatment and expected outcomes? What, if any, misconceptions do they have about the disease?

6. Possible changes in life-style that may occur as a result of diagnosis and treatment. Does his role within the family change? Has he had to change jobs? Are there any residual physical limitations?

Assessment, then, is a comprehensive examination of a wide variety of factors affecting all aspects of the individual. It is important for the nurse to recognize that it may have been very difficult for the person to seek information from a health care professional. Nurses should be aware that many factors went into the decision-making process before care was sought (e.g., age; socioeconomic level; culture; educational and employment background; previous experiences with the health care system; the person's and family's illness experience; the real or imagined consequences of a diagnosis of breast cancer; peer pressure; and whether one has confidence in the decision to meet his or her own health care needs). The data obtained from a careful assessment lead to the identification of treatment options, the beginning of the decision-making process, and the movement toward treatment.

Decision Making and Legislation

Historically, people have not known about or exercised their rights to information about options regarding diagnosis and actual breast cancer treatment approaches. As stated earlier, women are exercising these options more frequently, seeking information about one- versus two-stage procedures, mastectomy versus lumpectomy and radiation therapy, chemotherapy, or hormonal therapy. One factor that has fostered this approach has been the legislation addressing the need of women with breast cancer to be informed about choosing between a one- and a two-stage procedure. In the late 1970's, California was one of the pioneers in this effort, mandating not only that a woman has a legal right to have such information but also that she can choose between a one- and a two-stage procedure. In addition, standardized brochures describing treatment options must be given to all women newly diagnosed with breast cancer prior to treatment.

Nurses, therefore, must first be aware of the current status of legislation in their area of practice, so as to counsel patients concerning their rights and to answer questions on the appropriateness of an option. Second, a nurse must be aware of the current treatment options available to an individual diagnosed with breast cancer. Knowledge of the stage of disease at presentation is essential to appropriate counseling; in addition, knowledge of the woman's age and previous medical condition and of other factors that might influence the choice of a treatment approach is essential. Only with this kind of information can the nurse provide guidance and appropriate referral for patients.

Psychosocial Aspects

Studies have addressed such issues as the anxiety produced by a breast biopsy and by a diagnosis of cancer or breast cancer. Collectively, these studies identify such times as highly stressful. Interestingly, at a time when an individual is being required to make very difficult and often life-altering decisions, her ability to discriminate, critically assess a situation, and make a decision is significantly impaired because of high anxiety.

A diagnosis of cancer is known to generate a wide variety of reactions, including fear, shock, disbelief, anger, depression, hopelessness, hostility, guilt, grief, avoidance of reality, and thoughts of being punished for past acts. Patients facing a biopsy have fears related to unknown potential outcomes, including the fear of possible loss of a body part. It is important for the nurse to be aware that this is a time of crisis for the patient and that assessing the degree of crisis produced by the diagnosis of cancer enables the nurse to more successfully structure interventions. At the time of initial diagnosis, the nurse must assess what the diagnosis of cancer means to each patient. A comprehensive assessment should elicit the following information:

1. The length of time that the individual has been aware of the presence of a lump.
2. Any delay between initial discovery of the lump and seeking advice from a health care provider.
3. If there was a delay, the reason(s) for this delay, which may provide insight into the patient's perceptions of a diagnosis of breast cancer, the patient's attitudes toward his or her own health, and other factors that might might have future significance.
4. Identification of any inconsistencies in the time interval between discovering the lump and seeking medical attention (e.g., a tumor that is large and ulcerated, while the patient states that it has been there only a month).
5. The patient's understanding of the medical situation, what perceptions he or she has concerning breast cancer, and whether these are consistent with the patient's knowledge.
6. The patient's knowledge of treatment options and their appropriateness for his or her individual case.

As an outcome of this assessment, nurses will have many clues to aid them in designing care appropriate to the individual. The nurses' reactions to the patient who has not delayed in seeking treatment is important. All people with a breast problem go through a difficult decision-making process before presenting to the health care system. That a person has sought immediate advice does not preclude the possibility that he or she may have intense feelings about what is happening. The existence of a suspicious lump alone generates a host of fears, guilt, and anger. These emotions are real and must be recognized and addressed rather than brushed aside. These deeply rooted emotions are related to any or all of the following: having a family member or friend who developed breast cancer; fear of alterations in the individual's womanhood or manhood or in his or her role as wife, husband, mother, father, or lover; potential changes in sexuality and body image; potential role changes within and outside the home; and finally, fear of the unknown and of the potential loss of life. The guilt may be related to a multitude of factors, many of which are outside the individual's control. Guilt may be experienced because of previous poor health care behaviors (e.g., dietary habits, inconsistent practice of BSE, and not having physical examinations regularly).

The nurse will care for individuals who have delayed seeking treatment as well as those who requested health care advice immediately upon discovering a breast abnormality. Delay in seeking health care for a breast problem, especially if cancer is suspected, is a serious problem, one to which the nurse may react adversely. Therefore, it is essential that the nurses caring for people who delay seeking treatment be cognizant of their own attitudes, biases, and feelings, which may affect their ability to interact with and care for these persons. Whether an individual has been slow in requesting medical advice or not, nurses may encounter views toward health care and acceptance of treatment that differ from their own; for example, the individual who delays in seeking medical care often reports that the mass or lesion has been present for a short period. In discussing the issue with the individual, the nurses must carefully evaluate this information to avoid causing the patient to become defensive. In addition, the nurse must recognize that an individual's denial of his or her condition may be serving some important psychologic function.

Whether individuals have delayed seeking treatment or not and regardless of the explanations offered for the delay, the nurse must provide support for patients and their decisions to seek medical care. This support must be positive and nonjudgmental. The nurse should empathize with and assist patients in focusing on the positive steps that they are taking by seeking medical advice and treatment. The issue of the delay should be minimized. Therefore, the nurse should strive to emphasize that it is now time to deal with the issues related to the diagnosis and the initiation of appropriate treatment. At the same time, the nurse should encourage the patient not to expend energy on past events that cannot be changed. Nurses play an important role in caring for the individual whose condition has been newly diagnosed as breast cancer. Specifically, nurses must recognize that feelings of guilt, anger, and fear are not easily cast away and must identify mechanisms that the individual can use to deal with stressful events. Nurses must help the individual to identify strengths and to minimize limitations and must aid patients in designing strategies for effective coping throughout the diagnostic, treatment, and follow-up phases. Part of the nurse's responsibility is to identify the patient's degree of ability to cope with a situation; to recognize those mechanisms that the patient has used effectively in the past; and to accept the individuality of each person. This, perhaps, is one of the most difficult tasks that nurses face in their practice. It is well recognized that people rely on past experiences and use previously successful coping strategies in a new situation. Nurses must clearly distinguish their goals for the patient concerning adjustment and acceptance of breast cancer and its treatment from the patient's goals. Nurses must assist patients in recognizing which goals may be unrealistic and in channeling their energies appropriately and effectively.

Summary

A comprehensive assessment provides the nurse with the data essential to addressing these issues. Therefore, successful evaluation of the factors outlined in the assessment presented in Table 18–2 may provide information explaining an individual's behavior and assisting the nurse in care planning. Reviewing the results of the assessment with the patient and significant others, as appropriate, provides both the nurse and the patient with the opportunities to jointly establish health care goals in concert with the medical treatment plan. It also provides an opportunity for the patient, family, and health care team to agree on the identified problems and suggested solutions. This approach lays the groundwork for establishing a trusting relationship and for future planning. The components of assessment presented here are applicable throughout all phases of care of the person with breast cancer. The rest of the chapter will focus on the specific care needs of the breast cancer patient throughout the treatment and follow-up phases.

SURGERY

Mastectomy

The loss of a body part is never easy. The patient's response to such a loss is dependent on a number of factors, including visibility of the loss, the functional loss, and the emotional investment in, or the meaning of, the part affected.[7] Persons undergoing surgery for breast cancer have to deal with their losses. They must face the loss of a psychologically and sexually significant body part, a functional loss, an alteration in their body image, and the threat that cancer will kill them or leave them with unmanageable pain. In addition, the person with breast cancer may have the same preoperative fears as do other surgical patients. These include the fear of postoperative pain, anesthesia hazards, vulnerability while unconscious, and separation from loved ones and former activities.[8]

Patients undergoing breast surgery provide a special challenge for nurses. As part of the health care team, a nurse can contribute to the patient's well-being by preparing the patient psychologically and physically for surgery, providing the operative and postoperative teaching, and providing thorough postoperative care.

Preoperative Period

Preoperative preparation should begin with an assessment of the quality and availability of the patient's social support, the patient's perception of the quantity and quality of that support and the patient's willingness and ability to enlist such help. Current theories suggest that social support may have a protective function and may serve as a stress buffer or moderator following major illness and surgery.[9] Women with breast cancer who perceive significantly more understanding and emotional support from their spouses, their children, and their physicians and nurses reported better emotional adjustment following mastectomy.[7] The nurse can help a patient explore her support system and can provide counseling as to how the patient can best utilize her supports.

Preoperative preparation should include an assessment of the patient's perception of her past surgical procedures. Patients who expect a significant number of complications or who recall difficulties with previous surgeries may relate their past negative experience with their present surgery. By providing clear, concise information about the procedure and how this surgery differs from previous experiences, nurses may alleviate some preoperative anxiety. During the preoperative assessment, it is important to elicit the patient's perception of the procedure she is about to undergo. Although the procedure may have been explained in detail by the physician, the patient may have a limited understanding of what the procedure entails. This limited understanding may be due to anxiety, information overload, or denial, or it may be caused by an inadequate initial explanation. If the patient's understanding of the procedure is inadequate or inaccurate, the nurse should assist the patient in obtaining accurate information. When the nurse gains a clear understanding of the patient's knowledge, expectations, and attitudes toward the surgical procedure, he or she can then use this information as a base from which to begin preoperative teaching.

Preoperative teaching prepares the patient for the physical and sensory experiences of surgery and can also help prepare the patient to take an active role in her postoperative recovery. Teaching begins with a description of preoperative procedures. The patient should be informed of any presurgical tests or skin or bowel preparations that will take place and the patient's role in performing the procedure. Including the patient in the scheduling of tests and procedures may give her a sense of control over these events. The nurse can help the patient prepare by providing her with a detailed description of what will happen on the day of surgery. It is helpful if the experience is described in terms of what the patient will see, hear, and feel in the operating and recovery rooms and in her room as she regains consciousness from anesthesia. Often a preoperative visit to the recovery room and an introduction to the nurse who will be caring for the patient will alleviate some anxiety. The patient should be told what kinds of drains, dressings, and tubes will be in place after surgery, what their functions are, and how long the patient can expect them to remain in place. The patient should be made aware that pain is an expected side effect of surgery and that pain medicine is available. Instructions on how to obtain pain medication, and on the effective ways of using it, should be discussed. The patient may benefit from an exercise in role playing in which the nurse assists the patient in imagining how she might cope with the discomforts of surgery. Community resources, such as Reach to Recovery, should be identified and used during the postoperative period.

The importance of postoperative respiratory exercises should be emphasized. Coughing, deep breathing, and use of the Triflow should be demonstrated by the nurse, and the patient should be requested to give a return demonstration. Patients who understand the need for, and can perform, respiratory exercises correctly preoperatively will be more compliant with respiratory exercises postoperatively.

The nurse can help decrease preoperative anxiety by giving patients and their significant others the opportunity to talk about the impending surgery and their fears and to ask questions. Family members should be given information such as where to wait during surgery, where to meet the physician after surgery and when they can see the patient.

Postoperative Period

Postoperatively, nursing care for patients undergoing breast and axilla surgery should focus on maintaining an optimum level of comfort, preventing complications related to wound healing and altered respiratory function, facilitating the patient's acceptance of her altered body image, and teaching the patient care of the compromised extremity.

Patients vary immensely in the amount of pain they experience postoperatively. The pain experienced is often related to the specific nerves that have been severed during surgery. Initially, the patient may experience acute pain on the chest wall, axilla, and arm, radiating through the back. As time passes, the acute pain becomes a numbness or a dull ache, which may extend down the arm. Some patients experience hyperesthesias of the surgical area, and others may report pain or sensation in the absent breast similar to phantom-limb pain. The type, location, intensity, and frequency of the pain should be assessed. The nurse should discuss factors that precipitate pain and mechanisms the patient can use to cope with pain.

Many postoperative complications relating to wound healing and altered respiratory function can be prevented or detected in their early stages by frequent nursing assessment and vigorous nursing care. Meticulous assessment of the skin in the surgical site is essential. Complications in wound healing increase the probability of occurrence of negative psychologic reactions to the mastectomy site.[10] Delayed wound healing may also interfere with the use of an external prosthesis, and, therefore, women may feel isolated and unable to resume participation in social contacts and nonfamilial roles.[11] The nurse should observe the surgical site for redness, swelling, drainage, odor, and tenderness. The incision and flap should be assessed for temperature, blanching, and duskiness. Care should be taken to avoid pressure to the flap or suture lines from the patient's gown, bed clothing, tape, and dressings. When flap viability is in question, the use of a bed cradle is indicated. Postoperative assessment of the patient's respiratory status should include the rate, depth, and character of respirations, the characteristics of sputum, and auscultation of the patient's breath sounds. The nurse should ascertain that breathing exercises are correctly performed at adequate intervals. Scheduling and administering pain medication before breathing exercises may increase patient compliance.

One of the most difficult postoperative tasks for a patient who has undergone breast and axilla surgery is viewing the surgical incision for the first time. The earlier the patient views her incision, the more content she usually is with the cosmetic result at a later time.[2] The role of the nurse is paramount in helping the patient cope with her changed body image. One study by Maguire and colleagues[12] showed that counseling by a nurse resulted in significantly more satisfaction with the mastectomy incision in patients who were counseled compared with patients who were not counseled.

Some patients who have undergone a mastectomy may accomplish the task of viewing the surgical incision and the chest wall with minimal assistance. In other cases, the patient may require desensitization before actually viewing her incision. Desensitization requires cooperation between members of the health care team. To accomplish desensitization, the patient should first be shown pictures of chest walls and incision lines following mastectomies—both recent postoperative pictures and pictures of well-healed surgical sites. The patient should be told that her incision will appear red, bruised, and prominent but that the redness and bruising will fade over time. If the patient is unwilling to look at the incision, it should be verbally described to her during dressing changes. The patient should be encouraged to touch and explore the site even if this is accomplished with her eyes closed. The nurse and the physician should continue to encourage the patient to glance at the incision when the dressing is changed, until the time when the patient views the incision. Although nurses may suggest strategies to assist a woman in viewing her incision, the patient should always be encouraged to participate at her own pace. When viewing the incision with the patient, it is important to emphasize the positive aspects of her physical appearance. Specific suggestions about the types of clothing and lingerie that can be worn to minimize the surgical defect can be helpful. These may include a one-piece bathing suit with a single shoulder strap or summer shirts with capped sleeves.

Patients who have undergone a limited breast or axilla procedure, such as a lumpectomy, segmental mastectomy, axillary sampling, or axillary dissection, will also require support when viewing their surgical incision. Although their surgical defect may be minimal in comparison with patients who have undergone more extensive procedures, it still represents an alteration in the patient's body image and should be addressed by the nurse. The nurse should ascertain that all patients have the opportunity of viewing their surgical incision with the support of a health team member prior to discharge. Patients who return home without completing this task will not have the resources of the health care team available to assist them with this task. Additionally, information and psychologic support should be given to the patient's partner.

Psychologic recovery after breast surgery is difficult to achieve if a patient is constantly reminded of the physical defect caused by surgery. A patient's recovery can be enhanced by the use of a comfortable, well-made external breast prosthesis that is secured in place by a pocket sewn inside her bra. Prostheses are now available in a number of shapes, sizes, and differing materials. Discussing with the patient the advantages and disadvantages of the various types of prostheses will help her make an informed decision about the type of breast form she should purchase. A patient who knows the limitations of her prosthesis will be better prepared to cope with the reality of her deformity.[13]

Prostheses

The first prosthesis the patient should wear is a temporary, lightweight, breast form made of soft material, such as Dacron. These temporary forms can be worn as early as several days following the surgery, as they are light enough to allow the mastectomy incision to heal while still providing some chest wall contour. Because these forms are lightweight, they tend to "ride up" on the chest wall when placed inside a bra. Pinning the form inside clothing or lengthening the bra strap on the contralateral side to allow for a more equal balance can be helpful. Some hospitals provide these temporary prostheses to their patients. These forms are also available through the American Cancer Society's Reach to Recovery program. Although a woman may not be psychologically ready to wear it, every person undergoing a mastectomy should be offered a temporary prosthesis before she is discharged from the hospital.[14]

When the skin over the mastectomy site has healed, usually in about four to eight weeks following surgery, the patient may be ready to be fitted with a heavier, more permanent external prosthesis. This fitting can be a traumatic event for the patient. Often, the patient has not shown her chest to anyone except health care personnel and, possibly, her partner. Now, she must allow a saleswoman to see her surgical defect and to fit her with a prosthesis. Many people are uncomfortable during the fitting and often choose the first prosthesis shown to them in order to hasten the fitting. The patient should be encouraged to try different types and shapes of prostheses until she finds the one that fits well and feels comfortable. It is reported that 50 percent of women who wear a prosthesis have problems with the prosthesis: Either it fits poorly, or there is skin sensitivity or actual pain from their initial fitting.[11] Taking the time to assure a good initial fit may help alleviate these problems.

LYMPHEDEMA

Patients who have undergone axillary dissection or sampling procedures will have learning needs with respect to care of their lymphatic-compromised extremity. The reasons for the limitations and specific recommendations for care of the arm should be addressed. Table 18–3 summarizes the recommendations that should be given to patients who have had axillary surgery. All patients having axillary surgery should be encouraged to use their arms as normally as possible. The implementation of an early rehabilitation program, close patient follow-up care, and patient education are of primary importance in reducing the incidence of lymphedema.[15] It is best for all patients who have undergone an axillary procedure to be seen by a physical therapist for development of an individualized rehabilitation program.

TABLE 18–3. Arm Care Following Axillary Surgery

Contact your physician if your arm becomes red, warm, or unusually hard or swollen.
Whenever possible, have all injections, vaccinations, blood samples, and blood pressure tests done on the other arm.
Wash all cuts or abrasions promptly, cover with a sterile dressing, and monitor for signs of infection. This includes cuts that do not heal, redness, warmth, and drainage.
Wear sunblock number 15 containing PABA on the arm to prevent sunburn.
Wear protective gloves when gardening, working with harsh chemicals, or reaching into hot ovens.
Use an electric razor for underarm shaving to minimize the risk of nicks and scratches.
Avoid tight elastic cuffs and tight jewelry on the axillary dissected arm.
Carry heavy packages and handbags on the other arm.
Use a hand cream several times a day.

BREAST AND CHEST WALL SELF-EXAMINATION

Breast and chest wall self-examination practices should be reinstituted following the healing of the chest wall incision. The steps in performing BSE following mastectomy are the same as for persons who have no history of breast cancer. Table 18–1 illustrates the guidelines and steps in performing BSE that are recommended by the National Cancer Institute. Several physical changes can be observed and include chest wall asymmetry and redness of the incision, which may persist for weeks to months following surgery. This redness usually decreases over time. Small ridges or internal sutures may be palpated. The development of new lumps or ridges on the suture line or chest wall should be reported to a physician.

Reconstruction

Breast reconstruction is a surgical area in which great technical strides have been made. Some type of breast reconstructive procedure is now available to virtually every patient who has undergone a mastectomy. People with breast cancer who are at high risk for having recurrence or those with metastatic disease should not necessarily be excluded from the option of having breast reconstruction. Counseling those people who have had or who are facing mastectomies about the availability of reconstruction can contribute to their emotional well-being. Surgical planning for reconstruction at the time of mastectomy gives an active, positive message to the patient that they will live and be able to correct their change in body image.[16]

Ideally, an assessment should be done on all patients who are undergoing mastectomy or have had a mastectomy, to determine their interest in reconstruction. During this interview, special attention should be paid to their purpose for having or choosing not to have reconstruction.

The nurse should look at the patient's motivation for the surgery. Their expectations are often varied. Does the patient desire to free herself from the external prosthesis in order to be able to wear more types of clothing or to feel more balanced, or is the patient looking at breast reconstruction as the panacea for all physical and emotional problems?

The reasons that women commonly give for desiring breast reconstruction include the need to feel balanced, to feel feminine, to feel whole again, to improve marital and sexual relations, to become less preoccupied with their physical state, and to be less preoccupied with cancer. Questions that health care providers must ask are, Will the patient be happy with a restored breast contour when clothed in a bra with prosthesis, or is the patient seeking an anatomic replacement of her surgically removed breast? Is the patient considering that the reconstructive technique may take several operations or stages to produce the final results, or does she want limited surgery that will provide her with results quickly? The type of surgery and any other treatments the patient has had, her knowledge of what can be done to repair the chest wall defect, and how extensive a procedure the patient wishes to undergo should also be assessed.

The use of pre- and postoperative photographs of breast reconstructions will give the patient a realistic idea of what some reconstructed breasts look like. Many people contemplating reconstruction benefit from talking with people who have undergone breast reconstruction. Veteran patients offer support and share information about their personal experiences. Occasionally, they will show their reconstruction to a patient considering the procedure.

People interested in breast reconstruction should be informed of recent changes in insurance payments for breast reconstruction. Historically, this surgery was considered cosmetic plastic surgery, and, as such, insurance companies would not cover the expense. The recent trend of insurance companies is to classify reconstructive surgery as "postmastectomy rehabilitation."[17] Some states are now requiring that every health insurance carrier providing coverage for mastectomy surgery provide benefits for reconstruction.[18] The nurse should encourage the patient to contact her insurance company to determine its coverage.

The principles of nursing care for patients undergoing breast and axilla surgery will also apply to the people who are undergoing breast reconstruction. The nursing assessment, preoperative teaching plan, and general surgical postoperative care, all of which were discussed previously, can be modified for the patient admitted for breast reconstruction.

It is easy to understand that an individual may be euphoric on her admission for reconstructive surgery, perhaps viewing the impending operation as "easy" surgery that is without side effects and complications. The nurse should help the patient develop a realistic understanding of surgical outcomes. For the patient experiencing extensive reconstructive procedures, such as the rectus abdominis procedure, the operation is often more physically debilitating than the original breast surgery.

Surgical Procedures

Simple Implant

Reconstructive techniques vary with respect to complexity, the tissues involved, the postoperative course, and the patient's learning needs. The surgical techniques can be divided basically into two categories, those utilizing the existing muscles and blood supply and those requiring a myocutaneous flap. An example of the former type, termed a simple implant, involves placing a silicone implant either into a pocket formed under the pectoralis muscle or directly under the skin. In addition to general postoperative teaching, patients who have undergone simple implants should be given information about the signs and symptoms of implant deflation, migration, and infection. They should also be instructed in the art of massage, as breast massage helps decrease the incidence of capsule formation around the implant. Patients should be instructed to massage their breast implants at least three times a day. The implant should be massaged in a rolling fashion, from the sides of the body to the center, and from the bottom of the breast. Massaging the breast will help keep the implant mobile and give the breast a more relaxed natural appearance.

Tissue Expander

Reconstruction using a tissue expander initially in place of an implant is a variation on the simple implant type of reconstruction. The tissue expander is an inflatable silicone envelope, which can be placed under the skin or pectoralis muscle. This is often done following the mastectomy, or the tissue expander can be placed months or years after the initial surgery. When healing of the incision over the tissue expander is complete, usually four weeks after surgery, the tissue expander can begin to be filled with saline, thereby stretching the skin over the mastectomy site. At a later date, during a second surgical procedure, the tissue expander is removed and a permanent silicone implant is placed under the stretched skin. These patients should be provided with information about their inflation schedule and what to expect from the inflation procedure itself. The inflation is usually performed with a large saline-filled syringe with a 1½ inch, 22 to 25 gauge Huber needle attached. The sight of the needle, combined with the sight of the physician forcefully pushing the saline through a small-gauge needle, often frightens an unprepared patient. Because the inflation port lies under skin in which the nerves have been surgically cut, the patient usually will not experience pain with the procedure but may experience feelings of fullness, tightness, and pressure in the inflated breast. Patients undergoing reconstructive procedures involving a tissue expander require general postoperative teaching as well as instruction in the signs and symptoms of implant deflation or infection. The patient should be instructed to notify the physician of any recurring paresthesias of the arm or hand after inflation. These paresthesias are caused by pressure on nerves surrounding the tissue expander and may signal nerve damage. The breast contour will be constantly changing throughout the inflation process. Patients should be advised to use a temporary prosthesis with removable stuffing to augment their expanding breast contour.

Myocutaneous Flap

Myocutaneous reconstructive procedures, which involve the transfer of skin, muscle, and subcutaneous tissue from other areas of the body to the mastectomy site, are the reconstructive procedures most prone to morbidity but often provide the best cosmetic results. Two examples of these procedures are the latissimus dorsi procedure and the rectus abdominis procedure. In the latissimus dorsi procedure, the latissimus dorsi muscle, located on the back between the shoulder blades, is raised and tunneled under the skin from the back to the front of the chest. The silicone breast prosthesis is then placed under the muscle, and a breast contour is formed. In the rectus abdominis procedure, one or two parallel vertical muscles that cover the abdomen, the rectus abdominis, along with fat and skin are released. The muscle and its blood supply are tunneled under the abdomen to the breast area, and a pad of fat and skin are contoured into the shape of a breast. Patients who have undergone tissue transfer procedures require general postoperative care and teaching as previously outlined. These patients experience significantly more pain than do patients who did not require tissue transfer.

Specific orders for care of the reconstructed site and the donor site will vary among physicians and procedures. Some physicians require the patient to wear an underwire bra 24 hours a day for several weeks to support the transferred tissue. Patients should be instructed to bathe or shower with tepid water, as bathing or showering with hot water may increase the oxygen demands of the transferred tissue. Patients who have had an abdominal procedure, such as a rectus abdominis procedure, may be required to wear an abdominal binder to help prevent herniation of the abdominal wall. Because these patients are at greater risk for abdominal herniation, they should avoid abdominal exercises until directed by their physicians or physical therapist. Patients should be given guidelines on how much weight they can lift without risking herniation.

Breast Self-Examination

The woman experiencing reconstruction should be informed that she will notice physical changes as she examines her reconstructed breast. The majority of these changes are in the area of her surgical incisions and breast contour. The incisions may be reddened for weeks to months after treatment. This redness usually decreases over time. Small ridges or sutures along the incision may be palpated. The development of new ridges or lumps should be reported to the physician. Depending on the type of reconstruction a woman has undergone, there may be additional observations that she will make as she performs BSE. These observations include asymmetry and varying densities and protrusion as well as changes in skin tone in the areas where new tissue has been brought to the reconstructed site. Despite these changes, women should resume monthly breast self-examination practices at the completion of their surgical wound healing (Table 18–1).

RADIATION THERAPY

Radiation therapy plays an important role in the treatment of breast cancer. It may be used as the primary cancer therapy to the breast and regional lymph nodes, or it may be used in conjunction with chemotherapy or to control metastatic or recurrent breast cancer.

The goals of radiation therapy depend on the stage of the disease and the overall treatment plan. Radiation therapy, like surgery but unlike chemotherapy, is a local treatment of breast cancer. The radiosensitivity of specific tissues and organs is related directly to the cell renewal requirements of the irradiated tissue or organ. Radiation has its maximum effect on the cell during cellular mitosis.[19, 20] Therefore, rapidly growing and dividing cells, such as skin, hair, and bone marrow cells and cells that line the gastrointestinal tract, are often most sensitive to radiation therapy. Because radiation affects all cells within the radiation field, both normal and cancer cells within the treatment field may be damaged or destroyed. As the normal cells within the treatment field are damaged or destroyed, specific side effects appear. The effect of radiation on normal tissue effectively limits the dose of radiation that can be safely administered.[21]

The side effects that occur as a result of radiation therapy generally are confined to the tissues and organs within the area being treated. These side effects may be divided into two categories. The side effects that occur during the course of irradiation or shortly thereafter are classified as early or acute effects, and those that occur months or years following radiation therapy are classified as late or chronic effects. Although the effects are often predictable, they vary substantially among patients as to onset, severity, and response to medical and nursing interventions. Not every patient will experience side effects in sequence. Additionally, patients experiencing a specific acute side effect during treatment will not necessarily experience a late effect in the same site. Accurate assessment by physicians and nurses facilitates early recognition of problems and prompt interventions, both of which may enhance patient comfort and prevent progression of symptoms and complications. Table 18–4 illustrates potential acute and chronic side effects in the various phases of radiation therapy for breast cancer. Early side effects include fatigue; skin, subcutaneous tissue, and muscle changes; and bone marrow depression. Late side effects include skin and subcutaneous changes, cosmetic changes, rib fractures, and radiation pneumonitis.

Nursing care of patients receiving radiation should be directed toward anticipating acute and chronic side effects related to the treatment. Nurses should instruct patients in general skin care of the treated area and should provide interventions to minimize discomfort and additional trauma of the tissue and to promote healing. Preparation of the patient and her family begins when the specific treatment is identified and the treatment schedule is determined. Because there are many myths associated with radiation therapy, it is important that the nurse identify these misconceptions and correct them early in the treatment process. Verbal instruction should be supplemented by written or audiovisual material. The presence of a supportive family member or friend may assist the patient in gathering information and asking questions. Information should include a summary of probable and possible treatment effects and the role of the patient in managing such effects. Simulation, or the treatment planning process, should be explained. Skin markings, or indelible freckles, called tattoos, are placed on the skin during simulation in order to identify the treatment field. Schedules for routine appointments with members of the health care team and follow-up laboratory evaluations can be reviewed at this time.

After explaining the treatment process, the nurse should give special attention to the physical and psychologic difficulties associated with radiation treatment. Patients may find that they are uncomfortable assuming the treatment position on a hard treatment table, particularly if they are recuperating from recent surgery. The use of analgesics, muscle relaxants, or muscle relaxation exercises, under the guidance of members of the health care team, may be required to decrease pain in the early days of treatment.

In caring for a patient receiving radiation therapy, much nursing intervention is aimed

TABLE 18–4. Acute and Chronic Effects Related to Radiation Therapy

Therapy	*Sequence of Treatment Steps*	*Possible Acute Side Effects*	*Possible Chronic Side Effects*
Primary radiation therapy Combined therapy for T_1 or T_2 tumors (some T_3 tumors)	Treatment follows lumpectomy (excisional biopsy) and axillary sampling or dissection External radiation is generally combined with iridium implant or external electron beam boost treatments to the tumor bed If axillary lymph nodes are positive, patients may receive adjuvant chemotherapy or hormone therapy. They may also have additional radiation to the regional lymph nodes or axillary lymph nodes	Fatigue Erythema Pigment changes Dry desquamation, pruritus Moist desquamation (especially in skin folds) Breast edema Nipple tenderness Chest wall myositis Paresthesias	Skin hyperpigmentation Skin appears thinner Pronounced hair follicles Persistent chest wall pain and tenderness Paresthesias Fibrosis in previous surgical sites Increased breast firmness, breast sits more erectly on chest wall Change in breast size: slightly smaller or larger or significant change in some patients Arm edema (if lymph nodes dissected and axilla is treated with radiation) Uncommon, but possible: rib fractures or radiation pneumonitis
Local treatment for advanced or inflammatory breast cancer	Initial treatment is often chemotherapy, especially with inflammatory cancer. Irradiation is begun following several cycles of chemotherapy or as local therapy with or without surgery for local tumor control. Specific techniques and timing of therapy need to be individualized	Same as for primary radiation therapy with the addition of brisk erythema; moist desquamation (which is common); or bone marrow depression (primarily due to concomitant chemotherapy)	Same as for primary treatment
Postoperative radiation therapy following mastectomy	Modified radical or Halsted radical mastectomy is performed as primary treatment. Radiation therapy is administered to the chest wall and/or regional lymph nodes, under special circumstances such as when node-positive patients have extracapsular extension of disease into axillary fat or when the surgical margins contain cancer. Patient may or may not receive adjuvant chemotherapy or hormone therapy	Fatigue Erythema Pigment Dry desquamation, pruritus, itching Moist desquamation Chest wall myositis	Skin hyperpigmentation Persistent myositis Fibrosis of pectoralis major Fibrosis of incision line Arm edema when axillary lymph node dissection is combined with axillary radiation therapy

Table continued on opposite page

at maximizing skin integrity to minimize additional trauma to the skin. Table 18–5 summarizes the general skin care instruction that patients should be given prior to or early in the course of treatment. Nurses instructing patients should be well informed as to their institution's practices, because all radiation therapy departments do not give patients the same skin care guidelines. These guidelines generally include information on bathing the irradiated skin; the use of mild, nonperfumed soaps and lubricants; avoiding exposure to extremes of temperature; and avoiding other external irritants. Symptoms requiring phy-

TABLE 18–4. *Acute and Chronic Effects Related to Radiation Therapy* Continued

Therapy	*Sequence of Treatment Steps*	*Possible Acute Side Effects*	*Possible Chronic Side Effects*
Radiation therapy for metastatic breast cancer *Bone* (e.g., femur metastasis) *Brain* *Other sites* of involvement	Radiation therapy is tailored to the site of disease, lymphatic drainage patterns, and symptoms (e.g., pain)	*Bone* Minimal but possible increase in bone pain at onset of treatment. Pain usually decreases during treatment Fatigue Erythema Dry desquamation Bone weakness (e.g., bone marrow depression for pelvic irradiation) *Brain* Hair loss Erythema Dry desquamation, pruritus Moist desquamation *Other* Side effects dependent upon irradiated area	Hyperpigmentation

sician or nursing attention and the telephone numbers of resource people should also be identified.

Specific Side Effects

Fatigue. Although radiation side effects are most often related to the organs and tissues being irradiated, fatigue, a systemic effect, is the most frequently reported sequela of treatment. The physiologic causes of fatigue are unknown, but they are thought to relate to one or more processes. One potential cause is the biologic effect of radiation on normal and cancer cells that causes a release of cellular by-products into the blood stream, causing fatigue. Another potential cause may be the anabolism necessary to repair the normal cells within the treatment field. This also may be associated with postoperative wound healing.

The onset, duration, and resolution of the fatigue associated with radiation therapy varies from patient to patient. Many factors may influence the extent of fatigue, including the overall health of the patient, the size of the treatment field, and the previous or concurrent exposure to other cancer treatment modalities. Radiation therapy to a larger body surface area causes damage and destruction to a greater number of normal cells and tissues. Therefore, well-nourished, otherwise healthy individuals generally are better able to withstand radiation therapy than poorly nourished, debilitated individuals.[22] Likewise, previous exposure to other cancer treatments, such as irradiation, surgery, or chemotherapy, may deplete nutritional and hematologic stores. Finally, fatigue also may be associated with the recuperation from sur-

TABLE 18–5. *General Skin Care Instructions for Patients Receiving Radiation Therapy*

- When cleansing the skin in the irradiated field, use tepid water and no soap or minimal, mild soap (e.g., Ivory, baby soap, Basis, and those without perfumes).
- Avoid washing treatment marks off your skin. Notify your radiation therapist or radiation technician if your marks begin to fade.
- Avoid extremes of hot or cold to the treated area (e.g., from hot water bottles, heating pads, and ice packs).
- Gently pat area dry after bathing.
- Wear loose fitting, comfortable clothing over irradiated skin; whenever possible, wear 100 percent cotton clothing.
- Consult with radiation therapist before using creams and lotions on irradiated area. Use only creams without metals, perfumes, or alcohol, such as baby cream or oil. Apply creams or lotions only after radiation therapy treatment.
- Avoid sun exposure to irradiated area during treatment and direct sun exposure to area for 12 to 24 months. Cover area with loose clothing. When sun exposure is unavoidable, liberally apply a sunscreen containing 5 percent PABA on irradiated skin. Avoid injury to irradiated skin (e.g., from venipunctures, adhesive tape, tight jewelry).

gery and the depression that often follows the diagnosis of a potentially life-threatening illness.

Although there are no known measures to prevent fatigue, routine nursing interventions may be helpful, including preparing the patient for the insidious onset of fatigue that may require limitation of daily activities. The nurse should emphasize to the patient that fatigue is a normal, expected side effect of treatment and is not progression of the disease. Scheduled rest periods throughout the day may increase a patient's energy level. Nurses can identify available resources and assist in encouraging family, friends, and community members to use these resources. Fatigue associated with radiation therapy resolves slowly during the weeks and months following the completion of treatment. Support from members of the health care team helps people cope with the physical and psychologic effects of the disease and its treatment.

Skin. Skin reactions are an unavoidable effect of radiation therapy and should be anticipated at the onset of treatment. Fortunately, with newer, skin-sparing equipment, radiation-induced reactions are less frequent and less severe than in the early days of radiation therapy. Accurate terminology should be used whenever discussing skin reactions. The word burn should *never* be used in reference to a radiation skin reaction. The word burn implies accidental exposure to an offending substance and not the anticipated effect of a planned treatment. Reference to a skin reaction can be made using words such as skin reaction and erythema. While there is some variation among individuals, the effect of radiation on the skin generally begins 10 to 14 days after the onset of treatment or after a total dose of 2000 to 2800 rad.[23] Fractionation, the daily dose of radiation, the total dose delivered, and the patient's nutritional status and concomitant cancer therapy may influence the onset and severity of skin effects. Daily doses exceeding 200 rad and total doses exceeding 5000 rad frequently do not allow for normal cellular repair between treatments and therefore are frequently correlated with more severe skin reactions that are less responsive to conventional nursing interventions. Individuals with fair, translucent skin may be predisposed to an early onset and to a more pronounced skin reaction.[22] Areas of high friction and moisture are susceptible to the effects of radiation therapy because of the constant rubbing and irritation of the skin surfaces. Those at high risk include the folds of the axilla, groin, vulva, breast, and buttocks,[21] which are potential sites of irritation and friction. Poorly vascularized skin, such as that on the back of the hand, on the tops and soles of the feet, and overlying bony prominences, also is highly susceptible to skin reactions. At times, the nature of a patient's disease requires that high doses of radiation therapy be given to the skin (e.g., inflammatory breast cancer). Thus, multiple acute skin reactions should be anticipated, and under these circumstances, patients should be told to anticipate a temporary break in their radiation therapy.

Patients receiving external radiation therapy should be given general instructions regarding care of the skin in the treatment field at the beginning of treatment (Table 18–4). Information should be included regarding cleansing of the skin, use of topical creams and lotions, and comfort measures and interventions to minimize further trauma and injury to the irradiated tissue.

Once interruption of skin integrity has occurred, nursing assessment and intervention should be implemented to facilitate healing, to promote comfort, and to minimize additional injury to the skin and underlying tissue. Skin reactions can be divided into three levels. The majority of radiation therapy patients experience Levels I and II reactions. A summary of the levels of impairment can be found in Table 18–6. All patients receiving radiation therapy have the potential for impairment of skin integrity and generally will exhibit a skin reaction during the course of treatment. These patients are classified as having Level I reactions. The skin color ranges from pink to red and may have a mottled appearance. The patient may complain of tenderness and tingling, as with skin recently exposed to the sun. Nursing measures for Level I reactions include promoting comfort and protecting the tissue from additional injury.

Once skin integrity has been impaired and the patient is experiencing dry or moist desquamation, or both, the patient is classified as having Level II skin impairment. As sebaceous glands in the treatment field are damaged, dryness and scaling of the skin occur. Topical creams and lotions may be used to lubricate and minimize the scaling and flaking of the skin seen in dry desquamation. Cornstarch and, occasionally, mild topical steroids may be used to decrease pruritus. Moist desquamation is characterized by painful, open, weeping areas within the treatment field. In Level II reactions, these areas are generally small. Moist desquamation is caused by the sloughing of the epithelial skin layers and may begin with or without blister formation. Treatment of moist desquamation may include regular use of wet to dry dressings, using combinations of water and diluted peroxide, saline, or Dakin's solution. Analgesics and narcotics administered at regular intervals often are required for the pain associated with moist desquamation. Frequent observation for secondary complications such as infection is essential.

Level III alteration in skin integrity is an extension of the moist desquamation of Level II. The areas of moist desquamation are large and may have have purulent drainage. These lesions are very painful, often preventing a patient from carrying on the activities of daily living and disrupting sleep patterns. The same nursing interventions as used for Level II should be employed for patients with Level III skin, with special emphasis on decreasing pain and discomfort. The patient should be closely monitored for progression of symptoms and infection.

Although skin reactions can be anticipated during radiation therapy, their progression from one stage to another is often unpredictable. Two or more levels of skin reaction may occur simultaneously, such as an area of moist desquamation in the breast fold surrounded by brisk erythema. Therefore, in addition to describing the various levels of skin reaction, nurses should use descriptive adjectives to describe skin reactions and the effects of nursing intervention.

Electron Beam and Radioactive Implant

The standard treatment of primary breast cancer with radiation therapy includes boosting the original tumor bed with additional external electron beam treatments or intersti-

TABLE 18–6. Levels of Skin Impairment*

Level	Physical Changes	Interventions
Level I		
Potential impairment of skin integrity	Mild to moderate erythema	Support (such as an athletic bra during breast irradiation) Analgesics
Level II		
Impaired skin integrity	Mild to moderate erythema Dry desquamation Scaling skin Edema Moist desquamation Sloughing of layers of skin, with or without blister formation	Cornstarch, topical steroids, Aveeno bath Lubricant (baby cream), Aquaphor, Lubriderm Support Expose moist areas to air as often as possible Use nonadherent dressings on open areas, secured by burn net (no tape) Wet-to-dry dressings, b.i.d. or t.i.d. with one of following: water 1/4 strength saline/water 1/4 strength peroxide/water Dankin's solution (Domeboro solution/water)
	Moderate to severe pain	Analgesics, narcotics at regular intervals 24 hours a day
Level III		
Impaired skin integrity related to radiation-induced large, open, draining lesions	All of the above Ulcerated areas are large Severe pain	As above Aggressive pain management with narcotics

*Adapted from Guidelines for Nursing Care of Patients with Altered Protective Mechanisms. Oncol Nurs Forum 9:115, 1982.

tial iridium implants. Treatment with an external electron beam requires four to seven additional radiation treatments, beyond the five to six weeks of external beam therapy. The majority of the electron beam treatments are focused on the superficial tissues of the tumor bed. The side effects of the electron beam treatments are the same as for whole breast irradiation, with the exception of an enhanced skin reaction in the boosted field. Erythema of the skin in this area will be moderate to brisk and subsides in the weeks following treatment. Skin in the electron beam field may exhibit increased hyperpigmentation compared with the remainder of the breast for months or years following treatment. Nursing interventions include informing the patient of the probable skin rections, monitoring for interruptions in skin integrity, and making recommendations for additional skin care measures.

As described in previous chapters, iridium (^{191}Ir) often is used as a radiation source in boosting the tumor bed. The iridium is placed in hollow plastic catheters that are implanted in the breast. This procedure is done in an operating room with the patient under local, or occasionally general, anesthesia. During this procedure, the tumor bed is marked, and hollow stainless steel needles are placed in a linear fashion. A medium- to large-breasted patient often requires two layers of catheters. Hollow plastic catheters are threaded through the needles, the needles are removed, and the catheters are left in the breast. After an interval in the recovery room, the patient is returned to her own room, where iridium seeds embedded in a strand of plastic are threaded into the hollow catheter and are secured in the catheter by plastic or metal snaps. The iridium remains in place until the desired dose of radiation has been delivered to the tumor bed, usually for 40 to 48 hours. Although this procedure looks painful, the patients feel only minimal to moderate discomfort, with most of the discomfort occurring with breast movement and rubbing of the catheters on bed linens. Analgesics and, occasionally, mild narcotics may be required during the implant period. After the desired dose has been delivered, the catheters and iridium strands are removed at the bedside. This is not a painful procedure and is described by patients as feeling like the removal of sutures. The patient is often discharged soon after the implant is removed. Once the iridium is removed, neither the patient nor her bodily fluids contain any residual radioactivity. The catheter insertion and exit sites should be covered by a dry sterile dressing for 24 hours. After that time, they can be open to the air, and the patient can shower.

During the actual time the iridium is in place in the breast, the patient should remain in a private room with the door closed and appropriate radiation safety warning signs posted on the door outside the room. In order to decrease exposure to the staff and others, movable lead-lined shields should be placed on either side and at the foot of the patient's bed. To avoid unnecessary radiation exposure of health care personnel, the number of workers having physical contact with the patient should be restricted to essential nursing and medical staff. In order to monitor exposure, personnel entering the room during the iridium implant period should wear film badges on their collars or carry pocket dosimeters. In addition, hospitals using iridium sources for implantation are required to have a radiation safety department actively involved in the monitoring of all sources of radioactivity. This includes monitoring personnel exposure on a monthly, annual, and lifetime basis. Regular educational programs should be available and should be required for nursing personnel caring for patients undergoing radiation implant. The fundamental principles of radiation safety should be included. Instruction should include the basic precautions of minimizing the *time* in the room, maximizing physical *distance* from the radioactive source, and, whenever possible, using lead *shielding* between the radioactive implant and the health care worker's reproductive organs.

With few exceptions, women undergoing an iridium implant are able to care for themselves during the implant period. The nurse providing preimplant teaching should prepare the patient for the various procedures, possible physical discomfort, and physical isolation. The patient should be reassured that apprehension about the implant is normal and that discomfort associated with an implant is easily managed. Encouraging her to take active measures to occupy her time and minimize her physical isolation is helpful. Planned telephone contact with family and friends during the implant period assists in communication with her community supports while decreasing her feelings of isolation. Information related to the radiation safety procedures for nursing staff should be shared with the patient in order to enlist her cooperation and participation in planning her care and minimizing staff exposure.

Breast Self-Examination

In performing BSE in the months and years following radiation therapy, the patient will probably observe differences in the skin color, texture, and physical size of the irradiated breast. Additionally, the person may notice slight to moderate hyperpigmentation and pronounced follicles. The skin may appear thinner than usual and may be sensitive. The size of the treated breast varies from person to person and may range from being slightly larger to being smaller and sitting more upright on the chest wall. The irradiated breast may feel denser or heavier. These changes in the irradiated breast tissue often fluctuate during the year after treatment is completed. Breast tactile sensation may be diminished for an indefinite period after treatment. Despite ongoing changes, monthly BSE should resume immediately following completion of treatment (Table 18–1).

CHEMOTHERAPY

The use of chemotherapy is becoming more prevalent in the treatment of breast cancer. Breast cancer patients may receive chemotherapy as an adjuvant to their primary treatment, as treatment for metastatic or recurrent disease, or as a debulking agent prior to their definitive therapy. The nurse can make a significant contribution to the quality of life of a patient undergoing chemotherapy by taking an active role as a teacher, a symptom manager, and a skilled intravenous therapist.

Education

The nurse's role as teacher should begin as soon as it is decided that the patient will receive chemotherapy. This role includes providing the patient with information about the treatment regimen, drugs, possible side effects, and management. By providing this type of concrete information, many of the fears experienced by the patient can be alleviated. Patients may have difficulty in focusing on the teaching because of their anxiety, their physical condition, or an information overload. A supportive family member or friend helping the patient to listen and ask appropriate questions can be comforting to the patient and should be encouraged. Because the patient will probably be unable to retain all the information presented, verbal information should be supplemented by written information.

Written information should include the treatment schema, names of drugs, major side effects, and written instructions for taking any medications and antiemetics. The nurse should also ascertain whether the patient has telephone numbers of appropriate health team members to contact for routine questions or in an emergency. Whenever possible, the nurse should instruct patients individually. Individualized assessment and teaching is especially important during the initial chemotherapy instruction. The teaching process should start with an assessment of the patient's current level of knowledge of, and past experiences with, chemotherapy. A patient may have family members or friends who have received chemotherapy, and their experiences may have left the patient with positive or negative impressions of chemotherapy. Therefore, patients may present with many misconceptions about therapy. They may fear that they will be totally incapacitated, bedridden, or unable to care for themselves. Patients must be made aware that there are many types of chemotherapy regimens for many different stages of disease and that each patient reacts individually to those regimens; for example, a patient undergoing ablative chemotherapy for leukemia will have a course that differs greatly from that of a patient who is receiving adjuvant chemotherapy for breast cancer. Additionally, a patient who is receiving hormonal manipulation will not be faced with the same side effects as the patient who is receiving chemotherapy. Clearly, distinguishing the type of drug therapy, its expected outcomes, and toxicities is essential to patient management.

Patients should be given a general explanation of chemotherapeutic principles in terms that are understandable to them. By providing an explanation that the patient can understand, the nurse can assist the patient in developing a positive perception of chemotherapy and its side effects; for example, cancer is described to the patient as rapidly developing cells that cannot turn themselves off, and chemotherapy is described as an agent that kills rapidly developing cells. The patient can then conceptualize how chemotherapy can kill her cancer cells and, at the same time, kill some of her normal rapidly developing cells (e.g., bone marrow and hair follicles cells and cells that line the gastrointestinal tract). Some patients are then able to look at the side effects that they are experiencing as outward signs that the chemotherapy is killing other rapidly developing cells, that is, cancer cells. When patients understand how drugs work against their cancer cells and why side effects occur, they may be more tolerant of the side effects.

The side effects of individual drugs should be discussed with the patient. The list of possible side effects from a drug can be overwhelming; therefore, the nurse should make the patient aware that these effects are only a possibility and that each patient experiences a different assortment of side effects of differing intensities throughout her treatment. Emphasis should be placed on the role the patient can play in managing and preventing side effects; for example, a patient who is going to receive cyclophosphamide as one of her chemotherapeutic agents is told that the drug may cause hemorrhagic cystitis resulting from irritation of the bladder wall. The nurse should instruct the patient that she can decrease the incidence of hemorrhagic cystitis by drinking eight to ten glasses of fluid daily, thereby diluting the cyclophosphamide that will come in contact with the bladder wall. By providing examples of how the patient can influence the effects of therapy, the nurse allows the patient to gain some control. Appendix I provides some general guidelines, which may be used when teaching patients receiving chemotherapy.

Many patients have the misconception that the actual administration of chemotherapy is painful. The patient can be assured that the sensory experiences of receiving chemotherapy are no different from those experienced during an intravenous infusion (IV). Explaining the process involved in starting the IV or in administering the chemotherapy prior to therapy, along with providing information about sensory experiences such as the coolness of the solutions, may help decrease the patient's anxiety. Many patients benefit from mental distractions during the administration of chemotherapy. By involving the patient in pleasant conversation, providing personal radios and audio cassettes for use, and encouraging relaxation by using visual imagery techniques, the nurse can help the patient to become less preoccupied with the physical aspects of treatment.

Venous Access

It is often technically difficult to treat women undergoing chemotherapy for breast cancer. Their venous access may be compromised because of obesity, advancing age, or hypovolemia. In addition, the majority of these patients have had axillary dissections or sampling procedures. These procedures may have caused impaired lymphatic drainage, decreased blood flow, and increased venous pressure in the affected arm.[25]

Ideally, the arm on which axillary dissection was performed should not be used for administration of drugs. Patients with limited or absent venous access in the contralateral arm or patients who have had bilateral axillary procedures present special problems. In these patients, it may be impossible to avoid using the affected arm. The amount of time since the axillary surgery, the presence and severity of arm edema, and the duration and precipitating factors involved in the onset of edema should all be considered by the nurse before administering chemotherapy in the affected arm.

The nurse should do a thorough assessment of the patient's venous access status before attempting venipuncture. The entire arm and hand, with jewelry removed and sleeves rolled up, should be assessed. The accessibility of veins may be enhanced by applying moist heat to the arms and hands. Heat dilates the blood vessels and also brings increased blood flow into the area. Alcohol applied over the veins of dark-skinned patients and a bright light assist in visualizing veins that are difficult to see. Dependent arm position and rubbing or tapping the skin over the vein will also make the vein more accessible. Palpation of the arms and hands is essential, as many veins can be felt but not seen. Palpation will also determine if a vein is sclerotic or rope-like and the vein's approximate diameter. Areas of compromised circulation, recent surgery, and pre-existing IV sites or sticks should be noted.

In choosing a venipuncture site, consideration must be given to the type of drug being administered and the drug regimen. Vesicant drugs, such as doxorubicin, are best administered in the forearm, away from joints or tendons. Prudent practice in this area will deter any major functional loss in the hand or arm should the vesicant extravasate into the surrounding tissues. Drugs that can cause phlebitis, such as nitrogen mustard, should be administered via large-diameter veins in the upper forearm. The drug can then be diluted in a large volume of blood and can assimilate quickly into the general circulation.

Careful observations of the needle site, the rate of flow of the intravenous solution, and the amount of blood return should be made during drug administration. When the nurse or drug administrator suspects drug infiltration or extravasation, the drug infusion should be immediately stopped and the subcutaneous tissue immediately assessed for leakage. Even though prudent practice is maintained, extravasation may occur during administration of a vesicant drug. Treatments for extravasation are controversial and diverse. Recommendations for treatment include applications of heat or cold followed by injections of the subcutaneous tissue with steroids, bicarbonate, or other antidotes often recommended by the manufacturer or institution.

It is important that the nurse have a clear-cut plan of action should an extravasation occur. All necessary medication and equipment should be readily accessible, and standardized physician's orders should be in place. Nurses should elicit the patient's assistance in detecting an extravasation by instructing the patient to report any changes in sensation during administration of a vesicant drug.

Safety precautions must be exercised to protect the drug handler during preparation of chemotherapy. The Oncology Nursing Society Guidelines for Chemotherapy Administration summarize these precautions.[25] All drugs should be prepared in a Class II, biologic safety cabinet, which recirculates air through a high efficiency particulate air (HEPA) filter. The drug handler should wear vinyl gloves and a protective garment with closed front and cuffed long sleeves. If a Class II, biologic safety cabinet is not available, a Plexiglas face shield or goggles and mask should also be worn. If drugs do come in contact with skin or mucous membranes, flush immediately and generously with water, following drug product instructions. Emergency eye care kits should be available. The drug handler should avoid eating, drinking, smoking, and using cosmetics while in the drug preparation area.

RECURRENCE

Breast cancer recurs in about 40 to 45 percent of all women with a diagnosis of breast cancer. Of those women who have recurrences, virtually all will die of the disease. This fact comes as a surprise to many. For years, women and health care professionals alike have equated the five-year survival rate described by the American Cancer Society (ACS) with cure. This certainly is true for many cancers, but not for breast cancer. The reason for the differing situation with breast cancer is that in order for a disease to be considered cured, the death rate resulting from that disease must equal the age-adjusted rate of death from all other causes. Unfortunately, this is never the case with the breast cancer death rate. Therefore, all women who have been diagnosed with breast cancer remain *at risk* for a recurrence for the remainder of their lives. The interaction of many factors determines whether a person has a recurrence, when the recurrence arises, in what site(s) the recurrence is located, and what, if any, response the person will have to medical therapy. Nurses must be cognizant of the factors that carry prognostic significance for breast cancer patients for the following reasons: (1) so that they are knowledgeable about the impact that prognostic factors have on the natural history of the disease and (2) to be able to formulate a nursing approach to patient care management that interfaces with the current medical plan.

The significance of prognostic factors in metastatic breast cancer has been well described in the literature. The most significant factors related to ultimate outcome include (1) the performance status of the individual

(Karnofsky); (2) the site(s) of the metastasis; (3) the bulk of disease at those metastatic sites (people presenting with an isolated site of recurrence or a nonemergent metastasis—that is, one not involving a visceral organ—have a better prognosis); (4) prior therapy; (5) age; and (6) disease-free interval (that time from initial therapy to first recurrence).[42]

Nursing management of the patient with recurrent breast cancer poses many problems for those persons directly involved with the care. Until recently, little research could be found that addressed the needs of the person with recurrent cancer, let alone recurrent breast cancer. Kubler-Ross's pioneering work dealing with death and dying provided the impetus for others to look at the issues surrounding the crisis of adjusting to a finite existence. Until the mid-1970's, what seemed sorely missing was work that addressed the group of patients who face adjustment to the crisis of recurrent breast cancer.

Psychosocial Issues

Schmale[27] addressed the psychologic problems of recurrence in general and delineated ways in which the physician could assist the patient in this phase of illness. He emphasized the need to identify the meaning of a recurrence to the patient and the need to recognize the pivotal role played by the physician in facilitating adaptation to the new state. Then, Scott[29] presented a case history that described the psychodynamics of multiple remissions in the patient with nonlymphoblastic leukemia. Four major behavioral indicators of the recurrent syndrome were identified: volatility of emotion, progressive redirection in stamina, resurfacing of unresolved issues, and urgent attempts to remain in control. The author identified the need to investigate these concepts further for their relevance in other situations dealing with recurrent disease.

Chekryn[26] investigated the psychosocial meaning of recurrence to the marital dyad. The study identified a number of problems experienced by the patients and their spouses, including difficulty in dealing with the issues associated with an expectation of cure or remission and repeated assault by the cancer; pervasive feelings of uncertainty; grief about present and future losses; feelings of injustice, anger, and fear; concerns about death and dying; and concerns related to coping with recurrence. Of significance, it was revealed that the impact of recurrence was of as much concern to the spouse as to the person with the disease. Also, the study found that it was difficult to identify adaptive or maladaptive patterns of communication. Finally, despite the variety of understandings regarding the meaning of recurrence to the patient and spouse as well as the differing communication patterns, the spouse was viewed as a major support. Chekryn's study suggests that it is beneficial to include the spouse (or other targeted significant other) in care-related discussions and decisions, as appropriate. This would facilitate the needed supportive environment described.[26] Northouse[28] reported the first study that addressed the fear of recurrence in the mastectomy patient. She reported that poor social support was linked with an increased fear of recurrence. The study attempted to determine whether there was any correlation between variables such as age, marital status, and time since diagnosis or last treatment and the woman's fear of recurrence. No such relationship was found. The major limitation addressed by the author was the questionable validity and reliability of the fear of recurrence instrument. It remains to be seen if the results of this study will hold up with future use of the instrument. The results of the study are similar to those discussed by Chekryn concerning the importance of spousal support as perceived by the patient. If these results can be replicated, nursing interventions can be designed to include some emphasis on assisting the cancer patient in strengthening her support systems.[28]

Assessment

Although limited, this research does provide some guidance for the nurse responsible for the care of the person with recurrent breast cancer. In addition to accurately assessing the physical needs of the person, the nurse should also determine the significance of factors related to the initial diagnosis and treatment of the person's breast cancer. Obtaining information about the person's experience with the primary disease may shed some light on how she might adapt to this recurrence. In addition, unresolved issues might emerge, which, if not addressed, could

TABLE 18–7. Patient/Family Adjustments: Nurse's Role (Assessment)

Psychosocial	***Physical***
Meaning of recurrence	Pain
Cure, control, terminal	Changes in mobility
Emotional Reactions	Appetite
Anger—volatility	Weight gain or loss (nutritional)
Fear	Use of ETOH and/or drugs
Depression	Skin changes—color, actual skin metastasis
Denial	Stamina
Intellectualization	***Support Systems***
Potential Behavioral Manifestations	Who comes with patient
Withdrawal	Who asks questions
Suicidal ideation	Ascertain tensions or conflicts (unresolved issues)
Changes in personal habits	***Treatment***
Loss of concentration, affecting job and home interactions	Collaboration with physician
Need to maintain control	Ascertain medical treatment
Knowledge	Present nursing treatment
Identify patient's and family's knowledge of extent of disease	
Identify patient's and family's knowledge of treatment	
Identify patient's and family's knowledge of expected outcomes of therapy	

impede acceptance of therapy and adjustment to recurrent breast cancer. The following factors related to the initial experience with breast cancer should be explored to determine their relevance to the current situation:

1. Who discovered the tumor
2. What, if any, delay was involved in seeking medical attention
3. What type of primary treatment(s) was given
4. What role the person played in choosing a treatment approach
5. What, if any, residual morbidity exists from primary therapy (e.g., lymphedema, limited range of motion, chest wall or breast pain from surgery or radiation therapy, or poor cosmesis)
6. What information the person was given about her disease, the chance for recovery, and the chance of recurrence
7. Whether the person has had breast reconstruction

Additional general knowlege is needed by the nurse in the area of the meaning of recurrence to the breast cancer patient. For many patients, the diagnosis of recurrent cancer is equated with death. While metastatic breast cancer is not a curable disease, it is not necessarily imminently terminal. This distinction is critical and should be emphasized soon after the recurrence is diagnosed. This can be accomplished by asking patients what they perceive their prognosis to be and what their understanding is of the goals of therapy. Having this information, the nurse or physician can correct any misconceptions. Clearly identifying a patient's understanding of recurrent breast cancer in terms of treatment objectives and establishing realistic goals are essential beginning steps in the management of this population.

Crisis Intervention

Breast cancer, like many other cancers, often follows a tortuous course marked by remissions and subsequent recurrences. It is certain that the diagnosis of a recurrence raises a variety of issues for breast cancer patients and their family members. Unresolved issues from the initial diagnosis of breast cancer, internal familial conflicts, or unresolved issues with health care personnel all have the potential of fueling a crisis. However, this crisis period is of varying duration. Generally, at least partial resolution of the crisis occurs within the first six weeks after its onset. Weisman and Worden[35] have described the crisis period and subsequent resolution as the existential plight in cancer, encompassing the first 100 days. Although their work was done on patients with newly diagnosed cancer, certain behavioral similarities with the recurrent cancer patient exist; for example, the patients' focus on life and death issues and physical symptoms.

Whether this is the first, the second, or a later recurrence is important, since the goals of the therapy planned may differ. Even more significant is that the desires and goals of the patient and her significant others may be changing with repeated recurrences.

For the patients coping with their first recurrence, this is a critical time. The fears surrounding the initial diagnosis of cancer come rushing back. Resentment at having their life once again interrupted is oftentimes striking. It is not uncommon for patients to tell nurses that the scheduling of diagnostic tests or treatment must be delayed because of some previously arranged personal or professional commitments. Under these circumstances, it is often difficult for the nurse to understand how a person with recurrent breast cancer could establish priorities in such a manner. Nurses ask, "How can this person not see that establishing a firm diagnosis and treatment approach and beginning therapy are of highest priority?"

An example of such a patient follows.

Mrs. B. is a 65-year-old woman who has had a recurrence of breast cancer metastatic to her skull. All her diagnostic work-up has been scheduled, extending over a week. She arrived from out of town, expecting to be away only a few days, and was not prepared to remain for an extended period. Complicating the picture was her husband's scheduled beginning of chemotherapy in the middle of all her scheduled tests. She requested a change in her last test so that she could go home to be with her husband. Her second request was not to return when all the results of the tests are completed. Finally, she requested that therapy be delayed for six weeks so that she could organize her life.

Several factors need to be addressed in this situation. It is realistic and reasonable for the patient to want to adjust the scheduling of her tests. Fulfilling her obligation to her husband as she perceives it is of the highest priority. Nurses can assist the patient in several ways. First, if possible, a simple change in schedule of diagnostic tests could be done. Second, if scheduling is a problem or if the test is extremely important, the nurse can help the patient identify other family members or friends who could accompany the husband for his treatment. Third, if neither of these options is possible, it may be necessary to delay the completion of the work-up so that the patient can accompany her husband. One must recognize that the psychologic comfort of the woman is as important as obtaining a complete diagnostic work-up. Allowing some flexibility at this stage allows for a smoother transition from this acute crisis phase to the longer chronic phase. It also allows the patient some control when aspects of her life seem out of control.

The other major issue is her request to delay therapy for six weeks so that she can organize her life. While an initial reaction by the nurse and other health care professionals is oftentimes negative, one must fully assess what the patient is really requesting. Does the patient have reasonable grounds for making this request? Is it essential for her to be with her husband? Are other personal issues pending? Only through continued investigation does it emerge that this request may be a delay tactic. The truly difficult task for the nurse is to separate the reasonable requests from those that are delay tactics. The nurse must discuss the issues with the patient and attempt to assist her in recognizing the importance of getting on with therapy.

Recognizing the complex set of emotions that could be expressed by the recurrent breast cancer patient is another task. Anger and fear are probably the two reactions seen most frequently, yet are the most frequently denied by patients. Patients with recurrent breast cancer can be helped by nurses who listen attentively to their concerns, provide clear and accurate information, and allow the patient time to assimilate this information.

Acknowledging a patient's anger must be done with care, as many people are not consciously aware of their feelings and therefore cannot see their anger. Anger, like denial, may be a defense mechanism serving a specific purpose. Saying to patients, "I hear your anger," or "I can understand why you are angry," is a possible way of helping them recognize their feelings. A negative response from the patient, such as *"I'm not angry,"* clues the nurse into the fact that the patient is not ready to deal with these angry feelings. Verbally or nonverbally accepting the person's anger and demonstrating active support may be all that can be accomplished. A reply such as, "I believe you don't think you're angry, but perhaps you could describe your feelings to me," might be yet another way of assisting the person in adjusting to her feelings. Good eye contact or physical contact may be appropriate here. When working with patients, it is important for the nurse to respect their current psychologic status and to avoid forcing them to face issues prematurely. Likewise, for the patient who continues to deny her feelings and is obviously making no attempts to work through the issues associated with the recurrence, additional professional intervention is warranted.

Fear felt by the patient can relate to the unknowns associated with the extent of disease, type of therapy planned, or effectiveness of therapy. Additionally, the patient can fear the loss of her current life-style, the loss of her job, changes in body image and sexuality, and the ultimate loss of life. For many patients who have had adjuvant chemotherapy, the thought of facing the side effects of this treatment again is awesome. Unlike an adjuvant chemotherapy setting, in a chemotherapy setting for recurrent disease, the manner in which an individual's disease responds is often the critical factor in determining when, if ever, she stops receiving chemotherapy. Facing the future from this perspective may be overwhelming and may make it impossible for the patient to effectively address the issues.

In the assessment, the nurse should ascertain the development level of the patient to identify any life tasks or hurdles that the patient is facing. It is possible that the person is adjusting to many other issues in addition to her recurrent breast cancer, including:

1. The fact that her children are leaving home
2. A change in her work status or that of her spouse
3. Approaching menopause
4. Decisions to have a child
5. Feelings of loss if she is childless
6. The presence of a significant other if she is single
7. The aging of her parents
8. The death of parents or friends

The role of the nurse is to provide the individual with complete and concise information about the treatment goals and requirements and to ascertain the patient's need for additional information. Nurses should not expect that all this information will be assimilated initially or that all needs will be immediately identified. It is, however, important that nurses actively assess their patients and be alert to behavioral clues that might indicate distress. Finally, the nurse must remember that patients always have the right to stop therapy and that their reasons might not be ones that we, as health care professionals, support. It is critical that the nurse fully assess the meaning of therapy termination to the patient, the patient's understanding of the potential consequences of this act, and what the patient's expectations for the future are. Clearly, every patient with recurrent breast cancer faces the issue of termination of therapy at some point. Likewise, there are times when termination of therapy is appropriate therapeutically and times when other options should be explored.

Therefore, before a patient terminates therapy, the nurse should explore the following issues with the patient and her partner and family members, if possible. The results of these discussions should be shared with the patient's primary physician and with appropriate multidisciplinary team members.

1. What is the disease status?
2. What is the patient's understanding of the extent of the disease?
3. What is the patient's understanding of the outcome of the disease and is this consistent with reality?
4. What is the patient's understanding of the therapeutic plan?
5. Does the family agree with the patient?
6. Does the patient have an understanding of the consequences of stopping therapy?
7. Does the patient want to stop therapy so she can die, and is this imminent?

Ascertaining answers to these questions is critical when planning care for and providing support to the breast cancer patient. Obviously, there are many reasons that a patient might want to refuse further therapy, death being only one of them; for example, a patient may be truly "tired" of therapy, being tied to weekly treatment, or may have disease that is indolent, and it may be entirely appropriate for this patient to seek a break in treatment. Understanding the consequences of such a decision by patients and their family is essential. Another situation is

TABLE 18–8. Nursing Actions for the Patient with Recurrence

Actions are dependent on patient's phase and patterns of recurrence and on individual factors
Actions are dependent on identified psychosocial and physical support systems
Discussion of medical and nursing treatment plans

that in which the patient no longer believes that the therapy is helping and desires to seek some alternative (e.g., an unproven method of treatment). The nurse can be helpful in this situation by being open with the patient, listening to the descriptions of treatment, and providing accurate information on the efficacy of the proposed approach in a nonjudgmental manner. Avoiding discussions between patients and their families concerning unproved methods of therapy only pushes them further away from the traditional health care system.

Some patients say that they want to stop therapy because they want to assess the reaction of their health care professionals without really intending to stop treatment. Patients may wish to experience how it feels to say, "I don't want any more treatment." Making that type of statement may identify issues related to control, or it may be related to preparing for future decisions. Again, it is important that nurses assess the full meaning of the patient's statement, in order to intervene appropriately.

When therapies are not controlling the spread of breast cancer, it is reasonable to consider terminating therapy. If the relationship between the health care provider and the patient has been one of open communication, often the patient and family will appropriately bring up the issue of discontinuing therapy. Sometimes, however, neither the patient nor the family are able to do this. They may want everything possible to be done, or perhaps they do not want to disappoint their physicians and nurses by giving up. It is then incumbent upon the nurse and physician to begin exploring the issue of terminating therapy. The overall goals of caring for the patient with breast cancer through all phases of the disease include building on a sound nursing data base and establishing oneself as a consistent, competent nursing resource, one who is open to challenge, comes through with clear and complete information, and can disagree with a patient's decision but still "stay" and offer support.

PAIN

Pain varies in occurrence, intensity, location, and duration in the breast cancer patient, depending upon the stage of the disease, the treatment method(s) employed, and the sites involved. Other factors such as age; sex; cultural, social, and ethnic backgrounds; and feelings of anxiety, guilt, anger, and fear have a significant impact on the occurrence of pain. These factors also significantly influence the management of pain.

The nurse must be aware that patients with breast cancer will experience pain at different times during the course of the illness and that the pain will have different courses; for example, the patient with early-stage breast cancer will experience pain that is *generally* related directly to treatment (i.e. mastectomy, axillary node dissection, radiation therapy, chemotherapy, or a combination of therapies). Pain of this sort is generally classified as acute (i.e., of short duration), is causing changes in normal routines, and will be resolved with healing or discontinuation of the therapy. The nurse must assess the pain, accurately ascertaining the standard parameters of location, intensity, description of type, frequency, and what may exacerbate or mitigate the pain. Generally, oral or intramuscular narcotics are prescribed for postoperative pain. For the patient experiencing pain from therapy, symptomatic relief can often be achieved by local measures, for example, the application of cold or hot packs, topical sprays, or ointments to the affected areas or the utilization of prescribed exercises.

Two specific types of pain are often experienced by the patient receiving local treatment for breast cancer. One is phantom breast pain following mastectomy. In this situation, the person actually experiences the sensation of the presence of the amputated breast. This can be a very distracting and frightening experience. Although this phenomenon has been described in women, it is not known whether it exists in men with breast cancer. During preoperative teaching, the nurse can alert patients to this potential occurrence, assuring them that it is normal and nothing to be fearful of and that it is generally temporary. Offering some brief physiologic explanation for this may be appropriate for some individuals, depending on how much information they seem to want. Follow-up in the postoperative phase should include assessing what, if any, sensations a person might be experiencing in the operative site and allowing time to discuss any concerns relating to phantom breast pain.[51]

The second occurrence of pain results from radiation therapy. This pain is caused by radiation to the skin and subcutaneous muscle and fat. Skin care, as outlined in the section on radiation therapy, is often sufficient for the person experiencing superficial skin discomfort during therapy. For the person whose pain is not relieved by these measures, oral narcotics or anti-inflammatory agents are often appropriate. The nurse must accurately assess each person and plan interventions accordingly.

Breast discomfort may also be a long-term complication of radiation therapy. This type of pain has only recently been recognized, because of the large number of women who are receiving radiation treatment as primary therapy for their breast cancer and because of the growing number of women with locally advanced cancer who receive radiation as local treatment for their cancer, in conjunction with chemotherapy. The nurse can do much to allay the patient's fear by (1) telling the patient in advance that such symptoms may occur and are typical and usually temporary; (2) answering questions regarding the resolution of the symptoms; and (3) acknowledging that the patient may be fearful that the symptoms are similar to those at the time of diagnosis.

The patient with recurrent breast cancer is a prime candidate for pain at the site of the recurrence that is the result of the actual tumor invasion or tumor encroachment on a vital structure, nerve, or blood supply. The pain can also be due to treatment, for example, from flare-up of pain occurring in the patient with bony metastasis. Knowing the sites of recurrence and the physiologic alterations that may occur is essential to understanding the type of pain experienced and designing appropriate intervention.

The philosophy underlying the management of pain in the case of recurrent breast cancer is different from that previously described for acute pain experienced during early-state disease. The pain of recurrent cancer is of a chronic nature, one whose cause is not likely to be removed. This does not mean that the pain cannot be relieved, only that curing the cancer, and thus the pain, is not the goal of therapy. An accurate pain assessment yields information necessary for appropriate planning. See the reference section for a more comprehensive discussion of pain management. In addition to having the basic information about the patient's pain, it is helpful and important to know what types of pain medications the patient has used in the past, for what pain and with what relief. This provides the basic information necessary to generate a pain management program. Some general principles should guide such a program. First, the overall goal is to relieve the pain as quickly and as completely as possible. Second, one should use non-narcotic analgesics first, starting with the smallest doses required to control pain. Third, the dose of the drug used should be increased as much as is needed to relieve the pain and then titrated downward to the minimum dose necessary to achieve pain relief. Fourth, oral administration of medications is the route of choice when feasible, for as long as possible. Fifth, medication should be taken at regular intervals around the clock and not on a p.r.n. basis. Finally, patients should participate in the management of their own pain, whenever possible.

It is critical that the nurse involved in pain management of the cancer patient fully explore his or her own beliefs, prejudices, attitudes, and possible misconceptions concerning pain. Nurses must recognize that fears of addiction are misplaced and that use of placebos is inappropriate. Only by understanding the underlying principles of pain management in the cancer patient and by being aware of their own beliefs will nurses be able to participate effectively in controlling the cancer patient's pain. Additionally, the management of metastatic breast cancer pain often requires a multimodality approach. This could be any or all of the following: analgesics, radiation therapy, surgery, biofeedback, TENS, relaxation, or distraction. The nurse must be aware of the applicability of each of these approaches and must be instrumental in seeking appropriate consultation.

The patient may also experience psychologic pain. This pain may result from many factors, such as the impact of the diagnosis, be it initial or recurrent disease; the loss of a breast; changes in cosmesis; and the fear of the loss of a previous life-style or of the actual loss of life. Finally, the patient's psychologic pain may be the kind that occurs when people lose control of certain aspects of their life and accept or adjust to their altered life-style. Psychologic pain cannot always be separated from physiologically based pain. It is important that nurses and patients recognize that both types of pain are important and equally real. Therefore, any approach to pain management must take into account both the physiologic and the psychologic states of the patient. Antidepressants or tranquilizers may be useful for some patients.

Achieving pain relief is complex and requires the coordinated approach of several disciplines, types of medications, and other noninvasive measures. The basic principles of pain management that have been presented are designed to assist the nurse in caring for the breast cancer patient with pain.

NUTRITION

The majority of the literature on nutrition and cancer focuses on anorexia, weight loss, cachexia, and malnutrition.[36–38] People undergoing surgery, irradiation, and chemotherapy report having a loss of appetite, early satiety, and changes in food tastes and body weight. The impact that the cancer or the treatment has on an individual varies according to disease types and treatment, the person's nutritional status prior to diagnosis, and the treatment. More often than not, patients with widely metastatic disease are reported as having moderate to severe cachexia.

Nutritional changes in populations of patients with breast cancer vary. Those patients presenting for evaluation of a suspicious breast mass or with a newly diagnosed case of breast cancer rarely report significant dietary or weight changes prior to diagnosis. Women with metastatic disease, however, often give a history of unexplained weight loss and dietary changes.

While there may be some fluctuation in weight during the postoperative and postradiotherapy periods, this is often explained by changes in eating habits, activity, and mood. Over the last several years, reports in the literature have appeared identifying weight gain as a significant problem for women with breast cancer receiving adjuvant chemotherapy.[39–41] Although the reasons for this phenomenon are unclear, possible explanations include changes in activity levels, increased food intake (frequent meals often decrease nausea), depression, and hormonal changes.

Firm data now exist in the literature that women with breast cancer who maintain their weight within normal ranges have an increased disease-free interval. These data emphasize the importance of maintaining normal weight for disease-related benefits.[42]

The role of the nurse includes obtaining an accurate nutritional assessment at the time of diagnosis and treatment. Included in the assessment is a weight and dietary history as well as a physical and psychologic assessment to evaluate the impact of the diagnosis and treatment. Following the nutritional assessment, the appropriate nursing diagnoses should be made—the development of realistic nutritional goals and a realistic treatment plan. Patient participation is essential during the planning, intervention, and evaluation phases of nutritional intervention.

FAMILY

Until recently, the literature contained few works on the needs of the families of cancer patients. Often, what did appear were statements that acknowledged the need to address the problems that families might experience. Families and their needs received attention in the context of the patient's needs, and family members were not seen as persons separate and distinct, with identifiable concerns requiring intervention. Beginning in the mid-1970's, studies targeted the crises with which families were faced during the terminal phase of a patient's illness and during the bereavement phases.[42–44] Hampe[43] noted the needs of grieving spouses during the terminal phase of illness. Those identified most frequently by spouses included the need to be with the dying spouse, the need for assurance that the dying person is comfortable, the need to be helpful to the spouse, and the need to be informed of the spouse's condition. Freihofer and Felton[44] attempted to identify what nursing behaviors are considered by families to be most helpful during a terminally ill person's disease. Their findings were similar to those of Hampe, previously described. In addition, they found that family members rated their own needs (e.g., the need to ventilate emotions and the need for comfort, acceptance, and support) much lower. Constantino[45] examined the effects of structured interventions that were designed to assist widows in reducing depression and increasing socialization. She studied two groups of women, one receiving the bereavement crisis intervention and one not. Although the sample size was small and the groups were not randomized, it was found that the experimental group exhibited significantly less depression and more socialization than did the control group, suggesting that structured intervention in a group of newly widowed women has beneficial effects.

Giaquinta[46] designed a model with phases through which the family member passes and "hurdles" within each phase that families must overcome to successfully adjust to the crisis of illness experienced by their loved one. Within each phase are nursing interventions designed to assist the family member in overcoming the hurdles in each stage of illness. A model for family adjustment to cancer can be found in Table 18–9. Similarities exist between the model proposed by Giaquinta and that described earlier by Kubler-Ross in her now classic stages of death and dying experienced by the patient. Both models are derived from clinical practice, and although they provide significant guidelines for designing interventions for both groups, they remain untested as theories governing practice.

Wright and Dyck[47] focused on the needs of families throughout the cancer experience, primarily identifying concerns that were related to dealing with symptoms and fear of the future and trying to obtain more information. Results of the study indicated the importance of these issues and that distress about symptom management increases with advanced disease. The time between identification of a problem, diagnosis, and institution of therapy was identified as being very stressful, with delays in scheduling causing extreme frustration. Specifically, families rated receiving current information about the patient's condition and being assured of her comfort as having the highest priority. The families consistently rated their own needs for support and comfort as having lower priority, stating that nurses should not be burdened with caring for them and taking time away from that given to the patient. These results are consistent with those found by Hampe[43] and by Johnson and Norby,[48] as reported in the development of the program entitled "We Can Weekend," designed to assist the family in their adjustment process. Finally, Northouse[49] studied problems experienced by family members coping with cancer and identified specific issues that they potentially fail to deal with during three phases of the illness. During the initial phase, the family may feel excluded from care and may have difficulties communicating with the staff. During the adaptation phase, how to live with uncertainty and changes in lifestyle and how to meet the needs of other family members become problems. Finally,

TABLE 18–9. Model for a Family's Adjustment to Cancer*

Points of Transition in Individual with Cancer	*Family Stage*	*Family Phase*	*Family Hurdle*	*Goal of Intervention*
Individual receives initial diagnosis of cancer, continues to carry out role obligations with the family, and functions in varying ways as a family member	Living with cancer	Impact	Despair	Fostering hope
		Functional disruption	Isolation	Fostering cohesion
			Vulnerability	Fostering security
		Search for meaning	Retreat	Fostering courage
		Informing others	Helplessness	Fostering problem-solving
		Engaging emotions	Competition	Fostering cooperation
	Restructuring in the living-dying interval	Reorganization	Anonymity	Fostering identity
		Framing memories		
Individual with cancer ceases to perform familial roles and is cared for either at home or in the hospital	Bereavement	Separation	Self-absorption	Fostering intimacy
	Re-establishment	Mourning	Guilt	Fostering relief
		Expansion of the social network	Alienation	Fostering relatedness

*Adapted from Giaquinta B: Helping families face the crisis of cancer. Am J Nurs 77:1585, 1977.

in the terminal phase, the issues are related to death and dying, separation and loss. Here, one can identify similarities between Northouse's work and the earlier work of Giaquinta concerning the phases families go through and the problems they must address.

Nursing Interventions

As a result of this research, several points can be identified that serve as a basis for designing nursing interventions for the family. First, the major areas identified by families as care concerns having highest priority are provision of accurate and current information about the patient's condition; ensuring that the care of the patient is efficient and is in accord with the disease and treatment plans; providing comfort and relief of pain; and giving emotional support. Second, it is clear that families rate their needs as having a lesser degree of importance. This issue will be discussed in greater detail. Third, one should be aware that the family and the patient experience problems associated with the illness that, although similar in content, will probably differ in degree, timing, and resolution. Finally, it must be recognized that the care of the patient does not occur in isolation. The care given to a patient has an impact on the family system, and it is important that nurses "treat" the family as a whole and not just the individual members.

A diagnosis of breast cancer significantly affects the entire family in many ways. First, the family is faced with adjusting to the diagnosis of cancer and what this actually means: Will the patient be changed by the disease, and if so, how? And more importantly, is the person going to live or die? This initial phase can lead to a crisis of significant magnitude, and this crisis, if unresolved, can prevent healthy adaptation. Actions by the nurse play a significant role in fostering healthy adaptation by the family. (The patient is a member of the family and must be included in the planning.) The first step for the nurse in fostering this adaptation is assessing the meaning the diagnosis of breast cancer has to the family and identifying who the significant person(s) is in the family system (e.g., husband, parents, all children). Ascertaining from patients who, if any, of these persons they wish to have participate in certain aspects of their care tends to shed light on some of the family dynamics and gives clues as to which persons will be available as resources. Establishing what the family knows about breast cancer equips the nurse with data necessary for accurate planning. The family should at least understand the implications of the stage of breast cancer, the proposed treatment approaches, the potential for toxicities, the proposed length of therapy, and the expected outcomes. In addition, the family should be assisted in trying to separate their needs to be supportive of the patient from their own needs to be reassured and to be fearful and angry. As the studies have documented, families tend to minimize their own needs, often stating that there will be time in the future for them. While this may be appropriate during the crisis of diagnosis, over a sustained time, not dealing with one's needs causes energy to be lost and thus not available for other responsibilities.

The partner of a person with breast cancer may be most profoundly affected. Their reaction may significantly affect the patient's adjustment to illness. The spouse often bears financial and family responsibilities, in addition to those of being a partner in the relationship. The times of transition, from outpatient staging to hospitalization and from hospitalization to discharge, are often the most difficult times. To assist the partner, the nurse should provide information, in advance when possible, about the physical changes to expect during the transition and about the type of care requirements anticipated. Preparation of the partners of patients who are being discharged after a surgical procedure includes providing information about the physical changes in the operative site. Using pictures illustrating similar surgical procedures may minimize the partner's fear of the surgical site and assist in preparing the partner for visualization of the incision lines and surgical defects.

The responses of the children of patients with breast cancer vary depending on their age and state of physical and psychologic development. Young children often are fearful of a permanent separation from their parent. They often have misconceptions about the nature of their parent's hospitalization or about specific aspects of the disease and treatment. When possible, they should be given information that is appropriate for their developmental stage. Their questions should be anticipated and answered by their parents. Attention should be paid to their underlying fears and worries, and information should be supplied to allay those fears. Children's books about hospitalization or a visit to the hospital prior to hospitalization will decrease their fear and allow them opportunities to ask questions. Decisions about when and if children should visit the hospitalized parent should be made thoughtfully and will depend upon institutional policies. Consideration should be given to the fact that the presence of tubes, drains, and equipment may be frightening to children. When visits during hospitalization are not possible, frequent telephone calls, letters, and small gifts may ease the period of isolation.

Maintaining routine family patterns, whenever possible, should be a family goal. Young children need the reassurance that the family is intact and that the parents are concerned about their specific needs. At the same time, adolescents may feel that they are being pulled back into the family at a time when they are seeking independence. Assisting patients to identify and address the issues of breast cancer treatment, while supporting individual family members, is a special challenge for health care professionals.

The nurse can assist the family in identifying specific activities for which members can assume responsibility; for example, some normal household tasks such as meal planning, shopping, cooking, and cleaning could be shared by several family members. If young children are involved, including them in the activities is also critical. The more the nurse can foster the family's assumption of routine family activities, stimulate an awareness of the importance of having all members, including the patient, participate in the planning and carrying out of such activities, and provide time for the identification and solving of potential and actual family problems, the greater is the potential for healthy adaptation. Specific nursing interventions are included in Table 18–10.

An example of successful adaptation is a grandmother with recurrent breast cancer, who returns to the clinic every three weeks for chemotherapy. A family member routinely accompanies her to assist her with the care of her Hickman catheter and the routine activities of daily living, including taking care of her four-year-old grandson. The care of this woman, the needs of the family, and the integrated functioning of the family system have been preserved by this arrangement.

A young husband and father of two children, aged two and a half and five, is facing the terminal illness of his 40-year-old wife from widely metastatic breast cancer. Realistic planning includes encouraging the husband to seek additional child care, such as a "nanny" immediately, so that both patient and children will have a chance to adjust. Although the husband's mother has been a frequent participant in child care, she does have her own job and family to return to. The husband seeks advice on how to approach his wife concerning her impending death. The patient has continually maintained a very hopeful attitude, exhibiting a great deal of religious and personal strength. This has provided her with an uncanny degree of positive coping skills, which are now unrealistic, given her rapidly deteriorating condition. Assisting the husband through role playing (in which his conversations with his wife are rehearsed) can maximally aid in the planning for the care of their children, while accomplishing meaningful activities for both husband and wife and allowing them to begin their termination process.

Stages of Adjustment

The diagnosis of breast cancer affects not only the patient but also the family and friends. The stage of a woman's breast cancer, the nature of treatment, and her response determine the challenges her family faces in adjusting to her disease. The impact of the disease and subsequent changes in her role within the family may greatly affect the family's style of coping.

Giaquinta[46] describes a model of four stages of adjustment to cancer. This model, which can be used to suggest professional interventions at each stage and function, is summarized in Table 18–9.

The first step toward coping with the changes in family life involves openly discussing the breast cancer diagnosis and its implications for the woman and her family. Nurses can assist family members in making adjustments by suggesting ways that various family members can assist the patient. Assigning specific responsibilities to each family member fosters the "team spirit." These re-

TABLE 18–10. Nursing Interventions for Family Members

Identify the significant other (s.o.) with whom the patient most closely relates.
Include that person in all discussions and conferences with the patient, as is appropriate and realistic.
Provide a time for that family member to meet with the nurse alone, so that their specific concerns can be discussed.
Help the family (s.o.) identify their most crucial problems in dealing with the diagnosis of breast cancer. Ask them to identify which aspects of everyday life will be most interrupted. Take advantage of social services and community resources.
Provide the significant other with the name and telephone number of the nurse with whom she or he can make contact, as future needs are identified.
Schedule a follow-up meeting.
Identify the pattern of communication and problem solving used by the family system in the past.
Emphasize the importance of open communication and sharing of fears and concerns among family members. Role playing can be used when practicing communication strategies.
Openly support the concept that family members have needs that require attention. Emphasize that by being selfish in seeing that their own needs are met, the family members are taking good care of themselves.
Remind the family that life goes on and that the family activities should be encouraged, and should be interrupted as little as possible. Encourage regular scheduling of fun activities for the family.
Establish a relationship with family members that promotes their growth and reliance on health care personnel, as needed.
Recognize the changing needs of the family with recurrent and/or terminal disease.
Assist the family in their adaptation to these changing needs.
Recognize the informational needs of the family that aid in their understanding the disease, the prescribed treatment and side effects, and eventual outcomes. Assist family members in the decision-making process regarding treatment options.
Provide the spouse or other appropriate significant other with an opportunity to view the surgical sites while the patient is hospitalized and health care personnel are available for additional support.
Provide the family with information regarding the physical changes that will occur and the adjustments to be made as a result of surgery, radiation therapy, or chemotherapy.
Encourage the family to treat the patient as normally as possible, while resuming prior activities.
In the case of the family adjusting to changes in the patient's condition resulting from treatment or progressive disease, encourage the family to allow the patient to participate in family decisions and activities. Taking away the patient's role in the family and the decision-making process is detrimental to the entire family system.
Help the family realistically plan for the future.

sponsibilities may include assisting with household chores, running errands, accompanying the patient for treatment, and initiating a "fun" activity that is not related to breast cancer or its treatment. Nursing interventions also include facilitating honest, open communication between family members and the woman with breast cancer.

COMMUNITY RESOURCES AND EDUCATIONAL MATERIALS

Beyond accurate diagnosis and effective treatment, many patients with cancer need psychologic, social, and economic assistance to cope with their disease and its effects.[50] Use of public education materials and community resources allays the public's fears of breast cancer and those of patients and their families.[14] Advances have been made in the areas of breast cancer detection and treatment, breast reconstruction, and the management of treatment side effects. In 1979, the National Cancer Institute sponsored and coordinated a study of public knowledge, attitudes, and practices related to breast cancer. With information gathered from the data, the NCI Office of Cancer Communication has developed patient education materials related to benign breast disease, breast biopsy, mastectomy, radiation therapy, breast reconstruction, adjuvant chemotherapy, follow-up after breast cancer treatment, and living with advancing disease. Additionally, other general cancer education materials have been developed and are available for distribution.

Since its beginning days, the American Cancer Society has been actively involved in educating the public about benign and malignant breast diseases. In addition to providing printed and audiovisual material related to cancer and cancer treatment, the ACS sponsors a wide range of programs designed to provide information and psychologic support to patients and their families.

Table 18–11 summarizes some of the larger national programs available to people with breast cancer. Additional educational materials and support groups are often available through community hospitals and health care agencies. Local civic, religious, and fraternal organizations or trade unions may offer financial aid and nonmedical assistance to members and their families. These groups are often listed in the Yellow Pages under "Social Service Organizations" and include the Salvation Army, the United Way, Jewish Social Services, and Catholic Charities. The local chamber of commerce also carries listings of community groups involved in the support of cancer patients and their families. Table 18–12 provides a list of these additional oncology resources.

As patients and their families seek information about breast cancer, treatment options, and side effects, they have come to expect health care professionals to have access to, if not to be suppliers of, printed educational materials. For health care professionals, keeping abreast of accurate cancer education material is not easy. Larger hospitals often develop their own patient education materials that are specific to the cancer programs they run. Developing these materials is time consuming and costly. Fortunately, there are nationally available education materials for people with cancer and a growing amount of printed material related to breast cancer. Written materials are available free of charge. Table 18–13 is a listing of some of these publications. Public libraries and well-stocked bookstores are also sources of scientific and nonscientific works.

APPENDIX*

ANOREXIA

1. Instruct the patient to eat small, frequent, attractive meals.
2. Encourage the patient to eat a diet high in calories and protein; provide high-protein supplements, as needed.
3. Instruct patients to weigh themselves routinely; frequency determined by patients' condition.
4. Advise the patient to avoid unattractive smells and tastes, with the understanding that taste alterations may occur.
5. Provide a comfortable, nonstressful environment; encourage rest before and after meals.
6. Use nutritional consultants.

CONSTIPATION

1. Institute a bowel regimen early in the course of a program of narcotic administration or of a constipation-inducing chemotherapeutic agent.
2. Encourage a high-fiber diet and increased fluids.
3. Instruct the patient to note consistency and frequency of bowel movements and to report changes in patterns.
4. Advise the patient not to strain with bowel evacuation.

BONE MARROW DEPRESSION

1. Discuss with the patient the etiology of bone marrow depression and the possible effects of leukopenia, anemia, and thrombocytopenia. Discuss the signs and symptoms that the patient should be looking for.
2. Monitor CBC, and differential and platelet counts.
3. When the patient experiences bone marrow depression, assess the patient for signs and symptoms of infection, bleeding, and anemia.
4. Discuss the importance of the patient's role in monitoring, preventing, and decreasing the severity of complications resulting from leukopenia, anemia, and thrombocytopenia. Encourage the patient to report signs and symptoms early.
5. Prevent trauma to skin and mucous membranes. Instruct the patient to:
   a. Avoid elective dental work or surgery
   b. Avoid enemas or taking of rectal temperature
   c. Use toothettes or alternative nonabrasive dental cleaning devices
   d. Perform mouth care as indicated

---

*Adapted from Oncology Nursing Society: Cancer Chemotherapy Guidelines and Recommendations for Nursing Education and Practice. Pittsburgh, PA, 1984, pp. 4–20.

TABLE 18–11. Organizations and Programs Offering Services to Persons with Breast Cancer

Organization	*General Description*	*Services Available*
AMERICAN CANCER SOCIETY 777 Third Avenue New York, NY 10017 (212) 371-2900 Local chapters across the nation	Voluntary nonprofit organization offering programs of cancer research, education, and patient service and rehabilitation	Programs to support physical and psychologic rehabilitation of patient Patient educational materials (written and audiovisual) Transportation for treatment Equipment loans Financial assistance in purchasing medical supplies and medication Financial assistance in obtaining nursing and homemaker services
	Provides rehabilitation and support for women who have had mastectomies. Volunteers will visit hospital or home pre- and postoperatively	Information and demonstration on rehabilitative exercises Psychologic support Provides temporary prosthesis
Reconstruction Education (RENU)	Slides and coordinated audiotape describing some breast reconstruction procedures, possible complications, and decision-making process for women considering breast reconstruction	Available for loan or preview at local ACS chapters
CanSurmount	Focuses on patient and family members. Groups are composed of patient, family member, trained volunteer (also a cancer patient), and health professional	Patient and family educational services
I Can Cope	Addresses the educational and psychologic needs of people with cancer Six-week educational program covering a range of topics	Provides information and psychologic support
CANCER INFORMATION SERVICES (CIS) 1-800-4-CANCER	Toll-free telephone information and referral service for the general public, cancer patients and their families, and health professionals	Information on local and regional treatment centers, programs, and resources Printed educational materials
THE NATIONAL HOSPICE ORGANIZATION 1901 North Fort Meyer Drive Arlington, VA 22209 (703) 243-5900	Organization consisting of groups providing hospice care via in-home care or hospital-based program	Direct patient care, utilizing family as team members Family counseling Emotional and spiritual support Bereavement support for family
VISITING NURSE ASSOCIATION (VNA)	Organization providing direct nursing care to individuals in the home	Home assessment Planning and implementation of skilled nursing care program
MAKE TODAY COUNT P.O. Box 303 Burlington, Iowa 52601	More than 200 chapters consisting of patients and family members with the overall goal of living each day as fully and completely as possible	Peer emotional support
CANCER CARE, INC. and THE NATIONAL CANCER FOUNDATION 1180 6th Avenue New York, NY 10036 (212) 221-3300 (212) 221-2400 (Social Services)	Voluntary social service agency that provides professional counseling and planning to patients with advanced cancer and their families	Professional consultation and education Public education Assists with providing nursing care, homemaker services, and equipment Financial assistance
Home Health Care Agencies	Public or private organization often designed to assist patients and their families when ill at home. Services vary	Nursing care, homemaker services
Drug Companies	Often have an educational division that focuses on the educational needs of health care professionals and patients.	Information about specific drugs

TABLE 18–12. Oncology Resources

Directory of human services
Civil organizations
State and local departments of health
State and local departments of social services
Local health care organizations (hospitals, home care agencies, visiting nurse associations)
American Cancer Society
Library (MEDLARS, PDQ)
Comprehensive Cancer Center Network
Cancer Information Service (CIS), 1-800-4-CANCER
Drug companies

   e. Perform perineal care
6. Instruct the patient to avoid possible sources of infection and trauma.
   a. Encourage the patient to avoid crowds and persons with known infections.
   b. Instruct the patient to use caution when handling sharp objects, such as knives, razors, and gardening tools.
   c. Instruct the patient to wear protective gloves when gardening or engaging in other potentially traumatizing activities.
7. Advise patients to adjust their activity level to include provisions for rest periods, as needed.

TABLE 18–13. Printed Education Materials

General
Clinical Trials: What Are They All About?*
The Breast Cancer Digest*
Detection
Breast Exams! What You Should Know*
Questions and Answers About Breast Lumps*
Breast Biopsy: What You Should Know*
Treatment
Breast Cancer: Understanding Treatment Options*
Mastectomy: A Treatment for Breast Cancer*
Radiation Therapy: A Treatment for Early Stage Breast Cancer*
Radiation Therapy and You*
Adjuvant Chemotherapy: A Breast Cancer Fact Sheet*
After Breast Cancer: A Guide to Following Care*
Recurrent Disease
When Cancer Recurs: Meeting the Challenge Again*
Advanced Cancer: Living Each Day*
Rehabilitation
Breast Reconstruction: A Matter of Choice*
Breast Reconstruction†
Coping With Cancer: Support for Patients and Their Families*
Nutrition
Eating Hints: A Guide to Healthy Eating During Cancer Treatment*
Pain
Questions and Answers About Pain Control: A Guide for People With Cancer and Their Families†
Health Care Professionals
Clinical Oncology for Medical Students and Physicians†

*Available through the NCI/Cancer Information Telephone Service 1-800-4-CANCER.
†Available through the American Cancer Society.

CYSTITIS

1. Discuss with the patient the causes of cystitis induced by chemotherapy (cyclophosphamide therapy). Emphasize the importance of the patient's role in decreasing the incidence and severity of cystitis.
2. Instruct the patient in the signs and symptoms of cystitis. Encourage the patient to report symptoms early.
3. Instruct the patient to increase fluid intake to 8 to 12 glasses of fluid daily—before, during, and immediately after cyclophosphamide therapy.
4. Instruct the patient to void frequently, especially at bedtime and once during the night.
5. Instruct the patient to observe urine for color (tea-colored or red-tinged) and to note amount and frequency of voiding.
6. Instruct the patient to take all oral cyclophosphamide early in the day.

NAUSEA AND VOMITING

1. Instruct the patient to use antiemetics on a scheduled basis.
2. Premedicate with antiemetic prior to chemotherapy; instruct the patient in the same.
3. Advise the patient of the side effects of antiemetics.
4. Monitor for evidence of nausea and vomiting.
5. Observe for signs of dehydration; monitor fluid and electrolyte status.
6. Instruct the patient to report any weight loss.
7. Consider alternative approaches in order to modify nausea and vomiting—relaxation techniques, visual imagery, self-hypnosis, and music therapy.
8. If nausea is anticipatory:
   a. Provide a comfortable nonstressful environment

b. Encourage use of an antianxiety drug prior to therapy
c. Utilize relaxation techniques prior to and during therapy

SKIN CHANGES

1. Discuss the possibility of skin color changes and nail changes with the patient.
2. Discuss the impact of skin changes on the patient's body image.

VENOUS FIBROSIS PHLEBITIS

1. Assess venous status before each treatment and avoid venipuncture in the infected site.
2. Apply warm, moist heat to the inflamed area.
3. Consider additional dilution of the irritating drug.
4. Encourage the patient to report signs of pain *early*.

STOMATITIS

1. Advise dental consultation for pre-existing problems before initiating chemotherapy as indicated.
2. Assess oral mucosa as needed.
3. Instruct the patient to report oral discomfort *early*.
4. Instruct the patient to avoid irritants (e.g., alcohol, tobacco, spices, acid foods, commercial mouthwashes, and temperature extremes in food or beverages).
5. Instruct the patient in oral hygiene as indicated.
6. Instruct the patient to use a mouthwash of baking soda and water (1 tsp to 8 oz) or saline (1 tsp NaCl to 8 oz H_2O) at first sign of mouth irritation.

ALTERATIONS IN SEXUALITY

1. Discuss with the patient possible alterations in sexuality. When appropriate, include the partner in the discussion.
   a. Dyspareunia
   b. Premature menopause
   c. Increase or decrease in libido
   d. Mood changes
   e. Hirsutism
   f. Vaginal dryness
   g. Hot flashes
2. Discuss possible changes in reproductive functioning
   a. Advise patient of uncertainty of reproductive capability during chemotherapy.
   b. Provide contraceptive information to patient before initiation of chemotherapy.
   c. Discourage pregnancy during chemotherapy.
   d. Advise patient of long-term side effects and possible return of reproductive functioning.
3. Refer the patient for counseling as needed.

POTENTIAL PHYSIOLOGICAL ALTERATIONS—CARDIAC TOXICITY, HEPATIC TOXICITY, METABOLIC ALTERATIONS, NEUROTOXICITY, OTOTOXICITY, RENAL TOXICITY

1. Advise the patient of the possibility of physiologic alterations.
2. Instruct the patient to report signs or symptoms of psychologic alterations.
3. Monitor the appropriate laboratory values.

ALOPECIA

1. Discuss with the patient the onset and duration of hair loss, regrowth patterns, and temporary changes in hair texture and distribution.
2. Discuss with the patient the impact of hair loss on the patient's self-esteem.
3. Advise the patient of measures to minimize trauma to hair follicles and to delay severity of hair loss; for example, encourage patient to:
   a. Use mild shampoos

b. Use wide-tooth combs
c. Have frequent haircuts
d. Shampoo infrequently
e. Avoid permanents, chemicals, and blow-drying

4. Encourage the patient to select wigs, scarfs, and hats before hair loss occurs. Advise the patient to select wigs similar in appearance and color to natural hair or to have her hair cut in a style and length similar to her wig.

REFERENCES

Introduction

1. Oncology Nursing Society and American Nursing Association: Outcome Standards for Nursing Practice. Kansas City, MO: American Nurses Association, 1979.
2. Donovan ML, Pierce SG: Cancer Care Nursing. East Norwalk, CT: Appleton-Century-Crofts, 1976.

Detection and Diagnosis

3. Algna SW, Reddy DM: Predictors of proficient technique and successful lesion detection in breast self-examination. Unpublished manuscript, 1982.
4. Trotta P: Breast self-examination: Factors influencing compliance. Oncol Nurs Forum 7:13, 1980.
5. Scott DW: Anxiety, critical thinking and information processing during and after breast biopsy. Nurs Res 32:24, 1983.
6. Frank-Stromberg M, Wright PS, Segalla J, et al.: Psychological impact of the cancer diagnosis. Oncol Nurs Forum 11:16, 1984.

Surgery: Mastectomy

7. Carroll RM: The impact of mastectomy on body image. Oncol Nurs Forum 8:29, 1981.
8. Luckman J, Sorenson KC: Medical Surgical Nursing. Philadelphia: W.B. Saunders Co., 1974, p. 317.
9. Lindsey A, Norbeck J, Carrier V, et al.: Social support and health outcomes in postmastectomy women: A review. Cancer Nurs 4:377, 1981.
10. Bard M, Sutherland AM: Psychological impact of cancer and its treatment; adaptation to radical mastectomy. Cancer 8:656, 1955.
11. Woods N, Earp JA: Women with cured breast cancer. Nurs Res 27:279, 1978.
12. Maguire P, Brooke M, Tait A, et al.: The effect of counselling on physical disability and social recovery after mastectomy. Clin Oncol 9:319, 1983.
13. Silverman JJ, Cohen IK: Psychological aspects of breast cancer and reconstructive surgery. Va Med 106:140, 1979.
14. Cage C (ed.): The Breast Cancer Digest. Bethesda, MD: U.S. Department of Health and Human Services, 1984.
15. Markowski J, Wilcox J, Helm P: Lymphedema incidence after specific postmastectomy therapy. Arch Phys Med Rehabil 62:449, 1981.
16. Morris T, Greer S, White P: Psychological and social adjustment to mastectomy. Cancer 40:2381, 1977.

Surgery: Reconstruction

17. Dowden RV, McCraw JB, Dibbell DG: The breast reconstruction patient and her health insurance carrier. JAMA 242:2779, 1979.
18. Kushner R: Why Me? Philadelphia: W.B. Saunders Co., 1982, p. 295.

Radiation Therapy

19. Hilderly L: Skin care in radiation therapy. Oncol Nurs Forum 10:51, 1983.
20. Phillips T: Principles of radiobiology and radiation therapy. *In*: Carter S, Glatstein E, Livingston R (eds.): Principles of Cancer Treatment. New York: McGraw-Hill, 1982.
21. Schwade J, Lichter AS: Management of acute effects of radiation therapy. *In*: Carter S, Glatstein E, Livingston R (eds.): Principles of Cancer Treatment. New York: McGraw-Hill, 1982.
22. Yasko JM: Care of the client receiving external radiation therapy. Reston, VA: Reston Publishing Co., Inc., 1982.
23. Hassey KM, Rose CM: Altered skin integrity in patients receiving radiation therapy. Oncol Nurs Forum 9:44, 1982.

Chemotherapy

24. Goodman MS, Wickham R: Venous access devices: An overview. Oncol Nurs Forum 11:16, 1983.
25. Oncology Nursing Society: Cancer Chemotherapy Guidelines and Recommendations for Nursing Education and Practice. Pittsburgh, PA, 1984, pp. 4–20.

Recurrence

26. Chekryn J: Cancer recurrence: Personal memo and communication, and marital adjustment. Cancer Nur 7:491, 1984.
27. Schmale AH: Psychological reactions to recurrences, metastases or disseminated cancer. Int J Radiat Oncol Biol Phys 1:515, 1976.
28. Northouse LL: Mastectomy patients and the fear of recurrence. Cancer Nurs 4:213, 1981.
29. Scott DW: The psychodynamics of multiple remissions in a patient with acute nonlymphoblastic leukemia. Cancer Nurs 6:201, 1983.
30. Frank-Stromberg M, Wright P: Ambulatory cancer patients' perception of the physical and psychosocial changes in their lives since the diagnosis of cancer. Cancer Nurs 7:117, 1984.
31. Lewis FM: Family level services for the cancer patient: Critical distinctions, fallacies, and assessment. Cancer Nurs 6:193, 1983.
32. Kübler-Ross E: On Death and Dying. New York: Macmillan Publishing Co., 1969.
33. Holland JC, Mastrovito R: Psychological adaptation to breast cancer. Cancer 46:1045, 1980.
34. Jamison K, Wellisch D, Pasnau R: Psychological aspects of mastectomy: I. the woman's perspective; II. the man's perspective. Am J Psychiat 135:432–436, 543–546, 1978.
35. Weisman AD, Worden JW: The existential plight in cancer: Significance of the first 100 days. Int J Psychiatr Med 7:1, 1976–77.

Nutrition

36. Donaldson DD, Lenon DA: Alterations in nutritional status. Cancer 43:2036, 1979.

37. Knox L: Nutrition and cancer. Nurs Clin North Am 18:97, 1983.
38. Donoghue M, Nunnally C, Yasko J: Nutritional Aspects of Cancer Care. Reston, VA: Reston Publishing Co., Inc., 1982.
39. Knopf MK, Mullen JC, Xistris D, et al.: Weight gain in women with breast cancer receiving adjuvant chemotherapy. Oncol Nurs Forum 10:28, 1983.
40. Huntington MO: Weight gain in patients receiving adjuvant chemotherapy for carcinoma of the breast. Cancer 56:472, 1985.
41. Dixon J, Moritz DA, Baker TL: Breast cancer and weight gain: An unexpected finding. Oncol Nurs Forum 5:5, 1978.
42. Lippman ME: An assessment of current achievements in the systemic management of breast cancer. Breast Cancer Res Treat 4:69, 1984.

Family

43. Hampe SO: Needs of the grieving spouse in a hospital setting. Nurs Res 24:332, 1976.
44. Freihofer P, Felton G: Nursing behaviors in bereavement: An exploratory study. Nurs Res 25:332, 1976.
45. Constantino RE: Bereavement crisis intervention for widows in grief and mourning. Nurs Res 30:351, 1981.
46. Giaquinta B: Helping families face the crisis of cancer. Am J Nurs 77:1585, 1977.
47. Wright K, Dyck S: Expressed concerns of adult cancer patients' family members. Cancer Nurs 7:371, 1984.
48. Johnson JL, Norby PA: We Can Weekend: A program for cancer families. Cancer Nurs 4:23, 1981.
49. Northouse L: The impact of cancer on the family: An overview. Int J Psychiatr Med 14:215, 1984.

Community Resources and Educational Materials

50. Blumberg B, Flaherty M: Services available to persons with cancer. JAMA 224:1715, 1980.

Pain

51. Christensen K, Blichert-Taft M, Giersing U, et al.: Phantom breast syndrome in young women after mastectomy for breast cancer. Acta Chir Scand 148:351, 1982.

Statistical Considerations in the Design and Interpretation of Clinical Trials

MARGARET N. WESLEY, Ph.D.
BRENDA K. EDWARDS, Ph.D.

A clinical trial is the application of the scientific method of controlled experimentation to clinical medicine. Patients are asked to undergo tests or treatments that may not benefit them directly. Because of the complexity of delivering a specified method of care and, most of all, the ethical considerations of using human beings as experimental subjects, we must make sure that the trial is properly conducted, addresses a question of clinical importance, and adds significantly to our knowledge. To accomplish this, the investigator must know not only the latest laboratory and clinical results but also the methods of design and analysis of clinical trials. Practitioners must understand many of the same principles if they are to evaluate reports of clinical trials and to make informed decisions of whether new treatments should be incorporated into standard patient care.

This chapter cannot present a comprehensive coverage of all the statistical issues involved in clinical trials. Instead, we hope to touch on the issues critical to understanding and evaluating clinical trials. The reader is referred to the appropriate references for technical and computational details.

DESIGN AND IMPLEMENTATION

Important questions concerning the appropriate treatment and management of patients with breast cancer have been posed and answered through conduct of clinical trials. Controlled therapeutic trials in breast cancer, including multi-institutional cooperative studies, have been conducted since 1950. However, the decade of the 1970's is recognized as the turning point in clinical trials history, especially for oncology and cardiovascular diseases, with the initiation of several large-scale studies funded by the National Institutes of Health.

19

The basic principles of such research studies can be found in several texts.[13, 25] The first step is to decide on a well-defined purpose for the study, usually stated in terms of a hypothesis to be tested. Once this has been accomplished, the study plan must be laid out, usually in the form of a written protocol, before any patients can be entered. The proper implementation of a clinical trial hinges on good planning and organization as well as a team of dedicated personnel. As the trial progresses to completion, the data are analyzed, results are interpreted, and conclusions are made, based on accurate and complete information.

The design and implementation issues discussed in this section will highlight contemporary concepts in the methodology of clinical trials, including certain controversial topics. Discussions of the basic principles of trial design and implementation can be found in the texts previously cited and in some oncology texts as well.[31] The concepts discussed here will be illustrated with examples drawn from studies of the treatment of women with early-stage cancer as well as with advanced disease.

Comparison Group

Implicit in the evaluation of a new treatment regimen is the need for comparison with a group of control subjects receiving another treatment, usually the standard or conventional regimen. For a trial to be fair and objective, the comparison must be of results obtained from treating patients who are similar in terms of the factors that affect response to treatment. Outcome must be measured according to similar definitions and procedures, so that any difference in efficacy can be attributed solely to the effects of the respective treatments. This idea is basic to a scientific method of study.

Historical Control Subjects. Frequently, clinicians compare results from patients being treated on a promising new regimen with those from historical control subjects, usually obtained from patients previously treated by the same group of investigators or from published results in the literature. Supporters of these studies believe that they can be of value if carefully conducted and properly analyzed; others cite numerous examples of how conclusions from such studies can be biased and are therefore invalid. The major problem is that one is unable to ensure comparability between the groups of patients and the methods of evaluating treatment response.

Sources of bias in historical studies arise from differences in patient selection, the external circumstances surrounding patient management, and the quality of information available for analysis as well as potential changes in the natural history of the disease. Differences in patient characteristics, such as extent of disease, performance status, and prior therapy, can account for differences in treatment response. Patients treated on a promising new regimen may have been selected consciously or unconsciously because they were less seriously ill and therefore more likely to respond to the new treatment. Circumstances surrounding patient management, such as improvements in supportive care, surgery, and surgical pathology, change over time, as do criteria for defining and interpreting patient characteristics and for measuring response to treatment. Retrospective abstraction of information on patient characteristics and management for historical control subjects is often difficult and yields incomplete data or leads to great uncertainty regarding the accuracy of the data.

Even in situations in which bias should be minimal (for example, using the same treatment in consecutive trials within the same organization), cautious interpretation of results is required. The extent to which changes in patient characteristics that strongly influence outcome can occur over time in the same study is illustrated by data from a large seven-year multi-institutional trial in prostate cancer.[5] For patients entered during the last two and one-half years of the trial, analysis of results showed no survival difference between placebo and estrogen therapy, but a comparison of placebo patients in the first two and one-half years with estrogen patients in the last two and one-half years showed a significant improvement in survival for the estrogen patients ($p < 0.01$)! The protocol had not changed, but the earlier half of the study had a greater proportion of older patients with poor performance status. A review[23] of studies from three cancer cooperative groups identified 19 pairs of trials with over 100 patients per treatment for which it was possible to compare the annual death rate of two consecutive groups receiving the same treatment. Differences ranged from −46 percent to +24 percent, and in four comparisons the change was statistically significant ($p < 0.05$). Farewell and D'Angio[11] used data from a subset of patients with a common treatment arm in the first as well as in the second National Wilms' Tumor Study to illustrate how substantial differences in conclusions can result from a fully randomized study compared with one using historical control subjects.

Complex statistical analyses that allow for differences in patient characteristics among treatment groups may be used to overcome some limitations of these studies. However, such statistical adjustments are usually unsatisfactory because of inadequacies in the quality of data and the inability to adjust for factors that have not been measured or are unknown (e.g., changes in circumstances surrounding patient management). To a lesser extent, the mathematical form and assumptions required for the analytical technique may detract from the clinician's intuition regarding, and confidence in, the interpretation of results. Techniques that match each patient on the new treatment with one or more historical control patients who are similar with respect to major prognostic factors have similar limitations; additional questions are raised by the subjective aspects of the matching procedures.

Studies with historical control subjects can never be interpreted with the same degree of confidence as a properly conducted randomized controlled trial. Use of concurrent control subjects is preferable in the design of clinical trials, with the possible exception of situations in which the disease progresses rapidly and is fatal and in which no effective therapy is available.

Randomized Control Subjects. Randomization is a method to ensure that the variability in patient characteristics, which may affect the outcome of treatment among the treatment groups, is distributed in a way that can be handled by statistical techniques. In clinical investigations, randomization refers to the assignment of treatments using a chance procedure that does not depend on the patient's characteristics. Randomization tends to balance experimental groups on all factors, known or unknown, that may influence outcome. Also, random assignment provides a firm basis for statistical evaluation of apparent observed treatment effects and eliminates bias in the selection of patients for the different treatments.

Randomization does not *guarantee* that treatment groups are balanced with respect to prognostic factors strongly associated with outcome or with respect to the number of subjects per group. However, imbalances in prognostic factors are due to random variability, not selection biases, and can be dealt with statistically.

Imbalances in the number of subjects per group can occur in studies with small numbers of patients; it is seldom a problem for moderate-size to large-size trials. If possible imbalances in the number of patients assigned to the treatment groups are anticipated, one can use *balanced block* or *restricted block randomization,* a technique for implementing random assignments that limits the extent to which such imbalances can occur. Within small blocks of patients (e.g., six or eight), the number of patients assigned to each treatment is forced to a specified proportion.

Stratification is a technique that can be used both in the design of randomized clinical trials and in the analysis of data from various study designs. Patients are first classified into subsets (or strata). Factors known to have a strong influence on response (e.g., menopausal status or extent of disease) can be taken into account by randomizing patients within strata defined by these factors, usually with a balanced block design. For multi-institutional studies, it is frequently useful to consider the institution as a stratifying factor.

When the number of factors and resulting combination of strata of patients becomes large relative to the total number of patients, the expected number of patients in any stratum is likely to be quite small. The randomization is likely to remain valid; however, the benefits of stratification are largely nullified. Unless stratification is limited to relatively few strata, preferably involving factors that have a strong impact on treatment outcome, significant imbalances in the number of patients on each of the treatments can occur across all factors as well as within each stratum. This problem can be overcome by using procedures that tend to correct imbalances in treatment assignments existing at the time of each randomization. The probability of assignment to a treatment group may depend on the number of subjects randomized to each treatment (*adaptive allocation*) or may depend on a function that measures the extent to which imbalances exist within each stratification factor (*minimization allocation*).

Although statistical gains in improving the precision of treatment comparisons are usually modest, a pragmatic reason for stratified randomization is that it improves the treatment balance in numbers of patients per treatment for the variables that are most commonly thought to influence outcome. Conclusions derived from a simple presentation of results for comparable treatment groups are often more convincing than a statistically complicated analysis and are also useful in situations in which many clinics contribute a few patients each. However, stratification according to factors that are either ambiguous or subject to error, such as the often quoted 30 percent error in assessment of clinical nodal status for breast cancer patients, should be avoided.

Unequal Randomization. There are situations in which it is appropriate to randomize patients to the various treatment regimens with unequal allocation, such as two to one, or three to two. Assignment in proportions of three to one or other assignments that are more extreme are undesirable because of considerable loss in the ability to detect differences in treatment groups when such disparities truly exist. Unequal allocation may be used in situations in which one of the treatments is a standard regimen, the therapeutic outcome is fairly well established, and interest is primarily focused on obtaining a more accurate estimate of efficacy and perhaps gaining a better idea of the toxicities of the new regimen. In trials with three regimens, including one therapy at two dose levels, or a third drug given to a portion of these patients, unequal allocation may be considered either because results of each of the two new regimens are to be compared with those of the standard or control group or because one wishes to minimize the number of subjects assigned to the standard regimen. In trials in which one treatment may be much more costly than the others, a smaller proportion of patients may be randomized to the costly regimen in order to conserve research funds. However, treatment groups of equal size usually provide the most efficient means of comparison and estimation of treatment effects. In general, unless there are compelling reasons to do otherwise, equal allocation is recommended.

Randomized Consent Design

Randomized controlled trials are not easy to conduct. Additional clinical effort is required to adequately describe the trial to potential participants, determine eligibility, obtain informed consent, manage the patient in accordance with protocol requirements, and collect data in a timely and consistent manner. Often, informed consent is viewed as an obstacle both for the clinician, who must admit ignorance regarding the best choice of treatment, and for the patient, who must agree to the trial without knowing which treatment she will receive.

Zelen[32] has proposed a study design called *randomized consent*, with the intent of making informed consent more acceptable to the clinicians and to increase the participation rate in randomized trials. Several variations of this design have been described; most involve the comparison of a standard or control treatment with an experimental regimen. On the surface, this design differs from the conventional approach only in the timing of randomization and obtaining consent to participate in the trial. Figure 19–1 provides three schemata for randomized trials: *A*, the conventional design, *B*, the Zelen design for randomized consent, and *C*, a variation of the randomized consent design used in some cancer therapeutic trials. Only the conventional design is applicable for blinded studies, but such studies are seldom possible for cancer treatment trials. In schema *A*, patients are first determined to be eligible for a specific protocol, and then treatment options are described by the clinician and consent to participate is obtained; randomization occurs only for those who agree to enter the trial, and these patients are then treated according to their assigned therapy.

For randomized consent designs, all eligible patients are randomly assigned a treatment. Then, the clinician explains treatment options to the patient, informs her of the therapy that she has been assigned, and seeks her consent to participate in the trial. She receives the assigned treatment only if she consents; otherwise she may choose an alternative therapy. As originally proposed, a typical situation for the randomized consent design would be that in which a standard treatment or patient management strategy exists and a method is needed for selecting patients who would be offered an

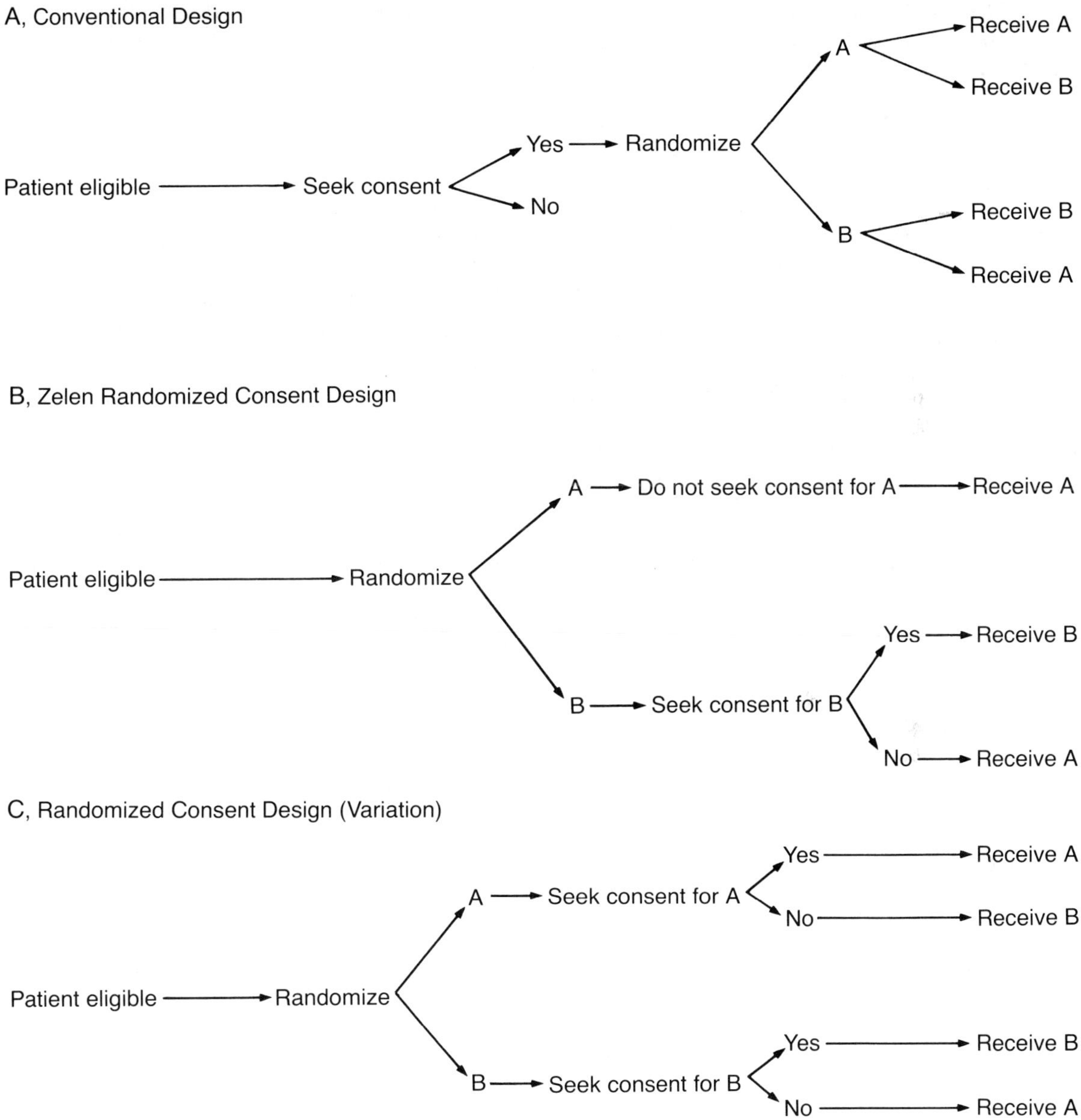

FIGURE 19–1. Schematic illustration for three types of randomized clinical trial designs.

investigational treatment or new management plan. The justification is that a patient's consent need be sought only after randomization has provisionally assigned her to the new treatment, since if she were not in the trial, she would have received the standard therapy anyway.

A breast cancer screening trial initiated in 1960 by the Health Insurance Plan (HIP) of New York[27, 28] illustrates the situation in which schema *B* has been applied, although the study was designed 20 years prior to published discussion of the concept. Approximately 60,000 women aged 30 to 64 years were randomized to receive either standard medical care or periodic screening with mammography and clinical examination. Consent to participate in the study was obtained only from those who came for screening.

Several large multi-institutional cancer therapy trials[10] have implemented schema *C*, in which patients in both treatment groups are informed of the regimen assigned to them and consent to participate is obtained from all patients. Clinicians tend to prefer explaining investigational studies when they know the treatment assigned for a patient; the decision to participate may be easier for the patient to make when she can focus on a known treatment assignment. This could result in accelerated patient accrual and could allow the trial to proceed to a timely conclusion. On the other hand, ethical concerns about the informed consent process have arisen; the physician may tailor the information regarding treatment options to emphasize the regimen selected for that woman, perhaps even omitting the fact that selection resulted from randomization.

There are other liabilities with the randomized consent design. Analysis of trial results is based on the treatment outcome for all randomized patients according to the *assigned* group, regardless of whether the patient actually received the assigned therapy. In many circumstances, those who refuse a treatment assignment receive the comparison therapy. The rule "analyze as randomized" is required as part of the theory for statistical inference and hypothesis testing. Thus, estimates of treatment effects are diluted, because of the inclusion of information on patients assigned to a treatment who never receive the assigned therapy. The magnitude of this effect depends on the proportions of patients who refuse their respective treatment assignments. This dilution also occurs in studies with conventional study designs, but the proportion is likely to be larger for studies with randomized consent designs. To offset the apparent blending of treatment effects requires an increase in the total number of randomized patients. Under some simplifying assumptions, it can be shown that the number of randomized patients is increased by a factor of

$$\frac{1}{(1 - r_s - r_t)^2}$$

where r_s and r_t are the respective proportions of patients assigned to the standard and test regimens who refuse to receive their assigned therapy. Thus, if as few as 10 percent of randomized patients in each group fall into this category, the number of subjects who must be studied increases by 56 percent, compared with having no dropouts or crossovers. Of course, there is the temptation to analyze individuals according to the treatment they actually received. This is likely to introduce bias into the results, since patients who accept a specific treatment option may differ in important prognostic characteristics from those who refuse the treatment. Those who refuse entry into the experimental arm of the trial may have either a better or a worse prognosis than those who accept, depending on whether the disease is minimal or advanced and on whether the treatment is aggressive or conservative.

The role of randomized consent design trials in cancer treatment has not been fully evaluated at this time. During the first year of patient accrual in the NCI randomized trial for treatment of early-stage breast cancer, serious consideration was given to switching to a randomized consent design in order to boost accrual. The underlying problem was a low yield of interested patients who would agree to randomization, reflecting contemporary attitudes of increased patient participation in decisions affecting patient management. However, careful discussions of potential benefits and limitations dissuaded the investigators from changing the design, because the anticipated proportion of patients refusing their assigned treatment would seriously compromise the comparison of true treatment effects and require substantial increases in sample size. Future experience with this design will provide insight into its usefulness in various clinical research situations.

Sample Size Considerations: The Scope of the Trial

A critical aspect of clinical trial planning is the calculation of the number of patients who must be studied to achieve certain goals. Sample size considerations are also relevant in the evaluation and interpretation of study results. Delegating this part of the study design to a statistician during the final planning sessions often leads to frustration and misunderstanding. Such considerations extend beyond merely using a formula to calculate a number; important decisions regarding the reasonableness of assumptions and parameter values, and the determination of a clinically meaningful difference in efficacy, need to be discussed among all the study investigators. These estimates are never absolutely correct because much of the information required for accurate calculations is not known when the estimation must be made. Such estimates can provide a reasonable guide as to what can be achieved by a clinical trial or whether a much larger effort will have to be mounted.

Sample size evaluation for a clinical trial tends to be a compromise between available resources and the study objectives. Resources, such as the number of available patients, medical personnel, facilities, and funds for implementing a clinical trial, usually influence the number of therapies to be compared and the total number of patients to be studied. Trials involving more than two regimens are more efficient than a series of two-treatment trials, since comparisons between any two treatments can be made. However, a simple comparative study of the two most interesting regimens requires the smallest number of patients, and these results are known at an earlier date.

Renewed interest in the use of *factorial designs* for clinical trials,[6] particularly cancer prevention studies, may lead to the application of more efficient designs in cancer treatment. Factorial designs, which investigate several factors in the same study, are efficient because every observation simultaneously provides information on all factors and on the relationship between effects of different factors. In cancer treatment trials, a factor may be chemotherapy, radiation therapy, immunotherapy, or other modalities. The trial may be designed to study the presence or absence of a factor, dose levels of a factor, or, perhaps, methods of administering a factor (e.g., intravenous versus oral). For a balanced factorial design to be feasible, it must be possible to administer each therapy simultaneously in some patients without alteration in intensity, a condition that may not exist when investigating multiple chemotherapeutic agents or chemotherapy and radiation therapy. Fractional factorial designs, which allow omission of certain combinations of factors, may prove useful in these circumstances.

Sample size considerations are illustrated here for the case in which treatment outcome is summarized by a simple proportion, such as the percentage of patients who achieve a partial or complete response. Suppose two chemotherapy regimens, a standard (S) and a test (T), are to be compared by a randomized clinical trial among patients with an initial diagnosis of advanced breast cancer. Sample size considerations begin by specifying relevant statistical procedures and parameter assumptions for testing a hypothesis defined by the main study objective. Suppose the primary end point is the proportion of patients who achieve a partial or complete response. A test statistic for two independent samples is chosen; the null hypothesis (H) is that there is no difference in response for the two regimens. The null hypothesis is never proved or disproved, but the study seeks to accumulate evidence that would make the null hypothesis appear highly unlikely.

Parameter assumptions are of two types. First are those substantive assumptions that quantitatively define a clinically meaningful result. For this example, assume that approximately 40 percent (p_s) of patients receiving the standard treatment S respond to therapy; further, assume that the test therapy T must yield at least a 60 percent (p_t) response, a 20 percent absolute improvement, to be clinically important. Implicit in this assumption is the alternative hypothesis (A): T is better than S; that is, only this one-sided difference is of interest. Second are those assumptions that quantitate the amount of error, associated with interpretation of the data, that investigators are willing to make. A Type I error (α) is made if we conclude that there is a difference in response to the two therapies when in fact they are equal. A Type II error (β) is made if we conclude there is no difference in the two therapies when in fact regimen T is better. The power of the test against the specified alternative of a 20 percent improvement in response for patients treated with regimen T is $1 - \beta$, the probability that the observations will result in a significant test statistic. Of course, it is desirable that both types of errors be very small, but this will increase the number of patients required. Typical, but nonetheless arbitrary, values are $\alpha = 0.05$ and $\beta = 0.10$. Sample size estimates for this example, using these assumptions and the formula presented in Figure 19–2, are approximately 103 women randomized to each regimen, for a total sample size of 206 patients.

Certain clinical trials are designed to show whether a new therapy is as effective as a standard therapy but not necessarily more effective.[3] An example would be the evaluation of a conservative therapy that is psychologically more tolerable or less debilitating but is similar in efficacy to the standard regimen. The NCI randomized trial in early-stage breast cancer was designed to investigate whether conservative treatment (lumpectomy, axillary dissection, and radiation therapy) is as effective as mastectomy with axillary dissection. Formulation of the hypothesis to be tested and derivation of the sample size are relatively straightforward, but confusion can occur. The usual null hypothesis of equality is inappropriate, since an infinite amount of information would be required to rule out the smallest imaginable difference in response between the two regimens. Such studies can only be designed to test whether the difference in response is less than some specified amount. The appropriate null hypothesis (H′) is that the standard therapy is better than the test therapy by at least some specified amount (d). One cannot show exact equality between the therapies, only that the difference is less than some specified amount.

Sample size formulas (Fig. 19–2) corresponding to the two null hypotheses (H and H′) differ slightly; sample size requirements may be larger for either of the strategies, depending on the chosen parameter values. If there is interest in rejecting a relatively small difference in treatments, the required sample size may be quite large. If the difference (d) is small but similar in magnitude to

Conventional Null Hypothesis (H)

$$\frac{(z_{1-\alpha} + z_{1-\beta})^2 \cdot [p_t(1 - p_t) + p_s(1 - p_s)]}{(p_s - p_t)^2}$$

for $p_t > p_s$

Hypothesis of a Specified Difference (H′)

$$\frac{(z_{1-\alpha} + z_{1-\beta})^2 \cdot [p_t(1 - p_t) + p_s(1 - p_s)]}{(p_s - p_t - d)^2}$$

for $p_s - p_t < d$

Example: $\alpha = 0.05$, $\beta = 0.10$

p_t	p_s	2n
0.9	0.7	130
0.6	0.4	206
0.4	0.2	172

p_t	p_s	d	2n
0.9	0.9	0.2	78
0.6	0.6	0.2	206
0.4	0.4	0.2	206
0.8	0.9	0.2	430
0.4	0.3	0.2	772
0.5	0.6	0.2	840

FIGURE 19–2. Sample size considerations for testing hypotheses of differences in two proportions under the null and the non-null hypotheses. The true response proportions for the standard and test regimens are p_s and p_t, respectively; $z_{1-\alpha}$ and $z_{1-\beta}$ are upper percentage points of the standard normal distribution; and 2n is the total sample size to be divided equally between the two groups.

the true difference in the two responses ($p_s - p_t$), the required sample size may also be quite large. Thus, in the prior example, if the two treatments truly have the same response rate of 60 percent and evidence is needed to rule out a difference in the two treatment responses of 20 percent (i.e., the standard therapy is not more than 20 percentage points better than the test therapy), 206 patients are required. However, if the true response rates for the two treatments are 60 percent for standard and 50 percent for test, 840 patients are required.

An assessment of the power of the test[16] is critical in the design phase, especially in small studies. If there is a clinically significant difference in treatment effects but an insufficient sample size, one might falsely conclude that there is no difference between the treatments because the test had power only when large differences existed.

Study Population

Every clinical trial needs to have a clear, precise, written description of the patients who are eligible for inclusion in the study and how eligibility is to be quantitatively documented. Exclusion criteria must also be explicitly specified. The clinician must be thoroughly familiar with the criteria for patient eligibility in a protocol, including the diagnostic and staging procedures required to evaluate eligibility.

Specification of eligibility criteria often involves judgments about the influence of patient attributes on treatment outcome. Restrictions placed on the subset of patients eligible for a clinical trial are aimed at defining a fairly homogeneous study population, thereby reducing the variability in treatment outcome resulting from extraneous factors and improving the probability of observing a treatment effect. For randomized Phase III therapeutic trials, the effect of patient heterogeneity can be minimized through stratification on prognostic factors, statistical analysis techniques that adjust for covariables, and increases in the sample size to allow for the inherent variability in outcome from unknown or uncontrollable factors. For Phase II trials in women with advanced breast disease, factors other than patient homogeneity must be considered. The extent of prior treatment and subsequent failures must be minimized; otherwise, the probability of a woman's responding to a new therapy will be negligible.

It is necessary not only to define the subset of patients who constitute the study population but also to clearly define which patients are to be included in the analysis of the study. Exclusion of certain patients from analysis is a matter of dispute among clinicians and statisticians.[14] Removal of cases from the analyzed data can lead to biases and can have an impact on the interpretation of study results. Generally, the exclusion of cases based on errors in objective data measured prior to entry—for example, the number of prior therapies, age, and receptor status—is seldom challenged. However, the deletion of cases because of errors in subjective data, such as performance status, or because of events that occur after entry, such as early recurrence, may be differentially related to treatment effectiveness and lead to biases. Published studies must account for *all* randomized patients—patients included in the analyses and patients excluded from the analyses—and for the reasons for each exclusion. Any published analyses based on a subset of patients should be interpreted with caution.

Outcome Measures

Assessment of each patient's disease state after therapy is started needs to be done in an objective, consistent, and accurate manner so that the trial provides meaningful results. Procedures that are used to measure treatment outcomes need to be defined in the protocol; attention should also be given to periodic review of the thoroughness with which these procedures are being followed. In general, patient evaluation in a clinical trial requires tighter control than would typically occur in general clinical practice.

Measurements must be taken prior to initiation of treatment and then at repeated intervals specified in the protocol. The frequency with which measurements are taken should be comparable for patients in each treatment group. The primary criteria that are used to define outcome should be stated clearly in the protocol and this definition applied to all patients. Typical measures of treatment efficacy and side effects include (1) tumor regression, a partial or complete reduction in tumor size, which requires measurable disease; (2) duration of tumor response; (3) time to disease progression; (4) survival time; (5) occurrence of toxicity; and (6) change in quality of life.

In some cases, reliable and reproducible measurements of patients are difficult to obtain because of inherent variations in measurements made by different observers. A study designed to investigate the accuracy and variability of clinical tumor measurements[20] illustrates some of these problems. Twelve solid spheres of varying diameters were arranged in random order on a soft mattress and were covered with a sheet of foam. There were two pairs of spheres of equal size. Sixteen experienced oncologists measured each sphere. When measurements of the two pairs of equivalent spheres were compared, a 5 to 10 percent objective response rate (using the criterion of a 50 percent reduction in size) was found.

Several approaches may be used to control observer variation, such as using the same individual to record all information, taking multiple measurements and reporting the average, and consensus review for the classification of outcome. One means for obtaining a fair and unbiased assessment is through blinded evaluation, in which those persons responsible for clinical assessment are kept unaware of which treatment the patient is receiving. Measures of treatment outcome that are difficult to quantitate or that have little or no meaningful benefit to the patient should be avoided entirely.

Factors such as nonadherence to the prescribed therapy, patient dropout before therapy is completed, lack of control of factors related to measurement of the outcome, and absence of a uniform standard procedure for assessment of the outcome will increase variability of the outcome measurement and reduce the power of the statistical test to detect differences. Clinical trials are complex research activities that require not only careful planning but also diligent execution.

Data Management

One of the less exciting features of implementing clinical trials is the design and development of manual and electronic systems for collecting information. However, data forms and procedures for capturing important information in a complete and thorough manner are essential to the conduct of a clinical trial. The approach to data management must become more formalized as the number of participating investigators and clinics increases. Training is required for individuals responsible for collecting and recording information, as is continuous monitoring of both the procedures at each of the clinical sites and the quality of data received from multiple sources. The primary purpose of these training and monitoring activities is to collect reliable and valid data in a timely manner and to correct any problems or errors as they occur. For a more detailed discussion of the coordination of clinical trials, see the work of Lavin.[17]

STATISTICAL ANALYSIS

In this section, a basic overview and understanding of the most commonly used statistical procedures are provided.

Many of the considerations of the previous section assume critical importance if we are to apply statistical techniques to the data collected. A typical clinical trial generates a large amount of data. The purpose of applying statistical techniques is to reduce the data to a smaller set of numbers, which is more readily comprehended. The goal of the statistical analysis is to summarize the data without distorting them and to provide an indication of how accurately these data describe the "real world."

Statistical analysis is based on a simplified view of the world. We assume that we are interested in drawing conclusions about a very large, in fact infinite, population. There exists a "true" state of nature, which we could discover if only we could observe the entire population. This true state of nature is usually given a mathematical definition in terms of a distribution. For any possible observation, the mathematical cumulative distribution function gives the probability of observing any value less than or equal to that observation. This distribution remains constant. However, we are limited to observing a small part of the population, called the sample. There is variability associated with sampling. As different samples are drawn at random, the observations change, and so do the results of the statistical procedures. If there were no variation, statistics would be unnecessary.

If our sample is selected in an unbiased (i.e., random) way, we can make good guesses about the general population or compare this population with others from which we have observed similar unbiased samples. If the sample is not random or unbiased, there is very little that can be said about the population as a whole, and we are limited to statements about the sample. It may be possible to make some inferences about the population from which the sample was drawn, but conclusions comparing this group with another may not be reliable. In real life, there are many sources of variation besides sampling, but the key to the validity of the statistical procedures is the absence of bias in the observations.

Another concept essential to an understanding of statistics is that the individual observations in the sample must be *independent* for most statistical procedures to apply. The term independence has a strict mathematical definition, but in rough terms, it means that an observation on one unit of the sample does not even partially determine another unit's value; for example, suppose we are trying to determine the probability that a chemotherapy regimen can be administered at full dosage. We have a small group of patients at various points in their therapy. What should be used as the unit of measurement? Observations on each cycle are clearly not independent. A patient who is going to receive markedly reduced dosage will probably receive reduced dosage on each cycle. If these patients tend to complete fewer cycles, the estimate could be biased. If individual patients are used as the sampling units, the assumption of independence is more accurate, although other issues may still affect the analysis.

A number of books for the general public[26] have emphasized that a well-informed patient who participates in her medical care will benefit by a better understanding of treatment decisions and outcomes. Similarly, the investigator who understands the statistical manipulations of the data and participates in the data analysis will be better able to interpret the data from a clinical perspective and to improve patient care. Patients should not view their physicians as gods, and physicians should not view their statisticians as gods. Data analyses performed should make sense to the study investigator. If they do not, a better explanation or a simpler analysis that verifies the complex one is in order.

Statistical tools can be divided into two categories: *estimation* and *hypothesis testing*. These tools are developed using various models of the real world. Parametric models assume a particular mathematical form for the function describing the distribution of values in the population. The method is developed to be optimal for this particular distribution; for example, the mathematical function describing the derivative of the normal cumulative distribution function, called the density function (the bell-shaped curve), is

$$f(x) = \frac{1}{\sigma\sqrt{(2\pi)}} \exp\left\{-\frac{(x-\mu)^2}{2\sigma^2}\right\}$$

where μ and σ are the true but usually unknown parameters defining this distribution. A nonparametric model does not assume a specific function for the distribution but instead relies on the order or the ranks the observations would take, given a general shape of the density function (e.g., symmetric and unimodal).

Estimation

In estimation, we seek to describe the population of interest, using observations of the sample. Some examples of parameters we might want to estimate are average age, estrogen receptor value not exceeded by 95 percent of the population, or average length of survival following initial diagnosis.

An estimate is simply a guess at the value of a parameter and, hence, cannot really be said to be right or wrong. However, statisticians have classified estimates as better or worse, according to the following criteria:

1. If we sample the same number of people again and again from a very large population, the average of these estimates should get closer and closer to the true population value.
2. If we increase the sample size to a larger and larger number, the estimate should get closer and closer to the true population value.

Occasionally an ad hoc estimate (for example, a new way of calculating the mean), often derived after examination of the data, is proposed for a particular set of observations. Such estimates have generally not been

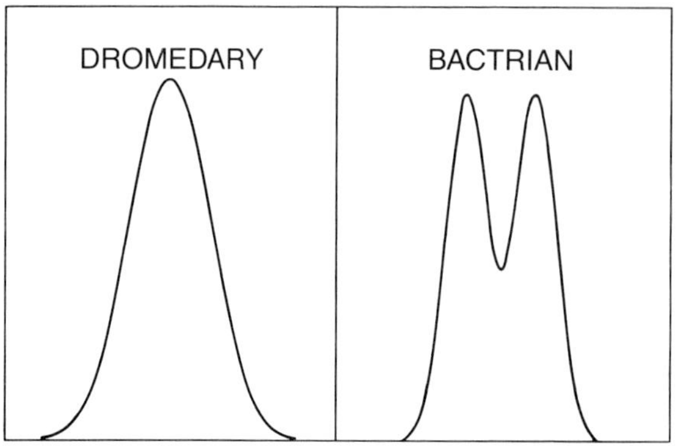

FIGURE 19–3. The general shape of a dromedary versus a Bactrian camel (also called unimodal and bimodal density functions).

compared with other standard estimates according to the aforementioned criteria and should be regarded with caution unless they have been shown to have good statistical properties. Otherwise, ad hoc estimates may or may not work well for the particular data set.

Care should be taken that the estimate provides an appropriate description of the population; for example, if we are measuring the mass of camels' backs (excluding the legs) and use as a summary statistic the point between the tail and neck that has a mass equal to that of the front and back, we would not be able to distinguish a dromedary from a Bactrian (Fig. 19–3).

Commonly Used Estimates

The Arithmetic Mean and Standard Deviation.[29] The mean is a parametric estimate that is used to estimate the center of a distribution. It is fine for a number of distributions, typically those that are symmetric and unimodal where the most extreme observations are not much farther from the mean than are the rest of the observations, such as the normal distribution. Often in clinical data and especially when dealing with people who are ill, the observations do not fall within a narrow range. There may be a few observations (called outliers) that are quite a bit larger or smaller than most. The mean is unduly affected by outliers. Consider, for example, the data shown in Figure 19–4. The data sets are identical, except for the last observation. Note the effect that this difference has on the mean.

When the data are distributed normally (gaussian, or bell-shaped, curve), the standard deviation provides an estimate of the narrowness of the distribution: A total of 68 percent of the population should be within one standard deviation of the mean, and 95 percent within two standard deviations of the mean. The population standard deviation is a mathematical construction. For some distributions, the standard deviation may be undefined. Like the mean, the standard deviation is unduly affected by outliers (as are measures derived from the standard deviation, such as the standard error of the mean).

The Median and Semi-Interquartile Range.[19] When outliers are present, the median or other nonparametric analogue is a more appropriate estimate of the center of the distribution. The median is the observation that has equal numbers of observations less than and greater than it. In the example in Figure 19–5, data sets 1 and 2 have the same median, although the means are quite

	Data Set 1	Data Set 2
	54	54
	116	116
	95	95
	108	108
	81	81
	94	94
	37	37
	119	230
Mean	88	101.9
Standard deviation	29.4	58.2
Median	94.5	94.5
25th percentile	67.5	67.5
75th percentile	112	112
semi-interquartile range	22.25	22.25

FIGURE 19–4. Example of two nearly identical sets of data, in this case values of creatinine clearance (ml/min), with corresponding effects on some standard estimates.

different. In clinical data, outliers are frequently observed. The long-term survivor in a group of patients with a rapidly fatal disease cannot be excluded from the data. In this case, the median survival will give a more accurate picture of how the group is doing than will the mean.

A nonparametric analogue to the standard deviation is the semi-interquartile range, half the distance between the twenty-fifth and seventy-fifth percentiles. Fifty percent of the observations should fall within one semi-interquartile range of the median. Unlike the standard deviation, the semi-interquartile range always exists.

Correlation and Regression.[4] The correlation coefficient is a measure of linear association between two variables. Pairs of observations are made on individuals in the sample. As with the mean, the Pearson correlation coefficient, which assumes that the observations are from a bivariate normal distribution, can be unduly affected by a few observations. A wise course might be to plot the data in a simple scatterplot. If they do not appear to be related, they probably are not. The Spearman correlation coefficient is a nonparametric estimate using the ranks of the observations and is less sensitive to extreme values.

The usual least squares linear regression and the Pearson correlation coefficient are closely related in that the test for a significant linear regression is equivalent to the test for a significant correlation coefficient. Keep in mind that the overall correlation may not be appropriate (e.g., you may be dealing with two distinct populations). Also, the relationship for which one is testing is *linear*. Therefore, if the relationship is parabolic (e.g., if higher values of a blood test are associated with a middle-aged group, while low values are associated with the very young or old), the correlation may not be significant, although there is a definite relationship between the two variables.

Rates and Proportions. A rate, or proportion, usually refers to the percentage of patients who have a certain characteristic. When all patients can be classified as being or not being in a special group, the calculation of a rate, or proportion, is very straightforward: the number in the special group divided by the total number of patients. The most common mistake is to count nonindependent events as though they were independent; for example, suppose we observed one patient for 20 cycles of chemotherapy to determine the probability of infection during a course. This is not an adequate estimate of the probability of infection during a cycle for the population as a whole. The "trials" are clearly not independent, even for this one patient. It would be better to observe many patients for a specified number of cycles, using patients as the basic independent units of the sample.

A statistic frequently used in clinical trials is the proportion of patients surviving a specified length of time (e.g., five years). Let

r = number of patients living five years or longer, and
s = number of patients who have died in less than five years.

Note that r includes patients who died at five years and one day. Then, an estimate of five-year survival is

$$q = r/(r + s). \qquad (19\text{–}1)$$

Patients who are alive but have not been observed for five years cannot be placed in either group and must be left out of the analysis.

Life Tables. A situation that frequently arises in clinical trials is that in which the variable is the time until a certain event occurs (e.g., time to death, time to relapse, and time to menopause). Since we are measuring a duration, it is important to define and record the start as well as the end of the time period. It is also important to record how long the patient has gone without the event being observed. If the event has not occurred, this is called a *censored observation*. Without loss of generality, death will be the event of interest, and survival will be defined as the time from our clearly defined start date to the death date or, if the patient is alive, the last follow-up date. A plot or table estimating the proportion of patients who will survive to an arbitrary time from the start date is called a life table or survival curve.

If we are willing to wait until all the patients in a trial have reached the end point (i.e., death), the calculation of the life table is straightforward, as described in the previous section. However, if some of the patients are still alive, we do not know where their death time might fall. As for all the estimates discussed so far, such patients would have to be excluded from some of the survival estimates.

There is information contained in the censored observations as well as the uncensored. We know that a patient who is still alive at 18 months did not die at 12 months. An estimate that can use all of this information should be more accurate than one that cannot (e.g., Equation 19–1).

In this case, a commonly used estimate is the Kaplan-Meier product limit estimator. The basic idea behind this technique is that the probability of survival to time t, which is hard to estimate directly without making assumptions about the shape of the curve, can be expressed as a conditional probability, which we can estimate easily.

Let P(t) be the probability of survival to time t, and let P(t | u) be the probability of survival to time t, given survival to time u, where t is greater than u. This is called a conditional probability. Then, we can write

$$P(t) = P(t \mid u) \times P(u).$$

This basic equation is used over and over again to calculate the life table. Thus, the probability of surviving three days is

$$P(3) = P(3 \mid 2) \times P(2).$$

We can continue to expand the right-hand side of the equation since

$$P(2) = P(2 \mid 1) \times P(1).$$

Hence, for any day t, the estimate of the survival curve will be

$$P(t) = P(t \mid t - 1) \times P(t - 1 \mid t - 2) \times \ldots \times P(2 \mid 1) \times P(1 \mid 0) \times P(0).$$

We can then estimate each of the conditional probabilities by

$$P(t \mid t - 1) = \frac{\text{number alive after t}}{\text{number alive up to time t.}}$$

Since everyone is alive at the start of the time period, P(0) = 1.0. Also, if there are no deaths on any particular day t, P(t | t − 1) = 1.0. Hence, the survival curve will start at 1.0 and at the first death, at time t[1], for example, will drop toward 0 proportionate to the number of deaths at that time, p(t[1] | t [0]) = the number alive after t[1] divided by the number alive before t[1]. At each death time, the survival curve is multiplied by a factor that causes it to drop the same proportion of the way to zero as there are deaths to number at risk.

Consider, for example, the life table and plot in Figure 19–5. At time 0, there are ten patients. At the first death on day 18, there are still ten patients at risk. The curve drops one tenth of the way to zero. Three patients have been observed only 20, 24, and 36 days. Thus, at the second death on day 47, there are six patients at risk, and the curve drops one sixth of the way to zero. On day 60, there is one patient at risk. When this patient dies, the curve drops to zero. If the patient had not died or if more patients had been followed past that point, the curve might have stayed the same or dropped a smaller percentage of the way to zero. This points out the extreme variability of the curve when there are just a few patients at risk, making the interpretation of the "tail" of the curve, especially the claim that a plateau does or does not exist, hazardous and subject to considerable error.

For an excellent discussion of the design and analysis of clinical trials involving censored data, see the work of Peto and colleagues.[21, 22]

Hypothesis Testing

So far, this chapter has discussed the uses of statistics to describe a population based on observations of a sample. Usually, we want to do more than this—we would like to compare two or more populations or to draw conclusions about the population that can be applied to future patients from a similar population. This area of statistics is called hypothesis testing.

First, a very simple hypothesis is set up, which we hope to challenge based on evidence from the trial. This hypothesis, usually that there is no difference between the two populations or that the difference is not more than a certain specified amount, is called the null hypothesis.

Let us take an example. Suppose a statistician on a street corner has an electric device that flashes either a red light or a green light when a button is pressed. He claims that the chances of getting a red or a green light are equal, at 0.5. To prove it to you, he presses

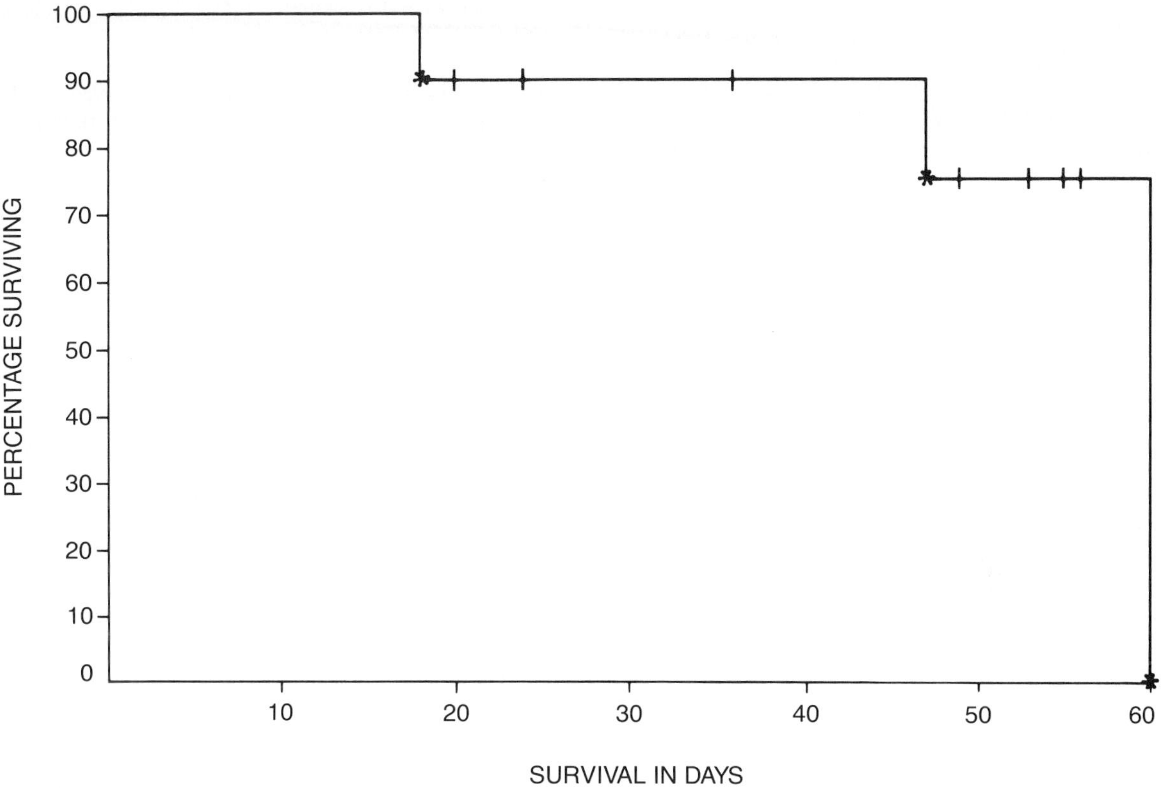

Time (t)	No. of Deaths	No. Censored	No. at Risk	Alive After t/ Alive Before t	Life Table
0	0	0	10	10/10 = 1.0	1.0
1	0	0	10	10/10 = 1.0	1.0
—	—	—	—	—	—
—	—	—	—	—	—
—	—	—	—	—	—
18	1	0	10	9/10 = 0.9	0.9
20	0	1	9	9/9 = 1.0	0.9 × 1.0 = 0.9
24	0	1	8	8/8 = 1.0	0.9 × 1.0 = 0.9
36	0	1	7	7/7 = 1.0	0.9 × 1.0 = 0.9
47	1	0	6	5/6 = 0.83	0.9 × 0.83 = 0.75
49	0	1	5	5/5 = 1.0	0.75 × 1.0 = 0.75
53	0	1	4	4/4 = 1.0	0.75 × 1.0 = 0.75
55	0	1	3	3/3 = 1.0	0.75 × 1.0 = 0.75
56	0	1	2	2/2 = 1.0	0.75 × 1.0 = 0.75
60	1	0		0/1 = 0	0.75 × 0 = 0

FIGURE 19–5. Computation and plot of the Kaplan-Meier estimate of a population survival curve. There have been three deaths at 18, 47, and 60 days. The other seven patients are still alive at 20, 24, 36, 49, 53, 55, and 56 days from their randomization dates.

the button five times and observes four red lights and one green light. His reasoning goes something like this: Suppose the box is fair. Then the chances of seeing four red lights during five trials is 5 × ½ × ½ × ½ × ½ × ½ (assuming that the trials are independent). This probability is 0.15. That is, if the box were really fair, we should see four red lights out of five trials about 15 times out of 100 repetitions of the five trials. The probability of seeing five red lights is $(½)^5$, or 0.03. Hence the probability of seeing four or more red lights is 0.15 + 0.03, or 0.18.

This probability, called the p-value, is a measure of the evidence against the null hypothesis. It is the probability that we would have observed a result as extreme or more extreme (farther away from the null hypothesis) if the null hypothesis were true.

This statistician claims that since the p-value in this case is greater than 0.05, you should not hesitate to bet on green. Whether you do or not (i.e., your interpretation of the p-value), depends on how much of a gambler you are. Although 0.05 has been considered to be the "magical" cutoff for statistical significance, it is just one gambler's choice. P-values exist along a continuum. Is 0.04 that different from 0.06? What about 0.049 and 0.051? In Figure 19–6, the two tables differ in the classification of one observation, yet this changes the p-value considerably. Should one observation change our conclusion?

The issue of a one-sided versus a two-sided test has been made into a bigger problem than it really is. Some argue that an investigator should not be doing a study if he does not expect the difference to be in a specific direction. Others claim that a one-sided test is an effort to make the differences look more significant than they are. Some statisticians privately admit doing only two-sided tests, as this lowers the probability of being challenged by a reviewer over this typically trivial matter. Basically, a p-value resulting from a one-sided test is half of that resulting from a two-sided test. One p-value can easily be calculated from the other. If you do not believe that one-sided tests should have been used, just double the p-value. Usually, doubling a significant p-value should not have any effect on the interpretation of the result. If a one-sided test gives a p-value of 0.3, would you believe it less if a two-sided test gave a p-value of 0.06? When reporting statistical tests of significance, it is best to report that exact p-value and whether the test was one- or two-sided, so that the reader can decide.

A p-value that is not statistically significant also needs to be carefully interpreted. More information is needed before a meaningful conclusion can be drawn. One can ask about the power of the test, the probability of detecting a difference of a specified magnitude when that is the true state of nature. Usually, the true mathematical distribution must also be stated in order to do a power calculation. When presenting an analysis, a more useful approach is to calculate a confidence interval for the parameter of interest. A c percent confidence interval (where c is a number between 0 and 100) is a pair of bounds on the parameter of interest such that if we sample repeatedly from the general population and calculate the confidence interval from the observed data, the interval

Study I		Survival Status	
		No. Alive	No. Dead
Treatment Group	A	13	7
	B	5	11

p-value = 0.046*

Study II		Survival Status	
		No. Alive	No. Dead
Treatment Group	A	13	7
	B	6	10

p-value = 0.096*

*One-sided Fisher exact test.

FIGURE 19–6. Example of 2 × 2 tables, which differ in one patient's classification. There is one more death in treatment Group B in Study I than in Group B in Study II. This has the effect of more than halving the p-value.

will include the "true" parameter c percent of the time. Any specific confidence interval either will or will not contain the "true" parameter, but it does give us an idea of how accurate the estimate is. For the example of the statistician and his electric box that flashes green and red lights, a 95 percent confidence interval for the probability of a red light is (0.284, 0.995). For comparing two groups, a confidence interval for the difference of the means or medians would be used.[4]

Commonly Used Statistical Tests

Paired Versus Unpaired Data.[4] When comparing two or more groups, the assumptions being made about the independence of the observations should be considered. The tests discussed in this section are for comparing two independent sets of data (e.g., measurements on two groups of patients with no individual belonging to both groups). Analogous tests exist for data that are paired (e.g., the same patient measured before and after a treatment).

T-Test. The t-test is used to test the hypothesis that the means of two distributions are equal. The variables should be continuous (e.g., age or actual estrogen receptor value) and should be distributed normally (e.g., height in adult white women). Age and estrogen receptor value may not be distributed normally, although height or IQ may. The t-test still works well even if the variable is not exactly normally distributed; however, the test may be disproportionately affected by a few outliers.[4]

Wilcoxon Test. The Wilcoxon test is more generally applicable than the t-test, since it is a nonparametric test that uses the ranks of the measurements rather than the actual observations, making it less sensitive to outliers. The test is based on the idea that if we have two groups of equal size that are drawn from the same population and we pool all the observations and rank them from smallest to largest, the sum of the ranks in each of the groups should be approximately the same. (The test is also applicable to groups of different sizes, with appropriate adjustments to the expected sum of the ranks in each group.) The probability that the sum of the ranks will differ by more than a certain amount can be calculated to yield a p-value.[4]

Chi-Square Tests and the Fisher Exact Test. The chi-square test is used to compare categorical data such as positive or negative nodes, stage of disease, or histologic type. The test is easy to compute, but the p-value is only approximate and can be misleading if the number of observations in a category is small. For 2 × 2 tables, the Fisher exact test provides an exact p-value. It simply enumerates all tables as extreme or more extreme than the one observed and sums the probabilities of all of these tables.[2]

Log-Rank Test. The log-rank test, also called the Mantel-Haenszel test, is one of several tests available for comparing survival curves. At each death time, the observed numbers of deaths are compared with the number of deaths that would have been expected if the probability of death at that time were the same in each group.[22]

The log-rank test weights each death equally. Gehan's generalized Wilcoxon test[4] weights deaths according to the number of subjects at risk. Thus, differences occurring in the earlier part of the curve, when there are more patients at risk, have a greater influence on the p-value.

Both of these tests assume that the difference between the two curves is always in the same direction. If the true survival curves cross (i.e., one treatment is superior in the beginning, but the other is superior later), these techniques do not apply, and ultimately a decision as to what is really meant by "better" must be made. In this case, adequate follow-up as well as a careful evaluation of the accuracy of the tails of the curves would be critical.

Multivariate Analyses

Multivariate analysis is frequently used to study the relationships among several variables at once or to adjust for the effects of some variables on the variable of interest. Many types of statistical procedures for multivariate analysis exist. Many cannot use censored data (e.g., multiple linear regression, analysis of variance, or factor analysis). Here, we discuss analysis of censored data.

A simple adjustment technique used in conjunction with the log-rank test is discussed by Peto and colleagues.[22] To adjust for a factor, such as axillary node involvement, we divide the patients into two strata—those with positive axillary nodes and those with negative axillary nodes. Observed and expected numbers of deaths are calculated within each stratum. The statistics for each stratum are then combined to give an overall comparison. If there are only a few factors to adjust for, this is usually the technique of choice. This technique is much easier to understand and involves fewer assumptions than does the Cox technique discussed later.

Most of the more complicated techniques are similar in that they assume a certain model for the data. We will discuss the Cox model[8]; the concepts and cautions apply to other models, such as the Weibull, as well.

Suppose there are two dichotomous prognostic factors: (1) presence or absence of certain sites of metastases that indicate bad prognosis (dire mets) and (2) positive or negative axillary nodes. The variables are coded as follows:

dire mets present:	mets = 1
dire mets not present:	mets = 0
nodes positive:	nodes = 1
nodes negative:	nodes = 0

Let $S_{[\text{mets, nodes}]}(t)$ denote the survival curve for this model. Assume the basic survival curve S_{00} (no dire mets, negative axillary nodes) is described by:

$$S_{00}(t) = \text{survival curve for patients with no dire mets and negative axillary nodes} = \exp\{-0.2 * t^{0.5}\} \quad (19\text{–}2)$$

We assume that the effect of dire mets or positive axillary nodes is to raise the basic survival curve to a power that remains constant over all values of t, and that the influence of prognostic factors is *additive* on the scale shown in Equation 19–3 following. This is an assumption that may not be true for a particular situation but that is required for most commonly used models of this type. Thus,

$$S_{01}(t) = \text{survival curve for patients with no dire mets and positive axillary nodes} = S_{00}(t)^{\exp\{\beta[1]\}}$$

$$S_{10}(t) = \text{survival curve for patients with dire mets and negative axillary nodes} = S_{00}(t)^{\exp\{\beta[2]\}}$$

$$S_{00}(t) = \text{survival curve for patients with dire mets and positive axillary nodes} = S_{00}(t)^{\exp\{\beta[1] + \beta[2]\}} \quad (19\text{–}3)$$

Note that in each case, the basic survival curve $S_{00}(t)$ is being raised to a constant power that is related to the specific prognostic factor present. When both prognostic factors are present, the parameters β[1] and β[2] are added before being exponentiated (Equation 19–3). These curves are illustrated in Figure 19–7 for β[1] = 0.2 and β[2] = 0.8.

$S_{00}(t)$ is given a specific form in Equation 19–2 for demonstration purposes. The Cox model does not require that we specify the form of the basic survival curve, whereas other models require that the shape of the basic survival curve be stated. β[1] and β[2] are called regression parameters, which reflect the influence of the associated variable and are estimated from the data. Tests of whether the β's are equal to 0 can be performed. If the test for β[1] is not statistically significant, it means that there is not enough evidence that the first variable has any influence on survival. This may be because β[1] is actually 0, because the sample is too small, or because we were unlucky and the sample does not reflect the true state of nature.

In this example, the variables were dichotomous. They may also be continuous (e.g., LDH) or may have more than two numeric categories (e.g., stages). The basic survival curve, S(t), is then raised to the value of the variable times a regression constant.

$$S(t)^{\exp\{LDH * \beta\}}$$

This makes sense only if survival decreases monotonically with values of the variable in a manner that is *linear* on the scale used. Clearly, this may not be the case for LDH. The relationship may not be linear or even uniformly increasing or decreasing.

In general, if you have k variables, z[1], z[2], . . . , z[k], and a particular set of values that z[1], . . . , z[k] may assume, the survival function is

$$S_z(t) = S(t)^{\exp\{\beta/[1] * z[1] + \ldots + \beta[k] * z[k]\}}$$

Multivariate analysis can be extremely useful if the proper amount of caution is used. In general, the more variables used in the model, the better the model will fit the data.

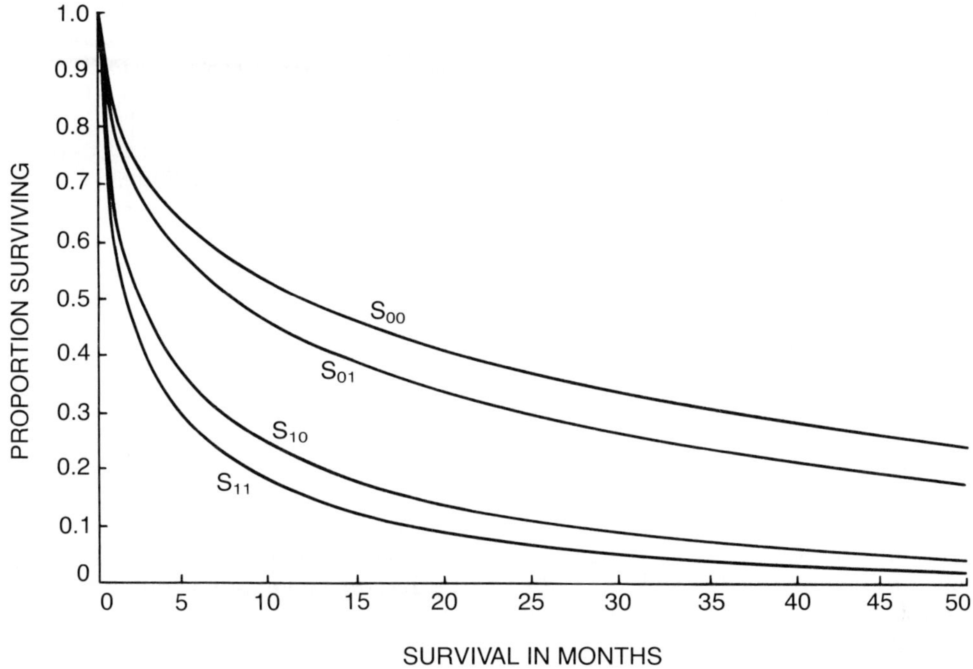

FIGURE 19–7. Plot of the population survival curves for Cox's proportional hazards model. The subscripts denote the presence or absence of the two prognostic factors: dire mets and positive axillary nodes.

This may be completely useless when applied to the general population. As an extreme case, if each patient is put in as a separate variable, the fit will be extremely good but totally useless, unless we run across a clone of one of the patients who has had the same life experiences! Indiscriminate entering of variables into a model may result in an equation that applies to the sample but that does not function well in the general population.

The order in which the variables are selected for entry into the model is an important factor in the final form of the model; for example, if we start with the presence or absence of dire metastases in the model and see what other variables add significantly to it to differentiate prognostic groups, we may end up with a different set of prognostic factors than if we had started with the variable describing axillary node involvement. This results from the methodology of selecting variables and the mathematics of model fitting rather than from some logical process.

There may also be two sets of variables that predict equally well but that cannot be combined in one model because of resulting overmodeling or because some of the variables are too highly correlated to allow the mathematical estimation of the regression parameters. In all cases, prognostic variables or relationships found by extensive examination of the data in a retrospective manner (a fishing expedition) will need to be verified in other data sets. There is a high probability that many prognostic factors found in this way are spurious, occurring in that particular sample just by chance. Verification of the model needs to be performed on a new sample of patients or by applying other statistical techniques such as the bootstrap or jackknife.[9] The basic idea behind bootstrapping and jackknifing is to use only part of the sample at a time to generate estimates, instead of getting a new sample. The variability of the estimates from subsample to subsample is used to give a better idea of how the model would perform if we were to sample a completely new group of patients.

Missing Data. There are no statistical techniques to replace missing data. Techniques that seek to "guess" the missing values so that other information will not be wasted are based on assumptions that the data are missing because of "random" phenomena, so that the mean or median of the known data is an adequate substitute. In many cases, this is not true. Data may be missing because they were "off the scale" (e.g., highly abnormal or too numerous for a count) or because the patient was too ill for a test.

Analysis of Response

There are a number of articles that discuss this topic.[1, 30] Most suggest that a comparison of survival in responders versus nonresponders is not appropriate and should not be done. However, this type of analysis is frequently presented, and it is important to know what it does and does not mean.

If an analysis of responders versus nonresponders is performed, the usual statistical analysis cannot be used. Technically, all patients start out as nonresponders and move into the responder category at later times as they meet the appropriate criteria. The eventual responders should be "at risk" as nonresponders until they are determined to be responders. At that time, they are censored in the nonresponder group and begin their survival time again (set the clock back to 0) in the responder group. This eliminates the bias that occurs because patients must live long enough for an evaluation of response; hence, they start out with an advantage of several weeks to several months.

Longer survival of responders does not mean that the treatment under consideration is effective. Other prognostic factors may be at work in selecting out a group that would have done better under any circumstances. Classification of patients into responders and nonresponders and comparing their survival curves may be useful as a prognostic factor and in patient care decisions, but only a comparative trial can answer the question of treatment efficacy.

Analysis of Subsets

The time and expense and patients involved in a clinical trial make it mandatory that we find out as much as possible from the data collected. This means looking beyond the main hypothesis that the study was designed to test. If there was not a significant overall treatment effect, analysis of subgroups of patients is performed to see if an effect exists in a subset that is not reflected in the group as a whole. If the overall treatment effect is significant, we want to know if the results hold for some subgroups but not for others.

When subset analysis is performed, especially when the overall test is not significant, the following points should be kept in mind.

1. Significant treatment differences in a subgroup may be spurious. Recall that the level of significance is an error probability for a single test. As we perform more tests, the chances that one of the tests will be erroneously significant goes up. If the experiment is repeated again and again at a 0.05 level of significance, approximately 5 of 100 will be statistically significant even when no difference exists.

2. Power is much reduced because of the reduced sample size; hence, a result that is not statistically significant may not mean very much. (Conversely, in very large samples, small differences will be statistically significant, although these differences may be of no biologic consequence.)

Crossover Interactions. Crossover interactions can occur in subset analysis when one of the treatments is better for some subsets, but the competing treatment is better in other subsets. True crossover interactions are very difficult to assess adequately. First, subsets should be specified in advance. This is rarely done. Most subset interactions are found by searching the data after the fact. Such results should be interpreted with great caution. Multivariate techniques such as the Cox model do allow for interaction terms; however, statistical tests for interactions and main effects will require more patients for adequate power; a nonsignificant test for interactions then means very little.

Interim Analyses and Trial Closure

Interim analyses are usually performed at specific intervals, the length of which depends on accrual rate, relapse rate, or death rate. The main purpose of such analyses is to monitor the study with respect to the major end points, in order to detect unusual results that might have an impact on a decision to stop the trial, either before the original number of randomized patients has been entered or before all patients have received the full treatment course.[12]

The problem of an appropriate stopping rule in situations in which the outcome measurement has not been made on all patients (e.g., survival) has not been satisfactorily resolved. Two decisions are required, one to terminate patient entry into the trial and another to terminate any continuing treatment that previously entered patients may be receiving. The goal is to minimize the number of patients receiving an inferior treatment; however, application of this principle is not always straightforward. In cancer treatment trials, study end points such as response, remission duration, and survival are not immediately observed, and patients enter the study sequentially over time.

In light of the increased error probability associated with multiple statistical tests, the investigator should require more evidence (i.e., a smaller p-value) before concluding that a specific difference exists. The p-value that will cause excitement and start people talking about early stopping is best agreed upon in advance. Its computation depends on the expected number of interim analyses. A conservative method is to take the level at which the final test will be done, say 0.05, and divide by the number of interim analyses to be performed. Hence, if five interim analyses are to be performed over the duration of the study, a 0.01 p-value would be required before a significant difference is declared at an interim analysis point.

As with the p-value, one should select in advance the statistic to be used to compare treatment outcomes at an interim analysis point. Interim data analysis should be limited in scope to simple tabulations of primary end points to see if there is any evidence of treatment differences sufficiently convincing to stop or change the trial. Measures of long-term treatment effects are of limited use in decisions that could lead to early termination of the clinical trial because this information is simply not available soon enough to be of use.

In other cases, interim analysis is used to monitor a specific aspect of the trial so that the protocol can be adjusted to correct what might have proved to be a confounding factor. In the NCI treatment trial of women with early-stage breast cancer, chemotherapy dose modification in node-positive women was monitored. Interim analysis of the data[18] indicated that irradiated patients required dose reduction more often than did mastectomy patients and that lymphopenia without substantial granulocytopenia might account for this observation. A decision was then made to change the criteria for dose modification from being based on total white cell count to reductions based on absolute granulocyte count. This change in criteria for dose reduction minimized the tendency for women managed with radiation therapy to receive slightly smaller amounts of drug than women treated with mastectomy, even when both groups were treated to an identical degree of bone marrow suppression. Although it is not yet certain that aggressive chemotherapy is associated with better disease-free or overall survival, this interim analysis permitted a refinement in protocol procedures that made the two modalities of primary therapy more comparable, with respect to the administration of aggressive systemic therapy.

For most cancer therapy trials, modest improvements in therapeutic outcome are more realistic than are extreme or large differences. These modest differences are usually more reliably established using a limited number of well-planned interim analyses, either at fixed intervals of time or at equally spaced numbers of patients (or outcomes) rather than on an ad hoc basis, such as when an investigator wishes to report on the study findings or requests an updated analysis. A rule of thumb frequently applicable is to plan on a maximum of five analyses, using *group sequential designs*[24] to define the criteria for repeated significance testing. These designs are an improvement on fixed-size trials if treatment differences exist, since they reduce the average number of patients who must be randomized. Likewise, there is a small increase in sample size requirements where there is no treatment difference.

Interim analyses must be based on data that are correct and complete. Analysis results can be influenced by reporting delays, especially differences in submitting information on patients according to their outcome (e.g., bad news may arrive early, or it may be delayed because additional time is required to document the failure). Consequently, interim analyses can be biased in one direction or the other; a therapy that delays early recurrence may later prove not to have a substantial impact on the number who eventually relapse or, ultimately, on survival.

Responsibility for reviewing interim analyses should be delegated to a specific group of individuals in whom the clinical investigators and patients have confidence. A certain amount of confidentiality of interim results is important while a trial is in progress because such information can influence the behavior of investigators in entering and treating subsequent patients. Premature disclosure and publication of interim results, especially those that could be inconsistent with later results, should be avoided.

An examination of interim and final analyses of a metastatic breast cancer trial comparing a five-drug combination chemotherapy with a single, sequential treatment illustrates some of these problems.[7] The original interpretation of the trial results was that of a survival benefit for combination chemotherapy. This was not supported by a final analysis seven years after the start of the trial, at which point 90 percent of the patients had died. Factors accounting for this inconsistency included delayed reporting of data in key cases, treatment effects that were limited to a subset of the patients, and a tendency to interpret interim results according to the expected outcome.

Ultimately, the decision to stop a trial is an ethical one. Statistical input is just a part of the decision-making process. However, keep in mind that stopping a study before there are enough data on which to base firm conclusions may mean that the trial will have to be repeated or that large numbers of patients will be treated with an inferior regimen.

Often, little attention is paid to procedures for *study closure* of cancer treatment trials, presumably because of the relatively short duration and small number of patients in most studies. Study closure refers to the final patient visits, final analysis of data and dissemination of trial results, and data storage. Orderly closure of a clinical trial requires careful planning and attention to detail. For therapeutic studies in women with advanced breast cancer, it is important to have accurate and complete information on initial treatment response and on subsequent survival status for all patients. For trials in women with early-stage disease, long-term follow-up with complete ascertainment of recurrence and death is extremely important, since fewer than half of the women will die of their disease.

INTERPRETING THE RESULTS OF A CLINICAL TRIAL

One of the main goals of the clinical trial is to provide information that can be applied to patient care. Even the best run and designed clinical trial differs from the real world in significant ways; therefore, the applicability of the trial and the extent to which its findings can be generalized must be carefully considered before a regimen is accepted for general use.

The trial should follow the basics of good design and execution. It must be determined whether the study was a clinical trial or a description of someone's experiences. Without the discipline of a formal clinical trial, data collection may not be complete and definitions (e.g., staging and eligibility criteria) may not be consistent. Conclusions drawn from a study that merely describes a population should be viewed with caution. Were appropriate controls used? Was the study randomized?

Evaluate carefully the main question being asked by the trial. The answer may or may not have an effect on patient care; for example, a study showing that a more invasive method of diagnosis is better than another should not influence patient care if therapy choices are not affected by the additional knowledge. Such studies are important for future clinical trials, which may yield applications to patient care.

The "real world" of the clinical trial is the world represented by those included in the trial. The eligibility criteria help to define this population but are generally not sufficient; it is usually impossible to accurately describe the population sampled. The best that can be done is to describe the sample, using summary statistics such as mean or median age, stage of disease, or ethnic background.

Good design and randomization between two treatments will eliminate unknown biases that would invalidate the trial but do not help to further define the population sampled. Clearly, a regimen shown to be superior in a clinical trial may be superior only in that somewhat undefined population that was sampled and may not apply to the next patient who walks in the door. There is no solution to this problem. The only way to evaluate the applicability of the results to another situation is through well-defined eligibility criteria, careful comparison with available descriptive statistics, thoughts on who did or did not participate in the trial, evaluation of who did not accept randomization, and so on.

The "real world" and even the population from which the trial participants were drawn are not static; for example, mortality from cardiovascular disease has been declining over the past few years for reasons that are not clear.[15] A study of a drug to reduce deaths from cardiovascular disease that used historical control subjects might find a significant improvement in the treated group that was entirely due to these unknown causes and was not at all related to the drug.

A study may be well designed and perfectly executed and still be wrong. The world is an uncertain place, and events of low probability (much lower than 0.05) do occur. Differences between treatments may have occurred simply by chance. The percentage of studies that show significant treatment differences when none exist is increased by the investigator's natural tendency to want to get exciting results into print quickly and a tendency on the part of journals to favor publication of significant results.[21]

Greatest attention should be paid to the methods and results sections of studies. Discussion and conclusions are irrelevant unless the methods of execution and analysis of data are correct. If crucial pieces of information are missing or explanations are not clear, the study cannot be adequately evaluated. Conclusions must be accepted tentatively, until their validity can be verified.

Watch denominators carefully to see if the sample size changes from comparison to comparison. Was the randomization undone by inappropriate exclusion of "inevaluable" patients? One example is a study of surgery versus no surgery, in which if operative deaths are excluded from the survival analysis, this might bias the analysis in favor of surgery. Similarly, in a study of a toxic versus a less toxic chemotherapy regimen, if early deaths, possibly resulting from therapy, are excluded, this might favor the more toxic regimen.

Technically, a randomized study should be analyzed "as randomized," with no exceptions. If errors (e.g., the patient did not get the correct therapy) or events of low probability (e.g., the patient was killed in an airplane crash) occur, these events should be distributed in an unbiased manner over all treatment groups. This added "noise" should not affect the conclusion in the long run. In reality, there is already enough extraneous noise, and we do not have the time or the resources to wait for long-run adjustments. Hence, some exclusions are acceptable, but they should be few in number and *clearly described*.

Large samples of several thousand patients, while unusual in cancer clinical trials, are not unknown, especially in breast cancer studies. With large enough sample sizes, even very minor differences will be statistically significant. In this case, the emphasis should be on the clinical significance of the differences found. A large sample will allow many subgroup analyses to be performed; the added probability of error should be taken into account. On the other hand, with small enough samples (or subgroups), even large differences become difficult to detect. A nonsignificant test means very little when the sample size is small.

Above all, keep in mind that the clinical trial is an application of the scientific method. The design should reflect the question being asked, and the conclusions should follow logically from the results. There is a place for intuition and clinical judgment, but in a clinical trial, the primary aim is to acquire knowledge that will convince other scientists and give us a glimpse of the "true" state of nature.

REFERENCES

1. Anderson JR, Cain KC, Gelber RD: Analysis of survival by tumor response. J Clin Oncol 1:710, 1983.
2. Armitage P: Statistical Methods in Medical Research. New York: John Wiley & Sons, 1971, pp. 126–138.
3. Blackwelder WC: 'Proving the null hypothesis' in clinical trials. Controlled Clin Trials 3:345, 1982.
4. Brown W, Hollander M: Statistics: A Biomedical Introduction. New York: John Wiley & Sons, 1977, pp. 110–117, 328–336, 346–350.
5. Byar DP, Simon RM, Friedewald WT, et al.: Randomized clinical trials: Perspectives on some recent ideas. N Engl J Med 295:74, 1976.
6. Byar DP, Piantadosi S: Factorial designs for randomized clinical trials. Cancer Treat Rep 69:1055, 1985.
7. Chlebowski RT, Weiner JM, Ryden VMJ, et al.: Factors influencing the interim interpretation of a breast cancer trial. Danger of achieving the "expected" result. Controlled Clin Trials 2:123, 1981.

8. Cox DR: Regression models and life tables. J R Stat Soc (B) 34:187, 1972.
9. Efron B: The Jackknife, the Bootstrap and Other Resampling Plans. Philadelphia: Society for Industrial and Applied Mathematics, 1982.
10. Ellenberg SS: Randomization designs in comparative clinical trials. N Engl J Med 310:1404, 1984.
11. Farewell VT, D'Angio GJ: A simulated study of historical controls using real data. Biometrics 37:169, 1981.
12. Fleming TR, Green SJ, Harrington DP: Considerations for monitoring and evaluating treatment effects in clinical trials. Controlled Clin Trials 5:55, 1984.
13. Friedman LM, Furberg CD, DeMets DL: Fundamentals of Clinical Trials. Boston: Wright-PSG Publishing Co., Inc., 1982.
14. Gail MH: Eligibility, exclusions, losses to follow-up, removal of randomized patients and uncounted events in cancer clinical trials. Cancer Treat Rep 69:1107, 1985.
15. Kannel W, Thom T: Declining cardiovascular mortality. Circulation 70:331, 1984.
16. Lachin JM: Introduction to sample size determination and power analysis for clinical trials. Controlled Clin Trials 2:93, 1981.
17. Lavin PT: Practical considerations in the coordination of clinical trials. *In*: Shapiro SH, Louis TA (eds.): Clinical Trials—Issues and Approaches. New York: Marcel Dekker, Inc., 1983, pp. 129–133.
18. Lippman ME, Lichter AS, Edwards BE, et al.: The impact of primary irradiation treatment of localized breast cancer on the ability to administer systemic adjuvant chemotherapy. J Clin Oncol 2:21, 1984.
19. McNeil D: Interactive Data Analysis. New York: John Wiley & Sons, 1977, p. 6.
20. Moertel CG, Hanley JA: The effect of measuring error on the results of therapeutic trials in advanced cancer. Cancer 38:388, 1976.
21. Peto R, Pike M, Armitage P, et al.: Design and analysis of randomized clinical trials requiring prolonged observation of each patient: Introduction and design. Br J Cancer 34:585, 1976.
22. Peto R, Pike M, Armitage P, et al.: Design and analysis of randomized clinical trials requiring prolonged observation of each patient: Analysis and examples. Br J Cancer 34:1, 1977.
23. Pocock, SJ: Randomised clinical trials (letter). Br Med J 1:1661, 1977.
24. Pocock SJ: Interim analysis for randomized clinical trials: The group sequential approach. Biometrics 38:153, 1982.
25. Pocock SJ: Clinical Trials, A Practical Approach. New York: John Wiley & Sons, 1983.
26. Robin E: Matters of Life and Death: Risks vs Benefits of Medical Care. Stanford, CA: Stanford Alumni Association, 1984.
27. Shapiro S, Strax P, Venet L: Periodic breast cancer screening, the first two years of screening. Arch Environ Health 15:547, 1967.
28. Shapiro S, Venet W, Strax P, et al.: Ten- to fourteen-year effect of screening on breast cancer mortality. J Natl Cancer Inst 69:349, 1982.
29. Snedecor G, Cochran W: Statistical Methods. Ames: Iowa State University Press, 1967, pp. 41–42, 44–45.
30. Weiss GB, Bunce H, Hokanson JA: Comparing survival of responders and nonresponders after treatment: A potential source of confusion in interpreting clinical trials. Controlled Clin Trials 4:43, 1983.
31. Wesley M, Wesley R: Biostatistics in clinical trials. *In*: Moosa AR, Robson M, Schimpff SC (eds.): Comprehensive Textbook of Oncology. Baltimore: Williams & Wilkins, 1986, pp. 346–354.
32. Zelen M: A new design for randomized clinical trials. N Engl J Med 300:1242, 1979.

Future Prospects in Breast Cancer Research and Management

JEFFREY SCHLOM, Ph.D.

The 1970's saw the introduction and utilization of two methodologies that represent quantum leaps in both molecular biology and immunology research: gene-cloning procedures and hybridoma-monoclonal antibody technology, respectively. The use of these methodologies in breast cancer research has led to investigations that may ultimately have an impact on the management of this disease. The areas of most intense investigation include (1) the utilization of monoclonal antibodies to define and detect breast cancer–associated antigens, (2) the identification and characterization of oncogenes, proto-oncogenes, and other cellular genetic elements that may play a role in breast cancer etiology, and (3) the role that growth factors, tumor factors, and other biologic response modifiers play in the maintenance of the transformed phenotype.

The precise etiology of human breast cancer is unknown. While factors such as genetics, hormones and, perhaps, environmental chemicals and radiation have some role to play in its etiology, the actual genetic elements involved in the initiation of the transformation event are still obscure. Another point that must be considered is that evidence clearly suggests that the pathogenesis of human mammary cancer is a multistep process consisting of (1) an initiation event, which may take place up to three decades prior to detection of a primary tumor mass; (2) promotional events (such as stimulation by hormones or growth factors), which also precede the classic transformed phenotype; (3) transformation (i.e., when cells take on the classic morphologic and biologic characteristics of cancer); and (4) early and late progression. Early progression can be defined as the invasion of cancer cells through basement membrane, while late progression involves the penetration of cells through vessels and soft tissues, subsequent growth in distal organs, and, perhaps, a second or third cycle of such events. This chapter will discuss selected examples of the role of cancer-associated antigens (proteins, glycoproteins, and carbohydrates), the role of specific genetic elements, and the possible role of growth factors in these multistep processes and how these concepts may ultimately be utilized in the management of mammary neoplasia.

20

MONOCLONAL ANTIBODIES

The identification of human tumor-associated antigens (TAAs) and the development of specific immunologic reagents directed against these targets have long been sought. In past decades, the classic method of generating antibodies to TAAs has been the hyperimmunization of an animal with an extract of a human tumor and the absorption of the resultant sera with a variety of normal tissues; for example, if an extract of human breast carcinoma were used as the immunogen, the sera would be absorbed with extracts of normal breast tissue or benign breast tumor as well as extracts of normal human red blood cells or liver. This absorbed hyperimmune sera would then be tested for its ability to react with the immunogen (in this case, breast carcinoma). All too often, only weak reactivity would be observed, and only enough sera would be obtained to complete a finite number of tests. At this point, the entire process would, of necessity, begin over again. Furthermore, since hyperimmune sera contain tens of thousands of different types of immunoglobulins, which differ in isotype, affinity, and specificity, reproducibility of results from laboratory to laboratory was difficult, if not impossible, to achieve.

The advent of hybridoma technology in 1975 represented a quantum leap in tumor immunology.[1] For the first time, single cell populations of B-lymphocytes from immunized hosts could be immortalized via fusion with drug-selected non–immunoglobulin secretor murine myeloma cells. These fused cell products could then be cloned and propagated indefinitely. The supernatant fluids of cultures from literally thousands of different cloned cell populations (termed hybridomas) could be assayed to select for homogeneous populations of immunoglobulins with the desired reactivity. As a direct result of this technology, numerous monoclonal antibodies have been generated, leading to the identification of novel TAAs from various human carcinomas, melanomas, leukemias, and lymphomas. At least a dozen monoclonal antibodies against human mammary carcinomas have been reported in the literature[2]; each one has been characterized with respect to range of reactivity and reactive antigen. In general, these monoclonal antibodies can be classified into four groups, based on the immunogen used to generate the monoclonal antibody. These immunogens include (1) breast tumor cell lines; (2) milk-fat globule membrane; (3) membrane-enriched extracts of breast carcinoma metastases; and (4) lymph nodes from mastectomy patients. Each of the monoclonal antibodies thus far described, including antibodies to milk-fat globule membrane prepared by several different groups, appears to be unique with respect to percentage of reactive mammary tumors, percentage of reactive cells within tumors, location of reactive antigen within the tumor cell, and degree of reactivity with nonmammary tumors as well as normal tissues.

An analysis of the monoclonal antibody literature as it relates to breast cancer reveals several important concepts: (1) Most breast cancer–associated determinants (as defined by monoclonal antibodies) are also found on other carcinoma cells (i.e., a large number of "pancarcinoma" antigens have been elucidated), (2) a great deal of antigenic heterogeneity exists in the expression of a given tumor antigenic determinant, both among cells of a given tumor mass and between different tumor masses of different patients, and (3) established breast cancer cell lines may not reflect the phenotype or even genotype of breast cancer biopsy material. The latter findings most probably reflect the enormous selective pressure exerted on cell populations in attempts to establish appropriate culture conditions and subsequent immortal cell lines. The monoclonal antibodies thus far characterized, and future generations of monoclonal antibodies, may ultimately find use in virtually all arms of patient management. The progress being made in several of these areas as well as the problems that have been encountered will now be discussed.

Serum Assays. The use of monoclonal antibodies to detect tumor-associated antigens in serum may eventually find a place in early detection of carcinoma lesions, monitoring for recurrence, and checking the efficacy of specific therapeutic regimens. Although no monoclonal antibody has yet been used as an early diagnostic test to follow large numbers of asymptomatic individuals, several monoclonal antibodies have been employed to monitor tumor burden in breast cancer patients; for example, one study describes the application of a monoclonal antibody (designated DF3)[3] in a radioimmunoassay (RIA) to check for the appearance of the 300,000d reactive antigen in serum. The results[4] indicate that 76 per cent of patients (33 of 43) with metastatic breast cancer had elevated antigen levels compared with 3 of 36 normal controls ($p < 0.001$). Further studies with this and other monoclonal antibodies, used either alone or as part of a MAb cocktail, are being evaluated to monitor the clinical course of patients.

Immunohistochemical and Immunocytochemical Methods to Detect and to Establish the Phenotype of Carcinoma. Perhaps the most immediate applications of monoclonal antibodies in the management of human breast cancer will be to detect occult tumor cells and to establish the phenotype of carcinoma cell populations; for example, a recent study[5] has shown that a particular monoclonal antibody (designated B72.3) can be used as an adjunct in the detection of breast carcinoma cells in pleural effusions. The reactive antigen (designated TAG-72 [tumor-associated glycoprotein]), which is a mucin-like molecule that is greater than 10^6d, was found on carcinoma cells in 22 of 23 samples from all 21 patients with metastatic breast cancer. Conversely, monoclonal antibody B72.3 failed to react with effusions from 41 patients without cancer. Since these studies were conducted retrospectively with formalin-fixed blocks of effusion material, the accuracy of diagnosis and the clinical outcome of each patient were already known. Most cytopathologists will admit to difficulties in the definitive diagnosis of carcinoma in approximately 10 percent of effusion samples, usually resulting from the presence of single cells that may be atypical or the presence of carcinoma cells among clusters of reactive mesothelial cells. Monoclonal antibody utilization appeared to complement standard cytologic procedures in those particular situations. These studies are being expanded by several groups to use various monoclonal antibodies as adjuncts to the diagnosis of mammary carcinoma with fine-needle aspiration biopsy and for the detection of occult carcinoma cells in specimens of bone marrow.

Monoclonal antibodies may also be employed in immunohistopathology to establish the phenotype of carcinoma lesions. This use of various monoclonal antibodies to estrogen receptor is being evaluated in comparison with immunoassays of tumor extracts. Immunohistochemical assays have the advantage of defining reactivity to specific cell types and overcome the criticism that values obtained from standard assays of tumor extracts may be more reflective of the percentage of tumor cells present in the sample than the actual amount of estrogen receptor per tumor cell.

Studies are also under way in several laboratories to use monoclonal antibodies in immunopathology and immunocytopathology for differential diagnosis; for example, monoclonal antibody B72.3 is reactive with breast carcinoma but is nonreactive with lymphomas. Thus, lesions in regional lymph nodes, in the absence of a primary breast lesion, will be assayed for the presence of B72.3 reactive antigen. It is envisioned that the pathologist will eventually use antibodies in concert to aid in a variety of such differential diagnoses.

Prognostic Studies. One future prospect is that a series of monoclonal antibodies will be employed to assay sections of the mammary carcinoma of a specific patient to help define the likelihood of metastasis (i.e., prognosis) of that tumor. There is a large body of evidence in the literature supporting the hypothesis that less differentiated tumor cells are more likely to metastasize. The degree of differentiation is, for the most part, determined on the basis of morphologic criteria such as nuclear and histologic grades, with estrogen receptor status showing some minor prognostic indication. However, it appears that more subtle changes in the levels of individual proteins or of the glycoprotein determinants (i.e., the degree or type of glycosylation of individual proteins) may eventually provide a more accurate assessment of the degree of (or lack of) differentiation of cells within a given tumor mass. The monoclonal antibodies eventually used in this situation may be directed against (1) tumor-associated antigens, (2) oncogene or proto-oncogene products, (3) differentiation antigens, (4) proteins associated with the metastatic process, or (5) normal cellular proteins or glycoproteins whose levels increase or decrease during the processes of dedifferentiation and early progression.

One example of the direction of this research is the finding that the expression of the determinant defined by monoclonal antibody DF3 has been shown to correlate with nuclear grade, histologic grade, and estrogen receptor status among breast carcinomas but is an independent marker of differentiation. Since monoclonal antibody DF3 also reacts strongly with lactating mammary epithelial cells, it can be tentatively hypothesized to be a novel differentiation antigen.[6]

Another set of hypotheses that can be considered toward this end involves the mechanism of attachment and invasion in the metastatic process: (1) Tumor cells that express high levels of exposed laminin receptor are more likely to bind to laminin in basement membranes, and (2) tumor cells expressing high levels of Type IV collagenase are more likely to invade through basement membrane via the dissolution of Type IV collagen. Thus, one could envision a panel of monoclonal antibodies such as DF3, anti-laminin receptor, anti–Type IV collagenase, and anti-oncogene products and growth factors (to be discussed later) as a means of better defining the probability of metastasis for a given carcinoma cell population.

Radionuclide-Conjugated Monoclonal Antibodies to Localize Tumor Lesions *In Situ*. A major concern in the evaluation of the primary breast cancer patient is the presence or absence of tumor in regional lymph nodes. The removal of the regional axillary nodes at the time of lumpectomy or mastectomy as well as subsequent histopathologic evaluation of individual nodes is standard procedure. The absence of tumor in the nodes is a favorable prognostic indicator, and in the vast majority of cases, no subsequent therapy is called for. Approximately 25 percent of node-negative patients, however, will eventually develop metastatic breast cancer. One reason may be that blood-borne cancer cells have already invaded distal organs at the time of mastectomy. Another, not necessarily nonexclusive, possibility is that tumor cells have spread via lymphatics to the internal mammary, interpectoral, or supraclavicular lymph nodes. Since the removal of these nodes would require thoracic surgery, they are not monitored for tumor involvement.

It is clear that direct visualization of nodes for the presence of tumor cells is optimal. However, in view of (1) the lack of accessibility of many lymph nodes and (2) the trend toward breast cancer surgery that is less invasive (perhaps leading to the question of whether axillary nodes need be removed in all cases), a less invasive way of monitoring the presence of tumor in axillary and other lymph nodes would be advantageous. A monoclonal antibody or a mixture of monoclonal antibodies to tumor-associated antigens, coupled with diagnostic radionuclides such as ^{131}I, ^{99m}Tc, and ^{111}In, could be used in lymphoscintigraphy toward this end. In this procedure, radiolabeled monoclonal antibody would be administered regionally (either subcutaneously or directly into lymphatics) and would thus migrate through regional lymphatic nodes. At appropriate intervals, the patient would be monitored via scanning with a gamma camera for localization (i.e., higher concentrations) of radionuclide-coupled monoclonal antibody in tumor-bearing lymph nodes. To evaluate the efficacy of such studies, they would first be conducted on patients prior to mastectomy or lumpectomy with axillary node resection. Then, the nodes could be weighed, their radioactivity assessed in a gamma counter, and sections subjected to autoradiography to determine if the radionuclide-conjugated monoclonal antibody had indeed efficiently localized in tumor and to more accurately quantitate such localization.

A major issue in the management of the breast cancer patient is defining the appearance and location of metastatic lesions. Regardless of the nodal status of the patient at the time of mastectomy or lumpectomy, the patient and physician must, in reality, wait at least ten years before ruling out metastatic spread. Radionuclide-conjugated monoclonal antibody to a breast tumor–associated antigen, administered intravenously at regular intervals, would potentially be quite useful in this situation. The state of technology is that several monoclonal antibodies are being evaluated and analyzed for optimal labeling conditions and for immunoglobulin fragmentation (for more rapid clearance from the blood). It will most probably take several years to define the right monoclonal antibodies and conditions for these purposes. Some of the parameters that must be investigated in the use of *each* monoclonal antibody include:

1. Dose and specific activity of the radiolabeled monoclonal antibody.
2. Affinity of the monoclonal antibody for the tumor antigen and the stability of the radionuclide–monoclonal antibody complex.

3. Route of antibody administration.
4. Whether intact IgG, Fab'_2, or Fab fragments are used.
5. Choice of radionuclides (they vary in energy and half life).
6. Metabolism (i.e., clearance) of the radiolabeled monoclonal antibody or fragment from the blood and lymphatics.
7. Location of the tumor (i.e., depth within the body).
8. Size of the tumor.
9. Degree of vascularity and other histologic properties of the tumor.
10. Degree of expression of the specific tumor-associated antigen in the tumor mass.
11. Presence or appearance of human antimurine Ig antibodies.
12. Presence of circulating tumor antigen.

Each of the preceding parameters must be evaluated as part of a network, since each is interrelated with many of the other parameters mentioned; for example, if one chooses to use a monoclonal antibody fragment that will clear from the blood faster, the monoclonal antibody dose, specific activity, and choice of radionuclide may have to be altered. It is emphasized that each monoclonal antibody or mixture of monoclonal antibodies may have to be evaluated in this manner, first, in experimental animal models using human tumor xenografts in athymic mice and, then, in controlled clinical trials. Thus, a systematic approach to these questions is necessary.

A related area of investigation will most certainly involve the use of monoclonal antibodies and nuclear magnetic resonance imaging (NMRI) to locate primary and metastatic breast cancer lesions. NMRI is based on the idea that static tissue protons, when subjected to a strong external magnetic field, will give off a characteristic "relaxation signal" when perturbed by a specific radio frequency signal. This signal can, in turn, be spatially localized into an image with the aid of computers. Heavy metals such as gadolinium can be coupled with monoclonal antibodies and administered intravenously to patients in an attempt to obtain an enhanced relaxation signal. It should be pointed out, however, that such studies are just now being initiated in experimental animals.

Therapy

Tumor therapy using monoclonal antibodies can theoretically be mediated via (1) effector cell mechanisms, (2) complement, (3) conjugation with toxin or drugs, and (4) conjugation with radionuclides. There are two major reasons that, in the opinion of this investigator, the radionuclide-conjugate approach should be pursued. The first is the vast amount of antigenic heterogeneity that has been observed in most tumor masses, using most monoclonal antibodies. When invoking drug conjugate–mediated or effector cell–mediated mechanisms, the monoclonal antibody must bind to all cells of the tumor mass for efficient killing. Thus, tumor cells not expressing cell surface tumor antigen would be unaffected. Since killer isotopes (alpha- or beta-emitters) have a killing effect that extends up to 50 or more cell diameters, the monoclonal antibody–radionuclide conjugate need not bind every tumor cell to kill all cells in a given mass. Second, many carcinoma-associated antigens have been shown to be stable components of the cell membrane.[7] Thus, monoclonal antibody–carcinoma antigen complexes on the cell surfaces have been shown not to internalize, as do many monoclonal antibody–lymphocyte antigen cell surface complexes. Since monoclonal antibody–drug conjugates must internalize to mediate cell killing, they may be ineffectual in these cases. Radionuclide–monoclonal antibody complexes, however, need not internalize for cell killing.

There is a unique situation in the use of monoclonal antibody–radionuclide conjugates for *in situ* diagnosis followed by their use for therapy. Since the same monoclonal antibody (coupled with different radionuclides) is used in both cases, one should be able to first define a "radiolocalization index" for a given monoclonal antibody and a given patient's tumor mass(es). This could be obtained from analyses of gamma scans and biopsy material (cpm/g) following monoclonal antibody–diagnostic radionuclide complex administration. This radiolocalization index can then be translated into a potential "therapeutic index," for use in that monoclonal antibody and that patient. In other words, analysis of the dosimetry of localization using the diagnostic radionuclide–antibody conjugate can serve as a predictor of the size of the dosage (monoclonal antibody coupled to killer isotopes) that will be delivered to given tumor masses versus normal organs for that patient. It should be pointed out, however, that any attempt at therapy using a monoclonal antibody is clearly a difficult task. The selective reactivity of the monoclonal antibody for tumor and versus adult normal tissues must first be carefully evaluated. Whether such monoclonal antibodies already exist or will be generated in the future is unknown.

As mentioned earlier, one of the major concerns in any attempt at immunotherapy of breast cancer involves the antigenic heterogeneity within many breast carcinoma lesions. Studies have shown, however, that much of this heterogeneity may well be due to a dynamic process of antigenic modulation (i.e., the turning on and turning off of the expression of given tumor antigens by factors such as cell cycle, environmental milieu, or spatial configuration of lesions).[8] One approach to this problem of antigenic modulation is the use of biologic response modifiers or drugs to selectively enhance the expression of tumor antigens on the surface of carcinoma cells; for example, a study[9] has shown that the use of low (noncytotoxic) levels of recombinant leukocyte interferon will enhance the expression of tumor antigens on the surface of breast cancer cells but not normal cell lines. Thus, administration of recombinant interferon, followed by administration of radiolabeled monoclonal antibody, could conceivably enhance efficiency of antibody binding in diagnostic and therapeutic trials.

A novel approach to potential cancer therapy involves the use of anti-idiotype monoclonal antibodies. Though still more or less in a conceptual stage, as far as breast cancer is concerned, preliminary studies using antiviral and antitumor experimental systems are intriguing. This approach involves the use of a monoclonal antibody to a tumor-associated antigen as immunogen, to prepare new monoclonal antibodies directed against the antigen-binding, or idiotypic, region of the first monoclonal antibody. The binding sites of these new anti-idiotype monoclonal antibodies should now contain an "internal image" of the original antigen. Thus, anti-idiotype monoclonal antibodies can potentially be used to immunize patients in an attempt to mount an active immune response against tumor antigens and, thus, tumor. Concerning long-term goals, an elucidation of the anti-idiotype network as it refers to specific antitumor immune responses will certainly aid in a better understanding of the reasons that tumor antigens have been classically poor immunogens.

Monoclonal antibodies may also have a use in monitoring conventional drug, radiation, and hormone therapies of breast cancer patients. Serum radioimmunoassays may be useful in monitoring tumor destruction (via a precipitous increase and then decrease in blood antigen) and tumor burden. Radiolabeled monoclonal antibodies inoculated intravenously or regionally may also be useful in visualizing tumor size prior to, and following, conventional treatments.

There has been some concern regarding the use of multiple inoculations of monoclonal antibodies for diagnosis or therapy, which may result in the development of human antimouse Ig immune responses in patients. Preliminary studies using intact IgG have shown that the vast majority of human antimurine IgG antibodies that develop in patients are directed against the Fc region of the molecule. One prospect for reducing this problem is to fractionate monoclonal antibodies to a very small size to obtain the minimum antigen-binding component available. This would most probably eliminate the more immunogenic constant regions on the Ig molecule. Another approach would be to clone the genes coding for individual monoclonal antibodies, reduce them in size via restriction endonuclease methodology, and if necessary, insert or ligate human Ig regions. A spin-off of this technology would be to ligate efficient metal-binding or drug-binding regions to the recombinant Ig molecule. Thus, recombinant DNA technology will, in the future, most probably play a larger role in monoclonal antibody research and in disease management.

ONCOGENES, PROTO-ONCOGENES, AND GROWTH FACTORS

One extremely exciting area of cancer research has been the elucidation of the existence of oncogenes and proto-oncogenes. Oncogenes and proto-oncogenes are usually defined by their ability to mediate transformation via (1) DNA transfection assays using the murine-established fibroblast 3T3 cell line as the target cell, (2) chromosome translocation, (3) gene amplification, and (4) promoter activation (i.e., the oncogene or proto-oncogene is located near a promoter sequence that regulates its level of transcription). Oncogenes usually have homology to the genomes of known RNA tumor viruses of animals. Proto-oncogenes are defined as endogenous elements of cellular DNA of a given species. Lists of the approximately 30 oncogenes and their proposed mechanisms of action have been detailed in numerous reviews[10, 11] and, thus, will not be addressed here.

The oncogenes and proto-oncogenes that have received the most attention as far as breast cancer is concerned are the *ras* family. The family consists of three major gene members: Ha (Harvey)-*ras*, Ki (Kirsten)-*ras*, and N (neuroblastoma)-*ras*.[11] Much attention has been focused on the fact that a single point mutation in any of these proto-oncogenes can lead to the formation of oncogenes with the ability to transform 3T3 cells. However, numerous studies in many laboratories have demonstrated that point-mutated *ras* is not involved in human breast cancer. Enhanced expression of the "proto" form of the *ras* gene, however, has been shown to mediate transformation in several experimental systems.[12] Other studies, moreover, have demonstrated that the majority of human breast carcinomas contain elevated levels of the *ras* 21,000d (p21) gene product compared with normal breast tissue and most benign breast lesions.[12] Studies are now under way in many laboratories to determine if other known or new oncogenes and proto-oncogenes are also associated with breast cancer. One prime candidate at this time is the *myc* gene, since the *myc* and *ras* genes have been shown to act synergistically in several experimental systems.[13] One concept quite prevalent in oncogene research is the fact that cell transformation may be the result of at least two, and possibly many, oncogenes or proto-oncogenes, or both, acting synergistically during the multistep processes involved in tumor initiation, promotion, transformation, and progression.

Oncogene research may well add to the elucidation of the etiology of breast cancer and the mechanisms by which cells become transformed; however, one is still faced with the question of how this area of research will directly aid in the management of human breast cancer. A far-reaching prospect, of course, is the identification of drugs that will selectively intervene in the action of specific oncogenes and proto-oncogenes, once they are identified. A more immediate application would be to use the techniques of *in situ* hybridization (using DNA probes to oncogenes) or immunohistochemistry (using monoclonal antibodies to oncogene products), or both, to identify RNA and protein products, respectively, of oncogenes in tissue sections of breast lesions. These techniques and reagents could potentially be used to identify early "preneoplastic" lesions not now detectable by conventional methods. The expression of a given combination of oncogene or proto-oncogene products could also potentially be used, as discussed earlier, to better establish a phenotype of a breast tumor cell population with regard to metastatic potential.

TUMOR GROWTH FACTORS

Tumor growth factors (TGFs) are defined as those substances secreted by cells that will mediate transformation via an autocrine (self-stimulatory) mechanism. Growth factors such as epidermal growth factor (EGF) are similar in many properties to TGFs but are mitogenic and not transforming. Both TGFs and EGFs act via a cell surface receptor mechanism and, in some cases, compete for the same receptor.[14] Findings have shown that some oncogene products are indeed growth factors; for example, the product of the *sis* oncogenes has been shown to be platelet-derived growth factor,[15] while the product of the *erb* oncogene is EGF.[16] EGF-like and TGF-like molecules have been isolated from rodent and human tumors and human milk. However, their role in either mammary cell differentiation or neoplastic transformation is unknown.

Two findings may have important implications in relating oncogenes, growth factors, and hormone receptors in breast cancer research. First, it has been shown that the insertion of the viral *ras* oncogene into the estrogen-dependent MCF-7 human mammary tumor cell line renders the line estrogen independent.[17] The second finding is the observation that there may be a relationship (inverse) between EGF receptor levels and estrogen receptor levels.[18] Thus, active research into the interrelationships of oncogenes, growth factors, and the action of hormones and hormone antagonists on breast cancer cells may ultimately lead to new approaches in the control of growth of mammary cancer cells.

Another set of endogenous human cellular

genes (termed HLM) has been shown to be related to the genomes of the Type-B mouse mammary tumor virus and Types A and D retroviruses of rodents and primates, respectively. These genomic homologies have been elucidated via restriction endonuclease analyses as well as by actual DNA sequence comparisons.[19] The human HLM genes have been shown to have the size and organization of a retrovirus (i.e., approximately 8.2kb in length with *gag, pol,* and *env* gene–homologous regions) as well as long terminal repeats (LTRs) at both ends of the genomes. It should be pointed out that it is the LTR region of the mouse mammary tumor virus that renders the virus under hormonal control. Studies have also shown that the human endogenous HLM sequences represent a family of different but related genomes. The role of any particular one of these genomes will most probably best be elucidated as follows: The DNA sequence has been or will be obtained for the various HLM genomes. From this information, synthetic oligopeptides can be constructed, which, in turn, will serve as immunogens for the generation of monoclonal antibodies. These monoclonal antibodies can then be used to assay tissues and body fluids for correlations with various disease states.

A similar course of research can be constructed for the various oncogenes and proto-oncogenes discussed earlier. Furthermore, in a reciprocal sequence, monoclonal antibodies to tumor-associated antigens can be used to select for, and identify, the genes coding for these antigens. In turn, more monoclonal antibodies reflecting determinants on other regions of these tumor antigens can ultimately be utilized. Thus, long-range prospects in breast cancer research, and potentially in disease management, will most certainly involve the integration of genetic engineering, cell biology (in particular, the exploitation of biologic response modifiers), and monoclonal antibody research and application.

REFERENCES

1. Kohler M, Milstein C: Continuous cultures of fused cells secreting antibody of predefined specificity. Nature 256:495, 1975.
2. Schlom J, Weeks MO: Potential clinical utility of monoclonal antibodies in the management of human carcinomas. *In*: DeVita V, Hellman S, Rosenberg S (eds.): Important Advances in Oncology, Vol. 1. Philadelphia: J. B. Lippincott Co., 1984, p. 170.
3. Kufe D, Inghirami G, Abe M, et al.: Differential reactivity of a novel monoclonal antibody (DF3) with human malignant versus benign breast tumors. Hybridoma 3:223, 1984.
4. Hayes DF, Sekine H, Ohno T, et al.: Use of a murine monoclonal antibody for detection of circulating plasma DF3 antigen levels in breast cancer patients. J Clin Invest 75:1671, 1985.
5. Johnston WW, Szpak CA, Lottich SC, et al.: Use of monoclonal antibody (B72.3) as an immunocytochemical adjunct to diagnosis of adenocarcinoma in human effusions. Cancer Res 45:1894, 1985.
6. Lundy J, Thor A, Maenza R, et al.: Monoclonal antibody DF3 correlates with tumor differentiation and hormone receptor status in breast cancer patients. Breast Cancer Res Treat 5:269, 1985.
7. Kufe DW, Nadler L, Sargent L, et al.: Biological behavior of human breast carcinoma–associated antigens expressed during cellular proliferation. Cancer Res 43:851, 1983.
8. Horan Hand P, Colcher D, Salomon D, et al.: Influence of spatial configuration of carcinoma cell population on the expression of a tumor-associated glycoprotein. Cancer Res 45:833, 1985.
9. Greiner JW, Hand PH, Noguchi P, et al.: Enhanced expression of surface tumor-associated antigens on human breast and colon tumor cells after recombinant human leukocyte alpha-interferon treatment. Cancer Res 44:3208, 1984.
10. Land H, Parada L, Weinberg RA: Cellular oncogenes and multistep carcinogenesis. Science 222:771, 1983.
11. Shih TY, Weeks MO: Oncogenes and cancer: The p21 *ras* genes. Cancer Invest 2:109, 1984.
12. Horan Hand P, Thor A, Wunderlich D, et al.: Monoclonal antibodies of predefined specificity detect activated *ras* gene expression in human mammary and colon carcinomas. Proc Natl Acad Sci 81:5227, 1984.
13. Land H, Parada LF, Weinberg RA: Tumorigenic conversion of primary embryo fibroblasts requires at least two cooperating oncogenes. Nature 304:596, 1983.
14. Heldin CH, Westermark B: Growth factors: Mechanism of action and relation to oncogenes. Cell 37:9, 1984.
15. Deuel TF, Huang JS, Huang SS, et al.: Expression of a platelet-derived growth factor–like protein in simian sarcoma virus transformed cells. Science 221:1348, 1983.
16. Downward J, Yarden Y, Mayes E, et al.: Close similarity of epidermal growth factor receptor and v-*erb*-B oncogene protein sequences. Nature 307:521, 1984.
17. Kasid A, Lippman ME, Papageorge AG, et al.: Transfection of v-*ras*^{H} DNA into MCF-7 human breast cancer cells bypasses dependence on estrogen for tumorigenicity. Science 228:725, 1985.
18. Sainsbury JRC, Farndon JR, Harris AL, et al.: Epidermal growth factor receptors on human breast cancers. Br J Surg 72:186, 1985.
19. Callahan R, Chiu IM, Wong JF, et al.: A new class of endogenous human retroviral genomes. Science 228:1208, 1985.

INDEX

Page numbers in *italic* type indicate illustrations; page numbers followed by *t* refer to tables.

Harris Methodist
Health Sciences Library
1301 Pennsylvania Ave.
Fort Worth, TX 76104